Theory and Practice of Nursing

Theory and Practice of Nursing

An integrated approach to caring practice

SECOND EDITON

Edited by

Lynn Basford, MA, BA(Hons), RN, NDN Cert, CPT, RNT
Dean and Professor of Health Sciences,
University of Lethbridge, Atlanta, Canada

Oliver Slevin, PhD, MA, BA, RGN, RMN, RNT, NTDip (London)
Senior Lecturer, University of Ulster, UK

First published in 1995 by Campion Press Ltd

Reprinted in 2001 by:
Nelson Thornes
Delta Place
27 Bath Road
Cheltenham
Glos.
GL53 7TH
United Kingdom

Second edition published in 2003 by:
Nelson Thornes

03   04   05   06   07   08   /   10   9   8   7   6   5   4   3   2   1

A catalogue record for this book is available from the British Library

ISBN 0-7487-5838-0

Typeset by Acorn Bookwork
Printed and bound in Great Britain by Ashford Colour Press Ltd

Contents

PREFACE

Theory and Practice of Nursing (2nd edition) is primarily a comprehensive textbook for those undertaking initial pre-registration education in nursing. However, it is also written for a wider readership of qualified nurses and students undertaking post-registration courses, and for the continuing professional development and updating of registered nurses. In this latter respect, the book is designed with those undertaking self-directed study in mind, and it will also be of value to those undertaking return to practice programmes following a career break.

Nurse education in the UK has undergone major changes in the past decade. All pre-registration education and an increasing amount of post-registration education is provided at higher education level within universities. There are now demands for students to undertake higher levels of learning that encompass the skills of analytical and critical thinking, the ability to procure, evaluate and utilise the best available evidence, and the capacity to adapt theory to real-world situations. The need now is for texts which facilitate individualised study and which are at a sufficient level to contribute to courses that demand more advanced levels of learning. This book meets these needs by virtue of its integrated approach and also by virtue of the level of knowledge acquisition and practice learning it facilitates.

The first major goal of the book is to facilitate the preparation of students as registered practitioners who can meet the demands of *Fitness for Practice*. That is, to be able to demonstrate that level of competence required for the safe and effective practice of nursing. In 1999, the United Kingdom Central Council for Nursing, Midwifery and Health Visiting (UKCC) published its report entitled *Fitness for Practice: The UKCC commission for nursing and mid-wifery education*. This report recommended what were probably the most significant changes to nurse education in the UK since the middle years of the last century. Following acceptance of the main recommendations by the Government, new pre-registration education programmes were introduced across the UK in the 2000/2001 and 2001/2002 academic years. These programmes introduced a new emphasis on the achievement of specified learning outcomes at the end of a 1-year foundation programme and the achievement of specified competencies on completion of 2-year branch programmes, at the end of the full 3-year course of study. While there will continue to be four different 'branches' and thus four pathways (leading to registration in adult, mental health, children's or learning disabilities nursing), and while the minimum level of academic award continues to be the Diploma of Higher Education, the new programmes mark a significant departure. The practice-centred nature of the new programmes declare an uncompromising commitment to meeting the profession's social contract for providing safe, competent and effective practitioners. This book is equally uncompromising in supporting this commitment to the primacy of practice. In this respect, the contribution of a chapter by the internationally renowned scholar Patricia Benner, whose work on practice development is influential far beyond the boundaries of the discipline of nursing, is an important aspect of this new edition.

The second major goal of the book is to facilitate the preparation of students to meet the demands of *Fitness for Purpose*. That is, the demands of contributing to a high-quality health service, committed to clinical excellence and responding safely and effectively to the changing health needs of society. In one sense, this relates to the need for practitioners to function adequately in roles that are essential to the safe delivery of high-quality health care. However, in its programme for modernisation of the health services, the UK Government recognises the rapidly changing patterns of demand, and the equally rapid development of health care knowledge and technologies. Thus, in *A First Class Service: Quality in the new NHS* (Department of Health, 1998), there is recognition that quality is dependent on a commitment to clinical governance (encompassing an acceptance of accountability for clinical effectiveness by managers *and* clinicians). This must be adequately underpinned by effective professional self-regulation and preparation for lifelong learning. This is emphasised by a chapter by David Davis on lifelong learning in the second module. In effect, quality will be dependent on effective research and development and appropriate education and training underpinnings. Indeed, in *An Organisation with a Memory: Report of an expert group on learning from adverse events in the NHS* (Department of Health, 2000), the vital importance of developing a learning culture that promotes active learning and positive attitudes to learning from mistakes is emphasised. This book reflects throughout the importance of learning that recognises and encompasses an attention to purpose. It also reflects a commitment to an evidence-based approach to health care and practice, and the demands placed upon practitioners to ensure their clinical judgement and practice are informed by the best available evidence. This commitment is recognised by the inclusion of a chapter on the development of evidence-based nursing and its contribution to clinical effectiveness by Alan Pearson, a distinguished nursing scholar whose work on practice development is widely acknowledged.

The third goal of the book is to facilitate the preparation of students to meet the demands of *Fitness for Award*. That is, to ensure that the pace and level of study are such that the outcome merits the appropriate academic award. In recognising this demand, the authors were

aware of the close collaborative working between our own professional and regulatory bodies and the Quality Assurance Agency for higher education, as the latter body proceeded towards establishing systems for the quality assurance of higher education, including the establishment of benchmarks for the discipline of nursing at diploma and degree level. The authors were also cognisant of the fact that, while the UKCC has set the Diploma of Higher Education as the minimal level of award for courses leading to registration, most institutions have been proceeding with course options at diploma and first degree levels. It is therefore recognised that students must learn at the appropriate pace and level, as required by the aforementioned benchmarks, up to and including first/baccalaureate degree level. The book is designed to respond to the challenges of learning to this level.

A fourth goal of the book is to facilitate the preparation of students to meet the demands of *Fitness for Professional Standing*. In implementing the new fitness for practice programmes (as referred to above), Nursing and Midwifery Council, the current regulatory body in the UK, has published guiding principles, outcomes and competencies to be met (NMC, 2002). Within these guiding principles, there is identification of this additional area of 'fitness'. It is recognised that nursing is not just about knowledge, skill, competence and clinical effectiveness, but also includes 'responsibility for the highest standards of professional conduct and ethical practice'. Within this book there is full recognition of the need to combine knowledge and skill with compassion and caring, and a recognition that this is an ethical imperative. In this respect, the nursing scholar Jean Watson, who also contributes a chapter, speaks of integrating these aspects in what she terms 'informed moral passion'.

This concept of integration is one that applies within the book on a number of levels. On one level, it is recognised that the aforementioned fitnesses – for practice, purpose, award and professional standing – are not separate and discrete concerns. They are in fact inextricably linked and complementary. Thus, to address *practice* at the level necessary within modern health care systems demands a concern for *purpose*, and can only be achieved if learning is at the *award* level of diploma or first degree. Similarly, the nurse's *standing* as a professional cannot be deemed ethical despite claims to caring and compassion, if the nurse has not taken care to ensure that she is fit to *practise*, i.e. competent and informed.

On another level, the book is integrative in its approach to learning. It is essentially designed to stimulate active study rather than passive reading. Each chapter carries a clear statement of learning outcomes, and the text is interspersed with relevant study activities. At the end of each module there are sets of self-test questions and seminar/discussion activities, which can be used with or without the teacher, as written assignments or as topics for debate. Attention has been given to the need to ensure that these activities are relevant and effective in terms of the chapter contents *and* in respect of the nature of modern-day practice. In this respect, there is an emphasis on activities that call the nurse to reflect on practice. This involves reflecting not only *before* and *after* practice, but that reflection *during* practice that involves a reflexivity between knowing and doing. This is realised by the inclusion of study activities that can only be carried through in practice situations – the student thus moving reflectively and experientially from text to practice and from practice to text. The activities not only promote personal reflection as an effective self-directed learning process, but where appropriate there are activities that encourage shared reflections with peers, clinical facilitators or mentors, and teachers. This interactive approach reflects a philosophy which subscribes to the notion that reading, thinking about what is read and doing something with it must be integrated to achieve optimal learning outcomes. The importance of this integrative, practice-centred approach to learning through reflection is recognised in the presentation of a chapter on reflective practice by Gary Rolfe, a distinguished nursing scholar who has worked in this area.

The book is also integrative in terms of its overall design. As indicated above, the book is designed on a modular basis. That is, it consists of 10 modules, each consisting of a number of chapters. Each module addresses a particular area of theory or practice. Within each of these modules, the chapters are complementary and cross-referenced to ensure that the module topic is covered in a comprehensive manner. This principle is carried through by establishing cross-linkages and continuity not only within but also between modules.

However, perhaps the most important integrative feature of the book is that of its total commitment to integration of theory and practice. It is certainly true that, in terms of sequence, the book commences with modules that have a greater theoretical orientation and then proceeds to those whose orientation is essentially practical. However, even where the primary concern is theory, this is firmly centred on the practice of nursing. Indeed, it is practice that is the core concern of this text. Even in Module 4, the module concerned with the evidence base of nursing, the final chapter is devoted exclusively to the interrelationship between theory, practice and research. The emphasis here is on the notion of a praxis of nursing in which theory, practice and research are integrated in such a way that nursing practice is in effect sound nursing knowledge in action.

The book is specifically designed to meet the needs of the nursing student in the first decade of the twenty-first century, not only by virtue of its integrated and interactive design, but also by the level of knowledge acquisition it facilitates and its uncompromising orientation towards practice. It must be noted that by knowledge acquisition we do not simply mean the supply of relevant and up-to-date information, important though this may be. The claim is that in nursing the requisite levels of knowledge must extend beyond the student's capacity to absorb and reproduce information in the same form that it is conveyed. If knowledge means 'to know', in the sense that there is insight and wisdom in knowing, then more advanced levels of knowledge imply not just knowing more, but understanding and insight, organising knowledge and linking concepts, critically analysing, evaluating and identifying the best available knowledge, reorganising and adapting, and applying knowledge in practice; in effect, moving from possession of a body of taken-for-granted facts to a comprehensive and organised body of sound knowledge that has validity in practice.

However, the knowledge that must inform nursing cannot be exclusively based upon factual information derived from a logical process of critical reasoning, whether as a problem-solving process or (in a more specific context) as a research process. It is recognised that nursing is a relational activity, lived out in an environment within which the complexity of human nature and its response to health and ill-health cannot be completely addressed by empirical knowledge. In this context, different forms of knowing are also acknowledged as relevant. Therefore, throughout the book, empirical, personal, aesthetic and ethical ways of knowing, those fundamental patterns of knowing originally presented in the work of the nursing scholar Barbara Carper, are addressed.

It is, of course, recognised that forms of knowledge that are classified as *'knowing that'* and derive from empirical research, are absolutely essential to safe and effective practice. But it is also recognised that *'know how'*, i.e. that knowledge derived from and immersed in skill mastery or the artistry of aesthetic knowing, often presenting in its more advanced forms as the tacit or intuitive knowing of nursing situations that emerges from the wisdom of experience, is also relevant. So too is that personal and ontological knowing of self, of the frailty and courage of human existence, of the meaning of pain and human suffering, of importance. Such personal knowing, which can only be approximated but never fully expressed in language, is an essential condition for reaching out to the patient in a

compassionate and healing sense. And it is also recognised that the form taken by moral reasoning in complex ethical dilemmas differs in notable ways from practical critical reasoning that is predicated by the laws and conventions of logic and science.

Importantly, recognition of the relevance of different patterns of knowing is not merely presented within the book as an extended epistemology of nursing knowledge. Rather, it is recognised that no one pattern of knowing is sufficient. All are essential and indeed complementary in developing a holistic understanding of the complexity of nursing practice. Exclusion of any one as irrelevant (and there are those who would and do so exclude) would result in an incomplete knowledge of nursing as an art and science. This book would surely fail in its mission if it excluded specific patterns of knowing relevant to the practice of nursing.

Thus far, we have spoken of the theory and practice of nursing, of the need to ensure competence and fitness, and of the different patterns of knowing that must inform nursing, all of which will be addressed in this book. But throughout the book we return again and again to the centre: to the practice of nursing. It is in this space, where the self of the nurse reaches out to the other of the patient or client, that the living praxis that is nursing lives. But this is not an insulated and static space. It is the dynamic space of a complex society and within it complex health care systems, constantly changing over time. And, as supersonic travel and high technology communications advance, it is an increasingly open and contracting space. We now find our nurse–patient space extending to families, communities, whole societies, and even into global and cosmic dimensions. We have grappled with the need to move from a mechanistic, role-bound nursing within inflexible health care systems to a need to acknowledge cultural influences on health and disease. Now, in increasingly multicultural societies, we must adopt new transcultural modes. We can no longer ignore or see as of no concern to us the global influences and risks to health and well-being. Nor can we choose to ignore inequalities that are detrimental to the health and well-being of those for whom we care. Nursing, in effect, occurs in context and it will only be successful if it is practised as a contextual undertaking. The nursing scholar Jacqueline Fawcett spoke of the *metaparadigm* of nursing (i.e. a concept that means identifying the fundamental phenomena of concern to nursing). She spoke of these as being person, environment, health and nursing. Others have proposed different conceptual framings; indeed, one of the current authors has suggested the metaparadigm elements to be person, environment, health and caring (as opposed to nursing). Throughout the book, this metaparadigmatic framing of nursing practice in context is recognised, and emphasised by a full module that addresses aspects of the social context of practice.

Many feel that there is a risk of nursing textbooks being too academic and too advanced. Nursing students, so the argument runs, will not be able to absorb such texts, which are far beyond the needs of ordinary pre-registration students. However, the complexity of nursing practice should not be used as an excuse to produce inadequate and simplistic texts. It should, conversely, present a challenge to produce a book that will facilitate the student in preparation for practice in a modern world. The authors argue that they have achieved this goal. In this book, students will find a comprehensive body of up-to-date, research-based knowledge that is applicable to practice. In this book, they will be challenged to grapple with the current status of nursing science and philosophy as applied to practice. In this book, students will be required to confront social, political and professional issues that influence practice. And, in this book, students will be required to reflect critically upon knowledge gained from these various sources and justify its application in nursing practice.

The latter comments should not be taken to imply a claim by the authors that this text provides everything the student will need for a full 3-year or more programme leading to registration in any of the branches of nursing. This is a generic textbook, providing a comprehensive theoretical and practical foundation, facilitating the student in developing generic nursing skills and therapeutic approaches relevant to any branch of nursing, and introducing the student to the main branches of nursing in the UK. It is not intended to include all the nursing knowledge necessary for all types of nursing practice. Indeed, the authors would reject the notion that a single course book for such programmes is a practical possibility. Each of the chapters carries a comprehensive list of references for up-to-date and seminal works, and students are encouraged to consult other books and journal papers, particularly with regard to primary sources. In this regard the book should prove a useful source for pre-registration students throughout their courses and for qualified nurses who are advancing their post-registration learning.

Due to the absence of a genderless singular personal pronoun in the English language, it is difficult to achieve political correctness in a book such as this with constant references to the nurse and the patient. For convenience, the authors refer to the nurse throughout in the female gender. Patients and clients are referred to as males. Where there is no distinction between patients and clients, the term patient is used rather than patient/client. No bias towards either sex is intended.

The authors of *Theory and Practice of Nursing* (2nd edition) have attempted to present a textbook on nursing which is up-to-date and relevant to the study and practice of nursing in the twenty-first century. They have started from the realistic premise that no such book will achieve perfection in all regards or be suited to the needs and personal tastes of all its potential users. The authors have been guided by their own experience and insights as nurse educators and by a desire to produce a book that will facilitate relevant learning for students of nursing. The needs of such students in developing and enhancing sound nursing practice, and the needs of patients or clients for effective nursing care, are paramount. The authors would therefore welcome any critical comment or advice, which may improve their future endeavours and strengthen subsequent editions of this text.

A respectful acknowledgement is made to the original authors of the first edition, with thanks for their contributions.

Oliver Slevin
Lynn Basford

REFERENCES

Department of Health (1998) *A First Class Service: Quality in the new NHS*, Department of Health, London

Department of Health (2000) *An Organisation with a Memory: Report of an expert group on learning from adverse events in the NHS*, Department of Health, London

Nursing and Midwifery Council (2002) *Requirements for Pre-registration Nursing Programme*, NMC, London

United Kingdom Central Council for Nursing, Midwifery and Health Visiting (1999) *Fitness for Practice: The UKCC commission for nursing and midwifery education*, UKCC, London

LIST OF CONTRIBUTORS

General editors

Lynn Basford, MA, BA (hons), RN, NDN Cert, CPT, RNT, is Dean and Professor of Health Sciences at the University of Lethbridge, Alberta, Canada. She was previously Professor of Nursing at the School of Health and Community Studies, University of Derby, and prior to that Head of the Community and Primary Care Nursing Department at Sheffield and North Trent College of Nursing and Midwifery, where she chaired the development of a preregistration advanced diploma in nursing studies, which contained a conpetency-based approach to assessment. Her previous roles included the implementation and delivery of the Adult Branch Programme (*Project 2000*) and a variety of clinical posts in medicine, surgery, gynaecology and community care. Her areas of particular interests are community and primary nursing care, and women's health.

Oliver Slevin, PhD, MA, BA, RGN, RMN, RNT, NTDip (London) is a lecturer in the School of Nursing at the University of Ulster, where he is Director of the Professional Doctorate programme in nursing. Oliver was previously Chief Executive of the National Board for Nursing, Midwifery and Health Visiting for Northern Ireland and Visiting Professor at the University of Ulster, and he has worked in clinical and educational posts in England, Scotland and Ireland. He is involved in postgraduate teaching and is currently completing a review of doctoral education. His current research projects include evaluation of international health care development projects in South Asia and health care ethics.

Authors

Claire Bale, BA(Hons), RGN, is Modernisation Manager at Greater Derby Primary Care Trust, Derby. She is also Secretary to the European Honours Society.

Lynn Basford, as above.

Patricia Benner, PhD, RN, FAAN, is a member of the faculty at the University of California San Francisco, School of Nursing, where she carries out research and teaches philosophy of nursing science, ethics, and interpretive phenomenology.

Denise Burgin, BSc(Hons), RGN, RSCN, RCNT, Cert.Ed. is an independent consultant at Solsgirth House, By Dollor, Kinross-shire.

Jo Cooper, BSc(Hons), RGN, Dip.Oncology, is a Clinical Nurse Specialist and Macmillan Nurse in Palliative Care at the North Devon Hospice.

Katie Dann, BSc, MSc, DPhil, is a research associate at the School of Health and Community Studies, University of Derby.

David Davies, BSc, MA, PGCE, Med, DProf, DPhil, FRSA is Director at Buxton College, University of Derby.

Dawn Freshwater, PhD, BA, RN, RNT, is Head of the Academic Research Centre at the Institute of Health and Community Studies and North Dorset NHS Trust, Bournemouth University.

Carol Kirby, Med, BPhil, RGN, RMN, RNT, Dip.N (London) is a Senior Lecturer at the University of Ulster, where she coordinates modules in the social context of mental health.

Ann Long, PhD, MSc (Counselling), BSc (Hons), RGN, RMN, RHV, Dip.N, RNT, RHVT is a Senior Lecturer at the University of Ulster, where she has directed the community nursing and health visiting programmes over a number of years.

Alan Pearson, PhD, MSc, Dip.Advanced Nursing, Dip.Nursing Education, SRN, Orthopaedic Nursing Cert., is Professor of Nursing at La Trobe University in Victoria, Australia, Adjunct Professor at the University of Adelaide, Director of the Australian Centre for Evidence Based Residential Aged Care, and Director of the Joanna Briggs Institute for Evidence Based Nursing and Midwifery.

Gary Rolfe, PhD, MA, BSc, RMN, PGCEA, is Reader in Nursing at the School of Health and Social Care, University of Portsmouth.

Marlene Sinclair, PhD, Med, BSc(Hons), DASE, Dip.N, RN, RM, RNT, is a Senior Lecturer at the University of Ulster, where she is also the Director of the Master's programme in Advanced Nursing and Midwifery.

Eamonn Slevin, DNSc, BSc(Hons), PGDip (Nursing), Adv.Dip.Education, RGN, RNMH, RNT, is a Senior Lecturer in Nursing at the University of Ulster and a Commissioner with the Southern Health and Social Services Board in Northern Ireland.

Oliver Slevin, as above.

Jean Watson, PhD, RN, FAAN, HNC, is Distinguished Professor of Nursing and Founder of the highly influential Centre for Human Caring, and holds an endowed Chair in Caring Science at the University of Colorado.

Paul Weller, PhD, MPhil, MA, CertEd is Head of the Division of Social Science, School Director of Research and Professor of Inter-Religious Relations at the University of Derby.

ACKNOWLEDGEMENTS

The authors and publishers would like to thank the following people and organizations for permission to reproduce material in this book:

Aspen Publications for Table 1.1 on page 5 and Table 40.2 on page 768; Ballière Tindall for Table 33.1 on page 614; Blackwell Science for Table 3.2 on page 50 and Table 5.1 on page 86 (Blanchfield, 1978); Cassell for Table 8.1 on page 129; Colorado Associated University Press for Table 3.1 on page 48; Constable for the quote on page 525 (Rogers, 1990); The Controller of Her Majesty's Stationery Office © Crown Copyright) for Table 20.1 on page 378, 20.2 and 20.3 on page 381, and Tables 20.4–20.9 on pages 382–4; David Gregory and Debbie Marshall/Wellcome Photo Library for the image (*E. coli*) on page 619; Decatur for Figure 40.1 on page 763; Elsevier Science (USA) for Table 35.1 on page 671; Heinemann for the poem on page 1; Hutchinson for the opening quote on page 519; Kluwer Academic Publications for the second quote on page 519; The Royal College of Nursing for Table 38.2 on page 742; Time Life Books for Table 1.2 on page 10; W.B. Saunders for Table 35.1 on page 671; Wellcome Photo Library for the image (*Straphylococcus aureus*) on page 616 and WHO for Table 30.2 on page 584 and Table 40.1 on page 763.

Every effort has been made to contact copyright holders and we apologise if anyone has been overlooked.

MODULE 1: FOCUS ON CARE

INTRODUCTION

The focus of Module 1 is framed around aspects of care, from its historical beginnings to contemporary structures, through which health care is delivered in the UK. It is a module that illustrates the many facets of care, which include the philosophical intent underpinning the commitment to care, the notion of self-care, altruistic and informal care, professional and organised care and a modern phenomena of empowered care.

It is reasoned that the philosophy of care is a principal through which humans interrelate with each other in sickness and health. It is the caring medium through which action is taken to protect each other and ourselves through all aspects of everyday living. It is when one's ability, or when informal caring interventions and support, are insufficient to restore and maintain health, that professional and organised aspects of care are required. This module comprehensively covers the concept of care in the belief that it is pivotal in nursing action and reason and that it should be the quintessential ingredient in providing nursing care for individuals and communities.

Module 1 is, therefore, the foundation of knowledge that you as a new student should acquire and understand as a basis to advance your knowledge, skill and understanding of the world of nursing in contemporary societies.

1 PRECEDENTS

Lynn Basford

Setting out on the voyage to Ithaca
You must pray that the way be long . . .
Many be the summer mornings
When with what pleasures, with what delight
You enter the harbours never seen before.

Do not hurry the journey at all.
Better that it should last many years;
Be quite old when you anchor at the island,
Rich with all you have gained on the way,
Not expecting Ithaca to give you riches.
Ithaca has given you your lovely journey.
Without Ithaca you would never have set out.

Ithaca no more to give you now.
Poor though you find it, Ithaca has not cheated you.
Wise as you have become, with all your experience,
You will have understood the meaning of an Ithaca.
                    (Cavafy, 1911, cited in Baly, 1980)

LEARNING OUTCOMES

After studying this chapter you will be able to:

- Discuss the historical developments of health and illness care from the period of antiquity to contemporary practice
- Understand that historical writings often reflect a specific view of health care
- Describe the philosophies and principles of health and illness care from different historical periods within different cultures
- Discuss the framework upon which contemporary medical practice operates
- Explain the political, social, cultural and gender-related influences on health care
- Compare and contrast eastern versus western ideologies of health.

INTRODUCTION

Cavafy's poem spells out, metaphorically, our journey in search of Ithaca (the meaning of life), and asks that we be enriched with our experiences and the knowledge we gain along the way. As a student of nursing your journey is just beginning in the search for explanations and understandings of the world and the essence of nursing in all its dimensions. Your journey of learning will focus on the knowledge and values of contemporary practice and will be enhanced through the experiences you will gain through caring for people from different cultures. The operative word here is 'care' and caring activities will be in promoting health, restoring health and maintaining the health of individuals and communities in a variety of health care settings.

The concept of care is a value-laden word that is central to our interactions and inter-relationships with each other, and should be understood within the context of the evolution of caring and healing relationships from different time periods and within different cultures. It is important to know about the past so as to understand the present and plan for the future, if mistakes are not to be repeated. As the old proverb states, 'Those who do not learn from history are doomed to repeat it'. The art and science of health care is no exception to this rule in that it has a dynamic relationship with the evolution of man, with cultural and social diversities, and with environmental, epidemiological and scientific discoveries. From this position, the history of care should not be seen in isolation from the present, but regarded as a 'seamless' interface that can inform the present through data, experience and collective wisdom.

This first chapter gives an overview of the evolution of care as a healing modality and the philosophical and therapeutic frameworks that were used in different periods in history from antiquity to the present time. It presents but a brief synopsis of major events and cultural and political influences, and you are encouraged to read other material, from wider political, socio-logical, anthropological and cultural perspectives, so that you can understand what has influenced health care in the UK.

Historical events can be recorded in many ways from the written form, books and diaries, or through oral communication, speech or song. The former mode is often said to be the most accurate, but feminists would strongly contend that history recorded in such a manner is male dominated and not grounded in theory. Based on these assumptions, they suggest that historical records cannot be considered to be a true representation of the past, but a record of selective and value laden facts (Davies, 1980; Versluysen, 1980). To suggest that any record is value free is a spurious position to take, given that philosophers would contend that nothing is value free. Nonetheless, feminists do have a particular point in that male historians would have placed their own values and assertions on the writing of history. Given this situation, modern historians suggest that if historical records are to portray a balanced view of health care that reflects the contributions men and women have made in the history of humanity, information should be recorded from data of different sources. These should include a review of historical records, oral history, personal diaries and letters, artistic representation, anthropology and archaeology (Davies, 1980; Versluysen, 1980). These views have a particular relevance if the historical writings on health care are to be believed and drawn upon to inform the future.

The dominance of male perspectives of historical events is especially salient when considering the historical position of women within the context of healing and caring. In her book, *Rewriting Nursing History*, Celia Davies (1980) has challenged the established view that women throughout most historical periods have only played minor and insignificant roles within the

constructs of healing and caring, pointing out that women have always been actively engaged in the work of healing and caring. In support of this argument, Ehrenreich and English (1973) assert that in the ancient world the provision of health care was a central feature of a woman's role. Women nurtured the young, cared for the sick and dying and provided healing care compatible with the scientific knowledge and folk wisdom of the day. This is a point the great nurse leader Florence Nightingale highlighted in 1859 when she said, 'God did not intend all mothers to be accompanied by doctors, but he meant all children to be cared for by mothers' (p. 33). Indeed it is this centralised and pivotal role women have within the context of caring that historians have overlooked and, according to Yeandle (1984), it is significant by its absence. Added to which, the phenomena of care is so internalised as a feminine characteristic and role that the significance of women's healing work has been massively underestimated, not least by women themselves. This is a point that Novarra (1987) and Watson (1989) make when they suggest that the continuity of women's work is one of the reasons for its invisibility.

These arguments are strongly biased towards the view that men have described health care from their own perspectives that reflect the stereotyping of masculine and feminine roles (De Beauvoir, 1952). Over time, this has influenced the development of the modern (female) nursing profession that has mirrored women's roles in society. This position is reinforced by the power relationships between nursing and the male medical profession and the historical focus of the advancements in medical science that have undermined the contributions nursing (feminine) care have made to the health and well-being of individuals and communities.

It may be argued that this position is reinforced by the power dynamics evident between the traditional feminine profession of nursing and masculine profession of medicine. Historically, the great importance modern society has placed upon medical and scientific advancements has undermined the contributions of nursing and caring upon the health and well-being of individuals and communities. Women, it is argued, have influenced caring activities and have advanced the knowledge and use of herbs through the process of trial and error (Alic, 1990), as opposed to scientific rationality.

While gender bias in the annals of the history of care has been noted it should be recognised that care and caring activities are a central function of human activity. This could be the sense of caring for things in a concerned manner, or caring for others, both in health and sickness, as a feature of social interaction that ensures the survival of humanity (Leininger, 1981; Dunlop, 1986; Buckman and Sabbagh, 1993). It is this intrinsic value of human caring that offers a unique contribution to the health and well-being of the individual at a micro level, as in a willingness to listen, or offering words of wisdom or health advice, or a helping hand in periods of sickness/disability. Conversely, caring can be at the global human perspective (macro) that engages different communities and countries to be concerned for each other with regard to the pursuance of health improvements and basic human rights. These two inherent philosophical standpoints do not have a priority with either gender and should be considered in a balanced way when reviewing the historical milestones of health care. For instance, if 'care' is a basic human function, then all men and women have the ability to care for others. Some, more than others, have used this characteristic as *a priori* or altruistic behaviour towards their fellow human beings.

PRIMITIVE HUMANITY

From the beginnings of humankind, people have been curious about the healing process. In many ways the desire to unravel the mysteries of health, illness and healing is a journey of discovery that has followed many different pathways, with each culture and each society in different historical periods developing new and diverse understandings. Keegan (1988) illustrates this in a table that provides a chronology of healing in antiquity (Table 1.1). Pearson (1991)

makes references to the evidence of early historical writings of primitive people engaged in caring and assisting in the healing process. It was an informal activity largely provided by a female member of the family. The informality of the arrangement, according to Edwards-Rees (1966), is due to the fact that the belief systems of health and illness were related to an act of displeasure from the gods, and restoration of health depended upon the charms, offerings and incantations that would appease them. Based on these assumptions formal aspects of care were unnecessary, with perhaps the exception of midwifery care.

Table 1.1 Chronology of healing in antiquity

Drawings and carvings signifying the recognition of the cyclic nature of time	35,000 BC
Cave depictions of shamanistic activities	20,000 BC
Necropsy (study of the dead and practice of mummification) in Egypt	3,000 BC
Egyptian literature on healing and magic	2,000 BC
Scientific classification and writings by Hippocrates in Greece	500 BC
The Yellow Emperor's classic of internal medicine: contents included anatomy, physiology, hygiene, acupuncture and moxibustion	200 BC
Rig-Veda: contents included philosophy and healing consciousness of India	200 BC
The materia medica of Shen-nung: contents included description of 365 pharmaceutical drugs	AD 200

(From Keegan, 1988, in Dossey et al., 1988)

While the assumptions made by Edwards-Rees (1966) are opinions that are shared by others and popular perception, they are not entirely congruent with the discoveries found by paleopathologists (those who study prehistorical evidence of disease). Paleopathologists have clearly demonstrated, by analysing bone and mummy remnants of primitive people, that they suffered from the same illnesses as their modern counterparts. For example, arthritis, sinusitis, bone tumours and osteoporosis were evident in the remains of ancient bones; while the tissue remains of mummies demonstrated the effects of diseases such as tuberculosis, appendicitis, smallpox and pneumonia. These illnesses would have required some care intervention other than appeasement of the gods. Nonetheless, evidence to prove the existence of primitive people's healing therapies has been difficult to establish with the exception of the science and art of trephination. Trephination (the process of boring into or removing a part of the skull) is a dangerous and complicated technical intervention but it is known that primitive people used this technique and some did survive the operation based on the evidence of ancient skulls from Europe, Peru and Mexico (Bullough and Bullough, 1979; Buckman and Sabbagh, 1993).

Other historians make the claim that primitive people would seek health care from the local wise man or shaman, who would have contextualised health and disease within a philosophical and mystical framework in an attempt to link people's interrelationship with the universe (Buckman and Sabbagh, 1993). Oakley (1976), however, makes the point that early people would have relied primarily on the services of women healers for their knowledge of the healing properties of herbs.

It is highly probable that primitive people would have adapted to a range of health care practices, particularly as they gained more knowledge and understanding of health care as and when societies became more sophisticated. These are hypotheses that historians, sociologists and anthropologists support in the knowledge that the pursuit of understanding disease would have increased within structured societies and continued to evolve over time within a dynamic framework.

This dynamic relationship with advancements in societies and the search to sustain and maintain health are both of vital importance. It is this concept that drives each culture within each era to respond to changes that reflects their cultural expectations and beliefs, scientific explanations and discoveries, and their response to new disease entities.

In recognising this fact it is clear that health care has evolved and developed in synchronicity with the evolution of humankind. Health care does not operate in isolation from developments in societies as historical records have portrayed.

Study Activity 1.1

- From a historical perspective, describe the concept of care.
- After some library research, describe a shaman and the role the shaman plays within the context of health care.
- Explore the notion that shamans still exist and describe the techniques shamans use to restore the health of the individual.
- Explain the reasons for the different patterns of health care within different cultures and different periods of time.

THE HISTORY AND PHILOSOPHY OF CHINESE HEALTH CARE

The Yellow Emperor said:

> Yin/Yang are the way of heaven and earth,
> the great principle and outline of everything,
> the parents of change, the root and source
> of life and death, the palace of gods.
> Treatment of disease should be based upon
> the roots of [Yin/Yang].
>
> (Nei Jing, first century BC)

Considering the above quote, Chinese philosophy of health care is clearly centred upon the balance of Yin and Yang (*see* Figure 1.1) that pervades every aspect of human beings' functioning and their interaction with their environments. The origins of such philosophy and teachings can be traced back 5000 years, drawing on findings from archaeology of the Neolithic period that provided evidence of medical (healing) care (Gao, 1999).

Embryonic beginnings towards a formalised structure that supports the provision of health care began in China with ancestral therapy, *wu* shamanism and magic practices. Principles for prescribing health care that were used in the Shang Dynasty (1766–1100 BC) and the Zhou period (1100–221 BC), relied heavily on ritualistic behaviour and divination as a central part of the healing process. The Shang culture had a simplistic interpretation of health and had catalogued certain illnesses that could be cured by praying. Illness, they perceived, had a direct causal relationship with the ancestors who were consulted to determine their will. Further to this, natural events such as 'wind-evil' were directly attributed to disease and disability. The Zhou period had a predominant view of demonic influences on health that had to be exorcised either through shamanic acts, herbal treatments, public exorcism or acupuncture. The legendary scientist Pien Chio (407–310 BC) is said to have been the first acupuncturist and is quoted as identifying 13 acupuncture points in the treatment against demons (Gao, 1999).

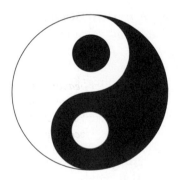

Figure 1.1   The Yin/Yang symbol

Following on from this framework of reference, there emerged a philosophy based on the observation of people's interconnections with health and disease that formed a basis for further scientific enquiry. However, there were several explanations and philosophical thoughts that are said to have influenced the development and understanding of health and disease in a significant way. Chief among these were the theories of Taoist alchemy, early empiricism (observation of nature), the astrological soothsayers who mapped out the course of seasons and celestial

events and the principles of the school of Yin/Yang and the Qi Vitalists (Porkert, 1982; Hoizey and Hoizey, 1993).

The empirical observation of nature became the process from which natural laws were founded and became the foundation for the development of the modern Traditional Chinese Medicine (TCM). While this is commonly known as the period of 'the hundred schools of thought', there were two classical schools that worked towards finding a scientific logic. These were known as the Logicians and Mohists. The Logicians, or schools of names, were developed in the fourth century BC and provided explanations of universals, such as oneness and twoness and ideas of change. The focus of concern for the Logicians was to provide dialectical rather than formal logic. By contrast, the Mohists (479–381 BC) identified a social philosophy based on the concept of universal love that also embraced a belief in spirits and demons. Their process of scientific enquiry was based on the exploration of phenomena within a social context. For example, verification of the 'truth' would come from community observers and terminology was defined as methods of explanation. These would include sensation, levels of causality, classification, the difference between first-hand and second-hand information, perceptions and deductive and inductive logic (Hoizey and Hoizey, 1993; Gao, 1999).

Taoist scientific influence

The Taoist alchemists were instrumental in seeking out knowledge and use of herbs in the field of prolonging life and restoring health. Life-prolonging activities for the Taoists centred around the belief that people should make use of their existence through life-enhancing activities such as meditation or special exercises, and/or the taking of medical substances. Each one of these health-promoting activities is said to promote the life giving energy known as 'Qi'. Qi is a term that considers the nature of universal energy that permeates through and within the human body. It is a similar concept defined by the Yogis of India in '*prana*' and the Greek idea of 'pnuema'. To make sense of this concept Porkert (1982) suggests that Qi is energy of a definite quality ordered in a particular direction in space and has a certain quality and structure within an energetic configuration. In essence, it is the vital force of all living matter and is essential for the homeostatic mechanisms of human functioning.

Confucian influence in the Han dynasty

In the first century BC Confucian philosophy and ideologies began to frame the scientific understanding that embraced a social and political theory based upon humanistic principles. These understandings were said to unify the various schools of thought towards directing future scientific enquiry that included health care. It was in the Han period that Confucian philosophy was adopted by the legendary Yellow Emperor and his line of successors, which embraced the philosophical notions of TCM (health care) to further advance knowledge and understanding. Their inquiry consisted of two parts: (1) essential questions that relate to anatomy, physiology and therapy; and (2) the notion of acupuncture and its effects (Gao, 1999). They used the knowledge of the existence of Yin/Yang with the perceived view that to maintain, restore and sustain health required the existence of a harmonious relationship that is inter-related with all aspects of human functioning. If human beings operated and functioned within these sets of rules then they would live beyond the three score years and ten to the full expectancy of life as nature intended.

Systematic correspondences

It was in the fourth century that the theories of Yin/Yang and the five elements began to emerge. They were collectively referred to as the theories of 'systematic correspondence', the notion being that the theories embraced concepts underpinning the universe and that human functioning had a dynamic inter-relatedness and interconnection with energy forces. Yin and Yang were the descriptions of polar opposites of inter-related phenomena. Yang represents the masculine ener-getic qualities of the universe while Yin represents the feminine structural, substantive and aesthetic aspects. While they are expressed in polar opposite dimensions one cannot exist without the other, for example, you cannot perceive night without day; nor can you go up without having the notion of down; you cannot have slow without the concept of fast (Porkert, 1982; Gao, 1999).

The above theories evolved through an understanding that the universal energy has a dynamic engagement with all that is within it and it is in perpetual motion or transformation through every passing moment. This feeling of perpetual motion or change is depicted in an old Native American statement that says 'We can never step into the same river twice'. This means that the river is in constant motion and the water itself will have changed as will the earth over which the water passed.

The notion of 'change' for the Chinese was a profound thought that led to the 'I Ching' or the book of changes. This book centres on the philosophy that life and death is a continually changing process. As a result guidance is extolled within the text of the I Ching that defines the rules enabling humans to exist with nature in this framework of constant universal change. The development of the ideas represented in the I Ching has formed the basis of Chinese scientific thinking and cultural expression. In health care the theory of Yin/Yang is the chief principle that guides the correlation of health information, for example, the differentiation of syndromes and pulse qualities. However, other important theories are considered, such as the five Transformative phases and Channel theories (Gao, 1999). The Transformative phases recognise five universal elements of wood, fire, earth, metal and water; elements that are considered to be inter-related for harmonious living, but can each possess an inherent property/influence in the process of change. The effect of these elements depends on the seasonal influence, their balance and connectedness with each other and their relative strength. Over time, each of these five elements has been associated with different parts of the human body. For instance, fire is symbolised by the heart and small intestines; earth, the spleen and stomach; metal, the lung and large intestine; water, kidney and bladder; and wood, the liver and gall bladder. The main premise hinges on the notion that health is a balance of harmony between all that is Yin and Yang, the functions of the body and between the body and the environment in which we live. Maintaining health within the process of dynamic change requires mechanisms that quickly restore balance. When this ability is weakened then ill health presents and can manifest into a diseased body.

During the Song Dynasty, around 1000 years ago, cause of disease was classified into three areas:

1 *External (exogenous) causes*: these included the external factors influenced by the climate.
2 *Internal (endogenous) causes*: these were caused by emotional distress, which had a profound effect on the visceral organs.
3 *Neither internal nor external causes*: effects on health were due to diet, trauma and sexual activity.

In the modern period, TCM considers the determination of disease by analysing the symptoms that have a causal relationship with the disease/syndrome, or differentiating the syndrome to find the cause or differential diagnosis to identify the pathogen.

The ancient ideologies of health and health care in Chinese cultures have had a significant and long journey of evolution. It is a seemingly very different journey to the developments and understandings of the west but they are no less scientific. The Chinese philosophers and scientists embraced rational thought using logical and deductive reasoning to explain the world in which they lived within a universal framework. Evolving from this was the notion of Yin and Yang and the five Transformative phases that represented the active universe that operated within a dynamic process of change. This signified the formal development of scientific and medical enquiry based on natural laws and empiricism. The philosophical teachings drawn together by Confucian social and political theories that underpinned humanistic principles were a significant milestone in the history of Chinese medical science that enabled a scientific framework that developed a distinctive Chinese approach towards health care (Hoizey and Hoizey, 1993; Gao, 1999).

THE AYURVEDIC SYSTEM OF ANCIENT INDIA

Ayurvedic (Hindu) principles and philosophical understanding of health and illness were developed some 2000 years ago. Fundamentally, Ayurvedic systems of health care were based on India's spiritual foundations that considered the inter-relationship between human health and humanity's connection with the heavens and cosmos. From this perspective, illness was a result of an imbalance, with the delicate and intricate relationship that was described in terms of an association with the five elements of ether, air, fire, water and earth. It is a philosophical concept that considers a person's health from an holistic perspective viewing a person's soul as being interconnected with the universe. It requires individuals to search for 'self' and the 'universal truth' as a basic requirement to achieve the purest state of health and longevity. On the other hand, life and the state of health is not a static entity but a dynamic process that continues in a cyclical manner through a life–death–life continuum. Consequently, the belief in reincarnation pervades every aspect of life and death.

Historians have classified Ayurveda as a system of medicine, but this can be misleading in that modern medical (western) systems are renowned for their particular systematic reductionistic view of health and illness. Ayurveda is much broader than this premise engaging in wider philosophical principles based on 'positivism'. The name is derived from two Sanskrit roots *'ayus'* or 'life' and *'veda'* or 'science'. Therefore, Ayurveda is the 'science of life'.

Caring for the ill person using Ayurvedic systems requires the practitioner to assess the patient using a multi-layered diagnostic process to gain information that relates to the current ailment and the person's constitutional type. This is a comprehensive undertaking prior to any prescribing of Ayurvedic therapy. Once the diagnostic findings are established the primary objective is to restore any imbalance between the vital life energies. This is followed by a maintenance plan that may require the individual to change lifestyle and behaviour to secure long-term stability and achieve optimum health. Ayurvedic healing is concerned with all elements of life and a person's harmonious interplay and interactions with them. The emotions, intellect, body, actions, general behaviour, societal influences and the environment in which we live are all significant to humanity's health and well-being. To focus on one element as a primacy for health intervention, according to Ayurvedic teachings, creates a further imbalance. This imbalance is dangerous in restoring the health of individuals in a manner that promotes a way of life and fosters a long life free from disease and suffering.

An integral part of Ayurvedic therapy is meditation to enable the person to free the mind from the influence of disease and to encourage a free flow of life 'vital' energy. These energies are controlled by 'doshas' that are maintained by the energy forces of vata, pitta and kapha. These three guardians of health function to provide homeostatic conditions that sustain health but when there is a blockage in either one or all of these energy fields then a process is activated in which illness occurs. This process has six distinct stages, as described in Table 1.2.

In acknowledging these stages, Ayurveda's prime function is to prevent the formation or build up of disease. The first four stages of imbalance are diagnosed and managed by therapeutic processes that are considered using the principles of holism. When illness has occurred, Ayurveda promotes healing so that the individual's health is restored to balance and harmony using or facilitating their life energy forces.

When the doshas become imbalanced health suffers. If the balance is not restored and the discord is allowed to continue, further deterioration of health manifests itself into an acute or chronic health situation.

Table 1.2 Ayurvedic therapy: The six stages leading to illness

1 The accumulation of negative influences on one or more of the doshas.
2 Negative influences continue that seriously undermine the flow of energy, which is known as 'aggravation'.
3 From a localised imbalance the effect permeates other parts and is known as 'dispersion'.
4 The spread continues, causing an accumulation of waste products that have a toxic influence.
5 The first part of the body to be affected by negative influences shows signs of illness.
6 This will manifest into an acute situation, or if left untreated, will become a chronic health problem (Schutt, 1997).

ANCIENT GREECE

The first major changes in health care provision began to occur when ancient civilisations concerned themselves with empirical observation and the quest for scientific reasoning. For many historians this point in history is said to have commenced with the ancient Greeks who, historians suggest, developed a profound interest in advancing scientific knowledge and philosophical reasoning. In terms of health care the ancient Greeks are credited as the founders of modern western medicine (Oakley, 1976).

The Greeks believed that a balance between the four identified humours of the body aided good health: blood, phlegm, yellow bile and black bile. For the ancient Greeks, restoring health depended on returning these four substances to a state of equilibrium. The Greeks further reasoned that there was a correlation between epidemics and the atmosphere, the environment and the behaviour of humanity. In response to this revelation they advocated principles of good hygiene and the promotion of public health (The Open University, 1985). This particular feature of health care superseded any knowledge and real understanding of the germ theory that came much later.

During the period of enlightenment and empirical study one notable Greek physician was Hippocrates. A philosopher and healer who lived in the period of 460 BC, Hippocrates is often cited as being the father of modern medicine. He formulated the principles upon which to base a code of medical ethics that included the following: a physician should be empathetic, calm and respectful to the patient, and, above all, incorruptible. Hippocrates also classified disease entities that emerged from his interest in systematic observation and recording of the disease process, the results of which he compiled into a comprehensive text. His technique of observing the patient in the clinical setting was emulated by others who collectively produced volumes of literature that 'became part of the medical library of Alexandria' (Baly, 1980, p. 15).

While these substantial literary works reflected the advancements and understanding of medical knowledge and the aetiology of diseases, there was no reference to either the nurse or nursing care. Historians have therefore concluded that nursing was the duty of Greek women and was considered to be of little interest to the advancement of medical science (Bullough and Bullough, 1979).

Historical writers do not all support the notion that ancient Greece was the birthplace of modern medicine, given that there is very little resemblance to the positions medical practitioners held in the old world and those positions and practices that reflect modern health care (King, 1991). In defence of this challenge King asserts that the Hippocratic corpus makes reference to 'Iatrois', usually translated as 'male doctors' or 'physicians', but which simply means 'healers'. She makes the point that it is difficult to establish the differences between the healing therapies offered by Iatrois and those offered by other healers in ancient Greek society. What is believed to have happened is that the Iatrois divorced themselves from other healers by focusing on the art of 'techne' that incorporated both drama and philosophy. Thus, the Hippocratic healer was seen to be an orator and actor, a necessary attribute to compete in the healing and health care markets of the day. For example, the Iatrois would travel and compete with other healers for trade, such as the shaman, wise woman, herbalist and bone setter. It is further suggested that the male Iatrois would not necessarily work in isolation but would employ female assistants to carry out the formal aspects of care, as they were skilled in the art of caring and drug administration (Bullough and Bullough, 1979). Power and authority would remain with the Iatrois so as to maintain credit and payment for cure (Holden and Littlewood, 1991).

The relationship between women healers and the use of drugs was often mentioned by the Greek historians, who frequently highlighted the knowledge and understanding women healers had of drugs both for healing and poison. This particular concept is considered to have a dual meaning, one pertaining to the caring qualities ascribed to women and the other supporting the notion that women are dangerous interlopers taking advantage of herbal knowledge to advance their own schemes (King, 1991).

From this perspective, women's knowledge of herbs was both revered and feared, and required a controlling factor operated from a male perspective (Brooke, 1993). If we examine this concept we can see history repeating itself during the witch-hunts throughout Europe, which occurred during the late Middle Ages.

ANCIENT ROME

From ancient Greece, the historical trail of healing and caring moves to ancient Rome. This process occurred so gradually that it is difficult to determine when one finished and the other commenced. Nevertheless, it is generally acknowledged that the influences of Greek science and Roman engineering permeated the ancient world and had a particular influence upon health care.

However, when Rome conquered Greece the two cultures held opposing views regarding health. The early Romans believed that health care was an individual responsibility to such an extent that to request help and assistance from others was seen as a sign of human weakness. Consequently the Romans saw no virtue in acknowledging the high status of the Greek physicians, nor their contribution to the science of healing. As a result, many of the Greek physicians became slaves of Rome, usually serving the élite. This enabled an interchange between Greek physicians and educated Romans that allowed substantial medical knowledge to be passed between individuals (Bullough and Bullough, 1979).

Nursing, in contrast, was an activity that was encouraged, especially within the framework of the armed forces. Evidence suggests that the Roman soldier was instructed in the art of first aid so as to assist his injured companions on the field of battle. Once a soldier was injured he would be removed to the safety of a portable hospital whereupon nursing care would be given by women who were skilled in wound care and healing the sick (Bullough and Bullough, 1979).

While caring for wounded soldiers was an acceptable practice that was encouraged, Rome's policy makers were not interested in advancing medical knowledge per se, but their focus of attention was on promoting and facilitating healthy lifestyles for both the individual and the community. To illustrate this point individuals were encouraged to maintain a positive attitude and responsibility for their own health by increasing their physical and mental well-being through physical training and relaxation programmes. This was a combination perceived by the Romans to be a prerequisite for the maintenance and promotion of good health (Baly, 1980; The Open University, 1985). Added to this, Roman policy makers adopted a more beneficent stance, which assumed that an abundance of clean water and good sanitation would benefit the health and well-being of the citizens of Rome. To achieve these aims they built elaborate works of engineering, which were the envy of the ancient world. Christ (1984) illuminates the point by citing the Greek geographer, Strabo, who describes the Rome of Emperor Tiberius (AD 14–37) as follows:

> *Their underground sewers, with vaults of jointed stones, would in many places allow entire hay carts to drive through them. The quantities of water brought into the city are so large that whole rivers stream through the city and its underground drains, and that almost every house has water cisterns and piped water and abundantly spouting fountains.*
>
> (Christ, 1984, p. 148)

This feat of engineering is still marvelled at by archaeologists and historians today. The evidence points to vast improvements in the health of the British community being directly attributable to clean water supplies and sewage systems that relate to modern day living. Pestilence and disease associated with poor sanitary conditions and clean sources of water in the third world are still a source of ill-health, morbidity and early mortality. Given the overwhelming evidence, Rome's policy makers could be seen to be visionary in pursuit of the common goal. Unfortunately, as Rome expanded, so did the health need of Rome's citizens and in particular the health of the Roman soldiers who were considered to be crucial in sustaining the might of the Roman Empire.

To facilitate the recovery of sick and injured soldiers, temple hospitals were constructed within an environment that radiated peace and tranquillity. These hospitals were often built near springs that were reputed to have healing properties (Edwards-Rees, 1966). Thus we see a considerable change in Roman philosophy towards health care that allowed the once enslaved Greek physicians to practise and extend their art of healing. During this period Roman noblewomen who perceived nursing to be a vocation and a high status occupation usually provided nursing care. Furthermore, historians suggest that the standards of nursing care were relatively high, addressing the needs of the patient from a physical, psychological, sociological and spiritual perspective, an approach that is currently embraced by contemporary nursing practice (Buckman and Sabbagh, 1993).

Study Activity 1.2 _____

So far a synopsis of understanding the evolution of health and health care has been described from the period of primitive humanity to antiquity, embracing both a western and eastern philosophy of prevailing ideologies of health and healing care of the time. It is evident that there are similar themes represented within different cultures and different periods of time. Reflect on the key issues emerging from the various themes on health and healing care to assess the following hypothetical clinical incident using each health paradigm:

- A six-year-old child is hyperactive and sleeps very little. His diet is based on seeds, nuts and fruits, when in season. Animal protein is eaten rarely and is often uncooked. He has frequent bouts of diarrhoea and sickness, together with poor memory. Sanitation is crude with raw sewage in the streets. Water supply is from the village well.
- A 20-year-old woman has been married for three years and has not yet conceived. She has been suffering from the effects of tuberculosis and has a significant weight loss. Her diet is poor and lacks protein and fresh fruits. She has consulted the village shaman for health advice.
- A young man has had cerebral convulsions over the past month. They started after a tree fell on his head six weeks ago. He is married with five children, but sexual relations have significantly declined since the birth of the couple's last child. He often visits prostitutes.

EARLY INFLUENCES OF CHRISTIANITY

The public health measures and engineering feats attributable to ancient Rome lost their impetus with the demise of the Roman Empire. For the next 1000 years health care became entrenched and symbiotically related to the doctrines espoused by Christianity. The reasons for Rome's demise have often been wondered about and answers have been provided from those theories based around theological debates to the notion that Rome was overextended and could

no longer support the health and well-being of the people it served. Evidence suggests that many of Rome's citizens repeatedly suffered from the ravages of poverty, disease and pestilence, with a resultant life expectancy of between 20 and 35 years (Pounds, 1974). The effect of this was quite devastating, resulting in social disarray and with it the demise of the existing political infrastructure. Disillusioned and disenchanted with the framework in which Rome operated the people of Rome drew solace and comfort from the teachings of Christianity.

Christian philosophies underpinning health care were antipathetic to those embraced by Rome. Early Roman Christians were advised to disengage themselves from any activities that were associated with pagan Rome, including the practices of health care performed within the constructs of the temple hospitals. As a result, many of the temple hospitals were destroyed and new models of health care were thereafter influenced by the teachings of Christianity. Teachings assumed that health was linked to one's fate, and only God could guide it. The Greek Galen, cited in Buckman and Sabbagh (1993), wrote 'all who drink of this remedy recover in a short time, except those whom it does not help will all die' (p. 20).

While the Christian Church held such a fatalistic view it did foster the notion that the sick and needy should not be ignored, but should be cared for as a humanitarian act of charity. This fundamental Christian principle inspired many of Rome's citizens to reject materialism and devote their lives to caring for others. Many were ordained as deacons and deaconesses, who were instrumental in delivering hands-on care within the patient's own home environment (Bullough and Bullough, 1979; Baly, 1980; Buckman and Sabbagh, 1993). Eventually, bishops were assigned responsibility for the sick and needy, and supervised the activities of the deacons and deaconesses.

However, historians' opinions are polarised on the actual input of the deacons and deaconesses on direct nursing care. There are those who suggest they were significant in the caring activity, and those who claim that the caring duties would be secondary to the charitable duties required by the Church. If the latter view is correct then it is assumed the central activity of caring for the sick would be by family members. If it is the former, it is reasoned that with the absence of hospital care the deacons and deaconesses would have provided care to the sick and needy (Seymore, 1957). Baly (1980) supports this argument by citing St Jerome (AD 340–420), who describes how Fabiola, a deaconess (AD 399), cared for the sick and dying by 'washing their putrid matter that others could not bear to look on' (p. 18).

MONASTICISM

As the voice of Christianity became stronger, the focus of providing care for the sick and needy changed direction from community to institutionalised care within the framework of the monastic system. Historians suggest the reason for this change was primarily because the deacons and deaconesses began to fear exposure and corruption from materialism (Edwards-Rees, 1966; Bullough and Bullough, 1979; Baly, 1980). The deacons and deaconesses therefore sought refuge away from the cities and formed small communities of like-minded people. These communities became enclosed in buildings that eventually became known as monasteries.

Adherence to strict rules and regulations was a principle feature of monastic life, which centred around work, prayer and self-flagellation. The notion of self-flagellation disappeared with the influence of St Benedict who established more lenient rules, one of which was the notion that each monk had a duty to care for his fellow brethren during periods of sickness. This principle was further extended to people outside the monastic order and resulted in sections within the monasteries being designated for the purpose of healing and caring for the sick and needy.

Throughout this period, advancements in understanding health and illness altered very little, despite the fact that monks and nuns were considered to be more educated than their lay counterparts. The reason offered by historians is that they maintained a total adherence to Christian philosophies relating to health and health care, models of care that were, at the very best, simplistic and, at the worst, barbaric. For example, the patients would receive basic hygiene care, they would often be purged and bled, and they would be constantly prayed over to prepare them for the afterlife (Baly, 1980). In short it was a framework of health care that assumed a passiveness and total acceptance of God's will.

To assume all health care during this period was within the confines of the monasteries is rather questionable, even though the focus of attention for historians is within this framework of reference. The sheer logistics of housing all those who were sick would be a task of considerable magnitude and made it not feasible. Added to this, the geographical distance between monasteries and villages would be too great for villagers to travel. From this position Alic (1990) makes the claim that most health care would be provided by family members and women healers.

THE MIDDLE AGES

Classic historians claim that the Middle Ages were generally devoid of any significant scientific advancement and have classified this period as the 'Dark Ages'. Such proclamations have significantly devalued any advancements or developments made throughout this period, particularly in the field of health care. This is a commonly held view that is challenged, based on the evidence that the Saracen physicians of Italy were contributing to the developments in health care influenced by the philosophies underpinning 'Vedic' medicine of India and the Arabian 'Saracens'. Vedic medicine combines the knowledge of the healing properties of herbs with the mystical incantations of song, while the Saracen physicians of Arabia concerned themselves with hygiene and developed advanced skills in surgery and anaesthesia.

The above philosophies and principles of health care were readily adopted and refined by the Italian physicians of the late Middle Ages, culminating in a framework that offered medical training within the hospices of Europe's first university (The Open University, 1985). One notable scholar from this Italian medical school was a woman known as Trotula, who was instrumental in advancing medical science with renewed vigour, bringing medical knowledge out of the Dark Ages. One of her major contributions to the scientific community was her classic text on 'the diseases of women' that surpassed anything previously written. The main focus of this text was centred upon midwifery care that included the care of the infant during the post-partum period (Alic, 1990).

Clearly, the end of the Middle Ages saw a renaissance of interest in the search for meaning and understanding of health care that was not solely centred on Christian values and beliefs. It was a return to the empirical observations and scientific enquiry that the ancient Greeks were familiar with. The difference was that the Saracen physicians of Italy were influenced by the Indian and Arabian philosophies of health and health care.

THE KNIGHTS OF ST JOHN

Throughout the period 1095–1271 Europe became embroiled in the religious wars known as the Crusades, which disrupted family life and disintegrated social order. Soldiers would be away from home for several years, leaving the burden of domestic responsibility on the shoulders of the women. The battles for the Crusades were fought across a wide area of Europe and the Holy Land of Jerusalem, and left many Crusaders sick, injured and dying (Baly, 1980). Public concern for the plight of the Crusaders was raised and this resulted in the construction of hospitals to house the sick and injured, and the encouragement of men to join the Order of St John, whose principal duty was to serve the sick and injured Crusaders.

The first hospital was built in Jerusalem and its architectural design established a precedent for others to be built. Nursing care within these hospitals was organised by the men who had joined the Order of St John, sometimes known as the Knights of St John or Knight's Hospitalier. Upon entering the order the knights were required to take the monastic vows of poverty, obedience and chastity, but added to these was the vow of serving the sick.

The knights were renowned for their skills in healing and their approaches towards nursing care that included the principles of asepsis and laws of quarantine. The latter concept was a model of nursing practice that was practised by the knights in times of epidemics. The main principle of quarantine practice was to isolate sick individuals and activate a form of nursing care that was to become known as 'barrier nursing'. The period of quarantine lasted for forty days with the view that any infection would have passed by then, and this would reduce the chance of infections spreading from one infected person to another (Bullough and Bullough, 1979).

This was a time in history where many people were displaced through the Crusades or pilgrimages. This situation facilitated the spread of diseases, such as syphilis, leprosy, typhoid and other related conditions that culminated in the need for nurses who were not family members. Many women responded to the need and worked in the hospitals or, as Alic (1990) points out, continued to provide care within the villages using traditional healing methods.

At the end of the Crusades, Europe was suffering from the ravages of war, disease epidemics, poverty and a lack of social order. On returning from the wars men wanted to restore social order, particularly from a male perspective. To achieve this aim, they colluded with the existing political mechanisms to devalue and deskill women. The Church contributed to this process by suggesting that women, particularly those who had healing skills, were in collusion with supernatural powers and should be opposed and feared (Brooke, 1993). This fear helped to fuel the witch-hunts that were an inherent feature of European life for almost four centuries. These witch-hunts were responsible for the loss of thousands of lives, mainly those of women, mentally ill and disabled people. Historians claim that many of these women were healers and with their death much healing knowledge that would have normally passed from mother to daughter was lost.

The reasons for these injustices remain inadequately explored, but historical literature suggests that they were induced by the many terrorising sermons preached by the Church and exacerbated by the use of hallucinogenic drugs (Brooke, 1993). Moreover, the condemning action of the Church undermined women's position in society and excluded them from the emerging medical schools. The result produced a healing service that had two tiers, with the male doctor at the top and women healers at the bottom. Both offered similar services, but the woman healer was considerably cheaper, a state of affairs that was considered intolerable by the male medical profession. As competition increased, the male medical fraternity constantly undermined the skills of women healers, suggesting that they were charlatans and quacks. Eventually, laws against women healers were enforced (Hall and Hall, 1964). However, this law was never fully enacted due to the fact that women were still the main providers of healing practices of an 'unorthodox' nature within village life (Oakley, 1976).

THE REFORMATION

European health care was derived from and influenced by the religious orders that were to proliferate throughout Europe between the sixteenth and nineteenth centuries. Most of these originated from the teachings of the Protestant and Catholic Church. The schism that eventually occurred between the two churches gave way to two schools of thought. The Catholic Church advocated a benevolent position suggesting that the art and science of caring was a vocation, a calling from God. Men and women were encouraged to become nurses within the auspices of the new orders, while the Protestant Church espoused the notion that each

individual had a clear responsibility to the community and the family unit. In England this concept became internalised as a central feature of the Elizabethan Poor Law Act of 1601, which stated that each parish was responsible for provision of care for its own sick and needy people; a philosophy of health care provision that was to remain relatively unchanged for three centuries. Critics of the Elizabethan Poor Law claim that it subscribed excessively to the concepts of paternalism, while others suggest that it was a formula that ensured the sick and needy were cared for in a structured manner across the country (Baly, 1980).

Throughout this period the advancements in medical science reflected, in a corresponding way, advancements made in other scientific arenas. Disease and human dysfunction was examined in microscopic detail by the male medical profession who asserted their dominant position in health care. Contemporary writers have questioned the quality of medical practice during these years, suggesting that improvement only began because of the experiences gained during the numerous wars, for example, the civil, religious, colonial, and revolutionary wars of the seventeenth and eighteenth centuries. These situations enabled medical practitioners to overshadow the more 'homespun' empirical observations of people's health made by 'wise' women (Parry and Parry, 1976).

Study Activity 1.3 —————

- The influence of Christianity strongly influenced health and health care for several centuries. What was its key philosophy regarding health?
- Why was care in the villages, by village people and family members, replaced with monastic infirmaries?
- What was the legacy of health care that the Knights of St John became famous for?
- Throughout the Middle Ages, was there any real advancement made in the knowledge of disease and therapeutic interventions?

THE EIGHTEENTH AND NINETEENTH CENTURIES

By the end of the eighteenth century sick and needy people were increasingly offered health care within the framework of institutions, such as charitable hospitals, workhouse infirmaries and asylums. Nursing care within this context was akin to the functions and duties of domestics and attendants and, as such, did not warrant any degree of intelligence or training. As a consequence the quality of nursing care was low. Nurses were recruited from the lower classes or they were patients themselves. Nurses had a very poor image and were described as sluttish, drunken and having dubious morals. Charles Dickens, who created the character of the nurse Sarah Gamp in his book, *Martin Chuzzlewit*, portrays one such image. The following quote epitomises the role of nurses in these institutions, 'What a blessed thing it is to make sick people happy in their bed, and never mind one's self as long as one can do a service'.

Smith (1988) contends that the above caricature may be unjustified, suggesting that in the absence of scientific medicine and knowledge about the importance of cleanliness, the comforting presence of a friendly nurse may have been as much as could be hoped for. In contrast, the medical profession was advancing in response to scientific and technological discoveries. Hospital institutions were thought of as places where doctors could observe their unsuspecting patients and experiment upon them in the pursuit of scientific knowledge. Edwards-Rees (1966) suggests that medical practitioners could see more patients in one day in a hospital than they could in one year in the community, thus facilitating greater opportunity to observe the disease process.

Clearly, dogmatically following such methods of scientific enquiry firmly established the judging of people's health through a reductionistic and mechanical approach. Nursing was not immune to such models of practice and was required to respond and develop new skills so as to operate within new health care organisations and provide new ways of thinking and changes to carry out care interventions. The medical practitioners now supported the nurse being well educated, developing the skills required in the art of caring and being able to dutifully record observations of patients and the effect of treatments prescribed by the doctor. In addition, the nurse must be sober, steadfast and demure. This is a striking difference from the caricature of Sarah Gamp, who was portrayed as a drunken, uncouth woman of low morals.

NURSING REFORM

The first influences on the reform of nursing came from France and Germany. The French were primarily instrumental in embracing new ideas regarding empirical observation in life and post-mortem examination. They designed tools to facilitate observation of health, such as the stethoscope and thermometer. By contrast, Germany formalised nursing care through the influences of the Protestant deaconesses. The deaconesses concerned themselves with a systematic nurse training that was underpinned by religious vocation. It is the German model of training nurses that was to have a significant impact on two English women: Elizabeth Fry and Florence Nightingale. Both women were to influence the education and training of nurses in England in a way that was eventually to form the framework of contemporary practice (White, 1978; The Open University, 1985).

Elizabeth Fry (1780–1845) was best known for her work within the prison services, but saw no distinction between the physical, psychological and moral welfare of her clients. She was known to have been an advocate of vaccinations and often performed this duty on the local parishioners. However, it was her work with the prison reform movement that brought her into contact with Pastor Fliedner of Kaiserworth in 1840. Pastor Fliedner had previously been impressed with the prison reform movement on his visit to England and upon his return to Germany inspired the deaconess movement to care for these unfortunate souls who had been discharged from the prisons. This influenced the recognition that the deaconesses needed to be prepared to undertake this role, and Pastor Fliedner and his wife organised the training scheme for deaconess 'nurses'. Their work in this field became renowned for its excellence and was the purpose of Elizabeth Fry's visit. The outcome of her visit enabled Elizabeth and her sister to organise a nurse training school in England. This became known as 'The Institute of Nursing'. Although the probationary nurses were carefully selected and received some elementary training, the venture was unsuccessful, primarily due to the lack of supervision and employment opportunities (Baly, 1980; The Open University, 1985).

Florence Nightingale (1820–1910) was a member of the English upper class, whose enforced idleness (the norm for society ladies) encouraged her desire to become a nurse. She maintained that this was a calling from God specifically, on 7 February 1837 (Seymore, 1957). This inherent desire to be a nurse came to fruition when she visited Pastor Fliedner at Kaiserworth in 1851 for a three-month period. During this time she admired the organised way in which the deaconesses cared for the sick, but failed to fully appreciate the training criteria for the probationary nurses. As a consequence, she chose to undertake nurse training with the Sisters of Charity at the Maison de la Providence in Paris. Her training as a probationary nurse was to be short-lived due to her grandmother's illness.

On her return to England she took up an appointment as a superintendent of a small hospital, where she diligently deployed the principles of nursing she had quickly learned. She was an ardent believer of the miasmas theory, whereby illness was due to the noxious smells and vapours in the air, and she never renounced this, even after the overwhelming evidence of the germ theory. Her codes of nursing care were therefore centred on the principles of good public health (Van der Peet, 1995). This did not affect her notoriety or her great influence on British nursing. The Crimean War offered Florence the opportunity to influence and improve the health

and well-being of the British soldiers. Her involvement in the Crimean War came about due to her friend Sydney Herbert who suggested that Florence and a few trusted and experienced nurses should go to Scutari in Turkey to assist the injured soldiers who were reportedly dying in their thousands due to neglect.

On 4 November 1854, Florence Nightingale and a small party of nurses set sail for Scutari. On her arrival, the horrors of the war were apparent. It was obvious that the British Army was in total disarray and the medical services non-existent. Further to this, there was no clean water provision, nor an adequate sanitation system, no dressings to cover the soldiers' wounds and food rations were minimal. The result of this was an unacceptably high rate of mortality among the injured soldiers.

After assessing the situation, Florence and her colleagues began to improve the cleanliness of the environment and gained access to clean water and food supplies. This was against a lot of opposition from the male military who believed these measures to be an unnecessary expenditure. While it is claimed that Florence did improve the health of the soldiers, it is the media who portrayed her as the 'lady with the lamp', who glided through the hospital at Scutari, providing comfort to the dying soldier (Van der Peet, 1995). Thus, on returning from Scutari, she was celebrated and adored as the saviour of the British soldier and became a legend in her own lifetime.

In recognition of her achievements in Scutari the public contributed to the Nightingale Fund established by her friend Sydney Herbert to create a training institution known as the Nightingale School for Nurses. Although she suffered from periodic bouts of ill-health, she was not deterred from lobbying her political supporters and writing about the practice of nursing.

Traditional historians contend that Florence Nightingale gave birth to modern nursing, a public portrayal that was readily and unquestionably accepted until recent writers began to reinvestigate her life. The result of this research clearly illustrates a different view. Contemporary writers point out that her nursing principles were influenced by her religious pragmatism and archaic models of sanitary implications that have served only to hinder the development of nursing (Have, 1983). Van der Peet (1995) supports this notion by citing Baly (1969):

> ... *living in the shadow of a legend is not an un-mitigating blessing. Exhorted to the 'Nightingale spirit', praised as 'ministering angels', sickled o'er with pale cast of sentimentality, nurses have tended to cling blindly to the tradition that raised them to such a pinnacle. To question the system was lese-majeste, and this bred orthodoxy; conformity operates against reform. In spite of some enlightened questioning, the profession has tended to look back to its days of glory and has chosen not reform, but a crown of thorns.*
>
> (Baly, 1969, p. 4)

Baly (1980) and Prince (1982) have convincingly demonstrated that the Nightingale School of Nursing never achieved independent educational status but was influenced and controlled by the hospital governors and the medical profession, a situation that was to persist in British nursing until the 1970s.

Study Activity 1.4 ———————

- The pursuit of scientific investigation within the context of health care enabled medical practice to assert its superior position in health care and this has remained the case ever since. Discuss this statement using the content of this chapter and your wider reading.
- What were the contributions to nursing care made by Elizabeth Fry and Florence Nightingale?
- On reflection, has the influence of Florence Nightingale been of benefit to modern nursing?
- The medical model followed a reductionistic approach to care. Why was this, and was it appropriate for nursing to adopt this approach when caring for the individual person?

Study Activity 1.5 ———————

A soldier in the Crimean War had gun wounds to the chest and leg. He was transported to the wards under the supervision of Florence Nightingale. His wounds were dressed regularly, and the ward was kept clean and tidy. Food, although rationed, was nutritious compared with that available on the front line. According to the doctor, his wounds should have mended, but he failed to respond. In your opinion, what were the reasons for this soldier's non-response to the care given?

CHANGING PARADIGMS OF HEALTH THROUGHOUT TWENTIETH-CENTURY EUROPE

The early twentieth-century health paradigms centred upon whether or not you were fit for work, or war, and you were categorised accordingly as 'healthy' or 'sick'. This was a black-and-white perspective embraced by the medical profession, which perceived people with disease or disability as being unable to work (Bergdolt, 1999). It became a mould embedded in policy and insurance laws that, until recently, was difficult to break. The physician, encapsulated within a legal and therapeutic framework, determined the legitimisation of a person's health. The predominance of this model was awe-inspiring to some, but it failed to recognise the fluid nature of health, the different dimensions the state of health engendered, or the individual relationship with one's health.

Medical health care was focused and entrenched in objectifying people's health in terms of physical or mental dysfunction without any correlation between the two. This explains the growth in specialised medicine that assessed, researched and treated the health of individuals from a system or compartmental approach. The environmental, spiritual and social factors were overlooked by the medical profession, apart from the public health programmes that were implemented by governments to produce clean air, water and sanitation.

Notwithstanding the above, the reductionistic approach used by medical physicians was viewed to be beneficial in seeking out new knowledge and understanding of health and disease. However, consensus with regard to the concept of health reached an impasse and continues to elude universal agreement. Nevertheless, moving from the classical medical perception that suggests health is when a person is free from disease, others have looked at defining the concept differently. For instance, Schnitzler (1967) suggests health is a positive function of human existence that serves to enhance the quality of life. By contrast, the World Health Organisation (WHO) proclaims that health is a state of complete physical, psychological and social well-being, and individual health is declared to be one of the basic laws of human existence. This is a well-intentioned proclamation, but its execution is over-ambitious, given that only a few Europeans would meet such criteria, and in the third world only a handful would comply. However, it would be foolish to ignore that optimising one's state of health is a dream humanity aspires to and as such health has become eulogised as a right and a virtue. In countries where a strong welfare state has emerged, the right to be healthy has become a principle of care. Whereas at the turn of the century, nursing was centred on providing care for the sick and needy, the modern day equivalent is concerned with the promotion of health to prevent illness or disability. It focuses on restoring health through using complex therapeutic interventions, and maintaining health throughout people's lives and thereby enhancing the quality of life.

Within these constructs patients are active participants in their own health care, taking responsibility for their own health and, wherever possible, encouraged to promote self-healing. Their lifestyles are examined in the context of health risk behaviour and they are encouraged to make choices based on the best evidence.

Nursing care has responded to reflect these changes, moving from the umbrella of the medical model to models that embrace a more humanistic and holistic approach towards health and illness care. This is not a static response as, with increasing advancements in health technology and health interventions, nursing (like the concept of health) will continue to evolve and adapt to societal and professional views of health and health care.

THE FUTURE

Societies are no longer small and simplistic groups, but complex, inter-related structures through which health care is delivered. The talk now is of global communities recognising the fact that actions or health care practices occurring in the western world have an effect in other parts of the global community, and vice versa. Technology is on the brink of major advancements in understanding the nature of human functioning and the disease potentiality through genetic make-up. Further to this we are, for the first time in human history, in a period of an ageing society. With advancements in age, increase in chronic ill-health is substantive and requires nursing care to facilitate the management of the chronic disease. Conversely, nursing care will also facilitate individuals' capacity to heal themselves by incorporating knowledge of health from the old worlds and the technology of the new. Deepak Chopra (1990) suggests that this can be done through *Quantum Healing*, which embraces mind/body medicine.

SUMMARY

The history of health and health care serves to remind us that health is never static, but a dynamic process of change influenced by external and internal factors. In this sense human existence cannot be summed up as being either health or illness. This has not stopped people's inquiry into the subject and this chapter shows how it is evident that through each different era and within different cultures health and disease has had a focus of attention.

The different perspectives from each culture offered have enabled a rich framework of understanding that can, combined, help to inform the future. Today, there is an explosion of seeking information from the eastern cultures, suggesting there is some dissatisfaction in the way medical practice operates within the west. This should not be seen as 'throwing the baby out with the bath water', but a recognition that both elements of practice can influence health care.

Study Activity 1.6 _____

- The historical journey of health and health care has followed many paths and defining health is complex. Offer four reasons to explain why this is so.
- If nursing is about promoting and restoring health, how can this be done if there is no universal agreement?
- Nursing has changed over time to accommodate changes in society, advancements in therapeutics and diagnostic reasoning, and scientific discoveries. Looking in your crystal ball, how might changes in nursing occur over the next 30 years?

REFERENCES

Alic, M. (1990) *Hypatias Heritage*, The Women's Press, London

Baly, M.E. (1969) Florence Nightingale's influence on nursing today. *Nursing Times* 65, 1–4

Baly, M.E. (1980) *Nursing and Social Change*, The Women's Press, London

Bergdolt, K. (1999) History of Medicine and Concepts of Health. *Croatian Medical Journal* 40, 119–22. *www.cmj.hr*

Brooke, E. (1993) *Women Healers Throughout History*, The Women's Press, London

Buckman, R. and Sabbagh, K. (1993) *Magic or Medicine*, Macmillan, London

Bullough, V. and Bullough, B. (1979) *The Care of the Sick: The emergence of modern nursing*, Croom Helm, London

Chopra, D. (1990) *Quantum Healing*, Bantam New Age Books, London

Christ, K. (1984) *The Romans*, Chatto and Windus, London

Davies, C. (1980) *Rewriting Nursing History*, Croom Helm, London

De Beauvoir, S. (1952). In: Miles, R. (1989) *The Women's History of the World*, Paladine Books, London

Dunlop, M. (1986) Is science of caring possible? *Journal of Advanced Nursing* 2, 661–700

Edwards-Rees, D. (1966) *The Story of Nursing*, Longman, Toronto

Ehrenreich, B. and English, D. (1973) *Witches, Midwives and Nurses: A history of women healers*, The Feminist Press, London

Gao, D. (1999) *The Encyclopaedia of Chinese Medicine*, Carlton Books, ??

Hall, A. and Hall, M.M. (1964) *A Brief History of Science*, New American Library, New York

Have, H.T. (1983) In: Van der Peet, R. (1995) *The Nightingale Model of Nursing*, Campion Press, Edinburgh

Hoizey, D. and Hoizey, M. (trans. P. Bailey) (1993) *A History of Chinese Medicine*, Edinburgh University Press, Edinburgh

Holden, P. and Littlewood, J. (1991) *Anthropology and Nursing*, Routledge, London

Keegan, L. (1988). In: Dossey, L., Keegan, L. and Gazzetta, C. (1988) *Holistic Nursing: A handbook for practice*, Aspen Publications, Gaithersburg MD

King, H. (1991) Using the past: nursing and the medical profession in ancient Greece. In: Holden, P. and Littlewood, J. (1991) *Anthropology and Nursing*, Routledge, London

Leininger, M.M. (1981) Leininger's theory of nursing culture: care diversity and universality. *Nursing Science* 1, 152–62

Nightingale, F. (1859, republished 1980) *Notes on Nursing*, Churchill Livingstone, Edinburgh

Novarra, N. (1987) *Women's Work, Men's Work*, Marion Boyars, London

Oakley, A. (1976) *A Social History of Medicine*, Longman, London

Prince, J. (1982) Florence Nightingale's reform of nursing 1860–1887 [unpublished PhD thesis], London School of Economics, London

The Open University (1985) *Caring for Health*, Open University Press, Buckingham

Parry, N. and Parry, J. (1976) *The Rise of the Medical Profession*, Croom Helm, London

Pearson, A. (1991) Taking up the challenge: the future for therapeutic nursing. In: MacMahon, R. and Pearson, A. (1991) *Nursing as Therapy*, Chapman and Hall, London

Porkert, M. (1982) *Chinese Medicine as Scientific System*, Henry Holt, New York

Pounds, N.J.G. (1974) *An Economic History of Medieval Europe*, Longman, London

Schnitzler, A. (1967) In: Bergdolt, K. (1999) History of Medicine and Concepts of Health. *Croatian Medical Journal* 40, 119–22. *www.cmj.hr*

Schutt, K. (1997) *Ayurveda – The Secret of Lifelong Youth*, Time Life Books, New York

Seymore, L.R. (1957) *A General History of Nursing*, Faber & Faber, London

Smith, P. (1988) Recruit and retain. The emotional labour of nursing. *Nursing Times* 84(44), 50–1

Van der Peet, R. (1995) *The Nightingale Model of Nursing*, Campion Press, Edinburgh

Versluysen, M. (1980) Old wives' tales? Woman healers in English history. In: Davies, C. (1980) *Rewriting Nursing History*, Croom Helm, London

Watson, J. (1989) *Towards a Caring Curricula: New pedagogy for nursing*, National League for Nursing, New York

White, R. (1978) *Social Change and the Development of the Nursing Profession*, Henry Kimpton, London

Yeandle, S. (1984) *Woman at Work*, Tavistock, London

2 COMMITMENT TO CARE: A PHILOSOPHICAL PERSPECTIVE ON NURSING

Carol Kirby

> As experience, the world belongs to the primary word I-It.
> The primary word I-Thou establishes the world of relation.
>
> (Buber, 1958)

LEARNING OUTCOMES

After studying this chapter you will be able to:

- Recognise care as a philosophical perspective within nursing
- Distinguish different uses for the term 'care'
- Appreciate that caring invokes commitment to others
- Discuss commitment in respect of its concern for others, which is in essence an ethical response
- Recognise that in a human context, caring occurs within relationships that are open to the giving and receiving of help
- Describe the processes involved within caring relationships.

INTRODUCTION

Caring is definitive of nursing. It is a moral ideal entailing commitment. Commitment is present in dedication to others, in personal allegiance, and in promises kept. With commitment we respond to peoples' lives, lives we are seeking to sustain, enhance and bring peace of mind to. Nursing generates healing; it creates hope and seeks to actualise dignity. The caring practice of nursing is based upon moral commitment, upon belief that people matter. When nurses say they care they are saying that *the person who is the patient matters;* that they want everything to be as good as it possibly can be for them, wanting what they consider and decide is best for themselves. Caring *with*, *for* and *about* is the essence of humanity. It makes a difference – the difference between being at home in the world or in exile, believing nothing matters anymore. Caring in nursing is both a moral and an energy source. Nursing identity is defined through caring for others. It is realised within informed, compassionate and skilled caring.

REFLECTIONS

Care

Heidegger (1962) spoke of human beings connected with one another and the world, intimately involved in their being-in-the-world concerned with their worldly nature, as *care* (Sorge). Thus, one cares to the extent that one cares about one's capacity 'to be'; is concerned with what one 'can be' and with the 'I who is' in union with 'for-the-sake-of-whom'. Gaylin (1976) believes that an impulse for caring is biologically programmed in human nature – 'caring and loving we are, and caring and loving we must be' (p. 180); we care because it is our nature to care, we survive because we care and are cared for; we are 'touched' by signs of caring and 'hurt' by signs of indifference. In speaking of caring Mayeroff (1990 [1971]) gave voice to what he perceived to be essential components of caring and to his belief that one experiences what is cared for as having a dignity and worth in its own right with potentialities and need for growth. Caring both evolves from and invokes commitment arising from within a deep source and dimension of our humanity.

Commitment

Commitment is regarded by Van Hooft (1995) as 'a stance towards the world or towards others on the part of an individual or group which defines what is important or imperative for that individual or group' (p. 13). Commitment, Clemence (1966) upholds, gives real significance to everything that the nurse does and is and she confirms that one lives nursing life authentically when fully committed, in open-eyed acceptance of and responsibility to life. Caring, she believes, is expressed within commitment through 'a willingness to live fully one's own life, to make that life meaningful through acceptance of, rather than detachment from, all that it may hold of joy and sorrow' (p. 500). Commitment gives testimony to nursing integrity, authenticity and faithfulness; it inspirits caring healing presence and is witness of our deepest ethical intentions.

Commitment to care

When we in nursing speak of a commitment to care we commit to action, to committed therapeutic action within relation. Caring is more than having concern or being concerned for others, it entails commitment – reaching to another intending to care. Care emerges from a deep moral source within; from a primordial concern for others we are compelled to act, willingly dedicating self through therapeutic use of self. In the caring moment we invoke and realise commitment. Caring ethically connects self with others and with the world. Care so understood is our way of being in relation to all people and all things; our connection with and interconnection in the world. It is the profound expression, the call at the heart of nursing.

We have looked to the beginnings of our profession in Chapter 1 and found commitment embodied in those dedicated to caring for others. While caring for others is not uniquely a nursing concern, nursing is unique in its origins – in its creation to care. In the remaining chapters of this module, we address the contexts within which caring takes place. A commitment to care underlies all of the endeavours discussed in the remainder of the book. In subsequent modules we consider how our profession has developed, its theoretical and empirical underpinnings, the frameworks within which practice is organised and realised through nursing intervention. All of this we dedicate to the fundamental purpose of nursing – caring for others. It is this fundamental purpose we address in this chapter.

BEING-IN-THE-WORLD-OF-NURSING: BECOMING

A link connects oneself with others – life lived in relation to others. The connection is not only being-in-the-world but also significantly being-*human*-in-the-world. Who I am and who I become, the meaning found in life, arises within the relationship. From within concerned involvement with others, a responsible relationship to others emerges. How we respond, our responsibility to another, defines how we stand ethically. Who we are and who we become depend upon the stand we take on being *self*. Moral action is brought about through engagement, emerging from within relation. Within a process of self-discovery we become authentic. Authentic being requires reflection, self-knowledge. The moral quest begins with experiencing, with reflection on experiences. The fundamental questions to be asked are: how should we live? and, what in life compels an allegiance to the *good*, the right *life*? Iris Murdoch (2001) believed that the 'love which brings the right answer is an exercise of justice and realism and really *looking*'. In addition, she tells us 'we act rightly "when the time comes" not out of strength of will but out of the quality of our usual attachments and with the kind of energy and discernment which we have available. And to this, the whole activity of our consciousness is relevant' (p. 89). Acting rightly in nursing requires integral knowledge and skill; it requires exercising the virtues of responsibility, honesty, courage, duty, obligation and the reasoning of justice. Importantly, it requires that we actualise possibility and potential; that we commit to care. The source of potential, of becoming, of being what one 'truly is', is put in focus by May (1983):

> *Being should be understood to mean potentia, the source of potentiality; being is the potentiality by which … each of us becomes what he truly is. And when used in a particular sense, such as a human being, it always has the dynamic connotation of someone in process, the person being something … We can understand another human being only as we see what he is moving toward, what he is becoming; and we can know ourselves only as we 'project our potential in action.' The significant tense for human beings is thus the future – that is to say, the critical question is what I am pointing toward, what I will be in the immediate future.*
>
> (May, 1983, p. 97)

Being-ethical-in-the-world-of-nursing is an obligation, a *must*. Attention to wholeness, to a consciousness of who one is and is becoming and to the ethical demands and difficulties of the 'good life' underpin the deliberative capacity essential to responsible choice and, to caring. Knowing who I am, becoming a question to myself – asking who and for whom I am – helps *me* to say with conviction: 'this is me, this is where I stand'. The examined life *is* worth living. Who we are and who we become, our selfhood, and 'good', are inextricably entwined.

Study Activity 2.1

Worth

'The examined life is worth living'. Discuss this statement in small-group formation, relating it to the importance of reflection in nursing practice.

Becoming self is spoken of by Dunne (1996):

> *Moreover, to be a self is to be involved not just in directional (i.e. ethical) questioning*

> *but also in a quest; for one cannot but care about how one is situated or is moving relative to the direction one discerns. If this is care about oneself it is at the same time care for the goods that determine the direction. These goods, in other words, are the objects of love as well as attention. 'Objects' is perhaps an unfortunate term insofar as it suggests that the power of the love comes from the self as subject or source – whereas it would be truer to say that these goods empower the self, by arousing its love, and are thus its sources (or resources).*
>
> (Dunne, 1996, p. 146)

In speaking of the sovereignty of good, Iris Murdoch (2001) commented that 'Good is the magnetic centre towards which love naturally moves and when the soul is turned towards Good the highest part of the soul is enlivened' (p. 100). When commenting on a difficulty in defining good, she reminds us that when Plato wanted to explain good he used the image of the sun. She believed this to be an extremely rich metaphor because it is real, is out there, gives light and energy and enables us to know truth; 'in its light we see the things of the world in their true relationship' (p. 90). In accepting that we often have difficulty putting into words exactly what we mean when we speak of 'a good person', when we speak of 'the good in nursing', it is easier to say with conviction – we speak of wisdom and of informed, compassionate, skilled caring.

The call *of* and *to* the 'good', the power of love and of powerlessness arouses and inspires caring and invokes a response in the face of human suffering. The significant is to know self, to care about oneself and others so that we can reach to and take hold of another when they are feeling fragile, powerless and in need. We grow, become *more* by becoming more self-determining, by choosing our values and ideals grounded in experience instead of simply conforming to prevailing values or compulsively rejecting them (Mayeroff, 1990 [1971]).

Certainly, in order to be able to go out to the other we must have the starting place, must have been, must be with self (Buber, 1958). Authentic being, authentic self requires that we are open to horizons of significance, to self-definition in dialogue: it requires creation, construction, discovery, originality, a challenging of moral views and the rules of society (Taylor, 1991). In speaking of authenticity, Taylor reflects:

> *There is a certain way of being human that is my way. I am called upon to live my life in this way, and not in imitation of anyone else's. But this gives a new importance to being true to myself. If I am not, I miss the point of my life, I miss what being human is for me.*
>
> (Taylor, 1991, pp. 28–9)

Study Activity 2.2

Authentic self
In speaking of authenticity, it has been said that the important thing is that we live life not in imitation of anyone else, but rather in being true to self. How easy or difficult is it to be 'true to self' in nursing? What dilemmas or tensions does it pose for you?

Being true to oneself has deep ethical intensity. It requires listening to and responding to inner voice; to one's unique existence. Responding to what is happening requires facing the unfolding moment attentively. 'What I am as a self, my identity, is essentially defined by the way things have significance for me' (Taylor, 1989, p. 34) and also for self within relation, in dialogue connected, discovering and understanding the significant together. Benhabib (1992) gives testimony to the importance of ongoing dialogue and to the communicative action essential to developing the capacity to assume the moral point of view:

> *To know how to sustain an ongoing human relationship means to know what it means to be an 'I' and a 'me', to know that I am an 'other' to you and that, likewise, you are an 'I' to yourself but an 'other' to me. Hegel has named this structure that of 'reciprocal recognition'. Communicative actions are actions through which we sustain such human relationships and through which we practice the reversibility of perspectives implicit in adult human relationships. The development of this capacity for reversing perspectives and the development of the capacity to assume the moral point of view are intimately linked.*
>
> (Benhabib, 1992, p. 52)

Such mutual relation, engagement, hearing and responding to multiple voices and multiple realities, acknowledging diversity and reciprocity, creates hope and engages care. It evokes and enables mutual understanding. Engaged care, inclusivity and relation are our source of moral wisdom and of love for one another. Relatedness is the important; 'the face of the neighbour signifies for me an exceptional responsibility, preceding every free consent, every pact, every contract' (Levinas, 1981, pp. 87–8). I respond with responsibility in full consciousness and attentiveness to the other:

> *Responsibility is what is incumbent on me exclusively, and what, humanly, I cannot refuse. This charge is a supreme dignity of the unique. I am I in the sole measure that I am responsible, a non-interchangeable.*
>
> (Levinas, 1985, pp. 100–1)

Within ethical nursing encounter, the bond of care is established. Within relation we 'constitute one another's world and destiny' (Løgstrup, 1997, p. 16). We commit to a compassionate journey with the other, the person who is the patient or client; a journey often of joy but also, at times, of sorrow. Saunders (1996) believes that:

> *The way care is given can reach the most hidden places and give space for unexpected*

development. We frequently see how both patient and family may find peace and strength for themselves when we know we have given so little. There are possibilities in people facing death that are a constant astonishment. We will see them more often if we can gain confidence to approach our fellow without hiding behind a professional mask, instead of meeting as one person to another, both aware of the depths of a pain that somehow has its healing within itself. In this discovery we might find out as much about living as dying. People at the end of their lives will then be our teachers.

(Saunders, 1996, p. 12)

Patients come to us as people in search of hope and of meaning; wanting to understand and to feel understood. Very often they feel powerless. We experience with them, to the degree possible, what they are going through. We are with them hoping to help them find meaning when things appear meaningless to them. We help them to pick up the pieces – to become 'whole' again. It is not easy, but it is always worth it. Barker (2000), speaking from nursing experience, points to possibility:

In my own practice I have come to believe that one of the central problems – in human terms – of most of the patients I have encountered is powerlessness (Barker, 1999). Caring needs to recognise and focus upon this sense of powerlessness, providing the necessary human, interpersonal and inter-subjective conditions for the development of the sense of security that the person not only seeks, but needs to continue. In my clinical work I often feel like Beckett's Unnameable, who pondered: 'Where I am, I don't know, I'll never know, in the silence you don't know, you must go on, I can't go on, I'll go on.' Such an attitude is, of course, an anathema to the evidence-based lobby that appears convinced that uncertainty is an inherently bad thing. If experience has taught

me anything, it is that there are few certainties in life – indeed much certainty has an illusory quality. What does seem certain is that people have the capacity to grow through experience, but awareness is a necessary ingredient. Maybe one of the virtues of caring is that it focuses the nurse's attention on her awareness of the person who is the patient, and in so doing fosters an increased awareness of the whole of that experience for the person.

(Barker, 2000, p. 332)

Study Activity 2.3

Hope

Patients come to us in search of hope, wanting to be understood. They very often feel powerless.

- Discuss from personal experience, one-to-one with a nursing colleague, the feeling of power-lessness. From such experiencing, determine how a nurse could respond meaningfully to *you*, helping you to feel understood.

We have the capacity to grow through experience, through remaining aware and attentive. We gain confidence; have faith in ourselves and others. 'Having faith' in ourselves and in what we are doing requires an awareness of self; awareness of 'a core in our personality which is unchangeable and which persists throughout life in spite of varying circumstances, and regardless of certain changes in opinions and feelings':

It is this core which is the reality behind the word 'I', and on which our conviction of our own identity is based. Unless we have faith in the persistence of our self, our feeling of identity is threatened and we become dependent on other people whose approval then becomes the basis for our feeling of identity. Only the person who has faith in himself is able to be faithful to others, because only he can be sure that he will be the same at a future time as he is today and,

> *therefore, that he will feel and act as he now expects to. Faith in oneself is a condition of our ability to promise, and since, as Nietzsche said, man can be defined by his capacity to promise, faith is one of the conditions of human existence. What matters in relation to love is the faith in one's own love; in its ability to produce love in others, and in its reliability.*
>
> (Fromm, 1995, pp. 96–7)

Having faith in one's self and in others is transformative, it realises possibility. It means that we can say with confidence to the patient and family –'you can count on me'. Being able to count on one to do one's best brings peace of mind. It is central to our ethical way of being and to becoming a nurse.

Study Activity 2.4 ⎯⎯⎯⎯⎯⎯

Faith

Having faith in oneself and what we are doing requires 'awareness of self'. Using literature to support your personal thoughts and reflections, write an account (approximately 400 words) of the importance of self-awareness in caring for others.

BEING A NURSE: CARING

The nurse is present in moments of healing, in movement to life and to death. Nurses are ordinary people in an extraordinary job, in a privileged and special relationship with another person, their family and the community. The human experience of nursing is extraordinary in that it involves a fullness of human responding. It is by its very nature a unique presence in the world and a most unique way of being with another person. The sustained intimacy of contact with another while they partake in their personal activeness – often activities only ever performed in the most private of situations – is a major element of nursing uniqueness. It is these moments, the experiencing of them with the other, which is the love, joy, often the sorrow, but always the dignity and beauty of nursing action, nursing care.

Human love and human care in their power and responsibility are the essential creative energies that actualise nursing care. The belief that love and care are central to nursing is not without controversy. Many nurses reject the belief that caring is a foundational or ethical basis of nursing. That loving is essential is even more controversial and often viewed as unprofessional. We ought not to love the people who are patients, because to do so would be to get emotionally (and dangerously) involved. Gadow (1980), in speaking of involvement, of personal versus professional, tells us that the movement of humanistic health has attempted to soften the distinction between the person and the professional. Professionals are encouraged to become involved with and attentive to patients as individuals. Patients have begun to assume some responsibilities formerly reserved for the professional. The dichotomy persists, nevertheless. In all health professions, new practitioners are warned that becoming personally involved with patients is unprofessional (in spite of patients' complaints that their care is too impersonal). The traditional view is maintained – the personal and the professional are mutually exclusive – behaving professionally entails avoidance of personal interactions and of behaviour expressing the professional's feelings, values, idiosyncrasies. If we accept this view, individuals are interchangeable – none of their individuality should enter interactions.

The importance of the personal engagement of the professional, of the need for the love and care that sources compassionate relation, is poignantly attested to in the plea, as he faced death, of Dr Jonathan J. King to health care professionals (quoted in Charon, 1996, p. 292). He spoke of the line that divides people who pass over into the condition he found himself in, and said 'there's no way I can convey to you the feelings of the death sentence and how it changes your life. In situations where odds are really very poor, how important it is for doctors and medical staff to foster a patient's feeling of control and hope. Empathise. Put yourself in the shoes of your patient as much as possible. Get as close to your patient as you can'. Jonathan King's cry from the heart for involved caring is echoed in the daily call of patients as they reach out, call out from their fragility, from their feeling of powerlessness. A powerlessness spoken of earlier by Phil Barker (see above). Often the cry is silent, the silent call given expression in the eyes of the patient as they face their fear and loneliness. Do we hear their cry, share their pain? Do we come from behind our professional mask, meet person with person, 'both aware of the depths of a pain that somehow has its healing within itself?' attested to by Cecily Saunders (see above). That often we do not hear nor heed the call is evident in the conditional, impersonal relating spoken of by Stevens (1967):

> '*I' am loved only if I let myself be pushed into a pattern which excludes me. I am not in any sense respected, and neither am I cared for, no matter how much may be done 'for' me. When a medical treatment is harmful to me, I can know this before it is apparent to others, but I am required to go on with it, and am 'troublesome' and 'unreasonable' if I protest, and 'unmanageable' if I refuse. I am subtly or unsubtly punished for my disobedience. I am placed in the position of having to fight, when what my body needs, to put itself in order, is to be at rest. This is not the place to go into all the other ways I do not feel respected by doctors and nurses. It can be lumped together into the statement that there is little or no interaction. I do not feel cared for, and when I do not feel cared for, I'm not – however much someone else may feel he is doing 'for' me. I am not consulted.*
>
> (Stevens, 1967, pp. 255–6)

The experiences described by Stevens some 35 years ago were not unique. Early works by Habenstein and Christ (1955), Peterson (1967)

and later in the UK by Stockwell (1972), illustrate how the person, the selfhood of the patient, is often viewed as an irrelevance, an irritation. Unfortunately this is not a condition of the past. More recently, Gerteis *et al.* (1993) vividly called attention to the failures within US health care systems to reflect adequately a caring for persons, and it is most unlikely that the upsurge of managed care will reverse this phenomenon. This is documented in a range of other studies (Mechanic, 1979; Szasz and Hollender, 1980; Thorne, 1993; Darbyshire, 1994).

Charon (1996) tells us that the most powerful response to suffering is compassion; 'the compassionate witness will be able to recognise the pain in another and thereby to act on behalf of the one suffering. However, suffering does not automatically call forth compassion. Rather, the witness must work very hard to achieve that state. Why is compassion sometimes absent in the face of suffering? What can we do to bring it about?' She answers:

> *The structure of hospitals and health care often thwarts our best intentions. Every time we have to deny people simple human services, every time we have to walk by a room with a distraught person inside calling out a part of our gentleness and kindness dies off. We steel ourselves against hurtful things about which we can do nothing. Our naive willingness to help and our innate human sympathy are replaced with executive necessity. Let us take a listen to our hearts. Let us acknowledge all that makes compassion so very difficult – the personal memories, the feeling of powerlessness, and the feelings of rage and defeat. Let us name the loss, the fear of death, and the fear of making mistakes. We, too, need to be heard as we tell of our pain, as we let ourselves come closer to the suffering of others.*
>
> (Charon, 1996, pp. 298–305)

It is necessary that we protest, take action against unconcerned, conditional, impersonal

relating and all-determining market force conditions, systems and practices. It is not always easy
to do something about such practices, in fact it
is more often than not very difficult when we
face indifference; it is indeed harder still in the
face of the power, confidence and sometimes the
arrogance of 'market enforcers'. Yet, it is essential that we try. It will be necessary that we
attempt to do so both individually and collectively, that we do so with the courage and creativity inspired by a belief in the 'power of one'
and, by passionate belief in the human and
humane wisdom inherent in nursing practice.

Study Activity 2.5

It is often easier to 'step out from' than to 'step into'
deep relating, to keep oneself at arms length rather
than to engage fully in the profound suffering of
another person. Reflect upon the following:

● How can nurses be enabled to remain deeply
engaged with patients and their families?
● Is there a possibility that we can engage too deeply
in the suffering of another?
● In what way can nurses be supported in coping
with the profound suffering of another person?

Through confronting authentic caring presence,
being open to what the present brings, meaning
becomes accessible. We have to name the
meaning emerging. We are faced with impulses
of concern, regard, compassion, giving and
receiving, unconditional acceptance and confirmation; in effect, with loving and caring. To
indulge in semantic arguments or facile claims
that loving and caring are not unique to – or
perhaps even justified within nursing – is to
move towards inauthenticity, to deny what in
essence amounts to nursing's social mandate.
Because, in all societies and at all times, when
nursing has emerged as a recognised activity, it
has been understood that nurses *care*, that is
what they do – 'the roots of nursing have

grounded the profession in a firm tradition of
enlightened and deliberate caring – an informed
compassion' (Bradshaw, 1997, p. 10). Jourard
(1971) makes the essential clear: 'hopefully,
nursing practitioners will soon learn that nursing
is a special case of loving' (p. 207).

What does it mean to love and to care in a
nursing context? Much of the difficulty in
accepting nursing as loving arises from the
problem of understanding what we mean to love
in that context. The problem arises because
there are in essence different yet overlapping
meanings and connotations to the term. In
Greek there are the separate words: *eros*, the
love of desire, of wanting for oneself; and *agapé*,
the love which gives, which is wanting for the
other and not for self and which is free of erotic
desire. It is the latter love that is significant in a
nursing context. Baelz (1982) reflects:

> *Agapé is a love which overflows. It gives
> rather than grasps, and seeks nothing for
> itself, everything for the beloved. ... (it is) ...
> the love which is advocated as the source
> and spring of morality. It has been described
> in a number of ways. It is regard for another
> person which is independent of that person's
> qualities, attainments or merits. It is
> therefore constant and unalterable. It is a
> turning from oneself to the other for the sake
> of the other. It is self-forgetful and self-
> sacrificial. What is the relation of such love
> to justice? Certainly it could never
> countenance injustice ... Ordinarily, however,
> we are inclined to contrast love with justice;
> justice operates within defined limits,
> whereas love does not. Even so, it is arguable
> that love cannot be content with anything
> less than justice, and in many spheres justice
> is the most that love can be expected to
> achieve.*
>
> (Baelz, 1982 p. 105)

The love and care of nursing are inextricably
interwoven with responsibility, responsibility to
love and to care for self and others; to discover

and extend potential and possibility with the person, family and community. Fromm (1967) believes that one's main task in life is to give birth to oneself, to become what one potentially is and he has said that if love can be defined as the affirmation of the potentialities and the care for and the respect of the uniqueness of the loved person, then, humanistic conscience can be justly called *the voice of our loving care for ourselves.* Humanistic conscience is self *being true* to self, the voice of our true self summonsing us to live productively, to develop fully and harmoniously, 'to become what we potentially are' (p. 159). Living productively in nursing is living with love, through care. Such love and care is foundational to the Nightingale command and counsel to do no harm. Love and care are nutrients sustaining and engaging life, helping to lift spirits. They arise from within as the nurse becomes involved in the fragility of sustaining life and helping to empower people to live their lives more fully. They are both the source and the spring of morality inspiring self and other; creating personal significance, contributing to nursing significance in movement that aims for growth and healing. If we accept the wisdom of Fromm (1995) that love is the only sane and satisfactory answer to the problem of human existence and that to speak of love is to speak of the ultimate and real need in every human being, we have discovered an understanding significant to rediscovering and reconnecting nursing spirit:

> If to love means to have a loving attitude towards everybody, if love is a character trait, it must necessarily exist in one's relationship not only with one's family and friends, but towards those with whom one is in contact through one's work, business, profession. There is 'no division of labour' between love for one's own and love for strangers. On the contrary, the condition for the existence of the former is the existence of the latter. To take this insight seriously means indeed a rather drastic change in

> one's social relations from the customary ones. While a great deal of lip service is paid to the religious ideal of love for one's neighbour, our relations are actually determined, at their best, by the principle of fairness. Fairness meaning not to use fraud and trickery in the exchange of commodities and services, and in the exchange of feelings. 'I give you as much as you give me', in material goods as well as in love, is the prevalent ethical maxim. But the practice of love must begin with recognising the differences between fairness and love. Society must be organised in such a way that man's social, loving nature is not separated from his social existence, but becomes one with it ... (because) ... to have faith in the possibility of love as a social and not only exceptional individual phenomenon, is a rational faith based on the insight into the very nature of man.
>
> (Fromm, 1995, pp. 101–4)

Nursing life is lived in an unfolding movement of expected and unexpected development, in relation with others and enabling them to realise their possibility and potential. Authentic being, being who we are, whole-hearted, present, consciously attentive to self and others is central to caring and relational responsibility. Being true to self is the core of being, of commitment and presence. It enables us to be there for another, to identify with and care for others. Boykin and Schoenhofer (1990) understood presence in caring to be 'the human expression of respect for and response to wholeness, an active engagement in the person-to-person of being and becoming' (p. 149). May (1989) believes that, while life comes from physical survival, the *good life* comes from what we care about, 'care is a state in which something does *matter* of identification of one's self with the pain or joy of the other; of guilt, pity, and the awareness that we all stand on the base of a common humanity from which we all stem' (pp. 289–90). Gaylin's (1976) view of the significant accords with May and he describes our caring nature as a fact of design: 'but social living is also a fact of design. We must trust ourselves and love ourselves for the primary purpose of loving others and caring for them' (p. 173).

Nursing requires the interdependence and involvement of one with other; the connection of feeling, consciousness and engagement. 'Human caring is not limited to an emotional response, much less is it merely an expression of the "touchy-feely" in human relationships. Human caring includes emotions and feelings, thinking and acting' (Roach and Sister, 1997, pp. 15–16). The nurse must be caring, knowledgeable and skilled, competent to effect informed, compassionate and skilled caring. Karl (1992) posed the question: 'being there: who do you bring to practice?' Initially, one would most certainly answer 'myself'. With further thought we might ask: who am I? Who do I bring to practice? In attempting to answer his question, Karl tells us that 'being there is difficult':

> *Being there is a very complex concept that involves several elements. (a) There are cultural and social norms and forms that shape the context, assign roles, determine legitimacy, and prescribe normative behaviour. (b) For the practitioner, a continuum of subjective evaluation exists which ranges from 'getting the job done' to peak experiences 'that make it all worthwhile'. A similar continuum of evaluation exists for the recipient. (c) At higher levels of performance and reception, 'being there' is a very complex human behaviour that involves maximum therapeutic use of the self. One is present, energetic, in-tune and has presence. 'Flow' is experienced, characterised by deep absorption in the task at hand and performance at optimal levels that couple intuitive and analytic knowledge . . . Therefore, 'being there' involves setting, role, evaluation, presence and complex competencies.*
>
> (Karl, 1992, p. 11)

Pearson (1988; quoted in Taylor, 1992), in a graduation address, deemed it important that nurses bring the ordinariness of human existence to nursing:

> *I passionately believe that nursing, and therefore helping, must draw on knowledge, understanding and insights which are part of good quality professional education. I also believe that it is important to marry this with the ordinariness of being a human being . . . Most of us are engaged in the process of helping people every day, often without conscious awareness of 'being helpful'. The foundation of genuine helping lies in being ordinary. Nothing special. We can offer ourselves, neither more nor less to others – we have in fact nothing else to give. Anything more is conceit, anything less is robbing those in distress.*
>
> (Pearson, 1988; cited in Taylor, 1992)

Pearson's thoughts inspire us to reflect upon the consequence of denying our ordinary self, donning the mantle of the expert and in so doing separating the unity of personal and professional. Taylor (1992) explored the phenomenon of ordinariness in nursing and found that ordinary nurses were perceived as being extraordinarily effective because they felt comfortable enough as professionals and people to be themselves with other people. It was the embodiment of that personal freedom which highlighted for patients the oneness of their shared humanity with nurses. Subsequently, Taylor (1994) wrote that ordinariness is sophisticated in its simplicity: that the shared human qualities of nurses and patients have within them the generative source of humanness, which is the ability to care for and cure one another. Oiler Boyd (1988) is concerned with the consequence of the reductive separation of the human from the professional:

> *Increasingly, nurses are instructed in the art of nursing through theoretical models which guide the nurse to practice the behaviours of*

a professional demeanour. Through a socialising process, concepts are used to transform the nurse–patient experience so that students learn to be professional. Empathy becomes technique: the individual, an object; holism, a multi-faceted approach; and humanism, a professional commodity. As human factors are professionalised in this way, a gap between role and person is created. Nurses can and do become estranged from the person that enacts the role. Student nurses tend to lose their natural access to themselves as an outcome of professional role requirements and the conflict between scientifically objective role and humanly involved person.

(Boyd, 1988, pp. 73–4)

Nurses can and do become estranged from the person enacting the role. This is testified in the writing of Menzies (1960), who identifies the various social defence mechanisms that nurses use to avoid close personal relationships and the potential personal trauma which results from such relationships. Her findings accord with Downie's (1971) presentation of the alienating influence of role and with Sartre's (1958) concept of 'bad faith'. These writings point to the depersonalising and restricting reality of acting out a role as opposed to engagement, person with person. Unwittingly we can betray possibility and potential, the oneness of humanity to the extent that we half-do in half-hearted ways.

One cannot question the need for professional knowledge and skill. They are essential to the safe and competent practice of nursing. That they should not be presented at the cost of de-humanising nursing goes without saying. People who come to nurses come in search of help, hope and understanding; seeking 'the generative sources of humanness'. Gadow (1980) tells us that it is a fundamental premise of nursing that a patient has the right to receive affirmation and acknowledgement as a human being, that human beings in their uniqueness and complexity transcend the categories of science. Thus, the reci-

pient of nursing care has more than a legal right to scientific and technically competent treatment – they have a moral right to humanistic care.

Being there, who then do we bring to practice? An honest answer may be that we do not always know, may not be entirely sure. We are alive to possibility, to remaining open, questioning; being human – a nurse. Parse (1989) is confident about who the nurse is and of their vital link in human healing. She helps in our quest, pointing the way to the fundamental essential for practising the art of nursing (*see* Table 2.1).

Table 2.1 Fundamentals for the art of nursing

- Know and use nursing frameworks and theories.
- Be available to others.
- Value the other as a human presence.
- Respect differences in view.
- Own what you believe and be accountable for your actions.
- Move on to the new and untested.
- Connect with others.
- Take pride in self.
- Like what you do.
- Recognise the moments of joy in the struggles of living.
- Appreciate mystery and be open to new discoveries.
- Be competent in your chosen area.
- Rest and begin anew.

Being a nurse requires a unity of person and professional. Nursing requires ordinary and extraordinary skills; directness and consciousness; the courageous presence of the nurse and the healing power generated through compassionate caring. Nurses need awareness, openness to experiencing and the knowledge generated from caring experience. The call to the nurse is to be alive to possibility and potential. The dynamic to discover is that: 'I am here, here with you'.

Study Activity 2.6

Presence

The nurse is with the patient in many of life's most significant moments. In these times of great intensity and intimacy, it is necessary to be fully with, involved, inside their shoes to the degree possible.

- Discuss with a colleague the significance that the entwined concepts of presence and empathy in nursing have. Are they empty words to be discarded or essential to a way of being that fosters hope and relieves suffering?

ENCOUNTER: THE DIALOGIC HEART OF RELATION

A wish to help others, to do so with compassion, knowledge and skill, is essential to the dialogical relation of nursing encounter: a relation of deep intimacy in which the person (patient or client) can have faith in the nurse to do their best to help them. Relation is mutual; in trusting in it the person gains the confidence to confide in the nurse what they are going through – their needs, fears, brokenness, suffering, joy or happiness. The nurse is with the other, involved; 'open' to encounter, to experience and responds with compassion, honesty, truth, responsibility and competence. Compassionate responding within the wholeness of an 'I-Thou' relationship creates freedom for growth and healing. Through attentiveness, awareness, acceptance and positive regard it upholds dignity and confirms personal uniqueness. Buber (1958) spoke of 'I-Thou' and 'I-It' relationships, revealing their significance. The 'I' in the primary word 'I-Thou' differs from the primary word 'I-It'. 'I-Thou' establishes a world of relation. 'I-It' belongs to the world of experience. The essential difference between these two relationships is not as is often thought inherent in the nature of the object to which one relates, rather it is inherent in the relationship itself. 'I-Thou' is a relationship of openness, directness, mutuality and presence. 'I-It' is, in contrast, a typical subject–object relationship in which one knows, observes, explores, uses and applies. They do not exist in exclusive duality. Rather, they are moments in necessary alternation with each other. Friedman (1972) explains:

> *Man cannot will to preserve in the I-Thou relationship. He can only desire again and again to bring the indirectness of the world of It into the directness of the meeting with the Thou and thereby give the world of It meaning. So long as this alternation continues, Man's existence is authentic. When the It swells up and blocks the return to the Thou, then Man's existence becomes unhealthy, his personal and social life inauthentic.*
>
> (Friedman, 1972, pp. xiv–xv)

Within an authentic relationship the nurse comes to understand, engages mutual understanding and confirms to the person that they 'matter'. It is a relationship in which the person feels understood and can attain peace of mind and healing. Jourard (1971) believes 'sincere attempts to know and to understand a patient and to help him be comfortable increase his sense of identity and integrity, and this experience seems to be a factor in healing' (p. 206). The importance of being with someone offering comfort and consolation has been spoken of by Nouwen *et al.* (1982):

> *It is often in 'useless' unpretentious, humble presence to each other that we feel consolation and comfort. Simply being with someone is difficult because it asks of us that we share in the other's vulnerability, enter with him or her into the experience of weakness and powerlessness, become part of uncertainty, and give up control and self-determination. And still, whenever this happens, new strength and new hope is being born. Those who offer us comfort and consolation by being and staying with us in moments of illness, mental anguish, or spiritual darkness often grow as close to us as those with whom we have biological ties. They show their solidarity with us by willingly entering the dark, uncharted spaces of our lives. For this reason they are the ones who bring new hope and help us discover new directions.*
>
> (Nouwen *et al.*, 1982, p. 14)

It is often the small things in life that are in reality the essential. They are often overlooked in a mistaken search for the significant. Mayeroff (1990 [1971]) reflects, 'there is a rock bottom quality about living the meaning of my life that goes, oddly enough, with greater awareness of life's inexhaustible depths; it is as if life is ordinary and "nothing special" when it is most extraordinary' (p. 104). If we pay attention to the little things, we become aware of the important; the essential manages to communicate itself to us – the touch of a hand, the silent presence of the nurse, the answer to the call, the comfort and consolation compassionately given. The tea and toast given to the person as they lie awake at night is important to them, truly significant. In essence, everything is spoken of in an anonymous letter from a client quoted by Godwin and Jameson (1991; quoted in Milligan and Clare, 1991):

> I remember sitting in your office a hundred times during these grim months and each time thinking, what on earth can he say that will make me feel better or keep me alive? Well, there was never anything you could say, that's the funny thing. It was all the stupid, desperately optimistic, condescending things you didn't say that kept me alive; all the compassion and warmth I felt from you that could not have been said; all the intelligence, competence and time you put into it; and your granite belief that mine was a life worth living. You were terribly direct which was terribly important, and you were willing to admit the limits of your understanding and treatments and when you were wrong. Most difficult to put into words but in many ways the essence of everything. You taught me that the road from suicide is cold and colder still, but – with steely effort, the grace of God, and an inevitable break in the weather – that I could make it.
>
> (Jameson, 1991, cited in Milligan and Clare, 1991)

Believing in the person, in their potential; feeling connection with them; involved, accepting, insightful; having confidence to create healing space with them, enabling their life to move forward, requires both courageous presence and listening, not only with one's head but with heart. When someone is on the cold 'road from suicide', the nurse must be with them, often in silent vigil, holding them with tenderness, listening heart with heart. With them, person with person in I-Thou relation, finding meaning through empathic understanding. Understanding spoken of by Rogers (1957):

> To sense the client's private world as if it were your own, but without ever losing the 'as if' quality – this is empathy, and this seems essential to therapy. To sense the client's anger, fear, or confusion as if it were your own, yet without your own anger, fear, or confusion getting bound up in it, is the condition we are endeavouring to describe. When the client's world is this clear to the therapist, and he moves about in it freely, then he can both communicate his understanding of what is clearly known to the client and can also voice meanings in the client's experience of which the client is scarcely aware.
>
> (Rogers, 1957)

The empathic and compassionate journey to understanding the world of another in the wholeness of their person can be, Buber (1972), believes 'directly known only in a living relation' (p. 205):

> Only a man who has communicated in his spirit with the pain of the world in the ultimate depth of his own pain, without any kind of 'apart from', is able to recognise the nature of pain. But for him to be able to do this there is a presupposition, that he has already learned the depth of the pain of other lives – and that means, not with 'sympathy', which does not press forward to being, but with great love. Only then does his own pain in its ultimate depth light a way into the

> *suffering of the world. Only participation in*
> *the existence of living beings declares the*
> *meaning of the ground of one's own being.*
>
> (Baber, 1972, pp. 192–3)

Responding to the pain and brokenness of another without any 'apart from' empathic understanding requires entering into the painful situation and experiencing the pain and suffering with the person. 'Those who do not run away from our pains but touch them with compassion bring healing and new strength. The paradox indeed is that the beginning of healing is in the solidarity with the pain. In our solution-oriented society it is more important than ever to realise that wanting to alleviate pain without sharing it is like wanting to save a child from a burning house without the risk of being hurt' (Nouwen, 1998, p. 38). Identification and solidarity with the pain of another, recognising and engaging with their suffering in our heart, invokes the image of the wounded healer and testifies to the wisdom spoken by Nouwen (1997) that 'in our own woundedness, we can become a source of life for others'. Wisdom resonant with Rogers' (1961) belief 'that what is most personal and unique in each one of us is probably the very element which would, if it were shared or expressed, speak most deeply to others' (p. 26).

Study Activity 2.7

Woundedness

'In our woundedness we can become a source of life for others'.

- Reflect upon the statement and upon the integral concept of 'wounded healer'. Discuss your reflection with a sensitive colleague, giving consideration to the pain and fragility of hope and dreams shattered, hearts broken.

Understanding from within, engaging with the suffering and joy of another as if it were our own requires feeling with, wholeness and connection. Another's world and experience cannot be understood from 'outside' or through the traditional subject–object duality that divides and denies. Gadow (1980) cautioned that 'for the patient's emotional complexity to be understood and supported, the emotional dimension of the nurse's own being cannot be excluded but must be consciously and directly engaged. The absolute prerequisite for advocacy – advocating the patient's own individually created values – is the participation of the advocate as an individual, a complete unity unfragmented by exclusion of any part of the self' (p. 92). In speaking of care as clinical subjectivity, Gadow (1989) affirmed caring and objectivity to be antithetical, believing that caring rests upon the moral principle of regard for persons as subjects and not as mere objects:

> *Pure subjectivity omits the reality of the*
> *body's objectness – its participation in the*
> *world of wounds and decay; the world of*
> *objectives and objects ... Objectivity*
> *unredeemed by subjective involvement is an*
> *assault when persons already are vulnerable*
> *through illness. Illness alters the person's*
> *relation to self and to the world; these are*
> *radical alterations. The last intervention can*
> *compound that vulnerability, and so must be*
> *offered only in the context of advocacy:*
> *caring which addresses the subjectivity of the*
> *patient through the subjectivity of the nurse.*
> *Addressing the person only as subject does*
> *not accomplish healing – there must be*
> *instruments and categories: the apparatus of*
> *cure. None of these constitute caring; often,*
> *the objectivity they entail is antithetical to*
> *caring. They can be redeemed, however, by*
> *the transcendence that subjectivity*
> *accomplishes.*
>
> (Gadow, 1989)

Transcending necessary objectivity is achieved through wholeness of relation, nurse with patient experiencing human with human, intending to realise potential. The significance of reaching out with and through wholeness of relation and participation is recognised by Parse (1981):

> *Being with is encountering or reflectively attending to the other. For the nurse, it is choosing to encounter the client in an open, authentic engagement. It is a way of reaching out to understand the client's experience. The nurse is authentically present in her/his wholeness to the wholeness of the client. The nurse as subject relates to the client as subject. The nurse bears a responsibility for choosing to participate with clients in the context of a health-related situation. Each experience of participation is a source of self revelation toward growth for both nurse and client.*
>
> (Parse, 1981, p. 31)

A dialogical relation, a caring liberating encounter, can empower both patient and nurse to actualise potential and, by protecting vulnerability, foster and enable growth. Care that achieves empowerment, liberation and growth is essential relation: it is without intention to dominate. Benner and Wrubel (2001) spoke of caring practices capable of transformation and growth:

> *Caring is dialogical, according respect for the other, shaped by the capacity of the other to receive or repudiate 'helping'. Caring practices require meeting the other in his or her particularity. The one caring does not get to determine the response of the other. Caring practices are fragile in that sometimes the one caring offers what they can, and the one cared for either cannot respond at all, or may elaborate the offering, transforming it into genuine growth, comfort or consolation.*
>
> (Benner and Wrubel, 2001, p. 173)

A caring relation creates possibility, discovers and confirms uniqueness. It recognises the value and dignity of the person, inspires hope and induces growth through the deep empathic engagement essential to healing. Engaged nursing care – healing relation – is rooted in receptivity, relatedness and responsible responsiveness. Caring is an ethic in and of itself. An ethic that begins with wanting to do one's best for another, striving to do what is right; it is realised in the moral action of dialogical relation. Noddings (1995) believes 'an ethic of care speaks of obligation, of *I must*. The I must is induced in direct encounter, thus it is thoroughly relational. At bottom, an ethic of care should be thought of as an ethical virtue of which dialogue is the most fundamental component'.

Study Activity 2.8

I-Thou

'I-Thou relation is an engaged way of being-in-the-world rooted in receptivity and connected in responsible response'.

- Reflect upon this statement, recording your reflections for a small group discussion attending to how such I-Thou relation diminishes feelings of isolation, objectivity and powerlessness while encouraging unity and a sense of belonging.

In the engagement of sincere dialogue we come to understand that we partake in and 'do indeed constitute another's world and destiny'. This privilege is essential ethical responsibility. It requires that when we face the interrogative challenge as to nursing's reason for being, we answer the inner voice that asks 'who are you?' and with confidence say 'I know who I am, what nursing is; I live nursing life my way and my way is "with" not "without" another'. The moral imperative is to respond with compassionate, committed care informed by virtues that not only sustain practice and enable us to achieve the good internal to practice, but which will also sustain us in the relevant quest for the good, enabling us to overcome the harms, dangers, temptations and distractions which we encounter and which will furnish us with increasing self-knowledge and increasing knowledge of the good (MacIntyre, 1985, p. 219). Being there, listening, willing to help, wanting to understand and be understood testify commitment and response to the moral injunction of responsibility to the other, to not turning away from suffering or human need. They are virtuous activities realised in dialogical relation through experiencing together a sense of unity, completeness and personal dignity. The virtues integral to caring and essential to informed, compassionate, committed caring are those of:

- *authenticity of being* – realising potential, renewing being
- *conscience* – consciousness of, engagement in, moral activity, awareness creation
- *commitment* – advocate with the other
- *presence* – being with, confirmation of, the other person, constancy and immediacy of the relationship
- *compassion* – the interdependence of feeling for and with and concern of care
- *empathy* – involvement with, acceptance of, understanding the way of the other
- *empowerment* – liberation, freedom to realise potential, mutual understanding and confirmation.

They are neither all inclusive nor are they in their realisation separable. They interconnect with virtues of honesty, courage, duty, obligation and with the reasoning of justice inherent in nursing relationships and decisions. They enable us to realise the good internal to nursing, to act rightly and, through compassionate commitment, to know and care about what happens to each wounded heart.

SYNERGY: UNITY OF BEING-ENCOUNTERING

We are together in a world of nursing in authentic caring presence. Within ethical relation and encounter we come together in dialogue; through mutual understanding and confirmation we recognise possibility and realise human potential. There is synergy, being-encountering, the 'one caring' with the 'one cared for' understanding diversity and reality,

expanding consciousness and competence through mutual enhancement. Through a unity of being and relation the nurse gains wisdom, synthesises knowledge, skill and compassion within a union of hearts and minds to realise one's commitment to care (*see* Fig. 2.1).

SUMMARY

In this chapter we have undertaken a journey of development in an attempt to discover the essential essence of committed care and its ethical significance for nursing relation. This is a journey that never ends – an exploration of life lived in nursing contexts that open us to care deeply experienced, felt at the core of our being yet not readily seen. We experience, reflect on and interpret our experiencing to find meaning in and through caring presence.

The journey began without controversy, with assurance that an impulse to care is a natural way of being-in-the-world, vital to humanity, present in the human heart and expressed in concern, compassion and commitment. As we journeyed forward we found that care and caring were not always simple. Rather, they could be profound and complex phenomena; we understood that within modern technologised health care systems care was very often institutionalised, standardised in the name of quality and safety and, as witnessed by many patients, too often absent. Technology, as Gadamer (1996) attests, could generate a service capable of, should it be carried to a possible and ultimate conclusion, being provided devoid of all human contact. We recognise that as the ever-increasing demand for evidence-based health care becomes an imperative, crucial to effect clinical governance, a command for measurable health care standards – measuring caring – may take hold. What will measuring caring mean? Is there an empirical means that can give expression to the nurse listening to and holding the fragile person whose heart is broken? Is there, Watson (2002) asks, a justification for having empirical objective measures about such an existential human relational phenomenon as human caring in nursing

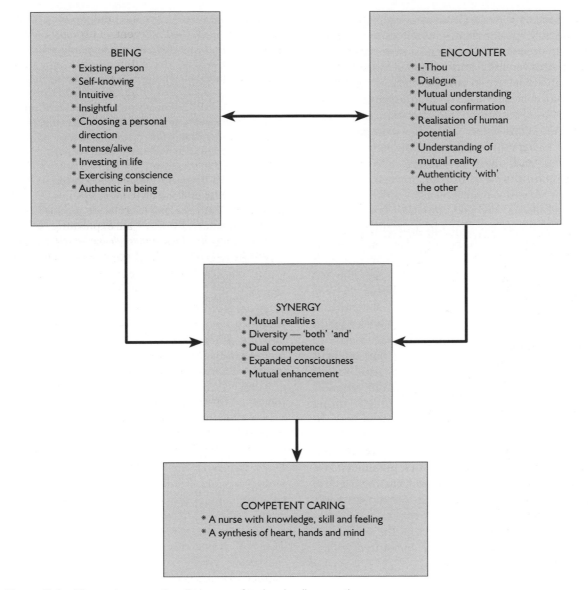

BEING
* Existing person
* Self-knowing
* Intuitive
* Insightful
* Choosing a personal
  direction
* Intense/alive
* Investing in life
* Exercising conscience
* Authentic in being

ENCOUNTER
* I-Thou
* Dialogue
* Mutual understanding
* Mutual confirmation
* Realisation of human
  potential
* Understanding of
  mutual reality
* Authenticity 'with'
  the other

SYNERGY
* Mutual realities
* Diversity — 'both' 'and'
* Dual competence
* Expanded consciousness
* Mutual enhancement

COMPETENT CARING
* A nurse with knowledge, skill and feeling
* A synthesis of heart, hands and mind

Figure 2.1 The pathway to the discovery of caring–healing practice

practice? These are among our essential questions; the tensions, ambivalences, conflict of value and beliefs to be faced with courage, then resolved.

Is one's hope that the inspiration, fragility and healing power of compassionate care – although not always visible or readily measurable – be recognised, celebrated and facilitated through sustained and effective resourcing a crazy hope? Will the oft-silenced voice of those who experience our caring be advocated for and will those voices critical of its absence be heard and heeded? Should the voice of compassionate care not be heard nor heeded, should nursing accept and collaborate with an alienating technologised service devoid of human care, we will have come to a dead end, to a deadening of inspirational source, an ultimate demise of the deep nurturing healing presence and compassionate committed caring that created and sustained nursing. The alternative is to recognise that a balanced connection and synthesis of indispensable technology and humanity, together with a convergence of knowledge, skill and compassionate ethical care, give credence to what is our constant and heritage – nursing's informed compassionate caring–healing practice.

If we should remain consciously attentive and while accepting the invitation in John Lennon's words 'you may say that I'm a dreamer, but I'm not the only one: I hope someday you'll join us and the world will live as one' we accord with and act upon the wisdom of George Bernard Shaw 'I hear you say "why?" always "why?" You see things; and you say "why?" But I dream things that never were; and I say "why not?"'', we will say with conviction 'why indeed not'. In so doing we commit to fostering our essential imaginative dreams and aspirations; true to self and others we will connect, solemn promises kept, with the person and through caring presence they will realise that they do matter. In becoming and living as one in the world of nursing we will have remained alive to and realised individual and collective possibility and potential; preserved human and nursing dignity. Significantly, we will not have cut ourselves off from nursing wisdom and conviction, from what we have known and know to be the all important – our caring source and committed endeavour to care.

REFERENCES

Baelz, P. (1982) *Ethics and Belief*, Sheldon Press, London

Barker, P. (2000) Reflections on caring as a virtue ethic within an evidence-based culture. *International Journal of Nursing Studies* 37, 329–36

Benhabib, S. (1992) *Situating the Self. Gender, community and postmodernism in contemporary ethics,* Routledge, New York

Benner, P. and Wrubel, J. (2001) Response to: Edwards, S.D. (2001) Benner and Wrubel on caring in nursing. *Journal of Advanced Nursing* 33(2), 167–71

Boykin, A. and Schoenhofer, S. (1990) Caring in nursing. *Nursing Science Quarterly* 3, 149–55

Bradshaw, A. (1997) The historical tradition of care. In: Brykczynska, G. (ed.) *Caring: The compassion and wisdom of nursing*, Arnold, London

Buber, M. (1958) *I and Thou*, T. and T. Clark, Edinburgh

Buber, M. (1972) *Between Man and Man* (trans. R.S. Smith), Macmillan, New York

Charon, R. (1996) Let me take a listen to your heart. In: Gordon, S., Benner, P. and Noddings, N. (eds) *Caregiving. Readings in knowledge, practice, ethics and politics*, University of Pennsylvania Press, Philadelphia, IL

Clemence, Sr M. (1966) Existentialism: a philosophy of commitment. *American Journal of Nursing* 66(3), 500–5

Darbyshire, P. (1994) *Living with a Sick Child in Hospital – The experiences of parents and nurses*, Chapman and Hall, London

Downie, R.S. (1971) *Roles and Values*, Methuen, London

Dunne, J. (1996) Beyond sovereignty and deconstruction: the storied self. In: Kearney, R. (ed.) *Paul Ricoeur. The hermeneutics of action*, Sage, London

Friedman, M. (1972) In: Buber, M. *Between Man and Man*, (trans. R.S. Smith), Macmillan, New York

Fromm, E. (1967) *Man for Himself: An enquiry into the philosophy of ethics*, Routledge and Kegan Paul, London

Fromm, E. (1995) *The Art of Loving*, Thorsons, London

Gadamer, H.-G. (1996) *The Enigma of Health*, Stanford University Press, Stanford, CA

Gadow, S. (1980) Existential advocacy: philosophical foundations of nursing. In: Spicker, S.F. and Gadow, S. (eds) *Nursing: Images and ideals*, Springer, New York

Gadow, S. (1989) The advocacy covenant: care as clinical subjectivity. In: Stevenson, J.S. and Tripp-Reimer, T. (eds) *Knowledge about Care and Caring: State of the art and future developments*, American Academy of Nursing, Missouri

Gaylin, W. (1976) *Caring*, Alfred Knopf, New York

Gerteis, M., Edgman-Levitan, S., Daley, J. *et al.* (1993) *Through the Patient's Eyes*, Jossey-Bass, San Francisco, CA

Habenstein, R.W. and Christ, E.A. (1955) *Professionalizer, Traditionalizer and Utilizer – An interpretive study of the work of the general duty nurse,* University of Missouri, Colombia

Heidegger, M. (1962) *Being and Time*, SCM Press, London

Jourard, S.M. (1971) *The Transparent Self*, Van Nostrand Rheinhold, New York

Karl, J. (1992) Being there: who do you bring to practice? In: Gaut, D.A. (ed.) *The Presence of Caring in Nursing*, National League for Nursing, New York

Levinas, E. (1981) *Otherwise than Being or Beyond Essence*, (trans. A. Lingis), Nijhoff, The Hague

Levinas, E. (1985) *Ethics and Infinity. Conversations with Philippe Nemo* (trans. R.A. Cohen), Duquesne University Press, Pittsburgh, Penn

Løgstrup, K.E. (1997) *The Ethical Demand*, University of Indiana Press, Notre Dame, IN

MacIntyre, A. (1985) *After Virtue*, Duckworth, London

May, R. (1983) *The Discovery of Being: Writings in existential psychology*, WW Norton, London

May, R. (1989) *Love and Will*, Delta Publications, New York

Mayeroff, M. (1990 [1971]) *On Caring*, Harper Perennial, New York

Mechanic, D. (1979) The growth of medical technology and bureaucracy: implications for medical care. In: Jaco, E.G. (ed.) *Patients, Physicians and Illness*, Free Press, New York

Menzies, I. (1960) *The Functioning of Social Systems as a Defence Against Anxiety*, Tavistock, London

Milligan, S. and Clare, A. (1991) *Depression and How to Survive it*, Methuen, London

Murdoch, I. (2001) *The Sovereignty of the Good*, Routledge Classics, London

Noddings, N. (1995) Care and moral education. In: Kohli, W. (ed.) *Critical Conversations in Philosophy of Education*, Routledge, New York

Nouwen, H. (1997) *The Wounded Healer*, Darton, Longman and Todd, London

Nouwen, H. (1998) *Reaching Out,* Fount, London

Nouwen, H.J., McNeill, D.P. and Morrison, D.A. (1982) *Compassion*, Darton, Longman and Todd, London

Oiler Boyd, C. (1988) Phenomenology: a foundation for nursing curriculum. In: *Curriculum Revolution: Mandate for change*, National League for Nursing, New York

Parse, R. (1981) Caring from a human science perspective. In: Leininger, MM. (ed.) *Caring: An essential human need*, Charles B. Slack, New Jersey

Parse, R. (1989) Essentials for practising the art of nursing. *Nursing Science Quarterly* **2**, 111

Peterson, D.I. (1967) Developing the difficult patient, *American Journal of Nursing* **67**(3), 522–5

Roach, Sister M.S. (1997) *Caring from the Heart. The convergence of caring and spirituality*, Paulist Press, New York

Rogers, C. (1957) The necessary and sufficient conditions of therapeutic personality change. *Journal of Consulting Psychology* **21**, 95–103

Rogers, C. (1961) *On Becoming a Person*, Houghton Mifflin, Boston, Mass

Saunders, C. (1996) Foreword. In: *Mortally Wounded: Stories of soul, pain, death and healing*, Marino Books, Dublin

Sartre, J.P. (1958) *Being and Nothingness*, Methuen and Co, London

Stevens, B. (1967) In: Rogers, C. and Stevens, B. (eds) *Person to Person – The problem of being human*, Souvenir Press, London

Stockwell, F. (1972) *The Unpopular Patient*, Royal College of Nursing, London

Szasz, T. and Hollender, M.(1980) A contribution to the philosophy of medicine: the basic models of the doctor–patient relationship. In: Flynn, P.A.R. (ed.) *The Healing Continuum: Journeys in the philosophy of holistic health*, Brady, Bowie, MD

Taylor, B. (1992) From helper to human: a reconceptualisation of the nurse as person. *Journal of Advanced Nursing* **17**, 1042–9

Taylor, B. (1994) *Being Human: Ordinariness in nursing*, Churchill Livingstone, Melbourne

Taylor, C. (1989) *Sources of the Self. The making of the modern identity*, Cambridge University Press, Cambridge

Taylor, C. (1991) *The Ethics of Authenticity*, Harvard University Press, Cambridge, MA

Thorne, S.E. (1993) *Negotiating Health Care: The social context of chronic illness*, Sage, Newbury Park, CA

Van Hooft, S. (1995) *Caring. An essay in the philosophy of ethics*, University Press of Colorado, CO

Watson, J. (2002) *Assessing and Measuring Caring in Nursing and Health Science*, Springer, New York

3 THE CONTEXT OF CARE

Lynn Basford

LEARNING OUTCOMES

After studying this chapter you will be able to:
- Describe the context of care within a variety of frameworks
- Give reasons why professional care should support and encourage self-care
- Describe the characteristics of informal care, voluntary care and professional care
- Describe the notion of altruistic care
- Analyse the professional relationship with regard to the concept of care
- Discuss the therapeutic caring relationship with the recipient and provider of care
- Describe the reasons why partnership in care is of paramount importance
- Evaluate professional responsibility and accountability within the context of assuring quality care
- Define the term quality as a feature of professional care
- Explain the reason for professionals operating from evidence of good practice
- Discuss the notion of empowerment as a caring concept
- Identify the process of professional reflective practice.

INTRODUCTION

The principle of caring for others is a central characteristic of being human. This caring concept is active during sickness and health, but is clearly observed during episodic or long-term illness of a loved one. It is reciprocal in nature in that in any given illness situation care is given and is exchanged when the health need is reversed. This type of care is recognised as informal care, which is undertaken within kinship, friendship or community frameworks. Over time, however, the business of maintaining one's health has become a complex intricate phenomenon that requires caring interventions and support systems that are reflected within organised professional care structures. The National Health Service (NHS) is one such organisation, with a plethora of professional health care workers and assistants, who are entrusted by societies with promoting, preventing, maintaining and restoring the health of individuals and communities. The question often asked is, 'What are informal care and formal care, and what are the differences between them?' This chapter will therefore discuss these issues as separate entities, but it should be noted that there are occasions when informal and professional care will occur as a simultaneous and complementary exercise. For example, an individual may have a progressive carcinoma that is being treated by the professional organisation with radiotherapy, but alongside this treatment there will be caring assistance given by the family and instrumental *caring* support by voluntary groups.

THE CONCEPT OF SELF-CARE

At a fundamental level care begins with the notion of self-care in that each person has the potential to undertake caring activities that will support their health and social well-being. Take, for instance, the caring intervention required when a person succumbs to the common cold, that person may decide to let nature take its course or treat the symptoms of the cold from home remedies. Conversely, they may decide that professional help is required and consult the nurse or doctor who in turn will make a judgement to give treatment or not. The delicate balance between caring relationships, the containment of independent self-care arrangements and professional care can be tenuous. Gormley (1995) draws on the notion that health and illness are a continuous entity and there is a point where the ability to continue with self-care arrangements becomes unmanageable and professional care is required. In this sense Haug (1986) suggests that self-care and professional care are polar opposites, but in reality this is a simplistic interpretation that does not give a comprehensive explanation. The intricacies and variable nature between self-care and professional care can be elusive in a sense of specific definition, nonetheless Banks *et al.* (1975) suggest that individuals transfer the *caring* responsibility to professional care agents when they believe (rightly or wrongly) that they are unable to maintain effective self-care and not necessarily at a fixed point in the continuum between health and illness. In addition, Banks contends that in the process of handing over caring responsibilities to the professional there is an accountability and liability on the part of the professional carer and, in turn, an increase of power and control over the *sick* person. The release of control over one's self-care ability creates a sense of helplessness and dependency on others (Gormley, 1995), which in itself is disempowering and has moral overtones within caring relationships. (The process of empowerment within caring relationships is discussed in Chapter 4, which you are encouraged to read to gain a full understanding of the dimensions of care.)

Characteristics of self-care

As mentioned above reference is made to the fact that each person has the potential to engage with self-care, which usually involves some degree of cognitive ability, physical functioning and to some extent social engagement to maintain health, prevent ill-health and, when illness presents, restore health. Dean and collea-gues point out that underpinning the notion of self-care is the need to make decisions based on the knowledge of one's health status, cultural norms and expectations, social support systems and the ability to evaluate health changes (Dean *et al.*, 1986). They go on to suggest that self-care has a two-dimensional framework that can either operate independently, or as a complementary activity between self-care and formal care. In this sense, Dean *et al.* contend that self-care can 'precede, substitute, influence, evaluate, and if so desired, comply with professional care' (p. 41).

In less complex or geographically isolated societies self-care is not only encouraged but it is a non-disclosed prerequisite for social life within the community. This is evidenced by the independent attitudes of people towards health and illness care. However, in modern western societies, particularly those societies that have engaged in social medicine and social welfare, a dependency on formal organised care has to a large extent replaced the self-care model. It has been suggested that this high level of dependency has not been wholly necessary (Cochrane, 1972; Mahler, 1975), and in a perverse way has increased the morbidity levels of society and the financial burden on the state. Take for example the NHS. Its underlying philosophy was based on the notion that all citizens had the right for quality professional care that was free at the point of use. Since its inception, the influence of technology, rising public expectation, epidemiological and demographic changes have constantly increased demands that are difficult to uphold. Successive governments have tried to address this by implementing various policies that have encouraged an increase in self-care to reduce state/public intervention (Department of Health, 1990).

Self-care models

There is no doubt that an empowered person is more able to undertake self-care and, in recognising this, nurse theorists have identified the importance of empowerment in sustaining, maintaining and restoring health (Rogers, 1980; Orem, 1985). On the other hand it is generally perceived that the relinquishing of self-care to the responsibility of professional carers can be detrimental to the health and well-being of patients and clients. The essence of the previous statement can be contested, given that many individuals owe their lives to professional caring intervention. Nonetheless, Illich (1976), in his much-quoted work, forcefully points out that the power asserted by the medical profession in the process and product of health care creates an unhealthy dependence, particularly by patients who from necessity require long-term care. The term he adopted was iatrogenic dependency, which, in his opinion, denied individuals the right to self-care. The organisational system, according to Illich, became so designed that it negated the opportunities of patients to use self-care and abused the rights of patients. If patients were seen to assert their rights in any way they were labelled deviants and, according to Stock-well (1984), became known as the 'unpopular patient'. Illich continued to illustrate the relationship between the advancement of medical involvement into a broader perspective of health, such as pregnancy and mental illness, which, in his opinion, has served to reduce the opportunity for self-care. However, the view expressed by Illich has been challenged by others who suggest that professional care does not always mean the demise of self-care (Dean *et al.*, 1986), given that there is a large percentage of care that continues without any intervention from health care professionals (Levin and Idler, 1981).

In a sense, family-centred care offers caring advice and interventions that are inherent features of everyday life. It is so intertwined with everyday existence that it is difficult to quantify. For example, take Joe, an 18-year-old, who comes home feeling ill and lethargic. His first task is to decide whether or not to tell his mother how he is feeling to get her expert opinion as she has taken on the role of assessing the health and well-being of the family members. On this occasion he decides to tell his mother and she makes an assessment as to whether his condition is minor or needs further expert assessment from the local doctor or nurse. Because there has been a spate of meningitis she decides Joe should seek further assessment from the doctor just to discount this disease. However, on another occasion she would tell Joe that it's nothing to worry about, he is just coming down with a common cold and he can manage this illness himself. Joe could well have come to the same conclusion also.

The identification of self-care deficits centres on the notion that humans are constantly making adjustments and self-regulation to maintain homeostasis (a stable health equilibrium). In this sense man operates in a dynamic interface with his physical, psychological, social self and his environment that requires a response within the guise of self-care. When the ability of self-care is diminished in any way, then that individual will benefit from formal health care interventions. Orem's (1985) basic principles assume that individuals operate from a self-care model and can evaluate and decide for themselves the existence of health or illness. Therefore the role of the nurse is to ensure self-care deficits are minimised so as to restore the individual's self-care ability and homeostatic stability.

Beneficence and self-care

Beneficence and the notion of self-care do not always go hand in hand in the context of nursing practice given nursing's historical patronage of the medical model and the notion of 'doing for others' in the interest of knowing what is best. Arguably, if nursing practice operates from a standpoint of beneficence, it can be contrary to supporting and advocating self-care. For example, dressing, feeding and making health goal decisions when patients are able to undertake these tasks themselves is both patronising and disempowering. Sometimes nurses make the excuse that they are undertaking a caring task for the benefit of the patient, but in truth, it is because the patient is slow and there are pressures on the nursing staff to complete numerous tasks in a short period of time. Such behaviour is inexcusable if the self-care model is to be encouraged. Nonetheless, there are occasions when the nurse must consider issues that conflict between acting in a beneficent manner and maintaining the health state and independence of an individual.

Study Activity 3.1 ——————————

Consider the following scenario and record in your portfolio the actions you would take, giving your reasons why.

Audrey is an 85-year-old living on her own. During the last year she has begun to suffer from senile dementia, and her once tidy home is unclean and full of excreta from her five dogs and three cats.

- Should the nurse act with beneficence, put the cats and dogs in a home and proceed to clean the house?
- Should she make alternative care arrangements without considering any adjustments that could be made to accommodate Audrey's chosen lifestyle, perceiving that she is a danger to herself and her neighbours from environmental factors?
- Or is there another solution to the dilemma?

—————————————————————

While it is understandable that the nurse would embark on a crusade to improve the circumstances of Audrey's situation, even though there is no obvious identified health problem except the Alzheimer's disease, it undermines the ability to support Audrey from a self-care standpoint. Dowd (1989) concludes that nurses frequently make decisions based on the concern for the patient, irrespective as to whether it is based on the wish or desire of the patient. Quite clearly, operating from a self-care perspective requires a degree of risk analysis, which requires a depth of understanding of the patient's life choices and preferences. From this position, the relationship between the nurse and the patient is built on trust and respect (Sherry, 1990).

INFORMAL CARE

There is often a misperception that voluntary care and informal care are one and the same. This is not the case, as informal care is determined as care given within the family or kinship structures, friends and neighbours. Such care can be either physical, emotional, financial and social in nature. In most societies there is a sense of a duty to perform informal care, which is often undertaken by women. The value of informal care has been significantly overlooked and taken for granted but changes in social roles for women and the growth in elder dependants has seen the need for governments to review the situation. The Community Care Act 1990 (CCA), which espoused 'care in the community and by the community', had a significant bearing on the nature of informal care. The CCA was seen as an instrumental driver for change, but at the same time it drew the attention of the plight of informal carers and a recognised aspect of the work that they carried out. The last decade has seen an increasing and welcome research attention on informal care in an attempt to provide frameworks that support the whole process of informal care (instrumentally and financially).

In a sense informal care draws on the notion of social capital and Green (1988) and Poon *et al.* (2003) have identified that a significant amount of informal care and social support is needed throughout the period of chronic illness and disability. The demand for informal care and support is set to rise given the projected figures for elderly people with chronic disease in the forthcoming decades. This demonstrates the need for the voluntary and formal care sectors to work in closer partnership with informal carers if the perceived health demands are to be met.

Providing informal care can be done under the notion of duty, but in a study by Nolan and Grant (1989), giving informal care could be a satisfying and a positive experience. They suggested that there is a bonding between the giver and receiver of care that is reciprocal in nature and is undertaken with trust and respect. On the other hand, some would argue that giving informal care is a stressful and negative experience, particularly so if the receiver of care has a mental health problem such as Alzheimer's disease (Seymour, 1991), or a physical dysfunction such as faecal incontinence (Sanford, 1975). The accumulation of stress within informal caring activities can result in breakdowns in family relationships. It is necessary for formal carers to work in a collaborative manner with informal carers to assess the levels of stress and offer help and assistance in forms that would prevent irretrievable family breakdowns. Respite care has been a positive service that has offered informal carers the chance to recoup their energies and allow them time to refocus on the caring activities that are meaningful to them out of concern and love for their dependent relative or friend. Nolan and Grant (1989) point out that informal carers express views that they are a helpful resource that is free, providing frameworks through which they become victims of exploitation.

Community nurses by the very nature of their place of work have opportunities to work in partnership with informal carers. Badger (1989) has suggested that community nurses are uncertain of the amount of support they should expect from informal carers and yet they are of central importance to the continuity of care given. In a sense, the whole situation comes down to relationship building, trust and mutual respect. If an informal carer is seen as giving inappropriate care that is detrimental to the health of the dependant then it is important that this issue is aired with great sensitivity. In addition it is also important that the care given by the informal carer is valued and respected. Any decisions made should be a joint initiative between the informal carer, community nurse and the recipient of care. Drawing on this issue the nurse theorist Leininger (1984) expressed the view that community nurses should have a wider remit than just giving direct care. She continued to state that their role should embrace empowering others either to help themselves or for informal carers to assist in the caring process.

Study Activity 3.2

- Describe the differences between informal care, voluntary care and professional care.

- Explain the need for partnership working, which includes the recipient of care, the informal carer and the professional.

VOLUNTARY CARE

So far the debate has focused on self-care and intervention through formal care. There is, however, an intermediary between these two known as voluntary care. Voluntary care operates from the concept of altruism, which refers to the fact there is concern for others as a principle of action (*Oxford English Dictionary*). There are many factors that impinge on altruistic caring behaviour that are both externally and internally driven. For example, many societies adopt a religious framework that recognises and rewards (in a spiritual sense) the principle of caring for others. In most societies this caring principle has been attributed as a feminine characteristic that is fulfilled by women's roles within the family and wider community. From this perspective, nursing care, a female role, is centrally seen as altruistic behaviour that is characterised by the desire to care for others. However, altruistic behaviour is a complex phenomenon that can operate from the level of unconsciousness and is viewed as an inherent feature of human characteristics. The underlying belief is that the survival and evolution of humanity has an affinity with the notion of altruistic care (Watson, 1988), and has been the subject of debate by anthropologists, psychologists and biologists (Gormley, 1998). One such debate is the notion of the selfish gene and as we move closer to understanding human genomes it will be interesting to note if there is such a thing as an altruistic gene as described by Malthus (1798), Ricardo (1817), Dawkins (1976), and Landsberg (1993). While their commentary is similar the explanations given have a different focus. For example, Malthus suggests that genes represent a selfish or egotistical personality trait that responds to the needs of survival. Dawkins draws on the notion of holism for his explanations of the selfish gene in that he contends the gene is the fundamental unit of evolution, while Landsberg makes the point that there is a need for large numbers of the population to have the altruistic gene if the human race is to survive. If people are biologically determined to act in altruistic ways towards each other as an innate sense of survival, the notion of free will becomes redundant in this argument. Drawing on this paradox, Wilson (1975) suggests that if the altruistic gene exists then there is the opportunity to respond and adapt to cultural and society values, thus operating a degree of choice.

Determining free will even though there is a latent altruistic gene can be activated through motivation or a sense of sympathy or empathy towards others. In a broad sense this could be the development of a social conscience and/or social responsibility. Batson *et al.* (1986) and Eisenberg *et al.* (1989) have suggested that altruistic behaviour can be activated from some internal trigger mechanism that responds to social circumstances or individual behaviour, or is based on altruistic personality characteristics that have evolved from previous experiences of caring for others.

Altruistic behaviour cannot be divorced from social expectations and norms, which support the notion of caring for others. Not to provide this care can create a sense of guilt and social isolation. Exploring this dimension Mauss (1966) proclaimed that caring for others was not solely altruistic but given in the knowledge of reciprocal need. In the UK the National Blood Transfusion Service relies on blood given as a gift in the knowledge it will do others good, but there is also an underlying awareness that one day the donor may need to be the recipient of blood. Titmus (1973) elaborates upon this point by suggesting that the blood transfusion service is, in fact, 'collective altruism'. Indeed, he contends that it is altruistic behaviour that receives no financial rewards in the knowledge that the blood is used at the point of need, irrespective of societal privilege or the recipients' ability to pay. The idea of giving blood is of social concern and free of external

influences. Drawing on this model, Barry (1990) points out that the welfare state as we know it is based on the principles of collective altruism and supports government direction in sustaining the NHS.

While health can be seen as framework for altruistic behaviour it is suggested that there are limitations and selectivity when altruism is used in other contexts and circumstances (Culyer, 1976). Limitations and selectivity are linked to the notion of envy, social standing and the ability to pay, and prevent or inhibit the notion of equality in all elements of social life. The UK population has, through the ballot box, successively supported the need for an NHS, but there are increasing indicators that the NHS will become a substantially privatised industry and the principle of 'collective altruism' may become a thing of the past.

In the absence of a national (collective) altruistic framework for health care, i.e. the NHS, the focus of altruistic care may once again turn towards the voluntary sector. The embryonic beginnings of the voluntary care sector were founded on Victorian philanthropic principles that have roots in three domains:

- the use of social power and class to exert pressure for social reforms that would benefit dependent members of society
- the development of mutual aid societies, from which trade unions, building societies, and co-operatives have their origins
- the recognition for the need of children's services, which were instrumental in the development of children's homes, such as Dr Barnardo's.

Voluntary care has played a pivotal role in the developments of services that have become mandatory, such as the district nursing or the home help service (*see* Table 3.1). Voluntary care is viewed as an unselfish act and an expression of collective responsibility that demonstrates a concern for others. In the founding of the hospice movement voluntary workers gave their time and expertise freely. Today, hospices are good examples of how the voluntary sector works together in harmony with formal care-givers.

Table 3.1 Examples of voluntary organisations

- Women's voluntary organisation
- Cystic Fibrosis Association
- Red Cross
- St John Ambulance
- Care of the Aged
- Oxfam
- Diabetes Association
- Alzheimer's Disease Association
- Multiple Sclerosis Association
- Housing associations

Study Activity 3.3

- Search the Internet and libraries and develop a list of voluntary organisations. Identify those that are useful to those of your patients with various chronic diseases, for those who are older adults and children.
- Identify activities undertaken by the voluntary organisation that could be altruistic in nature.
- Identify those activities offered that are different to professional activities.
- Identify the profile of a voluntary worker and analyse it. Record your findings in your portfolio.

THE CONCEPT OF PROFESSIONAL (FORMALISED) CARE

Throughout the modern period professional health care has played a pivotal role in the development and evolution of social medicine and the concept of a welfare state. Professional *care* workers have been instrumental in advising on policy and have implemented policy requirements through and in their practice arenas. Such interdependence by health care professionals and government agents has been further strengthened in the NHS Plan (Department of Health, 2000), in that the government has acknowledged the value placed on the *caring* skills and knowledge that professionals hold that will help solve health and welfare problems. Caring values, caring skills and caring knowledge are at the core of health care professionals' framework of reference. It is claimed that the professional is an individual who, through knowledge and skill in the *caring* arena, demonstrates a commitment to give care through professional rules and regulations (Hugman *et al.*, 1997). The duty to give care is a legal and binding concept, and is identified by the evidence of best practice, standards and benchmarks of caring practice.

The nature of care offered by different health care professional groups is often different in nature and design. For instance, those in nursing will engage in activities related to daily living, while others will share the common goal of commitment to give care in support of enabling health restoration and diagnostic interpretation.

Acting out a common *caring* goal unites all health care professionals and in one sense is part of the legal and binding duty to give care. Nonetheless, giving care and engaging in emotional caring activities is not a prerequisite for the provision of professional care as described previously. For example, the nurse who goes home at the appointed time regardless of a patient's imminent death will be thought uncaring, but this is very different to the fact that she will have undertaken her professional caring duties within the frameworks and standards of professional practice.

Giving care from a professional perspective requires a framework that embraces guiding principles through which education, research and practice are managed, organised and evaluated (Green-Hernandez, 1991). Adherence to procedural correctness is well established through moral and ethical frameworks that are contained within professional codes of conduct. Swanson (1991) enlarges on this point, suggesting that a caring consciousness guides nurses to respect, value, and take responsibility and accountability for their patients' care. While these are laudable principles upon which to base practice they are insufficient in themselves. Nurse theorists contend that professional caring is not just a reciprocal kindness, but a highly complex set of behaviours, patterns and processes, which are difficult to define.

Characteristics of professional nursing care

Kitson (1987) examined characteristics of both lay and professional care, and identified the similarities and differences. The similarities found were commitment, sufficient levels of knowledge, skill and respect for the person being cared for. The principal difference became evident when professional care was sought after lay caregivers reached the point when their skills and knowledge were insufficient, or when they became exhausted through the emotional interchange that caring sometimes demands.

The principles of care are therefore a necessary feature through which guidance is given to professional practice (Leininger, 1984; Watson, 1988). Nursing has embraced these concepts but there is a recognition that nurses do not have a monopoly on caring. To make this claim would undermine the millions of lay caregivers, and others in allied occupations and health professions who care for others as part of their everyday activities. In distinguishing professional care as central to professional identities, it is asserted that we should 'examine the motives for doing so and the intended and unintended consequences of our claims'.

While it is clear that the caring concept is not exclusive to the nursing profession, it is a feature used to enhance both professional knowledge and practice as exemplified within the ethical codes of conduct for nurses. For example, in 1982 the Council of National Representatives (CNR) identified a Code for Nurses, which stated that:

> *The nurse's primary responsibility is to those people who require nursing care. The nurse, in providing care, promotes an environment in which the values, customs and spiritual beliefs of the individual are respected …*
> (Quinn, 1989, p. 216)

Clearly, professional nursing must embrace caring concepts that take on the carative values of society but should extend these to address the caring needs of individuals that are protective, anticipatory, physically comforting and extend beyond routine care without obliging the patient to reciprocate. In so doing, the nurse must be knowledgeable relating to the empirical, aesthetic, personal and ethical dimensions of care.

From the above discussions there could exist a false assumption that the concept of care has always been a central feature of professional nursing. This, however, is not the case, as the caring value in nursing practice has only been a recent phenomenon within the context of a therapeutic relationship. As Davis (1976) notes, nursing was superimposed on a history of hygiene and order, a legacy from the Victorian era, the influence of Florence Nightingale and the dominance of the medical model. Not until nurse theorists such as Watson (1979) and Leininger (1981) came along were the caring principles that underpinned nursing practice identified in explicit terms. In each of these models the philosophies and principles of care were defined within the frameworks of holism that described health care from a physical, psychological, social and spiritual dimension.

HOLISTIC CARE

Holism, as described by Smuts (1926), assumes that people are individuals who always respond as a unified whole, and who are different from, and more than, the sum of their parts. Holism therefore asserts that there is a need to provide care and consideration for the whole person that creates a harmonious balance between the nature of people and their environment. Therefore, when illness occurs it is vitally important that all aspects of the person are assessed to ensure that the right care interventions are given to promote and restore health.

Holistic care is not a new phenomenon. It was recognised by the Greek physician Hippocrates in the fifth century and the ancient Chinese and Indian healers who stressed the need for harmony between the individual, social and natural world in diet, exercise, meditation and self-regulation as a whole. In this sense, holism and self-care have a symbiotic relationship with each other, whereby patients are encouraged and empowered to take control and responsibility for their own healing. This point, however, does not undermine or negate the value of scientific and technological input in health care. It is regarded as a complementary and necessary requisite if the promotion, prevention and restoration of health of the individual are to be achieved (Benner and Wrubel, 1989).

Nursing and holistic practice

Nursing practice based on holistic models takes account of patients in their broader socio-economic context, integrating a range of care characteristics in the field of practice. The essence of this is the development of the nurse–patient relationship, which is continued in degrees of intensity throughout the episode of care intervention. Such models of practice are common features with district nurses and health visitors, who have consistently demonstrated the development of such therapeutic relationships that are underpinned by trust and respect (Hiscock and Pearson, 1996; Quinney *et al.*, 1997). Other features include opportunities for non-threatening discussions relating to the care offered, the emotional fears and social issues that may be significant towards the healing process. In addition the primary care nurse can encourage the involvement of other carers within the family or kinship unit. Through delivering holistic care the primary care nurse is juxtaposed to understand the patient's total health needs and can more easily initiate the appropriate care intervention that meets these needs and encourages self-care and a speedy recovery.

Study Activity 3.4 ━━━━━━━━

- Explore the literature on holism and the relationship with contemporary health care practice.

- Compare the features of holism as distinct from the reductionistic medical model.
- From your nursing experience reflect on holistic care as it is used in everyday practice.
- Consider the following case study: Mr Young is a 53-year-old man whose physical health has been severely affected by the effects of heavy smoking. As a result he requires cardiovascular surgery. Psychologically he is heavily dependent on cigarettes, particularly since his wife of 30 years died three months ago. Socially he feels isolated and ill-prepared to cook properly for himself, as his wife attended to all his daily needs. Spiritually he is anti-religion, but he is also afraid of death.

Write a nursing care plan using:
  (a) a medical reductionistic approach; and
  (b) a holistic approach.

THE CARING MODEL

In an attempt to provide a model of care that is more sympathetic to contemporary nursing than the reductionistic, mechanistic approaches, Watson (1979) and Leininger (1981) have identified characteristics of care using a definitional approach that features the concepts of holism. Inherent within these models are identified lists that are categorised in order to promote the knowledge and understanding of the phenomena of care. Leininger gave recognition to a taxonomy of caring constructs, while Watson provided a list of ten carative factors that

Table 3.2 Watson's carative factors

1 Humanistic–altruistic system of values
2 Instilling faith/hope
3 Sensitivity to self and others
4 Helping–trusting human care relationship
5 Expressing positive and negative feelings
6 Creative problem-solving approach
7 Transpersonal teaching and learning
8 Supportive, protective, and/or corrective mental, physical, societal and spiritual environment
9 Human needs assistance
10 Existential–phenomenological–spiritual forces.

(From Watson, 1979)

reflected the humanistic and scientific principles underpinning nursing practice and the notion of human caring (Table 3.2). Such models have offered frameworks for nursing practice that have encouraged a change in direction. Change that embraces holistic assessments and partnership approaches to health care.

The caring model in action

Theoretical models in themselves do not enact changes in the ways professional practice is performed; it is how the models are used in action that determines change of a sustained nature. In 1986 the School of Nursing at the University of Colorado in the USA implemented the definitional model of Watson (1979). They believed that this model offered frameworks for new ways of working that included multi-disciplinary and multi-professional practice. Not only did this model reflect the basic tenets of a holistic caring philosophy, but it also embraced biotechnological concepts underpinned by relevant evidence and research findings. Evaluating the implementation of this model, it was determined that nurses had become more knowledgeable and competent to give medically supportive nursing services, while able to assess, plan, implement and evaluate a wide range of therapies in which to promote health and healing. Schroeder and Maeve (1992), in the Denver nursing project (1992), dissatisfied with the traditional models of nursing, adopted Watson's (1985) theories of transpersonal caring to enhance a caring partnership with persons living with human immune deficiency virus (HIV) and acquired immune deficiency syndrome (Aids). This approach was considered after consultations and requests from the client group who claimed that traditional methods of care were inadequate to meet their needs.

Reflecting upon Watson's carative factors, Schroeder and Maeve identified the need to add 'medically supportive care' to the list in order to document medically supportive nursing interventions such as medications and intravenous infusions. Having added these dimensions to the model, Schroeder and Maeve showed that the nurses who used this model in the caring environment had developed a greater sense of professional autonomy, accountability and responsibility within their sphere of practice. The nurses said that the change had affected their job satisfaction and increased their knowledge and understanding of the clients' needs. They also felt empowered to become more creative and innovative in clinical practice. The clients' evaluation of the partnership approach towards care was equally positive. They claimed that while they still felt cared for, they were still in control over their health care needs and gained a sense of empowerment and independence.

From these two examples we can believe that the definitional model offers explanations relating to professional care. However, this model is not without critics. For example, Clarke and Wheeler (1992) point out that the definitional model is insufficient in illuminating the caring concept identified and acted upon by practitioners. They believe that an approach that identifies the meaning and intuitive values of care, such as 'narratives' (Benner, 1984; Benner and Wrubel, 1989) and 'verbal descriptions' given by caregivers themselves (Forrest, 1989), are more relevant to nursing practice. These models centre around the notion that 'the spoken meanings of the carers themselves liberate the meanings and experiences of this phenomenon called "care"' (Clarke and Wheeler, 1992). Forrest's research (1989) undertaken in Canada provided the impetus for Clarke and Wheeler to identify professional caring characteristics from a UK perspective. They found that the commentators described care in terms of four categories, which were subdivided into theme clusters (Table 3.3).

These descriptions of care are clearly based upon a humanistic approach, which perceives that interpersonal skills are more central to the caring concept than the physical or technical elements of care. The descriptive prose to describe care was identified by Clarke and Wheeler as words that could justifiably be used to describe the concept of love. However, the term love is not commonly associated with

Table 3.3 The categories and themes of care

Category	Theme cluster
Being supportive	loving concern
	valuing people
	respect
	trust
	giving of self
	awareness of patients' needs
Communicating	prompting independence
	being firm
	talking
	information giving
	listening
	touching and hugging
	presence
Pressure	personal problems that affect caring
	frustrations to affect care
	difficult-to-care-for patients
	quality affected
Caring ability	origin of care
	coping

From Clarke and Wheeler, 1992

professional care and yet, according to McMahon and Pearson (1991), when love is used within the caring relationship it has a therapeutic effect on the provider and receiver of care.

PARTNERSHIP IN CARE

Partnership and collaborative working are features strongly recommended within the context of contemporary professional practice as part of improving the quality of care given (Department of Health, 2000). It is therefore necessary for the professional carer to develop a strong partnership approach with the patient and the patient's family so as to enhance the self-healing process that Watson (1985, p. 49) contends increases '... self-knowledge, self-reference, self-healing, and self-care processes while allowing increasing diversity'.

Developing partnerships requires a paradigm shift that moves away from traditional detached methods of practice that reduces the patients' control over their own health care. This requires

that the responsibility and decision-making of the health professionals are removed to models, which encourage a meaningful dialogue and involvement with the patient. In the first instance, giving away professional control can be a threatening experience, but the added value of an increased shared value and respect between both parties is an enriching experience that cannot be replaced (Watson, 1988). In recognising this fact the Royal College of Nursing stated that:

> *Each patient has a right to be a partner in his own care planning and receive relevant information, support and encouragement from the nurse which will permit him to make informed choices and become involved in his own care.*
>
> (Royal College of Nursing, 1978)

A caring partnership invites a sense of mutual responsibility, as does the notion of intimacy. McMahon and Pearson (1991, p. 8) contends that intimacy is an intrinsic value of a therapeutic relationship that can only be truly achieved if the nurse has first developed 'as a person and a member of the nursing team'. For example, students should be valued and respected as individuals who begin their education programme with a caring consciousness based on experience, values, philosophical beliefs and prior knowledge. As they progress through the course, the caring process guides and enhances theory and practice, and through the development of caring competencies a caring consciousness will develop. Thus, at the point of registration the students will have been exposed to and will have experienced the caring process, which will be internalised and empower them to engage in caring practice.

Study Activity 3.5

- List Watson's 10 carative factors and try to think of practical examples or illustrations of each one.
- Seek out your curriculum philosophy and identify references to the caring concept.

- Have you felt valued and respected as an individual since beginning the course? Write down your experiences.

PROFESSIONAL CARE AS A QUALITY ENTITY

In Clarke and Wheeler's study (1992) reference was made to the term 'quality' in terms of the caring concept. In the 1990s, quality and standards of care have become a central tenet of nursing. The term has become so internalised that reference to quality can be seen in most health care organisations' mission statements. Health care workers have fallen into two camps, namely those who have enthusiastically endorsed the concept and those who have openly resisted (Marr and Giebing, 1994). The White Papers, 'Working for Patients' (1990) and 'Caring for People' (Department of Health, 1989), have focused on the need for professional and financial audits to ensure professional accountability, responsibility and value for money. Quality assurance is therefore seen as a necessary requirement for professional practice and an essential ingredient of a total quality assurance system in the provision of health care (Koch, 1992). It is the measure of professional standards that will be examined periodically through audit by the Commission for Health Improvements (CHI).

In response to this initiative ways and means have evolved to evaluate care effectively, a process, which in the first instance has questioned the constitution of nursing systems, functions, staff performance and patient care (Marr and Giebing, 1994). The result of this activity has been the identification of standards upon which quality can be measured. The major impetus to produce standards was to provide an acceptable benchmark against which the quality of nursing care could be measured and improvements could be made. The task of setting standards has become an essential feature to the evaluation of nursing practice. Standard setting has been promoted by nurse theorists such as Kitson (1987), who has raised the debate on the quality of nursing care through her work. Kitson asserts that in providing professional care nurses are assuring their clients minimum standards of care or, as Kendall (1990) suggests, '... a professionally agreed level of performance' (pp. 32–3).

STANDARDS AND CRITERIA

Collins Dictionary defines standard as a 'level of excellence' or 'an accepted or approved example of something against which others are judged or measured', while criteria are defined as items or factors upon which standards can be measured or judged. Measuring standards of care and setting criteria is viewed as a complex mechanism. In an attempt to simplify the process, in 1980 Donabedian identified a strategy to enable quality to be measured. The process consisted of three inter-related components (see Figure 3.1).

Structure relates to the framework within which health care is delivered, i.e. the physical dimensions such as the building and equipment, the organisational elements, the written policies and procedures, the ratio of staff to patients, peer review mechanisms, continuing educational programmes for staff and the hierarchical delegation of decision-making.

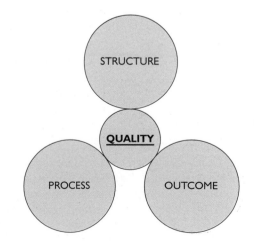

Figure 3.1 The inter-related components of quality

Process is the performance of the delivery of care from the initial stage to its resolution. It reflects the inter-relationship between patient and nurse. Process standards are the actions and behaviours required of the nursing staff in providing care, as well as the elements of care themselves.

Outcome is the result of the interaction of the structure and the process used, that is what is achieved in terms of improvement in health, attitude, knowledge or behaviour conducive to future health.

According to Donabedian (1980), these three phases are essential when preparing standards to ensure that the differences between the settings are identified to give the context within which the process is carried out. He goes on to suggest that to be able to compare the care given between two or more patients requires the standard to be described in terms, which are:

1 meaningful to the practitioners
2 achievable
3 observable
4 measurable.

Clearly standard setting is no easy task. But when collectively agreed upon it can provide a medium through which the strengths and weaknesses of professional care can be identified and improved.

Study Activity 3.6

- Define what quality health care means to you.
- If there were resource restrictions made upon your professional practice, would this impinge on your definition of quality health care?
- Consider the ethical implications of maintaining quality health care when resources are restricted.
- If your definition of quality health care equates to the quality of a Rolls Royce, but you can only afford a Mini, can you still receive quality? If so, how would you then redefine quality?

Through their codes of conduct, professional bodies have identified standards, which all practitioners must achieve. For example, the CNR code for nurses states that:

> *The nurse carries personal responsibility for nursing practice and for maintaining competence by continual learning. The nurse maintains the highest standards of nursing care possible within the reality of the situation. The nurse uses judgement in relation to individual competence when accepting and delegating responsibilities. The nurse when acting in a professional capacity should at all times maintain standards of personal conduct which reflect credit upon the profession.*
>
> (Quinn, 1989)

On a national basis the UK Nursing and Midwifery Council (2002) have similarly identified standards within the context of the Code of Professional Conduct. In effect, the Nursing and Midwifery Council (NMC) replaced the previous United Kingdom Central Council for Nurses, Midwives and Health Visitors (UKCC) and adopted the latter body's code (UKCC, 1992).

Study Activity 3.7

- Read the NMC Code of Professional Conduct (1992), and identify the professional standards. Professional codes ensure that nurses work within an ethical and moral framework, while being responsible and accountable for the quality of care they give. More recently it has been said that the nurse, in assuring quality, should utilise, initiate and be aware of research. This work can be accomplished via a systematic and reflective approach to the delivery of care.
- Access the Department of Health website and read about the newly established CHI activities as they relate to professional standards.

Reflective practice

The concept of reflective practice relates to the notion of 'reflection in action'. It is the process through which reflection can influence and inform practitioners about how to approach and respond to situations (Schon, 1987). It is considered to be 'thoughtful practice', whereby the practitioner can plan actions based on theories and then critically evaluate these actions (Jarvis, 1992). From this position, reflection can influence practice in three ways:

1 Questioning why outcomes occur
2 Extending the knowledge base
3 Informing research.

Moreover, the process of reflection occurs within a cyclical framework requiring the practitioner to reappraise the care given and in so doing analyse and evaluate the effectiveness of that care. Gibbs (1988) has defined five stages of the reflective cycle from the position of what has occurred:

1 Examine associated feelings.
2 Evaluate the experience.
3 Analyse the situation.
4 Reframe to consider alternative actions.
5 Identify what can inform future actions.

The notion of reflective practice will be discussed in greater detail by Gary Rolfe in Chapter 26.

Study Activity 3.8 ⎯⎯⎯⎯⎯

Consider the following caring activity and think about the situation using the reflective cycle.
• You are instructed to give a bath to Mrs Jones who is 83-years-old. Mrs Jones is suffering from a variety of health problems associated with the ageing process, and especially from reduced mobility and sensory deprivation. Mrs Jones expressed her reluctance to go to the bath and asked if she could have a bed bath. Her reasoning was because she was afraid she would fall. You more or less ignored her request and proceeded with the task you were given to do. During the activity Mrs Jones slipped in the bath and sustained a fractured femur.

⎯⎯⎯⎯⎯⎯⎯⎯⎯⎯⎯

By using reflection nurse practitioners can promote the skilled and flexible response of the expert (Benner, 1984), and continually improve the quality of care, which is underpinned by relevant research.

An integrated model of care

So far the debate assumes a position for self-care, voluntary care or professional care. However, there is another route that supports an integrated model between all three areas. It is a model that supports collaboration and partnership working, which relates to the notion of equality, while recognising the expert opinion of the professional (Gormley, 1995).

Expertise is not necessarily the domain of the professional. It could be contained within a voluntary organisation. Indeed some patients, who actually live day-to-day with their health problem, have learnt their own coping strategies and have therefore become experts in managing their own health situation. From this we can see how essential it is to allow patients to identify their own health care goals and decision-making. These should be based on the evidence of best practice and their own personal health journey and experience.

Managing care within frameworks of partnership has become the preferred model adopted by governments, professional bodies and users of the health care service. In 1990 the NHS and Community Care Act embodied the notion of working in partnerships through collaborative networks and team working. The Act offers guidance through which care will be delivered between health care agents, social services and the voluntary and private sector, and not least users and carers. The notion of integrated models of care will support the patient and empower them to maintain independence or, should they choose, transfer power and responsibility to the professional, based on informed choice (Funnel *et al.*, 1991).

Collaboration between the patient and the professional in the care situation is also based on reciprocal trust and respect. However, these two elements do not immediately occur and have to be earned and developed through relationship building. Long-term care situations afford the development of trust and respect between the patient and the professional, but there are instances that negate this opportunity. Examples include short episodes of acute care; fragmented care offered by a range of health care professionals; and the use of technology as a care intervention.

The use of technology is seen as a barrier to the integrated model between self-care and professional care and changes the power dynamics. Misener (1990), speaking of the overuse of technology, points out that there is a growth in the use of technology that is not always to the health benefit of the person and prevents their ability to self-care. He cites examples of inappropriate use of ventilators and diagnostic procedures that have no real bearing on the treatment regime or to the quality of care given. Drawing on this position, it is the responsibility of the nurse to assure that the patient is fully informed of the choices available, the discomfiture of the intervention and the perceived health benefits, so that self-care options are not compromised (Holzemer, 1992).

ORGANISED CARE

As with the growth and complexity of societies, the need for organised health care has evolved. Over time health care organisations have become highly sophisticated and complex, having emerged from humble beginnings without any planned consideration towards the changing needs or the continuous growth and expansion of the health business. In the UK there is both the private health care sector and the large complex organisation of the NHS. Caring

activity is divided between acute, community, intermediary and tertiary services, and is supported by the interface of the social service department, which provides domiciliary services for a range of clients. In addition, there is a growth of complementary therapy services that are poised to interface or wholly integrate with the mainstream business of health care.

COMMUNITY CARE

The notion of the community being involved in health care is not new. Historical policy from the 1601 Elizabethan Poor Law Act sets the scene for community involvement. More recently 'community care' in various guises has been embraced in policy documents and practice. In 1980, it was given a precise interpretation and meaning, which embraced beliefs and values that centred on 'individualism, familialism, voluntarism, managerialism and market accountability' (McBeath and Webb, 1997, p. 37). McBeath and Webb suggest that formulating principles on which care is provided 'in the community and by the community' is based on economic arguments in the face of escalating costs and not based on altruistic notions. In essence, the philosophies of community care are interlinked with the notion of individual responsibility or, during periods of diminished personal ability, to the family or friends. In the absence of family or friendship support, the individual is encouraged to engage with the voluntary or private sectors in the belief that individuals have a prime responsibility to care for themselves.

The Audit Commission (1992) called the political change in focus 'the community revolution', which continued throughout the 1980s and 1990s, culminating in the National Health Service and Community Care Act 1990. The principle aim of community care was to maximise the opportunities of health care that best served the needs of patients and their families. In essence, patients could choose health care that was either in their home environments or within the communities in which they lived.

From a much more sceptical position, community care could be viewed as a means of transferring responsibility to the individual away from the dependency of the welfare state, thus reducing public costs and increasing economic burden on the state. To illustrate the change in direction, community care was a means of de-institutionalising care, particularly with old, disabled and mentally dysfunctional people, in the inherent belief that they would prefer to live outside institutional settings, within the frameworks of family and community life. The latter concept, according to McBeath and Webb (1997, p. 38), is 'patient focused', while the former is 'institutional focused'.

The fear and imagery portrayed by Laing (1960), Garfinkel (1967), Goffman (1968) and Foucault (1979) of institutionalised living and health care, plus the legacy of the workhouse served to reinforce the notion that all institutionalised care is 'bad', therefore community care must be 'good'. However, little work has been undertaken with regard to the frameworks and services given that supports community care from an institutionalised perspective. For example, consider the elderly person who is supported on a 24-hour basis by a range of health and social care professionals. Breakfast is always at 8am, followed by assistance with daily activities. Drugs are administered as prescribed by the nurse or doctor at the same time each day. Meals are never individualised, but come from the meals-on-wheels service. In fact, there is no variant in daily activities and nor is there respect for individual needs and desires. The process becomes routine and change to this daily structure is unwelcome and threatening to the elderly person.

Policy makers have assumed that community care is a panacea for individuals, communities, societies and the state, which provides a framework for enhancing the quality of care given within manageable financial budgets. It is a bottom-up user-led service that is sensitive to local and individual needs (Department of Health, 1990). However, a decade on from the NHS and Community Care Act, we have a service with escalating costs and a growing dissatisfaction among members of the public on the range and disparity of services offered.

Community care by definition is a political ideal, but through the legitimisation and implementation of such strategies there is a purist interpretation that sees community care as a basis of 'folk wisdom and culture', and a failure of governments to implement quality care within an institutionalised setting. McBeath and Webb (1997, p.40), state that '... community care is a metonym for a reallocation of responsibilities of the modern state to a notionally separate part of human society, namely, what used to be called a civil society'.

The NHS and Community Care Act 1990 was a radical Act and a showed a shift in ideological thinking that set the blueprint for action. There was no precedence within the world health communities and the scale of the experiment was quite remarkable. While recognising a change in care philosophies the Act also encouraged the creation of a competitive internal market that shifted the balance of power between purchasers and providers of health care. As part of this framework general practitioners (GPs) became fundholders and were allocated budgets that would have previously gone to the health authorities. Nurses working in the primary care sector were afforded the opportunity to share in the decision-making, enabling them to increase their relationships with patients and other professional groups.

It was expected that within the resources to support community care would be the concentration and provision of highly skilled professionals who would be peripatetic. These would include doctors, nurses, clinical psychologists, physiotherapists, speech therapists and occupational health therapists. These specialist practitioners would complement the work of the primary health care team made up of GPs, community nurses, health visitors, general practice nurses, school nurses, community mental health nurses, midwives, community children's nurses, community mental handicap nurses and social workers.

PRIMARY CARE

The notion of a primary health care service has evolved since the embryonic beginnings of the NHS, recognising the fact that promoting and preventing the ill-health of individuals and communities was of pivotal concern for all societies. In 1978 the World Health Organisation and Unicef (United Nations Children's Fund) sponsored an international conference at Alma-Ata in an Asiatic republic of the former Soviet Union. At this conference attention was given to the basic health needs of all people, which culminated in the following declaration: '… a demand for radically modified health policies', which was encapsulated in the term 'primary health care'. Roemer (1986) described this as '… essential health care based on practical, scientifically sound, socially acceptable methods and technology made available to individuals and their families in the community … in spirit of self reliance and self determination' (Declaration of Alma-Ata, p.16).

The recognised need for societies to embrace such philosophies has been instrumental in reforming health and social care organisations to focus, as a major principle, on primary health care. The reforms aim to provide health care services to the total population while enabling maximum public participation in the planning and implementation of these services.

Since 1989 the NHS has significantly changed its organisational frameworks and structures, moving away from acute and institutionalised care to an increased focus on primary care. Such reforms have seen the development of internal market economies, as previously mentioned, and an expansion of health care services in the primary care sector. Philosophically, the change in emphasis was to support a preventive model of health care that supported and maintained independent living (Department of Health, 1989). In promoting and strengthening primary care, there has been a growth towards the development of primary care teams that can lead health care initiatives in a co-ordinated and cost-effective manner. The effectiveness of such

models has enabled an increased focus on the concept of a primary care-led NHS. Primary care practitioners will be expected to take forward strategic planning and purchasing of health services, and the continued provision of traditional primary care services, while coping with the expansion of health care services that respond to local needs and demands.

Primary health care nursing

The roles and responsibilities of primary care nursing have responded to the demands and changing nature of the work embraced in primary care. It is a diverse and often complex role comprising, on the one hand, nursing services provided by the community health and public health service, while, on the other, embracing general practice and emergency care interventions. More recently, new services such as Walk-in Centres and Nurse Direct are centred within the constructs of primary care.

Nurses working in primary care are said to be a heterogeneous group, when they were previously viewed as separate and disparate disciplines in their own right, having a discrete body of knowledge. This changed with the Cumberledge Report in 1986, which emphasised the need for all nurses working in primary care to work collectively as a nursing team and to substitute for each other as the need arose (NHS Management Executive, 1993). To support the change in direction in 1994, the UKCC identified new standards through which all community nurses would be educated and trained together, including public health nurses (health visitors), community nurses in the home (district nurses), school nurses, general practice nurses, community mental health nurses, community mental handicap nurses, community children's nurses and occupational health nurses. All of these nursing disciplines would be required to embrace the new public health agenda to enable them to engage in preventive medicine (Mahler, 1975). Emphasising this point, the Royal College of Nursing (1989) recommended that nurses should engage with models of health care that ensured disease was prevented and would empower individuals and communities to take responsibility for their own health needs.

EVIDENCE-BASED CARE

Contemporary nursing care has embraced the notion that professional caring should be underpinned by relevant evidence of best caring practice that is supported and underpinned by empirical research. The search for evidence-based care recognises the changing dynamics of practice, which is influenced by advancements in technological innovations and new paradigms. Stevens *et al.* (1993) identified three reasons why there is a growing interest in professional practice in the research process:

1 At the macro level there is an increasing relationship with professionalism.
2 At the collective level nurses are encouraged to utilise research in everyday practice and stimulate areas requiring further investigation (reflection-in-action and reflection-on-action).
3 At the micro level professional nurses are accountable for their actions in terms of knowledge underpinning practice that has been scientifically verified.

Thus, the principles of research practice have been firmly ensconced within the constructs of professional nursing care. It has become an inherent feature of nursing curricula promoted by Project 2000 (UKCC, 1986), which has identified the need to produce a practitioner who can be 'analytic in her approach, and be capable of applying critical thinking and a questioning attitude to her practice' (Stevens *et al.*, 1993).

Study Activity 3.9 ____

● Write down your own experiences/perceptions of care from both a lay and a professional perspective.
● Define the characteristics inherent within professional nursing care.

SUMMARY

In general it has been the norm for the female members of the family unit to provide lay *informal* care. It is a reciprocal arrangement privately organised and fulfilled. Professional care, on the other hand, is the result of organised education and training, carried out within defined parameters. It can be an emotional activity, which requires the practitioner to be flexible in responding to different circumstances as they present. In addition, professional care operates within a moral and ethical framework in which the nurse is always responsible and accountable for the care given. This accountability requires the nurse to be knowledgeable and skilled in the art and science of nursing practice, to respect human life and the quality of that life, and to give care that involves purposeful interventions underpinned by research and /or best evidence. In so doing, the nurse will critically evaluate the care given in a context of what Schon (1983) regards as reflection-in-action or a 'reflective conversation with the situation'.

Holistic care empowers professional nurses to engage in caring partnerships with their clients and through the inter-relationship and following discourse, restoration of health will occur more speedily and patients will become empowered through the process to take charge of their own health care needs. This process allows nurses freedom and autonomy but does not disengage them from their professional obligations or responsibilities. Indeed, holistic care increases professional responsibility and accountability.

The concept of care and the duty to give care should be an explicit value within contemporary nursing and, in recognising this, professional nurses should engage in consciousness-raising activities. In promoting a caring consciousness the profession of nursing should actively promote and reward outstanding care within the constructs of everyday practice.

Formalised (professional) care has evolved within complex structures that have changed to accommodate contemporary needs and demands.

Currently the focus and power dynamics have shifted to primary care fundamentally to increase individual and community participation in the prevention of health and in the provision of health intervention.

From 2002, the Labour Government is committed to initiating further radical changes that will reduce regional organisational structures in England, remove Local Health Authorities and in their place create Strategic Health Authorities. The power dynamics will change to increase the responsibility and authority of Primary Care Trusts. Similar developments are taking place in the other three countries of the UK. Much of the detailed planning is set to unfold, but it is evident that the effects of these changes will be far reaching and will change the face of professional practice in all areas.

Study Activity 3.10

- Search out the Department of Health policy documents that advise on health and social care reforms (1989, 1990, 2000). Identify how organised professional care will change with the implementation of these reforms.
- Analyse the role changes of nursing and allied professions within these changes.
- Identify how these reforms have been accommodated in clinical practice.

REFERENCES

Audit Commission (1992) *The Community Revolution: Personal social services and community care*, HMSO, London

Badger, F. (1989) The nursing auxiliary service and the care of elder patients. *Journal of Advanced Nursing* 14, 471–7

Banks, M., Beresford, S., Morrell, D. *et al*. (1975) Factors influencing demand for primary health care in women aged 20–44 years: a preliminary report. *International Journal of Epidemiology* 4, 189–95.

Barry, N. (1990) *Welfare*, Open University Press, Milton Keynes

Batson, C.D., Bolen, M.H., Cross, J.A. *et al*. (1986) Where is the altruism in the altruistic personality. *Journal of Personality and Social Psychology* 50, 212–20

Benner, P. (1984) *From Novice to Expert – Excellence and power in clinical practice*. Addison-Wesley, Merlo Park, CA

Benner, P. and Wrubel, J. (1989) *The Primacy of Caring: Stress and coping in health and illness*, Addison-Wesley, Merlo Park, CA

Clarke, J.B. and Wheeler, S.J. (1992) A view of the phenomena of caring in nursing practice. *Journal of Advanced Nursing* 17, 1283–90

Cochrane, A.L. (1972) *Effectiveness and Efficiency: Random reflections on the health service*, The Rock Carling Lecture, Nuffield Provincial Hospitals Trust, London

Council of National Representatives (1989). In: Quinn, S. (1989) *ICN: Past and present*, Scutari Press, London

Culyer, A.J. (1976) *Need and the National Health Service*, Martin Robertson, Oxford

Davis, C. (1976) Experience of dependency and control in work: the case of nurses. *Journal of Advanced Nursing* 1, 273–82

Dawkins, R. (1976) *The Selfish Gene*, Oxford University Press, New York

Dean, K.J., Hickey, T. and Holstein, B.E. (1986) Self-care behaviour: implications for ageing. In: Dean, K.J., Hickey, T. and Holstein, B.E. (1986) *Self-care and Health in Old Age*, London, Croom Helm

Department of Health (1989) *Caring for People*, DoH, London

Department of Health (1990) *The National Health Service and Community Care Act*, DoH, London

Department of Health (2000) *The National Health Service Ten-year Plan*, DoH, London

Donabedian, A. (1980) *The Definition of Quality and Approaches to its Assessment*, Health Administration Press, MI

Dowd, T. (1989) Ethical reasoning: a basis for nursing care in the home. In: Sherry, D. (1990) Autonomy versus beneficence: the dilemma and its implications in home care. *Home Healthcare Nurse* 8(6), 13–15

Eisenberg, N., Millar, P., Scaller, M. *et al*. (1989) The role of sympathy and altruistic personality traits in helping: a re-examination. *Journal of Personality* 57, 41–67

Finch, J. (1989) *Family Obligations and Social Change*, Polity Press, Cambridge

Forrest, D. (1989) The experience of caring *Journal of Advanced Nursing* **14**, 815–23

Foucault, M.(1979) *On Governmentality: Ideology and consciousness*, Tavistock, London

Funnel, M., Anderson, R., Arnold, M. *et al.*, (1991) Empowerment: an idea whose time has come in diabetes education. *The Diabetes Educator* **17**(1) pp. 37–41

Garfinkel, H. (1967) *Studies in Ethnomethodology*, Prentice Hall, NJ

Gibbs, G. (1988) *Learning By Doing: A guide to teaching and learning methods*, EMU, Oxford

Goffman, E. (1968) *Asylums*, Penguin Books, Harmondsworth

Gormley, K. (1995) Social graces . . . social policy in nursing curricula. *Nursing Times* **91**, 55–7

Gormley, K. (1998) Self-care. In: Basford, L. and Slevin, O. (1999) *Theory and Practice of Nursing*, Nelson Thornes, Cheltenham

Graham, H. (1983) Caring: a labour of love. In: Finch, J. and Groves, D. (eds) (1983) *A Labour of Love*, Routledge and Kegan Paul, London

Grant, G. and Nolan, M. (1993) Informal carers: sources and concomitants of satisfaction. *Health and Social Care* **1**, 144–59.

Green, H. (1988) *Informal Carers*, OPCS Series General Household Survey No. 15 (Supplement A), HMSO, London

Green-Hernandez, C. (1991) Professional nurse caring: a conceptual model for nursing. In: Neil, R.M. and Watts, R. (eds) (1991) *Caring and Nursing: Explanations in a feminist perspective*, National League for Nursing, New York

Haug, M.R. (1986) Doctor–patient relationship and their impact on elderly self-care. In: Dean, K., Hickey, T. and Holstein, B.E. (1986) *Self-care and Health in Old Age*, Croom-Helm, London

Hiscock, J. and Pearson, M. (1996) Professional costs and invisible value: the market in community nursing. *Journal of Inter-professional Care* **10**(1), 23–31

Holzemer, W.L. (1992) Linking primary health care and self-care through case management, *International Nursing Review* **39**(3), 83–9

Hugman, R., Peelo, M. and Soothill, K. (1997) *Concepts of Care*, Arnold, London

Illich, I. (1976) *Medical Nemesis*: *The expropriation of health*, Random, New York

Jarvis, P. (1992) Reflective practice and nursing. *Nurse Education Today* **12**, 174–81

Kendall, H. (1990) A strategy for Nursing. Monitoring standards of care. *Nursing Standards* **4**(37), 32–3

Kitson, A. (1987) Raising standards of clinical practice: the fundamental issue of effective nursing practice. *Journal of Advanced Nursing* **12**, 321–9

Koch, T. (1992) Review of nursing quality assurance, *Journal of Advanced Nursing*, **17**, 785–94

Laing, R.D. (1960) *The Divided Self*, Penguin, Harmondsworth

Landsberg, L. (1993) *Altruism in Medicine: Prescription for the nineties*, Pharos Honorary Medical Association, Winter **56** (1), pp. 9–10

Leininger, M. (1981) *Caring: An essential human need*, Charles B. Slack, Thorofare, NJ

Leininger, M. (1984) *Care: The essence of nursing and health*, Charles B. Slack, Thorofare, NJ

Levin, L.S. and Idler, E.L. (1981) *The Hidden Health Care System: Mediating structures and medicines*, Balinger, Cambridge

McBeath, G.B. and Webb, S.A. (1997) Community care: a unity of state and care. Some political and philosophical considerations. In: Hugman, R., Peelo, M. and Soothill, K. (1997) *Concepts of Care*, Arnold, London

MacMahon, R and Pearson, A (1991) *Nursing as Therapy*, Chapman and Hall, London

Mahler, H. (1975) Health – a demystification of medical technology. *Lancet* **2**, 829–33

Malthus, T.R. (1798) An essay on the principles of population. In: Fraser, D. (1982) *The Evolution of the British Welfare State* (1st edn), Macmillan, London

Marr, J. and Giebing, M. (1994) *Quality Care*, Campion Press, Edinburgh

Mauss, M. (1966) *The Gift*, Cohen and West, London

Mayeroff, M. (1972) *On Caring*, Harper and Row, New York

Misener, J.H. (1990) The impact of technology on the quality of health care. *Quality Review Bulletin*, June, 209–13

NHS Management Executive (1993) *Nursing in Primary Health Care: New world, new opportunities*, NHS Management Executive, London

Nolan, M. and Grant, G. (1989) Addressing the needs of informal carers: a neglected area of nursing practice. *Journal of Advanced Nursing* **14**(11), 950–62

Nursing and Midwifery Council (2002) *Code of Professional Conduct*, NMC, London

Orem, D. (1985) *Nursing: Concepts of practice* (3rd edn), McGraw-Hill, New York

Poon, L.W., Basford, L., Dowzer, C. *et al.* (2003) Coping with comorbidity in older adults. In: Poon, L.W., Hall-Gueldner, S. and Spouse, B. (in press) *Successful Ageing and Adaptation with Chronic Diseases in Older Adulthood*, Springer, New York

Quinn, S. (1989) *ICN: Past and present,* Scutari Press, London

Quinney, D., Pearson, M. and Pursey, A. (1997) Care in primary health care nursing. In: Hugman, R., Peelo, M. and Soothill, K. *Concepts of Care*, Arnold, London

Ricardo, D. (1817) The principles of political economy and taxation. In: Jones, K. (1990) *The Making of Social Policy in Britain 1830–1990*, Athlone Press, London

Roemer, M.I. (1986) Priorty for primary health care: Its development and problems. *Health Policy and Planning* 1(1), 58–66

Rogers, M. (1980) Nursing: A science of unitary man. In: Riehl, J.P. and Roy, C. (1980) *Conceptual Models for Nursing Practice* (2nd edn), Appleton-Century-Crofts, New York

Royal College of Nursing (1989) *The Duties and Position of the Nurse* (revised edn), Royal College of Nursing, London

Sanford, J. (1975) Tolerance of debility in elderly dependents by supporters at home: its significance for hospital practice. *British Medical Journal* 3, 471–5

Seymore, J. (1991) Pathological caring: a long term problem that must be solved, *Geriatric Medicine*, January, p. 17

Schon, D. (1983) *The Reflective Practitioner*, Temple Smith, London

Schon, D. (1987) *Educating the Reflective Practitioner*, Jossey Bass, San Francisco, CA

Schroeder, C. and Maeve, K. (1992) Nursing care partnership at the Denver nursing project in human caring: an application and extension of caring theory in practice, *Advances in Nursing Science* 15(2), 25–38

Sherry, D (1990) Autonomy versus beneficence: the dilemma and its implications in home care. *Home Healthcare Nurse* 8(6), 13–15

Smuts, J.C. (1926) *Holism and Evolution*, Macmillan, New York

Stevens, P., Schade, A.L., Chalk, B. *et al.* (1993) *Understanding Research*, Campion Press, Edinburgh

Stockwell, F. (1984) *The Unpopular Patient*, Royal College of Nursing, London

Swanson, K.M. (1991) Empirical development of a middle range theory of caring. *Nursing Research* 40(3), 161–6

Titmus, R.M. (1973) *The Gift Relationship*, Penguin, Harmondsworth

UKCC (1983) *Code for Nurses, Midwives and Health Visitors*, HMSO, London

UKCC (1992) *Code of Professional Conduct*, UKCC, London

Watson, J. (1979, 1985, 1988) *The Philosophy and Science of Human Caring*, Associated University Press, Colorado

Wilson, E.O. (1975) *Sociobiology: The new synthesis*, Harvard University, Boston, MA

World Health Organisation (1978) *Alma-Ata Primary Health Care* (Health for All Series No.1), WHO, Geneva

4 EMPOWERING CARE

Katie Dann

LEARNING OUTCOMES

After studying this chapter you will be able to:

- Appreciate how changes in care have resulted in a need for empowering practice from the perspectives of clients, informal carers and professionals
- Understand the long history of empowerment, appreciating how this has resulted in empowerment having many faces.
- Acknowledge the process and product elements of empowerment
- Appraise the concept of empowerment in relation to models of care and the issues of power distribution within the caring community
- Effectively transfer the theoretical and philosophical basis of empowerment to the practice arena, understanding the mechanisms of empowerment programmes
- Reflect on the structural and political implications of introducing patient and carer empowerment within the health care system
- Explore the realities of empowermrent – for client, professional, or informal carer – within the health care system of today.

INTRODUCTION

With a new millennium, a refreshed outlook on the conditions of optimum patient care in the UK health system is sought. Health care has not been immune to rapid change, therefore the fundamentals that epitomised the notion of care yesterday are markedly different to today's multi-faceted, multi-level and multimedia health care. This critical reflection on care has ignited controversial debate concerning the role of the professional, the informal carer and the patient. It appears that each member of the *therapeutic relationship* is searching for the Holy Grail of empowered care.

Therapeutic relationship describes the relationship in patient *care*. Generally speaking, there are two members of the relationship – the carer and the patient. However, the carer may be a professional or an informal carer, such as a friend or family member.

This chapter endeavours to introduce the concept, theoretical underpinnings and mechanisms of empowerment in the context of formal and informal care. The key objective is to promote the *quantifiable* approach to empowerment and prevent its abstract use. A *quantifiable* level of empowerment would help us measure change in empowerment programmes in a scientific and empirical way. Despite being a very emotive concept this chapter will illustrate that empowerment can be viewed from an empirical viewpoint, allowing measurement, evaluation and the development of programmes to enhance empowerment perceptions. Only when health professionals understand empowerment will it be possible to identify and enhance empowering practice. The bottom line is that we should first agree on the type of empowering practice before employing under-defined strategies.

WHY IS EMPOWERMENT SO IMPORTANT FOR CARE TODAY?

As indicated in the introduction to this chapter, health care is not immune to the external changes that have occurred in the last ten years;

changes that have been politically, socially and economically driven. For instance, in the previous decade there has been a radical shift in the way the patient and professional relationship is developed and maintained. Indeed, the health care system today has had to adapt to change, taking on a proactive rather than reactive role. In this dynamic society it is not so much about keeping up with the times but being in front, tracing new pathways in line with service user need.

Caring communities

As you will have observed in Chapter 1, when relating to precedents of care there has been a progression. Care, which once could have been described as a one-way path, from professional to carer, has diversified considerably. Today a network of caring communities supports health care. Membership of this network is not exclusive; indeed the core essence of the caring community is that it encompasses the notion of multi-agency. As with the most traditional perceptions of care there is the health professional and the service user. However, in conjunction with these two familiar identities are informal carers, user groups, and family and friends. It appears that the original duo now comes as part of a package, formally epitomised in the Community Care Act 1990 (Department of Health, 1990).

These developments run in parallel with the move towards empowering practice. Contemporary health care seeks to empower clients to take responsibility for their health, limiting the development of a dependency on the professional and the NHS. However, successfully moving away from a dependency model requires all parties of the caring community to perceive empowerment. The energy of the caring community should be harnessed in such a way as to improve health on an individual, community and societal level. It is argued that adopting an empowering approach to care avoids the philosophical minefield of whether caring is altruistic or indeed a duty of the carer and thus an expectation of the patient. Empowering practice advocates that all members of the caring community should strive for a satisfactory and self-determined level of empowerment. This final stage is only possible once the notion of empowerment has been fully clarified.

DEFINING EMPOWERMENT

Before beginning the immense task of defining empowerment, it is imperative to understand the reason for addressing the issue of definitions. Within the literature it appears that scientists and academics have an innate drive or perhaps hunger to conceptualise abstract terms, and for very good reasons. Arguably, it is only when an abstract concept, such as empowerment, is functionally defined can it be fully operationalised. Making a concept operational allows individuals to implement, measure and evaluate (*see* Fig 4.1). These steps are vital if empowerment is to become a reality in health care.

Study Activity 4.1

- Create a list of the various adjectives associated with the concept of empowerment.
- Using your list, write a working definition pertaining to the concept of empowerment. (Remember the definition of a definition: 1. A statement of the precise meaning of a word or phrase, or the nature of a thing; 2. Making or being distinct, clearness of outline.) Try to encompass notions of direction, any exchanges of power, antecedents and consequences, actors and recipients.
- Was this an easy task? Reflect on any difficulties you encountered while developing your definition. How might these difficulties impinge on developing an empowerment programme?

Despite the obvious need for a comprehensive definition of empowerment, an ultimate understanding is as yet not forthcoming. Perhaps we need first to consider the types of relationship in health care before we can begin to describe how

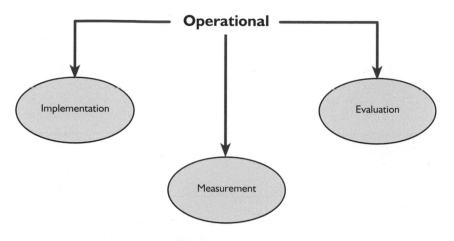

Figure 4.1 Why define empowerment?

each individual in that relationship can perceive empowerment. An exploration of models of care may help signpost the way.

MODELS OF CARE

The interactional process observed between professional and client is central to the application of empowerment in practice. A model of care describes the characteristics of a practice. The model of care attributed to a certain practice would offer information concerning the distribution of power between the players. Generally in the health care domain a service user and a service provider occupy the roles of player. There are three major models of care that aim to describe the distribution of power between the professional and the individual seeking care:

1 traditional medical model
2 transformed medical model
3 consumerist model.

Fundamentally the comparisons between these models is the extent to which the client takes an active or passive role within the dynamic (*see* Fig. 4.2). For a more detailed review of patient/professional relationship, *see* Ong *et al.* (1995) (Module 7).

Practitioners upholding the ethos of the tradi-

tional medical model approach would suffocate any attempts of their client to demonstrate an active role within their care. The traditional medical model advocates that the professional manages the power base within the therapeutic relationship. As such, the client maintains a passive role within the relationship, which essentially refutes the notion of client empowerment.

The extreme opposite to this relationship is observed in the consumerist approach to medical care. This model describes a relationship, which is dictated by the active client who elicits power through the choices their financial status permit. Consumerism is a strong feature in private health care, but there is also evidence to suggest that this model of care may become increasingly apparent in the NHS (Newton, 1995; Wiles and Higgins, 1996; Shepperd *et al.*, 1999; Eysenbach, 2000; Timmons, 2001).

The consumerist model addresses the obvious criticism directed at the traditional medical model with regard to professional dominance and patient rights. However, the shift to a purely consumerist model in certain circumstances is not the remedy for all ills. McCann and Weinman (1996) demonstrate that despite attempts to empower clients during a medical consultation, i.e. altering the relationship from a traditional basis to one where the client was active, did not always enhance perceptions of

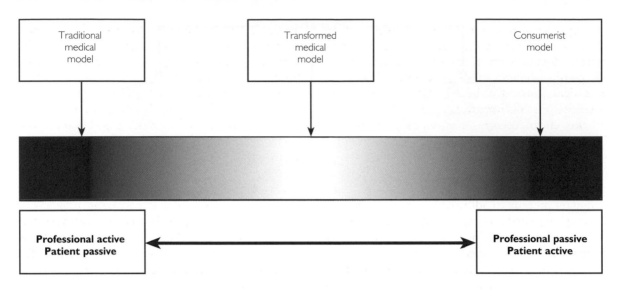

Figure 4.2 Models of care

empowerment. Essentially, consumerism was only empowering if the individual was comfortable with the shift in dynamics.

Clearly, both models demonstrate the polar extremes observed in clinical relationships, but the final model describes the ultimate professional/client partnership. The transformed medical model depicts a relationship in which a harmonious balance between professional and client has been struck. The relationship thrives through the expert contributions of each party. The professional claims expertise regarding clinical advice, whereas the client provides expertise concerning pain, symptoms and self-perceptions. This model recognises a truly equitable interaction and as such the balance of power is fluid throughout the exchange.

Any discussion of power appears to suggest that when one person gains power it is at the expense of another. Indeed, there is an implicit equation that a hierarchical system is in place and when power is transferred to one individual it is taken away from the other. However, the notion that appears most productive is one that pertains to the feminist stance of 'power to' as opposed to 'power over'. Rafael (1998) consid-

ered the term 'power to' to be the spirit of empowered caring. This rejects the notion that power is a commodity that is fed into an equation whereby the facilitator relinquishes power over to a receiver. Josefowitz (1980, as cited in Rodwell, 1996) reaffirmed the positive nature of power within empowerment. It was clarified that there is a negative form of power associated with forcefulness, i.e. a controlling, and in contrast there is power that infers ability, opportunity and the means to perform tasks. The latter epitomises the empowerment health care should strive towards.

The issue of *relativity* addressed by the transformed medical model is the key to empowering practice. A dictionary definition for *relativity* might describe the word as 'a state of dependence in which the existence or significance of one entity is solely dependent on that of another'. If we apply this to empowerment then it means that before merely reviewing the power dynamics we must take into consideration a client's previous situation and other aspects of their care, such as health status, age and gender. These additional characteristics are relative to that individual.

Empowerment is a relative construct; indeed what is empowering for one individual is ultimately disempowering for another. Addressing the possible repercussions of 'empowering all' is a critical move for health care professionals, necessitating consideration of the relative status of the client. Before empowering practice is implemented it is imperative that the professional considers the balance of power that would be most appropriate for that particular client. It could be argued that the rash decision to empower all fails to address the issue of whether passing responsibility on to all clients can be considered empowering. Arguably, in certain circumstances, this action can lead to the individual experiencing disempowerment. In addition to this, tarring everyone with the same empowerment brush ignores the core philosophy of empowerment that advocates an idiosyncratic approach to care, thus adopting a transformed medical model approach.

Study Activity 4.2

- Reflect on the three models of care. Which model does the NHS advocate today? To what extent has this been achieved?
- List the ways in which the following models act as barriers to empowering practice:
  - the traditional medical model
  - the consumerist model.
- What are the key elements of the transformed medical model that elicit empowering practice?
- Offer practical suggestions as to how the transformed medical model can be implemented in practice. Bear in mind how issues of communication, geography, resources, gender, ethnicity and socio-economic status may influence such initiatives.
- Offer four client examples where the relative empowerment approach may be necessary.

EMPOWERMENT AND ITS FAMILY TREE

The following section provides a historical snapshot of empowerment by reviewing the genealogy of the concept, from its philosophical routes to its present day application in health care. The family tree of empowerment described here is by no means complete. Tracing the roots of empowerment is much the same as locating relatives of a family in the traditional sense, as there are skeletons, black sheep and people who don't want to be found! Also, as you will gather from reading this brief history, there are many marriages, not in the traditional sense but in the way that disciplines such as philosophy, sociology, business management and psychology have influenced the evolution of empowerment. Like a family this has not been a completely harmonious amalgamation and progressing the construct has been plagued by battles of the vested disciplines.

Genealogy is a record of the descent of a person, family or group from an ancestor or ancestors. A common form of this is a family tree. In the context of this chapter we want to trace the roots of empowerment.

The aim of presenting a family tree was to illustrate how the modern day use of the term empowerment has evolved, influenced by numerous families (disciplines of knowledge). Indeed, it appears that the concept of empowerment facilitated in health care today is somewhat of a hybrid rather than a pedigree entity. However, as with most families, the empowerment family has a degree of linkage across generation lines; for instance you will note how the philosophical grandfathers contributed to the contemporary use and understanding of empowerment. As shown in Fig. 4.3 the philosophical forefathers form the roots of the family tree. From these solid foundations the tree has seen continuous growth. The top of the tree is made up of new foliage from contemporary research in empowerment. Inter and intra-family co-operation has resulted in a web of empowerment with contributions from all paradigms such as business, sociology and psychology. However, it must be questioned how the concept might have progressed if all factions were working harmoniously rather than in parallel. Indeed, mapping a concept development has highlighted

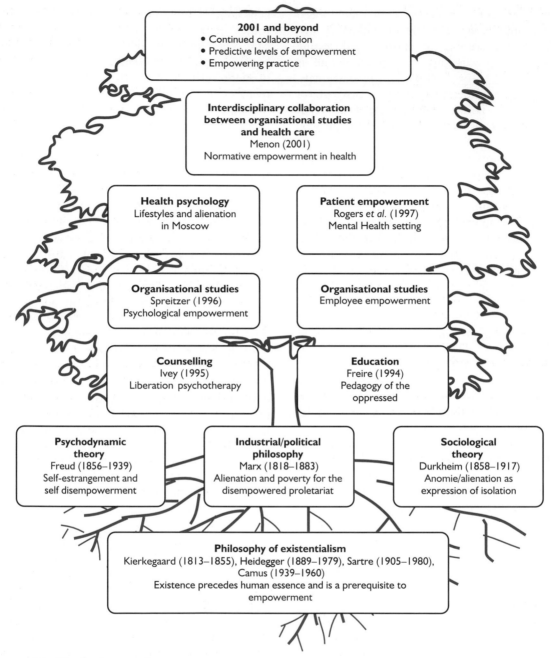

Figure 4.3 The family tree of empowerment

the need for inter-disciplinary action in order to harness the progression made by all of the contributing partners.

Starting with the roots, philosophers such as Søren Kierkegaard, Martin Heidegger, and Jean-Paul Sartre were existentialist commentators, sowing the seeds of the empowerment family tree. Reading through the basic assumptions of existentialism (*see* Table 4.1) will demonstrate the parallels of this philosophy with empowerment.

Table 4.1   Basic existentialist principles

- The individual is unique and has freedom to choose ways of seeing and being.
- The individual has free choice over and above the crowd and mass society (collective conscience).
- The individual has responsibility for their personality and existence.
- The main struggle for the individual is to attain self-definition and meaning in life through the choices available.
- Meaning and existence precedes essence.
- The only certainty in existentialism is death.

From these philosophical beginnings the notion of alienation was cultivated. Alienation is considered to be the antithesis or absolute opposite of empowerment.

As far as existentialism is concerned alienation is inauthentic existence where otherness and estrangement are recurrent. It was considered that alienation was synonymous with disempowerment, emphasising the notion of powerlessness over one's destiny as an inevitable part of the human condition.

The two poles of empowerment and alienation continued to have a huge amount of currency by the time social action theory emerged. This is a collective drive that is based on common understanding derived from everyday experience. For example, the Patient's Charter intended to rectify a deficiency in power relations based on recognised and collective need.

Empowerment in this context was associated with creating proactive community interests and with attempts to increase the power and influence of such oppressed groups as workers, women and ethnic minorities. Thus, the empowerment ideology concerned itself with enabling people to take action. Elsewhere, the same empowerment ideology and social action are perceived by social theorists, such as Durkheim (1897) and Radcliffe-Brown (1952), as the essence of society and collective conscience.

Emile Durkheim's social theory would have argued that alienation (anomie) might be a result of disempowerment. Durkheim (1897) saw alienation as a form of estrangement from oneself, other individuals, society or work. He saw this alienation or estrangement as a possible explanation for what he called anomic suicide. The term alienation is widely used in sometimes contradictory ways. Psychotherapists, for instance, consider alienation to be a self-induced blocking or dissociation of personal feelings, causing the individual concerned to become less effective socially and emotionally. The focus here is on the individual's difficulties in adjusting to society. Sigmund Freud (1930), on the other hand, asserted that alienation was self-estrangement caused by the split between the conscious and unconscious parts of the mind. Whatever the theoretical and philosophical debates, it appears that empowerment is about minimising the sense of alienation.

There was a further marriage in the family of empowerment connecting the psychoanalytic paradigm and a counselling perspective. The transfer and share of power between the two parties in a psychotherapeutic framework is a fundamental concern within emancipatory approaches to counselling. The goal of these paradigms is to strike a balance between professional-led and client-directed counselling. As such, the aim of counselling sessions is to allow the client to explore the social world in accordance with the client's experience and perception.

Within his liberation psychotherapy approach, Ivey (1995) contended that the client takes the lead. A key element to the process is for the client to nominate their 'resistance', which is essentially the features within their life that elicit some form of oppression of the individual. Discussion then progresses to analyse strategies for overcoming the oppressive force. From this brief account, it can be appreciated that empowering the client is the most significant and the primary goal of this form of anti-oppressive counselling practice.

Holland (1992) presented an additional example of this form of counselling, known as the social action therapy. This approach to counselling advocates the inclusion of all forms of the client's community and each representative is involved within the therapeutic alliance.

The theoretical origin of the social action therapy lies with the social action theory previously discussed. A shared notion is that there are oppressed individuals and the individual in isolation from his or her environmental, cultural and social factors cannot confront this notion of oppression. Acknowledging this, the social action approach states that individual psychotherapy is not enough to establish a sense of personal empowerment. The individual must progress through a transition from an individual-based therapy to a radical humanism and structuralism that encourages analysis of people and organisations that may oppress the individual.

As a distant relative in the empowerment tree there was empowerment work being conducted in the field of business and organisational management. The works of Spreitzer (1996), Menon (2001) and Sagie and Koslowski (2000) reflect this. This branch of the family has concerned itself with power relations, decision-making and organisational group dynamics in relation to perceptions of empowerment. The applicability of organisational models to the health domain may not be immediately apparent. However, in a later section of this chapter, concerning staff empowerment, the theories developed by these empowerment cousins raise pertinent questions regarding the reality of empowerment in a health system.

After this long and eventful history of empowerment we arrive at applications of empowerment in a health arena. Rogers *et al.* (1997) explored empowerment of individuals suffering mental illness. This application of empowerment runs parallel with the rise of user groups and the increase of representatives seeking advancements of patient rights. However, recent moves have endeavoured to review perceptions of empowerment in normative populations, i.e. individuals who do not suffer from ill health, as a means of identifying risk groups (Menon, 2002). This work

is largely based on the assumption that empowered individuals will take more responsibility for their health status, thus becoming an active agent in their health. There are parallels here with health-related locus of control, which describes the extent to which an individual believes they have control over their health status. For instance, how much control does an individual have over the maintenance of a healthy diet?

It is anticipated that a normative measure of empowerment would form the basis of a predictive model, allowing researchers to target specific populations. The research into the use of empowerment in a normative population is still in an embryonic stage, but it highlights the potential use of empowerment measures and strategies. The work also signifies interdisciplinary collaboration, as Menon's background is largely in business and organisational studies. The future use of empowerment is still unknown and thoroughly dependent on not only fully understanding the concept of empowerment but also in such a way that this understanding is shared across disciplines.

DEFINING EMPOWERMENT: REVISITED

There is no shortage of definitions attributed to the concept. In fact the overabundance of empowerment definitions can be accounted for through the lack of consensus as to whether empowerment qualifies as an acquired state or the transition from oppressed to perceived power. Indeed, it has become apparent that the most productive way forward is to view empowerment both as a process and as a product, but a comprehensive definition should portray the interaction between the product and process. To acquire this value-added definition it is necessary to revisit how empowerment can initially be viewed as either a product or a process.

Essentially definitions falling into this category view empowerment as an achievement, a commodity, or indeed something that can be obtained. The impression gained from definitions portraying empowerment as a product is that the empowered individual has reached an end state that is marked by an acquisition of some kind. This product can be concrete, for example clients gaining access to required information to make informed decisions concerning their treatment schedule or indeed as abstract as an enhancement of self-esteem.

EMPOWERMENT AS A PRODUCT

Rogers *et al.* (1997) state that an empowered individual has obtained self-worth, efficacy and acquired a sense of power. Clearly, this definition denotes empowerment as a product in that it is an element that the individual has gained (Fig. 4.4). Wowra and McCarter (1999) uphold the above definition of empowerment in terms of access and the uptake of skills, 'having access to information and resources ... (and) learning skills that the individual defines as important' (p. 960).

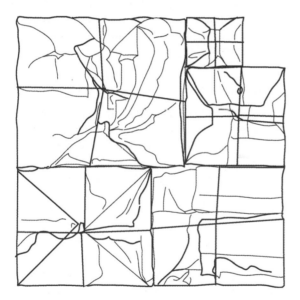

Figure 4.4 Empowerment as a product

EMPOWERMENT AS A PROCESS

The literature in this section, however, tends to describe empowerment as a journey, emphasising growth and transition. Essentially, movement

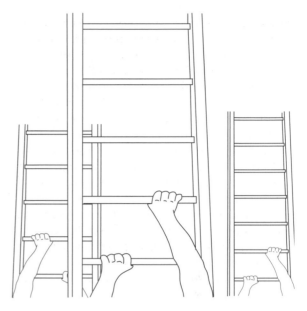

Figure 4.5 Empowerment as a process

towards empowering practice can be termed empowerment (Fig. 4.5).

Webb and Tossell (1995, cited in Jenkins, 1997) assert that empowerment should be viewed as a continuum. This appears to refute the notion of an end product and, in contrast, introduces the concept of relativity. The suggestion of relative empowerment is a useful idea within the context of mental health nursing, elderly care and paediatrics given that the clients within these groups are often significantly disempowered compared to other client groups. Within the above client categories there is incredible value placed on any small steps of progress. Relative empowerment would infer that a move towards empowering practice, no matter how small, would qualify as empowerment. This appears to suggest that the current situation and context of the individual alongside their idiosyncrasies are taken into account and contrasted against the previous history of the individual. In essence the growth and development determines what constitutes empowerment. As such, a definition under this subsection would contest the argument that state empowerment and service users are antagonistic concepts, thus refuting the comments made by Lamont (1999). If the definition of empowerment as a process of growth is accepted, then it is plausible to suggest that all individuals can achieve some level of empowerment.

The implications of relative empowerment are clear. If the process of empowerment itself is deemed empowering there is the chance that an additive momentum may be initialised, which will in itself produce an increased perception of empowerment. Furthermore, characterising empowerment as a process presumes that there is an endless resource for each individual. However, if the concept is deemed purely to be a product, empowerment will not be attained until the individual is in possession of the final outcome.

Staples (1993, as cited in Rogers *et al.* 1997) proposed a definition in which empowerment was depicted as a process through which the individual developed power. It was this development that allowed the individual to strengthen capacity. The latter section of the definition indeed suggests a relative stance to empowerment when capacity is viewed in terms of their previous capabilities.

According to Rodwell (1996) the process of enabling is equivocal to empowerment. Mason *et al.* (1991) build upon this distinction and assert that empowerment is the process of enabling individuals to acknowledge their existing strengths and encouraging the use of their personal power. Kuokkanen and Leino-Kilpi (2000) confirmed the process element of empowerment through reinforcing the dynamic nature of the concept. The authors reviewed the definition of empowerment in terms of three elected levels, namely community, organisational and psychological. In the community sense the term empowerment is the striving towards a shared goal. If, on the other hand, empowerment is viewed in the context of organisations it denotes a process of productivity. Kuokkanan and Leino-Kilpi (2000) stated that empowerment in the psychological context was the process of growth and personal development.

Finally, Kar *et al.* (1999) emphasise the notion of empowerment as a process, which addresses the concept in terms of health promotion. The authors state that empowerment is the 'movement towards the powerless to take proactive actions to prevent threats and to promote positive aspects of their lives' (p. 1433). Indeed, the authors confirm their assertions of empowerment as a process by arguing that empowerment is the means to gain a quality of life.

Study Activity 4.3

After reading through the list of characteristics of empowerment in Table 4.2, as identified by Rogers *et al.* (1997), try to assign each one to either a product category or a process category:

Table 4.2   The characteristics of empowerment

- Having access to information and resources
- Having a range of options from which to make choices (not just 'yes'/ 'no', and 'either'/ 'or').
- Assertiveness
- A feeling that one can make a difference (being hopeful)
- Learning to think critically; unlearning the conditioning; seeing things differently – for example, learning to redefine who one is; (speaking in one's own voice, learning to redefine what one can do, and learning to redefine one's relationship to institutionalised power'); learning about and expressing anger
- Not feeling alone; feeling part of a group
- Understanding that a person has rights
- Effecting change in one's life and one's community
- Learning skills (such as communication) that one defines as important
- Changing other's perception of one's competency and tcapacity o act
- Coming out of the closet
- Growth and change that is never-ending and self-initiated
- Increasing one's positive self-image and overcoming stigma

(From Rogers et al., 1997)

- Reflect on your practice and try to think of circumstances where you facilitate empowerment as a process and empowerment as a product.
- Return to this activity after reading the section on the cyclic nature of empowerment below. How has this representation altered the way you view empowerment? What does the cyclical representation mean for client types such as elderly people, children and sufferers of mental illness?

TOWARDS THE FUSION OF PROCESS AND PRODUCT: A CYCLICAL PHENOMENON

What began as a seemingly simple starting question ('What is empowerment?') has suddenly turned into a conceptual wrangle. It seems that defining empowerment is as difficult as defining love, because of the complex and diverse meanings attached to the concept. However, as previously discussed, to take the notion of empowerment forward and 'operationalise' the concept we must arrive at some level of communal agreement, which reflects context and time boundaries, and allows a flexibility of use. The above discussion credits empowerment being viewed as a process and a product. Indeed, the interchangeable nature implies that each perspective has credibility. Therefore, a comprehensive conceptualisation of empowerment would encompass the two, demonstrating a degree of energy and movement. Fig. 4.6 details a proposed conceptual representation of empowerment that highlights the process element, in conjunction with a representation of an end-state or product. The all-encompassing perspective of empowerment includes the notion of relativity, the additive nature of the concept and the interplay between process and product facets. If this is accounted for one could plausibly assume that empowerment is not merely on a continuum where there is a beginning and end point, but rather a cyclic phenomenon. Fig. 4.6 demonstrates how an empowering accomplishment would lead to a sub-product and catalyse the uptake of additional empowering tasks, essentially the empowering process. This would refute the idea that optimal empowerment can be achieved. Instead, a by-product of the previous empowerment process can be attained, which then fuels the subsequent empowering journey. In support of this is the commentary provided by Martin-Crawford (1999), who advocates that 'empowerment influences and is influenced by empowerment at other levels' (p. 19). Furthermore, incorporating the element of relativity implies that empowerment can be a reality in everybody's life.

Perhaps most English-speaking countries assume that empowerment is the process by which individuals or their communities gain knowledge and skills to influence and control their own activities of daily living (ADL). This position further assumes that everyone aspires for self-determination and power to control or influence their own quality of life. The reality might be that, for some people, empowerment has to be relative to their ability and context. In other words empowerment is not a unitary entity, but a kaleidoscopic entity relative to each person. People are likely to benefit from empowerment if they have the motivation and they value empowerment in relation to their perceived needs and aspirations. Look again at Fig. 4.6, which depicts a cyclic perspective of empowerment. This proposed model takes into account the fact that empowerment is relative to the individual and his or her circumstances. The model implies that empowerment is a metaphoric equation, in that it is a sum of the individual's prior status and the personal growth the individual has achieved during the empowerment transition. In essence, empowerment is a culmination of previous empowering experiences, yet remains specifically relative to the individual. This is qualitatively different to previous assumptions that consider an equation to represent empowerment. Previous assumptions tend to focus on a transaction between two individuals; the first individual transfers the ownership of power on to the second individual. This transaction clearly implies that the second actor is indebted to the 'empowerer', whereas the one who has empowered the receiver has ultimately lost the grasp of his or her power source. This equation is not a 'give and take' transaction, but is more closely associated with the interrelationship between the empowerment process and the empowerment sub-product in a fashion relative to the receiver.

EMPOWERING PRACTICE: CAN IT BE A REALITY?

The earlier sections of this chapter have provided theoretical backbone, dreamt up by scholars,

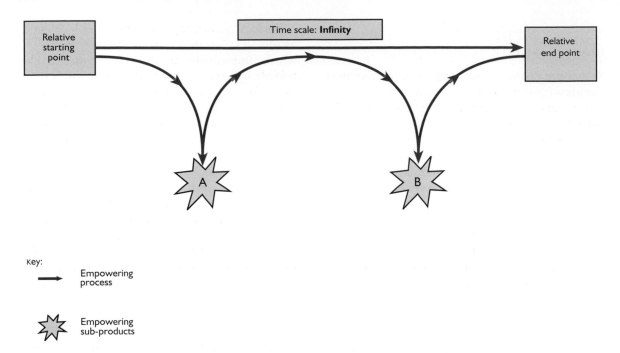

Figure 4.6 Relative and cyclical model of empowerment

historians and radicalists alike. However, these models, theories and ruminations only have currency if they can be applied in practice. Applying empowerment is unfortunately as difficult, if not more so, than producing definitions. The endless stream of empowerment programmes and governmental initiatives are testament to this implementation struggle. Empowerment programmes must have the momentum to absorb repressive organisational barriers by addressing not only practicalities but also philosophical issues of power relations. The following section of this chapter explores the historical distribution of power between the provider and recipient of care. It is argued that only when this distribution is rectified to suit both parties will empowering practice become a reality.

An analysis of empowerment would be incomplete without reference to the notion of power and would prove unrepresentative of the concept (Gilbert, 1995; Kuokkanen and Leino-Kilpi, 2000). As Webb and Tossell (1995, cited in Jenkins, 1997) suggest, empowerment is inextricable from the concepts of power and control. Power dynamics have been a familiar feature in the analysis of health care delivery and central to these commentaries has been models of care. It is argued that the adoption of specific models of care discussed earlier in this chapter can have a significant impact on user/provider empowerment.

EMPOWERMENT PROGRAMMES

It was evident from the NHS Plan (Department of Health, 2000) that empowerment targets extended both to client and carer. It is apparent that both parties of the clinical partnership should be striving towards communal perceptions of empowerment. Empowerment programmes comprise two methods, namely carer and client training, plus the creation of community networks, involving the increase of team working. Subsequent to all parties perceiving empowerment, the ultimate aim is to channel these perceptions in a collective manner, in order to enhance the well-being of the client. Below you will find a review of programmes that endeavour to enhance carer and client perceptions of empowerment, harnessing community spirit and collective motivation.

The majority of this chapter has been dedicated to discussing empowerment in terms of empowering the client or patient. It is, however, necessary to emphasise the importance of empowering the professional and informal carer with a view to providing the optimum environment for client empowerment. Chavasse (1992) confirmed this view when she stated that the only solution to patient empowerment was to offer the same means of empowerment to staff.

If we assume that the NHS is an organisational entity with status boundaries, targets and consumers, addressing the structural characteristics (*see* Table 4.3) could improve levels of empowerment (Spreitzer, 1996). In essence, an individual's sense of psychological empowerment can only reach an optimum if their organisational environment is conducive for them to reach their potential. The characteristics describe the optimum conditions for enhancing staff empowerment, tackling oppressive hierarchy and system barriers.

The characteristics identified by Spreitzer (1996) for formal staff networks should be appreciated in the context of informal carers. For instance, May *et al.* (2001) explore how gatekeeping by professional bodies can hinder the development of successful and effective relations. There must be a concerted effort to

Table 4.3 Characteristics of organisational empowerment

Spreitzer's characteristic	Description	Example
Role ambiguity	To empower the health care professional clear boundaries between consumers and staff must be reinforced, which in turn would minimise what Spreitzer (1996) has termed role ambiguity.	Continuous staff appraisal and re-evaluation of responsibility
Span of control	Spreitzer regards span of control as a parameter determined by the number of workers a manager has direct control over. More workers reporting to one manager reduces that manager's span of control. Rodwell (1996) considered autonomy in decision making and resources to be an attribute that was consistent to perceptions of empowerment.	Distance contact such as e-mail with managers for tasks that do not necessitate direct managerial intervention
Socio-political support	Jenkins (1997) maintained that for a nurse to feel empowered there are four emotional attributes he or she must experience. If an individual perceives that their organisational network values them, and offers support, safety and security, these feelings will lead to empowerment. This appears parallel to socio-political support.	Seek staff appraisals of the working environment
Access to information	Knowledge is a necessary medium of power, providing the individual with the capacity to predict their role and their duty within the organisation. For instance, if the individual had knowledge of the goals and targets alongside the current standing of the organisation, he/she would be better equipped to understand to what degree their individual input would attain the specified goals.	Monthly departmental report disseminated to all levels of staff
Access to resources	Rather than the resources being managed by a distant managerial board, resources including budgets, materials and space should be allocated from a local network. If this is the case, individuals will have more influence over and proximity to these resources.	Local budget holders
Participative unit climate	Within a participative work climate the individual diversity is valued, as opposed to an organisation environment, which promotes stringent and uniform input, monitored closely by line monitors.	Professional development programmes

(From Spreitzer, 1996)

include each member of the therapeutic alliance. Consideration of the expertise of lay carers may be critical to the well-being of the client, as the carer may offer a fresh perspective on treatment and care plans. It is imperative that the carer feels valued and supported in order to avoid carer burden and subsequent burnout, due to lack of resource availability. The notion of partnerships in care is echoed in the alternative form of empowerment programmes.

Study Activity 4.4

- Review the six structural elements proposed by Spreitzer (listed in Table 4.3). Spreitzer argued that not taking the above elements into account within the organisational context could lead to staff disempowerment. For each element, provide an instance of how disregarding them could lead to disempowerment within your practice. For example, limited representative at staff meetings would militate against participative climate.
- Reflecting back on your examples, what practical resolution can you suggest to heighten levels of carer empowerment? Remember to place your suggestions in a sphere of reality! Only proposals that lead to implementation can have an influence on empowerment perceptions.
- Consider how you would implement your suggestions, tackling the following barriers to implementation:
  - Finance, time and human resource constraints
  - Organisational layout of your department. How would you ensure all levels of your department benefited from your programme?
  - Sceptics of empowerment programmes. Don't be fooled, as change in a system often provokes anxiety and at times challenges to both parties.

DEVELOPING AN EMPOWERED COMMUNITY

Many interventions aimed at enhancing perceptions of empowerment have focused on a community element, encompassing the collaborative working of all parties in the clinical relationship. Working as a community necessitates acknowledging each member of the community and his or her role in the therapeutic process.

Machin (1998) explored application of teamworking strategies within community health care groups. Due to the nature of community health care teams being largely multidisciplinary the philosophy of teamwork is an ethos that does not exist naturally. Machin (1998) states that because of this overlap role ambiguity occurs, which arguably is parallel to the barrier to empowerment featured in the model suggested by Spreitzer (1996).

Musker and Byrne (1997) state that individuals should not be categorised by their role as client, informal carer or professional carer. The working relationship between carers and client needs to be readdressed to account for the power equilibrium to take place and for each party in the clinical partnership to refute the traditional and paternal roles of needy and provider. This ideal environment and, according to Musker and Byrne (1997), a catalyst for empowerment, can be achieved when the community philosophy is in place, as such carers and clients perceive membership to a network that is striving towards shared goals.

Musker and Byrne (1997) adopt the view that a notion of community must encapsulate a network comprised of individuals who perceive a sense of belonging (*see* Fig 4.7). Hand in hand with the concept of community is the feeling of membership. Within the programme presented by Musker and Byrne (1997), the clients were given the opportunity to complete a questionnaire regarding their experience in the ward. The authors claim that this implementation elicits a sense of influence from the point of view of the client, over the service provision. However, one must question whether the clients perceived this introduction as empowering or indeed whether the staff working within the ward paid any more than lip service to the client comments.

Kar *et al.* (1999) emphasise how community

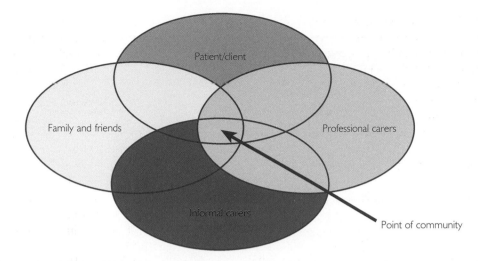

Figure 4.7 Necessary members of the empowered community

empowerment is a critical facet of any programme. Using a process analogy the authors present a stage programme with empowerment objectives and practical suggestions to attain these aims. Their stage programme acknowledges the essential step-by-step approach in order to encourage the optimum and nurturing environmental conditions to maintain any implementation (*see* Table 4.3 overleaf).

Study Activity 4.5

- Draft a proposed community web featuring all the members of a therapeutic alliance.
- Are there any barriers to your community web enhancing perceptions of empowerment at all levels? Reflect on the practicalities of your community web. How would these people communicate? Are the communication issues purely a matter of logistics?
- What kind of training would you offer your members so they could work as a community web more effectively?

BARRIERS TO EMPOWERMENT PROGRAMMES

In spite of the philosophy of empowering practice delivered in empowerment programmes

there are limitations concerning applicability and resource allocations. However, you will note that the primary barrier to empowerment programmes is overcoming the sceptics who continue to uphold traditional mindsets and perpetuate paternalistic care.

Anderson *et al.* (as cited in Snoek and Skinner, 2000) show that empowering practice can only be implemented if there is a revision of the traditional medical model of care. Essentially the authors advocate that a shift in thinking is required before empowering practice can become a reality. They state that there are two areas to target when initialising an empowerment programme, namely micro-empowerment, for instance the consultation, and macro-empowerment legislation (Morrall, 1996). The approach Anderson and colleagues discuss is parallel to the transformed medical approach that was introduced earlier. Essentially clients must be given the power to determine their programme of care and the health professional's role is that of a facilitator. With this objective in mind it is clear that the authors advocate the personalisation of consultation and health care that meets the client and carer needs. Lewis and Urmston (2000) and Edmonstone (2000), commenting on staff empowerment, reflect that quick fixes do not have a place in the struggle

Table 4.4 The empowerment process

Empowerment methods	Aim	Activities
Empowerment training and leadership development	Education of rights and opportunity, to develop leadership skills.	Conferences, symposium
Media use, support and advocacy	Influence the public	Press releases
Public education and participation	Promotion of public and leader awareness, support and action	Community advisory board
Organising partnership	To enhance negotiating power, self-reliance, resources and facilities within communities	Unions and coalitions
Work/job training and micro-enterprise	Promotion of economic self-reliance and employable skills.	Vocational training
Enabling service and assistance	Relief and critical services	Community out-reach
Rights protection and social action/reform	Protection	Delegation to governmental officials

(Adapted from Kar et al., 1999)

for empowerment. Bailey (1997) also advocates training to be on a multi-professional level and for implementation to adhere to a more systematic approach.

The second flaw of any empowerment programme is not addressing need but *assuming* need. McCann and Weinman (1996) demonstrate this in the study evaluating a programme aimed to empower clients during medical consultations. The authors primed the clients with a leaflet called 'Speak for Yourself' prior to their consultation. It was established that those who received this information leaflet had significantly longer consultations and directed more questions to the clinician. The authors point out several weaknesses, including the observed differences between client categories. It was noted that younger clients were more likely to assert their power within the consultation, compared to older clients. The authors attribute this finding to a generation hypothesis. It was argued that older clients were more satisfied with the traditional, more paternalistic relationship with their clinician due to their longer experience of this relationship. On the other hand the younger clients were more open to challenge this status quo and redirect the power.

McCann and Weiman (1996) accentuate the fact that the fundamental element in the success of any empowerment programme concerns the individual's desire to challenge oppression. Essentially the pursuit of empowerment will only be initiated if the individual perceives a need for change. Kar *et al.* (1999) state that the empowerment process will not commence until the first threshold of motivation and initiation has been satisfied, taking into account the individual's perceived need. Arguably, if the individual's point of view is not considered the spirit of empowerment is dulled along with the essence of active participation.

As discussed earlier in this chapter the recurring issue of defining empowerment has been a significant obstacle. This lack of clarity appears to have transferred into the realm of empowerment programme development. Indeed, if there are contentions in defining an entity this would present difficulties in acquiring an unknown state. Many programmes fail to offer clear guidelines for implementation, merely presenting descriptive analogies of empowering practice leaving the reader with the task to embellish on a means of introducing empowerment. This in turn creates a hindrance in terms of evaluation, leaving researchers unable to decipher whether empowerment has been achieved.

SUMMARY

This has been a long journey, but charting the history of empowerment is imperative to understanding the contemporary use of the concept. Significant moves have been made by the health service to break away from the dependent role the client plays, drawing in the informal carer into the partnership and encouraging the professional to act as a guide. This process necessitates the expert contributions of all members and harnessing the empowerment philosophy is the mechanism for productive and effective caring communities. The time is right to reflect on the concept and what it means for individuals of the therapeutic relationship. Health care has an opportunity to contribute to the empowerment family tree. For our contribution to be constructive we must not only understand the essence of empowerment but also the practicalities. As health professionals you need to ask several questions:

- What are the barriers to empowering practice?
- What is my role in this process?
- What level of care is most empowering for this client at this particular time?

The development of a caring community is not an overnight phenomenon but an initiative that requires nurturing and evaluating. This continuous evaluation is the way forward. Indeed the information here is only correct at this point in time. Empowerment is something that should be viewed in a context. This chapter was written as the first building block in a long line of re-evaluation. Today's empowerment may be tomorrow's disempowerment.

REFERENCES

Bailey, D. (1997) What is the way forward for a user-led approach to the delivery of mental health services in primary care? *Journal of Mental Health* 6(1), 101–5

Chavasse, J.M. (1992) New dimensions of empowerment in nursing – and challenges. *Journal of Advanced Nursing* 17(1), 1–2

Department of Health (1990) *The National Health Service and Community Care Act*, DoH, London

Department of Health (2000) *The NHS Plan: A plan for investment, a plan for reform*, DoH, London

Durkheim, E. ([1897] 1970) *Suicide: A study in sociology*, reissued Routledge and Kegan Paul, London

Edmonstone, J. (2000) Empowerment in the National Health Service: does shared governance offer a way forward? *Journal of Nursing Management* 8, 259–64

Eysenbach, G. (2000) Consumer health informatics. *British Medical Journal*, 320(7251), 1713–16

Freud, S. (1930) *Civilization and its Discontents* (in Standard Edition), vol. 21, 57–145

Gilbert, T. (1995) Nursing empowerment and the problem of power. *Journal of Advanced Nursing* 21(5), 865–71

Holland, S. (1992) From social abuse to social action: a neighbourhood psychotherapy and social action project for women. In: Ussher, J.M. and Nicolson, P. (eds) *Gender Issues in Clinical Psychology*, Routledge, London

Ivey, A.E. (1995) Psychotherapy as liberation: toward specific skills and strategies in multicultural counseling and therapy. In: Ponterotto, J.G., Casas, J.M., Suzuki, L.A. *et al.* (eds) (1995) *Handbook of Multicultural Counselling*, Sage, London

Jenkins, R. (1997) Issues of empowerment for nurses and clients. *Nursing Standard* 11(46), 44–6

Kar, S.B., Pascual, C. and Chickering, K. (1999) Empowerment of women for health promotion: a meta-analysis, *Social Science and Medicine* 49(11), 1431–60

Kuokkanen, L. and Leino-Kilpi, H. (2000) Power and empowerment in nursing: three theoretical approaches. *Journal of Advanced Nursing* 31(1), 235–41

Lamont, S.S. (1999) Patient participation cannot guarantee empowerment. *British Medical Journal* 319(7212), 783

Lewis, M. and Urmston, J. (2000) Flogging the dead horse: the myth of nursing empowerment. *Journal of Nursing Management* 8(4), 209–13

McCann, S. and Weinman, J. (1996) Empowering the patient in the consultation: a pilot study. *Patient Education and Counselling* 27(3), 227–34

Machin, T. (1998) Teamwork in community mental health care. *British Journal of Community Nursing* 3(1), 17–24

Martin-Crawford, L. (1999) Empowerment in healthcare. *Participation and Empowerment: An international journal* 7(1)

Mason, D.J., Backer, B.A. and Georges, C.A. (1991) Towards a feminist model for the political empowerment of nurses. *Journal of Nursing Scholarship* 23(2), 72–7

May, J., Ellis-Hill, C. and Payne, S. (2001) Gatekeeping and legitimization: how informal carer's relationship with health care workers is revealed in their everyday interactions. *Journal of Advanced Nursing* 36(3), 364–75

Menon, S.T. (2001) Employee empowerment: an integrative psychological approach, *Applied Psychology: An international review* 50(1), 153–80

Menon, S. (2002) Toward a model of psychological health empowerment: implications for healthcare in multicultural communities. *Nurse Education Today* 22(1), 28–39

Morrall, P. (1996) Clinical sociology and empowerment of clients. *Mental Health Nursing* 16(3), 24–7

Musker, M. and Byrne, M. (1997) Applying empowerment in mental health practice. *Nursing Standard* 11(31), 45–7

Newton, J. (1995) Dentist/patient communication: a review. *Dental Update* 22, 118–22

Ong, L., de Haes, J.C., Hoos, A. *et al.* (1995) Doctor–patient communication: a review of the literature. *Social Science and Medicine* 40(7), 903–18

Radcliffe-Brown, A.R. (1952) *Structure and Function in Primitive Society: Essays and addresses,* Cohen and West, London

Rafael, A. (1998) Nurses who run with the wolves: the power and caring dialectic revisited. *Advances in Nursing Science* 21(1), 29–42

Rodwell, C.M. (1996) An analysis of the concept of empowerment. *Journal of Advanced Nursing* 23(2), 305–13

Rogers, S., Chamberlin, J., Langer Ellison, M. *et al.* (1997) A consumer-constructed scale to measure empowerment among users of mental health services. *Psychiatric Services* 48(8), 1042–7

Sagie, A. and Koslowski, M. (2000) *Participation and Empowerment in Organisations: Modelling, effectiveness, and application,* Sage, London

Shepperd, S., Charnock, D. and Gann, B. (1999) Helping the patient access high quality health information. *British Medical Journal* 319, 764–6

Snoek, F.J. and Skinner, T.C. (2000) *Psychology in Diabetes Care,* John Wiley, London

Spreitzer, G.M. (1996) Social structural characteristics of psychological empowerment, *Academy of Management Journal* 39(2), 483–504

Timmons (2001) Use of the Internet by patients: not a threat to nursing, but an opportunity? *Nurse Education Today,* 21(2), 104–9

Wiles, R. and Higgins, J. (1996) Doctor/patient relationships in the private sector: patient's perceptions. *Sociology of Health and Illness* 18(3), 341–56

Wowra, S. and McCarter, R. (1999) Validation of the empowerment scale with an outpatient mental health population. *Psychiatric Services* 50(7), 959–96

MODULE 1: FOCUS ON CARE

REFLECTIONS

Throughout Module 1 you have been asked to undertake Study Activities requiring you to reflect in and on your practice to assist in either advancing your knowledge or in enabling you to relate the theory to the practicum setting. It is therefore useful now for you to reflect on the main tenets of the module to assess the level of knowledge and understanding you have gained.

The first chapter, 'Precedents', mapped the historical journey of care from the point of antiquity to a modern-day perspective and a glimpse into the future. While the evolution and frameworks of care have changed throughout historical periods, and the philosophical frameworks have been represented and interpreted differently within different cultures and time frames, at its very heart, 'care' is a phenomenon that has enjoyed universal understanding and application within human interactions throughout all historical periods.

Chapter 1 was followed by a 'Commitment to care', which explored the philosophical concepts that underpin the notion of care, recognising that in providing care, it awakens a social conscience and a collective responsibility. Other chapters augmented the latter statement by exploring the notion of self-care and altruistic care within informal and formal care settings.

Gaining an understanding of these caring issues and philosophical underpinnings enabled a further exploration of care within professional and organised frameworks, culminating in the final chapter that explored the notion of empowerment. Empowered care is a relatively new phenomenon and is a term that is often used in everyday professional language, and yet, it is a complex term that does not yet have a universal understanding or application. In this chapter we discussed the elements and diverse understanding of the word, culminating in a final analysis that empowerment is both a 'process and a product'.

It is important that you have understood the journey and evolution of care and enriched your learning and understanding from the chapter via further reading and reflections in and on your practice. It would be wise for you to reflect in your portfolio: what you have learned; how the caring philosophy is crucial for the individual nurse to adopt; and how the collective world of nursing uses the concept as a political voice and a quintessential ingredient of the code of professional conduct.

Your journey in your chosen caring profession will enrich your knowledge, skill and understanding, but they will have been strengthened through reading this chapter and internalising a caring principal throughout all aspects of your nursing actions.

MODULE 2: THE PROFESSIONAL DISCIPLINE OF NURSING

INTRODUCTION

The discourse and debates raised in Module 2 concentrate on the professional discipline of nursing, commencing with the notion of professionalisation. Professionalisation commences with a description that explores the notion and characteristics of a profession: What does membership of a profession involve? What is meant by professional responsibility? And what is the process of professionalisation? This is followed by the philosophical paradigms of nursing as a profession and what this means in practice. The practice of nursing within professional frameworks that embrace clinical supervision and leadership and expand the scope of practice through lifelong learning is explored.

Clinical supervision and leadership, continuing professional development and the skills of lifelong learning are necessary to ensure that all nursing practice is conducted from evidence of best practice in providing high-quality nursing care. It is for this very reason that we explore these domains in the context of nursing as a professional discipline.

Module 2 builds on Module 1 through the exploration of nursing as a professional entity and the requirements this calls for in practice. Knowledge and understanding gained within this module will empower you to take responsibility for your own learning, now and throughout your professional career.

5

PROFESSIONALISATION

Lynn Basford

LEARNING OUTCOMES

After studying this chapter you will be able to:

- Discuss the characteristics that underpin a profession
- Understand the sociological concepts that inform professional behaviour
- Reflect on nursing as a professional entity
- Understand professional responsibility and accountability
- Critically review new paradigms for future professional practice that engage partnership working with and between professional groups, users and carers.

INTRODUCTION

Being a profession, becoming a profession and having autonomous professional responsibility are issues that have been hotly debated within and outside nursing. It is therefore necessary for the novice nurse to understand:

- what constitues a profession
- what membership of a profession involves
- what is meant by professional responsibility
- the process of professionalisation.

Study Activity 5.1

Write down what you believe is meant by a 'professional person'. Compare your views with a colleague and, after reading this chapter, review your notes.

WHAT IS A PROFESSION?

Dictionary definitions of a profession provide some clarity, but they do not fully explain the fine nuances that are used in practice. To illustrate this point the *Little Oxford Dictionary* (1992) states it is 'an occupation, especially in the branch of advance learning or science' or, as the *Webster's Dictionary* (1980) points out, it is viewed as 'a calling requiring specialist knowledge and often long intensive academic preparation'. Neither of these explanations provides us with a universal explanation of the term or the relationship and need for standard setting and regulation. This has left opportunities for others to enlarge on the definitions and characteristics of being a profession to best enable others to understand the concept as a working framework.

In recent times lists of professional characteristics have been compiled that are generally framed around being in possession of a body of knowledge that draws on the evidence of practice and empirical research findings. This knowledge is gained through education and training that is conducted around the context of systematic principles and stated outcomes and regulated through a statutory body. In addition, there is a requirement that an altruistic attitude to service is of paramount importance, reducing the ability of professional people to abuse or misuse their 'professional power'. In 1978, Blanchfield compiled such a list, which can be seen in Table 5.1 overleaf.

While this list of characteristics is not exhaustive it demonstrates that being a profession does not exist within a static framework and should continue to evolve. This view is supported by Vollmer and Mills (1966) in their seminal text, *Professionalisation*, which states that professions should reflect the dynamic and evolutionary nature that occupations must possess if they are to achieve professional status. Vollmer and Mills also make the point that the term 'profession' is an ideal that occupations can emulate, moving from a position of non-professional to professional along an abstract continuum. As each professional criterion is achieved, then the occupation can locate its position along the abstract continuum. Full professional status is only achieved when all criteria are fulfilled (*see* Figure 5.1).

Table 5.1 The characteristics of a profession

- Its practice is based on a recognised body of learning.
- It establishes an independent body for the collective pursuit of aims and objectives related to these criteria.
- Admission to corporate membership is based on strict standards of competence attested by examination and assessed experience.
- It recognises that its practice must be for the benefit of the public, as well as that of the practitioners.
- It recognises its responsibility to advance and extend the body of learning on which it is based.
- It recognises its responsibility to concern itself with facilities, methods and provision for educating and training future entrants and for enhancing the knowledge of present practitioners.
- It recognises the need for members to conform to high standards of ethics and professional conduct set out in a published code with appropriate disciplinary procedures.

(From Blanchfield, 1978)

If the term professional is truly dynamic, evolving constantly in a sea of changing paradigms, the following question must be raised:

- Can any occupation be said to achieve full professional status and, if it does, can it be maintained?

Non-professional   Ideal

1 2 3 4 5 6 7 8 9 10 11 12
Criteria

Figure 5.1 Diagrammatical representation of an abstract continuum of a non-professional state to an ideal

This is a particular conundrum within the nursing profession that has never been successfully resolved.

Study Activity 5.2

- As a group, identify the professional characteristics can be associated with nursing.
- Where do you think nursing lies on the abstract continuum?
- Where do you think the profession of medicine lies on the abstract continuum?

NURSING KNOWLEDGE: A PROFESSIONAL CLAIM

For too long those in nursing have 'navel-gazed' in pursuit of recognition as a professional entity. During the late nineteenth century political struggles achieved the creation of a register of qualified nurses and, in the late twentieth century, full student status to new entrants and the creation of a body of knowledge that came out of practice and research. Underpinning all of this was nursing's quest to gain power and control of its own activities in order to shape the profession's direction in education, practice development and research resulting in the legitimate and unique body of knowledge that was nursing. In a sense, the search for nursing's unique body of knowledge remains unsubstantiated, despite universal acclaim given to the seemingly eclectic nature of knowledge that underpins nursing practice.

This eclectic nature of nursing knowledge draws on many scientific disciplines, such as life sciences, social science, psychology, philosophy, pharmacology and anthropology. From a purist position this eclecticism denies opportunities for nursing to meet the professional criteria. However, Pyne (1991) makes the point that although nursing knowledge may be eclectic, it is applied in the specific sphere of nursing practice and its uniqueness is claimed from this position. In addition, it is this application of knowledge upon which nurses are assessed to demonstrate their competence to practise. Given that the eclectic approach supports a claim to professionalism, not all nurse theorists support this concept. For example, Rogers (1970) claims that nursing has a systematic body of nursing theory, which is, to all intents and purposes, the science of nursing. All knowledge, according to Rogers, is in the abstract, formulated out of scientific research and logical analysis, which can be applied in a specific way to nursing practice. She goes on to suggest that nursing science is newly acquired, but has not arisen out of a vacuum, nor is the body of knowledge related only to nursing. While other nurse theorists concur with Rogers's sentiments, they assert that a profession is required not only to have a systematic body of knowledge but also a dynamic evolution. That is to say, the development and growth of the body of knowledge must evolve from the profession's own members through critical reflection and research into the validity of its abstract propositions (Buckenham and McGrath, 1981).

The growth of nursing evidence using a framework of critical reflection in and on practice is demonstrated within nursing and other related scientific literature. Evidence is drawn from research methodologies that engage in qualitative and/or quantitative research methods giving credence to the findings enabling nursing practice to be advanced and enhanced within the context of new paradigms or the identification of new ways of working. Further to which, the encouragement of nurses through professional re-registration frameworks and educational processes to be reflective practitioners is tantamount to this continued cyclical notion of practice informing the research question and research findings informing practice. Figure 5.2 illustrates these dynamic processes that provide a framework through which nursing can claim to be a profession.

PROFESSIONAL REGULATION

Nursing has not always had a regulatory body, as Emerton (1992) has pointed out. Throughout the modern period, nurse leaders and activists have consistently lobbied to establish a profession that was viewed separately from medicine. This goal was achieved in 1979 when Parliament endorsed the Nurses, Midwives and Health Visitors Act, which empowered nursing to govern itself. From this emerged the UK Central Council (UKCC) for Nurses, Midwives and Health Visitors and four National Boards for nursing, midwifery and health visiting (one for each of the four UK countries). In April 2002 the UKCC and National Boards disbanded, with a new Nursing and Midwifery Council emerging in line with the Labour Government's directives for all health care professionals.

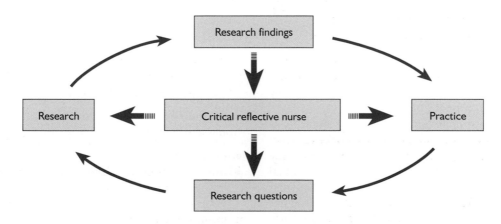

Figure 5.2 The dynamic processes of research informing practice

The purpose of gaining nursing's own regulatory body was a major landmark for the professionalisation of nursing. It was such a significant achievement that Reginald Pyne, Assistant Registrar of the UKCC, reminded the profession that:

> ... one of the hallmarks of a profession is that it accepts the onerous burden of regulating itself, but recognises that this is to be performed for the protection of the public and not for the prestige of its members. Such an arrangement exists for nursing, midwifery and health visiting in the United Kingdom. It is something precious which the members of the profession must safeguard.
>
> (Pyne, 1991, pp. 6–7)

The notion of regulation is made 'onerous' by the reality that it is in fact self-regulation and requires the profession to take responsibility and accountability in protecting the public. This does not mean, however, that a profession is totally autonomous and therefore totally self-regulating. A profession and its individual members are, as in the case of any other citizens, subject to the laws of the land:

- *Criminal law* – when an offence is committed against the state (e.g. as defined by the Criminal Law Act 1977). Thus, while nurses may be subject to professional regulatory sanctions if they deliberately injure a patient, they may also be tried in the criminal courts.
- *Employment law* – within employment law and the industrial relations regulations based upon it, employers may take action against a professional employee who in any way engages in misconduct.
- *Civil law* – civil law involves the obligations and rights individuals have towards each other. Under civil law an individual may sue others for compensation if that individual feels their rights have been infringed and that personal damage has occurred. Of particular relevance here is the law of tort (in England, Wales and Northern Ireland) or law of delict

(in Scotland). This is the law whereby if injury is caused through negligence or carelessness, the injured party can claim damages (usually in terms of financial compensation). Thus, while a nurse who injures a patient through negligence will be subject to professional regulatory sanctions, the injured party or their relatives may bring a civil suit against the nurse under the law of tort.

- *Public law* – this law regulates the relations between individuals and public bodies. A wide range of laws comes under this heading. However, those most relevant to nursing include administrative law, dealing with the power of government ministries and departments, and welfare law, concerning the operation of the welfare state. Public law comprises the types of laws that establish the social security system and the NHS in the UK. As most nurses are employed within the NHS they are required to abide by the wide range of legislation under the primary legislation, the National Health Service and Community Care Act 1990 (Department of Health, 1990), through to legislation and regulation concerning specific issues such as misuse of drugs, child abuse and mental health.

Clearly, nurses are subject to the internal regulatory mechanisms of their profession and also external regulatory mechanisms, which are mainly encompassed within the laws of the land. In the US it is not uncommon for patients, clients and others to take out civil actions against their nurses and this is already starting to occur in the UK. There is thus a dual onus on nurses to ensure that they adhere to high professional standards that are imposed by the profession and by the legal system in general. Nurses must therefore accept that in all their professional activities they must be aware of:

- public law
- nursing, midwifery and health visiting legislation (which in essence comes under public law)
- criminal law
- civil law, particularly the law of torts.

MAINTAINING PROFESSIONAL STANDARDS

Each professional nurse, midwife or health visitor must adhere to the legal requirements of maintaining professional registration through meeting the post-registration education and practice (PREP) standards laid down by the regulatory body, the Nursing and Midwifery Council.

These PREP standards are to protect the public and ensure that those nurses, midwives and health visitors who are registered with the Professional Council have demonstrated their competence to give care that meets professional requirements and standards in the context of health care that continues to change.

There are two PREP standards that are required to be achieved for the maintenance of registration:

PREP Continuing Professional Development (CPD)

In meeting this standard the nurse, midwife or health visitor must:

- undertake at least five days (35 hours) of learning activity relevant to their practice during the years prior to renewal of registration
- maintain a personal portfolio of this learning activity
- comply with any request from the Nursing and Midwifery Council to audit compliance with these requirements.

Registrants can choose in what manner or mode CPD is undertaken but it is essential that 'registrants must document their professional portfolio the ways in which their learning informs practice' (UKCC, 2000).

The PREP (Practice) Standard

- Nurses and health visitors need to have completed a minimum of 100 days (750 hours) of practice during the five years prior to their renewal of registration, irrespective of the number of their registrable nursing qualifications.

- From April 2001, practising midwives need to have completed a minimum of 100 days (750 hours) of practice during the five years prior to their renewal of registration.

Nurses, midwives or health visitors who fail to meet these standards must undertake a return to practice programme (UKCC, 2000).

Study Activity 5.3

Go to your library or search out on the Internet cases that pertain to public, civil and criminal law within the context of health care.

- How do these cases affect nursing practice and regulate practice?
- Write this information up in your portfolio for future reference.

SOCIOLOGICAL DISCOURSE

Medicine is one of the oldest professions that is theoretically recognised by all as fulfilling characteristics that give credence to being a professional body. Over time, the medical profession has developed a body of knowledge, which has enabled it to increase its power and authority within the context of health and illness at the expense of social models of health and lay perspectives (Friedson, 2001). Friedson argues that this process has existed between the perspectives of the doctor and client through which the doctor has successfully undermined the lay view of health and illness within the context of a technical and scientific model of disease. Further to which, the success of the medicalisation of health and illness is because of the ability of the medical profession to conduct its own affairs free from outside or lay interference, or from challenges from other occupational health groups.

Throughout the twentieth century the power of the medical profession has been enhanced by an increase in autonomy of practice, which has been sanctioned by the state. From this position the medical practitioner has been able to redefine and re-engineer the lay person's view within the context of scientific knowledge and therefore the process is socially constructed. It is a product of the 'doctor–patient relationship rather than a feature of the patient's organic state' (Friedson, 2001, p.129). In addition to this phenomenon, the medical profession has classified deviant behaviour, such as drunkenness, as 'alcoholism' and the patient an alcoholic. It is therefore suggested that the reinterpretation or labelling of deviant behaviour as illness reinforces the 'professionalised control institution' in which such illness is bad and the doctor becomes a moral custodian of social behaviour (Illich, 1976).

The medical profession's ability to put forward its views as absolutes has relied upon the acknowledgement and recognition from the public that 'doctor knows best'. Inadvertently, such attitudes and beliefs have created a dependency culture in which members of the culture are totally reliant on the doctor for all health and illness care and this is now deemed to be a unhealthy relationship.

The web of power and authority for medical practitioners has not stayed within the constructs of illness and deviant behaviours, but has encroached on new procedures or practice innovations that have been developed. For example, the medical profession have assumed a presence and authority as in the case of screening and surveillance services (Davies, 1998).

The medicalisation of all aspects of health and illness has not advanced individual or community health per se; indeed, Illich (1976) condemned medicalisation as a danger to health rather than a panacea. He went on to declare that medicine had created new health problems where none existed before and created a culture and society that were entirely dependent upon medical expertise to find solutions to all our health and illness problems. Illich labelled this 'iatrogenesis'. Throughout the intervening years, support has backed Illich's ruminations, clearly illustrating the dangers of the professionalisation of health under the auspices and guidance of the

'expert'. Governments have reinforced such expertise by calling on these 'experts' to direct policy and decision-making. Therefore the medical profession needed to determine or carve out its field of expertise, which was reaffirmed by government actions. In establishing this cycle the medical profession established a power base from which other professions within the health field would be directed. This, of course, included nursing.

In the pursuit of professionalisation nursing has tried to emulate the development of a body of expertise through which nurses can advise governments and play a major role in the direction of health care and the future of the nursing profession.

PROFESSIONALISATION AND GOVERNMENTALITY

The French philosopher Foucault (1979) has provided insights into the notion of professionalisation and 'governmentality'. He argues that the state and the profession are distinct entities; the profession having the complete independence and autonomy that denies state intervention. Professionals are experts who have undertaken a period of intense training within a particular occupational domain, fielding off any competition through legal claims and disputes. The inter-relationship and interdependence between professional power (because of their expertise), and the needs of governments to use this expert knowledge has been significant within the politics and directions of the NHS. Abbott (1988) suggests that because governments rely upon experts, they are continuously engaged in making claims and counter-claims to assert their expert knowledge in areas or fields of practice that have no recognised expert knowledge. It is the very same concern that Foucault (1979) has expressed in relationship to the enabling and empowerment of governments through the use of experts. For example, the medical profession, instead of avoiding politics in the name of neutrality, seeks to maintain a position of power and influence within the context of government politics and, as such, actively and competitively gets involved with government politics at every conceivable level. This enables the profession to assert its power and control over other professional groups in a cyclical nature. Government, by contrast, is a conduit for professional claims and an external agent contained within the framework of legislature, the courts, and the organisation frameworks through which professional practice will operate (Abbott, 1988).

The traditional dynamic relationship between government and the professions was slowly deconstructed in the Thatcher years through increased internal conflict and reliance upon market forces and has continued with growing scepticism over the succeeding decades (Dennis, 1972). While it is recognised that governments will call upon expert professional opinion the full impact of their influence depends on the season and governmental steer.

OLD PARADIGMS OF PROFESSIONALISM

Earlier in this chapter attention was given to the characteristics of a professional body and the medical profession has been cited as a successful professional group with power to shape and develop the direction of its related activities. Such exclusivity can be viewed as contradictory to contemporary practice that embraces team working, interprofessional practice and partnership working with others, especially the users and carers. It is a new philosophical approach that is endorsed by the government's National Health Service Ten-year Plan (Department of Health, 2000). The aim of this plan is to improve client care and make the NHS a more efficient service that is sensitive to users' needs and demands. In the broadest sense it sets an agenda to transform the NHS as a 'caring organisation' that has a commitment to ensure high standards of care for all. Thinking this through critically, the professionalisation of nursing could be argued to be perhaps the antithesis of such goals and ideals, given that professionalism centres on a masculine framework (Davies,

1998). However, the social model of caring that permeates the essence of nursing has the potential to nurture and support the government's agenda, while facilitating the growth of nursing as a profession.

Davies continues to suggest that new models for professionalism are required so as to better understand the modern world of health care and the professional groups that work within it. While accepting the sentiment expressed by Davies, some advise caution, given that nursing has already gained the status of a professional body. They suggest a period of debate and reflection, which will inform the new direction to ensure a marrying with the principles of the old world and the philosophies of the new. Considering the emergence of the new paradigms, Salvage (1985, pp. 95–101) has challenged the nursing profession to consider the following statements:

- *Professionalism is diverse* – the provision of nursing care is supplied by a wide group of people, many of whom are not nurses and have had no professional training. This inherent lack of training lessens the quality of care given, as does the maintenance of knowledge within the realms of an élite group.
- *Professionalism seeks to impose a uniform view* – there is undoubtedly a common goal of providing high quality care but some interests differ, as do those of individual patients and their families.
- *Professionalism denies the needs of its workers* – the needs of patients always take priority over the needs of nurses. Nurses do not take strike action to assert their needs.
- *Professionalism emphasises an individual approach* – there is an individualistic accountability and responsibility in the delivery of care, but in the absence of resources, human and physical, can individual nurses truly be called to account? Furthermore, can an individual nurse really be accountable to seek out the evidence of best practice from a wide range of sources?

- *Professionalism does not challenge the status quo* – is autonomy for the nurse necessarily better for the patient? Or, should all formal caregivers be given the opportunity for basic training?
- *Professionalism does not give strong support to the NHS* – a sweeping statement, which suggests that professionalism is about maintaining the needs of the professional group rather than the needs of the health care system as a whole.

Nurses, government officials and the public frequently express these concerns suggesting that professional élitism, power and autonomy negate the needs of the health service and its users. Where once the public gave resounding and unquestioning support to health professionals, frequent service failure and professional misconduct have seriously dented public opinion. More recently, the professions have been challenged openly for interventions they have used and the lack of evidence upon which they have practised. The government has called for changes that seriously call the professions to account publicly for their actions and to work within a framework of clinical governance. In recognising this fact, it seems foolhardy for those in nursing to continue to pursue professional recognition when that status carries so much historical baggage. Instead the stage is set for nursing to debate new professional frameworks that would best fit the new world order and enable nursing to claim its rightful position as a new profession model within the realms of caring and health.

NEW PARADIGMS OF PROFESSIONALISM

Margaret Stacey (1992) was an early proponent for change from old, outdated nineteenth-century custom and practice that was encased within the notion of 'professionalism'. Citing the activities of the General Medical Council (GMC), the interests of doctors were always paramount before the interests of the public or the state.

Stacey believed the cloak of professionalism had enabled doctors to practise without sound evidence in a defensive and restrictive manner, and with an air of professional arrogance. Such behaviour does not enable, nor empower, other professionals, users or their carers to contribute to clinical decision making at either the individual or community level. New political directions, such as the need for shared clinical governance, mean doctors must seek out and move away from traditional practice and find ways in which competence and qualification to practise can be assured in an open forum. They need to engage with skills for team and partnership working (Department of Health, 2000).

This new kind of professionalism places the interests of consumers first, or at least equal, to professional interest. This means embracing conceptual frameworks that move away from traditional medicine, accepting the knowledge base of others including lay frameworks. Indeed, the 1997 Public Health Agenda called for increasing levels of patient and lay practice, participation in health planning and decision making (Department of Health, 1997).

Stacey (1992) went on to predict a change from uni-disciplinary regulatory bodies to bodies that encapsulated the interests, needs and regulations of all health care workers. Such new models were set to emerge in April 2002 and over time will direct a change that engages new professionalism. Perhaps this new model of professionalism will be democratic, creating a kind of partnership that is empowering within the context of partnership working at the point of service delivery (Hugman, 1991). Jan Williams (1993), supporting the need for change, made the following suggestions:

> *Instead of a one-way transmission of knowledge from professional to client, there is a two-way transaction, building on existing knowledge and experience of the client, according to the client's perceived needs and the professional's response to these ... No longer is the professional*

seeking to impose her view ... Her role has changed from one of controlling to one of supporting and enabling, helping the client to draw on and think through his own experiences, and sharing her expert knowledge to help him develop understanding.

(Williams, 1993, pp. 11–12)

THE COMMISSION FOR HEALTH IMPROVEMENT AND CLINICAL GOVERNANCE

Commission for Health Improvement

In keeping with the spirit of partnership care and professional care giving, the Labour Government has provided a legal framework whereby professional groups, individuals and health care organisations will be accountable to the Commission for Health Improvement (CHI). This legal framework is contained within the 1999 Health Act and its associated regulations.

The main impetus for such a legal framework was the government's clear intention to improve the quality of care in the NHS across England and Wales. Numerous service failures, lack of professional competence and old models of organisational practices have contributed to this enforcement of governmental scrutiny and will be part of a continuous process of external review.

CHI commenced operation on 1 April 2000 and has a clearly identified rolling four-year programme, which aims to ensure every patient and client receives the same standard of care from competent professionals. CHI seeks to assure, monitor and improve the quality of patient care by undertaking clinical governance reviews. In addition, CHI is charged with the responsibility of investigating serious service failures, responding rapidly to minister's requests. CHI will base its findings on evidence and not subjective opinion.

There are six principles that will formulate the basis of the work that will be carried out by CHI:

1 *The patient's experience is at the heart of CHI's work.*
2 *CHI will be independent, rigorous and fair.*
3 *CHI's approach is developmental and will support the NHS to continuously improve.*
4 *CHI's work will be based on the best available evidence and focus on improvement.*
5 *CHI will be open and accessible.*
6 *CHI will apply the same standards of continuous improvement to itself that it expects of others.*

Clinical governance

At the heart of the investigation CHI's official investigators will examine every aspect of clinical governance. The question therefore to be asked is, 'What is clinical governance?' According to the government's White Paper 'A First Class Service' clinical governance is:

... a framework through which NHS organisations are accountable for continuously improving the quality of their services and safeguarding high standards of care by creating an environment in which excellence in clinical care will flourish.

(Department of Health, 1998, p. 1)

The examination of clinical governance activities covers the organisations, systems and processes for monitoring and improving services, as identified by the Department of Health (2001, p.1) and are replicated as follows:

- Consultation and patient involvement
- Clinical risk management
- Clinical audit
- Research and effectiveness
- Staffing and staff management
- Education, training and continuing personal and professional development
- The use of information about the patients' experiences, outcomes and processes.

The efficacy and effectiveness of clinical governance should therefore embrace:

- evidence of continuous improvement of patient services and care
- a patient-centred approach that includes treating patients courteously, involving them in decisions about their care and keeping them informed
- a commitment to quality, which ensures that health professionals are up to date in their practices and properly supervised where necessary
- the prevention of clinical errors wherever possible and the commitment to learn from mistakes and share that learning with others.

It is clear that the direction of government is to improve the quality of service for all patients irrespective of where they live. Health professionals who once enjoyed independent scrutiny within their own specific discipline must now be prepared to undergo external scrutiny by the agents of the CHI office. While there remains an individual need to undertake continuous professional development, there is also a collective responsibility engaging other health care workers and organisational managers. The new world order is definitely focused on partnership working, within the context of changing roles and responsibilities.

Study Activity 5.4

Use the Internet to examine the political directives and policy statements that support the agenda of clinical governance. Discuss with your colleagues the implications of this for nursing practice.

NEW NURSING ROLES AND RESPONSIBILITIES

Throughout the history and evolution of nursing the roles and responsibilities of nurses have continued to change in response to changes in practice, organisational structures, new services,

political directives, efficiency and economic gains and technological advancements. This position is no different to any of the other health care professions, including medicine. Nonetheless, these changes have more recently had a profound effect on increasing the independence of nursing in relation to some aspects of its role, which correlates more clearly with being a profession.

Through the 1960s to the 1980s nurse leaders strongly expressed the view that nursing should be fully recognised as a profession in its own right and not as an adjunct to the medical profession. They espoused the autonomous role of primary nursing and clinical development opportunities such as the widely acclaimed Oxford and Burford Clinical Development Units that were nurse led. Alan Pearson (1983, p. 5), speaking of the clinical development unit, said it was an important milestone in removing the 'shackles of bureaucracy and management' that have impeded the progress of nursing, and now enables and empowers nurses to develop a genuine, autonomous professional practice.

In the late 1990s and to the present day we have seen the emergence of independent nurse prescribers, nurse-led units employing doctors and other health care professionals, walk-in centres, NHS Direct, nurse triage and consultant nurses. While nurses can rejoice in these achievements and bask in the knowledge that nursing is a profession, there are critics of this position. Salvage (1985), for instance, asked the question whether nursing should be a profession at all, and, if so, what were the implications of this and what would it achieve? Certainly these are challenging and thought-provoking questions that serve to engage nurses in thinking through the issues and consequences of being a professional entity. Waerness (1992) similarly expressed concerns based on the premise of nursing's pivotal role in 'care giving'. Care giving, according to Waerness, has strong relationships between femininity and women's work, which contribute positively to health and healing that is somehow lost in the quest for professionalisation. From this view, nursing may celebrate being a professional entity, but does this serve the needs of society or the interests of the professional membership?

Study Activity 5.5

- Having read this chapter, do you now consider nursing to be a profession? Record your reasons for your answer in your reflective portfolio.
- Do old models of professionalisation fit easily with the government's agendas?

SUMMARY

The concept of a profession has been defined by a set of criteria and characteristics against which occupations can measure. For some theorists it is a dynamic state that can only be aspired to within an evolutionary process of change.

Some of these characteristics embrace the notion of autonomy and responsibility that is governed by a self-regulating body, as well as conforming to public law, civil law and employment law. A systematic body of knowledge underpins professional practice and members of the profession advance this knowledge through empirical research and clinical practice. Each professional person will use the skills of reflective practice, which will identify research questions to better inform practice.

Nursing has striven to gain professional recognition but has been working to old models of professionalism, when recently the government and the public have seriously questioned these characteristics and its associated use of power and influence. Moves have been made to change the notion of professionalism and nursing should engage with the new orders for professional practice and wherever possible influence the direction. Ultimately, the new professionalism should operate within partnerships that are about serving the public interest, instead of serving only the interest of the professional group as can be evidenced in the clinical govern-

ance agendas that will be examined in detail by the Commission for Health Improvement.

REFERENCES

Abbott, A. (1988) *The System of Professions: An essay on the division of expert labour*, University of Chicago Press, Chicago, IL

Blanchfield, R. (1978) In: Pyne, R.H. (1991) *Professional Disciplines in Nursing, Midwifery and Health Visiting* (2nd edn), Blackwell Scientific Publications, Oxford

Buckenham, J. and McGrath, G. (1981) *The Social Reality of Nursing*, Health Science Press, London

Davies, C. (1998) *Gender and the Professional Predicament of Nursing*, Open University Press, Milton Keynes

Dennis, N. (1972) *Public Participation and Planners' Blight*, Faber, London

Department of Health (1998) *A First Class Service: Quality in the new NHS*, Leeds NHS Executive, Leeds

Department of Health (2000) *The National Health Service Ten-year Plan*, DoH, London

Emerton, A. (1992) Professionalism and the role of the UKCC. *British Journal of Nursing* 1(1), 25–9

Foucault, M. (1979) On governmentality. *Ideology and Consciousness* 6, 5–22

Friedson, E. (2001) *The Sociology of Politics and Health*, A Reader (eds Purdy, M. and Banks, D.), Routledge, London and New York

Hugman, R. (1991) *Power in the Caring Professions*, Macmillan, London

Illich, I. (1976) *Limits to Medicine*, Marion Boyars, London

Pearson, A. (1983) *The Clinical Nursing Unit*, Heinemann, London

Pyne, R.H. (1991) *Professional Disciplines in Nursing, Midwifery and Health Visiting* (2nd edn), Blackwell Scientific Publications, Oxford

Rogers, M. (1970) *An Introduction to the Theoretical Basis of Nursing*, F.A. Davies, Philadelphia

Salvage, J. (1985) *The Politics of Nursing*, Heinemann, London

Stacey, M. (1992) *Regulating British Medicine: The General Medical Council*, Wiley, Chichester

Vollmer, H.M. and Mills, D.L. (1966) *Professionalisation*, Prentice-Hall, Englewood Cliffs, NJ

Waerness, K. (1992) On rationality of caring. In: Showstack Sassoon, A. (ed.) (1992) *Women and the State*, Routledge, London

Williams, J. (1993) What is a profession? Experience versus expertise. In: Walmsley, J., Reynolds, J., Shakespeare, P. *et al.* (eds) (1993) *Health and Welfare and Practice: Reflecting on roles and relationships*, Sage, London

UKCC (2000) *UKCC and PREP*, UKCC, London

6

NURSING AS A PROFESSION

Oliver Slevin

> *Their training is shorter, their status is less legitimated, their right to privileged communication less established, there is less of a specialised body of knowledge and they have less autonomy from supervision or control than 'the' professions.*
>
> (Etzioni, 1969)

LEARNING OUTCOMES

After studying this chapter you will be able to:

- Critically appraise the idea of a profession in relation to the occupation of nursing
- Review and explain the professional contract in terms of rights and obligations, and in terms of professional accountability
- Present the main arguments for and against recognising nursing as a profession in terms of the elements of the professional contract
- Identify alternative conceptualisations of professional standing that may more readily fit nursing
- Analyse common views and stereotypes of nursing, as witnessed in social, political and gendered discourses, and demonstrate how these may influence the professional standing of nursing
- Apply the concept of professionalisation, as presented in the previous chapter, to the development of nursing as an occupation
- Consider how nursing may emerge as a new health care profession in the future.

INTRODUCTION

In the previous chapter we considered the process of professionalisation. In one sense, this term relates to the process by which a group or occupational body becomes 'professional'. In a related sense, it can also allude to how the individual is inculcated into such a group or occupation; that is, it is a particular instance of socialisation. Socialisation processes involve the means by which individuals are actively inducted into the culture of a society, usually through social learning processes. By such means, we adopt the worldviews, norms and mores, social roles and even the artefacts that all go to make up the culture. Of course, professionalisation is a very special instance of this process. It is specifically concerned with how one learns the culture of a particular professional group. The professional group we are primarily concerned with is nursing. In this chapter we extend our consideration of these matters by examining the idea of nursing as a profession.

It will not have gone unnoticed that in the opening paragraph the word 'inducted' was used. This is perhaps not surprising. After all, when someone takes up a new post, or commences as a student on a course of study, there is often an 'induction' programme. However, the dictionary definitions of this term show different shades of meaning. In one sense it means to formally install someone in a position, and involves the giving of specific information about roles and expectations. However, in another sense, it involves not only introducing someone to new ideas, knowledge, beliefs, etc., but also ensuring that these are internalised (induced). Here there is a sense of something happening that is proactive, visible and formal in structure, which is clear and explicit in a professional education course. But there is also a glimpse of something much more subtle and passive that is happening. This other sense speaks more of subliminal or implicit socialisation (involving learning by exposure, influence and imitation that the learner is not even consciously aware of) than active guidance and instruction. This form of 'introduction' to membership *may* be subtler, but it is no less powerful for that. When experienced professionals are asked to reflect upon how they developed their professional ethos or worldview, they tend more often to point to mentors and role models than to codes of professional conduct or formal courses of instruction. Beyond this, there is a *consciousness* of being part of a culture and of identifying with it that is difficult to express in words. In this sense we can suggest that there is a *nursing* consciousness that is equally difficult to describe or explain in terms of its origins. Furthermore, we can question whether this is a *professional* consciousness in nursing and, if so, what this actually entails. This is part of the project in this chapter.

Of course, in the previous chapter, Lynn Basford has already spoken about the nature of professions, the process of professionalisation, and the position and influence of professions within our health care systems. It would be superfluous to reiterate detailed discussion of these issues here. This is especially the case as there are so many statements claiming to explicate the nature of professions that, while there is some degree of commonality, there is little prospect of arriving at a universally agreed position (Salvage, 1985; Davies, 1995; Nelson, 1997; Abbott and Meerabeau, 1998). The specific purpose of this chapter is to extend consideration of these matters in respect of the position of *nursing* as a profession. In the above opening quotation, Etzioni (1969), in his famous landmark publication, in a sense throws down the gauntlet. He is clearly seeing nursing, and other occupational groups such as teachers and social workers, as part-way to being professions or as half-professions. One issue is beyond dispute. This is the fact that professional status impacts powerfully upon how an occupational group carries out its occupational activities and the freedom or license it has to do so. It is

therefore, whether we like it or not, an issue of some importance to nursing.

PROFESSIONAL ETHOS, NURSING CONSCIOUSNESS AND SOCIAL STANDING

Professional retrospective

Without risking an extensive reiteration of our presentation in the previous chapter, it is worthwhile briefly reviewing the concepts of profession and professionalisation here. As is often the case, a consideration of the etymological roots of the terms is of help. There are two root terms of importance here, both from Latin origins. The Latin word *professio* refers to a public declaration. It is the root word of the term 'profess' or 'I profess'. The Latin word *vocatio* refers to a calling or calling out. Originally, it related to a calling from God to perform some duty or take up some position. Thus, we have the first great or high profession: that of divinity or the church. To a call from God, some professed publicly their response to enter into this service. Carr-Saunders (1928), in what is widely considered the most famous statement on the nature of a profession, added two other great professions that also emerged in antiquity: law and medicine. In respect of these three (church, medicine and law), we can say they consisted of learned men, devoted to the service of others. It may not go unnoticed that these were learned *men*, and that those who occupy Etzioni's semi-professions were (and still are to some extent) predominantly of the other gender. One further point is worthy of note here. While the etymological roots relate to a call from (or to) God in the first great profession, in a wider sense this involves a call to the service of others (whether or not this is seen as being an enactment of the Christian or some other religious calling).

Thus, this calling to a service and a professing to respond is in the nature of a social happening. It is, at least outwith narrow religious connotations, a social agreement or a social contract. That, in the final analysis, is what a profession is based upon. This social contract runs something like this: society delegates certain *rights*, and the profession accepts certain *obligations*. These delegated rights may be summarised as follows:

- *Autonomy* – to a certain degree society recognises that there are special knowledge and skills in respect of which the profession knows best.
- *Monopoly* – because the service meets important social functions (upholding the law, saving lives, etc.), the right to provide the particular service is only delegated to the profession, and often the status and activities are restricted to it by laws.
- *Rewards* – which usually involve high social standing and esteem, and financial rewards that are typically high.

Accepted obligationsmay be summarised as follows:

- *Expertise* – attaining, maintaining and advancing a high level of knowledge and competence in the particular field.
- *Integrity* – maintaining certain high moral or ethical standards, and ensuring that these are met through self-regulatory codes and frameworks.
- *Service* – providing the service the profession has 'professed' to provide to an accepted minimum 'level', as expressed in terms of standards, quality, or effectiveness.

We find in almost all statements about the nature of the 'true' or 'classical' or 'learned' professions some variations on these themes. Of course, as intimated in the introduction, the traits or characteristics identified as rights and obligations may vary in terms of number and content from authority to authority. Furthermore, the ways in which these characteristics are presented in reality vary to some extent across even the learned professions and indeed, for any one of them, across time. Such presentations of the (claimed) definitive rights and obligations are in effect *ideal types* or *heuristic models*. These are devices that, while they may never exist exactly as described in reality, nevertheless assist

us in recognising and analysing the phenomena they represent. In this respect, the above sets of rights and obligations are adequate for *assisting* us in our subsequent discussion of nursing as a profession.

Of course, meanings do in any case change with the passage of time. Today, we find the term 'professional' used with various shades of meaning. Thus, we find the term referring in some instances to simply the converse of *amateur*, meaning to do something well and expertly, as opposed to poorly and in a less effective manner. In a similar way, it may be used as a synonym for high standards or quality of work or service. In an old episode of 'Coronation Street', a well-known television soap opera, one of the characters, Hilda Ogden, the pub cleaning lady, states 'We *are* professionals, we are a family of professionals – professional cleaners'. Her husband, Stan, is a window cleaner. When people take pride in their work, and when they aspire to the highest standards, they allude to the professional level. In the previous chapter, 'profession' was viewed in the more specialised sense presented as an *ideal type* above, and it is this sense we are also concerned with in the current chapter. However, we should also note that there is now a more fluid approach to this concept, and a greater degree of social acceptance of occupational groups describing themselves as professions. As Lynn Basford points out in the previous chapter, there *are* laws in respect of specific professions. However, there are *no* laws that govern claims to being professional or being a profession. As we will see later, this has allowed for a number of variations on the theme of what a profession actually is.

A further point must be made here. It does not automatically follow that the social contract as presented in the above rights and obligations is a good or sound social contract. Indeed, in the previous chapter Lynn Basford referred to difficulties in respect of traditional professional orientations within modern health services. Two examples demonstrate this point. It will be noted that, in these two examples, where any of the six elements of our *ideal type* for a profession (autonomy, monopoly, rewards, expertise, integrity and service) are referred to, they are highlighted in italics.

1 *Autonomy*. A key feature – indeed, the primary purpose of the social contract establishing a profession – is *service*; that is, the provision of essential special services to minimum standards. However, as the contract delegates *autonomy* to the profession to be the 'expert' arbiter, by definition only it can determine if acceptable minimum standards are being met. The profession concerned may argue that this is necessary: only it has the *expertise* to make such judgements, and its *integrity* (obligation to maintain moral and ethical standards) guarantees it will do this in a truthful and impartial manner.

2 *Monopoly*. While modern health care may demand flexible working to achieve best outcomes within scarce resource situations, the *monopoly* granted to a profession may allow it to veto flexible working that impinges upon its area of practice. The profession concerned may argue that this is necessary. To allow others whose *expertise* (knowledge and competence) is not confirmed to provide this special *service* would breach integrity and place the client at risk. Furthermore (although the profession in question would not normally stoop to such arguments), as the profession is already being *rewarded* for providing the *service*, it is bad economics to pay others for an inferior *service*.

These two examples illustrate a vitally important point. By allowing professions to develop as autonomous groups with monopolistic control over increasingly large sections of social life, society has relinquished much of its capacity for self-determination and flexible working. This has been given particular clarity in the work of Ivan Illich. Illich (1973) described a particular form of monopoly that he termed *radical monopoly*. This involves not the monopoly of some particular brand or specific product, but the monopoly of a *type* of product or service. His

prime example was motor vehicles as a form of transport, which monopolises movement to a large extent in almost all modern societies (with the possible exception of countries such as China and the Netherlands). But he also included the example of a modern health service. This, he claimed, imposes a particular response to health, and by so doing excludes much of our natural capacity for self-help and healing. Later Illich (1976) extended this theme in his work entitled *Limits to Medicine*, but meaningfully subtitled *Medical Nemesis: The expropriation of health*. Here he argued that not only was there a radical monopoly centred upon the medical profession, but that increasing areas of life were being redefined as health (or ill-health) issues or problems. The implications of this are serious. Not only can a group (designated as experts) redefine parts of our life as illness or maladjustment, but they are also omnipotent in: deciding how we will be treated; excluding us from alternative treatment choices; in some instances (e.g. mental health) treating us against our will; delivering the said treatment; and, evaluating its effectiveness.

However, while in the age of modernity society was tied to the notions that science, technology and medicine were society's saviours, in the new post-modern age a more informed public is less naive, more critical and questioning, and less willing to relinquish individual freedom and choice (Slevin, 2002). While the professional arguments for maintaining the *status quo* have some merits, there is now a demand from both clients (the public) and their political representatives for more openness, more involvement, more choice, and more flexibility. As a consequence of these developments we now see the social contract as represented by the ideal type of the learned profession beginning to crumble. This has implications for the appropriateness of this model for nursing. It also raises the question of the need to search for more acceptable alternatives. And, as stated above, there is now greater social license to identify and define profession in different ways. We return to this matter later.

Study Activity 6.1

In this retrospective, we have reviewed the idea of a profession by placing it in the context of a social contract. At this stage it may be helpful to review the section on 'What is a profession?' in Chapter 5 and relate it to the above comments. In particular, you should consider, in your experience to date, the nature of the social contract between *nursing* and society, and the extent to which it contains the contractual elements under rights and obligations in the above 'ideal type'.

Nursing on a professional continuum

The previous section and the first Study Activity draw attention to another aspect of professions that is also alluded to in the previous chapter. There, it will be recalled that Lynn Basford refers to a continuum that extends from 'non-professional' to an 'ideal'. In this chapter, as will be noted above, we have used the concept *ideal type* or its synonym, the *heuristic model*. However, seeing this as a continuum begs two questions. First, there is the issue of what the 'ideal' is and whether or not nursing should aspire to this. Whether, in fact, we should embark upon a journey of professionalisation that has this ideal as its endpoint. This is a question we touched upon in the concluding paragraphs of the previous subsection, and we return to it in the next two subsections. Second, there is a related question about where nursing might sit on such a continuum. In this respect, Carr-Saunders (1955) made another notable contribution to this debate. He spoke of different levels or forms of profession:

- *The established or learned professions* – these being divinity (the clergy), medicine and law. Their characteristics being practice based on high learning (within universities) and a defined code of conduct.
- *The new professions* – these being similarly established upon practice based on high learning (within universities) in the new sciences (natural sciences, social and biolo-gical sciences, applied sciences of engineering, architecture, etc.). While codes of conduct are not always absent, they are not always central.
- *The semi-professions* – these being based upon technical knowledge and skills (not always and not at all until relatively recently attained within universities), which would not equate with high learning and the concomitant 'learn-edness'. As will be recalled from our opening quotation, Etzioni placed nurses, teachers and social workers in this category. Here also, it was argued, codes of conduct were not central characteristics and sometimes absent in any formal sense.
- *The would-be professions* – these not being based upon higher learning or technical knowledge and skills, and thus by definition not requiring a university preparation (as in the case of industrial managers, salespersons, estate agents, etc.). In addition, codes of conduct would typically be absent.

It is of course important to note that Carr-Saunders presented these views half a century ago, and that much has happened in the world since then. It is likely that many of the occupational groups referred to, particularly those associated with the semi-professional and would-be professional levels, would strongly dispute the relevance of this typology today. However, professional status, like beauty, is in the eye of the beholder and there is little doubt that while most people in modern-day society would accept medicine as a profession, they may look with distain upon the claims of estate agents in this respect. While this may be the case, as the old rigid definitions and classifications of professions become blurred, there are some groups who *do* seem to have a degree of social recognition and license to claim professional status.

Notwithstanding the latter position, the modern social world is characterised by rapid change and this affects those in professional configurations as much as other elements in society. In this context, a profession (or occupational group aspiring to professional recognition) can no longer be viewed in terms of occupying a *status*, but is always in a movement towards being and becoming. In this respect we might view nursing, using one shade of meaning to the term professionalisation we introduced above (a process of an occupational group moving towards professional status) as similarly being in a dynamic process of becoming. This might be viewed as a continuum along the lines presented in Fig. 6.1.

The rationale implicit in Fig. 6.1 is that nursing is progressing towards 'full' professional status, or has already more or less reached that point. The arguments that nursing has attained the status of a new profession are significant. Nursing is now (at least in the UK and almost all other Western countries) provided at the level of higher learning within universities, at either primary degree or higher education diploma level. It has also achieved a sophisticated level of theoretical knowledge, as is clearly attested to in Module 3. The research base of nursing's theoretical and practical knowledge is now extensive and equals if not surpasses other fully recognised professional groups. In the UK, particularly since the enactment of The Nursing and Midwifery

Order 2001 (Government of the United Kingdom of Great Britain and Northern Ireland, 2002), nursing has progressed to a sophisticated level of self-regulation in line with that in other recognised professions such as medicine and law. Under this legislation, the UK regulatory body, the Nursing and Midwifery Council, is empowered to regulate not only in respect of conduct (as previously), but also in respect of 'performance and ethics'. This in effect involves the capacity to regulate the competence of nurses and midwives, and this has been carried forward in a new Code of Professional Conduct (Nursing and Midwifery Council, 2002). This code is referred to further within Chapter 13.

It would seem that the latter comments provide a strong argument in favour of nursing having attained the status of a new profession [in the sense that Carr-Saunders (1955) defined this term]. However, this requires some further consideration, not least because of the fact that not all would agree with either the stages of progression suggested in Fig. 6.1 or indeed the claim to the point reached in the present. This has led to different means of viewing the

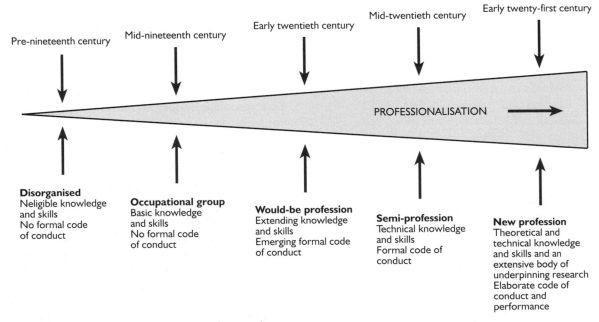

Figure 6.1 Nursing: the professionalisation continuum

progression, and variations in terminology, such as evolving, emerging and developing profession (Nelson, 1997). Implicit in such positions is the view that nursing has not yet reached the position of full professional status. Nelson (1997) and others (e.g. Catalano, 1996) attribute this to a number of factors of which the critical one seems to be that nurses do not work autonomously. As will be recalled, this is one of the important professional attributes referred to above, and it is a point of some significance. In this respect, Johnson (1972) referred to 'professions' such as nursing as *mediated* professions, and Parry and Parry (1979) similarly referred to *agency* or *bureau* professions. That is, groups who do not have the autonomy to direct their own practice but are under the ultimate managerial direction and influence of others. Hugman (1998) suggested that with the rise of managerialism over the last 20 years within the public services, this influence has been in fact strengthened. Indeed, it is often the case now that the immediate manager of the nurse is not another nurse and, as more structured managed care and clinical guidelines become common, even the extent to which clinical judgement can be applied is curtailed. Walsh (2000) is particularly insightful on this point, in respect of how nurses may advance the scope of their practice in response to patient need:

> ... the reader is struck by the dominant position occupied by medicine as it is the doctor's decision which new tasks will be delegated to nurses and also whether they are competent to perform them. There is no 'professional autonomy' here as clearly medicine is in control of nursing. Only those rather tedious tasks of which doctors want to be rid, such as giving intravenous injections of antibiotics or taking blood would be delegated to nurses. There is little scope for the nurse to take the initiative and decide how he or she would like to extend his or her role in response to patient need.
>
> (Walsh, 2000, p. 52)

It is, of course, the case, as Lynn Basford points out in the previous chapter, that nursing has autonomy in the sense of regulating itself in respect of conduct, education, maintenance of and entry to its register of practitioners, etc. But this is not the same thing as having autonomy of practice in the sense that Nelson, Hugman and Walsh speak of this. If we accept that *this* form of autonomy is an essential characteristic or trait of the 'true' profession, then nursing cannot be said to have attained this status. Indeed, unless there were to be radical shifts in how health services were to be managed in the future, it would be impossible for nursing ever to achieve what might be termed full professional status.

Study Activity 6.2

Reflect back to your initial entry to training or to nursing. At that time did you view this as entry to, or entry to preparation for, a profession?

- Having done this, consider what your views are now, in the context of the position presented above.
- Ask a qualified nurse (or if possible two or three) in your placement area (or if you are qualified, nursing colleague/s) if *they* consider themselves to be a 'professional' and, if so, upon what they base this assertion. Compare their position with your own.
- Do you feel this issue is of fundamental importance to nursing? If so, give your reasons.
- You may find it helpful to note down your responses and discuss these notes with your fellow students.

Between nursing consciousness and social standing

To consider where nursing may be going in terms of its professional standing, it is important to step back for a moment from these definitive and interpretive statements. To an extent, as a professional relationship is in essence a social contract, as argued earlier, the professional standing or otherwise of a particular group emerges as a social discourse between the group and society. It is in effect a social construction emerging from this discourse. This brings to bear issues such as image, power, and influence. In entering this discourse, nursing must itself have a clear sense of the direction *it* wishes to take – not in terms of its own self-interest but in terms of the interests of those nursing represents, its patients or clients. It is astonishing that this very question was begged almost 20 years ago by Salvage (1985), and we have not as yet succeeded in answering it. She stated:

> *Nurses should not go along with the assumption that winning professional status for nurses would mean nothing but good for nurses and patients. Even if it could be proved that nursing did fulfil the criteria, nothing would change. We would still be as badly paid, and powerless, and patient care would not change. The question we should ask is not 'Is nursing a profession?' but 'Should we want nursing to be a profession, and if so, what do we mean by it? What are we hoping to achieve, and is this the best way of going about it?'*
>
> (Salvage, 1985, p. 92)

There is of course a fundamental weakness in Salvage's statement. She is right to caution us about assumptions. But her own assumptions would require justification. That is, the assumptions that enhanced professional status (which by definition would include enhancement of professional autonomy) would *not* increase our power and *not* allow us to extend our care of patients. It is difficult to countenance any justification whatsoever for this aspect of her viewpoint. However, her fundamental question is valid, and indeed visionary in its impact. *Do we wish to attain the professional status and mirror the practices of these other 'professions'* such as medicine and law? In answering this question we must look to how these professions, and particularly medicine, have themselves evolved.

We see here, in medicine, a professional ethos that in its worst face has emerged as so drawn to a scientific and technological paradigm that its coldness of clinical practice has engendered wide social criticism. Such is the impact of this that even the term 'clinical' in our dictionaries and thesauruses is now defined as also meaning cold, dispassionate, disinterested, detached, severe, impersonal and unemotional. This negative image, and the reality of a medical practice indeed notable by such distant and uncommunicative relationships, led medicine's regulatory body (in the UK) to eventually amend its educational curriculum to include relational skills as compulsory learning. We see also an aberration of autonomy, to the extent that accountability becomes compromised. This is demonstrated, for example, in the unbridled clinical practices leading to such occurrences as the unacceptable high rates of mortality of young children reported in the Bristol Royal Infirmary inquiry (Kennedy, 2001). A profession that tolerates no questioning of its expertise, that turns in on itself for its values rather than to the society it is meant to serve, and that closes ranks against that society as its adversary rather than its sponsor, may not necessarily be our best model.

It would indeed be remiss of nursing, as a predominantly female profession, if we did not also acknowledge the feminist insights behind this discussion, as addressed by Savage (1987), Davies (1995), Slevin (1999) and Walsh (2000). There is a sense in which the clinical detachment and case orientation of the medical profession is part of a wider masculine orientation, and as such alien to the compassionate person centredness of the nursing project. There may of course be other professional groups who do not attach a premium to the caring dimension of their work. But for nursing, this is not an option. Caring is a fundamental issue for nursing, and as Carol Kirby demonstrated in Chapter 2, it amounts to our *raison d'etre*. A professional profile that engenders dispassion rather than compassion, clinical coldness rather than human warmth, detachment rather than connection, cannot be an option.

But here we must return to the notion of a social contract and the idea that our professional unfolding and subsequent enfoldment emerges from our social discourse. Our professional profile is not for us alone to determine, and in the final analysis society also participates in shaping what we will become, or rejects us if it cannot. However, the social voice is not easy to discern. In an insightful paper, provocatively entitled 'Handmaiden, battle-axe, whore: an exploration into the fantasies, myths and stereo-types about nurses', Muff (1982) identified what he found to be the three dominant public images of the nurse:

- *The handmaiden* – as the stereotype of the ministering angel to the patient and the servant or doctor's assistant, idealised in movie presentations of Florence Nightingale and Edith Cavell or the sweetness and light nursing heroines of the romantic novellas.
- *The battle-axe* – as the stereotype of the militaristic and domineering ward sister figure, feared by all; the Hattie Jacques of the old *Carry on Doctor* series of movies or more recently the brutal Nurse Ratched in the celebrated movie *One Flew over the Cuckoo's Nest*.
- *The whore* – as the stereotype of the nurse as a sex symbol, illustrated in the old *Carry On* films and the notable character of Hotlips Houlahan in the *M*A*S*H* television series.

The terminology in Muff's paper is shocking. But it is important to note that this is not some journalistic sensationalism. This is in fact the report of a scholarly study and it is chastening that these are the three dominant images that emerge. Nowhere among these is there any conception of nursing as a highly knowledgeable, highly skilled occupational group recognised for its wisdom and expertise. While the latter two of the above three images are fortunately indeed relegated to the realms of fantasy and chauvinism, it seems equally unfortunate that the image of a handmaiden is a fairly dominant image of how nurses are viewed.

However, we might reflect further on this situation. In a celebrated publication of over 20 years ago, Aroskar (1980) wrote of what she described as the 'fractured image', whereby the public images and stereotypes of the nurse do not in fact reflect the reality of nursing. Included as the most prominent of these fractured images, was the handmaiden role of the 'gentle sister', occupying the 'dependent functionary' position of supportive role to the physician. She suggested not only that this reflected a degree of inaccuracy in the actual role of the nurse, but also the view that nursing can be advanced by recognising the autonomy of the nurse in the area of care provision. However, in a response, Newton (1980) questioned whether the public view was indeed a fractured image. She argued that not only was the 'gentle sister' a prominent if not *the* prominent role of the nurse, but also that it was a role that many were indeed prepared to perform quite happily. We might beg the question as to whether this fundamental position has changed in two decades. Perhaps the question today may more appropriately be the following: is the real fractured image in fact that of the ruminations and fantasies of a small group of nursing scholars and malcontents who would make nursing what it is not, while to society at large, other health professions, and the vast body of nursing, the handmaiden role is accepted as the reality and purpose of nursing?

In her proposal for autonomous nursing practice based upon a caring orientation, Aroskar (1980) was in a sense anticipating the call to nursing as a profession established on the basis of its orientation towards human caring. This orientation has already been addressed by Carol Kirby in Chapter 2, and it is particularly reflected in the work of Watson (1985, 1988, 1999), Noddings (1986), Eriksson (1994, 2002), Roach (1997), and others. It is claimed that the nature of nursing is such that ministering to the other as a person in need demands a compassionate orientation. This extends beyond empathy (feeling *with* the other) and sympathy (feeling *for* the other) to a commitment to help. Such a commitment is in essence an ethical imperative to respond helpfully, and to do so we must not only have the will to help but also the capacity to do so through relational and technical skills. The claim here is that we can find our own professional space by virtue of attending to that which is at the core of nursing, its caring orientation.

It is useful to view this orientation as having been reached through a developmental and historical sequence. A helpful framing for this is provided in the work of Schulman (1958, 1972). In an original and controversial study, Schulman (1958) claimed that nursing was shifting from what he termed a 'mother surrogate' role to a 'healer' role. By 'mother surrogate' he was referring to the nurturing function of the nurse that encompassed acts of ministering to needs in a mother-like or womanly way; thus, the mother metaphor. By 'healer' Schulman was not referring to a holistic form of helping, such as the humanistic approaches to healing we refer to today. He instead was using this term to denote a disease- and case-orientated approach to procedural and technical nursing – an objective and scientific orientation in which the nurse is more a technician that a personal carer. In the USA, where the study was carried out, there was widespread outrage on the part of many nurses and nursing organisations, all of whom rejected his findings. However, Schulman revisited the topic after 10 years and in this second study (Schulman, 1972), he found that the trend was in fact continuing and indeed had become more accentuated. Some contemporary nursing authors (e.g. Kirby and Slevin, 1992; Mitchell, 1999; Watson, 1999) have claimed that this trend has continued. They suggest that seeking a firm foundation for nursing in an orientation that is exclusively or predominantly scientific–technical–rational fails to recognise the complex human nature of nursing work. Emerging from work such as that of Schulman, and more recent developments, the historical pattern broadly emerges as follows:

- *Prior to the final third of the twentieth century* – a traditional nursing role based largely on what was taken to be the natural nurturing–mothering traits in women, which was in line

with the handmaiden stereotype referred to previously.
- *Through the final third of the twentieth century* – an increasing orientation to a more technical–scientific nursing role, requiring specialist expertise and largely based on the rational medical model.
- *Over the past 15 years (approximately)* – a recognition, or claim, that a predominantly scientific–technical nursing carries the risk of distancing nursing from its caring roots, and a new orientation to informed compassionate caring, rather than a return to a less informed and passive handmaiden role; in effect, an autonomous caring orientation.

It can be seen that this pattern, emerging from discourses on the nature of nursing and nursing work, is largely parallel to and consistent with the discourse on professionalisation in nursing and the trends suggested in Fig. 6.1. However, we refer again, as we have done more than once in this chapter, to the fact that a profession is established on a social contract between that profession and the wider society. We have seen that the societal images or stereotypes of the nurse (that include handmaiden, battle-axe, whore) include only one of the images (that include traditional handmaiden, technical–scientific nursing, caring practice) within nursing's own consciousnesses. Furthermore, as illustrated in Fig. 6.2, in neither society nor nursing is there a definite consensus about any one of the images. There is a discourse within nursing, wherein the three images or nursing consciousnesses are still all in existence, each with their champions and detractors. Similarly, in society the three images or stereotypes are also present, again with their champions and detractors. It must also be recognised that the discourses extend to the interface between nursing and society. It is true that at least some if not all of the societal stereotypes are far removed from nursing consciousness, and indeed in some instances are considered highly offensive. But we cannot deny their presence and the need to correct them. It is also true that some of our

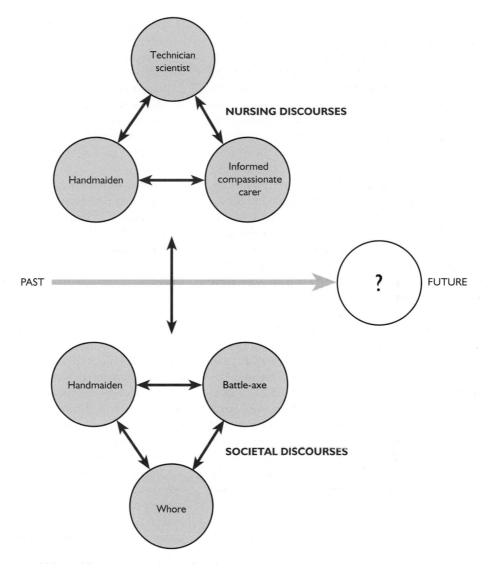

Figure 6.2 Discourses within and between nursing and society

own nursing images are far removed from societal awareness, and this must beg a question in respect of our failure to arrive at a consensus and convey this to the wider society. The most fundamental question of all is how we will emerge from these discourses within our profession and between it and the wider society, and indeed the health service community within that society. This is the issue we consider in our final section of the chapter.

Study Activity 6.3

In the course of your experience since entering training and/or nursing, have you encountered any of *society's* stereotypes or images of nursing as identified above? Reflect upon how such encounters made you feel, how you reacted, and whether or not the reaction was effective or appropriate.

SUMMARY

The above discussions cut to the heart of our one remaining dilemma – the resolution of the issue of autonomy. They also highlight the seriousness with which we must consider the image of the nurse, for this will indeed be important in determining how we will be acknowledged with seriousness as a profession. In the narrower confines of our health care world, this takes on a more sobering dimension. Within these systems, as indicated by Slevin (1999) we find, if anything, an accentuation of the wider social imagery and social influences. Because here we have, almost in a condensed form, that kind of clinical detachment, scientific thinking and objectivity to which we have alluded above. This is encountered in that particular brand of professionalism that is characteristic of the (predominantly male) medical hierarchy, and also in the particular brand of health economics-influenced managerialism that is characteristic of many in the (predominantly male) management hierarchy. In these circumstances the lack of nursing power and thus autonomy is actually institutionalised as a part of the fabric of our health care systems. How do we, or indeed should we, break out? No one who makes even a cursory exploration of nursing could fail to recognise the following position statements:

1 Nursing has advanced in very real and significant ways in terms of its theoretical and scientific knowledge and its technical skill.
2 It has similarly advanced significantly in terms of its self-regulatory and ethical code of practice, such that it can meet its commitment to maintaining high levels of conduct and performance.
3 However, it is framed within a social and political environment wherein power rests with others, such that self-determination and functional autonomy are limited.

To these three position statements can be added three related questions:

1 Should nursing remain as it is, occupying a role that is not independent, that still has vestiges of the handmaiden role, and that extends or expands its scope only at the behest of others?
2 Should nursing actively pursue the final bastion of 'true' or 'learned' professionalism, i.e. the establishment of full autonomy, and emerge as one of these established professions?
3 Should nursing search instead for a different model of professionalism that fits best with its mission of informed, compassionate caring?

It is suggested that in this chapter, and indeed the previous one, there are sufficient grounds for claiming that the first two of these questions *must* be answered in the negative. In a new and rapidly changing health care world we cannot stand still or indeed go back, as intimated in the first question. But, in recognising the valuing of the compassionate caring dimension that is at least one essential part of society's image of the nurse, and the fact that this is at the very heart of our *own* nursing consciousness, we equally cannot proceed towards a traditional autonomous professional standing, as presented in the second question. This leaves us with only one option, to proceed in a new and different way; we must respond affirmatively to the third question.

Here we find, in fact, that while some things appear *at present* not to have changed, this may not continue to be the case. We have already seen in the previous chapter that for all the professions there is a move away from self-interest and inwardness of thinking towards a more responsive and accountable professional model. The current author has referred to this elsewhere as a move towards a negotiated order in which the health professional role is empowering and facilitative and health choices are negotiated rather than imposed (Slevin, 1999). This same orientation is encompassed in statements such as Rosemarie Parse's (1998) 'theory of human becoming', wherein the role of the health professional is similarly viewed as 'co-creating' with the client his/her/their health choices. Suddenly we find in all this a shift that is not in fact so much a redressing of power across the professions, but a redressing of the power between the health care professions and society, as a more informed public demands its right to at least participate in health decisions (Slevin, 1999).

This latter aspect, considered briefly here and also addressed in the previous chapter, is of course only one facet of the new professionalism. To proceed to a more detailed discussion of what the nursing profession of the future may look like would involve another chapter in itself. Indeed, the concluding module contains just such a chapter. However, we can end here by drawing on what is possibly the most comprehensive examination of health professions within the last 100 years. This has been carried forward by a US public body, the Pew Health Professions Commission that has been chaired by Senator George Mitchell. Initially established to consider such issues as the dysfunctional effects of turf wars and divisions of labour and specialisations across and between the professions, the Commission has subsequently progressed to major definitive statements about the nature of the health professions. In its final fourth report (O'Neil and the Pew Health Professions Commission, 1998), the Commission has identified '21 competencies for the twenty-first century'. These clearly place the issue of professionalism in the arena of what service the professions provide in terms of the communities they serve. It may be that in statements such as this, the plea made by Salvage (1985) to which we referred earlier is at last reaching fruition. That is, what we want to achieve for those we serve is the important issue and it is this that should shape our future. Given the importance and relevance of the Pew Commission's competencies, they are presented in full in Table 6.1.

The suggestion here is that we disentangle ourselves from ancient arguments about what characterised the professions of the past. It is not our status, or our claimed traits, that are important, but the service we provide to our public. In

Table 6.1 Twenty-one competencies for the twenty-first century

1 Embrace a personal ethic of social responsibility and service.
2 Exhibit ethical behaviour in all professional activities.
3 Provide evidence-based, clinically competent care.
4 Incorporate the multiple determinants of health in clinical care.
5 Apply knowledge of the new sciences.
6 Demonstrate critical thinking, reflection and problem-solving skills.
7 Understand the role of primary care.
8 Rigorously practice preventive health care.
9 Integrate population-based care and services into practice.
10 Improve access to health care for those with unmet health needs.
11 Practice relationship-centred care with individuals and families.
12 Provide culturally sensitive care to a diverse society.
13 Partner with communities in health care decisions.
14 Use communication and information technology effectively and appropriately.
15 Work in interdisciplinary teams.
16 Ensure care that balances individual, professional, system and societal needs.
17 Practice leadership.
18 Take responsibility for quality of care and health outcomes at all levels.
19 Contribute to continuous improvement of the health care system.
20 Advocate for public policy that promotes and protects the health of the public.
21 Continue to learn and help others learn.

(From O'Neil and the Pew Health Professions Commission, 1998)

this respect, the Pew Commission gets close to the point in its carefully thought out listing of expected competencies for the new century. For our part, we can start where we began. That is, that a profession and its professional standing is established on the basis of a social contract. We can make this claim. If we can achieve a set of competencies such as those above, and let us now call them contractual obligations, we can say without fear of equivocation: we are a new profession.

Study Activity 6.4

We now leave this chapter and its concerns. We have ended with a possible framework – a set of competencies that can be construed as contractual obligations to be met by any health care occupational group that attains or claims professional status. The list in Table 6.1 may not be fully accepted by all, even if it clearly *is* comprehensive and the outcome of considerable experience and thought. But take it as to all intents and purposes, covering all that would be required as a profession.

- Reproduce the list and then tick against each competence (or contractual obligation) that you feel nursing already meets.
- For those you have ticked as being met, present a brief argument to justify your claim.
- For those you *have not* ticked, proceed as follows. If an item is not ticked because you do not know the answer, seek advice from your mentor or personal tutor. For those you feel nursing does not meet, present a brief statement to justify your claim.
- Finally, if there are any items you feel should not be included, or items you feel are missing, list these.
- If possible, discuss your own conclusions with your fellow students and/or personal tutor.

REFERENCES

Abbott, P. and Meerabeau, L. (1998) Professionals, professionalization and the caring professions. In: Abbott, P. and Meerabeau, L. (eds) *The Sociology of the Caring Professions* (2nd edn), UCL Press, London

Aroskar, M.A. (1980) The fractured image: the public stereotype of nursing and the nurse. In: Spicker, S.F. and Gadow, S. (eds) *Nursing: Images and ideals: Opening dialogue with the humanities*, Springer, New York

Carr-Saunders, A.M. (1928) *Professions – Their organisation and place in society*, Clarendon Press, Oxford

Carr-Saunders, A.M. (1955) Metropolitan conditions and traditional professional relationships. In: Fisher, A.M. (ed.) *The Metropolis in Modern Life*, Rooksbury, Garden City, NY

Catalano, J.T. (1996) *Contemporary Professional Nursing*, F.A. Davis, Philadelphia, IL

Davies, C. (1995) *Gender and the Professional Predicament in Nursing*, Open University Press, Buckingham

Eriksson, K. (1994) Theories of caring as health. In: Gaut, D. and Boykin, A. (eds) *Caring as Healing: Renewal through hope*, National League for Nursing, New York

Eriksson, K. (2002) Caring science in a new key. *Nursing Science Quarterly* 15, 61–5

Etzioni, A. (1969) *The Semi-professions and their Organization: Teachers, nurses, and social workers*, Free Press, New York

Government of the United Kingdom of Great Britain and Northern Ireland (2002) *Statutory Instruments 2002 No. 253. The Nursing and Midwifery Order 2001*, The Stationery Office, London

Hugman, R. (1998) Social work and de-professionalisation. In: Abbott, P. and Meerabeau, L. (eds) *The Sociology of the Caring Professions* (2nd edn), UCL Press, London

Illich, I. (1973) *Tools for Conviviality*, Harper and Row, New York

Illich, I. (1976) *Limits to Medicine – Medical Nemesis: The expropriation of health*, Penguin Books, New York

Johnson, T.J. (1972) *Professions and Power*, Macmillan, London

Kennedy, I. (Chairman) (2001) *Learning from Bristol: The report of the public inquiry into children's heart surgery at the Bristol Royal Infirmary 1984–1995*. Command Paper: CM 5207, HMSO, London

Kirby, C. and Slevin, O. (1992) A new curriculum for care. In: Slevin, O. and Buckenham, M. (eds) *Project 2000: The teachers speak*, Nelson Thornes, Cheltenham

Mitchell, G. (1999) Evidence-based practice: critique and alternative view, *Nursing Science Quarterly* 12, 30–5

Muff, J. (1982) Handmaiden, battle-axe, whore: an exploration into the fantasies, myths and stereotypes about nurses. In: Muff, J. (ed.) *Socialisation, Sexism and Stereotyping*, C.V. Mosby, St Louis, IL

Nelson, N. (1997) Images of nursing: influences of the present. In: Zewekh, J. and Claborn, J. (eds) *Nursing Today: Transitions and trends* (2nd edn), W.B. Saunders, Philadelphia, IL

Newton, L. (1980) A vindication of the Gentle Sister: comment on 'The fractured image'. In: Spicker, S.F. and Gadow, S. (eds) *Nursing: Images and ideals: Opening dialogue with the humanities*, Springer, New York

Noddings, N. (1986) *Caring: A feminist approach to ethics and moral education*, University of California Press, Berkeley, CA

Nursing and Midwifery Council (2002) *Code of Professional Conduct*, Nursing and Midwifery Council, London

O'Neil, E.H. and the Pew Health Professions Commission (1998) *Recreating Health Professional Practice for a New Century. Fourth report of the Pew Health Professions Commission*, Center for the Health Professions, University of California, San Francisco, CA

Parry, N. and Parry, J. (1979) Social work, professionalism and the state. In: Parry, N., Rusten, M. and Satyamurti, C. (eds) *Social Work, Welfare and the State*, Edward Arnold, London

Parse, R.M. (1998) *The Human Becoming School of Thought: A perspective for nurses and other health professionals*, Sage, Thousand Oaks, CA

Roach, M.S. (1997) Reflections on the theme. In: Roach, M.S. (ed.) *Caring from the Heart*, Paulist Press, New York

Salvage, J. (1985) *The Politics of Nursing*, Heinemann Nursing, London

Savage, J. (1987) *Nurses, Gender and Sexuality*, Heinemann Nursing, London

Schulman, S. (1958) Basic functional roles in nursing: mother surrogate and healer. In: Jaco, E.G. (ed.) *Patients, Physicians and Illness: A sourcebook in behavioural science and medicine*, Free Press, New York

Schulman, S. (1972) Mother surrogate – after a decade. In: Jaco, E.G. (ed.) *Patients, Physicians and Illness: A sourcebook in behavioural science and medicine* (2nd edn), Collier-Macmillan, London

Slevin, O. (1999) The nurse–patient relationship: caring in a health context. In: Long, A. (ed.) *Interaction for Practice in Community Nursing*, Macmillan, Basingstoke

Slevin, O. (2002) Valuing the past, embracing the future. In: McDaid, C. (ed.) *From Past to Future*, National Board for Nursing, Belfast

Walsh, M. (2000) *Nursing Frontiers: Accountability and the boundaries of care*, Butterworth Heinemann, Oxford

Watson, J. (1985) *Nursing: The philosophy and science of caring*, University Press of Colorado, Niwot

Watson, J. (1988) *Nursing: Human science and human care. A theory of nursing*, National League for Nursing, New York

Watson, J. (1999) *Postmodern Nursing and Beyond*, Churchill Livingstone, Edinburgh

7
CLINICAL SUPERVISION AND LEADERSHIP

Dawn Freshwater

LEARNING OUTCOMES

After studying this chapter you will be able to:

- Define the term 'clinical supervision'
- Discuss the principles of clinical supervision and their relationship to reflective practice
- Identify the personal, professional and practical factors involved in the implementation of clinical supervision
- Explore the links between clinical supervision and effective leadership skills
- Understand clinical supervision in the context of professional policies and national agendas.

INTRODUCTION

The provision of nursing care, and the role of nursing in the multidisciplinary health care team, has never been more complex. The demands on health care professionals to forge multiprofessional, multidisciplinary and interagency partnerships in the provision of that care are great. Added to the constant technological and medical advances, and set against the backdrop of an ever-increasing population, with constantly raised expectations, developments such as the New Deal for Junior Doctors and the Calman Report (Department of Health (DoH), 1993) have had an immediate 'knock-on' effect on nurse staff levels and nurses' responsibilities. These have had both a positive and negative effect. Never have nurses had more scope, or such a breadth of areas in which to work. On the other hand, they have never had as much possibility for 'burn out' and reduction in standards of care.

Current demands cannot be met without the health professional being able to understand and to develop from professional peer review. Clinical supervision offers a framework that encourages – indeed, is central to – this development.

Clinical supervision has been promoted as a method of ensuring safe and accountable practice in nursing (United Kingdom Central Council for nursing, midwifery and health visiting [UKCC], 1996; Butterworth *et al.* 1998; Department of Health, 1999; Bishop and Freshwater, 2000). While various attempts have been made to define and describe clinical supervision, with varying emphasis on standards, quality of care, patient safety and staff support, its implementation has to date been patchy and inconsistent. In addition, its value as a tool for developing skills of clinical leadership has not yet been fully realised. Where it is implemented successfully, available evidence indicates that a culture of caring critique, rather than a culture of blame, improves staff motivation and benefits patient care (Bishop, 1998; Bishop and Freshwater, 2000; Freshwater *et al.*, 2001). Integral to this process is the opportunity for cross-fertilisation of skills, professional development and support, and communication skills.

This chapter aims to explore the concept of clinical supervision, focusing specifically on the relationship between clinical supervision, reflective practice and practice development through clinical leadership.

BACKGROUND TO CLINICAL SUPERVISION

Contemporary developments in nursing have seen nursing practice assigned the task of implementing clinical supervision and evidence-based practice (DoH, 1993, 1999; UKCC, 1996; Bishop and Freshwater, 2000; Freshwater *et al.*,

2001; Rolfe *et al.*, 2001). While it is a fairly novel undertaking in nursing, with some specialist areas being more advanced than others, there is evidence to suggest that it is now a reasonably well-established concept in practice (Farrington, 1995; Butterworth *et al.*, 1998; Bishop and Freshwater, 2000). It is an important area of development, as much of the success of *The New NHS: Modern, dependable* (Department of Health, 1997) and the supporting strategies described in the publications *Information for Health* (Department of Health, 1998), *A First Class Service* (Department of Health, 1998a), *Working Together* (Department of Health, 1998b) and *Making a Difference* (1999), depend upon the ability of key players – identified, accountable, responsible and effective clinical leaders – to take the agendas forward.

Study Activity 7.1

Reflect on the term 'clinical supervision'. What does it mean to you? How does this differ from your understanding of the term 'supervision' in other professional and non-professional settings?

The skills of accountability and responsibility are deemed to be central to the practice of the professional practitioner and for many years have been part of discussions around the role of the nurse. The UKCC's *Scope of Professional Practice* (1992) encouraged the move towards nurses taking on more responsibility. This impetus was further supported by the most recent English nursing and midwifery strategy document *Making a Difference* (DoH, 1999), and the UKCC document *Fitness for Practice* (1999), both of which draw together all earlier moves to strengthen the role of nursing.

While the UKCC's 1992 document provided a set of principles to guide the development and expansion of professional roles and responsibilities in nursing and midwifery, and was widely welcomed by the nursing and midwifery professions, it did not offer any framework for self-regulation. Nonetheless, the document liberated the nursing and midwifery professions from their previous reliance on task-oriented practice with vicarious accountability through doctors, towards an acceptance that activities should be limited only by the individual practitioner's knowledge and competence. It sought to facilitate more flexible practice, and was intended to be advantageous to both patient and client needs, taking into account the fluctuating health care workforce and patterns of care.

WHAT IS CLINICAL SUPERVISION?

Clinical supervision provides a framework for self-regulation and developing informed deliberative practice, emphasising not only self-monitoring through reflection on action, but also encouraging reflection in action. This section examines the concept of clinical supervision in more detail, exploring its application and potential.

Originating from psychotherapy, counselling and social work, clinical supervision as applied to nursing is as yet a poorly defined and developed concept. While it is fair to say that clinical supervision is a relatively new concept to most branches of nursing, it is an established part of practice in some areas, for example, in mental health. It is well recognised in midwifery practice and is also used in child protection work. Much of the authenticated literature dealing with the theory and practice of clinical supervision has, however, emerged from within the disciplines of counselling, psychotherapy and social work (Casement, 1985, 1989; Kadushin, 1992; Holloway, 1995; Hawkins and Shohet, 2000). This is unsurprising, given that the notion of supervision evolved from the psychoanalytic work of Sigmund Freud in the 1920s. Freud advocated that supervision should be a formal requirement for trainee analysts. In 1951, Carl Rogers, the pioneer of person-centred therapy, expanded this idea to include all active counsellors and psychotherapists; that is to say, all those with a caseload, whether or not they were qualified.

Since the 1950s, clinical supervision has evolved rapidly, with several modes and models being built into the disciplines of counselling and psychotherapy as a prerequisite of training. Social work subsequently took its lead from these disciplines and developed its own strategy for caseload supervision.

Clinical supervision has been a part of midwifery practice for many years, although it has always been linked to appraisal systems and disciplinary procedures, taking more of a managerial route (Bond and Holland, 1998). Mental health practitioners probably engage more directly with the skills of counselling and psychotherapy in their everyday practice and so it is not surprising that models of clinical supervision in the arena of mental health draw upon tried and tested approaches within counselling and psychotherapy. However, while it is a well-accepted and widely acknowledged part of everyday practice in the field of mental health, there is evidence to suggest that it is not well established in practice (Farrington, 1995; Butterworth *et al.*, 1998). In addition, where it is practised, it is not always clearly defined, or linked to critical reflection and innovations in practice (Bond and Holland, 1998).

DEFINING CLINICAL SUPERVISION

Numerous definitions exist to describe clinical supervision. The DoH document *A Vision for the Future* (Department of Health, 1993) outlines clinical supervision as follows:

> ... a term to describe a formal process of professional support and learning which enables practitioners to develop knowledge and competence, assume responsibility for their own practice and enhance consumer protection and safety of care in complex situations.
>
> (Department of Health, 1993, p. 3)

However, one of the definitions most commonly referred to in the literature is that of Faugier and Butterworth (1994), who state that clinical supervision is 'an exchange between practising

professionals to enable the development of professional skills' (1994, p. 9).

Other definitions contain elements of the purpose of clinical supervision as identified in the UKCC (1996) position statement, emphasising standards, and quality of care, patient safety and protection. Bishop (1998), for example, says the following:

> Clinical supervision is a designated interaction between two or more practitioners, within a safe/supportive environment which enables a continuum of reflective, critical analysis of care, to ensure quality patient services.
>
> (Bishop, 1998, p. 8)

Other writers highlight the value of supporting of the practitioner and the role of learning from experience:

> Clinical supervision is a regular, protected time for facilitated, in-depth reflection on clinical practice. It aims to enable the supervisee to achieve, sustain and creatively develop a high quality of practice through the means of focused support and development.
>
> (Bond and Holland, p. 77)

What all of these definitions have in common is the fact that they acknowledge the dynamic nature of the shared experience in the process of clinical supervision. Some qualify this by adding the desired environmental characteristics, safety and support, but few of them relate clinical supervision directly to the notion of reflection.

This chapter is based on the premise that reflective practice is at the heart of clinical supervision; for an in-depth discussion of the concept of reflective practice, *see* Chapter 26. This does not mean that supervision is dominated by the use of a reflective model; rather, effective clinical supervision always involves critical reflection by the supervisee and, indeed, by the supervisor. Clinical supervision is therefore an environment within which critical reflection can be fostered (Johns, 1993; Rolfe *et al.*, 2001). As a result, the functions and tasks of clinical supervision are inextricably linked to the development of critical reflection; clinical supervision offers the formalised structure within which this can take place (Binnie and Titchen, 1995).

PRACTICAL CONSIDERATIONS

The effective implementation of clinical supervision will rely on mutual agreement in terms of definitions and expectations. This will enable both supervisor and supervisee to achieve ownership of the programme and appreciate its value and importance, to themselves, to the organisation and to their patients. Achieving ownership will not only help to allay some of the anxieties but also ensure clarity of information in relation to the choice of modes and models. But do professionals feel that clinical supervision is important for them and their professional practice, or is it something that they feel is imposed upon them? What are the anxieties and barriers to the successful implementation of clinical supervision? The problem of achieving ownership through shared aims and expectations is one. Linked to this is the perception of many practitioners that the drive towards clinical supervision is led by policy makers, rather than having emerged from within the profession.

Study Activity 7.2 ━━━━━━━━━━

Spend some time reflecting on the following questions:

- What is the most appropriate setting for discussing clinical practice?
- When might it be important to reflect on your practice?
- What would need to be in place in order for you to feel safe to discuss the details of your professional practice with another person?
- Can you imagine any barriers to this process?

━━━━━━━━━━━━━━━━━━━

Professional drivers

Initial interest in clinical supervision in general nursing developed as a direct result of two notable publications – the *Vision for the Future* document (DoH, 1993) and the Faugier and Butterworth (1994) position paper on clinical supervision. The Allitt Inquiry did much to raise the issue of professional standards in the public arena; the Clothier Report of this inquiry (Clothier *et al.*, 1994) subsequently highlighted the necessity for adequate standards of supervision, training and education. The UKCC (1996) responded to these documents by issuing a position paper advocating the implementation of clinical supervision within nursing. The document also recognised the importance of the role of clinical supervision and its contribution towards ensuring safe, effective care delivery through the process of lifelong learning.

It is increasingly included in the NHS trust-wide strategies, and there is a continued illusion (held by many) that it is being successfully undertaken in clinical practice, but clinical supervision is still not a reality in many areas of health care (Farrington, 1995; Bond and Holland, 1998; Butterworth *et al.*, 1998; Freshwater *et al.*, 2001). Implementation is generally sparse and a significant number of nurses are still not aware of the UKCC guidance on the issue (Bishop and Freshwater, 2000). This is particularly the case in non-NHS settings, the voluntary sector and prison health care (Freshwater *et al.*, 2001). Recent research suggests this is related not only to a perceived lack of ownership, but also to a lack of leadership within nursing. For example, a recent study undertaken in prison health care settings concluded that a lack of leadership and a subsequent lack of ownership were fundamental barriers to the successful implementation of clinical supervision. As such, these issues demand careful consideration prior to the development of local protocols (Freshwater *et al.*, 2001).

Clinical supervision and practice development

There are many different ways to take part in clinical supervision. As long as the key elements are in place, and understood, the specific format is up to the individuals concerned. Some of the areas for consideration include the following:

- Is clinical supervision to be voluntary or mandatory?
- Who will lead the implementation?
- How are the supervisors to be selected?
- What training will be provided for supervisors and supervisees?
- Which staff are to be involved?
- What support and resources will be needed?
- Will it be multidisciplinary or unidisciplinary?
- Will the supervisees be offered group or individual supervision?
- How should it be used and for what purposes?

There is some disparity of opinion about whether clinical supervision should be provided by nurses or by nurse managers within the local NHS, with a feeling that there is a lack of identified leaders who can drive these nursing agendas forward (*see*, for example, UKCC and University of Central Lancashire, 1999). In addition, there is also some confusion about how to maximise the potential of the clinical supervision relationship and, indeed, what sort of discussions should be taking place. The following vignette briefly typifies the sort of conversation that might take place in supervision:

> *Supervisor*: How would you like to use the time today?
> *Supervisee*: Well, I'm not sure. Things have been going pretty well on the ward recently, especially since I was able to discuss my professional development with my manager. It's strange. I know that clinical supervision is for working through positive incidents too ... but I found myself worrying about the fact that nothing really had 'gone wrong' since our meeting last month.
> *Supervisor*: Perhaps it's worth spending a few minutes talking about this ...
> *Supervisee*: Yes, we're not very good on the ward at congratulating ourselves. For example, we had our ward audit last week and before the auditors visited everyone was

> running around like headless chickens worrying about what we hadn't completed since our last audit. We have worked so hard since the audit last year and have improved our support for staff and students and many other things, but no one was thinking about how much we had achieved in that time. We seem to focus on our deficits.
> *Supervisor*: And now you're aware of doing that in clinical supervision?
> *Supervisee*: Mmm, but it's not good to blow your own trumpet, is it?
> *Supervisor*: Can you say a bit more about that?
> *Supervisee*: So much of what we do each day – ordinary practice that is – is taken for granted. I think we just get on and do it without even thinking about it. I don't expect anyone to thank me for that.

Barriers to success

The literature is full of anxieties, misconceptions and misunderstandings about clinical supervision, although it appears that one of the greatest causes of anxiety relates to the perceived lack of power ascribed to the supervisee (Kohner, 1994). Bond and Holland (1998) link this to the emphasis on the managerial component of supervision, although the UKCC (1996) quite clearly indicates that clinical supervision is not the exercise of overt managerial responsibility nor is it a system of formal individual performance review.

Nursing, among other professions, is well known for its defensiveness around the building of intimate relationships. Research undertaken by Isabel Menzies-Lyth in the 1970s and 1980s (Menzies, 1970, Menzies-Lyth, 1988) described the anti-emotional climate in nursing, highlighting the behaviour of nurses within social organisations and, in particular, their coping mechanisms. Menzies-Lyth discussed the difficulty of establishing professional relationships and both the fear of and the desire for control within personal, collective, social and organisational defence mechanisms. A number of authors link anxiety and defensiveness with the resistance to clinical supervision, arguing that Menzies-Lyth's research still holds true today (Bond and Holland, 1998; Briant and Freshwater, 1998).

Many reasons are put forward to explain the apparent lack of enthusiasm for clinical supervision, not least the argument relating to the lack of resources and finance, and also to some extent the difficulties with the term itself.

In order to influence the potential success of an implementation programme, it is essential to establish ownership of clinical supervision itself. Research has shown that, where an advocate was clearly in evidence, clinical supervision programmes were successfully implemented. Interestingly, the advocate does not necessarily have to be a senior member of the staff but should be someone who can demonstrate leadership skills and is able to overcome many of the real and perceived barriers to the management of change (Freshwater et al., 2001).

For clinical supervision to be accepted, the common purposes, functions and aims of supervision must be discussed and agreed. All concerned must be given an opportunity to discuss any anxieties, to clarify misconceptions and confusion, to concur, and then to determine an appropriate way forward.

CLINICAL SUPERVISION AND LEADERSHIP

Clinical supervision is not currently a formal part of clinical leadership programmes, neither is it specifically used to develop clinical leadership skills. It may be a useful tool for developing leadership skills but it also relies heavily on strong leadership for its success. Such skills have been identified as a priority for training in the nursing profession, with such organisations as the Royal College of Nursing and the Kings Fund establishing leadership programmes (Department of Health, 1999, 2000).

Making a Difference (Department of Health, 1999) recommends that practitioners use clinical supervision and statutory midwifery supervision to help identify, support and develop nurse, midwife and health visitor leaders and potential leaders. Much of the success of any individual in achieving his or her professional aims will depend on the vision and support of good management and careful career planning. The combined efforts of various professional nursing bodies have put clinical practice back into career advancement in nursing, a focus which the present government is more than happy to support; indeed, it is promoting it. The White Paper *The New NHS: Modern, dependable* (Department of Health, 1997) and, more particularly, *Making a Difference* (Department of Health, 1999) make it clear that the present government is committed to extending recent developments in the roles of nurses, and is encouraging and supporting developments in nursing practice, including the strengthening of leadership.

Study Activity 7.3

- What are the attributes of an effective leader?
- In what situations would you find yourself taking the lead? Or following a leader?
- Spend a few minutes reflecting on a change you decided to make in your life. How did you go about it? Did you need the support of others? If so, how did you gain it?

Historically, nursing may never have been better placed to take forward a new professional status, which will empower its practitioners to provide the care that they are well equipped to give, and to take their rightful place in society, at the bedside and at the policy table. This will not be achieved by innovation alone, however well publicised. It will be achieved, in the long term, only by nursing continuing to show its reflective and dynamic abilities, and by sound research to underpin its practice.

Clinical supervision, if properly implemented, will be the greatest driver in taking forward excellence in care, and will support the nurse's place in achieving effective clinical governance.

Butterworth wrote in 1998 of 'a future dream ... to see any absence of clinical supervision as a curiosity; when that is so, we can be sure that its [integration] into the profession is complete.' Once it is fully integrated it becomes a central component of the continuing professional development strategy and a tool for establishing the practice of lifelong learning.

CLINICAL SUPERVISION AND LIFELONG LEARNING

Clinical supervision is closely aligned to lifelong learning and continuing professional development (CPD) (Bishop and Freshwater, 2000). It is important to remember that clinical supervision will, as the UKCC (1996) states, 'assist lifelong learning ... throughout all registered practitioners' careers' (1996). To this end, it is important that supervisors as well as supervisees are receiving supervision. In relation to lifelong learning, clinical supervision is the formalisation of what has often been taking place informally, and it is about recognising that each nurse is responsible for his or her practice and ongoing learning.

SUMMARY

The heart of clinical supervision is the need for peer review, for staff support, and for public safety. Clinical supervision is about the profession entering into a relationship with itself, and having the confidence from that to enter into equal partnership with other health care professions. This empowerment is vital if nursing is to achieve its potential in making its contribution to health and health care. Quite properly, patients and their carers are moving into the centre of health care focus, and nurses, perhaps more than any other group of health care professionals, are required to meet patients' needs in as flexible a manner as possible.

Clinical supervision has been promoted as a method of ensuring safe and accountable practice in nursing. Various attempts have been made to describe and define clinical supervision,

each highlighting specific aspects of the concept. The emphasis is on standards, quality of care, patient safety and protection, and staff support. In essence, clinical supervision is widely agreed to be a process through which nurses can reflect on and review their practice, develop and enhance their skills and knowledge, while maintaining and improving standards of care.

Clinical supervision is intended, and generally emphasised, as a voluntary process, not as a management tool linked to performance targets or appraisal. However, as yet, the evidence suggests that its implementation is sometimes management-driven and not always linked to professional and practice development. In order to maintain the implementation of clinical supervision effectively it is essential that supervisors and supervisees have ownership of the programme, and are able to appreciate its value and importance, both to themselves and to their organisation. For the potential of clinical supervision to be realised it is essential that all participants receive adequate preparation.

The concept of clinical governance, the pivot on which successful implementation of NHS reforms rests, has to be a joint responsibility of all those in health care delivery:

> *Clinical governance is about openness, admitting and learning from mistakes to prevent reoccurrence.*
>
> (DoH, 1999)

Clinical supervision offers a formal structure in which openness and willingness to learn from mistakes can be fostered and nurtured. The successful implementation of clinical supervision requires some cultural as well as managerial change as already highlighted. Hence if clinical supervision is to be prioritised (and it must be for clinical practice to progress) then so must the development of clinical leadership skills.

REFERENCES

Binnie, A. and Titchen, A. (1995) The art of clinical supervision. *British Journal of Nursing* 4, 327–34

Bishop, V. (1998) Clinical supervision: what is it? In: Bishop, V. (ed.) *Clinical Supervision in Practice: Some questions, answers and guidelines*, Macmillan, London

Bishop, V. and Freshwater, D. (2000) *Clinical Supervision: Examples and pointers for good practice*, Report for University of Leicester Hospitals Education Consortium, November

Bond, M. and Holland, S. (1998) *Skills of Clinical Supervision for Nurses*, Open University Press, Buckingham

Briant, S. and Freshwater, D. (1998) Exploring mutuality in the nurse-patient relationship. *British Journal of Nursing* 7(4), 202–11

Butterworth, T., White, E., Carson, J. *et al.* (1998) Developing and evaluating clinical supervision in the United Kingdom. *EDTNA/ERCA Journal* 24(1), 2–8

Casement, P. (1985) *On Learning from the Patient*, Tavistock, London

Clothier, C., MacDonald, C.A. and Shaw, D.A. (1994) *The Allitt Inquiry: Independent inquiry relating to deaths and injuries on the children's ward at Grantham and Keskeyen General Hospital during the period February to April 1991 (The Clothier Report)*, HMSO, London

Clothier, *et al.* (1994) *The Allitt Inquiry* (The Clothier Report), HMSO, London

Department of Health (1993) *A Vision for the Future: The nursing, midwifery and health visiting contribution to health and health care*, HMSO, London

Department of Health (1997) *The New NHS: Modern, dependable*, The Stationery Office, London

Department of Health (1998a) *A First Class Service: Quality in the new NHS*, Leeds NHS Executive, Leeds

Department of Health (1998b) *The New NHS – Working Together: Securing a quality workforce for the NHS*, DoH, London

Department of Health (1999) *Making a Difference*, The Stationery Office, London

Department of Health (2000) *The National Health Service Ten-year Plan*, DoH, London

Farrington, A. (1995) Models of clinical supervision, *British Journal of Nursing* 4(15), 876–8

Faugier, J. and Butterworth, T. (1994) *Clinical Supervision: A position paper*, University of Manchester, Manchester

Freshwater, D., Storey, L. and Walsh, L. (2001) *Establishing Clinical Supervision in Prison Health Care Settings*. Report of a research study funded by Department of Health, UKCC and FONS, London

Hawkins, P. and Shohet, R. (1989; 2000) *Supervision in the Helping Professions*, Open University Press, Buckingham

Holloway, E. (1995) *Clinical Supervision: A systems approach*, Sage, London

Johns, C. (1993) Professional supervision. *Journal of Nursing Management* 1, 9–18

Kadushin, A. (1992) *Supervision in Social Work*, Columbia University Press, New York

Kohner, N. (1994) *Clinical Supervision in Practice*, Kings Fund Centre, London

Menzies, I.E.P. (1970) *The Functioning of Social Systems as a Defence Against Anxiety*, Free Association Books, London

Menzies-Lyth, I.E.P. (1988) *Containing Anxiety in Institutions: Selected essays*, Free Association Books, London

Rolfe, G., Freshwater, D. and Jasper, M. (2001) *Critical Reflection for Nurses and the Helping Professions: A user's guide*, Palgrave, Basingstoke

UKCC (1992) *The Scope of Professional Practice*, UKCC, London

UKCC (1999) *Fitness for Practice*, UKCC, London

UKCC for Nursing, Midwifery and Health Visiting (1996) *Position Statement on Clinical Supervision for Nursing and Health Visiting*, UKCC, London

UKCC and University of Central Lancashire (1999) *Nursing in Secure Environments*, UKCC, London

8 Towards a Learning Society

David Davies

LEARNING OUTCOMES

After studying this chapter, you will be able to:

- Explain the rationale for applying the principles of lifelong learning to the world of professional health care practice
- Describe the meaning of lifelong learning
- Discuss the exponential growth of lifelong learning
- Describe the reasons for political directives and policies that support the notion of lifelong learning
- Identify the process and learning opportunities as they relate to vocational practice
- Understand the changing emphasis towards work-based learning (WBL) as a central component of continuous professional practice (CPD)
- Recognise the skills required to undertake lifelong learning as a mechanism for ensuring competence to practise
- Understand the critical importance of reflexive learning.

INTRODUCTION

The focus of lifelong learning is the cornerstone of the UK's modernisation agenda (Department of Health (Department of Health), 2000) to improve working lives and the quality of care given within health and social care organisations. According to the Secretary of State,

> ... *lifelong learning is about growth and opportunity, about making sure that our staff, the teams and organisations they relate to, and work in, can acquire new knowledge and skills, both to realise their potential and to help shape and change things for the better*'
>
> (Department of Health, 2001, p. 1)

At the heart of all of this is the recognition that patients and their families will benefit from a workforce suitably qualified and fit to practise in a dynamic health care system. To assist this process it is envisaged that the National Health Service (NHS) will adopt changes in attitude and culture to become a learning community, which will enable individual, team and organisational performance.

Such radical change from traditional educational and training approaches has not emerged in a vacuum. There are some external influences that have influenced this ideological change:

- changes in work patterns
- expectations for professional learning and work competence
- changing patterns of health care delivery
- overall government policy on lifelong learning and the new technological revolution
- philosophies inherent within *The NHS Plan* (Department of Health, 2000)
- the government's commitment to ensuring equality of opportunity and valuing diversity. This requires the NHS to play a significant role in the economic, educational and social life of the communities it serves (Department of Health, 2001).

The government has a clear vision of lifelong learning. For the professional in the twenty-first century it will be embedded with continuing professional development and demonstration of the individual's competence to practise. It is envisaged that there will be a set of core values and skills that are pivotal to lifelong learning, which will enable practitioners to undertake their work with proficiency and quality. All learning, whether formal or informal, should be valued, recognised, recorded in a professional portfolio and, wherever possible, accredited. In addition, the infrastructure to support lifelong learning should exist in the workplace, to add relevance and meaning and provide greater opportunity and wider access to learning (Department of Health, 2001). Such change in emphasis requires a significant shift in educational provision to models that embrace the new technology, virtual universities and work-based learning.

The concept of lifelong learning is seen as a recent phenomenon, driven by government policies and philosophical thinking, but the English National Board for Nurses, Midwives and Health Visitors (ENB) document *Creating Lifelong Learners* (1994), which supported and encouraged lifelong learning, was quite clearly a forerunner of current ideology. The ethos of such philosophical thinking was drawn from the creation of a new preparation for professional nursing practice, known colloquially as Project 2000 (P2K). P2K was a radical shift from previous models of educating and training nurses, which had relied very heavily on 'learning with Nellie'. This was an apprenticeship model that did not encourage the enquiring critical practitioner, neither was it based on the principle of encouraging students to seek out evidence of best practice, so as to advance and enhance professional practice. Conversely, P2K was focused on preparing the new generation of practitioners who would become 'knowledgeable doers' and would be 'fit for practice', having the necessary skills to reflect in and on their practice within the context of learning throughout the life of their professional practice.

Juxtaposed with the changes in pre-registration nursing, concerns were expressed about the fact that, upon registration, nurses, midwives and health visitors were given the licence to practise for life, without any professional challenge as to the currency of their knowledge and their competence to practise. In the interest of public safety and the provision of quality care, the United Kingdom Central Council for Nurses, Midwives and Health Visitors (UKCC, 1994), set out regulations through which professional competence would be verified and audited. The UKCC framework for such regulation operates through the mechanisms laid down for the Continuing Professional Development standard and the Continuing Professional Practice standard (PREP-CPD and PREP-Practice); these standards are discussed more fully in Chapter 5.

This chapter has a single overall focus: the important and far-reaching factors that have brought about change in the learning opportunities within higher education and in the wider context of the workplace. Under this theme, three specific aspects are considered for learners within higher education:

1 The exponential growth of lifelong learning
2 Charting the vocationalisation of learning opportunities
3 Increasing our understanding of the changing nature of work in relation to education, which is conceptualised in the notion of 'fitness to practise'.

Following on from this, innovative practice in lifelong learning is mapped as an aid to our understanding of the whole picture and the critical importance of reflexive learning is explored.

PROSPECTS FOR LEARNING

Learning is in the air we breathe and the food we eat; learning is what makes us what we are, as social beings and as members of the wider human family. Each individual must learn to be a part of the society and culture in which they grow and live, and into which they are socialised. However, the twenty-first century offers us a radically changed prospect for learning. Some say that our very existence and future depends upon our capacity to create a 'learning society' (Coffield, 1995). We are, many argue, forced to engage with the crucial issues impacting upon life, through the 'prism' of learning. This means that our understanding of how modern society is organised depends upon a different approach to how we learn, when we learn, where we learn and, vitally, how learning cannot be limited or compressed within what we know as schooling. We are moving, arguably, towards a 'learning society' but this term itself covers a large number of individual themes. We need to consider these in order to be clear about what such a concept may mean:

- The industrially developed nations throughout the world had developed mass higher education systems by the end of the twentieth century and several are predicting universal higher education for their citizens as the norm early in the twenty-first century.
- Knowledge, and 'knowledgeable workers', have come to represent a major world industry.
- A nation's economic performance can be closely related to the levels of education the majority of its people achieve.
- Lifelong learning has become a generalised 'positional good' in modern society in that learning opportunities are valued by many throughout all stages and ages of life. Many people will pay for and invest in learning for themselves, their children or their families.
- Lifelong learning embraces concern with both social policy and educational change and with personal growth and learning.
- Investment in lifelong learning is now increasingly undertaken by individuals (as it always was by adult learners) and by corporations, firms and public authorities (such as health and social welfare agencies).
- The idea of a 'graduate job' or graduate career is being replaced by the reality of a constantly moving market for a flexible and adaptable 'skills mix', where nearly all worthwhile jobs demand high levels of skill, adaptability and appropriate specialist qualifications.
- Traditional distinctions, once made between 'academic' and 'vocational' learning, are

breaking down in favour of a view that knowledge, wherever it is generated or acquired, is the key to opportunity and change, which can benefit the many rather than the few.
- Distinctions between further and higher education are disappearing as institutions such as universities and colleges seek to provide continuity and progression for their students.
- As the global economy develops, and as products, services and lifestyle choices appear to become more uniform throughout the developed world, a more commonly shared culture of knowledge and shared aspirations can be said to be emerging (although not always in predictable ways or with predictable consequences).
- As both working and learning patterns change in response to economic change, opportunities for learning are transformed. Part-time work and work-related learning, for example, have moved from the margins of concern for many employees and employers to be a central part of their businesses.

Study Activity 8.1

- Consider your own learning style and approaches; what circumstances would lead you critically to challenge traditional practice, or to accept the status quo?
- What is the purpose of using a portfolio of learning?
- What is the purpose of providing evidence of advancing your knowledge of practice within a professional portfolio?
- In your learning sets, identify the skills and knowledge required for lifelong learning. Write these up in your portfolio with supporting references.

All of these factors are part of what has been called the 'providential' part of the learning society equation (Davies, 2000). This view assumes the generally beneficial and progressive nature of learning. Learning itself, it may be argued, never harmed anyone and a vision of continuous social improvement, the growth of economic prosperity and the continuous expansion of individual opportunity are conceptually linked with the opportunities for learning throughout a person's life. Whenever we see high standards of living for the majority, civilised social welfare systems, respect for individual freedoms and an open and democratic political system, we also see mass literacy and schooling, mass access to modern communication systems and an increasing recognition that individual and collective learning must go on throughout a person's life.

Extended educational opportunity through lifelong learning is, however, not a simple panacea for the problems of modern life. As Anthony Giddens has argued, as we move into the state of society that he calls 'modernity', we are also moving into a more fragmented society, where the social bonds and shared values and traditions that held us together in the past are breaking apart or dissolving (Giddens, 1990). In contemporary society, there exists a tendency for groups to develop an identity focused on ethnicity, faith, and on 'local' factors such as regional or communal life, and these may serve to set communities apart. It has been argued that we are moving towards a more fissile and fragmented society where, under the impact of globalisation, many seek refuge in potentially destabilising social formations such as fundamentalist religious beliefs (Castells, 1997). Perceived threats to modernity are also thought to undermine the forces of stability and prosperity and include the following features:

- the impact of uneven industrial development and also de-industrialisation, where, globally, whole industries can come into existence and/or disappear within a relatively short period of time – this process is not strategically managed on a global scale but is part of a generalised 'marketisation' of productive capacity and social life, which has unpredictable consequences
- a need to manage the semi-permanent cycles of employment growth and unemployment and consequent rises in social deprivation and need
- in the heartlands of traditional industrial societies, the decay of some inner-city, urban centres, leaving a 'hollow' core of abandoned and decayed neighbourhoods
- the breakdown of law and order, where typically urban social and economic problems have erupted into violence and destruction, necessitating 'containment' and intervention, at great economic and social cost
- emerging divisions and tensions between ethnic, religious and social groups and even social movements against globalism, which have led, in many documented cases, to violence and armed conflict (Castells, 1997).

The world of learning, despite all its diversity across schooling, within further and higher education and as part of adult and continuing education, is an element in a wider social milieu. Within this we can observe both the explosion of opportunities and access to life-enhancing work and education, and a breakdown of traditional forms of social life, which once guaranteed continuity and a sense of belonging for many. Giddens (1990) has referred to this process as a 'disembedding' of personal life from the social roles and activities, which historically gave a structure to life, and offered shared understandings and meanings through commonly experienced and shared lifestyles and cultures. It involved the acceptance of traditional authorities – people and institutions whose word was authoritative and was accepted as such. In the modern world, however, there is unlikely to be any such source of unchallenged authority. We experience many sources and types of ideas and explanations of our behaviour and life patterns. Modern electronic communications enable us, for example, to find many diverse sources of information and knowledge on almost any aspect of modern or past life. Giddens argues that we now have a world of 'multiple authorities', where the traditional and monopolistic sources of authority, which delivered common experiences and expectations in the past, have broken down in the present. The 'reflexive modernity' of today's 'risk society' (Giddens, 1990, 1991; Beck, 1992) involves an increasing knowledge-based capacity for intervening in the world's social, economic and political problems, but also leads to new risks and uncertainties.

Clearly, modern social reality offers no single explanation or model for the plethora of perspectives on how life might be lived. We can safely say that it is a matter of contested terrain. What is clear is the fact that learning occupies a central place in the growth and sustained existence of modern economies. The needs of modern economic and social systems for highly educated and skilled labour are matched by the personal and professional demands made by individuals themselves for expanded and flexible learning opportunities. This imbrication of the social and individual levels of expectation signals the eventual end of some divisions that have bedevilled education for many generations. These are the distinctions once held to be valid between education and training, and between what was thought to be 'vocational' (in other words, involving skills acquisition) and 'professional' education (in other words, the education thought necessary to follow a profession). The compartmentalisation or separation of learning for work or at work, from learning for individual self-development, is breaking down. This is happening as the capacity for lifelong learning evolves and transforms the aspirations of millions who in the past would have had no such expectations of access or use for such learning. Teachers and providers of learning are confronted by new techniques and methods of learning through a myriad of information and communication tools, such as mobile phones, digital recording and video, interactive computing and wireless technology, and the massive release of resources through the Internet. This vast range of technical resources can only continue to expand exponentially, and the challenge of change is therefore a tangible reality for teachers and learners.

LIFELONG LEARNING

Learners in higher education

A key objective for the growth of opportunities in the UK has been the improvement of social life, which, it is argued, results from an increase in the type and range of students successfully entering and completing higher-level education. All sections of the community have been involved in this, but particular groups have been targeted, including mature people, members of ethnic groups, women and employees needing re-skilling. Nursing has been at the forefront of these developments, encouraging a wider access and increasing the percentage of mature individuals through pre-registration programmes. With nursing's assimilation to higher education, nurses have been able to influence the dynamics of change within higher educational structures, which have in turn recognised the needs for professional nursing practice and professional award.

Of course, such changes are not the sole influence on nursing; the higher education system has also been influenced by political and economic factors and it is now able to offer a variety of contexts from which both younger learners and mature adults can benefit. Educational variety through an increased diversity of academic programmes is available by subject, award, mode of study and location. Broader learning programmes based on generic skills as well as academic subject knowledge are available, as are a variety of staged awards achieved by students demonstrating effective performance rather than by length of the period of study. Continuing education offers opportunities for flexible and accessible study, increasingly linked to accredited courses. Educational mobility and exchange are now realities offering transfer between levels of achievement and across the learning experiences of differing sectors of provision and institutions and even across national boundaries (Robertson, 1994).

These developments signal a radical change for higher education, which must re-shape and re-conceptualise its conventional courses. This part of the chapter attempts to chart some of the processes and demands involved in these changes, especially in respect of modular and credit-based academic courses, which are often delivered off-campus and in work-based situations.

Study Activity 8.2 ⎯⎯⎯⎯⎯⎯

- Examine curricula opportunities within your local higher education providers and identify those that have a work-based activity and any programmes that are delivered through the process of accreditation.
- Identify the advantages and disadvantages of a work-based learning curriculum.
- Compare your list of programmes for nursing with such learning experiences for other student groups.

⎯⎯⎯⎯⎯⎯⎯⎯⎯⎯⎯⎯

The response of British universities to the growth of demand for learning has been varied, with some developing towards becoming lifelong learning centres. On the other hand, it can hardly be denied that much that is new and innovative flourishes on the margins of institutional activity rather than at the centre. The argument is, essentially, that the contours of a new paradigm can be seen to be emerging in higher education, connecting what might appear to be disparate areas. These include the university's role as a centre of recurrent learning and teaching, its role within a regional community and the variable pacing of study and flexibility in course provision that it offers to its students. The key to these developments is access, by which is meant the widening of participation via 'Access' schemes, the development of credit accumulation and transfer schemes (CATS), the modularisation of courses enabling greater student choice and the onset of new technologically-based learning systems such as that offered by the Internet. All of this has occurred in the context of an expansion of professional and vocational education on campus and within a wide variety of workplaces. Both the rise in attainments and the expectations of mature adult students have been matched by a growth in the number of students requiring qualifications and/ or formal recognition of their learning achievements. Many such students are almost exclusively off-campus in terms of their physical or geographical location, studying in local neighbourhood centres, and have, until very recently, been viewed as a marginal cohort of university students.

For pre-qualifying health care practitioners the model is similarly reflected, with the new models and attitudes to learning challenging traditional teaching and learning models. Current curricula in response to *Making a Difference* (Department of Health, 1999) have enabled universities to embrace much more flexibility, with 'stepping on' and 'stepping off' programmes, which allow students to leave the course for a period of time and return at a later date.

Vocation and work

In the UK, the growth of a mass-entry higher education sector is based on increasing vocationalism and specialisation. It challenges previous concepts of the university's role by incorporating a broad range of learners at several levels of previous education, and offers higher learning to many who were previously excluded.

This new provision is for people well beyond the traditional categories of age and qualification. It represents a response that corresponds to the changing nature of employment, leisure and social patterns, which are themselves part of a constantly changing labour market.

The intention here is to signal some key aspects of this process. There is little doubt that fundamental changes are taking place in the labour markets of western societies, and that these have great significance for education. We are now in a 'Post-Fordist' (Piore and Sabel, 1984; Scott, 1998) and modernising society, where the pioneering mass production techniques of the Ford Motor Company, first used to manufacture cars in the 1920s and 30s, are declining due to technological developments. Manufacturing industry has a diminishing role, service sector industries are growing, old skills barriers in the workforce are breaking down and new divisions between 'core' and 'peripheral' workers are being created. New forms of work and integration of productive processes are being created by the growth of the global economy (Giddens, 1990; Sherman, 1995; Castells, 1996).

These changes demand new responses from educators; a flexible relationship between work and education is called for, which is more creative and less divisive than the vocationalist perspective prevalent in the 1980s and 90s. The imperatives of modernisation imply the coming together of education for personal growth and education for work. It is work that connects us with so many aspects of our market-oriented, consumer-driven society, with its emphasis on personal satisfactions and life chances.

The end of work (as we know it?)

The nature of work as we know it is undergoing profound change. Work for many people is no longer simply about the nature of occupations, the labour market and employment. Rather, it is about the way in which individuals transform themselves and their environment both practically and intellectually, through creative and fulfilling activity. Work is increasingly about how 'knowledge' comes to be defined as 'useful' and education itself is increasingly viewed as a form of work, which can lead to self-realisation and self-fulfilment at an individual and existential level (Teare *et al.*, 1998; Davies, 2000).

For developed industrial societies, the movement from labour-intensive production to capital-intensive high technology has profound implications for employment and the organisation and distribution of work. Job loss, de-skilling of individuals and whole groups of people, the emergence of temporary work on a permanent basis, and the emergence of career loss and executive unemployment all signal the need for a different approach to education in respect of work and career in modern society (Sherman, 1995).

With regard to educational institutions such as schools and universities, work can no longer be seen as something that happens at a later stage in life. Increasingly the higher education curriculum is embracing the world of work. The meaning of work is shifting under these new circumstances, which demand learning renewal throughout a working life. Such learning is, increasingly, focused on work itself and is 'action learning' in that it involves 'real time' and 'real place' problem solving. Work as an educational principle (Wittmann, 1989) is being increasingly recognised so that knowledge and practice are being brought together to form a new curriculum. Knowledge is being constructed by learners in ever more open systems rather than being assimilated through existing subjects and modes of delivery in conventional educational settings.

Work is increasingly the site where pre-formulated and 'textbook' knowledge is being transformed into new knowledge and where new paradigms for knowing and learning are emerging. Perhaps this is not so surprising if we see new knowledge as part of a task and problem-solving environment, where an individual's own lifestyle, understood as a 'reflexive project' (Giddens, 1992), may need to be developed. Work is the site where the learner must be a primary actor, acting on the conditions and opportunities that shape experience and personal opportunity and identity. This perspective is 'constructivist' and places the management of self-learning competence at the centre of educational development (Scott, 1998; Teare *et al.*, 1998).

In practical terms in the world of work, this means that companies have now set great value on corporate learning. Increasingly they are declaring themselves to be learning organisations, which actively seek to identify the high-level competencies upon which success in a competitive economic environment depends. Work-based learning is now seen as a means of capturing corporate learning and its recognition by the academy is increasingly demanded. The learning organisation generates knowledge of its own practice as well as its own product. Such knowledge requires academic and professional recognition, which is the point of contact and interface between the world of corporate learning and that of higher education. It is where the credit given for learning achievement crosses the boundary between work and education.

Study Activity 8.3 _____

- Investigate how many Primary Care Trusts and Acute Trusts are also labelled as Educational Trusts.
- Examine their educational portfolio and see if they fit with the notion of advancing clinical practice.
- How many of their programmes are accredited by the local university?
- Reflect on your understanding of work-based learning, CATS, advanced standing and modular curricula.

Work can be viewed as part of a 'progressive' curriculum and it must be stressed that work is no longer viewed by many just as paid employment. Work is about future employment in the labour market but it is also about work as leisure, work in the home, gift work, voluntary work, and self-employment. If we look at work in this way, then we need to conceptualise work as a new way of looking at the curriculum, which includes all these aspects as the basis for the development of knowledge, understanding, skills and qualifications.

Indeed, work is central to how personal identities are constructed in modern life. The nature and organisation of work is a key structural feature of our social system, which, however, distributes educational access unevenly and unequally. It is a generalisation, but contemporary society everywhere appears to demand greater expertise and professionalism in an era of continuous economic de-construction/re-construction and its attendant threat of mass unemployment and social instability.

This is the overall context of socio-economic trends of our times, in which the skill-based and knowledge-based functions of lifelong learning and post-school provision have been expanding. The response to the demands of new technology, and the need of masses of individuals to adapt to the changing nature of work and the ever-evolving division of labour, help to account for the uptake of opportunities in both the liberal learning tradition and the vocational education sector. This is an agenda for change shared by the 'vocational' further and higher education providers – and their basis is worldwide, since no modern economy is isolated from the effects of economic and cultural globalisation.

Study Activity 8.4 _____

- Consider the impact of a globalised educational service in respect of:

  - the individual
  - the team
  - the organisation
  - global health care
  - ethical dimensions.

- Consider how far the new modern and dependable NHS has come with regards to learning opportunities and widening access for all.

EDUCATIONAL INNOVATION

Our understanding of what is happening in the world of work and learning may lead us to be critical of the professionalisation and specialisation of academic life and to wish to re-assert the values of the older academy and of the validity of separate and unequal provision. Alternatively, this issue may force us to define new and emergent values, which allow us a culture of inclusion for the world of higher education on a basis other than specialisation and expanded vocationalism. The populations and individuals who now participate in this learning culture have emerged into the stream of higher and further education provision in the UK in recent years, and there is now mass participation – but participation in what and to what eventual end? These questions signal a continuous debate about educational change and innovation.

The start of the twenty-first century has seen an explosion of innovative teaching and learning systems, which have been at the heart of post-school education (Davies, 1997). In one sense the development of 'Access' and accessibility to further, adult and higher education has been co-terminus with the increased openness, flexibility and responsiveness to a wide variety of student learning needs; these needs were poorly served and largely invisible in previous eras.

The flexibility available to students is a touch-stone for identifying the different levels at which innovation and change occur. Innovative systems use flexibility and responsiveness to meet the specific need of individuals. It is inconceivable, for example, that the flexible needs of indivi-duals will be met without innovation in manage-ment, financial, personnel, quality and curricular systems and practices.

The flexibility available to students can be separated into two fundamental categories (Spencer and Wynne, 1990). The first is that of open access arrangements, which have been targeted at students for whom conventional qualifications for entry to higher education have been thought to be appropriate. There has been a huge expansion of 'Access' courses within the last five years with much provision being made by the British further education sector and by conventional 'old' and 'new' universities. The second category concerns schemes that allow students to choose the pace of study and to negotiate significant parts of the curriculum for themselves.

There is an increasing demand for learning situations that give students genuine flexibility and have organisational procedures that facilitate its growth. Student choice and flexible methods of acquiring and using knowledge are at the centre of educational innovation.

The framework shown in Table 8.1 (overleaf) is an attempt to bring into a diagrammatic form the major dimensions of innovation and learning.

The distinctive – perhaps unique – feature under scrutiny here is the credence given to student-centred learning. In this view, learning is student-centred not only in terms of allowing students some control over curricula and teaching methods, but also in what Squires calls the 'profound' sense: that is to say, the whole activity of education turns on the student, rather than on the organisation of the curriculum or on the formal certification of learning (Squires, 1987). This approach yields a number of possible components of individual and collective experience:

- adult learning
- adult thinking
- adulthood itself, and
- adult development.

These components can contribute to the indica-tors of flexibility and innovation. The first is concerned with the way in which teaching and learning occurs with adults, and is distinctive. The second is concerned with the kind of 'dialectical' and transformative thinking of which adults are capable, while the third and fourth categories are focused on adulthood itself, its roles and life experiences.

The implications of this are that the curri-culum for lifelong learning and the learning society is more diverse than anything that precedes it in the formal system of schooling and in further and higher education. This diversity supersedes the limitations of what is taught as the formal curriculum, since everything from archaeology to zoology is included, as is personal, professional and vocational learning. The form and content of continuing, lifelong education are more diverse than those offered by any single sector of education, testing to the limit some conventional distinctions between life and learning. Experience and experiential learning are central therefore to the perceived learning outcomes and processes to be fostered. There is no possibility of role closure, where individuals can be excluded from learning by virtue of their previous experience, or lack of it.

Table 8.1 An index of innovation

From individual to social-centred provision	Curriculum content	Assessment methods	Learning	Resources	From openness to access
Recognition of individual experience	Fixed curriculum and subjects	Traditional end-of-course examination	Formal class-based-didactic	Teacher/subject	Campus-based
Recognition of group experience	Narrow choice of options	Continuous course assessment	Plus informal classes	Centrally allocated	Home-based
Accreditation of prior learning (APL)	Wide choice of options	Ad hoc testing of individual objectives	Seminars, tutorials	Interactive resources available on demand	Information technologies
Accreditation of prior experiential learning (AP(E)L)	Content negotiated by students	Self-assessment	Projects and problem solving	Resource centres – libraries	Multimedia
Recognition of potential	Modularity and inter-disciplinarity	Group assessment	Open-ended learning	Student-based	Ongoing student support
Modular system to reflect life experience	Individually negotiated programmes (experience)	Accreditation and credit accumulation and transfer schemes (CATS)	Learning outcomes demonstrated	Community resources	Output-related audit
Social-collective experience	Deconstruction of the formal curriculum	Criteria: contents, skills, personal growth	Academic, professional and vocational learning	Partnership	Work-based learning
Social transformations	New curricula and new knowledge	Personal learning statement and professional skills	Action learning/self-managed learning	Learning organisations and the illusory classroom	Virtual learning

(Adapted from Teare et al., 1998, p. 35)

Across the diversity of higher education and lifelong learning there is undoubtedly a transformation under way, building upon the growth of flexible learning opportunities and the movement for greater access to education. It is possible to discern new and emergent categories of educational experience and aspiration, though it is a far from complete process.

The charting of themes for innovation within an 'index' is a simplified and schematic device, which cannot do justice to a complex reality. Nevertheless, it may be possible to derive benefits from its use by bringing a range of potential characteristics of innovation into juxtaposition and thereby creating a repository of ideas and concepts to act as a resource for practice. This process may enable the role of teachers, schools, colleges and universities involved in innovation to be underpinned by a classification and rating of the extent and pace of change. This in turn should facilitate the application of the model as an audit mechanism, as an applied 'theoretical' framework for innovation and as a practical tool for development. An index of innovation is not a completed product, but rather an aid to thinking through common issues facing those who wish to innovate in the field of continuous learning.

Open and closed systems for learning

What kind of knowledge and learning is emerging from innovatory sites at which education is delivered? The focus of the answer to this central question is the way in which, across time and geographical space, personal learning, previously strongly connected with personal development, is now beginning to articulate with wider, professional learning, especially that related to the workplace.

Fundamentally, two contrasting viewpoints relate to the way in which we think about knowledge (Gibbons *et al.*, 1994). First, cognitive and foundational understandings of knowledge assume both the objectivity and externality of knowledge. External reality and objective facts are taken to exist and are complemented by a second cognitive entity that we commonly call the subjective self or the inner world. An alternative understanding relies on the assumption that knowledge has no absolute foundations, either internal or external. People construct knowledge out of the paradigms (Kuhn, 1970) or discourses and languages available to them, whether these are spoken languages or symbolic languages such as algebra or computer languages, or paralinguistic forms such as music and dance. Knowledge is seen as neither absolute nor universal; it is local, historically changing and has to be reconstructed time after time on the basis of lived, individual and social experience. In this sense, knowledge is understood in the dynamic of each generation and, as a result, the 'wheel of knowledge', as it were, has to be re-invented by every generation wishing to use it.

The implications of this approach for learning and teaching are significant. For example, if we assume education or learning is 'given' to learners, teachers help students to assimilate and absorb knowledge. Students perform to arrive at pre-determined answers, which are validated by the disciplinary paradigm or knowledge community to which the teacher belongs. On the other hand, if we assume teachers help students to construct or reconstruct knowledge, there are no pre-determined answers. Learners therefore can begin to break the dependency upon received wisdom and a received curriculum. This has profound implications for our concept of lifelong learning. It must now be re-connected with experience and the curriculum must reflect the 'real time' and 'real place' and 'real problems' and needs of learners. Students must be trusted to perform in ways not determined ahead of time by teachers. Their knowledge must not be disconnected from experience. It is the argument of this part of the module that such experience can be characterised as moving historically from closed to open systems, and from a monopoly of knowledge (held by the academic disciplines and their practitioners) to a shared and collaborative system of knowledge production. Perhaps surprisingly for traditional classroom-based teachers, the world of work and management development has provided some key elements of a new paradigm – that of action learning, based on the work of Revans (1982, 1984) and his followers (Wills, 1997). Here insightful questions plus requisite individual and relevant objective and corporate learning are brought together so that 'expert knowledge' is re-appropriated by ordinary people who need to gain and apply new knowledge to their everyday lives.

Innovation and diversity

The growth in diversity within British higher education can be considered in the context of growth in innovatory practices, and a key feature of this has been the emergence of credit and credit accumulation systems (Robertson, 1994; Davies, 1995). The expansion in recent years of modular schemes and qualifications frameworks can be explicated in terms of their impact on the wider learning culture and growth of mass higher education in Britain and beyond. The following sections, building upon the ideas of innovation, flexibility and 'open' learning, are intended to provide an indicative overview of some key themes of change, which are having an impact on lifelong learning, and direct attention towards a vision of greater learning opportunity.

A range of innovations has been evolving since the 1980s, particularly in Britain, including the following starting points:

- the growth of learner-centred knowledge and action learning
- the development of open systems of accreditation and the movement from 'closed' to 'open' knowledge systems
- the growing significance of adult learning (andragogy), as opposed to child-focused learning (pedagogy) and teaching methods
- the development of a national credit framework
- the growth of credit accumulation and transfer (CATS) within higher education
- modular courses and the unitisation of the curriculum
- growth of independent learning opportunities and recognition of prior learning and experience
- accreditation of previous learning and of experiential learning, known as APEL
- a focus on learning outcomes (learners) rather than on inputs (teachers)
- recognition of work and work experience as a key source of learning
- the growth of continuous learning available to all
- an increasing recognition of the need for lifetime learning opportunities and of their social and economic benefits
- the explosion of new computer-based communications technologies, which are capable of revolutionising teaching and learning practices.

These diverse, yet related, aspects of the education system have had an impact on the wider world of management development, as has the converse, where industry-based innovation has radicalised, in some cases, what further and higher education institutions do.

Perspectives on learning and teaching

The list of starting points above suggests a plethora of fruitful themes, which contribute to the shaping of learning in modern higher educa-tion. However, to grasp the way in which lifelong learning is beginning to be a reality for a mass population of learners, who will be prepared for the new and ever-evolving communications technologies, we need to consider how open learning and open systems of knowledge are merging. These open systems and the kind of knowledge they sponsor are at the heart of the current transformation of teaching and learning.

For lifelong education, debates covering the validity and nature of knowledge, and how it is to be transmitted, have had profound implications for the curriculum. This has been especially the case where formal, classroom-based didactic methods have been challenged by self-managed, action learning paradigms (Mumford, 1996).

One of these conceptions of teaching has been variously described as 'student-centred', 'progressive', or as 'open' pedagogy. The term 'pedagogy' refers to the principles and methods of teaching – the ways in which a teacher carries out the task of presenting new knowledge and experience and generally manages the learning environment. Progressive and 'open' styles of pedagogy might be seen as peculiarly character-istic of adult teaching and learning, which claims a distinctiveness of its own (Squires, 1987).

There is a historic and contemporary tension between the view that asserts the primacy of didactic teaching, with its emphasis on the trans-mission of socially desirable and approved knowledge required for the order and control necessary to preserve social life or culture, and the view that teaching is concerned with personal growth and development.

The argument is that there are two different views of classroom relationships, based in turn on two very different conceptions of the nature of teaching/learning. Disputes relating to this issue are not new. The philosophical and prac-tical elements of 'progressive' teaching methods can be traced back to the work of Dewey (1959), for instance, in the early decades of the twentieth century (Skillbeck, 1970). 'Progress-ivism' represents an expression of the liberal ideology of schooling, which has become deeply embedded in the principles of educational theory. The first approach is consistent with the view of education as necessary for establishing social control, and the successful induction of the young into the industrial-political system. The second accords with the liberal-democratic ideal, which emphasises the potential of education for personal development.

Study Activity 8.5

- Prior to entry to your nursing programme you will have experienced a range of learning and teaching strategies. List those that empowered you to be an independent learner and those that disempowered you. Give your reasons, backed up by empirical studies that enabled you to arrive at your conclusions.
- Now consider your current learning and teaching experiences. In your opinion are they student-centred? Do they offer a partnership between you the learner and your teacher? If not, can you explain the power dynamics?
- Do you encourage your teacher to be facilitative and operate a student-centred approach towards learning, or do you and your group encourage lots of hand-outs and straight delivery of knowledge?

Paradigms for teaching and tearning

Two contrasting perspectives or paradigms can be identified and used to inform debate on this issue. The traditional paradigm has fundamentally an objectivist orientation, which focuses on the *products* of learning. The second paradigm is much more orientated to the subjectivity of the student and focuses on the *processes* of learning. In their organisational forms they are sometimes described as 'closed' and 'open' types of pedagogy. These concepts refer not simply to the classroom structure in which learning takes place, but also to the boundaries between subjects and areas of teaching responsibility. In other words, they have contrasting perspectives as to what constitutes the 'proper' basis for the curriculum and what counts as knowledge.

Underlying each of the paradigms are different psychological assumptions, different conceptions of curricular knowledge and different vocabularies and beliefs about the status of the student in the interaction of the classroom. They contain different conceptions of teaching and learning. They also offer very different possibilities for learner identity.

The closed or conventional paradigm

Within this paradigm, ability is viewed as the result of a number of prior 'factors' in the genetic make-up and personality of the individual. These factors are not really known, but it was thought that their effects could be 'scientifically' assessed through intelligence (IQ, or intelligence quotient) tests, which were thought to provide an 'objective' measure of ability. IQ is not necessarily static; it is generally conceded and may vary over a limited range.

Under the premise of this paradigm, achievement is defined in terms of mastery of specific bodies of knowledge, which are mapped out to coincide with particular stages of the learning career. It is the task of the teacher to arrange and present these bodies of knowledge to students. The focus of interest of the teaching tends to be in the products of learning – not in the process. Learning is thought to be most effective when a teacher-expert, who knows the subject matter, structures and imparts it to those who do not. The higher status of the teacher is maintained during interaction by a teacher's definition (taken for granted) of what counts as 'worthwhile knowledge', and the teacher's right to exclude what is not.

The classroom interaction that embodies the principles of this paradigm reflects an 'objective' view of both knowledge and the student. The teacher imparts knowledge to recipient learners. Learning is collective in the sense that a nominal pace, sequence and structure for the subject content of a lesson are imposed on all the students in the group together.

The open paradigm

A different paradigm has emerged in opposition. One version of this is rooted in the social sciences and takes as its central concern the power of the mind to organise experience and meaning. This paradigm emphasises an active rather than a static notion of the mind. The processes of thought are not taken to be reducible simply to the possession of 'intelligence', nor to the performance of standardised routines characteristic of, for example, IQ tests. They are, instead, seen to be part of a highly complex personal system of interpretations, intentions and recollections. This paradigm upholds a view that cognition is a growth process and that the mind is capable of unlimited development.

This could be described as the phenomenological or humanistic paradigm. Deriving from a philosophical tradition, which differs in a number of respects from the positivistic tradition (Mead, 1962; Allen, 1975), it has become established in several areas of social scientific enquiry. In educational psychology, its major representatives have been Jean Piaget (1955), George Kelly (1955), Jerome Bruner (1962, 1968) and each of whom has been involved in exploring theoretically and empirically the constructive processes of the mind. The work of Malcolm Knowles (1970, 1981, 1983) applied a similar perspective to the theme of adult learning and teaching, or what became known as andragogy. It is not possible to memorise here even a fraction of the work of these social theorists and psychologists. However, they do have a particular orientation towards the study of human society and humankind – one that is concerned with the ways in which subjective experience is ordered and understood.

The main focus of this paradigm rests on the processes of knowing and the learner's organisation of meaning into larger schemes of knowledge and experience. This kind of enquiry has led to a view of learning in which the structuring of knowledge and the processes by which it is acquired are seen to be fundamental to the development of understanding. For the teacher, the essential problem is to understand the logic of the learner's processes of knowing – to understand how the learner interprets and accommodates new knowledge. The relationship between the structures of meaning that the learner habi-

tually uses and the structures that are presented by the teacher is critical.

A central part of the argument asserts that, because all knowledge is external to the self, its meaning has to be reconstructed in terms of the life-world and the existence of the individual approaching it. In other words, it needs an 'internal dimension'.

As an aspect of her 'phenomenological' viewpoint, Maxine Green (1971) suggested that any act or process of learning involves three distinct states of consciousness: disclosure, reconstruction and generation. The act of disclosure is the bringing of self to the object to be learned; reconstruction is the process of interpretation whereby the newly acquired knowledge becomes incorporated with existing knowledge; generation refers to the creative potential that arises in the fusion of the two.

Learner-centred perspectives

The learning and teaching interaction that follows from an acceptance of a broadly conceived 'phenomenological' paradigm is likely to allow the learner more control than the alternative 'closed' paradigm over structuring the learning process and experience. The teacher is more of a guide than an instructor. Expertise is seen to reside in the ability to stimulate learning rather than in the communication of a body of knowledge. The individual is given or takes increased responsibility for his or her own learning.

The prevalence of the 'closed' pedagogy in many educational institutions is particularly due to the reification of subject specialism, as well as departmental separation based on subject expertise. This can lead in the context of higher education to the magnification and inflation of the content of specialist subjects. By pursuing individual interest, however, the learner is very likely to move into areas of knowledge that do not fit conveniently into existing curriculum subjects and specialism. This perspective leads us to consider the significance of choice and of the 'thinking student' in the development of teaching and learning strategies. The development of open systems and lifelong learning appears to sponsor the growth of an open and 'liberal' approach to what can be learned, with the students' choice playing an increasingly significant role.

In the open pedagogy paradigm, the teacher's status as the provider of knowledge is significantly reduced. Control by the teacher is potentially weakened and the learner gains much more control over the pace of learning. The paradox is, however, of the existence of a liberal pedagogy in a wider hierarchical social structure and educational system, which may contradict most of the principles of open access to learning.

Applying the 'open' paradigm

The belief that alternative methods of teaching and learning are particularly appropriate to lifelong learners has found expression in several different yet related contexts. The work of Malcolm Knowles (1981, 1983) and Carl Rogers (1974) focused on adult learners' own projects for learning; Reg Revans (1982, 1984) explored action learning and stimulated the foundation of global business-orientated 'open learning' (Wills, 1997); the Open University gave impetus and organisational form to mass 'open' higher education; and the concept of independent learning (Spencer and Wynne, 1990) connected with the emerging notion of 'Access'. This wide process, embracing many streams of change, involved essentially a de-constructed curriculum, which questioned the authority of traditional knowledge and asserted that knowledge was something that could be constructed independently, between learners and teachers (Bruffee, 1995). Above all, these developments chart the recognition of the fact that there is now in existence what Teare (1998) refers to as the 'dynamic curriculum'. This curriculum embraces the open paradigm; its pedagogy is similarly open to student experience and it insists that knowledge is crafted from learning experiences, wherever and whenever these occur. Since the role of work and the need for lifelong, work-related learning has changed so radically for so many people, surely the time has come for the notion of a dynamic curriculum!

LIFELONG LEARNING AND REFLEXIVE THINKING

Adult learners

The 'macro' theme of this chapter concerns lifelong learning, which can be taken to refer to the undoubted potential we all have to acquire learning from the cradle to the grave. It is often assumed that learning is most beneficially and easily acquired by the young and, until recently, formal learning, including schools, colleges and universities, has been devoted almost exclusively to children and young people. However, there is a body of writing, research and evidence that points to the specific importance of the way in which adults learn. Gagne (1965) and Wilson (1980) have assessed theories of learning, based respectively within biological and psychological 'conditioning' paradigms, while Bruner (1962, 1968) focused his work on the way learners organise their conceptual and cognitive experiences. These are only three from many competing and sometimes complementary perspectives, most of which do not address the specific nature of adult learning.

Following the work of Knowles (1981), it is possible to identify four major assumptions that distinguish adult learning from childhood learning:

1 As 'lifelong learners', adults have a strong need to be self-directing. As we get older the self-concept moves from dependency on others to self-direction and autonomy.
2 Maturity brings experience, which is a resource for learning.
3 As life proceeds, readiness to learn becomes associated with a person's social role. We therefore internalise learning needs in response to our need to know, and not because we are told to learn.

4 As a person grows older and matures, problem- or project-centred learning takes over from subject-centred learning.

If it is assumed that there is a distinctive pattern of adult learning over the life span of an individual, then there are implications for the way in which that learning should be organised. The following principles are therefore required to be embodied within the social learning process for adults and they will shape the conditions under which lifelong learning can flourish:

- Adult learners are less dependent upon teachers as they get older. They are more self-reliant and develop self-learning competency; they can decide on their own direction for learning and become more autonomous.
- Individual differences need to be acknowledged. A learning group will always have a range of abilities, which can be both a benefit and a problem in a learning situation.
- Whenever new knowledge is acquired it has to be adapted to and assimilated with existing knowledge. The recognition of existing knowledge and experience in all its potential variety represents a challenge to teachers and learners.
- Learners in later stages of life require rewards and recognition for their achievements. These may vary, but where failure has previously been encountered, individuals may need to have positive reinforcement.
- Active learning and practice and participation should characterise adult learning. At later life stages, time for learning may be at a premium and the sequencing and organisation of learning periods needs to be highly relevant to the learner.
- Students who have experienced previous failure or simply indifference to learning may require sensitive and appropriate guidance. The significance of personal experience cannot be ignored, but it may provide challenges to the assimilation of new knowledge.
- Adult learners display a greater range and stability of cognitive structure and experience

which in turn makes them more likely to adopt idiosyncratic approaches to learning. Getting adults to focus on learning techniques is important and these must be meaningful if they are to be effective aids to learning and motivation.

The concept of knowledge embodied in adult and lifelong learning insists that thinking and understanding develop as people interact, consciously and critically, in their social context. It insists that there is no fixed or final stage of development and that the teacher-learner relationship is changed within an andragogical approach to learning. There are thus hugely significant implications for continuing learning and higher education when we consider that knowledge quickly becomes out-dated and that the context in which it applies rapidly changes. Where there is continuous change, there must also be continuous learning. The learning society that is emerging will enjoin us actively and consciously to lead these developments, as subjects in the process, rather than as objects in a process beyond and outside our understanding and control. If the learning society is to deliver its promise in full it must surely do so through an open and innovative set of values and practices, which are of concrete use and value to learners.

Reflexive learning

The theme of lifelong learning incorporates many facets of education and study. One central theme has been that of individual, reflexive activity, undertaken in a variety of settings, sites and contexts. Experience is always a combination of individual and social aspects of life, interacting and being in dynamic tension with one another. However, it is when experience is reflected upon in an 'adult' context that change takes place. Anthony Giddens captures this idea of learning as follows:

The reflexivity of modern life consists in the fact that social priorities are constantly examined and reformed in the light of

> *incoming information about those very priorities, thus constitutively altering their character . . . . In all cultures, social priorities are routinely altered in the light of on-going discoveries, which feed into them. But only the era of modernity is the revision of convention radicalised to apply (in principle) to all aspects of human life.*
>
> (Giddens, 1990)

The argument is that thinking in and about everyday life, in work or in the home or in the classroom, can be a radical experience. It is also apparent that, in modern society, institutional reflexivity is a key to the way in which life and human action is organised and experienced.

Reflexivity is central to an understanding of lifelong learning, but we need to grasp its meaning within the contexts outlined earlier. As society fragments and becomes increasingly differentiated and individualised, and as more aspects of life are marketised and become part of a globalising cash nexus, then aspects of social and collective or community life are transformed and, in some cases, abandoned. As more and more individuals seek 'edutainment', in self-instructional videos, fitness and body training centres and computer-based individual learning, there may be less and less engagement with organisations devoted previously to broad social aims and improvement.

The value of the reflexive, autonomous learner is therefore paramount and we need to conceive of learners creating knowledge in a learning society, which demolishes the barriers to learning. The school or college can no longer be the epicentre of learning it once was. Formal institutions of learning now compete with informal and 'edutainment' learning via fax, journals, TV, radio, video, text messaging, satellite broadcasting and a panoply of multimedia gadgets and Internet-based data, and entertainment.

These developments throw into relief the historical privileging of teaching rather than learning. Under the new learning opportunities, teaching has become more pro-active and learner-centred in order to retain its impact and potency. Teachers need therefore to be creators of support systems for autonomous and reflexive learners. The ways in which individuals learn, and transmit to each other what they have learned, becomes a vital element of a learning society. Personal autonomy, choice and the application of reasoned and critical insightful questioning do not arrive simply on time, like the daily rising of the sun. It is always part of a struggle to create and transmit understanding and meaning in social life.

It seems self-evident that the current freedoms and autonomy on offer demand committed learners who are themselves prepared to sacrifice some of their autonomy and choice, for the rewards of longer term achievement. As we move towards the reality of lifelong learning, and can see the outlines of a learning society emerging, we may need to admit to ourselves that we are all apprentices in the learning game. The chances of achieving mastery, however, are greater for most people than they have ever been.

REFERENCES

Allen, V.L. (1975) *Social Analysis*, Longman, Harlow

Beck, U. (1992) *Risk Society: Towards a new modernity*, Sage, London

Bruffee, K.A. (1995) *Collaborative Learning: Higher education, independence and the authority of knowledge*, John Hopkins University Press, Baltimore, MA

Bruner, J. (1962) *On Knowing*, Harvard University Press, Cambridge, MASS

Bruner, J. (1968) *Toward a Theory of Instruction*, Norton, New York

Castells, M. (1996) *The Rise of the Network Society*, Blackwell, Oxford

Castells, M. (1997) *The Power of Identity, Volume II: The information age – economy, society and culture*, Blackwell, Oxford

Coffield, F. (ed.) (1995) *Higher Education in a Learning Society*, University of Durham on behalf of DFEE, ERSC and HEFKIE, Durham

Davies, D. (1995) *Credit Where It's Due*, University

of Cambridge/Employment Department, Cambridge

Davies, D. (1997) From the further education margins to the higher education centre? *Education and Training* 39(1)

Davies, D. (2000) Lifelong learning in a global society; providential or pathological? In: Thomas, L. and Cooper, M. (eds.) (2000) *Changing the Culture of the Campus*, Staffordshire University Press, Keele

Department of Health (1999) *Making a Difference*, The Stationary Office, London

Department of Health (2000) *The National Health Service Ten-year Plan*, DoH, London

Department of Health (2001) *Working Together – Learning Together: A framework for lifelong learning for the NHS*, DoH, London

Dewey, J. (1959) The child and the curriculum, In: Dworkin, M.S. (ed.) *Dewey on Education*, Teachers College Bureau of Publication, New York, p. 91

English National Board (1994) *Creating Lifelong Learners*, ENB, London

Gagne, R.M. (1965) *The Conditions of Learning*, Holt Rheinhard and Winston, New York

Gibbons, M., Limoges, C., Nowotny, H. *et al.* (1994) *The New Production of Knowledge: The dynamics of science and research in contemporary societies*, Sage, London

Giddens, A. (1990) *The Consequences of Modernity*, Polity Press, Cambridge

Giddens, A. (1991) *Modernity and Self Identity*, Polity Press, Cambridge

Giddens, A. (1992) *The Transformation of Intimacy*, Polity Press, Cambridge

Green, M. (1971) Curriculum and consciousness. *Teachers College Record* 73(2), December 1971, Columbia University, New York

Kelly, G. (1955) *The Psychology of Personal Constructs*, Volumes 1 and 2, Norton, New York

Knowles, M. (1970) *The Modern Practice of Adult Education*, Associated Press, New York

Knowles, M. (1981) *The Adult Learner: A neglected species*, Gulf, Houston, TX

Knowles, M. (1983) An andragogical theory of adult learning. In: *Learning about Learning: Selected readings*, Open University Press, Milton Keynes

Kuhn, T. (1970) *The Structure of Scientific Revolutions*, University of Chicago Press, Chicago, IL

Mead, G.H. (1962) *Mind, Self and Society*, University Chicago Press, Chicago, IL

Mumford, A. (1996) Creating a learning environment. *Journal of Professional Human Resource Management*, July 1996

Piaget, J. (1955) *The Construction of Reality in the Child*, Routledge and Kegan Paul, London

Piore, M. and Sabel, C.F. (1984) *The Second Industrial Divide: Possibilities for property*, Basic Books, New York

Revans, R. (1982) *The Origins of Growth of Action Learning*, Chartwell Bratt

Revans, R. (1984) *The Sequence of Managerial Achievement*, MCB University Press, Bradford

Robertson, D. (1994) *Choosing to Change: Extending access, choice and mobility*, HEQC, London

Rogers, C. (1974) *On Becoming a Person*, Constable, London

Scott, P. (1998) Mass higher education: a new civilisation. In: Jary, D. and Parker, M. (eds) (1998) *The New Higher Education: Issues and directions for the Post Dearing University*, Staffordshire University Press, Keele

Sherman, B. (1995) *Licensed to Work*, Cassell, London

Skillbeck, M. (1970) *John Dewey*, Collier Macmillan, London

Spencer, D. and Wynne, R. (1990) *Embedding Learner Autonomy in Further Education in Wales*, WJEC, Cardiff

Squires, G. (1987) *The Curriculum Beyond School*, Hodder and Stoughton, London

Teare, R. (1998) *Developing a Curriculum for Organisational Learning*, MCB University Press, Bradford

Teare, R., Davies, D. and Sandelands, E. (1998) *The Virtual University*, Cassell, London

UKCC (1994) *Continuing Professional Standards for Nurses, Midwives and Health Visitors*, UKCC, London

Wills, G. (1997) *Engendering Democratic Action*, MCB University Press, Bradford

Wilson, J.P. (1980) Individual learning in groups. In: Boyd, R.D., Apps, J.W. *et al.* (eds), *Redefining the Discipline of Adult Education*, Jossey Bass, San Francisco, CA

Wittmann, L.C. (1989) *Working Class Education: Towards a relevant relationship between work and education*, University of London Institute of Education, London

FURTHER READING

Department for Education and Skills (2001) *Education and Skills: Delivering results. A strategy to 2006*, Annex C, DfES Publications, Suffolk

Finegold, D. *et al.* (1992) *Higher Education – Expansion and reform*, IPPR, London

House, D. (1991) *Continuing Liberal Education*, NUCEA, New York

Perkins, H. (1990) *The Rise of Professional Society: England since 1880*, Routledge, London

Spours, K. and Young, M. (1988) *Beyond Vocationalism*, University Institute of Education, London

MODULE 2: THE PROFESSIONAL DISCIPLINE OF NURSING

REFLECTIONS

Through reading the scholarly musings in Module 2 you will have gained a useful insight into the demands of being a member of the nursing profession, which requires you to take responsibility for your learning at the point of entry to the profession and throughout your professional career. Current governmental policies have called for all professional groups to work within a framework of evidence-based practice, which is underpinned by continuing professional development, lifelong learning and clinical supervision. The essence of all of this is to ensure that all health care professionals operate within frameworks of clinical governance that assure clinical competence and the provision of quality health care.

So far you will have gained knowledge and understanding of the political and theoretical frameworks that relate to these issues. It is, however, essential that you gain the necessary skills of lifelong learning, acknowledge your knowledge and skills deficit and seek to amend this through continuing professional development and through meaningful and wise clinical supervision, which will facilitate your ability to reflect in and on your practice. In addition, the use of your professional portfolio can become a conduit that enables you to advance your level of knowledge and skill congruent with your roles and responsibilities.

Having gained the knowledge and skills discussed throughout Module 2 you are now set to advance your own learning and professional development in the true knowledge that you are fit and competent to practise.

MODULE 3: THE PILOSOPHICAL AND THEORETICAL BASIS OF NURSING

INTRODUCTION

In this module, it is fully recognised that while knowledge does inform our practice, that practice in turn also informs the knowledge of nursing. However, notwithstanding this recognition, it is vitally important to recognise that there is a growing body of best available knowledge at any given time, constantly being modified, refined and extended, that informs practice. Indeed, this provides the basis for our practice, even though it is constantly subject to challenge and review, not least by that very practice it informs. Keep this in mind as you read through the chapters in this module.

To provide information about knowledge, it is necessary to address the nature of knowledge and how it relates to nursing. To do this, it is necessary to adopt an approach that 'breaks' consideration of this knowledge into manageable 'chunks'. However, this is not how knowl

edge 'exists' in practice. There, within each nursing act, different elements of knowing come to bear upon the practice and are in turn influenced by that practice. Patterns do exist, such that we can see similarities between situations and make predictions about how we must respond. But it is also important to recognise that each nursing situation has its own uniqueness. We know that practice is a dynamic and developing phenomenon. Not only does knowledge influence practice and is in turn influenced by that practice, but the knowledge and practice that is integrated in this way today are different to the knowledge and practice which will be integrated next year or even next week. As you read this module, remember that although knowledge and its different forms are presented to you here in a sequential and structured way, it is a necessary step towards ultimately understanding that knowledge and practice are integrated.

9

AN EPISTEMOLOGY OF NURSING: WAYS OF KNOWING AND BEING

Oliver Slevin

> *You must keep your knowledge and skills up-to-date throughout your working life. In particular, you should take part regularly in learning activities that develop your competence and performance.*
>
> *To practice competently, you must possess the knowledge, skills and abilities required for lawful, safe and effective practice without direct supervision. You must acknowledge the limits of your professional competence and only undertake practice and accept responsibilities for those activities in which you are competent.*
>
> (Nursing and Midwifery Council, 2002)

LEARNING OUTCOMES

After studying this chapter you will be able to:
- Explain the term 'epistemology' and demonstrate the importance to nursing of establishing its own practical epistemology
- Define the term 'knowledge' and relate this to nursing
- Outline how knowledge is constructed and justified
- Describe the elements that make up the nursing metaparadigm and thereby identify the parameters of nursing knowledge
- Provide a definition of nursing in the context of its main metaparadigm
- Discuss the different patterns or ways of knowing that may inform the practice of nursing.

INTRODUCTION

When you get out there, you had better know what you are doing. As a reader of this book you are probably either preparing to be a member of the nursing profession, or you are already a practitioner. We have already discussed professionalisation and nursing as a profession in Module 2. In the modern world, the meaning of the term profession has broadened and its features are less sharply defined. Nowadays members of all occupational groups would claim to function as professionals. Irrespective of the status, and arguments about whether this is a legitimate claim, there is one fact we can hold to. When you say you are a professional, you are in effect saying the words 'I profess'. This phrase means, 'I proclaim', or 'I confirm', or 'I assert'. As nurses, we are in effect saying 'I *know* how to care for you, and I am *competent* in this activity'.

This is what marks off any profession (in the classical sense of this term) from any other occupational group. It is the fact that there is a claim to be able to serve by virtue of expertise and competence. This is a special expertise and competence that only the particular profession can provide, safely and to a high quality. Others who are not in membership of a profession may claim to be able to *do* law, or *do* medicine, or *do* nursing. Indeed, this may be to a greater or lesser extent true. But they would seldom be able to claim the profession's level of knowledge and proficiency. Nor would they be recognised through any social, regulatory or legal contract as meeting such guaranteed levels of knowledge and proficiency. The need of society for such guaranteed expert knowledge and skill is in effect the profession's *raison d'être*, its reason for being. The above opening quotation, from the current UK Code of Professional Conduct (Nursing and Midwifery Council, 2002) for all nurses and midwives states this requirement as a regulatory imperative. If you cannot live up to this requirement, you cannot practise as a nurse or midwife.

This requirement, to be in some way *knowledgeable*, does of course beg some questions. What *is* this knowledge that we require? What forms does it take, how much of it do we need to know, and what ways can we put it to use? These are the matters we address in this chapter.

There is one final opening consideration. As a statement on epistemology, this chapter is a little unusual. Knowing is, as we shall discuss below, a cognitive process. That is, it involves mental processes of a 'rational' or 'reasoning' nature. A case has been made, and indeed extensively argued, that a very rational, logical, objective and almost clinical approach to knowledge construction is a masculine trait. Indeed, so strong is this orientation, that the commonly used thesauruses give as synonyms for the word 'clinical', words such as dispassionate, disinterested, detached, disengaged, scientific, quantifiable, etc. On this basis, it has been suggested that there are alternative ways of coming to know that are subjective and passionate, contextual and engaged, and that stress experiential and intuitive ways of coming to know. It has been suggested that these alternative approaches to knowledge reflect a feminine trait. This begs the question of the possibility of a *feminist* epistemology, a case that is addressed by a number of authors, e.g. Gilligan (1982), Longino (1990), Code (1991), Lazreg (1994), Hartsock (1997) and Jagger (1997). One of these authors (Hartsock) has proposed a 'standpoint' theory, alluding to ways of looking at the world, and identifying a specifically feminist standpoint (in this chapter, the metaphor of lenses and how we view the world through a particular lens is used as a similar device). This chapter does not identify any allegiances to either of these apparently opposing positions. But it does (perhaps unusually) address them, and it does present a case for a more inclusive approach.

EPISTEMOLOGY: A FIRST GLANCE

The term is one of those words that puts almost everyone off. Most people cannot even pronounce it (it should sound something like *epp-iss-tem-ology*). However, it is vitally important for all that. Furthermore, as a term it is clear, concise and useful. It derives from ancient Greek language, with the following roots: *Epistéme* (knowledge) + *Lógos* (study, science or discourse) – or putting these together – *Knowledge about knowledge, or the science or study of knowledge*. In a nutshell, epistemology is the branch of philosophy concerned with defining and classifying knowledge. It may be useful in this context to place epistemology in the broader context of philosophy (a term which itself means the pursuit of wisdom or knowledge). Generally, philosophy can be divided into four broad areas.

Epistemology. The study of what knowledge is, how we come to know, and the nature and forms that knowledge takes. It deals with the matter of justification, the arguments we can present to justify our belief that the knowledge is in some way true or accurate. And, it deals also with how we accumulate a body of given or acceptable knowledge, and how we classify this knowledge.

Metaphysics. The study of the being of things, in their essence. The term is sometimes misinterpreted to some extent as transcending or being a higher order than physics, which is the study of observable, concrete things in our world that properly come within scientific study and informs our epistemological knowledge of the material world. However, the term simply derives from the fact that the ancient Greeks studied its topics *after* the physics. The philosopher Martin Heidegger (1959) more appropriately defined metaphysics as a study that goes beyond physics. He spoke of the things that make up our world as being *essents* or *existents*. Metaphysics asks not what these things are (knowing about them would be an epistemological issue), but rather how they come to be and the nature of this being. In studying *being*, metaphysics is contrasted with *knowing*. It is concerned about how we experience the world we are thrust into, and draws a contrast between knowing about the world and living in it. The issues it addresses can be crudely divided into ontology (the nature of being in the world, and how we experience this being) and cosmology (how our world came to exist in the first place, or what is beyond our world – particularly the origins of the universe and how it was created, by a Supreme Being or otherwise).

Ethics. The study of how we live as moral beings in the world. The concern here is not what we know (epistemology), or indeed the matter of our existence as knowing beings in the first place (metaphysics), but the way we live as responsible and moral beings (ethics). It concerns matters of what is good as opposed to bad, and how we *ought* to live as responsible human beings. It is this moral dimension (discussed more fully in Chapter 13) that is significant here. The concern is primarily *evaluative* in the sense that ethics is about values: how we value something as good, right or virtuous; or, their converse as being bad, wrong or vicious. Clearly, such knowledge can be more controversial as it firstly often depends on opinions in respect of good–evil, right–wrong, or vice–virtue, and, secondly as it often presents not simply as an assertion of true or sound knowledge but as a prescription for action.

Aesthetics. The study of how we appreciate beauty and form, and their creation. This is a perceptual activity, as is epistemological knowing referred to above. It is also evaluative, as we observed was the case for ethics. However, it is specifically to do with how we *appreciate* that which we perceive. Such appreciation of beauty and form is, as far as we can ascertain, a uniquely human capacity. A further extension of this aesthetic dimension is the appreciation of the *doing* of art, the actual *artistry* that is involved in the production of a work of art. In its most common manifestation, aesthetics is taken to relate to things that are considered within a particular culture as works of art (fine art, music, literature, etc.). Of course, as our modern cultures become more diversified, those things that we conceive of as works of art also become more diverse. Furthermore, we can recognise the qualities of artistry or masterly skill in all areas of human endeavour. This area

of philosophy therefore becomes increasingly interested in issues of *doing* as well as issues of how the product is evaluated or appreciated. Such artistry or mastery involves, as we suggest below, a specific form of knowledge that is embedded in practice, which is sometimes termed 'know-how'.

At this point, the question the reader as a nurse begs comes easily to mind. It almost reverberates from the page! What possible use can all this abstract thinking be for someone who expects, for most of the time, to be nursing the sick? But this study is in fact essential if we are to become good and effective nurses in any real sense of these terms. To illustrate this point, take a young patient in your care who has just been informed that he has an advanced form of cancer and that life expectancy, for him, is now six months rather than 40 years. What important issues will influence how we will respond to him? The following are among the most important considerations in our response.

1 We must bring to our care of this person the most appropriate and soundest knowledge at our disposal. All the valid research evidence or knowledge, all the body of knowledge built up through experience and reasoning, will be essential to help us in supporting this person through the course of his illness (Muir Gray, 1997; Sackett *et al.*, 2000; Freshwater and Broughton, 2001).

   Epistemology is the study that critically addresses this knowledge and enables us to accumulate the best knowledge available.

2 We must enter into a relationship with this person at a time when their existence as such is now in question. He is now beset with questions of his being as a person: he is *experiencing* in a very acute way his very existence or being in the world and the prospect that this is soon to come to an end. From this emerge extreme experiences of angst, feelings of desolation and despair. There is a desperate calling to understand, to establish the meaning of his life and what is now happening to him. It is not enough for us

to *know* what to do for him, as under 1 above. We must also now *be* with him, as he faces this ordeal (Watson, 1985, 1999; Paterson and Zderad, 1988). We are, in effect, now in the realm of a very personal and existential mode of knowing.

Metaphysics, or more specifically ontology, is the study that informs our insights into how we may enter into this relationship of being with the patient in such circumstances.

3 In the course of our care of this person, we will be confronted with many questions about what is the best, or right, or good thing to do. Matters such as giving or withholding information become problematic from the very initial stages. Other issues such as truth telling and allowing the patient to determine what interventions will take place will become important. Major moral dilemmas may arise in respect of the use of radical surgery or chemotherapy and, ultimately, issues pertaining to euthanasia may emerge. As members of the health care team, we will have no option but to participate in such moral choices (Seedhouse, 1998).

Ethics provides us with the moral theories and frameworks that will assist us with our part in making such choices.

4 Beyond knowing, being with, and acting morally towards this person, we are also called to *do*. That is, we must bring our practice and its incorporated skills to bear on the care of this person. In this sense, we are confronted with a wide range of technical and interpersonal skills, all of which are of vital therapeutic consequence to this person we are caring for. There is a skill in how we will manage the administration of highly dangerous chemotherapy. There is a skill in how we will deliver bad news. How we do these things may range from gross incompetence through mechanical baseline competence to a level of proficiency that is fluid and effective in its mastery and incorporates a high level of clinical or practical wisdom (Benner, 1984; Benner *et al.*, 1999; Flaming, 2001).

Aesthetics provides us with the insights necessary to know and develop the clinical wisdom and mastery essential to our practice.

This example could have been invented for our purposes. In fact, it was not. The author was confronting this exact situation on the day he drafted this example. It should by now be clear that all four of these orientations are of vital importance to nursing. On this basis, the four chapters that follow this one address the important areas of empirical, personal, aesthetic and ethical knowing in more detail. This reflects a shift from considering nursing knowledge in terms of specific adaptive theories and borrowed conceptual models (which unfortunately continue to proliferate to the extent that hardly anyone is familiar with all of them) to a more fundamental consideration of knowing in nursing. Indeed, in the fifth edition of their celebrated text on *Theory and Nursing*, Chinn and Kramer (1999) parallel this significant shift, and their text indeed serves as excellent further reading on these issues. However, in the remainder of this chapter we give further attention to epistemology, which considers how all this 'knowledge' can be framed.

Study Activity 9.1

In this section we have attempted to arrive at definitive statements about what epistemology actually is. This is a complicated concept.

- To help you grasp the meaning, now (immediately on finishing your initial read) write down your understanding of the term. Then re-read the section in more detail and, as you go, make any strengthening amendments necessary to your written statement.

Study Activity 9.2

- In the Introduction, we included a sort of proviso, drawing attention to the possibility that gender may be a factor in how we come to know, and how we view the world. Go to your library and search literature on Gilligan's (1982) thesis that women *do* think and know 'in a different voice'. You may not find the original research works, but Gilligan's thesis (or theoretical viewpoint) is widely cited and discussed in the literature.

- Having considered this work, and the different approaches to knowledge discussed above, reflect upon whether *you* feel such gender differences exist, and the possible implications of this for nursing. You might find it useful to discuss this with fellow students who are also undertaking the activity, and it might be particularly enlightening to include both male and female colleagues in the discussion.

THE NATURE OF KNOWING

Thinking

To know something, we must be aware of it, and this involves a mental process we term thinking. Knowledge is being in possession of information, insights or understanding. It is more than a perception or an idea. When we perceive something, in essence what happens is that we observe or take in a sensation, we form a mental image of the phenomenon we are observing and attach a meaning to it. This *mental image* (perception) *plus attached meaning* is in fact an *idea*. When we organise ideas into interrelated systems that explain the phenomena in our environment, we are forming knowledge. Often, we see interrelationships and connections between perceptions, such as that a living organism that has four legs, a tail and barks, is a dog. Such groupings of ideas we term *concepts*. We often in turn see interrelationships between the concepts. Thus, we may see one concept that is a patient. We see another concept (albeit indirectly) that is pain or discomfort. We observe yet another concept that is a body of information that we can communicate. We might then observe certain connections or associations between these concepts. For example, we might observe that by giving the patient the

information, the pain and discomfort is made more endurable or even reduced. This association of concepts to describe, explain or even predict is what is often termed a *theory*. This process – this ordering, organising and interrelating of ideas – is called thinking, and theory construction is an example of its more sophisticated form (*see* Walker and Avant, 1995). Essentially, thinking can be divided into two types.

- *Concrete thinking* – here, tangible, observable phenomena are experienced in reality, i.e. within time and space. These phenomena – persons, things or events – are out there to be seen, heard or felt. We observe them and we attach specific meanings to them: a child is screaming and holding her finger; we perceive a person with a sore finger and in acute pain.
- *Abstract thinking* – here, the ideas we string together are not directly observed. They are not out there in time and space. The ideas here are mental images, which we ourselves manufacture and in regard to which we attempt to apply meaning, patterns and relationships. Thus, we may consider pain as a general phenomenon, reflecting on its physical, emotional and situational characteristics. In such circumstances, what we do is in fact abstract or single out characteristics and put them together in classes or patterns, so that we arrive at generalisations. This is in fact what is happening in the example of theorising above.

While the two types of thinking are fundamentally different, their objects are the same. In each case they attempt to organise ideas into meaningful wholes, whether in regard to specific situations (concrete thinking) or in regard to the general nature of things (abstract thinking). It is important to recognise that these are not 'either/or' approaches to thinking; one is not an alternative to the other, but both are in effect necessary. As we observe and attach meanings to things in our environment (concrete thinking), we reflect on them and try to understand their more fundamental nature, characteristics and relationships. We in fact search for the meanings behind the things we perceive. In doing this, we posit explanations, generalisations or predictions about such phenomena (abstract thinking). When possible, we may design a means of systematically observing and measuring the phenomena and proceed to do this (concrete thinking). In analysing this 'concrete' data (abstract thinking) we may confirm the explanations, generalisations or predictions, or come up with further 'abstract' ideas which may require further 'concrete' data to carry them forward. Thus, by the interaction between concrete and abstract thinking, we may extend our knowledge.

Knowing

Knowing implies the possession of knowledge, and knowledge is the product of thinking. However, it is insufficient to state that knowledge is simply the outcome of thinking. Not all thinking leads to the construction of new knowledge or the verification or refinement of current knowledge. Sometimes our thinking is simply directed at coping with day-to-day living activities or relationships and we give its knowledge base little thought. Sometimes it is even more free-flowing and undirected at anything in particular, and we use terms such as stream of consciousness or flight of ideas to describe such fanciful thought. Of course, a Freudian psychoanalyst may see all sorts of meanings and interpretations in such thinking! However, a large amount of our thinking is to do with the processing of knowledge in some way, involving the concrete and abstract thinking processes described above. We are always adding to our store of personal knowledge and reviewing and refining it. Indeed, sometimes if we think carefully about something, we arrive at the conclusion that what we took to be factual and correct is not true at all. Here, of course, we are getting to the heart of what 'knowledge' actually means, for the more we question 'facts' or 'held truths' and refine or modify them, the sounder our knowledge is.

Knowledge can therefore be defined as facts or information that we believe to be true on the basis of, on the one hand, thinking involving empirical testing (of directly observed phenomena), or on the other hand, thinking processes such as logical reasoning or problem-solving (that can be done without direct observation, and even in respect of things that cannot be observed at all, such as moral ideas about what is good or evil). This draws attention to one of the great controversies of epistemology. Some, essentially those who subscribe to a scientific orientation, feel that empirical knowing is the only valid form of knowledge. Others feel that knowledge derived from reasoning by rational minds is equally valid. We return to this controversy presently. For now, we may note that the use of the word 'we' is relevant here, as it suggests knowledge that is held to be true by a group as opposed to an individual. It is important to distinguish between something that only the individual believes to be true and public knowledge, i.e. things held to be true by the group, or society or culture as a whole, on the basis of the best evidence or reasoning available to it. According to the distinguished British philosopher, A. J. Ayer (1956), for knowledge to exist in the real sense, the following conditions must apply:

- What we claim to know must be true – we must be sure it is true.
- We must establish this right to be sure, by testing our claim or belief in a publicly accepted way (e.g. through empirical research or logical reasoning).
- As a result of establishing truth, we must all share and accept this knowledge.

On the same argument, Adler (1985) states that data or information must be *communal* before it can be accepted as knowledge. Until its status has not only been validated but also accepted as credible by the group, it is mere opinion. This position begs some fundamental questions, of course. Some beliefs a society or group holds to be true are 'known' by another group or society to be false. Some things that are later accepted as true are at the time rejected by the society and those who propose them are sanctioned or even martyred. Some things may be found to be true, but it may take quite a long time for the information to be disseminated and accepted by the society or the group. For example, in respect of research-derived knowledge about health care, Baker (1998) states that the body of research knowledge is so vast that even if we had a mark-time for 10 years, all of it could not be evaluated as valid knowledge. By that time much of it would be out of date in any case. Yet other things may exist, but we have not yet even discovered them. For example, penicillin did exist and possessed its antibiotic properties before we discovered it. It is important to remember that knowledge is not the actual existence of things; it is in fact our awareness and understanding of these things, and our acceptance as a group that this understanding is true.

Study Activity 9.3

It was previously claimed that by rubbing surgical spirit over pressure areas (bony prominences on the body) the occurrence of pressure ulcers or bed sores could be prevented.

Using your library resources, answer these questions:

- Do nurses still claim that this is true (or sound knowledge)?
- Has the right to claim that this is true (sound knowledge) been established by any acceptable method?

A useful distinction is that between reality (the world out there) and mind (what we perceive of it). It is implicit that *knowledge* about the world we live in, the environment, is within us and not 'out there'. Such knowledge is in fact the outcome of processes by which we in our minds ascertain that things 'out there' exist, that the relationships between these things and the laws and patterns that govern them also exist. Thus, so the argument runs, the closer this knowledge within us approximates to reality, the sounder that knowledge is. This notion of a split between the mind or soul and the body (and

thus, in turn, the 'out there', or reality, or external world) was originally put forward by the seventeenth-century French philosopher Rene Descartes. Drawing on his name, it is referred to as Cartesian dualism. The concept is useful for helping us to attend to the fact that knowledge is within us and as such is not necessarily the same as what exists in nature. Two terms sometimes used in philosophy, derived from Greek terms, are useful here. The actual things in our world are *noumena*, things that as we noted earlier Heidegger (1959) termed *existents* or *essents*. But in our perception or experiencing of them, they are mind-things or *phenomena*. Thus, we can never fully access or 'know' the *noumenon* (using the singular form) but only our experience of it, or the *phenomenon* (again using the singular).

The concept of dualism is limited, however, when we consider knowledge at a more fundamental level, particularly when we are addressing knowledge about non-material things, things which we cannot in fact see 'out there'. Here we may be concerned with issues such as good and evil, right and wrong, beauty and ugliness, mathematical number patterns, etc. We then begin to realise that all knowledge is to a greater or lesser extent subjective and the result of our thought processes and the meanings we attach to things. In this sense there is no objective 'out there' at all, but a total world of which we are an inextricable part. This subjectivity is a significant factor not only in subjective things such as good and evil, but also to a greater or lesser extent in regard to things that we see as objective and obvious and (apparently) matter-of-fact. The logical corollary of this is that we can never claim a total objectivity. The best that we can hope for is a degree of objectivity. That is in fact the greatest closure of the gap between *noumena* and *phenomena* that we can achieve.

In an extreme extension of this form of thinking, the Irish philosopher George Berkeley begged the question of there being a real world at all! How can we be certain, the question runs, that everything we are conscious of holding to exist and to be true are not simply mental constructs in our minds (or indeed the mind of some higher being) and as such do not exist at all outside of such a mind? That is, that there are phenomena but *no noumena* at all! There is, of course, no way of disproving this (although many scientists and philosophers disagree on this point). The discussion marks the debate concerning *idealism,* the notion (of which Berkeley's views are a part) that ideas do not necessarily confirm or equate with the external world and *realism,* which claims that our ideas are conditional on the external world and reflect accurately to a greater or lesser extent that reality. Descartes, who we introduced above, writing many years after Berkeley, penned his now famous Latin phrase: *Cogito ergo sum.* Translated literally this means, 'I think, therefore I am'. The argument here is that because we are conscious of our thinking, we *must* logically exist. Berkeley's extreme idealism in essence turns this claim on its head. It states, on the contrary, that 'Someone or something else may have thought you up, and your thoughts and indeed your existence may not extend beyond their imagination'. Such notions may seem interesting in the tranquil halls of academe. However, in our nursing world, when the blood is hitting the ceiling or someone cries out in agony, we cannot hedge our bets. We must assume the realist position, and we usually have no problem in doing so.

This does not mean, of course, that we proceed without some caution. In nursing, where the nurse often holds the life or death of their patient in the palms of their hands, sound knowledge is essential. Yet, can we always be certain that our knowledge is a true, objective reflection of reality? Remember that once most people knew with absolute certainty that the Earth was flat and that those who heard divine voices were either saints or witches. Nowadays, of course, we all know or think we know that if someone hears a divine voice, he is suffering from a mental illness! In our situation, we cannot afford to incorporate in our thinking the extreme idealism of Berkeley. But at the same time we cannot be courted by a naive acceptance of extreme realism that accepts unquestionably all that we at first perceive. It is important that we are always sceptical of the knowledge we are confronted with. This does not imply a mindless or immovable rejection, but it *does* call us to bring critical reflection to the knowledge that we would apply to the bodies and minds of our patients.

This requires going beyond accepting knowledge as simply that which the group accepts to be true. We must attend to how this acceptance has arisen. Russell (1995) has suggested that there are three characteristics to anything we would adjudge to be true:

1 First, it must meet a deductive reasoning process, or have a *logical premise*. In *deduction* we are moving from some general, basic or taken-as-given premises 'inwards' or 'down' to reasoned conclusions. For example, all persons have two legs; this individual is a person; therefore he/she has two legs.
2 Second, it must meet an inductive test based upon empirical or perceptual experience, or have a *psychological premise*. In *induction* we are moving from some specific empirical experience 'outwards' or 'up' to generalisations on the bases of these experiences. For example, all the persons I have observed have two legs; therefore, all the people in the world have two legs.
3 Third, it must meet an analytical test or have an *epistemological premise*. In the case of deduction, we arrive at our conclusions on the basis of logical reasoning; in the case of induction, we arrive at our conclusions on the basis of observation and experience. But, as can immediately be seen from the above two examples of deduction and induction, they are both incorrect: there are in fact a number of people with deficits in the leg category and – in the case of infrequent congenital deformity – some who may have more than the norm in this category! Deductions depend on the accuracy of their base premises, and induction depends to some degree on a leap of faith. Therefore, we need to be sceptical of the

results of our inductions (empirical generalisations) and deductions (logical reasonings). This analysis or critique of knowledge is what Russell termed the third or epistemological premise, in respect of which he stated: 'We assume that perception *can* cause knowledge, although it *may* cause error if we are not logically careful' (p. 133). In another sense (although not one articulated by Russell), our analytical scepticism is a mindset that causes us to use the term 'probably'. In the above examples, we would therefore say that the conclusions could at best be reflected as (under the logical-deductive premise example) that he/she *probably* has two legs, and (under the psychological-inductive premise example) that all people *probably* have two legs. Probability (sometimes referred to in modern science as 'probability theory') refers to the degree to which we can make a claim, or the strength an assertion we make holds. The term *abduction* is sometimes used to identify this concept.

One of the primary functions of epistemology is thus the need to *analyse* and *justify* what we hold to be true. Indeed, some say that this is its sole purpose. In the case of nursing, therefore, *nursing* epistemology is also involved in justification: ensuring that the knowledge we apply in our practice is relevant and accurate (or at least as sound as we can humanly make it).

Justifying

If we accept for the present that knowledge is something we accept as being true or a valid construction of reality, we are still left with a problem if we subscribe to the counsel to be critical and questioning in respect of this knowledge. This raises the issue of justification, which is accepted as a fundamental issue in epistemology. It concerns the basis upon which our claims to truth or our belief in the validity of any knowledge are based. Generally speaking, this involves two perspectives that are essentially polarised; these are most commonly described as foundationalism and coherentism.

- *Foundationalism* – the essential position here is that there are certain fundamental beliefs, which, if held to be true, form the basis or foundations for all other beliefs. On the basis that these foundational or basic beliefs are true or justified, we can build other conditional beliefs upon them. Thus, if we hold the foundational belief that the Earth is round we can have confidence in the other related beliefs associated with this, such as if we continue to travel west we will eventually circle the globe and arrive where we started. Of course, if the Earth was flat, we would be in for a rather big fall. The usual metaphor here is that of the inverted pyramid, as summarised in Fig. 9.1. The whole body of knowledge rests on a single or few foundational beliefs. But if these are found to be false, the whole knowledge pyramid comes toppling down. Prior to the first centuries BC, it was believed that illness was caused by the entry of harmful spirits into the body. But Galen, one of the fathers of modern medicine, presented 'the doctrine of the four'. That is, that illness is related to the balance between four bodily humours or

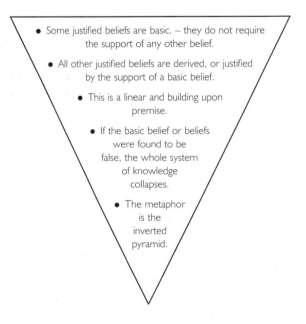

Figure 9.1 The foundationalist inverted pyramid

- Some justified beliefs are basic. – they do not require the support of any other belief.
- All other justified beliefs are derived, or justified by the support of a basic belief.
- This is a linear and building upon premise.
- If the basic belief or beliefs were found to be false, the whole system of knowledge collapses.
- The metaphor is the inverted pyramid.

substances: blood, choler (yellow bile), phlegm, and melancholy (black bile). The foundations of the spirit theory crumbled and the doctrine of the four held sway as the dominant medical knowledge almost through to the nineteenth century. However, with the discovery of the germ theory (the idea that actual living micro-organisms caused infection), the foundations established by Galen in turn crumbled and were replaced by new and different approaches.

Such instances are unusual but not necessarily rare. Thomas Kuhn (1970), in his famous work entitled *The Structure of Scientific Revolutions*, describes a phenomenon termed *paradigm shift*. A paradigm is a particular perspective, or world-view, or theoretical framework that establishes how we view and understand the world. Of each science or discipline, we can say that it has one or more dominant paradigms, which represent its way of looking at the world. These are that discipline's particular lenses, through which it sees and then explains the world or a part thereof. Kuhn found that while a paradigm or worldview can grow and develop over time, as its body of knowledge is developed, in some instances this reaches a point where its validity is challenged. In such circumstances, if the challenge is successful, a major shift may take place and a very new and different paradigm replaces the old as our way of understanding the world.

Another foundational problem is particularly relevant to the human sciences and those professions (including nursing) that primarily draw on their knowledge. If different disciplines or even different subdivisions within the same discipline have different paradigms or worldviews that they use to explain the same reality, how do we judge which is best? The discipline of psychology, and in particular its application to therapy, is a good example of this. An individual may present with an anxiety illness, characterised by symptoms of compulsions, phobias and emotional distress of various sorts. From a behavioural psychology perspective, the issue is one of dealing with conscious cognitive patterns and behavioural aberrations caused by stress and anxiety. Behavioural and cognitive processes are the foundations upon which this perspective is based. A therapy such as cognitive behavioural therapy is indicated. Were the same person to present to a psychodynamic psychologist, the roots of the illness may be explained in terms of repressed desires and unconscious conflicts and urges that are emerging as distressing symptoms. In this perspective, the foundational beliefs are based upon unconscious motivation. A therapy such as psychoanalysis is indicated. How can it be that two such different perspectives, based upon foundations that are in fact not only different but also strongly incompatible, each claim to be the best or true knowledge? And this may not be the only two conflicting psychological perspectives that would purport to give the only or best explanation and posit the only or best therapeutic intervention. We may even find other disciplines beyond psychology claiming *their* explanation for this *exact same* situation. For example, from the discipline of biology, a biological or neurochemical explanation may be suggested, and the treatment adopted by a psychiatrist may not be psychological therapy at all, but the use of drugs and physical therapies.

This diversity of explanations for the same 'object' or phenomenon is a problem widely recognised and it is not exclusive to foundationalist matters. For example, David Bohm (1980) describes this phenomenon as follows:

> *Thus art, science, technology, and human work in general, are divided up into specialities, each considered to be separate in essence from the others. Becoming dissatisfied with this state of affairs, men have set up further interdisciplinary subjects, which were intended to unite these specialities, but these new subjects have ultimately served to add further separate fragments ... The notion that all these fragments are separately existent is evidently an illusion, and this illusion cannot do other than lead to endless conflict and confusion ... What will be emphasized ... is that fragmentation is*

continually being brought about by the almost universal habit of taking the content of our thought for 'a description of the world as it is'. Or we could say that, in this habit, our thought is regarded as in direct correspondence with objective reality … it follows that such a habit leads us to look on these as real divisions, so that the world is then seen and experienced as actually broken up into fragments.

(Bohm, 1980, pp. 1–3)

Bohm suggests that this fragmentation of the world leads to theories that result in specific ways of looking at the world. He emphasises this by drawing on the Greek origins of the word *theory*, which originates from the same roots as the words *theoria* and *theatrum*, indicating 'to view' and 'to present a spectacle'. The consequence of this is that for each theoretical perspective we are viewing a fragment of the world through a particular lens. We are furthermore assuming this corresponds to the reality. This is an important distinction to make in our nursing knowledge. As nurses, we are concerned with the totality of the person in his or her social and physical environment. This is a complex situation that calls our attention to the totality. We must therefore be cautious (as will be argued more fully in the final chapter to this module) that we do not elect to base our nursing entirely on a single theory position, or indeed upon the insights of a single scientific discipline.

- *Coherentism* – this alternative to foundationalism argues that basic beliefs can never be the foundation for all knowledge. This reflects a scepticism that any one belief or small set of beliefs is of a higher order (or more basic) than all others. Instead, it views all beliefs to be of equal value, at least in so far as they merit critical attention. Justification is seen as the extent to which the various beliefs fit together, or are confirmatory in respect of each other. This introduces a collaborative or reinforcing principle. In so far as a set of beliefs hangs together and has consistency, and in so far as any belief confirms or supports all the others and is in turn confirmed or supported by them, we can have confidence in the full set as a sound body of knowledge.

The usual metaphor employed here is that of the ship, as summarised in Table 9.1. This is often referred to as Neurath's Boat (after the Austrian social theorist, Otto Neurath). The image here is that of a ship at sea. All of its parts are essential in keeping the vessel afloat. If any part becomes defective, it can be repaired by using other parts, or reorganising the parts, as long as the whole stays afloat. Similarly, with a set of beliefs is a coherent and interdependent whole. As it proceeds some beliefs may come into question and be discarded and others may be added. When the set comes into question, there is a reappraisal and reorganisation. As long as the set of beliefs holds together in a confirmatory cohesiveness, the body of knowledge endures. It is when they all come apart that there is a threat, not when any single belief or small subset of beliefs adjudged to be foundational is disproved.

Table 9.1   The coherentist ship metaphor

- A belief is justified if it belongs to a coherent set of beliefs.

- No one belief within the system has a distinguished 'epistemic' (point of first origin) status.

- No one belief within the system has a distinguished 'importance' (being more vital than others to the system) status.

- This is a premise based upon consistency, and comprehensiveness of the system, and relations between beliefs rather than linearity.

- If the consistency and comprehensiveness were to break, the belief system would collapse.

- The metaphor is the ship, with its interdependent and self-correcting whole (Neurath's Boat).

The problem with such a perspective is really the converse of its strength. That is, while coherence gives the knowledge its justification and strength, this in itself may be a powerful resistance to correction and the development of knowledge.

As the coherent body of knowledge builds up, and as the commitment and investment of the social group becomes more deep-rooted, it becomes more difficult to reject. In effect, the coherence becomes an end in itself. This is reflected to an extent in the fable of the Emperor's new clothes. When he was presented with a suit so fine that it was invisible and paraded in this, only one soul seemed to be prepared to say 'But he's naked!' Nobody wanted to point out that the Emperor was in fact naked; the repercussions were unthinkable. The problem here is a very human one. When we are faced with the emptiness and futility of all that we may perhaps have held to be true, perhaps for generations, being overturned, it is difficult to countenance the future.

Study Activity 9.4

- Do you feel the situation in the first years of our new century is stable?
- If not, what do you feel the issues are that concern people today? Are we in any sense experiencing a lack of cohesiveness in our beliefs and knowledge, or are we confident in our systems of beliefs?
- It is claimed by some (who are often termed 'modernists') that we are now in a new golden age, wherein science and technology are answering all our questions and solving all our problems. Others (who are often termed 'post-modernists') feel that this is not so and have grave concerns about how the modern world is impacting on our health, well-being, and even survival. With the assistance of literature searches (using keywords such as 'post-modernism', 'risk society', 'scientism') explore such concerns and reflect on the extent to which they may be real threats.

Eclectic integration

There is no specific perspective recognised by this title, but a number of authorities have suggested that there is no reason why the two opposing perspectives of foundationalism and coherentism cannot be combined in some way to enhance the level of justification for our belief in a body of knowledge. Indeed, it has been suggested that this is an imperative. Essentially, this may involve some degree of acceptance of some of the beliefs as foundational but requiring also that there is cohesion between all the beliefs within a body of knowledge. Susan Haack (1993) invented her own term to explain this: *foundherentism*. Robert Audi (1998) similarly described such an orientation but, seeing coherence as a means of strengthening the foundational premise, he described it as *moderate foundationalism*.

Study Activity 9.5

'Aids is a disease caused by the HIV virus.'
'Aids is a punishment from God for evildoing.'

- Which of these pieces of 'knowledge' is 'accurate' or most justified in believing? Write down which of these statements *you* adjudge to be correct, explaining why. Express your arguments in foundationalist and/or coherentist justification terms.
- Then write an argument supporting that the other view is incorrect, that it is in fact faulty knowledge. Remember: if you cannot show that it is wrong, how do you 'know' that it is wrong?
- Your write-up should be about 250 words (one page). When you have read Kerlinger's classification of knowledge below, return to your write-up and decide which type of 'knowing' your response best reflects.

Confirming

Thus far we have spoken of what knowledge is and how we justify it. There is an assumption in all of this that knowledge is of a particular nature or takes a particular form. That is, it is to do with what we believe to be true (or at least the soundest knowledge available). In this sense, knowledge has a propositional nature: we propose a particular set of facts to be true, and we believe it to be so. However, in everyday life, we often use the terms knowing and knowledge in different ways. In some instances we are simply saying that we recognise something we perceive: we remember seeing it before, as we would recognise the man who delivers our milk each morning. Or, we speak of a knowing person as a person of wisdom. Often we do not see these rather common-sense turns of phrase as having much to do with knowledge in its real sense. Indeed, many authorities, particularly those who subscribe to the natural science perspective, only view propositional knowledge derived from empirical evidence and subjected to stringent and robust tests as valid knowledge. However, it may be a mistake to see these other forms of knowing as simply weak knowledge or not knowledge in any real sense. Underlying such ideas are indeed valid and important forms of knowing that must be recognised. It is therefore important that we can confirm or accept that knowledge may be of different forms.

Generally speaking, epistemological philosophers classify knowledge into the following forms.

- *Knowing of, or acquaintance* – this identifies all matters about which we have *some* knowledge. In simple terms, we know of its existence and we know something about it. We may not be able to describe or justify it in propositional terms but we recognise things and patterns in our world. This is more to do with conscious logic and reasoning, and more to do with that way of knowing that we described as ontological earlier, it is knowing by existential experience rather than description. It is also in line with what Michael Polanyi (1967) describes as tacit knowing and what nursing scholars such as Benner (1984; Benner *et al.*, 1996, 1999) describe as intuitive knowing. In such circumstances we may see patterns or recognise situations and how we should respond to them without being able to explain how this is so. Thus, knowledge of this form can extend from simple recognition to a more intuitive and tacit knowing. Clearly, however, such tacit knowing extends far beyond mere acquaintance in its sophistication.

- *Knowing how, or 'know-how'* – this refers to knowledge about how to do something. It is what we mean when we say someone has 'know-how'. For example, a diplomat may be able to speak several different languages, or a nurse may be able to pass a nasogastric tube – she in fact 'knows how' to do this. This is very much in line with that aspect of aesthetics that we described as artistry or mastery earlier. It has an integrative quality in that it blends a capacity to utilise propositional knowledge skilfully, respond to tacit or intuitional cues, and integrate this wisdom in high degrees of proficiency. This idea of a separate type of knowing that is in fact a practical wisdom (Benner *et al.*, 1999; Flaming, 2001) was first famously proposed by Gilbert Ryle (1949). He argued that this form of knowing, which he termed 'know-how' is in itself sophisticated and important, but in western (as opposed to Eastern) philosophy it has been largely ignored or undervalued.

- *Knowing that, or belief about what is true* – this refers to knowledge in the sense of understanding something, in terms of what it means, what its properties are, how it 'works', how it relates to other things, etc. This is essentially that form of knowledge referred to above that is sometimes referred to as propositional knowledge. That is, it is based upon reasoning or empirical evidence, and subject to justification in line with our description of this earlier. Such 'knowing that' can be divided into the following:

  A priori *knowledge* refers to knowledge derived from a self-evident axiomatic basis. That is, it is produced by a process of reasoning and deduction without any external stimuli or evidence contributing to the conclusion (thus, the term *a priori*, or 'coming before'). We say this or that is true because 'it stands to reason' or is self-evident. Thus, for example, we believe that solving an ethnic problem by genocide is wrong without needing concrete evidence to support this position.

Empirical knowledge is knowledge derived from sense perceptions, i.e. observations we make about phenomena in our environment. From things we observe we arrive at knowledge by a process of induction. Here we are not inferring that conditions exist; we actually observe the conditions and 'know' they exist. We then proceed to confirm knowledge by induction, i.e. generalising from the specific to the general. For example, if by testing and re-testing we find that mercury expands at a particular rate when heated, we conclude that this is a general property of mercury. We can then use this knowledge to measure temperature.

In recent times the nursing profession has increasingly valued the application of propositional knowledge, which is scientifically derived from research. For example, a leading British nurse Lisbeth Hockey (1987) has stated that:

> *Legally, a professional nurse in the UK is held responsible for his or her actions and has to be able to defend them on the basis of the latest knowledge. The latest available knowledge must be based on research because this is the only way by which the body of knowledge can be changed or extended.*
>
> (Hockey, 1987)

The suggestion that research is the only valid source of nursing knowledge is one that would be disputed by many nurses and indeed is a matter of concern to some (e.g. Kirby and Slevin, 1992; Flaming, 2001). However, the increasing emphasis on responsibility and accountability demands that nurses can point to sound scientific evidence as a justification for their actions. This preoccupation with research-derived knowledge is also understandable in a profession closely aligned with a medical profession that bases its practice on a predominantly scientific perspective. In addition, as nursing aspires to full professional status, it leans towards the respectability of the natural sciences.

Notwithstanding this apparent preoccupation with the scientific, there is an increasing tendency for nurses to try to establish the meaning of nursing in a more fundamental manner. This is quite different from concrete, scientific thinking and involves abstract and philosophical reflection on nursing practice. Irrespective of whether we utilise concrete thinking and scientific enquiry (research), or abstract thinking and reflection (philosophy), or indeed a mixture of both, the goal is the same. We are trying to understand nursing and the phenomena which surround and influence it, and by doing so explain, generalise, and possibly make predictions about the nursing world and the practice of nursing. In effect, we are systematically attempting to explain the phenomenon of nursing, describe its parameters and practices, and predict the outcome of our nursing interventions. This is in fact the process of theory-building, and statements which describe, explain relationships between concepts, or predict outcomes of such relationships are called theories.

FRAMEWORKS FOR NURSING KNOWLEDGE

Establishing parameters to nursing knowledge

Clearly all knowledge is not of major relevance to nursing. If we accept that to practice well we must have a sound knowledge base, it is important that we know, at least in broad terms, what the parameters of nursing knowledge are. That is, we need to know what sources of knowledge can inform our practice, or which knowledge from the total body of what is known is relevant to our practice. There are basically two ways we can go about this: from the top down, or from the bottom up:

1 In the top-down approach, we are adopting what we will in a later chapter refer to as a classical *theory-testing approach*. That is, we would survey the world of knowledge, identify what from the total body of

knowledge *may* be relevant to nursing, proceed to *adapt* it to nursing if necessary by making any relevant modifications, and then *test* its relevance in practice (Meleis, 1997). Of course, if the knowledge we need is not there, we may formulate our own theories and test them.

2 In the alternative bottom-up approach, we would in essence move in the opposite direction. That is, on the basis of our knowledge of nursing gained through practice insights, we would know, tacitly and experientially, the nature of the knowledge we must seek. On this basis, we would either go out seeking the specific knowledge we need or, if it were not actually available, we would construct it ourselves from the field of our practice. In a later chapter we refer to this specific nursing knowledge derived from the field as *grounded theory* – theory that emerges from the ground or the situation so to speak (Glaser and Strauss, 1967).

Whichever of these approaches or combinations of them we utilise, we must strive to establish the parameters or extent of knowledge that is necessary. One way of doing this is to attempt to condense or distil this body of knowledge into a relevant framework. This may be achieved by identifying the key elements or features of the dominant nursing paradigm. As noted earlier, one meaning Kuhn (1970) suggested for paradigm was that it is the worldview or lens through which a discipline views the world, and includes the methods and language it uses to achieve this. According to this view, a discipline can have only one *dominant* paradigm. If there is more than one competing for this dominance, the discipline is in fact unstable or has not yet attained full maturity as a discipline in its own right. An alternative view is that a practice discipline, such as nursing or medicine, may draw on different paradigms that inform different aspects of practice. Whichever of these views we accept, it is important that we can identify the key elements that make up the paradigm (or paradigms) of nursing.

The metaparadigm view

Two useful concepts for achieving this end are *metaparadigm* and *domain*. In nursing, Fawcett (1993, 1995, 2000) uses the term metaparadigm and speaks of abstract concepts that delineate the discipline's concerns. Meleis (1997) and Kim (1983, 1987) prefer the term domains, which identifies the domains (discrete sets of related concepts) encompassed in the practice of nursing. For our purposes, we can see these two terms as broadly similar in meaning.

The term metaparadigm seems to have achieved great popularity in academic nursing, and therefore merits particular attention. However, it is problematic in that different authorities define it rather differently. Some see it as a different and discrete term to paradigm, dealing with the broad areas of concern for the discipline. Others see it as simply the main or dominant paradigm of the discipline, but similarly reflecting the main concerns in its language and methods. A third view sees the prefix 'meta' as important. We will recall that in metaphysics this prefix identifies a study that goes beyond physics or knowledge about the actual or observable world, to the essences or meanings implicit in the existence of this world. On this basis, a metaparadigm looks beyond or behind the dominant paradigm/s of a discipline to determine the elements or fundamental concepts emerging from them that establish the areas of interest (and thus knowledge areas) of a discipline. Indeed, Masterman (1970), who is credited with inventing the term, was bringing together the notions of metaphysics and paradigm to create the word 'metaparadigm'. This 'metaphysical paradigm' is not the specific scientific orientation of the discipline, but is rather an attempt to establish the ways we see the world or the elements that constitute our worldview. In this sense, it is an analysis of paradigm 'content' into its constituent parts. Ideally, this should reflect a degree of parsimony, in that we work towards the most concise set of *discrete elements* that are still representative in terms of including the *totality of concerns* for the discipline.

Beyond the latter choice of terminology, there are a number of competing views about what the metaparadigm or set of domains should include. McKenna (1997) presents a clear and useful overview of these. However, for the purpose of this study, that proposed by Fawcett (1984, 1995), which is by far the most widely recognised, is presented here as the best example. She proposed that nursing encompasses four elements or abstract concepts, as follows:

- *Person* – the individual who is being nursed, who must be recognised as a person in his/her totality.
- *Health* – the conceptual field within which nursing takes place, and drawing attention to the fact that nurses care in the health context (as opposed, for example, to teachers who primarily care in the educational context, or the clergy who primarily care in the spiritual or religious context).
- *Environment* – the total environment, both physical and social, which impacts upon the person, upon the nurse, upon health and even upon the caring relationship.
- *Nursing* – the actual activity that takes place when nursing care is given.

Fawcett saw these elements as associated with four propositions indicating linkages between: person and health; person and environment; health and nursing; and person, environment and health.

The Fawcett metaparadigm is not without its difficulties. For example, the current author (Slevin, 1995, 1999) and others (e.g. Conway, 1985; Meleis, 1997) have suggested that including nursing as one of the central elements within a metaparadigm *of* nursing amounts to a tautology. That is, a description of nursing cannot logically include 'nursing' as one of the descriptive elements: this is tantamount to saying nursing is nursing. Slevin (1995) suggested that the term nursing within the metaparadigm should be replaced by the term 'caring', which more accurately reflects the action mode within nursing. He furthermore (Slevin, 1999) suggested that a metaparadigm encompassing *person,*

health, environment and *caring* reflects the dynamic relational aspect of nursing and as such links directly to a definition of what nursing is. This might be worded as: nursing is a caring relationship between nurse and patient that takes place in the health context.

The key metaparadigmatic elements caring (nursing), patient (person), health and context (environment) are all contained within this statement, as presented in Fig. 9.2 opposite.

It is important to recognise Fawcett's response to the above criticism. She points out that the term nursing *within* her metaparadigm is intended to reflect the actual activity of nursing. It thus is meant in a different context to the *title* of the metaparadigm, which is in fact designating the discipline of nursing. However, this has not been accepted as adequately resolved by many nursing scholars (Rawnsley, 1996). It is furthermore not the only difficulty that has been identified.

The other main concern about the Fawcett metaparadigm is the extent to which it claims to encompass the unique or specific elements that make up nursing. This concern can be demonstrated by drawing on Fawcett's own work. The strength of a metaparadigm depends on a number of things. Fawcett (1996) identified four requirements for a metaparadigm as follows:

> *First, a metaparadigm must identify a domain that is distinctive from the domains of other disciplines. That requirement is fulfilled only when the concepts and propositions represent a unique perspective for inquiry and practice. Second, a metaparadigm must encompass all phenomena of interest to the discipline in a parsimonious manner. That requirement is fulfilled only if the concepts and propositions are global and if there are no redundancies in concepts or propositions. Third, a metaparadigm must be perspective-neutral. That requirement is fulfilled only if the concepts and propositions do not reflect a specific paradigm or conceptual model, or a combination of perspectives. Fourth, a*

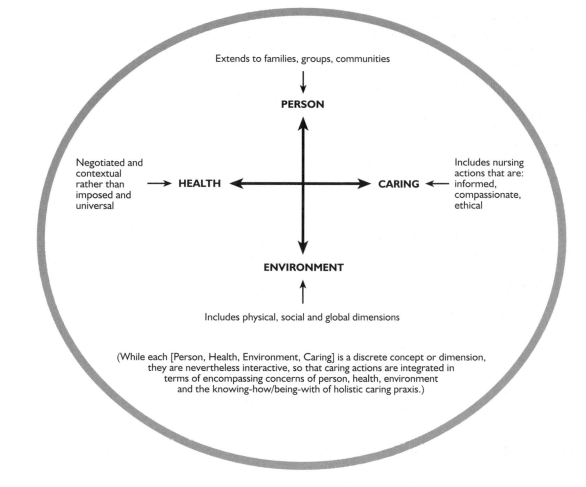

Figure 9.2 A nursing metaparadigm. Adapted from Slevin (1999)

metaparadigm must be international in scope and substance. That requirement, which is a corollary of the third requirement, is fulfilled only if the concepts and propositions do not reflect particular national, cultural, or ethnic beliefs and values.

(Fawcett, 1996, pp. 94–5)

The fundamental notion that a metaparadigm presents a *distinctive* domain with a *unique* perspective (in this case nursing) immediately calls into question the other three elements – person, health and environment. This is powerfully stated by Cody (1996):

The simple tetrad of 'person, environment, health, and nursing,' for over a decade now, has been and still is being touted repeatedly, like a mantra, in serious discussion on nursing philosophy and theory as 'the metaparadigm' or the central focus (or is that foci) of nursing ... After due reflection on the claim that the four concepts taken with the four propositions reflect the unique focus (or foci) of nursing, this author finds the claim unmerited in that many disciplines besides nursing study three of the four concepts – person, environment, and health – and many disciplines study the relationships

> *described in the four propositions with the exception of those including nursing per se.*
> (Cody, 1996, pp. 97–8)

It is perhaps a fundamental difficulty of the Fawcett metaparadigm that it is established upon a perception of nursing grounded in abstract rather than real world premises. This is understandable when its origins are noted. Fawcett's work draws from a survey commissioned by the National League for Nursing in the USA to determine the common concepts in the nursing curriculum (50 nursing curricula that expressed nursing concepts were examined). This survey identified four common elements: man, health, nursing and society (Yura and Torres, 1975). In her own extension of this into person, health, nursing and environment, Fawcett based her arguments upon conceptualisations reflected in 11 theoretical examples from the literature that mentioned nursing concepts. In both cases, it might be argued that there are two significant considerations:

1 First, the metaparadigm might be argued to be particulate and mechanical, failing to recognise the adage of the whole being more that the sum of the parts. This attends to what Parse (1987) described as the two separate paradigm perspectives. There is the *totality paradigm*, which attempts to explain the nursing situation – and the person/patient/client – as being made up of interrelated but still separate parts. By even referring assiduously to the human makeup as being 'bio-psycho-social' or as being concerned with biological, psychological, social and spiritual dimensions, there is an attention to parts rather than the whole. Then, there is the *simultaneity paradigm*, which views these matters in a more holistic way, seeing the person as a unitary whole, responding, changing and becoming. Here, the person is irreducible to his/her parts, and where we countenance such reduction we are losing the sense of the dynamic whole that is 'more than the sum of its parts'.

2 Second, in both their origins and structuring, both the Yura and Torres and the Fawcett metaparadigms are grounded in rational thought and logical reasoning rather than practice and the lifeworld of nurses and their patients. This may be a basis for the fact that these metaparadigms have been more influential in the lecture theatre and student dissertation than at the caring interface.

Indeed, this explication of the nursing metaparadigm is far removed from its alternatives, such as that proposed by Kim (2000). Kim (now also using the term metaparadigm as opposed to domain) proposes a metaparadigm that is not only firmly based upon the practice situation, but also centred upon the person/patient/client. She suggests three interrelated elements in her metaparadigm:

1 *Human living of oneself* – this recognises the person/patient/client as not only a physical living organism, but also an existential being that experiences living in the world. By definition, this includes living of oneself where health is compromised – including both the biological imbalance and the conscious or existential experiencing of ill-health.

2 *Human living with others* – this recognises the sociality and communality of human beings. We influence others and are influenced by them, we depend upon them and they depend on us. By definition, when health is compromised this impacts on others, and when we are in ill-health our dependence on others (family, friends, health professionals) is increased.

3 *Living in situations* – both ourselves and those we 'live with' are influenced by contextual factors. The environment in which we live can be relatively enduring, and includes physical and cultural factors that influence how we live. Alternatively, it can be rapidly changing, e.g. as a result of wars or great natural disasters such as floods, famine, earthquakes. By definition, the situation cannot only influence our health and well-being, but also presents

the resources and opportunities (or lack of them) that may influence our return to health.

The relevant orientation is therefore *human living* and the concern of nursing becomes helping others to live in the context of health problems and health care.

Why Fawcett endures

In all of this, a question is begged as to why we give so much attention to the metaparadigm concept here. This can be answered by addressing the issues of weakness or threats and strengths or opportunities at stake in committing to a particular metaparadigm. The most vital issue is whether the particular metaparadigm we choose encompasses fully and comprehensively all aspects of the discipline of nursing and thus nursing knowledge (and by definition excludes all that is irrelevant). The risks involved must be viewed in the potential costs and benefits. The benefits of a metaparadigm that effectively marks out the parameters of our professional knowledge and practice are clear. They allow us to focus on developing an epistemology or body of knowledge that will inform our practice. The costs of an inadequate metaparadigm are equally clear. They involve the possible inclusion of knowledge that does not inform our practice or, of equal importance, the exclusion of areas of knowledge that may be essential to safe and effective practice.

Assuming that Fawcett's metaparadigm achieves the purpose of delineating the parameters of our knowledge, we can use it to establish and indeed justify any knowledge that is claimed to be *nursing* knowledge. Thus, if a particular theory is proposed to describe or explain nursing (or indeed predict the effects of our nursing interventions), we can examine the extent to which person, health, environment and nursing (as a caring activity) are successfully addressed in that theory. If they are not, the argument runs, there is something amiss in the theory, and it cannot fully inform our practices. This is a tall order and, as indicated above, the consequences are significant.

In these circumstances, it is still important to cast a critical eye on the Fawcett metaparadigm. As noted above, there have been numerous criticisms. It is important to acknowledge, as do Rose and Marks-Maran (1997), that Fawcett's metaparadigm has withstood the test of time, retaining its popularity against competing views. However, this is not in itself a rational argument for committing unequivocally to this metaparadigm. It is also important to note that some nurses (e.g. Rawnsley, 1996) have suggested that there is little evidence to demonstrate any real utility of the Fawcett metaparadigm in nursing practice. While the above example of how the metaparadigm might validate or confirm the usefulness of a theory has got a clear logic to it, it seems that this particular metaparadigm (after 20 years of promotion) has not become a major influence in the day-to-day work of the nurse.

Given the assertion by Rawnsley (1996) and the critiques presented earlier, the reason for the Fawcett metaparadigm enduring for almost 20 years is itself an enduring question. Textbook after textbook and journal paper after journal paper refer to the person–health–environment–nursing metaparadigm in an uncritical and taken-for-granted way. Nurses, many of whom have never read (sometimes not even heard of) Fawcett, not less critiques of her work, pay lip service to the framework indiscriminately. How can this be so?

One explanation may be implied in the reference by Cody (1996) to the Fawcett tetrad as a mantra. That is, by simple repetition and ritualistic allusion it has become embedded in our nursing culture irrespective of (or in spite of) any inherent weaknesses. This is not an empty or trivial explanation. The evolutionary scientist Richard Dawkins (1976) developed a *meme* theory to complement the *gene* theory of evolution. The term *meme* refers to a unit of knowledge that is remembered and passed on in a way broadly similar to genetic transfer (conveniently *meme* rhymes with *gene*). Applying this theory to the Fawcett metaparadigm, using Dawkins' criteria, it clearly fits the bill as a meme in that it has:

- *Copying fidelity* – it has been clearly explicated and copied precisely and relatively permanently (in textbooks, journal papers, lecture halls, by word-of-mouth). By its nature, it is a simple framework that is easily replicated.
- *Fecundity* – it has been disseminated widely via the communication channels referred to so that many nurses are aware of it (and certainly many more than for the competing metaparadigms).
- *Longevity* – it has endured the passage of time. By being the first major reference to a nursing metaparadigm and as such creating much interest, it continued to be a topic of interest. Even the number of critiques that questioned it contributed to the enduring attention being paid to it.

Of course, the existence of a meme as an element of cultural knowledge that is transferred across time and space says nothing about its validity or accuracy. There *are* 'bad' memes as well as 'good' ones. Coca Cola or Big Macs are not necessarily the best soft drinks or food in the world, but the 'copying fidelity' of their branding and the 'fecundity' of their availability make them central international cultural elements. Experts widely agree that the video medium Betamax was superior to VHS, but VHS got into the market place first and became rapidly and widely available, leading to the demise of the superior Betamax. In a similar sense, we must recognise the Fawcett metaparadigm as the dominant meme (at least within nursing scholarship). Meme theory may explain how this has come to be. But it does not confirm that it is a *sound* knowledge framework or even that it is the *best* metaparadigm.

What does all this say about the Fawcett metaparadigm and about nursing knowledge in general? We can perhaps summarise the position as follows:

1 There is little doubt that unlike other nursing metaparadigms proposed, Fawcett's metaparadigm functions as a meme: it is by far the dominant position on this issue within the discipline.

2 Given its situation as a point of reference, we can use this metaparadigm (possibly adapted as in Fig. 9.2) as a source for establishing the parameters of our nursing knowledge.

3 It is reasonable to claim that the metaparadigm has a degree of face validity. It clearly identifies important parameters and those who consider it often have a tacit feel for its degree of fitness: it seems right and it does provide a clear and precise way of establishing the field of nursing knowledge and practice, or at least the greater part of that field.

4 By conceiving it in terms of meme theory, or memetics, and by awareness of the critiques of it, we can adopt a critical and indeed sceptical orientation towards the metaparadigm. That is, we can recognise it as potentially identifying significant boundaries to our knowledge, but not allow it to restrict the advancement of the boundaries of our knowledge. In essence it can be a facilitative starting point rather than a restriction to progress.

5 Beyond a consideration of the metaparadigm, meme theory helps us to appreciate the potency of information sharing and information transfer in respect of the *totality* of nursing knowledge. In that moment that a claim is made about knowledge it becomes a prospect. In so far as it is repeated without challenge it becomes embedded in our culture until at a certain point it is accepted uncritically. This phenomenon enables us to cast a wary eye on other nursing memes, such as the Nightingale image of nursing (van der Peet, 1995) or the Henderson definition of nursing (Henderson, 1966). Such scepticism, questioning *what* our knowledge is, *how* it is constructed, and *why* or on what basis we feel it is justified, is at the very core of a nursing epistemology. This is not simply negativism and dogmatic rejection. As the physicist and philosopher Karl Popper (1989) famously stated when he dragged empirical sciences into the new modern age, it is by a continuous process of conjectures and refutations (posing descriptions, explanations or predictions, and

then challenging or testing them) that we establish and extend sound knowledge.

Retrospective

Thus far we have defined epistemology as the study of knowledge, and justified our attention to it by arguments for the importance of a nursing epistemology. Such an epistemology involves an awareness of what it is *to know,* and how we can *justify* what we know or claim to be valid, or true, or sound knowledge. It also requires that we attend to the nature of knowledge (including *nursing* knowledge); in this respect we differentiated between knowing by acquaintance, knowing-how, and propositional or knowing-that knowledge. This, of course, begged a further question. Assuming that all three of these are relevant in the nursing context, what – in all the world of knowledge – can we claim as *nursing* knowledge?

The Kuhnian notion of paradigm started us off here. Our *nursing* knowledge will be determined by what Kuhn (1970) termed our paradigm or paradigms (worldviews or ways of examining our nursing world). In effect, we view or examine the world through particular lenses we have adopted, and these determine how we perceive and interpret the world, thereby constructing our nursing knowledge. It was then suggested that, whichever paradigm we use, it will be directed towards certain fundamental or essential concerns that are common to the study of nursing across all paradigms or theoretical frameworks. This is the discipline's most abstract and yet most fundamental discerning characteristics or concepts, its metaparadigm. The most common presentation of this was identified as the Fawcett metaparadigm, which established the concerns of nursing knowledge and practice as being: person, health, environment and nursing.

Here, we can again allude to the nature of epistemology. It requires that we critically examine and seek justification for the knowledge we claim. In applying this orientation to the Fawcett metaparadigm we utilised meme theory, interpreting the metaparadigm as a notion that has become reified and incorporated in our nursing culture as the dominant accepted framework for establishing the parameters of our nursing knowledge. But this device (meme theory) also assisted us in viewing this metaparadigm in a balanced and critical manner. What we must address in the final section of our chapter is how we actually formulate the knowledge that is within our metaparadigm.

Study Activity 9.6

In a recent journal paper, Thorne *et al.* (1998) presented a case for concern about how nursing theory and the nursing metaparadigm debates have become polarised and reflect extreme positions of nursing theorists. They claimed that this is in fact putting nursing's mandate (or support and acceptance by society) at risk. It is perhaps regrettable that they advanced their arguments by assuming the above Fawcett metaparadigm and also by referring to this as nursing's 'main metaparadigm' as if this is taken for granted, and as if there are other metaparadigms that are subsidiary to the 'main' metaparadigm. However, in their conclusion they stated:

> . . . we can no longer tolerate our theorists standing apart from the whole of nursing knowledge and from each other. In our view, it is the job of mainstream nursing to challenge the theorists to show how the projects underway in their own theory development will contribute to epistemological holism.

- Do you feel these theoretical debates, as outlined above, including those advanced by the supporters *and* detractors of the Fawcett metaparadigm, *do* reflect a standing apart from the real world of nursing?
- What are your views about the possibility of arriving at an epistemological 'holism', a metaparadigmatic framework that all nurses will be aware of and will subscribe to?
- If we *do* not manage to achieve this, what do you think may be the implications for the future of our profession?

WAYS OF COMING TO KNOW AND TO BE

Sources of knowledge

One approach is to consider how we come to know in terms of *sources* of knowledge. Kerlinger (1986) identified four sources of knowledge, which were essentially based on the means by which knowledge is derived.

- *Tenacity* – here we believe something is true because it has always been held to be true. Such knowledge is often culture-bound and as such is often also termed traditional knowledge. Because it is so embedded in a culture, it is believed in and held to with a high degree of persistence. Thus, in one society we 'know' that it is wrong to eat pork, while in another this is not the case and pork is considered a delicacy. Similarly, in one society we 'know' that Jesus was the Messiah while in another he may only be recognised (if at all) as having been a minor prophet.
- *Authority* – here knowledge is held to be true simply because a person or body in authority says it is true. This type of knowledge also has strong societal influences, in terms of social pressures to conform to the dominant view and in terms of real or imagined sanctions for those who do not conform. As a result, people often accept something to be factually correct simply because the authority says this is the case. If people operated with a degree of independent reasoning, they might question such authority, and indeed sometimes do. For example, a government may state that there are not enough resources to provide all the health care that everyone needs. But this *may not* be the case if resources were not also being allocated to other activities such as nuclear armaments or Millennium Domes. However, the sheer power of authority is its underpinning. There is a tendency to assume that those in authority are the experts, that they have more knowledge, that they *must* know. After all, they *are* an authority on the matter! By this process, the position of the 'authority' becomes *reified;* that is, what the 'authority' values, aspires to, or actively promotes as the true position becomes interpreted not as their *view* of the world, but in fact the *real* world.

However, there is sometimes a tendency to view authority with suspicion. This is not always entirely unfounded. For example, the French scholar Michel Foucault (1972) drew attention to the close relationship between knowledge and power. In effect, not only does knowledge *give* power, but those *in* power also have the capacity to control the distribution of knowledge and even to construct knowledge in dominant discourses. This is particularly important in the modern information age where communication networks are now subject to unprecedented scrutiny. On the one hand, our own privacy is invaded and 'authority' knows about us and what we do. But at the same time, under an illusion of access to an exponentially expanding mountain of knowledge, some vitally important knowledge can be withheld. Indeed, even in respect of our own health care systems, there are numerous examples of medical error and pharmaceutical disasters being suppressed by governments and multinational corporations. It is probably the case that those exposed by investigative journalists are but the tip of an iceberg.

- *Empiricism* – here knowledge is gained by direct observation of the external world. By observing phenomena in the world, describing, measuring, searching for relationships, making predictions, generalising from the specific instances we have observed to similar situations, a process we defined earlier as induction, we arrive at knowledge of the world. When we replicate our investigations and come to the same or very similar findings, we are strengthening the reliability of this knowledge. We can then make claims for its validity as a true reflection of the world or a part of that world. This is in fact the application of the scientific method and such activities we term research. Of course, a part of the argument behind this process is that if you cannot measure it, cannot test and re-test its authenticity, it does not exist. It is not real knowledge. For most people, and this is certainly the view expressed by Kerlinger (1986), empirically derived knowledge is the most reliable and that which should be strived for in the quest for true knowledge.

- *Apriorism* – here, as noted earlier, knowledge is arrived at *a priori*, i.e. prior to and without any experience to base it upon. Such knowledge is the product of internal processes of reasoning and the deductions made in the course of such reasoning. The argument here is that we can arrive at knowledge through discerning patterns, or logical reasoning from premises to conclusions (which is in effect a deductive process). We do not *need* experience or prior knowledge to reach our conclusions. This is in direct contrast to the view that knowledge is *a posteriori,* i.e. always based upon some previous knowledge or experience of the real world. On the basis of such previous experience, such as observing liquids expanding when heated, we can propose (or hypothesise) that this is factual information (knowledge), and indeed generalise from this to other situations where heat is applied to liquids. This process of moving from the particular to the general is, as noted earlier, the opposite to deduction, a process of *induction*. Those aligned to the empirical perspective (that is essentially inductive as well as deductive) find it difficult to accept the notion of apriorism. It is of course recognised that in mathematics and deductive logic it is possible to see numerical patterns and relationships, and logical progressions, that are apparently not dependent on experience, but are a characteristic of the way humans think. A capacity to intuitively recognise such patterns and make deductions from them seems to be a facet of our humanity. But even here, the empiricists either claim that the product of such processes is not real knowledge, or that it is in fact the product of past experiences of which we are unaware.

Immanuel Kant (1938/1781) viewed *a priori* knowledge as of the highest order, not resulting from experience and not susceptible to it in any way. Thus, we know or deduce in an *a priori* way that to wantonly kill another human being is wrong. We do not need to observe the external world and derive 'proofs' from it to arrive at this conclusion. We just know that there is no justification for killing another person when they have done us no harm and are not threatening us in any way. It is self-evident from our internal reasoning that this is correct.

Kerlinger (1986), conversely, places apriorism at a lower level than empirical knowledge. The scientist might suggest that if you cannot test the reliability and validity of a piece of knowledge, then you can never prove it is correct. Some philosophers will of course argue, like Kant, that it does not have to be proved: it is in fact self-evident. These arguments become less important in practice due to the fact that the two viewpoints usually address different kinds of knowledge. In general, empirical knowledge concerns external objects we can perceive. In *a priori* knowledge we often address non-material notions, sometimes of an ethical or moral nature, which could not in any case be directly observed even if we did want to utilise an empirical approach. For us, there is no 'either/or' argument here. We need them both.

In nursing, therefore, it is important to recognise that the development of empirical knowledge is essential to safe and effective practice. But it is not the only source of relevant knowledge in what is fundamentally a complex humanistic activity. In the absence of empirically derived knowledge, we may be justified in applying traditional knowledge, which in our professional experience has been found to be sound. It is only a problem if we hold on to this knowledge with tenacity when our experience or sound empirical evidence disproves its validity. Furthermore, we are often equally justified in following our *a priori* reasoning in adopting ethical stances in regard to nursing or wider health care issues.

In an occupation which is essentially practice orientated, 'knowledge of doing' or 'know-how' is also highly important. Benner (1984), in her work involving mapping nurses' development from the level of novice to that of expert, found that novices required concrete rules and procedures but that experts operated on a level of intuitive knowing, being able to know exactly what to do in complex problem situations without even being able sometimes to explain why they made exactly the correct decisions. Polanyi (1967) has labelled such deep know-how as *tacit knowledge,* a high degree of capacity to function with expertise without having to think, explain or problem solve, indeed often being unable to explain why it is 'just known' that something is right in a particular situation. There is a close affinity between 'just knowing' and apriorism. Given the importance of each of these different forms of knowledge, an approach such as Kerlinger's (1986), which ranks types of knowledge and by definition devalues some of these, is open to criticism.

Study Activity 9.7

Do you feel that Kerlinger (1986) is justified in prescribing empirical knowledge as the most important form of knowledge? What are the arguments for and against?

Patterns of knowing in nursing

Perhaps the most influential contribution in this area is that by Carper (1978). Carper reviewed the nursing literature and found that four discrete patterns of knowing emerged. Each of the patterns is recognised as a valid way of knowing in its own right and none is viewed to take precedence over the others in the way suggested by Kerlinger (1986). The four patterns of knowing identified were as follows.

- *Empirics: the science of nursing* – this is essentially the same as the empirical dimension identified in the previous section. The empirical or scientific perspective, as empha-

sised by Carper, is similarly derived from observation and experience that is subjected to the scientific method for confirming the knowledge claim.

- *Ethics: moral knowledge in nursing* – this is similar to the notion of *a priorism* discussed in the previous section. Ethics, however, is concerned specifically with notions of moral right and wrong. Much of nursing literature on ethics and the knowledge contained within it addresses not only the formal principles of ethics and moral philosophy, but also the practical nature of decisions of a moral nature, which nursing demands from the individual nurse on a daily basis (e.g. Tschudin, 1993a, b).

- *Personal knowing in nursing* – this way of knowing does not really find a close equivalent in Kerlinger's (1986) scheme. Personal knowing concerns the capacity to be introspective and to become aware of one's inner being. It thus does not fit in at all with Ayer's (1956) view of knowledge as by definition that which is shared and accepted by the group, as it is by definition personal, idiosyncratic and internally reflective by nature. However, it is increasingly recognised in nursing that in order to be able to reach out and help the other person on a highly personal and intimate basis, we must first have a deeper knowledge and acceptance of ourselves as individuals. This intensely personal and deeply subjective form of personal knowing is at the very heart of our capacity to care for others, as discussed in Chapter 2. In the phenomenological experiencing of self and other by the two people involved in a nurse–patient relationship, it can be experienced, it can be alluded to, but it cannot in its actuality be described. It is to do with the personal wisdom of knowledge of self, of knowledge of and empathy with the other, of *being* with *and for* the other at a time of need. While such personal knowing cannot be readily explicated, its vital importance as a capacity that grows and must be nurtured, as the very essence of the nurse's therapeutic presence, must never be overlooked.

- *Aesthetics: the art of nursing* – in many regards this form of knowing equates with what the epistemologists refer to as knowledge of doing or 'know-how'. This refers to the spontaneous expression of the art/act of doing nursing. Aesthetic knowledge at its most developed is the capacity to know what to do at a given moment without having to consciously deliberate on what needs to be done. The nurse who has achieved this level of aesthetic knowledge, which we might term artistry or mastery, just knows what to do in the instant, even though she may not be able to explain why the particular course of action was taken. This is in effect the tacit knowledge of Polanyi (1966) or the intuitive expert practitioner described by Benner (1984) at work. Aesthetic knowledge, like the tacit knowledge described by Polanyi, would also not fit in with the highly prescriptive explication of public knowledge as presented by Ayer (1956). However, as in the case of personal knowledge, it is a vital and central element in the practice of nursing.

There are perhaps two important things to note about Carper's 'patterns of knowing' in nursing. First, unlike Kerlinger's classification, there is no reference to knowledge based on tenacity or authority here. Does this mean that these forms of knowledge are missing from Carper's classification? This is in fact not necessarily the case. What Carper describes as personal and aesthetic knowledge will often include knowledge that nurses hold with tenacity and perhaps pass on to each other in an authoritative way. These nurses just know something is right, it does not have to be *proved* empirically and they hold on to this knowledge with confidence and certainty – some would say tenacity. Those who see such knowledge as unscientific and invalid will reject it. To them, notions of intuition or tacit forms of thought that cannot be explained and broken down into their component ideas or conceptual frameworks cannot be depended upon. But increasingly, writers like Polanyi and Benner have shown that personal knowledge and tacit

understanding *are* in fact sound ways of knowing, no less valid because they cannot be observed and explained easily in mechanistic terms.

Second, Carper recognises that these are not alternative ways of knowing. Rather, in the complex field of nursing practice there is an interrelationship and indeed interdependence between the four patterns. Inherent in this perspective is an understanding that in relating as whole person to whole person, as self to self, one narrow approach to knowing would be inadequate. During the enactment of nursing practice, the nurse brings to bear all these ways of knowing. Empirics which provides objective knowledge about the disease process and its treatment cannot be excluded; safe practice depends on such knowledge. At the same time, the nurse needs sound ethical knowledge to guide her practice. This is not a mode of knowing dissociated from empirical knowledge. New knowledge and technologies emerging from it raise new moral questions – about allocation of resources, genetic engineering, euthanasia, etc. Furthermore, the need to keep up-to-date with the latest evidence is itself an ethical imperative. Personal knowledge is at the heart of all nursing action; the nurse must know her innermost self as she goes out from this knowledge to knowledge of her patient in the intimate interpersonal act of nursing. In high technology health care systems there is a great risk of depersonalising and objectifying the patient or client. There is a need to ensure that evidence-based health care takes account of the individual and their choices, and our own ethical choices, which also impact upon real persons. Finally, we must not as nurses ignore or disvalue our tacit and intuitive knowledge of nursing practice simply because it cannot be explained and justified on a scientific basis. We recognise the feel of the artist for his brushwork and the sensitivity of the airline pilot to the functioning of his aircraft, which extends far beyond what his instruments are telling him. We must also recognise that in the complex human endeavour that is nursing practice, nurses too have an aesthetic feel for their art, a degree of intuitive know-how that extends beyond mere following of rules and procedures.

Increasingly you will hear debate about the notion of nursing as art or science. The message implicit in Carper's conceptualisation is that of nursing as *art and science*, as practised within an intimate personal relationship.

Study Activity 9.8

Consider the following vignette taken from memos in a qualitative study.

Four in the morning
It is 4 a.m. The hospital is quiet. The nurse enters a single-bedded ward. In the bed is a 12-year-old girl. She is fine-featured and attractive; the first touch of womanhood is upon her. But she is frail and wasted, an almost skeletal form on the bed. The girl is wide awake and stares almost pleadingly at the nurse. She is pale and drawn. Most of her hair is missing, her scalp unsightly with bald patches and lifeless wisps of hair. An intravenous infusion is running. There is a sour smell of sickness, cloying and sweet in the warm room. Beside the girl a woman slumbers in an armchair; she too – the girl's mother – has a pinched and exhausted appearance.

The nurse 'knows' this girl and her mother. She 'knows' the lethal condition and the almost as lethal chemotherapy the girl is enduring. She knows other things too. At this time, in this place, there is only the girl and the nurse. The physicians and pathologists, the hospital pharmacists, the administrators – all are at home in their beds, asleep. Here, now, in the hours before dawn, in the mutual gaze between nurse and girl, there is also a knowledge. The nurse 'knows' pain and distress here and she recognises the unspoken fear of death here. She knows too her own feelings of compassion and fear, her urge to leave and forget about this room of pain and its desperate occupants. With all this knowledge – of disease, of treatment, of pain and nausea, of hopelessness and desperation, of the begging for deliverance contained in a gaze – the nurse moves toward the bed and into the presence of the patient. All this knowledge the nurse must bring to bear in this moment of being

with the patient. There is only her; she must do what she can as knowledge and doing become one.

- It should be apparent that some of the patterns of knowing identified in Carper's framework are related to passages in this account. Identify the passages so reflected and the particular knowledge pattern in each case.
- Clearly, in this brief time sample, not all four of Carper's patterns would be fully reflected. However, using each of her four patterns as side-headings, identify how each (empirical, personal, ethical and aesthetic) might serve as knowledge underpinnings in the care of this young patient.
- When you are next in a clinical placement area, consider the care of a patient with whom you are directly involved. In a similar manner, establish the extent to which each pattern is informing the care of this patient.

SUMMARY

The intention in this chapter was to provide the reader with an overview of that branch of philosophy entitled epistemology. There was an attempt to present this topic as essentially being the study of knowledge. More specifically, it is concerned with what knowledge is, how we come to know it, and how we justify claims in respect of it. It also includes a consideration of the different forms that knowledge takes, and how we may develop frameworks or taxonomies of knowledge.

An important consideration is, of course, the relevance of all this for nursing. In the very first opening sentence of this chapter it is stated that: 'When you get out there, you had better know what you are doing'. However, the word 'know' is in question here. This followed an opening quotation from the Code of Professional Conduct established by the UK regulatory body for nursing and midwifery (Nursing and Midwifery Council, 2002). This opening quotation draws attention to requirements in respect of knowledge acquisition and updating for nurses in the UK. In that same Code the following is also stated:

> *As a registered nurse or midwife ...*
> *You have a responsibility to deliver care*
> *based on current evidence, best practice and,*
> *where applicable, validated research, when it*
> *is available.*
>
> (Nursing and Midwifery Council, 2002)

This is the only place in which the Code is specific about the nature of knowledge that should inform our practice. In referring to 'current evidence' and 'validated research' (which are essentially the same thing), the Council is clearly attaching priority to that which we have termed empirical knowing in this chapter. We can assume (and this would only be an assumption) that the requirement to base care on 'best practice' implies other forms of knowledge or wisdom are also important.

This issue of forms, or types, of knowledge in respect of nursing is also addressed in this chapter. In a recent publication, Watson (1999) speaks of the need to view our world through Venus's mirror, i.e. from our feminine side as well as from the more rational and logical perspective that is often viewed as emerging from our masculine side. In this, Watson and others (Gilligan, 1982, 1997; Belenky *et al.*, 1997) are alluding to the more intuitive and contextualised form of knowing that we have addressed earlier. It is indeed important that in the complex human undertaking that is nursing, characterised by demands for highly sophisticated technical intervention *and* a need for highly personalised caring, we can draw on a range of ways of knowing. Put simply, there are things about the care of people that can *never* be known through empirical knowledge (based upon objective observation). Equally, in a highly objectified and technical health service, there are things that can *only* be known through empirical knowledge. There are no either/or choices here. There is in fact a moral or ethical imperative to integrate all such forms of knowing in our practice. Clearly, we must recognise that there is a need for a *nursing* epistemology, and justifying this claim was a major aim of the chapter.

In addressing such issues, the chapter has in essence two further broad aims. First, it is intended as an introduction to the four chapters that follow. In considering a *nursing* epistemology, we gave considerable attention to how nursing knowledge may be framed. This included a consideration of the nursing meta-paradigm (the essential conceptual elements that are a common feature in nursing knowledge and practice). In this context, we attended in particular to Fawcett's (1984, 1996) metaparadigm, with its elements of: person; health; environment; and nursing. We also considered Carper's (1978) patterns of knowing, which included: empirical knowing; ethical knowing; personal knowing; and aesthetic knowing. Each one of the following four chapters address one of Carper's patterns. Second, by presenting such frameworks, it is hoped that the reader will be able to evaluate knowledge in terms of how it reflects or measures up to the metaparadigm and the patterns of knowing. By so doing, we may indeed move towards that best practice that is alluded to in the above Code of Professional Conduct (Nursing and Midwifery Council, 2002).

Within the chapter we have met difficulties in respect of what are essentially divisions between the sciences and the humanities, between the ascendancy of the empirical or scientific claims on knowledge, and a nursing world that also calls for other ways of knowing. We have also met the need to be sceptical or critical of all ways of knowing, including the empirical. Indeed, as we have moved beyond the scientific world of modernity we are faced with a new post-modernism that sensitises us to the relativity, contextuality, culture-boundedness and transient nature of our knowledge. In answer to our opening sentence stating, 'When you get out there, you had better know what you are doing', your response must be: 'But how are we to know?' If this *is* your question, and if you *care* about the answer, then this chapter has succeeded and you are on the right path. The problems have not gone away, but you are now a nursing epistemologist and you will participate in the solutions.

169

REFERENCES

Adler, M. (1985) *Ten Philosophical Mistakes,* Macmillan, New York

Audi, R. (1998) *Epistemology: A contemporary introduction to the theory of knowledge,* Routledge, London

Ayer, A.J. (1956) *The Problem of Knowledge,* Penguin, Harmondsworth

Baker, M. (1998) Challenging ignorance. In: Baker, M. and Kirk, S. (eds) *Research and Development for the NHS* (2nd edn), Radcliffe Medical Press, Oxford

Belenky, M., Clinchy, B., Goldberger, N. *et al.* (1997) *Women's Ways of Knowing: The development of self, voice, and mind* (10th anniversary edn), Basic Books, New York

Benner, P. (1984) *From Novice to Expert: Excellence and power in clinical practice,* Addison Wesley, Menlo Park, CA

Benner, P., Tanner, C. and Chesla, C. (1996) *Expertise in Nursing Practice: Caring, clinical judgment, and ethics,* Springer, New York

Benner, P., Hooper-Kyriakidis, P. and Stannard, D. (1999) *Clinical Wisdom and Interventions in Critical Care: A thinking in action approach,* W.B. Saunders, Philadelphia, IL

Bohm, D. (1980) *Wholeness and the Implicate Order,* Ark Paperbacks, London

Carper, B.A. (1978) Fundamental patterns of knowing in nursing. *Advances in Nursing Science* 1, 13–23

Chinn, P.L. and Kramer, M.K. (1999) *Theory and Nursing: Integrated knowledge development* (5th edn), Mosby, St Louis, IL

Code, L. (1991) *What Can She Know? Feminist Theory and the Construction of Knowledge,* Cornell University Press, Ithaca, NY

Cody, W.K. (1996) On the requirements for a paradigm – response. *Nursing Science Quarterly* 9, 97–9

Conway, M. (1985) Toward greater specificity in defining nursing's metaparadigm. *Nursing Science Quarterly* 7, 73–81

Dawkins, R. (1976) *The Selfish Gene,* Oxford University Press, Oxford

Fawcett, J. (1984) The metaparadigm of nursing: present status and future refinements. *Image: The Journal of Nursing Scholarship* 16, 84–7

Fawcett, J. (1993) From a plethora of paradigms to parsimony in world views. *Nursing Science Quarterly* 6, 56–8

Fawcett, J. (1995) *Conceptual Models and Contemporary Nursing Knowledge* (3rd edn), F.A. Davis, Philadelphia, IL

Fawcett, J. (1996) On the requirements for a paradigm – commentary. *Nursing Science Quarterly* 9, 94–7

Fawcett, J. (2000) *Analysis and Evaluation of Contemporary Nursing Knowledge: Nursing models and theories,* F.A. Davis, Philadelphia, IL

Flaming, D. (2001) Using *phronesis* instead of 'research-based practice' as the guiding light for nursing practice. *Nursing Philosophy* 2, 251–8

Foucault, M. (1972) *The Archeology of Knowledge,* Tavistock, London

Freshwater, D. and Broughton, R. (2001) Research and evidence-based practice. In: Bishop, V. and Scott, I. (eds) *Challenges in Clinical Practice: Professional developments in nursing,* Palgrave, Basingstoke

Gilligan, C. (1982) *In a Different Voice: Psychological theory and women's development,* Harvard University Press, Cambridge, MA

Gilligan, C. (1997) In a different voice: women's conceptions of self and morality. In: Meyers, D.T. (ed.) *Feminist Social Thought: A reader,* Routledge, New York

Glaser, B. and Strauss, A. (1967) *The Discovery of Grounded Theory,* Aldine, Chicago, IL

Haack, S. (1993) *Evidence and Inquiry: Towards reconstruction in epistemology,* Blackwell, Oxford

Hartsock, N. (1997) The feminist standpoint: developing the ground for a specifically feminist historical materialism. In: Nicholson, L. (ed.) *The Second Wave,* Routledge, New York

Heidegger, M. (1959) The fundamental question of metaphysics. In: Heidegger, M. (ed.) *An Introduction to Metaphysics,* Yale University Press, New Haven, NY

Henderson, V. (1966) *The Nature of Nursing: A definition and its implications for practice, research, and education,* Macmillan, New York

Hockey, L. (1987) Issues in the communication of nursing research. In: Hockey, L. (ed.) *Recent Advances in Nursing: Current issues 1987,* Churchill Livingstone, Edinburgh

Jagger, A.M. (1997) Love and knowledge: emotion in feminist epistemology. In: Meyers, D.T. (ed.) *Feminist Social Thought: A reader,* Routledge, New York

Kant, I. (1938/1781) *The Fundamental Principles of*

the Metaphysic of Ethics, Appleton-Century-Crofts, New York

Kerlinger, F.N. (1986) *Foundations of Behavioural Research,* Holt, Rinehart and Winston, New York

Kim, H.S. (1983) *The Nature of Theoretical Thinking in Nursing,* Appleton-Century-Crofts, Norwalk

Kim, H.S. (1987) Structuring the nursing knowledge system: a typology of four domains. *Scholarly Inquiry for Nursing Practice* 1, 99–110.

Kim, H.S. (2000) An integrative framework for conceptualizing clients: a proposal for a nursing perspective in the new century. *Nursing Science Quarterly* 13, 37–44

Kirby, C. and Slevin, O. (1992) A new curriculum for care. In: Slevin, O. and Buckenham, M. (eds) *Project 2000: The teachers speak,* Campion Press, Edinburgh

Kuhn, T. (1970) *The Structure of Scientific Revolutions,* University of Chicago Press, Chicago, IL

Lazreg, M. (1994) Women's experience and feminist epistemology: a critical neo-rationalist approach. In: Lennon, K. and Whitford, M. (eds) *Knowing the Difference: Feminist perspectives in epistemology,* Routledge, London

Longino, H. (1990) *Science as Social Knowledge,* Princeton University Press, Princeton

Masterman, M. (1970) The nature of a paradigm. In: Lakatos, I. and Musgrave, A. (eds) *Criticism and the Growth of Knowledge,* Cambridge University Press, Cambridge

McKenna, H. (1997) *Nursing Theories and Models,* Routledge, London

Meleis, A. (1997) *Theoretical Nursing: Development and progress,* Lippincott, Philadelphia, IL

Muir Grey J.A. (1997) *Evidence-based Healthcare: How to make health policy and management decisions,* Churchill Livingstone, Edinburgh

Nursing and Midwifery Council (2002) *Code of Professional Conduct,* Nursing and Midwifery Council, London

Parse, R. (1987) Paradigms and theories. In: Parse, R.R. (ed.) *Nursing Science: Major paradigms, theories and critiques,* W.B. Saunders, Philadelphia, IL

Paterson, J. and Zderad, L. (1988) *Humanistic Nursing,* National League for Nursing, New York

Polanyi, M. (1966) *The Tacit Dimension,* Routledge and Kegan Paul, London

Popper, K. (1989) *Conjectures and Refutations* (5th edn), Routledge, London

Rawnsley, M.M. (1996) On the requirements for a paradigm – Response. *Nursing Science Quarterly* 9, 102–6

Rose, P. and Marks-Maran, D. (1997) A new view of nursing: turning the cube. In: Marks-Maran, D. and Rose, P. (eds) *Reconstructing Nursing: Beyond art and science,* Baillière Tindall, London

Russell, B. (1995) *An Inquiry into Meaning and Truth* (revised edn), Routledge, London

Ryle, G. (1949) *The Concept of Mind,* Hutchinson, London

Sackett, D., Straus, S., Richardson, W., *et al.* (2000) *Evidence-based Medicine: How to practice and teach EBM* (2nd edn), Churchill Livingstone, Toronto

Seedhouse, D. (1998) *Ethics: The heart of health care* (2nd edn), John Wiley, Chichester

Slevin, O. (1995) Theories and models. In: Basford, L. and Slevin, O. (eds) *Theory and Practice of Nursing: An integrated approach to patient care,* Nelson Thornes, Cheltenham

Slevin, O. (1999) The nurse–patient relationship: caring in a health context. In: Long, A. (ed.) *Interaction for Practice in Community Nursing,* Macmillan, Basingstoke

Thorne, S., Canam, C., Dahinten, S., *et al.* (1998) Nursing's metaparadigm concepts: disimpacting the debates, *Journal of Advanced Nursing* 27, 1257–68

Tschudin, V. (1993a) *Ethics – Nurses and patients,* Scutari, London

Tschudin, V. (1993b) *Ethics – Aspects of nursing care,* Scutari, London

Van der Peet, R. (1995) *The Nightingale Model of Nursing: An analysis of Florence Nightingale's concepts of nursing, and their impact on present day practice,* Campion Press, Edinburgh

Walker, L.O. and Avant, K.C. (1995) *Strategies for Theory Construction in Nursing* (3rd edn), Appleton-Lang, East Norwalk, CT

Watson, J. (1985) *Nursing – The philosophy and science of caring,* University of Colorado Press, Niwot, CO

Watson, J. (1999) *Postmodern Nursing and Beyond,* Churchill Livingstone, Edinburgh

Yura, H. and Torres, G. (1975) Today's conceptual frameworks within baccalaureate nursing programs. In: National League for Nursing (ed.) *Faculty Curriculum Development, Part 3, Conceptual Framework – Its meaning and function,* National League for Nursing, New York

10 EMPIRICAL KNOWING: A KNOWLEDGE BASE FOR NURSING PRACTICE

Eamonn Slevin

> 'What the Devil Does it all Mean?'
> A person may be supremely able as a
> mathematician, engineer, parliamentary
> tactician or racing bookmaker; but if the
> person has contemplated the universe all
> through life without ever asking 'What the
> devil does it all mean?' he (or she) is one of
> those people for whom Calvin accounted by
> placing them in the category of the
> predestinately dammed.
>
> (George Bernard Shaw, *The Adventures of the*
> *Black Girl in Her Search for God*,
> cited in Silver, 1998)

LEARNING OUTCOMES

After studying this chapter you will be able to:

- Demonstrate an understanding of empirical knowledge
- Define and explain the concepts induction, deduction, retroduction, and also verification and refutation
- Comprehend the value of 'science' to knowledge generation
- Develop a critical stance to the question of certainty in knowledge
- Discuss the issue of 'contemporary nursing empirics' in a way that demonstrates an understanding of:
  - theories as empirical nursing actions
  - nursing science
  - conflict between nursing and traditional empiricism
  - how empirical knowledge for nursing emerges
  - the value of empirical evidence in nursing.

INTRODUCTION

Barbara Carper (1978), in her seminal work, identified four main 'ways of knowing' in nursing: empirical, ethical, personal and aesthetic. The four patterns do not inform nursing knowledge in isolation from each other but rather nurses draw on each in the care they provide. However, this chapter is mainly concerned with empirical knowledge and its benefits, as well as limitations, to nursing.

TRADITIONAL EMPIRICS

Empirics is aligned with the quantitative research tradition, referred to as natural science, and the systematic modes of knowledge development valued within this paradigm. This is one of the oldest paradigms of knowledge discovery and it can be traced back to the philosophy of Rene Descartes (1596–1650). Prior to Descartes there were beliefs in magic, myths and various other forms of knowing. Descartes may be considered the forefather of what became known as 'science'(although one could argue that the work of Aristotle in Ancient Greece was perhaps the beginning of science). A British philosopher, John Locke (1632–1704), who was influenced a great deal by Descartes, is recognised as one of the founders of empiricism. There are two basic tenets of empiricism. One is that what we know is learned from our senses, knowledge is derived from observation and the observer must maintain distance and objectivity in order to discover an unpolluted truth. Second, the truth must be able to be tested or verified by strict scientific criteria.

There are various types of empiricism, for example classical, radical, critical and logical. One of the differences in the various types of empiricism is the 'extremeness' with which the tenets are adhered to. In respect to this chapter, only two forms are considered, one is the extreme paradigm known as 'logical positivism' and the other is referred to here as contemporary nursing empiricism.

Logical positivism

In the early 1920s, a group of philosophers known as the 'Vienna Circle' gave birth to the extreme form of empiricism referred to as 'logical positivism'. This group of philosophers presented thoughts on knowledge development, many of which are still intrinsic to the positivist (quantitative) research paradigm. These views still underpin much of the 'traditional scientific' approach to knowledge acquisition. With respect to knowledge, logical positivism is underpinned by a number of tenets:

- the belief that truth is only truth if it can be objectively experienced (or at least indirectly perceived) through observation of the natural world.
- the belief that truth can be verified or tested by a process of systematic steps
- the use of quantitative methods to verify truth or falsity.

The presumptions of the members of the Vienna Circle are not considered extreme only because of the methods of inquiry (many are still used today) but because of their objection to almost all other forms of knowledge. Silver (1998) states 'logical positivism is empiricism taken to extremes'. To illustrate this, Silver cites Ayer (an English follower of the Vienna Circle) who stated 'a sentence is factually significant to a given person if, and only if, he knows how to verify the propositions which it purports to express'. Silver (1998) goes on to cite the philosopher David Hume, who stated the following:

> Does it contain any abstract reasoning concerning quantity or number? No. Does it contain any experimental reasoning concerning matter of fact existence? No.

> Commit it then to the flames: for it can contain nothing but sophistry and illusion.
>
> (Silver, 1998)

As you will gather from the above comments, there is little room within logical positivism for knowledge that is generated by means other than the traditional scientific method, and this most often involved quantitative experimentation. The notions and ideas of logical positivism have few who rigidly adhere to all these principles today, but many of the underlying premises are still held. Richard Dawkins is one of our most influential academics. His book, *The Selfish Gene* (Dawkins, 1976), is well known to many as a popular science classic. He has a distinguished academic record and is certainly one of the leading proponents of evolution in the latter third of the twentieth century.

Dawkins is a confirmed scientist of the traditional positivistic science kind. He sees the project of science as the establishment of truth or sound and incontrovertible knowledge on the basis of observation and measurement. Note these comments he made in 1993, in response to a plea for science and theology or religion to work together in the growth of knowledge and wisdom:

> ... you remark that people want to know as much as possible about their origins. I certainly hope they do, but what makes you think that 'theology' has anything useful to say on the subject. Science is responsible for the following knowledge about our origins. We know approximately when the universe began and why it is largely hydrogen. We know why stars form, and what happens in their interiors to convert hydrogen to other elements and hence give birth to chemistry in a world of physics ... It is science, and science alone, that has given us this knowledge and given it, moreover, in fascinating, overwhelming, mutually confirming detail. On every one of these questions theology has held a view that has been conclusively proved wrong. Science has eradicated smallpox, can

immunise against most previously deadly viruses, can kill most previously deadly bacteria. Theology has done nothing but talk of pestilence as the wages of sin ... When has 'theology' ever said anything that is demonstrably true and is not obvious? ... I have listened to theologians ... I have never heard any of them say anything that was not either platitudinously obvious or downright false. If all the achievements of science were wiped out tomorrow there would be no doctors but witch-doctors, no transport faster than a horse, no computers, no printed books, no agriculture beyond subsistence farming. If all the achievements of theologians were wiped out tomorrow, would anyone notice the smallest difference ... What makes you think that 'theology' is a subject at all?

(Dawkins, 1993)

Dawkins may well apply his criticism to any non-scientific discipline: the humanities, philosophy, perhaps even the qualitative social and human sciences. It is unlikely that the claim for alternative sources of knowledge, such as that proposed by Carper (1978) or Slevin (1995), would carry much weight with Dawkins. His view would clearly be very much in line with the proposition that research or empirically derived knowledge is science and all else is conjecture.

Dawkins sees the project of science as being the production of *verifiable evidences* and the establishment of consistencies within and between theories or emerging 'proven' hypotheses. This is, of course, the position of classical natural science. In very simple terms, *truth* is established on the basis of evidence that *verifies* the relationships, and indeed often the cause–effect relationships, between variables.

Study Activity 10.1

Reflect on the ideas of logical positivism and those of Dawkins cited above. Discuss with colleagues whether or not you agree with the ideas that only knowledge

that emerges from a rigorous scientific method is of value.

Deduction and induction

Inductive reasoning is a process of knowledge development that involves making specific observations of a number of cases and then inferring this to further instances of the phenomena, or drawing a general conclusion. Early empiricists and philosophers suggest this method is associated with quantitative research and experiments. However, contemporary views are that inductive reasoning is most often associated with qualitative research. Moody (1990) suggests that many nurses use qualitative research methods to inductively develop theories. Put simply, inductive knowledge development involves observing multiple occurrences and then combining these multiple occurrences into the whole picture. The approach is often used in nursing to generate theory, for example Glaser and Strauss's (1967) grounded theory research approach (Moody, 1990; Chinn and Kramer, 1995).

One of the most famous examples of induction cited in many texts is that of the 'black raven'. If a number of ravens are observed that are black (these observations are premises) then inference can be made that the next raven that is seen will also be black, or that all ravens are black. However, the truth of inductive premises can never guarantee the truth of the outcome to the premises. This is because the premises predict something that is beyond them, i.e. that the next raven seen will be black, or that all ravens are black. All it takes to overturn this is for someone to see a white raven and then the conclusion is dismissed. A main difference between induction and deduction is that in deduction the truth of all the premises is held to guarantee the outcome or conclusion, whereas in induction this is not so.

Deductive approaches usually involve quantitative research methods – a researcher begins with a theory or hypothesis and then tests these by the collection and analysis of empirical data

(Moody, 1990). Deductive approaches are thus aligned with traditional (or natural) science. Deductive reasoning involves making specific conclusions from general premises. The following is an example:

(premise)   all A is B
(premise)   all C is A
(conclusion)   all C is B

(Powers and Knapp, 1995).

We can use the above premises to come to the conclusion that all C is also B based on the two preceding premises.

Deduction is also called the hypothetico-deductive approach, i.e. the premises may be stated as hypotheses (statements about relationships between variables) and deductive reasoning is used to test the outcome to the hypothesis statement. A problem can arise, however, if one of the premises or hypotheses is not correct – for if a premise is incorrect then the conclusion on which it draws will also be incorrect. Silver (1998) illustrated this well with the following:

> All homosexuals are evil (hypothesis).
> Benjamin Britten was a homosexual (true).
> Therefore, Benjamin Britten was evil (false).
>
> (Silver, 1998)

As Silver states, by all accounts Benjamin Britten was not evil, so the hypothesis is wrong. But, if all the premises are true then it follows that the conclusion on which the premises are based should be true.

In the case of induction, how far can a universal or inductive statement be justified on the basis of a finite number of observations, whereby on the basis of specific instances we draw conclusions that allow us to see the total picture or phenomenon? How do we know for sure that there are no exceptions to the rule? In the case of deduction, how much credence can we place on specific or deductive statements made on what we may perceive to be deducible from a number of objective observational facts? All inductive-deductive processes are established

on the basis of foundationalism, the premise that a body of knowledge in any discipline rests on a single or small set of foundational 'truths'. If the foundations are untrue, the castle comes tumbling down (see, for example, Haack, 1993).

Study Activity 10.2

With a group of colleagues, organise a discussion in which you identify a list of outcome statements, based on inductive and deductive reasoning, related to nursing care, health in general or any aspect that relates to nursing. Initially just develop the list. Then, when you have the list completed, debate whether you feel each statement is based on inductive or deductive reasoning. You will probably find this quite difficult, but do not worry, there is not total agreement among all theorists as to what constitutes induction and deduction.

Retroduction

There is another type of knowledge development referred to as 'retroduction' (also called abduction) that combines induction and deduction. It is often the case that research involves deductive and inductive approaches used together within a single study (McKenna, 1997). Retroduction involves a number of steps:

- Empirical data infer a relationship between phenomena.
- A hypothesis is developed that supports the possibility of the inference.
- Data are collected at several points (there is movement in this process between deduction and induction).
- The outcome is verification of the probability that the inference is true (probability will be discussed later).

In relation to theory or knowledge generation, some suggest that as retroduction begins with deduction, moves to induction and then again to deduction (perhaps a number of times) it can be considered a variation of deductive knowledge generation (Kim, 1996).

Is there certain knowledge?

The above discussion on induction and deduction and the critical questions that can be raised about each, may lead you to ask the question – how can we really 'know' anything for sure? Is there certain knowledge? And if not, then how relevant is Carper's (1978) empirical knowledge at all to nursing? In order to answer these questions, we need to consider a number of aspects. First, it can generate a great deal of debate if we say there are no 'certain' truths in life (even though logical positivism as discussed above strived to achieve certitude). One aspect that will always make this statement difficult to disprove is 'time'; no matter how certain we are of something *now* there is no guarantee that it will remain certain at a given time in the future. It can be argued that at a given time and in a given place something is true, and if it is 'facts' we are referring to it seems reasonable to do this (a fact might be something like the statement that 'man sees through his eyes'). In nursing there are many facts that are accepted as true. In order to answer the question – is there any certain truth? – scientists utilise two main approaches 'verification' and 'falsification'.

Verification or falsification

The issue is whether science is in the business of proving the undeniable truth or *verification* of knowledge, or showing that it has not been proven to be false, that it has withstood some test of *falsification*. This problem can be illustrated with the example of the black and white ravens (see above). From the point of view of *verification*, we can state that having observed a large or sufficient number of ravens and found that in all observed instances they were black, we can reasonably claim that ravens are black birds. But, from the point of view of *falsification*, the statement can only be accepted as true until disproved. The reasoning here is that, as study after study fails to show any falsity in the claim, it is reasonable to claim (at least tentatively) that ravens are black birds *until it is*

proved otherwise. What is being said here is that the *probability* is that all ravens are black until this is shown to be otherwise. It is worth noting this difference. Verification attempts to establish certain truth, on the other hand falsification establishes that the truth is probable (never certain).

The important point here, and the difference between verification and falsification in their extreme forms, is that falsification never assumes unassailable truth. It always involves recognition that the claim it makes may be disproved; indeed, such a possibility is at the core of its philosophy. Both verification and falsification address the same problem, but from different perspectives. These issues of verification and falsification, and the related issues of deduction and induction, are at the very heart of debates on the nature of science and the soundness of the evidence it presents.

The difficulty is that even when we utilise large samples, we are making what is essentially a leap of faith to some extent. However, in reality we can never be entirely sure that the final *truth* we generalise is sound. This is in fact what is commonly behind the claim that someone is making a gross generalisation. The message here is clear: ultimate and definite truth is unachievable.

Refutations

For the greater part of 2000 years and more, indeed up to the present century, the approach to the acquisition of knowledge was predicated on the concept of verification. The quest was to show or prove the unequivocal truth or falsity of any proposed body of knowledge. However, in the twentieth century, and primarily through the work of Karl Popper (1939, 1963), this idea was turned on its head. Popper argued that science could not be based on proof of truth by verification. The notion that certain truth could be arrived at was unsafe. Even if something was found to be true, Popper's view was that this was an improper course of action. He believed this to be flawed because accepting the original premise on which the truth was based was reliant on faith. Popper's premise was that no matter how often an assertion of truth was shown to apply, there is always the possibility of the alternative appearing.

On the basis of the latter argument, Popper proposed the concept of *falsification*. He claimed that science could only proceed by a process of *conjectures* and *refutations*. Popper suggested that the scientist makes conjectures or theorises about the nature of phenomena. The process then proceeds whereby research is carried out, not to verify the theory, but in fact to refute it. If repeated attempts to refute the theory fail to show it to be untrue, it has withstood the test of falsification. According to Popper, even then we would not claim verification. We would, conversely, recognise that the theory holds tentatively true until and if at some future time it is refuted.

When scientists set out to test their theories, they formulate hypotheses. A *hypothesis* is a statement indicating that there is a relationship between two or more variables. An example might be: giving children multivitamins each day for 10 years (from 2 to 12 years of age) will lead to an increase in their IQ levels. It is argued here that there is a relationship between the two variables – multivitamins and IQ level. One could set up an experiment involving an experimental group of children receiving multivitamins and a comparison control group who do not for the 10 year period. However, nowadays scientists seldom state the *experimental hypothesis* that postulates the conjectured relationship. Instead they state a *null hypothesis*, which in fact refutes the experimental hypothesis. Using the above example they will state: 'multivitamin supplements given to children each day from when they are aged 2 years until they are 12 years old will not lead to an increase in their IQ levels'. The extent to which the null hypothesis is *refuted* gives strength to the original conjecture about multivitamins increasing the children's IQ levels. This practice is recognition of the principle of refutation as opposed to verification.

Study Activity 10.3

With a group of colleagues organise a debate. The question to be debated is: 'Truth has to be certain or else it is not truth'.

CONTEMPORARY NURSING EMPIRICS

Having considered the historical philosophical movements in empirical knowledge, we now move on to what is referred to here as contemporary nursing empirics. Empirical knowledge in nursing is a systematic way of knowing that allows nurses to understand, explain and predict what the outcome to their actions will be. It is one type of evidence that nurses use to support the nursing care they provide. Nursing should base its practice on the evidence that is best suited to achieve the outcomes that are desired to help patients (patients here refers to patients in hospital or clients who receive nursing care in any setting). From the above discussion you will gather that evidence is never certain. Even in the most rigorous types of experimental research the best that can be said is that an outcome is probable. In this type of research you may see an outcome stating that the finding is 'statistically significant: $P < 0.05$'. What this means is that it is probable (P) that in less than five times in 100 (<0.05) this outcome will not occur again. Therefore, it is probable that in the future, all things being similar, 95 times out of 100 the outcome will occur again. This is not definite proof, but a probability. However, it is as near to certain as we can get. Strong rigorous empirical evidence should guide nursing practice. Such practice is underpinned by nursing theory and science.

Theories as empirical nursing actions

In nursing, theories have particular relevance. Theories here are not speculative. The reason for this in nursing is obvious, in that nursing is concerned with caring for people and, therefore, a nursing theory needs to be more than speculative, it should have a scientific basis. Frey (1995) acknowledges this when she states:

> nursing, as a profession, is responsible for its scientific basis, which documents its distinctiveness and separateness from, as well as its interrelatedness with, other disciplines [and] ... as a science ... nursing should have an identifiable theory base.
>
> (Frey, 1995, p. 3)

In nursing, theory informs (or should inform) professional practice (Cody, 1994; Parse, 1995a; Roy, 1995; Smith, 1995), so it follows that it is essential for nurses to define what they mean by theory. Here the term theory is used to refer to nursing theory of scientific origin. There is a consensus on definitions of nursing theories in that they either *describe*, *explain*, or *predict* relationships, responses or events related to practice. Meleis (1997) uses the additional term '*prescriptive*' as a type of nursing theory that has a clear orientation to nursing practice (words in italic above indicate the function of the theory). So theory in nursing is used to predict what will happen when nurses do something for a patient. This is most visible in 'practice theory', i.e. theory related to what a nurse actually does in a practice encounter (here the focus is on practice-level theory, other chapters in this book discuss types of theory referred to as mid-range and grand). Some examples are presented in Table 10.1.

Table 10.1 Nursing actions based on empirical knowledge

- Checking a person's temperature, pulse and blood pressure indicates whether their body is functioning within normal limits and changes in these can predict something in the future, i.e. infection, blood loss, or a cardiac problem.
- Changing the position of a frail old person each 1–2 hours can prevent them developing decubitus ulcers.
- Talking to someone and explaining things to them before an operation can lower their anxiety levels.
- Use of pressure bandages by a district nurse will hasten the healing of a leg ulcer.

- Early mobilisation post-operatively can prevent the development of a deep venous thrombosis.

Taking the listed statement in Table 10.1 regarding the development of a deep venous thrombosis as an example, we can look at the knowledge that allows us to make this prescriptive statement. Knowledge acquirement, as discussed in the first part of this chapter, allows us to demonstrate the basis on which the statement regarding the prevention of a deep venous thrombosis can be made. Table 10.2 presents this.

Table 10.2 One causative theory in the development of post-operative deep venous thrombosis

(A) Prolonged immobility during and following surgical operation; muscle relaxant medications, anaesthesia and lowered cardiac output with subsequent reduction in blood pressure during surgery

↓

(B) Stagnation of blood; increased likelihood of thrombosis

↓

(C) Development of a deep venous thrombosis

In addition to the premises in Table 10.2 we may have additional knowledge that indicates a person is at increased risk of a deep venous thrombosis, for example they might smoke, be obese, have a cardiac problem, have a history of a previous deep venous thrombosis, etc. What sort of empirical knowledge allows us to make the theoretical prediction that the assertion (A) (B) (C) is probable? Because of ethical reasons we cannot of course set up experiments to determine the degree of probability in this relationship. However, the empirical knowledge that allows us to make this prediction is nonetheless based on science, i.e. biology, physics and movement, pharmacology, anatomy and physiology. Thus, nurses know that early mobility combined with anticoagulant medication can reduce the probability of a deep venous thrombosis developing.

In Table 10.1 we could continue to list many things that nurses do. Nurses frequently do not reflect on such everyday actions, and in fact may not see them as being underpinned by theory, but there is no doubt that these and many other actions are 'practice theory' driven.

Study Activity 10.4 ────────────

Reflect on the statements in Table 10.1 and continue adding to this list until you have around 10 things that nurses do. Look at the list and ask the following questions:

● As a practice theory, what is the intended outcome to this action?
● What is the evidence to support this action? Take some of your listed actions and identify the empirical rationale, as in the logical sequence in Table 10.2.
● How certain is it that this action will lead to the desired outcome?

Nursing science

The term 'scientific' (or science) relates to 'a unified body of knowledge about phenomena that is supported by agreed on evidence' (Meleis, 1997). Empirical knowledge in nursing is related to 'science', but some criticise empirics and thus science because they view nursing as an art. Such a critical perspective sees the humanistic caring side of nursing as being incompatible and in conflict with what is perceived as 'hard' science (Playle, 1995). But there is a growing recognition that art and science combine in a unique way within nursing (Rose and Parker, 1994). In addition, nursing science differs from traditional science because it is a 'caring' science. In a dialogue on nursing science, Zanotti (1997) states:

> The science of nursing is an emergent new product in the universe of human knowledge ... it requires the application of rigorous, distinct procedures and methods to observe, classify, and relate the processes by which persons change their health status. The

> body of nursing knowledge is enhanced by these methods. Nursing science responds to compassionate concern for maintaining and promoting health, preventing illness, and caring for and rehabilitating the sick and disabled ... Thus, nursing science can provide conscious and consistent criticism to popular explanatory myths, and it challenges many traditional scientific truths.
>
> (Zanotti, 1997)

Here, Zanotti's definition of nursing science calls for the use of rigorous methods to be used to inform nursing knowledge but to do so in a caring way. This can be seen as nursing science that leads to the generation of nursing empirical knowledge. Many nurse theorists view nursing as a 'caring' science (Rogers, 1985, 1990; Watson, 1988, 1996; Parse, 1995b).

Addressing the conflict between nursing and traditional empiricism

In this second part of the chapter I am suggesting that there is a *nursing empiricism* and that one of the fundamental differences between it and traditional empirics is that which, although not unique to nursing, is central and unique in nursing *'caring'*. There are different languages, different modes of enquiry and different worldviews between traditional science and the humanistic caring science of nursing. The differences are most manifest in debates within and without nursing on: art and science; quantitative and qualitative research; rationalism and humanism and so on. The question is whether or not these differences can be combined within an empiricism for nursing. You will note that the discussion above on deep venous thrombosis uses as its rationale empirical evidence that originates in a number of disciplines. Silva (1999) suggested five possibilities for reconciling nursing and other sciences. These are presented in Table 10.3 overleaf.

The five ideas suggested by Silva (1999) and presented in Table 10.3 would allow nursing to access and utilise a wide range of empirical knowledge to underpin its practice. In doing so, nursing need not lose its uniqueness, but rather it can lead to richness for the discipline.

Study Activity 10.5

- Read and reflect upon the five possibilities for reconciling nursing suggested by Silva (1999) and presented in Table 10.3; also obtain Silva's article and read it. As you read the article, make notes on whether or not you agree with the ideas forwarded by Silva – are they in keeping with your beliefs about nursing?

Table 10.3   Possibilities for reconciling nursing and related discipline sciences

- *Synchronising* – nursing science and related discipline sciences coexist . . . but retain separate identities.

- *Overlapping* – nursing science extends over and covers part of the related discipline sciences and vice versa . . . [each] maintain a part of themselves that is unique.

- *Overlaying* – nursing science is attached to and placed over and/or under the related discipline sciences.

- *Synthesising* – combining the parts of nursing science and the related discipline sciences into a whole.

- *Blending* – to combine smoothly nursing science with related discipline sciences so that they are inseparable and indistinguishable from one and other.

(From Silva, 1999)

It was stated at the beginning of this chapter that the focus here is on empirical knowledge but that in the real world of practice, Carper's (1978) four patterns of knowing integrate to guide practice. To illustrate this point and address the conflict between nursing science and other science disciplines, let us return to the example above of the deep venous thrombosis and apply this to a practice vignette:

Margaret is a 72-year-old lady who is admitted to hospital for cardiac surgery. She is weak and ill from years of heart problems, but she is looking forward to her operation, hoping life will be more worthwhile when it is over.

Margaret's nurse is Ann. Ann is an experienced nurse with expertise in pre- and post-operative cardiac surgery. She knows that the development of a deep venous thrombosis is a real possibility for Margaret, due to a number of factors, especially her previous cardiac history and the extremely long operation she will have (empirical). She also knows, based on past experience, that some people of this age are reluctant to mobilise early after their operation and that they often require a great deal of coaxing and encouragement (personal knowledge). So, even before the operation, Ann begins to gain the trust of Margaret – she sits and talks to her and tells her everything she will need to know about her operation. Ann is a highly skilled communicator and she relates well to people of all ages, all the patients like her.

Margaret returns from surgery and when she gains consciousness she hears the reassuring voice of Ann. She also receives comfort from Ann gentling holding her hand. The calm and effective fluidity with which Ann cares for Margaret is a hallmark of her 'expertise' (aesthetics). As time progresses, Margaret becomes more conscious but she is weary and weak, and she is in pain – too much pain to want to move. It would seem kinder not to encourage mobility, but Ann knows the danger of a possible deep venous thrombosis. Above all Ann must not by her actions or lack of actions cause any harm to Margaret (ethical). So Ann encourages Margaret to begin mobility as soon as possible: moving her toes in bed, then moving her legs, getting her to sit up as soon as possible. She also ensures that Margaret's fluid intake is adequate to encourage a return to homeostasis, and she uses the tilting bed position as appropriate to discourage stagnation of her blood (empirical). Ann works with her colleagues to help Margaret: the physiotherapist to help with mobilising, the physician to ensure pain relief and anticoagulant medications and members of Margaret's family to help encourage her to become mobile.

Through these endeavours and the combination of empirical, personal, aesthetic and ethical knowledge, Ann is successful in her and Margaret's aim of an uncomplicated post-operative recovery. Ann has used theory, practice, research, knowledge to provide the best possible care.

Study Activity 10.6 _____

The next time you are on clinical placement, observe a nurse who you think is experienced and expert in her practice. Can you identify Carper's patterns of knowing in this nurse as in the vignette above? And do these ways of knowing appear as transient patterns, i.e. do the nurse's actions move back and forth between each pattern?

How the empirical knowledge for nursing emerges

The uniqueness of nursing as a caring science gives credence to the use of empirical knowledge from many sources. Qualitative as well as quantitative research may underpin practice, the process of 'reflection' may be used (Johns and Freshwater, 1998; Ghaye and Lillyman, 2000; Bolton, 2001) and philosophical reasoning may be appropriate when research is not feasible. Knowledge, and so theory, development in nursing can be through a philosophical discourse process – theorising, or what Holden (1996) refers to as non-propositional knowledge development. Or, nurse theorists such as Watson (1996) would suggest that in keeping with post-modern constructivist perspectives, literature such as poetry can be utilised to gain 'truth' – what Heidegger (1971, cited in Watson, 1996, p. 128) refers to as 'aletheia' 'the unconcealment of beings'. It is emphasised here that following the formulation of such theories they should be verified by theory testing research before implementing them in practice. Theory testing research is associated with the positivistic paradigm and approaches related to quantitative

research, such as experiments, will usually be utilised to achieve this objective.

The important thing to remember is that the method used to gain knowledge must be that which provides the *best possible evidence*. Quite often the best evidence will be research. Research can be considered the fuel of knowledge and this fuel when it is collected is that which brings light to theory. Fawcett and Downs (1992) suggest that research 'is neither more nor less than the vehicle of theory development'. And, it is asserted here that there are many different types of such vehicles. To consider a simple analogy, contemplate a commuter travelling from point A to point B. He/she has a number of modes of transport to select from – car, bus, train, taxi, etc. These are the tools used to move from A to B. It would seem absurd to suggest to this commuter that you cannot arrive at point B unless you use a train, when this person is fully aware that one of the other modes of transport, i.e. car, bus, or taxi, is a better means of transporting them to point B. To suggest that one type of research is best to generate empirical knowledge in all situations is suggestive of a 'methodological imperialism' (Sayer, 1992) in nursing, which it is argued here should be countered.

The value of empirical evidence in nursing

If one was to argue the case for a core element in nursing, it would be that the main aim of all nursing is to 'care for patients'. Nursing is a science, but it is an applied (practical) science, the very reason for nursing is to promote health, heal, or care for people when they have a progressive disability or illness. Therefore, the nature of nursing is a 'caring' applied science (Whelton, 2000).

Clinical effectiveness and evidence-based practice

In caring for human beings, nurses must minimise any errors, there is no room for chance. We need empirical evidence to guide our practice. Chapter 17 discusses evidence-based practice, so it is not discussed here in detail. However, as empirical knowledge is an integral aspect of evidence-based practice, it is important to mention it briefly here. A very simple definition that can apply to clinical effectiveness and evidence-based practice is forwarded by the Royal College of Nursing (1996): 'Doing the right thing in the right way for the right patient at the right time'. This is quite a simple definition and, thus, it is difficult to be critical of it.

Clinical effectiveness is an outcome to the use of evidence-based practice. One of the most widely used definitions of clinical effectiveness is that it is practice that is measured by the extent that interventions achieve intended outcomes (National Health Service Executive, 1996). Regan (1998) suggested that this definition can be difficult for nurses, as the outcomes are frequently medically orientated. However, it is argued here that a medical orientation does not need to be at odds with nursing. In relation to evidence-based medicine, Sackett *et al.* (1996) provide the following definition: 'the conscientious, explicit and judicious use of current best evidence in making decisions about the care of individual patients'.

Although this relates to evidence-based medicine, it is a quite useful definition for most caring professions because the terms used provide key features of evidence-based practice, i.e.

- *Conscientious* – this implies a moral obligation to provide evidence-based practice, not merely a financial and management efficiency-driven rationale.
- *Explicit* – the practice needs to be explicit so that practitioners can clearly follow and implement care.
- *Current and best* – in any care that is guided by evidence-based practice it is essential that interventions that are *best* according to *current* knowledge are used.
- *Individual* – Sackett and colleagues recognise that evidence-based practice should be individual-directed and this is commendable; they also recognise that individual judgement is an aspect of evidence-based practice along with external systematic research evidence.

The idea of individual clinical judgement could be considered quite similar to Benner's (1984) view of individual (and even intuitive) expertise in nursing.

Study Activity 10.7

With regard to Sackett *et al.*'s definition of evidence-based medicine above, I suggest it is applicable to, and so could be used in, nursing. Organise a class discussion in consultation with your lecturer and discuss your views on using a medical definition like this one for nursing.

Moral reasons for the use of empirical knowledge

Moral or ethical reasons for the use of empirical knowledge may seem quite straightforward. There are a number of moral principles that have relevance, but perhaps the most fundamental to nursing are:

- *Beneficence* – this means that nursing care should do good;
- *Non-maleficence* – this means that care or acts that are maleficent (harmful) should be removed or avoided;
- *Justice* – this means that care should be provided for people in a fair and unprejudiced way, and they should not be stigmatised against on any grounds.

It is suggested here that very good reasons for the use of empirical knowledge as discussed in this chapter are the three principles above. The first two are aspects that should, and in fact must, be achieved. The third, 'justice', is a much more difficult principle. Archie Cochrane, who was influential in the establishment of the Cochrane Collaboration Centres for evidence-based practice, identified three main aims of these centres:

1 *Effectiveness* – health care interventions should be based on evidence-based empirical interventions;

2 *Efficiency* – relates to how well resources are being used, i.e. cost-effectiveness;

3 *Equality* – this relates to access to health care and resource allocation (and the ethical principle of justice above).

These three aims are easy to remember as the three 'Es'. But it is interesting that the third 'E' (equality) is often forgotten by health care services, even though, as Dingwall *et al.* (1998) suggested, Cochrane intended it to be as important as effectiveness and efficiency. Equality relates to justice and all health care providers do and will continue to face dilemmas in this area. For example, a nurse may be faced with having to provide an intervention for cost-effective reasons when she has knowledge that there is empirical evidence to support an alternative more clinically effective practice yet there are inadequate resources to allow provision of this care practice.

Study Activity 10.8

In relation to the ethical dilemma indicated above, i.e. not having adequate resources to provide the most empirically based practice, discuss with a group of colleagues any such dilemmas that you are aware of, or that you feel could potentially occur. Given the power to do something about the dilemma of resources, what would you and your colleagues do?

Adapting a critical stance

Empirical knowledge is not just about observing and taking what we 'see' for granted. It is about submitting what is observed to the scientific rigour of critical appraisal (Parahoo, 1997; Crookes and Davies, 1998). And, it is not about absolute truth, but about the soundest knowledge/best available evidence we can claim until/ unless (in Popper's terminology) it can be refuted. We must acknowledge that science cannot give us absolute truth, that our nursing practice too must be guided by a science of conjectures and refutations. In awareness of this

knowledge, our disposition must always be one of critical appraisal: we must also seek to refute, to question our evidence, and to be open to change in our knowledge.

Our goal must be the development of a dynamic and evolving body of theory that informs nursing practice and indeed is informed by that practice. We must recognise too that the knowledge of empirics, of evidence, is not the only knowledge that may inform our practice. Stajduhar *et al.* (2001) stated that 'using such techniques as critical thinking ... nurses can be guided towards not only understanding scientific understanding but also its epistemological alternatives'. By such processes we are building up – by processes of conjecture and refutation – a body of the 'best available evidence'.

SUMMARY

There are dangers in taking a firm stance on knowledge or seeing the world through the lens of a favoured worldview. One danger is that we refute empirical or 'evidence-based' knowledge because of its narrow assumptions. That is, the assumptions that it and only it is the source of valid and reliable knowledge. The second danger is that we are enchanted by the narrow empirical viewpoint into rejecting other ways of knowing.

The message in all this is fairly simple. It is about the need to approach that which is presented as evidence in a critical and cautious manner. In a sense much of this chapter may seem to question the validity of scientific evidence. But, as the work of Karl Popper has illustrated, such evidence is given its true strength by being constantly exposed to tests of refutation. The nursing profession must recognise that there is a case for evidence that has withstood such stringent tests.

And, finally, Popper (1963) illustrates, with resounding strength, the extent to which science is indeed about theory and theorising. In Popper, conjecture is not a dirty word, a non-scientific postulation. It is in fact at the core of science and essential to its very strength, giving it its creativity and vitality. An equally distinguished scientist, Sir Peter Medawar (1967) said this, many years ago:

> Let me turn now to two serious but completely different conceptions of science ... According to the first conception, science is above all else an imaginative and exploratory activity, and the scientist is a man taking part in a great intellectual adventure. Intuition is the mainspring of every great advancement of learning, and having ideas is the scientist's highest accomplishment. The alternative conception runs something like this: science is above all else a critical and analytical activity; the scientist is pre-eminently a man who requires evidence before he delivers an opinion, and when it comes to evidence he is hard to please. Imagination is a catalyst merely (and) must at all times be under the censorship of dispassionate and sceptical thought.
>
> (Medawar, 1967)

Medawar decried this dichotomy, arguing that science needs both its imagination and creativity, and its rigour and critical disposition, its theorising and its researching. Indeed, Thomas Kuhn (1970) has argued strongly, in his influential work, that a discipline without a growing body of theory derived from research to guide its practice is pre-paradigmatic. That is, it has no basis, no worldview, it is in fact not a discipline in any real sense at all. In nursing, our discipline must also have its theory to guide practice, and empirical knowledge is an essential source of such theory.

REFERENCES

Benner, P. (1984) *From Novice to Expert: Excellence and power in clinical nursing*, Addison-Wesley, Menlo Park, CA

Bolton, G. (2001) *Reflective Practice Writing and Professional Development*, Paul Chapman, London

Carper, B.A. (1978) Fundamental patterns of knowing in nursing, *Advances in Nursing Science* 1, 13–23

Chinn, P.L. and Kramer, M.K. (1995) *Theory and Nursing: A systematic approach* (4th edn), Mosby-Year Book, St Louis, IL

Cody, W.K. (1994) Nursing theory-guided practice: what it is and what it is not. *Nursing Science Quarterly* 8, 144–5

Crookes, P.A. and Davies, S. (eds) (1998) *Research into Practice Essential Skills for Reading and Applying Research in Nursing and Health Care*, Baillière Tindall, London

Dawkins, R. (1976) *The Selfish Gene*, Penguin, Harmondsworth

Dawkins, R. (1993) Letter to the Editor, *The Independent*, 20 March, p. 20

Dingwall, R., Murphy, E., Watson, P., *et al.* (1998) Catching goldfish: quality in qualitative research. *Journal of Health Service Research Policy* 3, 167–72

Fawcett, J. and Downs, F.S. (1992) *The Relationship of Theory and Research* (2nd edn), F.A. Davis, Philadelphia, IL

Frey, M.A. (1995) From conceptual frameworks to nursing knowledge. In: Frey, M.A. and Sieloff, C.L. (eds) *Advancing King's Systems Framework and Theory of Nursing*, Sage, London

Ghaye, T. and Lillyman, S. (2000) *Reflection: Principles and practice for healthcare professionals*, Mark Allen, Dinton

Glaser, B.G. and Strauss, A.L. (1967) *The Discovery of Grounded Theory: Strategies for qualitative research*, Aldine, New York

Haack, S. (1993) *Evidence and Inquiry: Towards reconstruction in epistemology*, Blackwell, Oxford

Holden, J.R. (1996) Nursing knowledge: the problem of the criterion. In: Kikuchi, J.F., Simmons, H. and Romyn, D. (eds) *Truth in Nursing Inquiry*, Sage, London

Johns, C. and Freshwater, D. (eds) (1998) *Transforming Nursing through Reflective Practice*, Blackwell Science, Oxford

Kim, S.H. (1996) Identifying alternative linkages among philosophy, theory, and method in nursing. In: Kenney, J.W. (ed.) *Philosophical and Theoretical Perspectives for Advanced Nursing Practice*, Jones and Bartlett, Sudbury, MA

Kuhn, T. (1970) *The Structure of the Scientific Revolutions* (2nd edn), University of Chicago Press, Chicago, IL

McKenna, H. (1997) *Nursing Theories and Models*, Routledge, London

Medawar, P. (1967) *The Art of the Soluble*, Penguin, Harmondsworth

Meleis, A.I. (1997) *Theoretical Nursing: Development and Progress*, J.B. Lippincott, Philadelphia, PA

Moody, L.E. (1990) *Advancing Nursing Science through Research*, Vol. 1, Sage, London

National Health Service Executive (1996) *Promoting Clinical Effectiveness: A framework for action through the NHS*, National Health Service Executive, London

Parahoo, K. (1997) *Nursing Research Principles, Process and Issues*, Macmillan, London

Parse, R.R. (1995a) Nursing theories and frameworks: the essentials of advanced practice nursing. *Nursing Science Quarterly* 8, 1

Parse, R.R. (1995b) The human becoming theory in nursing. In: Parse, R.R. (ed.) *Illuminations: The human becoming theory in practice and research*, National League for Nursing Press, New York

Playle, J.F. (1995) Humanism and positivism in nursing: contradictions and conflicts. *Journal of Advanced Nursing* 22, 979–84

Popper, K.R. (1939) *The Logic of Scientific Discovery*, Unwin, London

Popper, K.R. (1963) *Conjectures and Refutations*, Routledge and Kegan Paul, London

Powers, B.A. and Knapp, T.R. (1995) *A Dictionary of Nursing Theory and Research*, Sage, London

Regan, J.A. (1998) Will current effectiveness initiatives encourage and facilitate practitioners to use evidence-based practice for the benefit of their clients? *Journal of Clinical Nursing* 3, 244–50

Rogers, C. (1985) Toward a more human science of the person. *Journal of Humanistic Psychology* 25(4), 7–24

Rogers, M.E. (1990) Nursing: science of unitary, irreducible, human beings: update 1990. In: Barrett, E.A.M. (ed.) *Visions of Rogers' Science Based Nursing*, National League for Nursing, New York

Rose, P. and Parker, D. (1994) Nursing: an integration of the art and science within the experience of the practitioner. *Journal of Advanced Nursing* 20, 1004–10

Roy, C.L. (1995) Developing nursing knowledge: practice issues raised from four philosophical perspectives. *Nursing Science Quarterly* 8, 79–85

Royal College of Nursing (1996) *Clinical Effectiveness: A Royal College of Nursing guide*, Royal College of Nursing, London

Sackett, D.L., Rosenberg, W.M.C., Gray, J.A.M., *et al.* (1996) Evidence-based medicine: what it is and what it isn't. *British Medical Journal* 312, 71–2

Sayer, A. (1992) *Method in Social Science: A realist approach* (2nd edn), Routledge, London

Silva, M.C. (1999) The state of nursing science: reconceptualizing for the 21st century. *Nursing Science Quarterly* 12, 221–6

Silver, B.L. (1998) *The Ascent of Science*, Oxford University Press, New York

Slevin, O. (1995) Knowledge and theory. In: Basford, L. and Slevin, O. (eds) *Theory and Practice of Nursing: An integrated approach*, Campion Press, Edinburgh

Smith, J.A. (1995) Qualitative methods, identity and transition to motherhood. *The Psychologist* 8, 122–5

Stajduhar, K.I., Balneaves, L. and Thorne, S.E. (2001) A case for the 'middle ground'; exploring the tensions of postmodern thought in nursing. *Nursing Philosophy* 2, 72–82

Watson, J. (1988) *Nursing: Human science and human care: A theory of nursing*, National League for Nursing, New York

Watson, J. (1996) Poeticizing as truth in nursing enquiry. In: Kikuchi, J.F., Simmons, H. and Romyn, D. (eds) *Truth in Nursing Inquiry*, Sage, London

Whelton, B.J.B. (2000) Nursing as a practical science: some insights from classical Aristotelian science. *Nursing Philosophy* 1, 57–63

Zanotti, R. (1997) What is nursing science? An international dialogue. *Nursing Science Quarterly* 10, 10–13

11 PERSONAL KNOWING: NURSING AS A CARING AND HEALING PROCESS

Oliver Slevin and Carol Kirby

> *... we can know more than we can tell.*
> (Polanyi, 1967, p. 4)

> *Behind your image, below your words, above your thoughts, the silence of another world awaits. A world lives within you. No-one can bring you news of the inner world.*
> (O'Donohue, 1997, p. 13)

LEARNING OUTCOMES

After studying this chapter you will be able to:

- Recognise that a discrete pattern of knowing termed *personal knowing* is a vital element in the knowledge that underpins nursing practice
- Demonstrate that there are different meanings that may be attached to the term 'personal knowing', by detailing the differences between the orientations presented by Carper and Polanyi
- Describe the notion of personal knowing as a knowing of self and other through the process of coming into relation
- Recognise that the alternative orientation that sees personal knowing as a tacit cognitive dimension rather than a relational concern is also an important source of how nurses come to know
- Demonstrate that the alternative orientations described as personal knowing can in fact be complementary to each other
- Discuss in an informed way how Carper's pattern of personal knowing may be particularly relevant in modern health care systems.

INTRODUCTION

You will be aware that this chapter comes within a module that considers different patterns or ways of knowing relevant to the practice of nursing. In adopting this orientation, the patterns originally proposed by Carper (1978) have been taken as a framework, and we thus consider (in separate chapters) empirical, aesthetic, ethical, and personal patterns of knowing. It is, of course, the latter which is the concern of the current chapter. However, it is the latter, *personal* knowing, that is in some senses the most problematic of the four. This is not to say that empirical, aesthetic or ethical patterns of knowing are straightforward and without controversy. As will have been noted in the preceding chapter (on empirical knowing) and the two chapters (on aesthetic and ethical knowing) that follow the present chapter, each of these other patterns has its own sophistication and complexity. And each is beset to some extent by controversy in terms of meanings and relevance to nursing practice. However, it is in the range of meanings and the controversy surrounding each of these that personal knowing stands out as something of a special case.

The aforementioned state of affairs presents, for authors and readers, a particular set of challenges. We must recognise different connotations of the term personal knowing, relate these to the other 'patterns' of knowing presented in the module, and take from these considerations insights that will inform the practice of nursing. This is the primary purpose of this chapter.

DIFFERENT WORLDS USING SIMILAR WORDS

We end our Introduction above by indicating that we are in search of insights. This may be a fortunate (or indeed unfortunate) choice of words. There is a sense in which *personal* knowing refers to knowledge that derives in some way from within the person, as something that comes to light apparently spontaneously and without conscious deliberation. In this respect we come across terms such as insight, intuition, tacit understanding. The philosopher Michael Polanyi (1967) spoke of this, as presented in the first opening quotation above, as a situation wherein 'we can know more than we can tell'. This is a matter to which we will return presently. However, for now, we can note that what Polanyi was concerned with was a form of cognitive knowing, an apprehension or understanding of an object or phenomenon. The issue here is the state of knowing, and it has been termed *personal* knowing by Polanyi (1958) and others because it emanates from the person; essentially, we can tell something, we can demonstrate that we know it tacitly, without necessarily being able to explain *how* or *why* we believe as we do.

In his thesis, Polanyi (1958, 1967) does not suggest some magical or mystical power to know that we may see as a sixth sense. In our secular society people in general would now look critically upon the notion that there are some who have a supernatural power to know. It is true, of course, that some aspects of 'new world' thinking subscribe to such ideas: the writings and predictions of Nostradamus are still read, astrology is big business, and there are still some who speak of 'women's intuition'. However, in the objective and scientific world of modernity, such views are castigated and we are aware that most serious empirical studies of astrological predictions have demonstrated no significant variation from what would have occurred by mere chance in any case. Nevertheless, there is one sense in which there is in each of us an awareness of our existence, of being a person prior to our reception of all those experiences that lead us through rational thinking to something we might think of as objective or empirical knowledge. This awareness of existing as a being, that may be described by some as the life-force, or soul, or archetypal self, is in a different sense a form of personal knowing. The emphasis here shifts from knowing things to knowing self or person, and we might also term this *personal* knowing. It is this awareness to which O'Donohue refers in the second of our opening quotations. This inner self is not disjointed from the world about us; it is receptive to it and in turn is the lifeforce that leads us to a creative enjoining and imprinting of ourselves upon that world. The archetypal psychologist and psychotherapist James Hillman (1989) explains that 'Knowledge is received by the soul as understanding, in exchange for which the soul gives to knowledge value and faith' (p. 67).

The view of personal knowing taken by Carper (1978) in her seminal paper is to an extent an extension of the latter meaning. She states:

> *Personal knowing is concerned with the knowing, encountering and actualizing of the concrete, individual self. One does not know about the self; one strives simply to know the self. This knowing is a standing in relation to another human being and confronting that human being as a person. This 'I-Thou' encounter is unmediated by conceptual categories or particulars abstracted from complex organic wholes (Buber, [1939] 1970). The relation is one of reciprocity, a state of being that cannot be described or even experienced – it can only be actualized. Such personal knowing extends not only to other selves but also to relations with one's own self ... Certainly empirical knowledge is essential to the purpose of nursing. But nursing also requires that we be alert to the fact that models of human nature and their abstract and generalized categories refer to and describe behaviours and traits that groups have in common. However, none of these categories can ever encompass or express the uniqueness of the individual encountered as a person, as a 'self'. These and many other considerations are involved in the realm of personal knowledge, which can be broadly*

characterized as subjective, concrete and existential. It is concerned with the kind of knowing that promotes wholeness and integrity in the personal encounter, the achievement of engagement rather than detachment; and it denies the manipulative, impersonal orientation.

(Carper, 1978, pp. 251–2)

By now the difficulty we refer to should have become transparent. Carper is not speaking of a cognitive phenomenon at all. She is speaking of an awareness of self and more specifically the issue of personal relating between self and other. In the final analysis, Polanyi (1958, 1967) was speaking of cognitively knowing something tacitly or intuitively. Such intuition, according to Hillman (1997), is:

... direct and unmediated knowledge, immediate or innate apprehension of a complex group of data. Intuition is both thoughtless and also not a feeling state; it is clear, quick, and full apprehension, the significant feature being the immediacy of the process. Intuitions occur to a person without any known process of cognition or reflective thinking ... Intuitions occur; we do not make them. They come to us as a sudden idea, a definite judgement, a grasped meaning. They come with an event as if brought by it or inherent in it. You say something and I 'get it,' just like that ... I suddenly find myself gasping 'Aha' in front of a painting on the wall. I've been struck.

(Hillman, 1997, pp. 97–8)

Carper, conversely, is speaking of a knowing that is subjective and relational. It is not about apprehending or understanding at all; indeed, as in the above quotation from her paper, she describes it as 'a state of being' rather than a coming to know in a cognitive sense. For this reason, her position has been criticised as confusing. Indeed, Egan and Beckstrand (1979) suggest that as Carper quotes Polanyi as a source

of her thinking there may be a discrepancy in that she proceeds to describe something entirely different. Furthermore, while her emphasis is on self there is a sense in which Carper moves quickly to self-in-relation without a specific consideration of the nature of self as referred to by Hillman (1989) and O'Donohue (1997), or how we may, as individuals, know our own selves.

Subsequent significant contributions relating to Carper's work, such as White (1995) and Chinn and Kramer (1999), address the issue of personal knowing in some detail. However, the fundamental difficulties in respect of meaning, as identified by Egan and Beckstrand (1979), are notably absent in such contributions. These difficulties can be summarised as follows:

- Carper's treatment of personal knowing concentrated primarily on the existential or ontological issue of knowing of self and other, and is thus essentially relational.
- The issue of tacit or personal knowledge treated by Polanyi and others is conversely concerned with a way of acquiring knowledge or coming to know that is about apprehension or understanding, and thus is essentially cognitive.
- By referring to the influence upon her of Polanyi's work, and speaking of personal knowing as being something that cannot be described or explained (a position close to Polanyi's assertion that 'we can know more than we can tell'), Carper's treatment of personal knowing has the capacity to confuse.
- The situation may become even more complex when we recognise that even in the context of self and other, tacit knowing (as a cognitive element) may occur. That is, we may have tacit *cognitive* knowledge of self and other (in the sense meant by Polanyi) that is not relational knowing in any sense.

There are perhaps some useful conclusions that can be drawn from the above discussion. One is that personal knowing, whether it is a cognitive or relational phenomenon, is of importance to nursing. Another is that, as will be demonstrated below, both emerge from an embeddedness and engagement in the practice situation. A third is that the apparently polarised positions are in practice more interconnected than may at first appear to be the case. These assertions are addressed in the subsequent sections.

Study Activity 11.1

In the opening paragraphs we have begun to become acquainted with the vocabulary of personal knowing. In one sense in which the term personal knowing is used, there is a tendency to see a particular group of words frequently used, and sometimes used interchangeably. These are: insight, intuition, and tacit knowing.

- Do a library or Internet search on these three terms and write a brief (250 words) definitive statement for each term. Reflect upon differences and similarities in uses of the terms.

THE RELATIONAL DIMENSION

This is the form of personal knowing proposed by Carper (1978), and is in line with her statement as quoted above, in the previous section of this chapter. This is essentially a view that is largely founded upon a phenomenological ontological view that is concerned with our being in the world, as referred to in Chapter 9. As such, it is essentially existential – to do with how we exist in the world and in relation to others. In taking this position, Carper shares an orientation proposed by Paterson and Zderad (1988) in their presentation of humanistic nursing and subsequently by Parse (1992, 1998) in her science of human becoming. Also in line with Parse, Carper presents personal knowing as an integrative perspective that views self and other as holistic beings rather than in a fragmented way. The individual, both self and other, is approached as a whole person. The orientation is furthermore relational and Carper cites the particular existential perspective of Martin Buber ([1939] 1970) by referring to an *I-Thou*

relation within which the 'self' enters into relation with the 'other' in a spirit of true relation that is an opening of one to the other in an unmediated and non-judgemental manner. This contrasts to an *I-It* orientation, within which the 'other' is viewed objectively and the connection is mediated by observation, reflection, judgement, etc. In essence, in that moment that we view the other as an it or an object we have left the *I-Thou* relation. We move also from the subjective, tacit, passionate and intuitive knowing of self in relation to other to an objective, reasoned and dispassionate countenancing of the other that is in that instant a movement to an entirely different empirical pattern of knowing (as presented in the previous chapter).

In the relational sense, personal knowing is about self and others. Each one of us is a body–mind–spirit unity dwelling in the world in intuitive, knowing, understanding connection. Within interdependent relationships we come to know and to understand who we are, what our life is about and what is of value in and to it. Through being present to self, present *to, for* and *with* one another we are ceaselessly becoming. In life together, inextricably bound to each other, we express our humanity. With one another we create and realise possibility, search for what is meaningful in life's experiences and mysteries, and come to know what it means to '*be*'. A world lives within us, as suggested by O'Donohue (1997) in the second of our opening quotations. It is our individual task to understand our inner world, to create inner and outer balance, coherence and wholeness. No-one else can do this for us. We have each to know and to understand *self*, to live life true to self and other. In dialogue with self and with other we experience; in consciousness we discern, understand and act. Our act is personal – our unique responsibility and significance.

Nursing values wholeness – the whole person, the whole of human experience and consciousness, holistic thinking and knowledge. Through holistic nursing care and the integral knowledge that informs it we concentrate on this wholeness

– on possibility, potential and all that can be. The gift of nursing is the whole-hearted commitment and compassionate action that unfolds the innate healing potential of each person. To nurse, to participate in this activity we call nursing, is to make this gift of self. In therapeutic use-of-self, we are potentiating healing and bringing peace-of-mind to people when they need it most.

This view of the nurse as therapeutic self is an issue we return to again in Module 7. But it will be clear that it is essentially embedded in how we relate to the others we care for. In this sense, personal knowing is situated and contextual. When we are caring for the other our attention is centred exclusively on that person; we are in a state of constant intentional openness to their predicament, constantly taking from them the direction of our nursing actions. This is not an argument for discarding other ways of knowing. As intimated in the opening chapter to this module, all the patterns of knowing are of vital importance to an integrated approach to holistic care. We do, of course, attend to the best available evidence to inform our practice, as contained within the empirical pattern of knowing. But this must not be at the cost of excluding by fiat the personal ways that we know self and other. We must endeavour to ensure that these too influence how we care. It is often easier to attend to other forms of knowledge that are propositional, objective and factual. In doing so, there is sometimes a tendency not to attend to the inner voice or indeed to the voice of the other. Indeed, sometimes just because this is not based upon observable fact or rational thinking it is deliberately devalued and excluded, often to the extent of not being deemed knowledge in any real sense at all!

Munhall (1993) proposes a way of approaching Carper's view that in personal knowing we must set aside generalisations and assumptions and attend to the unique situation of the other. Munhall proposes a state of *unknowing*, where we suspend our awareness of externally constructed knowledge, and indeed our own

preconceptions and views, and attend to the experience of the other as he or she is living this. This openness is akin to the process of *bracketing* or suspending other knowledge and judgement that is proposed as a technique in transcendental phenomenology. It allows one to as great an extent to enter into the world of the other, to experience it as they are experiencing it (or at least to have a degree of insight into what they experience). This is close to what the psychotherapist Carl Rogers (1990) proposes when he speaks of empathy. Of this, Paul Solomon (1991) states most powerfully:

> *If I want to know what you're thinking right now, all I have to do is care more about what you're thinking than what I'm thinking ... As soon as I care more about what you're thinking than what I'm thinking I will give up my thoughts and I will absorb yours, and I will understand you.*
>
> (Soloman, 1991, p. 28)

Solomon adroitly draws attention to a facet of Carper's pattern of personal knowing that is implicit in her emphasis on personal knowing as a relational phenomenon. That is the fact that the 'personal' element in personal knowing is also about coming to know the other person. It is this sense of personal knowing – the knowing of the other's personal knowledge (their thoughts *and* the feelings these engender) – that makes it essentially and necessarily relational. The implication of this for the nurse is clear. If we choose to ignore the personal call from the other, if we operate exclusively on the level of object and fact, if we fail to enter into relation with the other in a holistic and caring sense, there will be a major and dangerous omission in our caring practices.

Study Activity 11.2

In October 2002, following a number of controversial events within the British educational system, the Secretary of State for Education, Estelle Morris, resigned. Over the preceding months, difficulties had emerged over examinations, when following modifications to the system, large numbers of pupils' examination papers required re-marking. Accusations were made that the Secretary of State had behaved inappropriately in respect of an inquiry set up to investigate the cause of these difficulties, and a senior public figure resigned in protest at her actions. Immediately following this, allegations were made that the Secretary of State had reneged on commitments made previously in respect of educational targets. Morris took the unusual step of stating that she felt she was not competent to carry out the duties of Secretary of State, and following deep reflection had determined that she must resign.

Obviously there may have been *evidence* to suggest to Morris that she was not managing, and at the time she was under considerable pressure from political opponents, the media, and possibly within her own government.

- Is there an indication that Estelle Morris may have 'come to know' tacitly that she was unable to cope? Consider any similar situation you may have been in, where you also may have come to a realisation of your inadequacy in that situation. How do you think you came to know this, and what did *you* do?
- Many of the commentators analysing Morris's decision commented on the pressures of politics, and the need for great personal strength of character. In effect, it is not enough to be competent, there must also be a confidence in who one is before one can go out to others. Do you think Morris may have lacked a confidence in her own sense of personhood and identity, as a person with strengths and limitations?

THE TACIT DIMENSION

We have already noted the controversy that surrounds the idea of personal knowing. That described in the previous section is an essentially relational concept that derives in large part from phenomenological and existential philosophy and humanistic psychology. It is concerned with the ontological nature of self and how this emerges through and in relation with other. The alternative view is essentially a cognitive concept that derives in large part from the philosophy of mind and cognitive psychology. It is concerned with a particular way of coming to know that, as referred to earlier, Polanyi (1967) described as a knowing that we cannot tell. This is not about an awareness of self, but rather about a tacit knowing of things whereby we often cannot explain adequately how we come to know.

There is within this particular perspective, a controversy in respect of how we *do* come to know something tacitly or apparently intuitively. Bastick (1982) conveniently presents two opposing explanations. From the behavioural psychology perspective, the explanation is that through experience and doing, and by trial and error, we gradually move towards a capacity to recognise patterns more quickly (indeed sometimes instantaneously) apparently suddenly coming to a realisation of what something is or how something works. From gestalt psychology comes the view that the capacity to see patterns in things is an innate and essentially human characteristic (although shared to some extent by some of the higher primates). There is a capacity for the human to see unity in things, to recognise patterns, whereby the parts make up a whole that is more than the sum of those parts (the term 'gestalt', as a word of German origin, refers to a configuration that has 'wholeness' or unity).

However, the literature on tacit or insightful knowledge is, as indicated by Bastick (1982), characterised by a failure to arrive at anything approaching a consensus on defining this meaning of personal knowing. About the only thing that seems to achieve any sort of universal consensus is the extent to which as we come to tacitly know something we are to a large degree not attending to any sort of process. We are consciously unaware of the means that leads us to this knowledge. For this reason, Reber (1995) has referred to a *cognitive unconscious* that suggests that the mechanisms we use in arriving at what we call an intuitive knowing, are outside of our consciousness but nevertheless active.

This may explain why it is often the case that if we leave a problem for a period and return to it we see the solution in a flash.

Notwithstanding the difficulties of definition and expression, there is a general agreement that the tacit dimension is a valid source of knowledge. Patel *et al.* (1999) express this effectively, when they state:

> It is commonly accepted among scholars in diverse fields that there are two types of knowledge: knowledge that can be verbalised, such as knowledge of facts and concepts; and knowledge that cannot be made verbal, such as intuition and knowledge of procedures. The former type of knowledge has received a great deal of attention in cognitive research. This research has addressed the role of domain-specific knowledge in problem-solving and reasoning in diverse fields. However, after many years of investigating the effects of domain-specific knowledge, cognitive researchers have realised that informal knowledge is as important as, and sometimes more important than, formally acquired knowledge ... We can relate the distinction between verbal and nonverbal knowledge to the one, originally made by Ryle, between 'knowing that' and 'knowing how', and to the more recently made distinction made by cognitive scientists between declarative and procedural knowledge. Declarative knowledge is characteristic of explicit, verbalised knowledge, and procedural knowledge is exemplary of tacit or implicit knowledge.
>
> (Patel *et al.*, 1999, pp. 77–8)

The reference by Patel *et al.* (1999) to the seminal work of Gilbert Ryle (1949) draws attention to the notion that propositional knowledge or 'knowing-that' (which relates to knowing about something, *what* it is, *how* it works, etc), is different to 'know-how' (which is the knowledge implicit in *doing* something). This usefully draws attention to the fact that tacit knowledge is to do with something in our world,

that is always in some way contextual. However, it may also be misleading in that it appears to deny the possibility that it is also possible to arrive at 'knowing-that' forms of knowledge (knowing *about* something, rather than how to *do* something) through tacit and insightful means.

There is nevertheless a widely held view that tacit or intuitive knowing emerges from our experiencing of the world and attends to how we function within that world. This is in keeping with Sternberg's (1999) definition, that '[T]acit knowledge is procedural knowledge that guides behaviour but that is not readily available for introspection'. It is on this basis that some nursing authors such as Benner (1984), Benner *et al.* (1999) and Carlsson *et al.* (2002) present the view that expert practitioners are those who through extensive experience have come to tacitly know patterns which emerge in the course of practice and tacitly know how to respond to these. It is not the intention to dwell further on these ideas in the present chapter. In the chapter which follows, on aesthetic knowing, attention is given to the issue of skilled know-how, or mastery that is relevant to what might be termed the artistry of nursing practice. Also, in Chapter 27, Patricia Benner considers the notion of clinical wisdom or reasoning that draws upon the tacit knowing that occurs in clinical practice. But what is important to note at this stage is that, while the two apparently opposing views of personal knowing derive from radically different positions, they are nevertheless in some senses complementary. Personal knowing as a tacit cognitive process is an important adjunct to an increased awareness of the world, how we exist within it, and the patterns of knowing by which we come to know self and other. Similarly, an awareness of self, and an openness to the knowledge that may emerge from such awareness, reflect a greater willingness to accept tacit cognitive knowledge and a lesser likelihood that such knowledge would be rejected simply because it is not the product of empirical experience or conscious rational processes.

Study Activity 11.3 ━━━━━━━━

In a novel by John Le Carré (1974), a traitor has caused great damage, leading to the death and imprisonment of a number of people and, as he is about to be discovered, bringing ruin to those who trusted him. In the moments before the traitor falls into a trap wherein he will be exposed, the main protagonist, George Smiley, who has led the investigation leading to this exposure, lies in waiting; and his reflections are described:

> *He had no sense of conquest that he knew of. His thoughts, as often when he was afraid, concerned people. He had no theories or judgments in particular. He simply wondered how everyone would be affected; and he felt responsible ... He wondered whether there was any love between human beings that did not rest upon some sort of self-delusion; he wished he could just get up and walk away before it happened; but he couldn't ... He thought about treason and wondered whether there was mindless treason in the same way, supposedly, as there was mindless violence. It worried him that he felt so bankrupt; that whatever intellectual or philosophical precepts he clung to broke down entirely now that he was faced with the human situation.*
>
> (Le Carré, 1974, p. 322)

- Consider the way in which Smiley reflects by looking in upon his own psyche and his self-doubts, and also outwards to the implications of what is just about to happen for the others concerned. Do you see any value in such reflection, and has it any correspondence to circumstances within nursing activities?
- In his final comment, Smiley says in effect that in the face of the human situation all his knowledge (or intellect) and sense of values and meanings (philosophy) were of little avail. Clearly this is a reflection made at a moment of great duress and it may indicate a less than level-headed position. However, might this be an example of the coming to Smiley of a heightened self-awareness, of the frailty of his own self and also of others?
- Do you think nurses may face situations where all that is known and valued may be in some way insufficient for dealing with the situation? When this happens, what can we fall back upon to carry us through?

━━━━━━━━━━━━━━━━━━━━

THE REFLEXIVE DIMENSION

A particular issue that emerges in consideration of personal knowing is that of the phenomenon of reflection, and its operation within professional work in the form commonly referred to as reflective practice. (This issue is discussed in more detail by Gary Rolfe in Chapter 26.) It may seem at first that reflective practice and personal knowing (at least in that sense in which it is related to tacit cognitive knowledge) are incompatible. If we accept Polanyi's famous phrase that personal or tacit knowledge is that which we cannot tell, that we are in fact knowing 'more than we can tell', it would appear that by definition there is nothing that we can consciously reflect about. If we do not know *how* we have come to know something, then obviously we cannot reflect in any meaningful sense upon the process that was involved. All we can reflect upon is the result of this tacit knowing – that is, on what we have come to know. However, here again we might present an argument that reflection and personal or tacit knowing are not necessarily incompatible but can indeed be complementary.

A useful approach to this premise is to consider the product of tacit knowing. As we have already noted, this is characteristically intuitive or insightful knowing. We have also noted that in making this claim we are not necessarily claiming some mystical or magical sixth sense with which some are gifted. On the contrary, these terms usually imply (at least within the perspectives discussed in this chapter) simply that we come to a realisation, sometimes quite suddenly, without being aware of how we got there. However, we often find that our intuitions or insights turn out to be ill founded and inaccurate. Indeed, it is accepted that such possibility is a characteristic of such forms of knowing; in this respect, knowledge that emerges intuitively does not differ from that emerging from other forms of knowing, such as empirical knowing, that is also frequently found to fail tests of its validity. A question therefore emerges for this as for other forms of knowing: how do we ascertain its validity?

A helpful view is proposed by Bernard Lonergan (1957) in his extensive study of 'insight'. He spoke of insight as a form of self-appropriation of knowledge involving three processes of experiencing, understanding, and judgement. Through experiencing the phenomenon we come to an understanding of it, which is of course subject to error. However, by a further process of judgement we then come to the realisation, sometimes suddenly, that the explanation we have derived does in fact fit. Lonergan recognises that such insight has about it an epiphany of knowledge, a coming to realise, sometimes in an instant, what something is, how it works, what is happening here. This judgement stage is essentially reflective in nature. It involves thinking critically about the emerging understanding, drawing not only from our intuitive fitting of explanations but from our observations and prior experiences. There is, of course, a sense that this cuts across the idea of tacit or intuitive knowing as something that is an epiphany, a leap to understanding without a conscious awareness of how we got there that is central to Polanyi's thesis. However, whether we do or do not agree with Lonergan's view that judgement and reflection are part of insight, it is wise to reflect upon the outcome of our insights. Sometimes, as we have noted, they can be wrong and in the course of caring for vulnerable others there is little margin for error.

Study Activity 11.4 ————

In the arguments above, we have presented a case for the relevance of reflection in personal knowing that is essentially cognitive rather than relational. However, in that relational pattern of knowing described by Carper (1978), it might be argued that reflection is an essential aid to the achievement of self-awareness. This may be seen as a necessary step

towards awareness of, and entering into relation with, the other. Sometimes we term this self-reflection introspection. But even when we enter the relation with the other, we often feel the need to step back from the relation, and our highly subjective immersion in it, so that we can reflect more objectively about the other and how we might best help them. This is the movement between Buber's (1970) *I-Thou* and *I-It* states introduced earlier. It might be argued that if we are to be successful in our helping of others, there always needs to be this reflexive movement of moving out from the relation to observe and reflect, and then moving in again to be and to do. So understood, the form of personal knowing described by Carper, by definition, not only allows for reflection, but such reflection is an essential aspect of the progress towards understanding our tacit knowing of self and other.

- Re-read the statements earlier in the chapter on the idea of *I-Thou* and *I-It* relating. Supplement this by considering Carper's original work and how she interpreted Buber, and also by searching out and considering Paterson and Zderad's (1988) adaptation of Buber's work in psychiatric nursing.

- Present an argument demonstrating how reflection is an essential element of the *I-It* position, but by definition cannot occur in the *I-Thou* position. If you cannot present this argument, return to the readings listed above, extend your consideration of these, and revisit this activity.

- Explain why it may be necessary to maintain a degree of reflexivity in terms of movement between the two relational states described by Buber. Use a nursing context to demonstrate your argument and present this in a brief written account (about 400 words/one A4 page). You may seek the help of a fellow student or personal tutor to obtain a critique of your work.

SUMMARY

In this chapter we have addressed what is perhaps the most difficult of all the patterns of knowing presented in this module. The difficulty is particularly characterised by the different ways in which we can approach an idea of personal knowing. In her seminal work, Carper (1978) addressed such knowing as an essentially existential way of knowing self and other, and of the characteristic emergence of such knowing in the relationship between self and other. But even at the time her paper was published, the difficulty of conciliating this perspective with the equally influential view presented by Polanyi, of personal knowing as a tacit cognitive dimension, became apparent. In this chapter we have recognised and highlighted these differences. But in doing so we have argued that there is a complementarity between these perspectives, that an awareness of self is informed by a tacit form of cognitive knowing of that self, and that in turn an awareness and openness to self as a source is an important prerequisite to an openness to tacit cognition.

Carper has spoken to us of a need to attend to our awareness of self, and through this an intentional commitment to an awareness of the other that can only emerge in the course of a personal and caring relationship. When Carper wrote her seminal paper, there appeared a sound argument for attending to the personal in the nurse–patient relationship. She would not have known a quarter of a century ago the extent to which modern technology would impose its potentially alienating influence upon modern living. Nor would she have appreciated the full extent to which health care systems themselves would become enslaved to technology and the impositions of scarcity and economies reflected in managed care and the rationing of resources through formulae such as that for quality adjusted life years. In the intervening years, the places of asylum and healing have become, to many, places of depersonalisation, alienation and threat, as identified in the writings of Fromm (1999) and Gadamer (1996). At every turn the nurse is pushed towards science and procedure, and the highly objective and complex processes of modern health care interventions. The remarkable achievements of science and technology must, of course, not be devalued; millions who in the past would have succumbed to disease and death now live longer and healthier lives. But these are not recipes or excuses for turning away from the person. Now, more than ever, there is a call for the nurse to engage with persons, to convert what might otherwise be a barren and alienating space to one that is compassionate and caring, within which healing and sustenance that are at the heart of nursing are available to those in need.

REFERENCES

Bastick, T. (1982) *Intuition: How we think and act,* John Wiley, Chichester

Benner, P. (1984) *From Novice to Expert: Excellence and power in clinical practice,* Addison Wesley, Menlo Park, CA

Benner, P., Hooper-Kyriakidis, P. and Stannard, D. (1999) *Clinical Wisdom and Interventions in Critical Care: A thinking in action approach,* W.B. Saunders, Philadelphia, IL

Buber, M. ([1939] 1970) *I and Thou,* Scribner, New York

Carlsson, G., Drew, N., Dahlberg, K. *et al.* (2002) Uncovering tacit caring knowledge. *Nursing Philosophy* 3, 144–51

Carper, B. (1978) Fundamental patterns of knowing in nursing. *Advances in Nursing Science* 1, 13–23

Chinn, P.L. and Kramer, M.K. (1999) *Theory and Nursing: Integrated knowledge development* (5th edn), Mosby, St Louis, IL

Egan, E.C. and Beckstrand, J. (1979) 'Personal knowledge' versus 'self knowledge' – reaction. *Advances in Nursing Science* 1(4), viii–ix

Fromm, E. (1999) *On Being Human,* Continuum, New York

Gadamer, H-G. (1996) *The Enigma of Health,* Stanford University Press, Stanford, CA

Hillman, J. (1989) *A Blue Fire,* Harper and Row, New York

Hillman, J. (1997) *The Soul's Code: In search of character and calling,* Bantam Books, London

Le Carré, J. (1974) *Tinker, Tailor, Soldier, Spy,* Hodder and Stoughton, London

Lonergan, B. (1957) *Insight: A study of human understanding,* Longman, Green and Co, London

Munhall, P.L. (1993) "Unknowing": toward another pattern of knowing in nursing. *Nursing Outlook* 41, 125

O'Donohue, J. (1997) *Anam Cara: Spiritual wisdom from the Celtic world*, Bantam Press, London

Parse, R.R. (1992) Human becoming: Parse's theory of nursing, *Nursing Science Quarterly* 5(1), 35–42

Parse, R.R. (1998) *The Human Becoming School of Thought: A perspective for nurses and other health professionals*, Sage, Thousand Oaks, CA

Patel, V.L., Arocha, J.F. and Kaufman, D.R. (1999) Expertise and tacit knowledge in medicine. In: Sternberg, R. and Horvath, J. (eds) *Tacit Knowledge in Professional Practice: Researcher and practitioner perspectives*, Lawrence Erlbaum, Mahwah, NJ

Paterson, J. and Zderad, L. (1988) *Humanistic Nursing*, National League for Nursing, New York

Polanyi, M. (1958) *Personal Knowledge: Towards a post-critical philosophy*, University of Chicago Press, Chicago, IL

Polanyi, M. (1967) *The Tacit Dimension*, Routledge and Kegan Paul, London

Reber, A. (1995) *Implicit Learning and Tacit Knowledge: An essay on the cognitive unconscious*, Oxford University Press, New York

Rogers, C. (1990) A client-centred/person-centred approach to therapy. In: Kutach, I. and Wolf, A. (1986) *Psychotherapist's Handbook*, Jossey Bass, San Francisco, CA

Ryle, G. (1949) *The Concept of Mind*, Hutchinson, London

Solomon, P. (1991) Paul Solomon speaks on spiritual roots and the journey to wholeness. *Human Potential Magazine* 16(3), 28–32

Sternberg, R. (1999) What do we know about tacit knowledge? Making the tacit become explicit. In: Sternberg, R. and Horvath, J. (eds) *Tacit Knowledge in Professional Practice: Researcher and practitioner perspectives*, Lawrence Erlbaum, Mahwah, NJ

White, J. (1995) Patterns of knowing: review, critique, and update. *Advances in Nursing Science* 17(4), 73–86

12 AESTHETIC KNOWING: NURSING AS SKILL AND MASTERY

Oliver Slevin

> *What art is should be inferable from the work. What the work of art is we can come to know only from the nature of art. Anyone can see we are moving in a circle.*
>
> (Heidegger, 1971, p. 18)

LEARNING OUTCOMES

After studying this chapter you will be able to:

- Explain aesthetic experience as a pattern of knowing
- Recognise the difference and relationship between that which is aesthetic and that which is art
- Identify the different ways in which aesthetic experience as conveyed through art impacts upon nursing
- Differentiate between art as a product and art as a process
- Identify characteristics that differentiate artistry or mastery from other levels of human activity
- Recognise and explain how nursing can be recognised as art work involving artistry and mastery.

INTRODUCTION

On one of the mornings during the time this was being written, in early autumn, the author is driving out to an appointment. At this time of year, mists clear late in the early mornings amidst the boglands in this part of Ireland, with the bracken appearing to float on shifting waters. It seems as if this mistiness creates a great silence, as if there is no other living thing on the very face of this landscape. But now the half-seen forms of grazing cattle seem to move into view in slow motion and total silence. At a later time of day these beasts would go unnoticed, but now the driver watches with wariness as they lumber in and out of visibility amidst the shifting mists. This all gives a sense of timelessness to this scene. And indeed there is a sense of timelessness in this locality, where the Irish High Kings and Queens dwelt under the protection of their Druids and Royal Knights before the time of Christ. The driver thinks of this and looks across the bogland again, half expecting to see the Knights of the Red Branch once again appear out of the mist. In this seemingly timeless scene the mists hide much, but the mind completes the image, extends the meanings. Yes, knights could appear here; anything could happen here. The watcher is ever-so-slightly discomfited and would break out of this time warp, but the scene seems to draw him in.

All this, of course, lasts mere seconds. But during this time, although the car continues its course, for a short time this scene has called out to the driver, as shapes and forms conjure up meanings and feelings that seem to suffuse the very being of the watcher. We might say of this, that here was an aesthetic experience. But how do we describe it? And, more importantly, how do we move from an Irish bogland at dawn to an aesthetics of nursing at the dawning of a new century? This is what we must achieve in this chapter.

TOWARDS AN UNDERSTANDING OF THE AESTHETIC

In Chapter 9 we identified aesthetics as one of the main branches of philosophy. We described it as the study of how we appreciate beauty and form, and their creation. We, of course, also recognised that 'beauty' in this context was problematic. Indeed, it is so problematic that some who study aesthetics desist from using it as a concept, and prefer alternatives such as 'sublime' (a term meaning awesome, or wondrous, or invigorating and enlivening). But more frequently beauty *is* recognised as central to what we understand by aesthetics. Not, however, as some stereotypical notion that is taken as the norm of what is beautiful in our modern cultures. Rather, it is recognised as a quality that calls an appreciative response from the observer. By any mechanistic and objective criteria this object may be categorised as ugly and unsightly by others, but to the individual it may stimulate responses that are compelling rather than repulsive, enlivening rather than deadening. One may attempt to convey this meaning in a rational and objective manner, but words will often not suffice to convey the meaning of something that is felt rather than known. This is perhaps one instance where the old adages are best, as demonstrated here in the assertion that 'Beauty is in the eyes of the beholder'. This statement indeed stands true to the original Greek meaning of aesthesia as being sense perception, or feeling perception, or taste perception. In our field of health care we are familiar with one of its opposites, that of *anaesthesia*, or lack of sense perception – the making of the patient senseless in order to perform surgery.

Study Activity 12.1

Aesthetics, and indeed philosophy, of which it is a part, is problematic in terms of its meaning. Beyond being aware that it is not a science – indeed it is very different to a science – we are already encountering difficulties. The term is closely associated, as we shall presently see, with the term art – both are to do with expression, meaning, form, beauty, etc. This seems to place them in the domain of something called the humanities rather than the sciences.

- Look up the term humanities. Seek at least two or three statements on what this term means. Having done this, indicate whether you feel aesthetics comes within the humanities and the arguments for sustaining this viewpoint.

- As we are embarking on a consideration of aesthetics and art as orientations within an aspect of health care (nursing), a question is begged as to how much the humanities in general inform health care. Do a library search using keywords such as humanities, health, medicine. Identify at least three instances where the literature demonstrates a humanities input to our approaches to care.

Drawing on how we sense or experience something, we further noted in Chapter 9 that aesthetics is a perceptual activity, to do with how we sense or view the things in our world. In this sense, aesthetics has some common ground with epistemology (another branch of philosophy), which is concerned with how we come to know and explain the things in our world. However, the subtle difference here is that aesthetics is not in the business of constructing knowledge, but concerned with how we experience and appreciate form. Therefore, aesthetics is concerned with an evaluative rather than confirmatory project. In this sense we saw in turn some common ground with ethics (another branch of philosophy), which is also concerned with making evaluations about things and actions in our world. However, the subtle difference here is that aesthetics is not concerned with evaluative judgements about what is good or bad, virtuous or vicious. What is being evaluated in aesthetics is our direct experience of that which we perceive and the response it stirs in us. This takes the form of a direct cognitive–emotional response to the object of our aesthetic experience. As a whole, the object of our attention calls out this response in us. This shows yet another link, this time with metaphysics, or more specifically ontology (yet another branch of philosophy), which is concerned with existence and the meanings we attribute to things.

The subtle difference here is that the aesthetic experience is not one of *attending to* the existence of that phenomenon which we address with intentionality, and from which we *derive* meaning. It is rather a particular way of *responding to* something that calls such a responding from us, and in respect of which we see meaning *in* the object. This is a rather complex differentiation but it is worth grasping. In ontology we are *deriving* meaning *from* the experience, or *through* our experiencing of it. In aesthetics we are *responding* to meaning *in* the experience, and we are *appreciating* that which is shown to us. This is at once immediate and existential and has no purpose beyond this appreciation. To illustrate this point, imagine that someone explains the meaning in a poem we have not yet read. They have attempted to derive meaning, to interpret the poem. But we cannot confirm agreement or acceptance of their interpretation. When we, in turn, read the poem, it may open to us in a particular way. How *we* respond to what is *in* the poem and the meaning *we* discern may be quite different.

We might summarise the latter paragraph by suggesting that philosophy in general is concerned with truth, beauty, good, and existence. These areas of concern are in fact the branches of philosophy that we termed, respectively, epistemology, aesthetics, ethics and metaphysics (or more specifically, ontology). Each of these is a particular way of looking at the world. In aesthetics, this is commonly spoken of as *the aesthetic attitude* (Scruton, 1994; Janaway, 1995). This, as Janaway states, is:

> ... *a particular way of experiencing or attending to objects. It is said to be an attitude independent of any motivations to do with utility, economic value, moral judgement, or peculiarly personal emotion, and concerned with experiencing the object 'for its own sake'.*
>
> (Janaway, 1995, p. 8)

It can be seen why the point is made above that in aesthetics there is no purpose of deriving meaning from the exper-iencing of an object. We are, after all, concerned with how we, individually, experience the object. This was what Kant (1969) described as the *judgement of taste*. This highlights three fundamental aspects of any experience that we can define as aesthetic:

1 The meaning of an object is within it and indissolubly a part of it; it can only be experienced when we experience the object directly and with immediacy.
2 Only the individual can directly experience the object and make his or her 'judgement of taste'; there is no sense in which this meaning can be extracted and expressed as a common or generalised meaning, at least in the aesthetic sense.
3 The objective or goal of the experience has no motive other than an appreciation of the object itself; we are not surmising whether the object is valuable, or if it would make a good present, or serve as a doorstop; we are simply adopting the 'aesthetic attitude' and seeing in it a beauty, or sublime quality (or indeed their opposites).

There is perhaps one further important point to address in this consideration of aesthetics as a judgement of taste. This is related to the second and third bullet points above in particular, and it raises a question in respect of whether an aesthetic experience has any value beyond the immediacy of the experience. Kant (1969) is again a useful source here. He spoke of the 'antimony of taste' (or in modern language, the paradox of taste). The argument runs as follows. Given the aesthetic properties of any object, any rational person, using the universal faculty of reason, will discern the aesthetic qualities contained in that object. If they do not, they are not paying it full attention, or operating from some other motive (e.g. self-interest or profit, rather than responding to the intrinsic aesthetic properties of the object). However, if we claim the *aesthetic* meaning is indissolubly a part of the object and can only be experienced directly by the individual who experiences his/her reaction and sense of meaning in it, there can be no objective deriving of meaning from the object that can in any true sense be successfully transmitted second-hand to others. This was the case in our earlier example of how different people may derive different meanings from a poem. These two contrary claims amount to the paradox or antimony. It is akin to saying aesthetic experience is objective judgement and at the same time it is impossible to claim for it common objective criteria. That is, of course, what a paradox is: two opposite statements or claims, both of which cannot be correct at the same time. Philosophers are, of course, fond of mental gymnastics for resolving such paradoxes. We have neither the time (nor, perhaps, the inclination) to follow suit. It is sufficient for us to recognise that while an aesthetic experience is one that is a subjective response and specific to its object (the entity to which we are attending), we can nevertheless gain insights from recognising common or reasonable responses to it.

Taking these various notions of the nature of an aesthetic experience, we can attempt to summarise its main elements. This is not necessarily an easy project, as there is little agreement about what the elements are. However, Carroll (2002) provided what is at least a comprehensive and easily conceptualised framing for the elements of anything we might term aesthetic. This framing suggests the following elements:

1 *An affective element* – this relates to the *emotional* or affective response the object engenders in us. We may see it as something beautiful, or wondrous, or awesome. The significant point here is the extent to which the experience lifts us to a different level, or transports us out of the mundane, or releases or liberates us (even momentarily) from the everyday. We might say that the 'watcher' in our opening paragraph to this chapter was briefly lifted out of the car and 'taken hold of' by the wonder of the passing landscape. (Sometimes people who combine the muse with the act of driving end up in roadside ditches, but that is an entirely different aesthetic experience!)

2 *A content element* – this relates to the *form* of the object of our aesthetic experience. That is, the way in which its parts come together to construct the whole, and the sense of unity or integrity of the object. In this form we may be drawn to the cohesiveness of the object, how its structures, shapes, sounds, colours draw us to it, and even convey to us a meaning that emanates from the overall form. We might say that the 'watcher' in our opening paragraph to this chapter was not only 'taken hold of' but 'transported towards' the nature of the landscape and how its elements came together to form an otherworldly and even mystical quality.

3 *An axiological element* – this draws from the Latin root of the term axiom (which relates to something that is self-evident). However, its meaning in this context is that the object stands on its own merits and is *valued* in and of itself. In this almost existential sense, the immediacy of the object of the aesthetic experience and the contingency (or immediate presence) of the observer is important. The object is therefore seen to be a thing of value, but its value is contained within it and it alone, and it is experienced uniquely by each of us. We might say that the 'watcher' in our opening paragraph to this chapter was not only 'taken hold of' and 'transported towards' the passing landscape, but that he 'experienced' a sense of appreciation of the potency of this landscape and the meanings that for him were enfolded within it. Of course, the 'watcher' passed on, and the mists lifted and the sun came out, and the scene as it was also disappeared. In the once tremendously popular and multi-Emmy award winning television series, *The Rockford Files*, James Garner played the hapless private detective whose run-ins with the underworld often brought him into conflicts with the police and his acquaintances. As he repeatedly tried to explain his constantly recurring predicaments, he resorted in frustration to what became his catch phrase: 'Well, you woulda had to've been there.' In this sense, to have something

even remotely akin to the 'watcher's' axiomatic experience (or indeed any other reaction to the landscape described), you would, literally, have had to be there.

Study Activity 12.2 _____

Consider the following verses from the music of a current popular songwriter:

> I want to sing this song for you
> I want to lift your spirits high
> And in my soul I want to feel
> The beauty of the days gone by
> The beauty of the days gone by
> It brings a longing to my soul
> To contemplate my own true self
> And keep me young as I grow old
>
> Van Morrison (2002)

Of course, as an aesthetic object, this being a song has much missing from it. You cannot hear, on this written page, the plaintive melodies and wistfulness of diction that add to the celebration of days gone by and the gift that is offered here by the author. However, going on what you have to work with here:

- Do you feel this *is* an aesthetic 'object' and if so, how does it meet the three attributes of an aesthetic experience proposed by Carroll (2002)?
- Can you think of any ways in which this song might be used as an aesthetic experience that would help in the care of patients?

WHERE ART COMES IN

In modern scholarship it is the case that aesthetics (as a discipline) devotes much of its time to a critical study of art. However, this is not a necessary condition, and not all aesthetic study is tied to this perspective. It is equally acceptable to attend to the aesthetic qualities of things that exist in our social and natural world that are not termed art, or indeed not a manmade object at all. The aesthetic experience of the early morning driver is an example of this. It is possible to see beauty in, and to appreciate, a rainbow, the Grand Canyon, or indeed an Irish bog at dawn. The fundamental principle that seems to apply here is that not all that is aesthetic is art, but all that is art is aesthetic. However, this assumes that all artists subscribe to a view that their work should only produce aesthetic experience and this is not necessarily the case. Sometimes artists intend that their work will make a social statement, or exert political influence, or even have a therapeutic effect. To the extent that this is so, aesthetic philosophers may make the point that these motives have nothing to do with specific aesthetic concerns. This, of course, has no impact upon the aesthetic qualities of such works of art, and it is unlikely that anyone would claim as a work of art something that is not also aesthetic. As for the philosophers in question, their concerns with such fine distinctions are unlikely to be of interest outwith their own academic community. This distinction does, however, allow us to recognise art as extending beyond the aesthetic, as demonstrated in Fig. 12.1 overleaf.

This, of course, brings us to the question of what *art* is. It may be simplest to claim here (perhaps with tongue in cheek) that art is to do with the act of creating something of aesthetic merit, or the aesthetic product of such activity. The term itself arises from Latin origins of the words *ars* meaning (roughly) the skilful putting together of something (the word articulate meaning joining having similar roots) and the word *artem* or creative product. Of course, if we view the product of art as being aesthetic, this is (if we accept our earlier definitive description of aesthetics) an object that exists for its own sake and which calls us to nothing other than an appreciation of its beauty, form or sublime qualities. This was notably expressed in the motto of the movie organisation Metro-Goldwyn-Mayer which states *ars gratia artis* – 'art for art's sake'. However, as noted above, not all artists would subscribe to this notion and, as illustrated in Fig. 12.1, there may be other motives behind the product of the artist's work. On the basis of these comments and Fig. 12.1 we can say that a

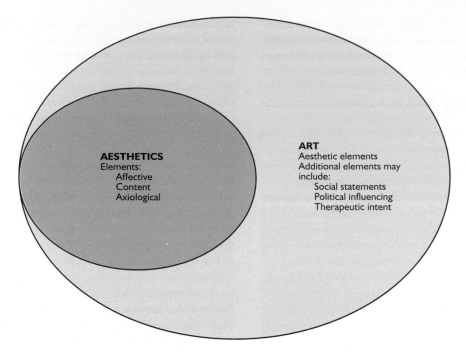

Figure 12.1 The relationship between aesthetics and art

work of art is a product that:

- is a composition in form that represents some physical entity or psychic idea
- intends to have definitive aesthetic qualities – that is, to have a quality inherent in it and specific to it that is capable of engendering appreciation of properties of the beautiful, sublime and meaningful that are enfolded in the work
- may in addition have additional aspirations – which may include educational, political, social, or therapeutic intentions
- can be produced in a variety of media – extending from paintings and sculpture, through music and literature, to drama and dance (and other instances of what are known as the performing arts), and even beyond this to a variety of modern media such as photography, film, architecture and a virtually limitless list of other artefacts.

While in the past distinctions were made between what were termed the fine arts and other compositional works, in the post-modern world this distinction is no longer meaningful, beyond giving a general pointer towards sculpture and paintings as reflecting what is commonly understood as the fine arts. What is suggested in such a term is something like this: the product of the artist's mastery or artistry is something of high aesthetic value, having the rarity of refinement and form to be appreciated for its own sake. This is different to the mastery of the master craftsman (such as the cabinet maker, the stonemason, or the French polisher) whose product, while frequently having almost equal aesthetic appeal, is nevertheless primarily motivated by utility and is seen as 'lower' for that (we even refer to such a person as an 'artisan' rather than an artist). On this basis, we might even consider nursing as such a coming together of skill and utility, and think of the nurse as an artisan rather than an artist.

The latter outline of the product of 'art work' throws light upon what is *recognised* as art work. In a narrow sense, it can of course be claimed that 'art work' is restricted to that which aims to produce products that meet the above criteria. By this argument, work that is not specifically aimed at producing a composition in form that has definitive aesthetic qualities, would not in effect be 'art work'. However, implicit in this notion of art work is the view that there is artistry or skill involved, and we would expect of the gifted artist a degree of mastery that indeed produces something we find beautiful or awesome or wondrous in that it speaks to us with meaningfulness. But two questions are begged here. The first is as follows. If that which is aesthetic is in the eye of the beholder, then is that which is art equally in the eye of the beholder? This is what Heidegger was alluding to in the opening quotation to this chapter. What art is can only be taken from knowing it when we see it, when we appreciate it as such. It is in turn only when we know this that we know what the *work* of art is: one determines the other in a circular manner. The second question is as follows. What do we term other areas of human endeavour which do not aspire to the above four bullet points for the product of their labours, but nevertheless display high levels of skill, or artistry, or mastery? Are they examples of non-art, or some form of non-aesthetic art, and can we (as suggested above) use some other term such as 'artisan' to describe the creator of such work? This is relevant to us, because we speak in our profession of 'the art of nursing'.

THE AESTHETIC DIMENSION IN NURSING

We must ask ourselves what the relevance of all this consideration of aesthetics and art is for the practice of nursing. In this respect, our quest may address the two interrelated conceptualisations addressed in this chapter so far: aesthetics and art.

Let us first turn to the issue of aesthetics. Assuming we accept the earlier suggestion that an aesthetic experience involves affective (emotional), content, and axiological elements, can such experiencing inform nursing in any way? There are two ways in which we might

respond positively. First, we may recognise that in the situations we address, health care situations peopled by those who need our help, there may be merit in developing the capacity to respond to particular and complex situations with a capacity for openness and receptiveness to what the situation is telling us. Second, we may recognise that what we discern from such receptiveness is a meaningfulness that is enfolded in such complex situations, wherein elements may behave in patterns that have a coherence within the situation as a whole. That is, we may look beyond the parts (the observations, instruments and gauges) to what the situation as a whole *means;* in essence the meanings *enfolded* within the situation become unfolded and available to our evaluation and determinate action.

Let us now consider the issue of art. This again depends on the interpretation we place upon art. If we accept that it involves those aesthetic elements identified in the previous paragraph, but can extend beyond this to having a degree of utility, there may again be two ways in which we can respond positively. First, we can consider ways in which we can bring such art or its utility to bear on our practice of nursing. That is, we can utilise paintings, sculpture, music, literature, drama, etc. as diagnostic and therapeutic devices. Second, we can recognise in our own nursing practice an artistry that can be extended to mastery in terms of how we utilise our relational and technical skills in the practice of nursing. However, if we are to proceed in this manner, we do need to have a clear view of what we mean by art and how this term *is* used in nursing circles.

In all walks of life, and nursing is no different, the word art is used in many different ways. We indeed find the term utilised in senses that are often unclear and frequently overlapping. Thus we have, to identify just some of these differences in meaning or emphasis, the following:

- *Nursing as art as opposed to or as well as science* – thus, we hear talk of 'The art and science of nursing' and this is usually taken to mean some combination or apposition of that which is subjective and humanistic, and that which is objective and scientific.

- *Nursing as the art of responsiveness and interpretation* – this relates to how nursing practice essentially commences with a process of 'coming to know' that is in fact akin to the aesthetic experience of being open to and receptive of the objects of our attention. It relates specifically to our capacity for seeing patterns and meanings in the patient-centred situations we confront. From this insightful capacity to intuitively grasp situations (which is in fact an expertise that grows with experience) we develop the ability to see nursing needs unfolding and even to anticipate these. This is a process akin to what in medicine is termed the art of diagnosis and some nurses (e.g. Benner *et al.*, 1999) refer to as clinical wisdom.

- *Nursing art as skilful activity* – this relates to the artistry or mastery that is to be found in the expertise of nursing actions, and it may or may not be included in some people's understanding of nursing as 'art and science'. We may tend to think of these as physical or psychomotor skills, and these are of course important. But there is also the issue of mastery in terms of relational skills (that is very close to the performing arts) and the expressive skills of safe and effective report writing (that bears some relationship to expressive arts such as literature).

- *Nursing as the art of aesthetic presentation* – this recognises how nursing practice can have a grace and meaningfulness about it that can, as with any aesthetic experience, be enlivening, and raise us above the ordinary. While it incorporates the aspect of art as mastery, it is this experiential aspect – that can be healing and therapeutic – that is the emphasis in this case.

- *Nursing art as form and content* – this again relates to nursing as mastery, but the mastery here is to creatively see, and indeed innovatively construct, the nursing frameworks within which we operate. This would cut across the former division of nursing into art and science, because in nursing science and also theory construction, the influence of insight and creativity is an essential element.

- *Art in nursing* – here we are recognising that art as it is normally understood – the fine arts, the expressive arts, the performing arts – can be harnessed to the nursing purpose. Thus, we can see, for example, how nursing may use literature as an educational tool in nurse training. Similarly, we can see how fine and expressive arts (painting, sculpture, writing) or performing arts (poetry, drama) can be used as therapeutic devices, as, for example, with psychodrama in mental health nursing.

The message in all of this is straightforward. When we hear of nursing as an art or of art in nursing, we must beg a question: what exactly is the speaker alluding to? In their helpful text on nursing knowledge development, Chinn and Kramer (1999) make a useful distinction. They see the two main relevant connotations of art and nursing as follows:

- Knowledge of the experience towards which the art form is directed.
- Knowledge of the art form itself.

In respect of the *experience* of nursing as an art form (in essence what we earlier referred to as the aesthetic experience or aesthetic attitude), they state as follows:

> *In nursing, knowledge of experience encompasses knowledge of the lived experience of nursing and the experiences of health and illness. It is the lived experience of nursing, and of health and illness, towards which our aesthetics is directed, and it is the experience itself that our* art *is intended to transform.*
>
> (Chinn and Kramer, 1999, p. 186)

In respect of nursing *as* an art form, they proceed to state the following:

> *Knowledge of nursing's art form is the focus ... We will explore a definition of the art of*

> *nursing, the elements that form the whole of the art as a product, the technical skills involved in creating the art-act, and the processes by which those elements can be shaped to form a satisfying, artistically valid whole.*
>
> (Chinn and Kramer, 1999, p. 187)

We should perhaps turn here to the views of Carper (1978). It was her famous seminal work that first placed the aesthetic dimension in the nursing arena. Indeed, her classification of nursing's patterns of knowing into the empirical, the ethical, the personal and the aesthetic, is the basis for how our chapters are presented in this module. It is predominantly on the area of knowledge of the lived experience that Carper (1978) centres her aesthetic perspective. In this respect she states:

> *The more skilled the nurse becomes in perceiving and empathising with the lives of others, the more knowledge or understanding will be gained of alternative modes of perceiving reality. The nurse will thereby have available a larger repertoire of choices in designing and providing nursing care that is effective and satisfying.*
>
> (Carper, 1978)

Chinn and Kramer (1999) extend this project by considering the skilful response to this aesthetic knowing. In doing so they are proceeding beyond aesthetic knowing to the artistry or mastery of effective interventions. Their project, that of nursing practice as an art form or, to use a less pompous term, as artistry or mastery, is one that has been advanced by a number of nursing authorities. Among these, two examples are of particular value.

The first of these is the work of Patricia Benner and her colleagues, carried forward over the past 15 years or more. While Benner is not particularly given to the language of aesthetics, there is a notable similarity between her conceptualisation of the nursing situation and that of Carper (1978). Benner *et al.* (1999) speak

instead of 'clinical grasp', a capacity to intuitively see situations and emerging patterns which is born out of experience and tacit knowing. While Carper (1978) has spoken of an empathic understanding of the patient in his situation, Benner *et al.* (1996) speak of emotional attunement to the whole situation. For example:

> *Whereas the new graduate suffers from the inability to recognize situations, and the competent nurse overdefines the situation, the proficient nurse's practical grasp of the situation is increasingly accurate, and thus when a practical grasp is missing, the nurse feels uncomfortable or a vague uneasiness ... These feelings are not just a self-reference to internal emotional states. They point to what nurses notice in the situation. To have a perceptual grasp of the situation is to have an emotional tone related to the situation. Emotional responsiveness and tone are central to having an embodied skilled know-how and signal an understanding of the situation as well as a way of being in it.*
>
> (Benner *et al.*, 1996, p. 118)

While Benner and her colleagues proceed to speak in their work of the actual nature of expert practice, their concepts of clinical grasp and emotional attunement correspond with both Chinn and Kramers' (1999) description of knowledge of experience and Carper's (1978) description of perceiving and empathising with the lives of others.

The second notable contribution is that of Johnson (1994, 1996). As with Chinn and Kramer (1999), Johnson extends the consideration of art in nursing into the domain of nursing actions. In identifying meanings attributed to the art of nursing in nursing literature, Johnson (1994) presents five meanings that have a progressive sequence in terms of emerging patterns of meaning, as follows:

- *Nursing art as the ability to grasp meaning from encounters with patients* – this is similar to the ideas of perception and empathy expressed by Carper (1978) and that of clinical grasp, suggested by Benner *et al.* (1999).

- *Nursing art as the ability to establish meaningful connections or relationships with patients* – this is in line with the idea of relational skills referred to earlier.
- *Nursing art as skilful doing, the carrying out of procedural activities with confidence and mastery* – this is in line with the idea of technical skills referred to earlier.
- *Nursing art as the ability to determine rational courses of action* – this meaning would appear to be at odds with the notion of aesthetic knowing that has a degree of holistic existential immediacy to it, as it may seem to imply a distancing from the object of our attention and a more particulate problem-solving approach. However, it does have some degree of similarity to that idea of nursing art as dealing with form and content in creative ways to recognise patterns of meaning that may lead to successful framing or theorising of nursing action, as presented earlier.
- *Nursing art as the ability to conduct nursing practice morally* – this meaning would be at odds with the idea that in an aesthetic sense we evaluate the object of our perception on its own merits (beauty, form, qualities that set it above the everyday, etc.). The evaluations involved in this moral dimension would typically be ethical values that by definition look beyond the thing itself to values of goodness, utility, etc.

Here we find a set of meanings that again provides some insight into how we might view art in nursing, but we find also that some of Johnson's meanings may not easily fit into any common understanding of aesthetics or conception of art as a product or process.

Study Activity 12.3

One art form that is recognised and often described as an expressive art, is that of literature. This can take various forms extending from poetry to prose, encompassing fiction and non-fiction, and extending from narrative (or story-telling) to more modern forms of aesthetic expression. You will be aware that there is much talk of the importance of empirical knowledge in health care, and we speak of evidence-based health care. However, in recent times, there is also talk of something called narrative-based health care.

- Using your library resources, look up this term and note down its major characteristics. Useful starting sources may be Greenhalgh and Hurwitz (1998) and Frank (1995).
- Consider whether this narrative-based health care is art or science, or some mix of the two.
- Write a brief case for the development of narrative-based nursing as an extension of the art and nursing debate. This should take up no more than one A4 page and you should ask a fellow student or your personal tutor to critique the case you have made.

SUMMARY

In this chapter we have attempted to consider the relevance of an aesthetic way of knowing to nursing. Not unexpectedly, we found that there is a variety of views about how something is viewed as aesthetic. However, we proposed that in most, if not all, of these there are at least three possible aspects of an aesthetic experience: an affective aspect, that relates to how we appreciate or respond to the object; a content aspect, that concerns a recognition of form and cohesiveness in the whole, from which meaning is taken to emanate; and, an axiological aspect, that concerns a valuing or appreciation of the object in its own right. It was recognised that all things may have such aesthetic qualities in their own right, whether they are objects that occur naturally in the physical world or artefacts that are the product of cultures. However, among the latter we recognised that particular class of objects that are created specifically for their aesthetic merits and are termed works of art.

Even here we found that determining what qualifies for such a distinction is no straightforward task. In this context, we noted in particular the divergence between those who claim that art should have no function beyond the aesthetic, and the alternative view that it can also incorporate a degree of utility (as when it is utilised for social, political, educational or therapeutic purposes).

The possibility of extending art in this way can of course be taken as an opening for a discussion of the relevance of art in nursing. In our penultimate section of the chapter we addressed this issue, both from the point of view of an aesthetic of nursing and from the related point of view of art in, of and for nursing. Of course, no easy answers were advanced, for the simple reason that, here again, there are none. There is instead a range of ways in which aesthetics and art may impact upon the nursing situation. It is hoped that, in touching upon most of these, you are at least aware of the potential for a variety of applications of aesthetic thinking and knowing, and artistic expression, in the theory and practice of nursing. However, to leave the subject in this way, with nothing more than a *pot-pourri* of ideas, many of which are in contention, may create a feeling of business left unfinished. This may be alleviated to some extent by two concluding messages.

The first of these messages relates in a sense to one aspect of the aesthetic premise, i.e. that we look to the thing itself. In a health care system that is characterised by empirical science and high technology, and within which precedence is given to evidence-based approaches and rational thought, we should give a thought to the weaknesses that hide behind the strengths of these important foundations. We refer here to weaknesses in the bias towards the objective and away from the subjective, and towards the general with its standardised cases and away from the particular and its personal contexts. We might simplify this by speaking of an art as well as a science of health care. But, if we reflect again upon the aesthetic project, this takes us back to a countenancing of the thing

itself, to the particular. This is the first of our final messages. It asks us to look for the meanings and patterns contained within the particular as opposed to the general case. We shall call this message the message of *enfoldment* and *unfoldment*. This orientation and its terminology find their origins in the work of the physicist and philosopher David Bohm (1987). Bohm applied his concept not only to the physical world but also to the world of human consciousness. The light metaphor serves to clarify the meaning. As all the light from images in a room radiate, they are *enfolded*, thus to pass through the pupil of the eye. They are then *unfolded* by the retina of the eye and the visual areas of our brain. In a similar manner, when we consider this person we would call patient, there are meanings enfolded here – within the person, his history, the present context, the contexts of health and illness, etc. We can of course look elsewhere for our understanding. But if we attend to this situation in all its particular circumstances, if we really attend in the immediacy of this situation as, in an aesthetic sense, the thing or person in itself, we can find that meaning which is enfolded now unfolding. This, therefore, is the first of our two messages: to look for the meanings that are enfolded. This is close to what Benner *et al.* (1999) spoke of as the clinical grasp referred to earlier. But we perhaps speak more here of a grasp of the holistic person and what he means to us.

The second of these messages relates to how we respond when such meaning unfolds. We are, of course, here speaking specifically of the aesthetic or artistic response. We have seen in our discussions in the previous section of the chapter that the possible responses are many and varied. And we might ask the question: Which is the best or right response, in the context of an art *of* nursing, or art *in* nursing, or art *for* nursing? There are perhaps two aspects that would be important in a balanced response. The first of these is that we would not respond in an either/or sense in which 'art' has precedence over 'science', or vice versa. Rather, we would respond by an integration of different ways of knowing – in Carper's (1978) terminology, by an integration of empirical, ethical, personal and aesthetic ways of knowing. The second aspect is, that we would respond in terms of the context. That is, the knowledge and skills upon which we would draw are dependent on the needs of the situation. Extrapolating from this to the issue of the aesthetic domain in nursing or the application of art to the nursing situation, we would not be exclusively guided by any one of the interpretations of nursing art presented in our previous section. Rather, we would choose from and adapt such means as suits the specific context. Here we might call on the notion of the *bricolage* as presented in the qualitative human and social sciences by Denzin and Lincoln (2000). The *bricoleur* (a French word meaning handyman or Jack-of-all-trades) is adept at seeing what is called for in problem situations, and his particular forte is the adaptation, or modification, or alternative use of tools and devices, using in turn adapted or modified methods, to solve the problem that presents in the particular context. Applying such a *bricolage* to aesthetic nursing, we do not tie ourselves to ascendancy of a particular orientation, whether it be nursing art as appreciation, or nursing art as skill mastery, or nursing art as the therapeutic use of art, or indeed whatever other orientation is advanced. Instead, we draw as necessary from all such orientations to serve our caring purpose in the particular situation. This, then, is the second of our messages. That as our nursing aesthetics unfold for us the meanings to which we must respond, our nursing art response is a skilful and creative *bricolage* formed in response to the unfolding situation.

In leaving the chapter now, these two messages may form the basis for your reflections on what we have discussed. Specifically, they may assist you in forming a vision of what aesthetic knowing and artistic mastery means in nursing. In the final analysis you must make up your own mind. Is the nurse an aesthetic unfolder of the enfolded, and is her response most appropriately established as a skilful *brico-* lage that is shaped by the emerging needs of the situation?

REFERENCES

Benner, P., Tanner, C. and Chesla, C. (1996) *Expertise in Nursing Practice: Caring, clinical judgment, and ethics*, Springer, New York

Benner, P., Hooper-Kyriakidis, P. and Stannard, D. (1999) *Clinical Wisdom and Interventions in Critical Care*, W.B. Saunders, Philadelphia, IL

Bohm, D. (1983) *Wholeness and the Implicate Order*, Ark Paperbacks, New York

Bohm, D. (1987) *Unfolding Meaning: A weekend of dialogue*, Routledge, London

Carper, B. (1978) Fundamental patterns of knowing in nursing, *Advances in Nursing Science* 1(1), 13–23

Carroll, N. (2002) Aesthetic experience revisited. *British Journal of Aesthetics* 42(1), 145–68

Chinn, P. and Kramer, P. (1999) *Theory and Nursing: Integrated knowledge development* (5th edn), Mosby, St Louis, IL

Denzin, N. and Lincoln, Y. (2000) *Handbook of Qualitative Research*, Sage, Thousand Oaks, CA

Frank, A. (1995) *The Wounded Storyteller: Body, illness, and ethics*, University of Chicago Press, Chicago, IL

Greenhalgh, T. and Hurwitz, B. (1998) *Narrative-based Medicine: Dialogue and discourse in clinical practice*, BMJ Books, London

Heidegger, M. (1971) The origin of the work of art. In: Heidegger, M. (ed.) *Poetry, Language, Thought* (trans. A. Hofstadter), Harper and Row, New York

Janaway, C. (1995) Aesthetic attitude. In: Honderich, T. (ed.) *The Oxford Companion to Philosophy*, Oxford University Press, Oxford

Johnson, J. (1994) A dialectical examination of nursing art. *Advances in Nursing Science* 17, 1

Johnson, J. (1996) Dialectical analysis concerning the rational aspect of the art of nursing. *Image: Journal of Nursing Scholarship* 28, 169

Kant, I. (1969) *Critique of Judgement* (trans. J. Meredith), Oxford University Press, Oxford

Morrison, V. (2002) The beauty of the days gone by. In: Morrison, V. *Down the Road*, Exile Publications, London (CD music media)

Scruton, R. (1994) *Modern Philosophy*, Sinclair-Stevenson, London

13 ETHICAL KNOWING: THE MORAL GROUND OF NURSING PRACTICE

Carol Kirby and Oliver Slevin

> *Because work for health is a moral endeavour it must be thoughtful. And because careful thinking matters so much it is not acceptable that healthcare decision-makers hide behind status, codes of practice, ethical biases dressed up as truths, or even the law. Whenever you ask – how does what you are doing create better health? – nothing less than honest, reasoned answers will do.*
>
> (Seedhouse, 1998, p. 4)

LEARNING OUTCOMES

After studying this chapter you will be able to:

- Define and explain the term 'ethics'
- Recognise the difference between moral and non-moral ideas
- Outline major ethical theories and their strengths and weaknesses
- Describe the dimensions or features that characterise ethical theories
- Discuss the basis of our moral thoughts, intentions and actions by reflecting on the nature and possible sources of what we deem morally good or right
- Discuss personal and professional accountability and responsibility for moral decisions
- Explicate care-orientated approaches to ethics, as presented in empowering and compassionate nurse–patient relationships
- Consider an eclectic approach to ethics that draws on the strengths of the various ethical perspectives addressed in the chapter.

INTRODUCTION

This is a book about the theory and practice of nursing. As a student of nursing you have much to learn. There are the biological and life sciences and also the behavioural and social sciences, each with their growing body of empirical research that must underpin evidence-based practice. There is a wide range of technical, communication and relational skills that must be learned if nursing interventions are to be safe and effective. With all this to cope with, it may seem reasonable to question why we should spend scarce time on often complex and difficult discussions of ethics and moral philosophy. Surely, the argument runs, such matters are of little interest to anyone other than those occupying the dusty halls of academe. In the real world, common sense tells us what is right or wrong, and our professional codes of conduct tell us how we should deport ourselves.

However, it is precisely because real life is complex and difficult, and because we so often fail to make the right moral choices, that we need to address such matters. This is particularly the case in respect of health care, where not only is life complex and difficult, but almost every decision has implications for the well-being and perhaps even the survival of the recipients of that care. An error in moral judgement can maim or kill every bit as much as an error in treatment or technique. Ethics, therefore, is an essential aspect of health care. Any decision on our part as nurses to exclude it from our deliberations would be tantamount to an act of professional misconduct.

In Chapter 9 it was noted that ethics is recognised as a branch of philosophy and that it properly falls within the broad area of moral philosophy. This branch of philosophy concerns itself not so much with the existence of knowledge or phenomena (ontology) the form or beauty of phenomena (aesthetics) or the nature, structure and form of such knowledge (epistemology), but the moral values we ascribe to our knowledge or thoughts (ethics). The concerns here are with attributes or intrinsic values such as right versus wrong, good versus bad, beneficence versus maleficence, or virtue versus vice. But ethics differs from other branches of philosophy by its emphasis on action as well as knowledge. It is the study not only of how our *thoughts* are good or right, but also how our *actions* or their *consequences* are good or right. This area of concern, which we might term the moral ground, has a long pedigree. It emerges (at least within western cultures) from ancient Greek concerns about what is moral – what Aristotle referred to as 'the good life', the concern with how we should live. The concern in this chapter is in line with this: it addresses how we should live as nurses. It is, therefore, not simply about a particular pattern or way of knowing, but also about how this guides our moral choices and actions.

This concern is relevant to every nursing act. Being in the world as a nurse is essentially about being in relation. This is most obvious in terms of being in relation with those others we see as our patients or clients. It is they who we see primarily as having a call upon us, as being those to whom and for whom we are responsible. In every nursing act there is some moral dimension, some call to do what is the good or right thing. And this is not only a commitment to the immediate other who is at any moment the individual patient in our care. It extends to that person's family and friends, to their wider community, to society as a whole, even to the wider environment. This extension of concern is not simply a human orientation extending from self to humanity as a whole. It is also multidimensional in its concern for environment, for all the things that co-exist in a world of persons, other living organisms and things (see also the discussion of a global ethic in Chapter 44).

Thus, the International Council of Nurses states, in its Code of Ethics for Nurses (2000), that 'The nurse also shares a responsibility to sustain and protect the natural environment from depletion, pollution, degradation and destruction'.

Study Activity 13.1

Consider the following. This is a fictional case, but in our health services almost identical situations are being confronted every week of the year.

> *A female patient who is 68-years-old is in renal (kidney) failure. If she is provided access to renal haemodialysis (an artificial kidney machine), the patient will survive, at least for the present. If she does not receive the treatment, she will almost certainly die in the near future. The care team (including doctors and nurses, but with the final accountability for treatment decisions resting with the doctors) decide that haemodialysis will not be made available. Within a week the patient dies. The team who made the final decision are confident that they made what they view as the 'right' decision.*

Of course, you do not know the circumstances in full. You have no factual information on how the decision to withhold access to the life-saving intervention was made, other than to know that those who made the final decision feel it was the 'right' choice. And even after the patient has died they hold to this view. Reflect on the circumstances in this example.

- Consider how anyone, in any circumstances, could withhold a treatment that would almost certainly save or prolong a life, and claim that it was a 'good' thing to do, that it was the right or only moral choice.
- Reflect upon how you might feel if such a decision was to be made about your own mother, or your child, or even some day yourself. Bear in mind that there may be other persons, perhaps even another single person, who may be making the decision that affects your survival.
- Write down your reflections, including all possible explanations and justifications you can think of for the choice that was made. Reflect further on

whether you feel any or some of these – in your opinion – might in any circumstances be valid reasons for the choice that was made. Keep your notes, as you will be asked to refer to these in Study Activity 13.2.

It should be clear to you, even on the basis of the latter brief excursion into the nature of decisions in health care settings, that this is a serious and indeed sometimes deadly serious area of concern. It will also be noted that this term 'concern' is much used in these opening comments. This is because ethics is at its heart about concern. It is about caring about people and things, about what happens to them, and about how our actions affect them. It is about accepting a responsibility for the other (person or thing), and a commitment to ensuring that our actions benefit rather than harm them. This is no less important in the caring professions. In his treatise on caring, Van Hooft (1995) speaks of caring in terms of 'caring for' and 'caring about'. This matter of caring has already been addressed in Chapter 2, and is returned to again below, where an ethic of care is discussed. For now, we attend to the notion of 'caring about'. It relates to how we have concern about the people and objects in our environment. It is only when we value these others, when we have a disposition in which we genuinely care *about* them, that we recognise the responsibility to care *for* them. In effect, we are predisposed to do good and do no harm, to act rightly in their interests.

This is essentially what ethics is all about; indeed, this is why ethics is so essential in a profession that professes to do good and avoid harming. However, as will be noted from a close consideration of the above opening quotation from David Seedhouse (1998), ethics is not about formulae that are handed to us, providing prescribed ways of being 'good' or doing the 'right' thing. We can never claim that our actions were justified because we were following rules or orders; this did not work for the Nuremberg war criminals and it will not work for us. In matters of ethical or moral choice, the

responsibility rests with each of us. Ethics challenges us to recognise that we are moral agents, that we are indeed responsible for our own ethical comportment in all we do as persons and as nurses. As Yeo and Ford (1991) state:

> In some ways, life would be easier if we were not moral agents. Nurses might simply adapt themselves to the realities of the workplace and confine their activity to whatever was expected of them or whatever they were told to do. Some nurses do just that. This is not a moral option. Nurses are moral agents in their professional role, and as such are accountable for conducting themselves in accordance with personal and professional values and principles.
>
> (Yeo and Ford, 1991, p. 212)

ETHICS DEFINED

In the introduction it is suggested that ethics is concerned with notions of right versus wrong and good versus bad. However, the terms ethics and ethical are often used in different ways and have different meanings in different contexts.

Ethics as positive values

Here the term ethics is reserved for values or acts that are exclusively good or right. Thus, it is often claimed that 'our professional ethics consist of such-and-such'. These statements are our positive values, which we aspire to as high professional ideals. In this context it is often said in regard to some idea or act that it is or would be ethical (good or right) or, conversely, unethical (bad or wrong). In exactly the same way people speak of some positions or actions as being morally correct and others as being immoral. We return to the terms ethical and moral later. For some, ethics is to do with how we *think* about such issues, while morality relates to our *actions* or way of being in respect of them. That is, the former is about 'theory' or thinking, the latter is about 'action' or doing. However, there is no general agreement about such differentiations, so for the purpose of this chapter we shall use the two terms interchangeably. This is indeed the most common modern practice.

Ethics as rules

Ethics can also be viewed as highly empirical or action-orientated rules of conduct. The values attached to ideas or phenomena are usually socially derived from within a group's culture, and the individual member is expected to learn and abide by these rules. At their most sophisticated level, such systems of rules are illustrated in professional codes of conduct or charters of ethics, as discussed later in this chapter.

Ethics as etiquette

This case is very similar to the definition of ethics as rules. However, the rules here are not exclusively, and sometimes not at all, concerned with moral values. They are essentially rules about what are the correct or appropriate forms of behaviour. As in ethics as rules, the rules of etiquette are socially constructed systems which are part of a group's culture. There are society-wide rules of etiquette. For example, the knife and fork are normally held in the right and left hands, respectively. There is nothing wrong or bad, in the moral sense, about holding the fork in the right hand; it is simply not the 'done thing', not the correct conduct (at least, in British as opposed to American society). Etiquette is, therefore, a rightness or wrongness based on manners, conventions and social preferences. In this sense the serious student of ethics may argue strongly that etiquette has little to do with ethics at all.

Ethics as moral thinking and acting

Here ethics is about moral values that are attached to ideas or acts. It is firstly about thinking, which attaches a value to something. But it also includes anticipatory thinking, i.e. thinking about choices of action, about how we should behave in a situation. The first type of thinking is about what '*is*'; the second type is about what '*ought*'. Ethics is secondly about doing, and it thus has a practical dimension

concerning what we do and why we do it; in this context, the issue is one of motive. In the sense described here, ethics is essentially a study of values and there is no positive or negative inference in the term itself. Here the converse of ethical is not *unethical* or *immoral* (as in the case of ethics as positive values discussed above), but *non-ethical* or *amoral* (i.e. nothing to do with ethics or morals at all). At a simple level the inference is that all thinking and acting can be divided into that which is and that which is not of an ethical nature. The *study* of ethics, therefore, involves establishing exactly what falls within the parameters of moral or ethical thinking and acting, the nature of the ethical or moral thoughts (constructs) that may guide our actions, and the fundamental essences, arguments or foundations upon which these 'constructs' are based (Johnstone, 1994).

It is this latter sense of the word ethics that is the meaning intended in this chapter. That is, we are defining ethics as the study of moral thinking, the values we attach to thoughts or actions; it is also the study of how we determine what we ought to do and what we actually do when we make moral choices.

It will be noted that ethics is not just about how we are right–wrong or what we ought–ought not to do; being right could simply mean being accurate, and doing what we ought to do may be simply to comply with etiquette or social convention. Ethics is about values which are specifically *moral values*. These are values that have a sense of goodness or badness attached to them, where goodness equates with notions such as virtue and praiseworthiness and badness equates with notions such as vice and blameworthiness. To obtain a fuller sense of the specific meanings, we must address ethical theory and the dimensions of morality itself.

ETHICAL THEORY

Theory for action

We consider the notion of 'theory' as a topic in its own right in Chapter 14. However, for the purposes of the current chapter we view a 'theory' as something that not only describes or explains an aspect of our world (or our conscious understanding of it), but also provides a framework for action. That is, theory guides our practice. In an early but influential publication, Dickoff and James (1968) described such theory as 'situation-producing theory', and in an equally influential publication Argyris and Schön (1974) spoke of 'theories-of-action' and 'theories-in-use'. Of course, the theory of action we are concerned with here is specifically ethical, as opposed to being concerned with other aspects of our practice. Such theory is the basis for making sense of our moral positions and, importantly, it provides us with a framework upon which to base our ethical decisions. It is vitally important that this is recognised. It is never the case that a person acts without some theory or guiding framework. This is the case even when we are not *aware* of having a theory at all! There is always some framework, or theory, or worldview, or set of beliefs and values, that guides our actions. Irrespective of our level of awareness of these, we live by them implicitly or explicitly. However, as suggested above, in health care our decisions and actions can have the most profound impact upon others. It is, therefore, essential that we develop *effective* theoretical frameworks that assist us in making the *best possible* moral choices.

There are many ethical theories that purport to explain moral matters and offer guidance on how we should live morally, and there is insufficient space here to deal with all of them. However, the majority of these fall within two broad perspectives. These different ways of viewing how thoughts and actions possess ethical values are referred to in terms of teleology (more commonly referred to nowadays as consequentialism) and deontology. They present more or less opposing viewpoints on ethics, as indicated below.

Teleology: ethics as consequences

The teleological viewpoint is essentially what is known as an 'outcomes' theory of ethics. It involves deciding on whether something is right or wrong, good or bad, on the basis of its consequences. Indeed, *consequentialism* is the more modern term in ethical theory today, although the term teleology is still sometimes used. This involves considering the consequences of some act in terms of whether on balance it is better to do one thing than another in terms of the outcomes the action will produce. This is the only and overriding principle in all consequentialist theory, unlike deontological theory (discussed below) which is essentially based upon duties and principles, such that it is often contrasted to consequentialism by virtue of its reliance on principles. Consequentialism is sometimes divided into two forms.

Teleological egoism

Here the judgement is made on the basis of whether the act in question will on the whole produce the greatest good for the individual. This involves deciding if doing one thing will, on balance, be better for the person in the long run than if they do another. What is being said here is that an action is good or bad, right or wrong for the individual him/herself on the basis of actual or anticipated outcomes. It is the result or consequence of any act *for the individual* which determines if it is good or bad, right or wrong to perform that act. This does not necessarily mean that the egoist ignores the well-being of others. Such egoists will most commonly desist from theft, assault, murder, etc. However, they are motivated primarily by an awareness of the negative or punitive consequences for themselves if they perpetrate such acts. In a similar vein, a nurse may carry out her duties assiduously and to an acceptable standard, but her motivation may be to stay out of trouble, or to avoid losing her job, rather than a concern for the well-being of those in her charge.

Teleological universalism or utilitarianism

Here the same type of judgement is being made. That is, the important principle is again whether one action will produce greater good than another. However, here the decision is made on the basis of whether the act will produce *the greater general good*. The motto of utilitarianism is 'the greatest good for the greatest number of people'. The notion, first explicated by eighteenth- and nineteenth-century philosophers such as David Hume, Jeremy Bentham and John Stewart Mill, is a society-orientated rather than an individual-orientated ethic, and is an important underlying principle in a society's legal system. Within this perspective, choices are made on the basis of the utility or benefits for the group, community or society as a whole. According to this viewpoint, teleological egoism (as discussed above) would not be an ethical theory at all, but an example of selfishness. For this reason, many people see utilitarianism as the only valid consequentialist theory, the terms consequentialist and utilitarian thus being more or less synonymous in their eyes.

It is, of course, possible to have variations along a continuum that relates to the beneficiaries of the outcomes from such moral choices. Thus, between teleological egoism and teleological universalism may range different levels extending from self through chosen groups to everyone except the self (the ultimate sacrifice of putting all before the self) to the universal level where all (the total society, including oneself) are taken into consideration. Such a continuum may be as illustrated in Fig. 13.1.

Deontology: ethics as duty irrespective of consequences

The deontological viewpoint is one that explicitly excludes the notion of consequences from ethical decisions. It takes the view that an act is intrinsically good or bad, right or wrong irrespective of its outcomes or consequences. That is, when we consider a phenomenon or situation, we should by intuition be able to discern the rightness or wrongness of how we should respond or act in the situation. This evaluation is the act of making a decision on the basis of *a priori* knowledge (i.e. where we either can see intuitively, or reasonably deduce without the need for any empirical confirmation, what the decision must be). Some ethicists (philosophers who specialise in ethics) also speak of this as being a *prima facie* case (that is, one that appears *on the face of it* to only have one clear choice at

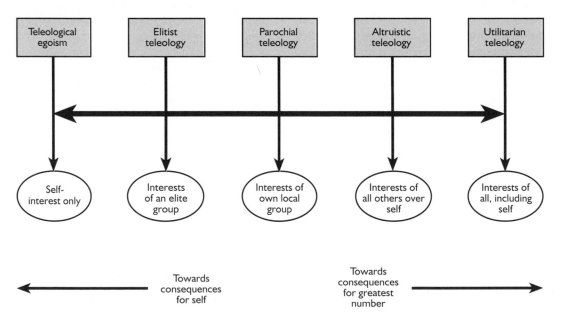

Figure 13.1 The consequentialist continuum

the time). Therefore, we do not determine if an act is right or good by drawing upon present or past empirical experience – which would be termed *a posteriori* knowledge. We just intrinsically know or reason that it is the right thing to do before the act, or *a priori*. In essence, it is good or right in and of itself (and its converse is bad or wrong in and of itself). We might feel that it is our duty to save the life of another, irrespective of whether they are felt to be deserving (indeed, the term deontology derives from the ancient Greek as duty-science: the science or knowledge of duty). This is usually established as a *principle* – a fundamental truth or assumption that we should always hold to. Deontological ethics are by definition ethics of duty and principle and, as they relate to that which is intrinsically good, they are also often seen as encompassing virtue ethics (i.e. an ethics of good or virtue versus evil or vice). However, deontological decisions can also be identified as being of two different forms.

Act-deontology

This is a situation-specific deontological theory. Here, while it is accepted that a decision can be reached on the basis of intuitive or *a priori* knowledge, it is argued that this relates to the specific situation. The act-deontologist says, 'I know intuitively that this is the right choice in these particular circumstances, but it may not be correct in a different situation'. The decision is still, however, based on intuitive or *a priori* values of rightness or goodness, not on any consideration of consequences. Today this is often described as *situation ethics*, and it is the view of ethics which would be shared by many existentialists (see Chapter 9).

Rule-deontology

Here ethical decisions are not dependent on consequences, as suggested by teleological theorists and cannot be situation specific, as suggested by act-deontological theorists. Rather, the submission of rule-deontologists is that universal rules apply on the basis of the *universal* intrinsic value or goodness of an act. The rule-deontologist says, 'It is *always* by definition right to do this thing, in any like situation, irrespective of the consequences'. This is the interpretation of ethics promoted by Immanuel Kant, who was probably the greatest of all moral philosophers, and whose work we return to below. It is the underlying principle adopted by most people who claim to be guided by conscience.

Unlike consequentialism, deontology is not only more difficult to explain in rational terms, but in its purist form it is uncompromising in its rejection of an ethic of consequences. These two characteristics have made it the subject of much criticism, particularly within that tradition that largely emerges from the logical-positivist movements, i.e. science and analytic-rationalist forms of philosophy. Furthermore, the two main forms of deontological ethics are uncompromising in respect of each other. Indeed, as demonstrated in Table 13.1, the characteristics of act-deontology and rule-deontology are by definition opposites, sharing only the rejection of consequences as a basis for ethical decisions.

Table 13.1 The deontological divide

Act-deontology	Rule-deontology
Particularistic	Generalised
Situational	Universal
Plastic/flexible	Immutable/binding
Relativistic	Deterministic
Personal choices	Universal principles

Study Activity 13.2

A doctor determines to prescribe a rare and expensive medicine for his elderly patient. He explains that his decision is made exclusively for the good of his patient, and that the benefit of this medicine is clearly superior to an alternative therapy that, although cheaper, is less effective and has more side-effects.

The Chief Executive of a Health Services Trust advises his Trust Board to limit access to major open heart surgery to patients who meet certain stringent criteria (which involves excluding heavy smokers, people with certain levels of learning disability, and people over a certain age). He advises that by doing so, the Trust will be able to free up resources to treat many more people who need hip replacement operations.

- Determine which of the two main ethical theories just discussed (or their two subsets in each case) best describes each position, explaining your reasons.
- Re-read your reflective notes on Study Activity 13.1. Which of the above ethical theory positions might best describe the choice made in the circumstances described in that Study Activity?
- In Study Activity 13.1 you also recorded your feelings about such choices being made. Do you feel this indicated where you might have stood then on the utilitarian versus deontological dimension (even though you may not have used those terms)? Finally, do you think this brief overview of ethical theory has so far altered how you might perceive such situations?

Prescriptivism

It was acknowledged earlier that there are other ethical theories but that in general the majority of these are also based upon consequences (or outcomes) or conversely upon rules (or principles) irrespective of outcomes. One notable exception is the theory of prescriptivism, a more recent ethical theory postulated by the philosopher R.M. Hare (1993, 1997). Hare argued that it is inadequate to simply be *descriptivist* (i.e. identify objectively through careful analysis what is on balance the basis for the good or right choice). In the final analysis, an ethical statement must give some guide (or prescription) in respect of ethical action. It is equally inadequate to be non-descriptive (i.e. expect, as do most deontologists, that the right or good choice is subjectively, intuitively or emotively obvious). It is, of course, important that we do attempt to reason or critically determine what is the best choice in terms of objective consequences or considerations. That is, we must have a universal *prescription* for so determining our actions – one that can be applied in any like situation.

However, simply adhering to a prescribed method based exclusively on a critical consideration of consequences may in some instances lead to questionable moral choices. In short, the method of critical reasoning is not enough. For example, it may be determined that the greatest good for the greater number can be achieved by overcoming an opposing political group (situations which occurred in countries such as South Africa and Chile in the recent past). A radical consequentialist position would claim that *any* means of achieving this end are justified for the greater good of society. However, if we reflect upon deontological concerns about what is fundamentally good or right, we are informed by such views. In this example, *some* means, such as torture, may be adjudged to be breaches of human conduct that are unacceptable in any circumstances. In one sense, Hare's theory is a bringing together of the consequentialist and deontological viewpoints, one informing the other in our final ethical choices. We shall return to this notion of complementary use of these two main and apparently opposing perspectives later.

Study Activity 13.3 _____

Clearly, Hare does not feel that it is necessary to settle for either a consequentialist or a deontological position, and that indeed we can bring both together in the real world of ethical decision-making. Indeed, some have viewed his approach as a consequentialist or utilitarian theory that is moderated by checks that are essentially deontological principles of duty. However, the distinguished social scientist Max Weber (1991) presented two opposing views of ethics, which he saw as polarised and incompatible. One of these – the ethics of responsibility – is simply another term for utilitarianism. This involves taking account of circumstances within situations and the ultimate consequences of our actions, which become the guiding influence in our decisions. The other – the ethics of conviction – is simply another term for deontological ethics. This excludes taking account of circumstances or allowing consequences to determine or modify our behaviour. If it is wrong to kill, no justification – even the possibility of saving more lives in the longer term – is acceptable. What is different in Weber's thesis is that he felt that an ethics of responsibility was the only practical alternative in the real modern world. He identified the ethics of responsibility as being the characteristic position of the politician, and the ethics of conviction as being the characteristic position of the saint. In effect, in their extreme forms, the two positions and those who occupy them are irreconcilable. Because his thesis seems to intimate that an ethics of conviction has no place in the real world of politics and modern society, Weber's position has been viewed with some hostility by religious groups and theologians.

- Having considered the two main ethical theories (consequentialism and deontology), do you agree with Hare or Weber? That is, do you feel the two very different theories *can* be brought together to inform our moral choices?
- Review Study Activity 13.1 again, in particular your own responses. If we determine that because of scarce resources we will withhold treatment from someone who needs it (who may indeed possibly die without it), is there any way that we can truly claim we are also taking account of a fundamental deontological principle that requires us to do no harm?

Ethical relativism

One final ethical theory of importance in a sense transcends the issues of ethics based on outcomes *and* ethics as a duty or end in itself. A significant criticism often made in respect of the former ethical theories and all variations of them, is that they are in a sense ethnocentric (Wong, 1993). That is, they are based on what is to be valued in a particular culture (in this case, Western culture). Therefore, it is assumed that the principles derived from such ethics are either universal or absolute. They are claimed to be valid in any place and at any time. However, largely through anthropological studies we know this to be a weak position, and the reality is that there is diversity in moral norms across places

and time. Two examples, commonly presented in ethics texts, demonstrate this.

- Within our Western culture it is commonly held as a universal principle (certainly within the deontological perspective) that we should not kill. In a particular Inuit culture, it was the practice to kill people before they advanced into old age. To us, this seems horrific. Yet, within the native culture, the belief was held that we carry the body we die with into the hereafter. To them, it was equally horrific to allow an old person to deteriorate and thus in the hereafter be imprisoned in a frail body.
- The ancient Greek Darius asked fellow Greeks how much money they would accept to eat their deceased fathers rather than (as was the custom) cremating them. He received the universal response that no money would induce them to such an act. He then asked certain Indians whose custom it was to eat their deceased fathers, how much would induce *them* to burn their dead fathers. The universal response was one of horror and a plea to not even mention such a horrible thought.

Such examples indicate how moral values can vary across cultures. But even in our own culture, things that were once viewed as immoral or sinful, such as suicide or homosexuality, are now often (although not universally) held to be acceptable. The position in this perspective is, at a simple level, that morality is relative to or contingent upon other factors. Usually, this is taken as being relative to the culture that is dominant at that time and in that place. Putting it another way, morality, or what is adjudged as being 'good' or 'right', is influenced by the context.

The natural extension of this line of thinking, and indeed a major criticism of extreme relativist moral theory, is that as there can be no universally accepted morality, no moral position carries an absolute imperative. On this basis, we can – or so such a line of thinking would argue – make up our own morality, or even discard moral concerns altogether. This is the view much aligned with some versions of existential ethics.

The existential perspective is no doubt illuminating. It draws attention to the extent to which we must indeed be sceptical of formulae that purport to solve our ethical dilemmas. If such formulae are unsound foundations (and this is the important contribution that relativism also makes), we are indeed thrown back on our own resources. It is important that we as nurses also recognise this. In the final analysis, *our* moral decision is the one *we* make, and it is this which we must live with. Furthermore, in the complex field of health care, we will be constantly confronted with new and different ethical dilemmas so that we too, every moment, have to construct a response. Against this, no health care system can survive in an anarchic state in which there is not at least some degree of common ground in respect of how we make ethical choices.

Another extension of the relativist perspective is that approach which we refer to under act-deontology above as situation ethics. In this case the argument also runs that in making our moral choices we must base our decisions on the circumstances as they present in the particular context. On this basis, the following premises may hold:

- In one situation, we may support a choice for abortion, while in another we may withhold our support, because the particular circumstances differ.
- In one situation, we may support abortion, while a colleague may withhold such support, and we can adjudge neither to be wrong as such. If we accept that there is no absolute principle or set of rules that we must follow, each has a right to choose.

Here also, the prospect of a world in which there are no general moral principles or rules presents major difficulties. In attempting to overcome these fundamental problems, those who subscribe to relativist ethics tend to present two main practical resolutions. This is sometimes referred to as the *soft relativism* perspective.

The first of these resolutions is to attempt to identify some foundational universal principle or law that would inform decisions while allowing for consideration of contextual matters. This is the position taken by Christian approaches to situation ethics. This is most notably argued in the famous contribution by Joseph Fletcher (1966), who in fact coined the term situation ethics. In this case, the underlying foundational principle is love, as intended in the biblical Christian commandment known as the *Golden Rule*, i.e. to love your neighbour as yourself. Within this Christian formulation of situation ethics, the argument runs that if we have love, or concern, or compassion, or care for others, we would not knowingly do them harm. With this underlying good will, and the commitment to having a concern for the other in *their* situation and faced with *their* problems, we are therefore in a position to determine the best ethical choices. With a caring concern for the other, we enter the situation, we do take account of maxims or principles that may assist us, but our decision finally depends on what is relevant and right in the particular situation. This perspective has much in common with the idea of ethics as caring in relation, which we discuss later.

The second resolution is similar in its recognition of the need for some core principles to which we should adhere. There is a recognition here of a respect for the positions of others and the need to relate moral positions to their cultural norms. But this does not mean that where we have strong moral convictions that we feel are universal, we should not attempt to convince others of this position. This is particularly important in the modern world, where global boundaries become blurred and where what affects one society also impacts on others, particularly as these societies become more multicultural. Of course, moving forward in this way involves going beyond recognising the moral positions of others to a dialogue that not only promotes understanding but also may lead to consensual resolution of ethical dilemmas. This also has much in common with a perspective we address later, that of communicative ethics.

Study Activity 13.4 ———

Female circumcision is a part of the culture of many mainly Moslem societies throughout the world. It involves various degrees of excision of the female clitoris and vulva and then the occlusion of the opening by use of sutures (ranging from threads to acacia thorns) and pastes (ranging from beaten egg to animal excreta). The purpose is to reduce the vaginal opening to a tiny aperture at a very young age so that men can be sure that their brides are virgins. Of course, this necessitates a re-opening at the time of marriage, and this is sometimes accomplished by the husband, using a dagger and maintaining frequent and painful intercourse for several days to ensure the wound does not heal over again. In some of these cases there is no use of anaesthesia and as a consequence physical restraint and binding of the limbs is essential. In these 'societies', female circumcision is a vital part of the culture, and nowadays female circumcision and re-opening are often performed under safe surgical conditions by competent medical and nursing staff. However, in our Western culture most people view it as totally unacceptable. The alternative title female genital mutilation is used, and it is viewed as a form of child abuse. To those social groups who practise female circumcision, this may be viewed as offensive and intrusive.

It may be assumed that this procedure only occurs in far-off African and Asian countries. However, in multicultural Britain, there is evidence that female circumcision is in some cases practised here, or in other cases the young girls are sent 'home' to Somalia or other countries to have it performed. The incidence is hard to indicate precisely, because of the closed nature of the ethnic groups and the secrecy that prevails (see Dorkeno, 1994).

- In the course of your community experience within a Moslem community, you may encounter parents who are contemplating having their daughter circumcised. Using the above ideas on relativist and situation ethics, reflect on how you might react to this information.
- What advice would you contemplate giving these parents?

- Assuming they indicate that they are going to proceed, what ethical decision and subsequent action do you think you would take? Explain the ethical theory or theories that would have informed your decision.

THE MORAL DIMENSION

Ethical and non-ethical values

It was suggested earlier that ethics is about thinking and doing in regard to values that have a specifically moral sense. In general, values may be expressed in terms such as good or bad (some prefer the terms good and evil), virtue or vice, right or wrong, etc. However, as noted earlier, not all values are ethical values. For example, we may say that an apple is good, or it is wrong to insert a capital letter after a semicolon. However, these are not normally taken to be ethical 'goods' or 'rights'. They are values, of course, but they are in essence *non-ethical* values. This begs a question, therefore, as to what are and what are not ethical values. In general, values are ethical if they have attached to them a moral dimension.

It should by now be apparent that ethical evaluations are of a special form. They are evaluations that have a moral dimension and centre around the notion of what is good. What is good is by definition morally right. And, similarly, what is right is by definition morally good. Thus, we have repeatedly referred, in this chapter, to ethics in terms of good versus bad and right versus wrong. Ethicists or moral philosophers do not always agree on this line of argument. For example, they often argue that 'right' (or rights) are to do with issues of equity or justice, while good is to do with issues such as compassion and love. They may even argue that there are instances wherein what is the good thing to do and what is the right thing to do can be different. To ease our way through these difficult concepts, we hold to the position that, if not synonymous, the two notions are at least inextricably related.

However, it may not be enough to explain such evaluations in terms of tautologies – that good is good, or right is right, or good is something right, or right is something good. Nor is it sufficient to assume the consequences we aim for are by definition good without justifying or demonstrating *how* they are good, and *for whom* they are good. It is important to establish the foundations upon which ideas, people or actions are established as having goodness or rightness. One way of establishing this is to consider the moral thinking that informs these ethical theories.

The moral basis of teleological or consequentialist theory

As will be recalled, most teleological theory is based on the principle of utilitarianism. In what is often taken as the definitive explanation of utilitarianism, Mill (1969) described the right choice as any course of action that *as a consequence* leads to the greatest happiness for the greatest number of people. This idea is known as the *Greatest Happiness Principle.* In simple terms, a thing is morally right or good to the extent that it produces happiness and avoids sadness, distress or pain. Unlike earlier utilitarians, Mill did not view happiness as simply hedonistic pleasure. He viewed it as a condition of well-being under which humans could flourish. That is, a situation of happy or optimal circumstances necessary for a good life, as opposed to happiness as a human emotion of pleasure. In this, Mill was following the ethics of the ancient Greek master Aristotle, who spoke of *eudemonia,* a term describing the good life as being a flourishing, meaningful, rewarding life.

The problem with such approaches is that of determining what *will* produce happiness for the greatest number and who, in effect, is to make the judgement. When individuals in society have the power to determine this, there is always the risk that those who speak for society (political leaders, totalitarian governments, etc.) will decide on egoistic or self-interested principles. Of importance here is the notion of *altruism,* i.e. a concern for the well-being of others, which is

sometimes put forward as an essential element in utilitarianism. The argument here is that actions are carried forward not for egoistic reasons, but because they lead to good (happiness or well-being) for others – the good, in fact, of the greatest number of others. This is perhaps the weakest element in the utilitarian thesis. The assumption that people will be prepared to relinquish their good or the good of those close to them for the good of others (particularly when this may not even be a certain outcome) may represent a naive understanding of human nature. For this reason, Mackie (1977) described utilitarianism as 'the ethics of fantasy'.

The argument is also one of egalitarianism or democracy, because there is an assumption here that what is good is that which is good for the majority. We usually think of the majority as being the greatest number of people, but it may in fact be the group with the most power. If the ultimate aim is the greatest utility, it is implicit that the best educated, most healthy and by definition most prosperous offer the greatest likelihood of maximum utility. This would, of course, fly in the face of principles of fair and just distribution that are part of egalitarian democracy.

Another problem with utilitarianism is the situation in regard to the minority. The greatest good for the greatest number may sound a laudable principle, unless you happen to be a Jew in Nazi Germany or a black person in a white-dominated society. It is obvious that if an act is done because it benefits *most* people, this means that it *may not* benefit all or some of the minority. There is one further consideration here, which may have worrying, if not indeed sinister, consequences. If 'the good', or happiness, or flourishing is the ultimate ethical or moral goal, what about those who may not be able to flourish? If we accept that people with severe disability or the very old cannot flourish, then do they become part of a minority for whom there is no moral obligation? Taken to its extreme, might an argument run that such people may be discarded in some way, for the greater good of the remainder? Indeed, in some times and places, such positions have indeed led to extreme solutions, such as the extermination of people with learning disabilities in Nazi Germany, or the incarceration of such people in other societies.

This may seem an extreme area to be delving into, with little other than historical interest today. However, in our modern health services, decisions are already made on similar premises. One example of this is the notion of quality-adjusted life years (QALYs). Proponents of the QALYs approach (e.g. Weinstein and Stason, 1977; Williams, 1985, 1997; Euroqol Group, 1990) argue that it is possible to apply weightings to certain health-related aspects such as mobility, capacity for self-care, level of pain, degree of anxiety or depression, etc. (Williams, 1995). On the basis of this, the benefits of giving someone added years (quantity) of healthy life (quality) through health interventions can be calculated and balanced against the costs to others who by definition forfeit these scarce resources. In such a system, if it is 'calculated' that QALY benefits which outweigh costs cannot be attained, then the health care may be withheld and redistributed to others with better QALY expectancy.

Those who have been critical of such economics-driven decision-making (e.g. Chadwick, 1993; Elhauge, 1994; Seedhouse, 1998) have not always presented convincing alternatives about how scarce resources are to be allocated. Nevertheless, they are right to be concerned about how those who will be assisted to flourish are identified. Indeed, in a recent critique, Heller (2002) points to the lack of reproducibility of measures and other inconsistencies across QALY studies. He suggests that this may be attributable to underlying assumptions about meanings assigned to quality of life, and the moral values that may be imposed by those determining the measures to be applied. In this context some critics have raised questions about equity, e.g. in respect of wealth and gender (Hanson, 1999). For example, if the costs to informal carers of older people (usually female relatives) are not included, such approaches may already have built-in inequities.

All this highlights the difficulty in determining the greatest happiness conditions to be applied. In the cold hard light of day, the happiness, well-being, or even survival of some trumps that of others; someone always has to be the loser. The health economists argue that the scarcity of health care resources is a constant, and must be confronted. Their critics claim that in a world of plenty, if our priorities are based on different values, we can aspire to helping all.

Study Activity 13.5

At the end of the Second World War many Americans claimed that the dropping of atomic bombs on Japanese cities was justified. Although a large number of civilians were killed or injured, it was claimed that many more lives were saved in the longer term by bringing about the early end to the war.

● Was the killing and injury of thousands of civilians justified because it led to the possible saving of many more lives in the longer term? Make your decision and write down your answer and its justification before you read on.

The moral basis of deontological theory

In answering the above Study Activity you may have subscribed to the teleological 'greatest good for greatest number' viewpoint. That is, you may have supported the bombing on the Greatest Happiness Principle. Alternatively, you may feel that it is never right to kill people irrespective of what good could come out of it. As indicated earlier, this is the deontological view, the view that some acts are in themselves good or bad, right or wrong; they have a special type of goodness (or lack of it) attached to them. They are on the face of it irrefutably good or right. Using the terminology we introduced earlier, the claims are recognised on *a priori* grounds, as reasonable and rational in their own right without needing empirical justification. We may use terms such as rectitude, rightness, virtue, or purity to describe this goodness, but all such terms are simply synonyms for goodness. In the final analysis we cannot fully describe 'good'. If we take this deontological view, we often claim to 'know' it intuitively.

The notion of ethical values as something we recognise intuitively gave rise to a particular perspective in ethical theory known as *intuitionism*. Intuitionists claim that all ethical values are known intuitively. However, the most well-known proponent, G.E. Moore (1903) argued that *good* is the fundamental ethical value which we intuitively know and other ethical values can be explained in relation to this. Thus, if an act is right it is good, and if it is wrong it is by definition bad in the moral sense. However, that which we term *good*, the fundamental ethical essence, cannot itself be observed, described and analysed in the same way as can other phenomena using scientific or naturalistic observational methodologies. Good was defined by Moore as the fundamental essence underlying other qualities such as right, honesty and duty, but not in itself visible as are these manifestations of itself. Thus, to attempt to observe, measure or describe good (in the way we scientifically seek, describe and explain knowledge of our physical or natural world), is a fallacious premise. Moore defined such attempts as '*the naturalistic fallacy*' (the fallacy of assuming that we can treat 'the good' as some empirical, observable or even measurable part of the natural world).

The intuitionist movement in philosophy is no longer a significant force. However, their notion, that of intuitively knowing what is good and what is bad or evil, still stands as an important idea for explicating the deontological viewpoint of which it is part. In more recent times, Iris Murdoch (1970) and Raimond Gaita (1991) have presented influential studies recognising the importance of goodness. They argue that, while it is difficult to isolate and describe other than through acts or characteristics emanating from it, it is nevertheless recognisable as a fundamental moral source. Indeed, one of the most influential ethicists of modern times, Alisdair

MacIntyre (1985), is credited with returning attention to the idea that ethics can be approached from the point of view of traits or characteristics which are accepted as 'good', such as benevolence, love, caring, concern, courage, etc. Those who are possessed of or embrace such virtues have the capacity for living moral lives.

The problem, however, is to convince the cynic or the empirical scientist that intuition is a valid way of knowing anything, including ethical truths. This situation led some of those of a deontological persuasion to look elsewhere for an insight into how we arrive at our moral values. It was the philosopher A. J. Ayer (1936) who suggested that moral judgements emanate from the *feelings* of the individual. Thus, when a person adjudges that child sex abuse is bad, this value judgement arises from *feelings* of disgust or disapproval. The argument originally put forward by Ayer and others who subscribe to this perspective, known as *emotivism*, is therefore that moral action arises not so much from intuitive thought as from our feelings about phenomena. This is the philosophical equivalent of the 'gut-reaction' that people explain as the basis of their evaluations in everyday life.

The problem with the intuitionist and emotivist stances is that they both, to a greater or lesser extent, depend upon acts of faith. That is, there is no way in which a logical and rational argument can be made to support these positions. Intuition is by definition a tacit dimension, neither arrived at through analytical deliberation nor explainable in such terms. Similarly, the project of explaining our emotional positions in response to some phenomena is beyond such logical defences. This is a bit like the old adage: 'I can't explain what I like, but I know it when I see it'. For even the most hardened professional criminals, given to armed robbery and extortion, there is a common bond that states there are certain things they will not do and certain things they will not stand for. Thus, within our criminal justice system, a whole system of regulations and prison isolation facilities are needed to protect the child molester and the rapist from the professional criminals within the prison population. Were these professional criminals to be asked to explain their positions, they would be amazed at their attitudes even being questioned. There is, it would seem, no explanation: what is good, right, virtuous or acceptable is self-evident. And so too are their converse.

Study Activity 13.6 _____

Read the following excerpt, drawn from the account by Gaita (1991), presenting a diary entry written by a Jewish man during the Nazi occupation. Have a pen and pad ready before you begin.

> A rabbi in Lodz was forced to spit on a Torah scroll that was in the Holy Ark. In fear of his life he complied and desecrated that which is holy to him and his people. After a short time he had no more saliva, his mouth was dry. To the Nazi's question, why did he stop spitting, the rabbi replied that his mouth was dry. Then the son of the 'superior race' began to spit into the rabbi's mouth and the rabbi continued to spit on the Torah.

- Immediately, and without taking time to reflect, write down your *feelings* about the passage. Work quickly, as if you were brainstorming – single words or phrases will do. Spend no more than 1 minute on this.
- Now, reflecting on the words and phrases you wrote down, consider whether you feel this account was of a particularly bad or evil act by a bad or evil man.
- You may by now come to a decision (although perhaps you have not), on the basis of a fairly immediate reaction. Is it best explained as an intuitive or emotional reaction, or can you explain it differently? Is this a moral or ethical decision you have arrived at?
- Having considered this example, what is your view about the existence of something in the world that we might call good, and its converse that we might call bad or evil?
- In the era of this example, a number of German nurses actively killed many hundreds of adults and

children with (alleged) learning disabilities by poisoning and lethal injection (as witnessed in the trials of nurses such as Margarete Ratajczak and Luise Erdmann). Do you think that there could be people working in health care who reflect such evil, or is it impossible for nurses to be like this today?

Morality based upon the rational application of a good will

For those who view a deontological ethic based upon intuitionism or emotivism as irrational, the German philosopher Kant offers a more acceptable alternative, a deontology which is based upon rational thought. When Kant (1938) spoke of the fundamental principles of ethics he was proposing a predominantly rule-deontology perspective. His premise was that if a particular choice (e.g. that it is wrong to kill another human being) is truly right in one situation, it is right in all situations and it is right that each and every person should make this same choice in those situations. It is in fact a matter of principle or a general rule that this is so. It would be irrational, so the argument runs, that such a rule applies for one or some situations but not for others. In line with Kant's thinking, the principles of ethics therefore operate according to the following rational formula: if it is right for you to act in a particular way towards someone in a particular set of circumstances, then you must accept that it is right that in similar circumstances they should act towards you in a similar way.

Study Activity 13.7 _____

As an example of this principle, refer back to Study Activity 13.5 on how some Americans justified the atomic bombing of Japanese cities on the moral grounds that this shortened the war and saved more lives. In line with Kant's thinking, if you accept this as morally right, then you may also have to accept that it would have been morally right for Germany and Japan to drop atomic bombs on London and New York, for exactly the same reasons, i.e. to shorten the war and save more lives in the long term.

- Reflect upon this proposition. Do you feel it is acceptable that a principle can apply in some situations and not in others, or for some people but not others?
- If so, is it (in the form it takes) a principle at all? You might find it useful here to explore what the term 'principle' actually means.

It is possible to identify a number of principles and propose these as the basis of dispositions to act that are intrinsically virtuous, i.e. good or right, in all circumstances. Such examples may be respect for life, duty, love, justice, honesty, etc. However, often we may adhere to such principles because of social injunctions to do so, or because of some advantage doing so may bring to us. In the Kantian view, we adhere to such principles because it is good or right to do so, rather than because of such injunctions or rewards. Kant (1938) suggested that what made anything fundamentally good or right was the existence of a *good will*, and he stated that:

> It is impossible to conceive of anything anywhere in the world or even anywhere out of it that can without qualification be called good, except a Good Will ... The good will is good not because of what it causes or accomplishes, not because of its usefulness in the attainment of some set purpose, but alone because of the willing, that is to say, of itself. Considered by itself, without any comparison, it is to be valued far more highly than all that might be accomplished through it in favour of some inclination or the sum of all inclinations. Even though by some special disfavour of fortune ... if with the greatest of efforts nothing were to be accomplished by it, and nothing were to remain except only the good will (not, to be sure, as a pious wish

> but as an exertion of every means in our power), it would still sparkle like a jewel by itself, like something that has its full value in itself. Its usefulness or fruitfulness can neither add nor detract from its worth.
>
> (Kant, 1938, pp. 9–10)

In illustrating this, Kant used the example of duty. He suggested that we might do a number of things because we are inclined for various reasons to do so. Such inclinations may be brought about by the anticipation of reward or the threat of sanctions. But in these situations there is no moral sense of duty. A person performs these acts because of some external forces acting upon him. However, if a person takes on a *duty* when there is no inclination or pressure upon him to do so, if he does it because he wishes to do it, because he feels morally bound to do it and can do no other, then it is a truly moral choice. Nothing impels this person other than his good will. The notion here is not dissimilar to the principle of 'good' explicated by Moore (1903), as discussed earlier. Indeed, the latter's work, as was the case for most moral philosophers in the last 200 years, was influenced to a greater or lesser extent by Kant's seminal work in this field. Implicit in this view is the notion that a good will is within a person or that any capable person can act from a good will. But is it within every person to so act? Did Hitler or the murderer Charles Manson have a good will? These are questions we will return to presently.

Kant's work also suggests that a number of fundamental ethical principles have universal application, and can function as ethical rules. In Kantian terms, each area of principle if acted on by a 'good will' is implicitly a good or right decision. This is tantamount to saying that if you act with a good will, you always make a particular decision or behave in a way which is morally right, irrespective of the consequences. You do this or that because, in acting with a good will, you cannot and would not wish to do other than this and, furthermore, you accept that this is also a universal maxim.

This universal position in regard to moral actions is what Kant described as the *categorical imperative*. The categorical imperative produces statements that are taken to be universally self-evident and correct. The following would be an example of such an imperative: always explain the treatment to your patient.

The opposite of this is the *hypothetical imperative*, which is always stated in consequential terms. The above example, restated as a hypothetical imperative, might therefore read: explain the treatment to your patient, if you want to ensure his co-operation.

The first statement says, simply, to always explain to the patient because it is universally right and your duty to do so. The second statement says to do it because of the anticipated consequences. The hypothetical imperative, unlike the categorical imperative, is not a universal law. According to its logic, you would not explain to the patient at all if his co-operation was unnecessary and if you did not want a causal relation between *explanation* and *co-operation* to operate. Here, explaining to the patient is not deemed *universally* right, you are only doing it in *certain* circumstances because you have to. This would, of course, negate the deontological nature of Kant's rational ethics and convert it to a consequentialist or teleological ethic.

A major problem in Kant's approach lies in the apparent rational basis of his arguments. It would seem that here is a dispassionate, almost mathematical or mechanical, formula for moral choices. For example, if a person using their good will genuinely believed as a universal principle that killing for pleasure was acceptable, and if they genuinely felt that all should apply this principle, then they would appear to be applying the categorical imperative and thus living ethically. By this line of rational thinking, an argument that Manson and Hitler were making good or right ethical choices could be sustained. However, Kant did have one additional element in his categorical imperative. He did recognise *one* end, that is that humanity as represented by the individual and by all people must never be a means to an end, but an end in themselves. Thus, the sacredness of the person excludes from Kant's rational ethics any choices that would treat people as mere means to ends, to be manipulated or harmed for some other advantage to be procured (such as Manson's pleasure derived from killing or Hitler's mass extermination solutions to what he viewed as threats to purity of race).

Study Activity 13.8

Read the following two statements:

Statement A. We (nurses) put the elderly patients in our ward to bed at 5.30 p.m. each afternoon. It is necessary to do this to ensure that they are all comfortable, clean, and 'tucked in' for a good night's sleep. If we did not do this, with our current staffing levels, many of the patients would not be settled down properly for the night and the nurses would not be able to get their work schedules completed and have a well-earned coffee break. It has been suggested that some of the patients might like to stay up later each evening. However, under the circumstances this would just not be feasible and would play utter havoc with the ward schedule. We have to think of the majority, and the nurses need their time to unwind too.

Statement B. We (nurses) feel it is wrong to be putting elderly patients to bed at 5 or 5.30 p.m. each day. Most of them just lie there awake for hours. It is a fundamental right of any person to make a decision about when to go to bed at night! If we were patients, would we like to be herded off to bed so early? Letting the patients go to bed when they wish, assuming they have the capacity to make this decision, is a lot better. It makes life much harder for us. But what else could we possibly do? It is just totally wrong to herd old people about like animals, just to suit our tidy little ward routines and make life easier for ourselves

- Which of the above group of nurses, those in statement A or those in statement B, are operating in accordance with a categorical imperative?
- In about 200 words write arguments for and against the position taken by the nurses in statement B.

Morality based upon principles or virtues

As will have been noted, the various deontological perspectives presented, including that of Kant, have a common feature of identifying some form of characteristic or rule that establishes our ethical duties or obligations. Most commonly these are expressed in terms of principles (which in this context refers to rules or maxims that guide action) or virtues (which in this context refers to personal attributes or characteristics that are valued, laudable, good). The terms are not mutually exclusive, as one can also speak of a person who is one of principle, who adheres to certain standards (virtues). In general, it is more common to speak in terms of principles than virtues.

Unfortunately, there is little agreement not only about the difference between principles and virtues, but also about the principles and virtues that are important. This, as suggested by MacIntyre (1985), is more often a consequence of history and culture. Notwithstanding such difficulties, there are various sets of ethical principles put forward, although all bear similarities. If we accept Kant's philosophy, these principles are universal maxims, and the categorical imperative applies to each one of them, i.e. they are adhered to on all like occasions irrespective of consequences because we hold them to be universal. One such example is that of Thiroux (1980), who suggested principles of:

- the value of life
- goodness or rightness
- justice
- honesty
- individual freedom.

Writing specifically of ethical principles relevant to nursing, Yeo and Ford (1991) presented principles of:

- beneficence
- autonomy
- truthfulness
- confidentiality
- justice.

It is perhaps wise to avoid here the difficulties arising from the terminology. However, irrespective of whether we see honesty or truthfulness as a principle that guides us or a quality of the virtuous person, and even after we address the issue of what is the most comprehensive listing, certain practical problems remain. These largely centre around the problem of what we do when, in particular situations, the principles conflict. For example, if a male patient has a sexually transmitted infectious disease, we may wish to respect his right to confidentiality and autonomy in respect of who is or is not informed of his illness. But, what if his wife asks about the nature of his illness, which in this instance may have implications for the health of both her and their children? How do we then meet the principles of truthfulness and justice? There are two main ways around such predicaments that are commonly suggested:

1 We simply have to work out what is best in the context of the particular situation. However, while this is central to that contextualised form of ethics termed *situation ethics* discussed earlier, it obviously makes a nonsense of claiming that each one of the set of principles is universal and subject to a categorical imperative (i.e. being principles we *always* adhere to).

2 We can accept that one or more of the principles has, as a general rule, priority or precedence over the others. That is, that there is in fact a hierarchy of principles. The best-known example here is John Rawls' (1971) *A Theory of Justice*. Rawls argued that justice is the primary principle, and he viewed this as being fairness in the collective distribution of liberty. That is, that each person should have that maximum amount of liberty that does not impinge upon the liberty of others. Within such a situation, Rawls recognised that there may be inequalities, with some better off than others. However, he argued that such inequalities are acceptable if they advantage society, including those less well off. The problems here may seem obvious and include:

how we determine the priority of principles (e.g. setting justice over love); how we define them (e.g. whether justice is fairness, liberty or equality); and, what place or weighting we give to other principles in terms of making our choices.

Biomedical ethics and the Four Principles Approach

Still within the perspective of establishing universal principles as the foundations for what is good or right, and therefore largely within the deontological perspective, is the dominant medical ethic described as the Four Principles Approach. This is an important and highly influential ethical framework. While developed within the medical profession, it has had a remarkably wide range of influence and is the framework of choice also adopted by many nurses. The approach was developed primarily by Tom Beauchamp and James Childress (1979, 1994, 2001) and extended in many publications by these two authors (e.g. Beauchamp, 1994; Childress, 2000). One of the main proponents over many years in the UK is a physician and philosopher, Raanan Gillon (1985, 1994). The four principles postulated are as follows.

- *Beneficence* – the commitment to do good or to act in the person's best interests. This encompasses the responsibility to do only what benefits the person or to ensure that the benefits to be accrued outweigh the risks.
- *Non-maleficence* – the commitment to avoid harming the person, and to take no action where the risks clearly outweigh any benefits. This is in line with the Hippocratic Oath which is taken to include 'First, do no harm' (although historical evidence to support this source is inconclusive).
- *Autonomy* – the commitment to respect the capable individual's right to self-determination and to be involved in decisions affecting themselves.
- *Justice* – the commitment to ensure equality of treatment and a fair distribution of time and resources, taking adequate account of the

benefits and risks of such decisions for the individual and for others.

Such is the clarity, precision, and apparent ease of use of the Four Principles Approach, that it has attained universal recognition, often cited and used by doctors, nurses and others who have never read, or in some cases even heard of, Beauchamp and Childress. For this reason, it is often described (sometimes pejoratively) as the *Georgetown Mantra* (an allusion to the authors' university affiliations – Georgetown University hosted their original work).

Of course, the same problems apply in respect of these principles as for those other systems or listings of principles addressed in the previous section. That is, there are problems of how conflicting claims between the principles are resolved, and also of determining whether some have precedence over others and how such precedence might be ranked or weighted. On the basis of such difficulties, some (e.g. Seedhouse, 1998) have been highly critical of the Four Principles Approach, seeing it as little more than a checklist of principles with no deeper consideration of how they should be applied, and furthermore no recognition of the fact that not all may find those chosen as the four to be acceptable. This is perhaps an unfair criticism. The approach does, of course, have its difficulties, as acknowledged here. However, both of its original authors (Beauchamp and Childress) have recognised the potential weaknesses and over the years have openly and willingly responded to criticism. Most notably, they have responded by proposing ways in which the principles can be contextualised to real-world situations and, in the case of Childress (2000) and Beauchamp and Childress (2001), how the principles can be extended to encompass such areas as truth telling, acting faithfully, and respecting privacy and confidentiality.

Study Activity 13.9 _____

In 1947, the famous *film noire* entitled *Odd Man Out* was released. Starring many mainstream movie 'stars', it was widely acclaimed as the best film of its year. Directed by Carol Reed (1947) and based on the novel by F.L. Green (1945), it tells the story of Johnny McQueen, a fugitive on the run during a night time snow storm in a city. Although the city is clearly not explicitly stated, it is Belfast in Northern Ireland, and Johnny (played by James Mason) and his 'friends' are obviously an Irish Republican group. Johnny has been fatally wounded in a robbery to raise funds for the 'cause', during which he also killed a man. The film follows his course through the frozen and snow-swept city in his final hours, from place to place, and from person to person. It is a dark and allegorical tale. Good and evil are always in the balance and Johnny is presented at times as an ogre, as a pitiful creature, or as a Messiah constantly on the point of betrayal by those he encounters, as the police dragnet tightens inexorably. Each character in the film is a set piece, and with a powerful script and magnificent performances it has become a classic of the *film noire* genre.

Consider the characters:

1 An English man and his wife and daughter are newly arrived in the city. When they find Johnny semiconscious in their home, the husband argues that he has broken the law and that they must hand him over. His wife and daughter show compassion. They see the fugitive as a poor wounded creature who they must help. Eventually, they wrap him warmly and help him out of the house and back into the night. As he leaves, the husband offers him whiskey to drink.

2 Shell, a down and out, finds Johnny and goes to the local priest, offering to deliver up Johnny for money. He is clearly afraid to betray him to the police: Johnny's friends are powerful and their revenge would be terrible. But he has to eat and he sees in this an opportunity to gain.

3 The old priest, Father Tom, has no financial reward to offer, but he convinces Shell to bring Johnny so that he can hear his confession and save his immortal soul. He knows the police well, and their call for law and order. He knows also the members of the political organisation, and their cause. But his cause is to fulfil God's will, to bring Johnny back to God and his mercy. All he

can offer Shell and Johnny's girlfriend is the gift of faith.

4 Johnny's girlfriend, Kathleen, has no such aspiration. Faith has no hold on her, and when the old priest cajoles her, she responds that she has only love for the fugitive and if she cannot save him she would die with him rather than live on without him (which she eventually does).

5 Along the way, Johnny falls into the hands of Lukey, a deranged artist who lives with Shell and the medical student Tober. Lukey is obsessed with the desire to paint Johnny with the moment of death in his eyes. He is completely unconcerned about the legal and political viewpoints, and he casts aside pleas for compassion or indeed using the situation for profit. He sees in all of this only the unique opportunity for himself as an artist.

6 Tober, the medical student appears equally dispassionate. However, he insists on treating Johnny's wound. Shell, in exasperation, states the obvious futility of this, as Johnny will simply be tried and executed in any case. Tober's response is that this is no concern of his, he is obliged to treat Johnny and (as he states) it is none of his responsibility what others do afterwards.

7 The police inspector leading the manhunt is at once a spectre hovering over Johnny and at the same time someone who understands what Kathleen and Father Tom feel. However, his position is clear. Johnny has killed a man and he must be apprehended and brought to justice. While he is clearly a man of some human understanding and compassion, he is immovable in his sense of duty.

Consider each of the seven positions adopted by the characters. In each case, identify:

– the ethical theory that best describes the character's position
– the dimensions of the moral theory, or moral framework, that explains the character's position.

The moral basis of relativism

At first glance, the dimensions that underpin relativist ethics may seem nebulous to say the least. At its extreme, radical relativism appears to be simply saying 'anything goes'. Given the diversity of cultures, the moral schema of each is relevant only in its context, and there are therefore no universal moral laws. Furthermore, if this is the case, it reflects ethnocentrism to assume that *our* moral standards (whoever we may be), are the right or only relevant moral standards. The extension of this is that the primary underlying dimension of relativism is that of individual freedom and diversity.

However, as globalisation progresses, and as each 'society' becomes more multicultural, it becomes increasingly difficult to maintain an orderly and efficient society, if a multitude of vastly different and often conflicting moral codes are accepted. The natural response to this is that which we described earlier as soft relativism. That is, a minimalist approach is adopted whereby some minimal universal principle or principles can be identified which allow for some common ground but permit maximum diversity. Two examples are of note. The first of these is that which we earlier described as situation ethics. In the form known as Christian situation ethics, as explicated by Fletcher (1966), the foundational principle is the Christian principle encompassed in the Golden Rule: that of agapistic love, to love thy neighbour as thyself. In considering ethnical dilemmas in context, taking account of the situational factors of circumstances and actors, we are guided by this commitment to help through our concern for the other. Indeed, the quest to derive our decisions from considering the context is seen as a fundamental requisite if we are *really* concerned for others; as Fletcher (1966) states, 'It is entirely possible to be calculating without loving, but it is *not* possible to be loving without calculating' (p. 141). The second example, deriving from the liberal tradition of individual freedom, looks instead to principles that underpin human rights to self-determination. According to Dworkin (1977), others, including the state, cannot impinge upon the rights of the individual to make their own choices, excepting in those circumstances where there are clear justifications (predominantly where the rights or well-being of others are seriously threatened). The most well-known example of such an orientation is Rawls' (1971) 'theory of justice' as discussed earlier. Of course, where such principles (love, individual freedom, justice) are held to be *universal* principles, the question is begged as to whether we have moved from relativism to deontology.

From dimensions to essences

So far in this chapter we have considered the nature of ethics, common ethical theories, and the dimensions or underpinning features upon which such theories are based. The range of such dimensions is outlined in Fig. 13.2 overleaf. But little has been said so far about the fundamental concepts (whether we use terms such as good–bad, right–wrong, virtue–vice, etc.), which are at the very centre of our moral thinking. The dimensions in Fig. 13.2 present the ethical perspectives or devices we may utilise in our ethical theories, but they do not help us in establishing the source or sources of what is 'good' or 'right'. We may incorporate such dimensions or features as maximum 'utility' and the 'greatest happiness principle' in a consequentialist theory, or indeed apply a 'categorical imperative' with a 'good will' in a deontological theory. But in a sense these are devices we use in our quest for the good. The question here is how something comes to be *accepted* as good, or what exactly it is that *makes* something admired or sought after as being morally desirable. Whether we use generic terms such as 'good' or 'right', or other terms that are agreed to encompass them (as principles or virtues), such as beneficence or honesty, it is important that we know their sources. Particularly in health care, where our ethical choices affect people's well-being or even survival, it is important that we know the root source from which our choices ultimately emerge. We need to be prepared to place our moral choices very clearly on the line in respect of such sources. But more importantly, we need to have confidence in the source from which our valuing of something as good or right derives.

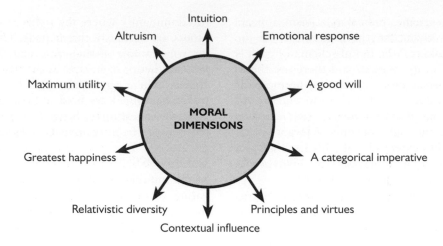

Figure 13.2   Moral dimensions: the underpinning features of ethical theories

THE ORIGINS OF GOOD AND RIGHT

A question of source

The question put simply is: where does morality come from? Is it something genetically built into us, like our hair colour or our temperament? Is it something we learn and internalise as we take on social roles? Or, is it something in our very being which is akin to soul or spirit, which makes us different from lower animals that appear to have no moral sense, and respond only to bestial instinct and similar needs and drives? And, if so, does this ethereal and peculiarly human property derive from simply being human or does it derive from a higher power? These are fundamental questions often avoided in moral philosophy and there are no easy answers. There are, of course, various *tentative* answers to some of these questions.

It can be suggested that in the broadest terms the sense of what is good or right and their converse come either from within or without. That is, either they are in or a part of the person as some intrinsic quality, or their source is outside the person and as such acts upon him, causing him to think and act in particular ways. We have variously used terms such as good, or

right, or virtue to describe those moral positions that we value. Likewise we have spoken of principles for achieving these valued positions. We can use 'good' not simply as an adjective to delimit that which we value, but as the representative term to describe the essence of all that we value morally. We can then search for its source accordingly.

Good as a social construction

It can be argued that society rather than the individual is the source of what is good or right. Here, whether based on teleological notions of meeting the general good, deontological notions of choices being good or right in themselves as a 'self-evident' fact, or a conglomerate of both, moral values are in the social domain and a part of a society's culture. Effectively, our understanding of what is good or right is constructed as part of our culture – it is valued as such by the whole society and we are required to internalise and accept it as such. By definition, what is good or right can therefore differ from culture to culture and even change over time. That is, cultural definitions of 'the good' are subject to *time* and *space* variations. Thus, something like individual liberty is recognised as a good in Western modern society, while its converse, communality is valued in Chinese society. Similarly, while in the UK in the years of Conservative Thatcherism individuality was valued, in recent years under Labour Governments there has been some shift towards a more communitarian set of values.

The establishment of what is 'good' through social construction is of course dependent on the incorporation of agreed norms within a culture. In earlier times, this was not problematic, as culture was tightly defined within church and legal systems, and maintained through highly structured and close-knit communities. However, with progression into modernity, traditional norms were rejected and the new religions of science and technology were looked to as the source of our salvation. This was accompanied by an increasingly individualistic Western world, within which liberalism and individual freedom became the modern patterns (Bellah *et al.*, 1985; Taylor, 1991). An increasing disillusionment with the impact of science and technology and their impingement upon private lives led to what became known as post-modernism. In this post-modern turn, both the old religions and the new (science, technology, modern bureaucracies and political systems) became subject to a critical reflection. This recognised the failure of the old religions and the new sciences to provide absolute answers. It led to what in effect was a deconstruction of social norms and their replacement by a new openness or relativism that says there is no one right way and we all have the right to choose. We have, of course, already met this in the section on relativistic ethics discussed earlier in this chapter. In his celebrated study *The Closing of the American Mind*, Allan Bloom (1987) stated:

> There is one thing a professor can be absolutely certain of: almost every student entering the university believes, or says he believes, that truth is relative. If this belief is put to the test, one can count on the students' reaction: they will be uncomprehending. That anyone should regard the proposition as not self-evident astonishes them, as though he

> were calling into question 2 + 2 = 4 ... The students, of course, cannot defend their opinion. The best they can do is point out all the opinions and cultures there are and have been. What right, they ask, do I or anyone else have to say that one is better than the other? If I pose the routine questions designed to confute them and make them think, such as, 'If you had been a British administrator in India, would you have let the natives under your governance burn the widow at the funeral of a man who had died?,' they either remain silent or reply that the British should never have been there in the first place.
>
> (Bloom, 1987, p. 25)

This trend presents us with two possibilities. One is that what is 'good' will, at least within our own culture, be socially constructed. We, as part of our social contract to that group, will be expected to internalise, value and live by this view of what is good. To an extent, this is still the case. But for some of the time we are in fact socialised into the relativistic orientation of acceptance of diversity and the view that we can determine our own position on what is good. This freedom is, of course, an individualistic freedom, much in line with the notions of egoistic teleology and ethical relativism discussed earlier in this chapter. It states, more precisely, that we can do what we will as long as it does not impact upon others. Therefore, the second possibility is that we are socialised into a conception of the 'good' that is pluralistic. Our egoistic interests become paramount, and the new 'good' is in fact the individualism and freedom that allows us to achieve such ends, as long as they do not limit the individualism and freedom of others.

Morality is often seen as a function of the social roles we enact rather than a function of the person who takes these roles. This view is explained by Emmet (1966) when she states that:

> The notion of role has built into it a notion of some conduct as appropriate ... (social

> *behaviour) is informed by expectations to which people have been taught to conform, as to how they should behave in certain relationships and situations; this may come to seem 'natural' where the expectations are so strongly grounded in custom and so widely accepted that they have come to seem self-evident. (This may lie behind the claim to 'self-evidence' of intuitionist views of moral principles) ... The notion of role, therefore, I suggest provides a link between factual descriptions of social situations and moral pronouncements about what ought to be done in them.*
>
> (Emmet, 1986, pp. 40–1)

In this sense, the moral decision of right–wrong or good–bad would appear to be taken out of the hands of the individual. According to this argument, moral behaviour is to a greater or lesser extent prescribed by the role in which we are placed. It is in fact part of a social contract between the person and society: for the benefits or rights accrued by being a member of society, we have the responsibility or obligation to live by its agreed norms. Tschudin (1992) speaks of a nurse's duties as being those prescribed by the institution, an idea not dissimilar to Emmet's notion of role-based prescribed behaviour. The nurse is contracted to carry out duties in a way in which the health care institution (e.g. hospital) considers right and proper. If he or she feels on a personal level that the prescribed position is bad or wrong, and if he or she follows his/her personal convictions rather than the official line, there is the likelihood of major conflict occurring between the nurse and the institution's agents. Referring back to Weber's (1991) categories, in a political world dominated by an ethics of responsibility, it may be difficult and costly to live by an ethics of conviction that calls us to keep faith with our own conscience. In recent years, how such concerns have been carried forward, and the consequences of doing so, have been shown to be problematic.

Study Activity 13.10

Graham Pink was a nurse at Stepping Hill Hospital in Stockport, UK. After having made various efforts to report staff shortages and have these remedied, Pink expressed his concerns publicly in the press. He was dismissed for 'breach of confidentiality' in September 1991, and subsequently reported to the UK regulatory body for nurses, midwives and health visitors for alleged misconduct. The employing authority subsequently settled with Pink before an industrial tribunal heard the case. The regulatory body did not uphold the allegation of professional misconduct.

Dr Helen Zeitlin, a medical consultant at Alexandra Hospital in Redditch, UK made public statements about nursing shortages, and following this was made compulsorily redundant by the West Midlands Regional Health Authority in February 1991. Subsequently, a Department of Health inquiry vindicated Dr Zeitlin and the employer was instructed to reinstate her. The Chairman of the Regional Health Authority and the General Manager and Chairman of the District Health Authority managing the hospital resigned.

After expressing concern about what he felt was an unacceptably high level of mortality among children undergoing cardiac surgery at Bristol Royal Infirmary in the UK, Dr Stephen Bolsin, an anaesthetist at the hospital, proceeded to express concerns to external agencies including the Department of Health, all without much success. He subsequently made his concerns public, and a major Government inquiry (Kennedy, 2001) vindicated his concerns, confirming that over a number of years (possibly extending back to the mid-1980s) the number of such deaths had been much higher than they should have been, according to accepted yardsticks. In the course of his attempt to have his concerns acted upon, Bolsin met with significant hostility from a number of sources, such that at one stage he had contemplated claiming constructive dismissal against his employers (an employment term describing circumstances being made so difficult that continuing in the post becomes untenable). In the aftermath of 'going public' he was unable to obtain a post in the UK, despite the fact that his professional work was exemplary, and he had to move to Australia to find employment.

- Do you feel these individuals were justified in their decisions to act in the ways that they did?
- Clearly, the brief facts presented above only touch upon the personal distress and damage to health and career they and their families suffered. In view of this, do you feel it is right to expect anyone to carry their moral convictions this far?
- Consider the outcomes of the actions in respect of the patients and their relatives. Taking the Bristol case in particular, given that the children could not be brought back, might it have been better to keep quiet and avoid the distress and heartache to parents that ensued? Using the consequentialist and deontological theories considered earlier, present your view of this proposition in around 200 words or one page. Test your position by discussing your response with your personal tutor and/or student colleagues.

Irrespective of how you responded to the Study Activity above, it does raise the premise that the individual is responsible for his/her actions and he or she alone is accountable for them. It is unacceptable to simply rely on what society or any group within it says. The 'good' as this was socially constructed by some at Bristol Royal Infirmary, clearly centred upon notions of confidentiality and loyalty to the group. But for Stephen Bolsin the 'good' was something quite different and in the end he followed his own conscience. Hunt (1992) has stated that:

> *Moral responsibility means accepting and carrying the burden of judgement and decision in matters of right and wrong. It means a preparedness to accept guilt and blame for wrongful actions and for any wrong that results from one's action. Morality, like your bus ticket, is non-transferable: I cannot do what is right simply by doing what others want me to do. Of course, I may do what another tells me believing it to be right, in which case I do it because it is right and not simply because I have been told to do it ... Morality is non-transferable because each of us is his or her own source of morality.*
>
> (Hunt, 1992, p. 100)

It is not the place of this book to judge whether, in the examples presented above, the individuals concerned were right or wrong. However, if they *thought* what was happening was wrong and threatened the well-being of their patients, they were right to recognise that they had a *personal* responsibility to do *something*. After all, most people have rejected the Nazi war criminals' rationale that they were only 'following orders'. It is generally accepted, paradoxically, that even if society or a group demands certain values and behaviour, we have a duty not to conform if it is wrong. In the aftermath of cases such as those presented above, legislation has been introduced in the UK to protect people who speak out – the so-called 'whistleblower' legislation. However, the risks even today of doing so speaks to the courage demanded of individuals in taking such actions. Beauchamp and Childress (1989) spoke of this in terms of *supererogation* (a word meaning to pay, or do, or perform more than is required or can be reasonably expected). Their view here was that in meeting an ethical requirement such as non-maleficence (i.e. not knowingly doing harm), there are certain lengths that we can be reasonably expected to go to. What sets the limits of this normal range is the personal risk to ourselves, which might be considered in terms of low-risk or high-risk levels of supererogation. This is perhaps best viewed as a continuum, as presented in Fig. 13.3 overleaf.

For some, extending responsibility supererogatively is a reflection of courage, and as such is viewed as an unusual virtue: we may admire such people for making their stand and envy them in the knowledge that we would not have the courage to do the same. For others, this is viewed as an unavoidable demand: irrespective of the costs, the ethical demand is so strong that they feel they could take no other course of action despite the risks involved. In extreme cases, historical figures such as Sir Thomas More

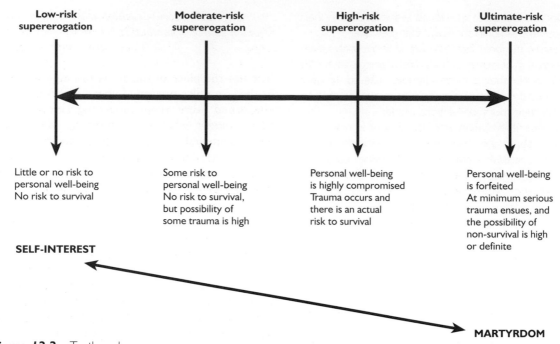

Figure 13.3   Truth and consequence

or Martin Luther felt called to pay ultimate penalties for their moral stands and it was a matter beyond courage. Indeed, while they appeared to be most fearful of the consequences, they could not go on living with the less threatening choices that were seemingly available to them.

Study Activity 13.11

Consider yourself in the following position. You are allocated to a unit for the care of people with learning disabilities. Most of your colleagues are well known to you and some of the staff nurses and your fellow students share a communal residence and social life with you. It soon becomes clear to you that a number of the staff physically abuse the patients on a regular basis. You observe patients being tied in chairs and smacked. In addition, some of their private property and gifts have been stolen. While some of your colleagues also seem unhappy with this situation, they are afraid to speak out. Having been concerned about this, you raised the matter with the unit manager, but

nothing was done about this. You now find you are being shunned by colleagues, not only on duty but also in the residence where you live.

- Consider what options are now open to you. Determine where the action that you feel most appropriate would place you, on the continuum presented in Fig. 13.3.
- Anticipate possible consequences of the action you contemplate, and reflect upon how you might respond to these consequences.

Study Activity 13.12

You are working in the community psychiatric nursing service in a densely populated urban area of the north of England. There have been violent riots that seem to be directly related to issues of race and ethnicity. This has caused great distress to large numbers of the Asian community in the area, some of whom have developed anxiety and depressive illnesses – thus your involvement. The local community feels that the police have not been impartial and that this has greatly increased the problems. Dissatisfied with the response to their complaints, they have decided to set up their own local community-based 'Truth Commission' to investigate their complaints and determine subsequent action. A local non-Asian politician has agreed to chair the Commission. The local community leaders invite you to sit on the Commission. Your manager has not actually forbidden you to accept this invitation, but her reaction is clearly negative and she has questioned whether this would be appropriate activity for a nurse. Furthermore, she has expressed the view that while there may indeed be substance in the community's concerns, this action will only rekindle tensions and it would be better for everyone in the long run if the matter was just dropped.

- First, recognise that the parameters of your responsibility as a nurse are set by nursing's concerns with health and well-being. But health and well-being are not necessarily simple and clear concepts. Before you proceed, look up modern definitions of these concepts as they apply to individuals and communities.
- What is your opinion – do *you* feel you have a moral responsibility as a nurse to get involved in such activities?
- If you have reservations about this, what are these and how do they relate to your commitment to the health and well-being of this community?
- You are aware of your manager's view that it would be best if this whole matter was dropped. Do you feel society (or elements within it) may have *constructed* reservations about what is the 'good' thing to do in such instances? If so, what might be the reason for this?
- Where do you think involvement in this Commission might place you along the continuum presented in Fig. 13.3? If you have identified a different level of risk than in Study Activity 13.11, consider why this may be so.

Good as a personal way of being

In the previous section, we considered the strength of social pressures to comply with socially constructed positions on morality and

also instances where individuals have stood against such positions. One explanation is that irrespective of what others may demand of us, we have a built-in personal capacity that is for each of us the source from which we recognise what is good or right. That is, in the final analysis we have some source of moral knowledge or consciousness within us, which will guide our actions. It is in effect a facet of being human, and the movement within society that is called *humanism* is based partly upon the idea that people are naturally drawn to see the worth in each other (and indeed all living things). This, in essence, is close to what Kant (1938) meant when he spoke of a *good will* and respecting others as '*ends in themselves*'. It is also to what Moore (1903) spoke of as the good that we know intuitively. It can also be posited as the source from which our natural emotional recognition of what is morally right stems, in the emotivist theory of ethics proposed by Ayer (1936) and others. And, it may relate to what Sartre (1993) spoke of as existential morality, a fundamental part of our existence as a person thrown into the world, confronted with moral choices from moment to moment, but – as Heidegger (1967) postulated – faced with a demand to respond with intentional care to what we confront in that world.

According to some, morality – the capacity to think and behave with goodness and rightness – is a kind of inner spirituality which we can open ourselves up to; in this sense it is within each person if we are prepared to receive and nurture it. Fox (1990) views this in terms of *compassion*, a concern and caring for others and for the world in general, and a living of this caring. For Fox, compassion is not simply pity for another, or even a sense of altruism or love towards others. It is at once an inner way of being that calls us as persons to respond to others, a movement from this inner tendency to its outer realisation in moral action. He states that:

> ... *compassion without joy and celebration, without action and public justice, without ideas and ideals, without passion and caring,*

> *without a consciousness or a way of living,*
> *without cosmic and divine awareness and*
> *interaction, is not compassion at all. It is a*
> *co-optation of compassion. It is a demonic*
> *substitute for compassion. It is death-dealing,*
> *not lifegiving. All these elements of*
> *compassion are themselves interconnected,*
> *and to fail in one of these is to threaten*
> *compassion altogether for each energy*
> *depends on the others, much like the spokes*
> *on a wheel.*
>
> (Fox, 1990, p. 34)

Thus, by living a compassionate life, one is living the good or right life. When asked why they made what they believed to be 'good' moral choices, people often allude to a call from their *conscience* (some inner voice or mind-set by which we naturally know what is 'good' or 'right'). This can, of course, draw us back into controversial and circular arguments. Some Freudian psychodynamic psychologists recognise conscience as the *superego*, the mind's moral watchdog which is derived from being socialised into and internalising social values. In this sense, morality, or what is good, is in its origins a social construction, as described in the previous section. This, of course, suggests a mechanistic and reductionist interpretation. When Saint Paul spoke of the conscience of the Gentiles, he said it was 'written on their hearts' such that they required no laws requiring them to instinctively obey its calling, giving this notion of conscience a particularly human connotation. In the sense intended here, conscience is a fundamental way of being human, that sets us apart from other creatures and is more than just an automatic submission to social norms and rules. Indeed, it is often the case that we stand on our conscience *against* the dominant values, as in the case of the conscientious objector or the whistleblowers Pink, Zeitlin and Bolsin considered in the earlier Study Activity.

Study Activity 13.13 ────────

In May 2002, a father who had previously refused to allow his 3-year-old daughter, who was HIV positive,

to receive drug therapy and had taken her to Australia, returned with her to the UK. The child's mother who was also HIV positive, had died of Aids in the interim. The father had apparently expressed a strong preference for alternative medicine, and was concerned about the toxic side-effects of the potent drug therapy (which may include serious liver, bone and blood damage, particularly in young children). Furthermore, there is a dearth of research evidence on the efficacy and longer-term side-effects of such treatment on young children. However, the prognosis for children with HIV proceeding to full-blown Aids is also extremely poor.

In one of the usual television news-time debates, a bioethics expert and a childcare spokesperson were invited to speak. The bioethics 'expert' expressed the view that in these circumstances, the welfare of the child took precedence and that society had a responsibility to overturn the father's decision and impose therapy.

- Reflect upon the application of the Four Principles Approach of biomedical ethics (as discussed earlier) in this situation, and identify which, if any, of the four principles may be in conflict here.
- Reflect upon the conflict between good as a social construction and good as a personal way of being in this case.
- On the basis of your reflections, think carefully about your position in this controversy. In about 200 words (one page) present your position, and include in this the ethical theory that influenced your decision.
- Ask a fellow student or your personal tutor to read your written statement and then ask them to act as a devil's advocate (someone who challenges your viewpoint). Consider whether their viewpoints have added any new considerations that have altered your position in any way, and add notes on these to your written statement.

───────────────

The third bullet point in the above Study Activity asked you to commit yourself to a position in respect of the personal way of knowing what is the good or best position, as perhaps was adopted by the father of this child.

In doing so, you probably became acutely aware of the difficulties in defending his case. One reason for this is that a rational defence involves, by definition, a naturalistic approach (i.e. treating it as a problem of logic and reason). But this (or so it is argued by the intuitionists) is to commit the naturalistic fallacy discussed earlier. By the same token that we cannot argue this personal and intuitive ethical perspective from a naturalistic base, we cannot defend the position against those who hold it to be fundamentally irrational and lacking in a sound empirical base.

In the sense intended in this section, the 'good' is a fundamental part of what it means to be human. It cannot be attributable to any religious or cosmic force acting upon us: it is just the way humans are in their natural state, and when they fail in this regard – through less good or even evil acts – they are to that extent denuded of their humanness. This 'goodness' is a natural compassionate state, a way of living as a human person to which we are all called by a natural concern or conscience. Its presentations may be numerous: a loving care for others; a sense of justice that may incorporate equity and freedom of choice; courage in the face of inequity or threat; truthfulness and fidelity, etc. These characteristics (some would call them virtues) are indicators of this human state of goodness. But, as we noted earlier, it is not some concrete or observable thing, like a limb or human organ [although the heart, as Midgley (1983) and others indicate, is its symbolic metaphor]. We are aware of it tacitly and intuitively (as in intuitionism, discussed earlier) or emotionally (as in emotivism, discussed earlier). Therefore, we can recognise the good (or its converse) in all things, and through our humanness we are aware when we are living by it authentically or relinquishing it inauthentically. However, the modern health service values naturalistic science and technology, managerial utilitarianism based upon ethical reasoning, or universal principles and formulae that guide ethical decision-making. Holding that moral choices can be based on personal ways of knowing that are tacit, intui-

tive or emotive may have little currency in such systems.

Good as a divine command or a gift from God

This *living* of *goodness* is also espoused by Smith (1985), who suggests that what differentiates man from other animals is the capacity to reflect upon himself and by so doing to possess a conception of life and living. To Smith, *good* is an essential way of being which is not by definition within us, but something we must open ourselves up to, something we can in fact choose. In explaining this viewpoint, Smith (1985) states that:

> Were we merely desiring, self-seeking creatures, the answer would have to be that life has no meaning. The truth is, however, that reality contains the Good, which is not our creation and to which we are called to respond ... I take it ... that this same vision of the good life is enshrined in St. Augustine's injunction: dilege et quod vis fac, where it is understood that what you want to do arises in and through the love which is openness and attention.
>
> (Smith, 1985)

Smith suggests that this state of goodness is achieved by the individual avoiding self-deception and reflecting upon and evaluating his or her own self and through this the selves of others. By doing so, the illusion of self-deception which obscures and prevents the emergence of *good* in the person is avoided.

While still being highly personal, this view of goodness has distinct theological or religious connotations. Unlike the humanist perspective, which might suggest that there is a natural goodness in people, here goodness is a state of being which is available to us (from some outer cosmic or spiritual source) but which we must strive for. In an increasingly secular and science-orientated world, such almost mystical explanations of the basis of good or right have become unpopular. Yet even the most rational of individuals find it difficult to explain a Mother Teresa or a Martin Luther King, other than to suggest the existence in them of a quality of true goodness which, some have observed, seemed to shine from them like a light.

This does not go far in explaining what the 'good' *is*. There are, of course, various religious principles put forward within religious movements. We have already identified the Golden Rule, which is attributed to Jesus in the Sermon on the Mount, but the principle of 'do to others as you would wish they would do to you' is also found in many other religious movements, extending back into antiquity in Chinese, Hindu, Jewish, Buddhist and Islamic cultures. Smith (1985) refers to St. Augustine's famous admonition of '*Dilige, et quod vis fac*' (Love, and do what you will). That is, if we follow God's example in loving the other, we cannot knowingly or willingly do them harm. All of these rest on an assumption that God (or *a* God, or some other cosmic presence or principal) wills that we do good. In essence, the good or right is what God intends us, or requires us to do. We are following His will and His example.

For unbelievers, this is of course a problematic position: there is first the question of whether there *is* a God, and, if there is, then the question of how we know what He intends that we do. If we get past this problem, there is the pitfall posed by the ancient Greek philosopher Socrates: is something right because God commands it or does He command it because it is right? Thus, even the religious claims to the foundations or essences of 'good' or 'right' are problematic, unless we can accept them in blind faith. Furthermore, the apparent admonishments of a God or supreme being may seem to many cold and sometimes even inhuman. This is particularly the case in respect of the more fundamental and uncompromising movements within Judaism, Christianity and Islam. The humorous, yet quite serious message within George Bernard Shaw's (1903) reworking of the Golden Rule is enlightening in its veiled attack upon the imposition of immovable principles upon individuals who have their own humanity and personal preferences: 'Do not do unto others as you would they should do unto you. Their tastes may not be the same'.

As in the case of 'Good as a personal way of being', sustaining ethical decisions as based upon divine will may be particularly difficult within highly scientific and technological health care systems founded almost entirely upon naturalistic premises.

Good as caring in relation

Such views as those expressed by Smith (1985) are not dissimilar to the earlier work of the French philosopher Simone Weil (1952). She suggested *love* as the fundamentally authentic way of being, stating that it is: 'Belief in the existence of other human beings as such ... Among human beings, only the existence of those we love is fully recognised' (p. 52).

Such vocabulary rests uncomfortably with our modern ways of thinking and is often alien to our professional nomenclature. In our Schools of Nursing we are not encouraged to *love* our patients. This possibly would be viewed as a dangerous concept, as love has various connotations, some of which are rightly seen as having no place in a professional relationship. However, the notion of love conceived by Weil is different to that usually understood by romantic or familial love, or similar forms of emotional attachment. We must accept here that the use of this word has different, although sometimes overlapping, connotations: *eros*, or love as an erotic and passionate sexual relation; *philia*, or brotherly love as exists between family members, and close friends, as a reciprocal (giving and receiving) relationship that does not have erotic elements; and, *agapé*, or a benevolent love that draws its origins from the Christian ethic of love of neighbour, which is the ethical call to be concerned for all persons. This not only demands no reciprocity but also actually draws its strength from the compassion for all beings it involves, and the concomitant commitment to help others without any thought of acknowledgement, reciprocal response or reward. It is this agapistic love that is primarily an ethical stand, by virtue of its call to action even when we do not know or perhaps even like those for whom we accept an ethical responsibility.

This agapistic ethic concerns an openness to the reality of one's own self and through this a receptiveness to the reality of the other person. There is here an appreciation of the self as one exists in the world. And an intentional going out to the other as a person, a willingness to experience and accept the other non-judgementally, irrespective of that other's goodnesses and badnesses or strengths and weaknesses. This is in keeping with the notion of *care* or *concern* which the existential philosopher Martin Heidegger (1967) identified as an essential aspect of authentic as opposed to inauthentic being in the world (*see* Chapter 2). Heidegger suggested that through an intentional awareness of our existence we experience a concern about how we live in the world and how we relate to others in this world. Where Heidegger speaks of care or concern and the psychologist or psychoanalyst speaks of conscience, the moral philosopher speaks of ethics.

It has been claimed that such a capacity for relating to others is an essential aspect of ethics. We can, of course, have ethical stances in regard to a number of phenomena. For example, we may view euthanasia as bad. However, such views are enacted in the real-life situation of our relationships with others. We cannot relate to another person with compassion and respect if we do not first relate to that individual as another human being in the fullest sense. If we relate to others as roles or, in the nursing or medical context, as cases, issues such as euthanasia are viewed rather differently.

It is indeed a common assertion that nurses and doctors have a tendency to see their patients as cases or conditions rather than seeing them as individuals; even the term patient imposes a role which can be depersonalising. In such situations it is not unusual to see treatment and nursing being carried out without regard to the patient as a person. Values such as autonomy and choice, confidentiality, respect, honesty, and compassion – often presented as important

ethical principles – are totally disregarded. It could be argued that compassion [as Fox (1990) views it] or love [as Weil (1952) views it] are not only ethical principles in themselves, but essential prerequisites for moral decision-making. Indeed, it may be argued that *caring* for others is not merely a precondition for morally good thinking and acting, but that caring is *the* implicitly ethical way of *being*. That is, if we care for and respect others, if we have regard and compassion for them as persons, we can in effect not knowingly do them harm. This caring disposition (a non-reciprocal, unconditional concern for the other as a person) can therefore be proposed as the source of the good within us. It has much in common with the powerful appeal of St. Augustine which we addressed in the previous section: '*Dilige, et quod vis fac*' (Love, and do what you will). Of this, Gaylin (1976) states: 'We must respect the goodness *in* ourselves; to do so we must recognize its presence. The caring nature of human beings is so self-evident as to escape our observation if we are not careful' (p. 179). The risk of this happening is increased within a modern health care system that is not only sometimes obsessed with the technology and mechanics of health intervention, but adopts a positivistic and hard scientific outlook that actually speaks against unscientific notions such as love and care.

Care is a value, caring a virtue. Mayeroff (1971) is instructive in relation to the value of care (despite the dated gender-biased nature of his writing) when he states:

> To care for another person in the most significant sense is to help him to grow and actualise himself ... In the context of a man's life, caring has a way of ordering his other values and activities around it. When this ordering is comprehensive, because of the inclusiveness of his carings, there is a basic stability in his life; he is 'in place' in the world, instead of being out of place, or merely drifting or endlessly seeking his place. Through caring for certain others, by serving them through caring, a man lives the

meaning of his own life. In the sense in which a man can ever be said to be at home in the world, he is at home not through dominating, or explaining, or appreciating, but through caring and being cared for.

(Mayeroff, 1971, pp. 1–2)

Meeting the other person morally is central to ethical nursing care (Watson, 1988, 1990; Greene, 1990). Noddings (1984) sees ethical caring as something which arises out of a natural caring for others. This natural caring she identifies as:

... the human condition that we, consciously or unconsciously, perceive as 'good'. It is that condition toward which we long and strive, and it is our longing for caring – to be in that special relation – that provides the motivation for us to be moral. We want to be moral in order to remain in the caring relation and to enhance the ideal of ourselves as one-caring ... It is the ethical ideal, this realistic picture of ourselves as one-caring, that guides us as we strive to meet the other morally. Everything depends upon the nature and strength of this ideal, for we shall not have absolute principles to guide us. Indeed, I shall reject ethics of principles as ambiguous and unstable. Wherever there is a principle, there is implied its exception and, too often, principles function to separate us from each other. We may become dangerously self-righteous when we perceive ourselves as holding a precious principle not held by the other. The other may then be devalued and treated 'differently.' Our ethic of caring will not allow this to happen ... our efforts must ... be directed at the maintenance of conditions that will permit caring to flourish.

(Noddings, 1984, p. 5)

What Noddings appears to be saying is that principles cannot provide formulae for ethical actions, and also that they can become a source of people taking high moral ground positions which serve to cause divisions. It is fundamental to the nature of moral principles that they are universal. That is, an attempt is made to reduce a moral dilemma to the status whereby we can say that when A applies we should always do B. This is close to Kant's notion of the categorical imperative discussed earlier. However, according to Noddings, this completely ignores situational and contextual factors which must be taken into consideration and which must influence a moral decision.

Primary within the contextual frame is the regard of each person for the other. If we care for the other, our relating to and with them is by definition morally good. In such situations, principles and rigid rules of conduct become obsolete and moral behaviour exists in the consciousness of caring individuals. As Noddings (1984) says:

To behave ethically is to behave under the guidance of an acceptable and justifiable account of what it means to be moral. To behave ethically is not to behave in conformity with just any description of morality ... an ethic of caring locates morality primarily in the pre-act consciousness of the one caring ... human love, human caring, can be quite enough on which to found an ethic.

(Noddings, 1984, pp. 27–9)

This perspective of caring in relation, or *care ethics*, or *an ethic of care*, is not without its critics. It is beyond the remit of this chapter to delve too deeply into this controversy. However, one significant facet of this is the view that the controversy is to some extent part of a wider gender discourse. According to this argument, ethics based upon rational discourses tend to be part of a wider male discourse that emphasises dispassionate problem-solving and logical argument. Thus, we found that utilitarian ethics involved weighting costs and benefits, determining whose happiness or well-being trumped others on various 'objective' criteria. Similarly, we found that some deontological ethics involved the systematic identification of principles (such as the biomedical Four Principles Approach), and sometimes the ranking of these in terms of their superiority as a call on ethical choices (such as in Rawls' theory of justice). Such thinking would appear to be in direct opposition to a more feminine ethic which emphasises compassion, love, and the foundations of ethics in caring relationships within specific contextualised situations, wherein the subjective experiences of those affected are important considerations.

To identify this latter perspective as an exclusively feminine discourse is inaccurate, but there is some evidence to support the argument that it is a position more commonly adopted by women than men. The most significant example of this derives from what has become known as the Kohlberg–Gilligan controversy. Laurence Kohlberg (1973) proposed a developmental system of moral development, as presented in Table 13.2. His systematic and rational exposition of moral development is typical of that approach which is characterised by an attempt to apply objective and empirical thinking to the understanding of moral and ethical issues. This device, using rational arguments, empirical evidence and scientific methods, is what we

earlier referred to as a naturalistic approach. It contrasts with the non-naturalistic perspective which views ethics and its concerns as not amenable to such analysis. However, Carol Gilligan (1977, 1982), who had been a student of Kohlberg, noted that all his subjects were male and in her own research on female subjects she identified a different way of thinking and moral decision-making that essentially reflects the ethics of caring in relation as described in this section (her research publication was, significantly, entitled *In a Different Voice*). Her female subjects tended not to operate in terms of general or universal rules and maxims, but saw the moral problems they encountered as highly contextualised situations in which they responded empathetically to the individuals with whom they were relating.

It will be seen that the controversy involved here is at its core a conflict between what Mary Midgley (1983) described as ethics of the mind and ethics of the heart. That is, a conflict between a view that ethics can be resolved as if the issues at stake are akin to factual knowledge of the natural world, through rational, problem-solving approaches; and, the alternative view that such issues are different and can only be

Table 13.2 Kohlberg's stages of moral development

Level A	Pre-conventional
Stage 1	The stage of punishment and obedience. One obeys in order to avoid being punished.
Stage 2	The stage of instrumental purpose and exchange. The objective is to advance own interests.
Level B	Conventional
Stage 3	The stage of mutual interpersonal relationships and conformity. Doing what is right is conforming to the expectations of close ones, to obtain their approval.
Stage 4	The stage of social system and conscience maintenance. Doing what is right is being loyal to particular social institutions and meeting duties and obligations to these entities.
Level C	Post-conventional – the level of principle
Stage 5	The stage of prior rights and social contract. It is acknowledged that there are values and rights which must be upheld in any society or social institution. Here society is the source of what is right, and this in turn is based on the greatest good for the greatest number.
Stage 6	The stage of universal ethical principles. There are universal ethical principles which all should follow, and which take precedence over all legal, institutional and social obligations. One does the right thing because this is the rational and reasonable thing to do in all situations.

(From Kohlberg, 1973)

approached intuitively or at the level of emotional response to real people in real situations. There are, of course, the critics on each side. Those who subscribe to an ethics of the heart point to such weaknesses in ethics of the mind as the naturalistic fallacy which we discussed earlier, and sometimes also in terms of gender bias (as in the Kohberg–Gilligan controversy). Those who subscribe to an ethics of the mind point to such weaknesses in ethics of the heart as its extreme contextuality, lack of universal application, and failure to withstand rational argument. Indeed, Seedhouse (2000) suggests that philosophy (of which the study of ethics is a part) is characteristically an analytical discipline, devoted to the use of logic and rational argument to clarify issues. He argues that, in general, nursing has failed to address *its* philosophical concerns at this level, and (as a rule) promulgates 'philosophies of life' fashionable among a small group of nursing philosophers. Paradoxically, when he proceeds to present cases that are critical of, for example, the caring dimension in nursing, his arguments discount such concepts as care and intuition without a depth of analysis in respect of such matters as the ontological and tacit dimensions of these concepts. Indeed, it has been suggested that Seedhouse's own approach to ethics is also of a particular analytical persuasion that seems to emphasise a naturalistic approach, seeing ethical matters as those that can be resolved through similar rational arguments to those seeking explanations of the natural or physical world (Cassell, 1998). In doing so, he excludes fundamental aspects of a deontological perspective that would be essential to a full understanding of such approaches as the ethic of care discussed here. This is also apparent in his own generally admirable text on health care ethics referred to several times in this chapter (Seedhouse, 1998).

Study Activity 13.14

There is no writing to be done in this Study Activity. Instead you are asked to step back from the text for a while, to contemplate and to reflect.

Mothers love their children. There are, of course, the exceptions of the bad mother, of loveless parenting, even of child abuse. But mothers are generally so connected to their children that it might appear to be humanly impossible for a mother to do her child harm. This caring of one person for another exists in different types of relationship. Lovers also appear unable to knowingly harm each other. When this togetherness is destroyed, and when in acts of passion wrong is done, the hurt is compounded by the intimacy of the relationship. One partner says, 'How could he possibly do this to me?'; such is the expectation of non-maleficence in these situations. The implication is, if we care, if we really care for others – our children, our spouses, our friends, or our patients – it is not possible to knowingly do them harm. This is what Simone Weil meant when she spoke of love as an openness, an appreciation and an acceptance of others.

- Think of nursing in these terms. What do we mean when we care for our patients? Is it enough to do things for them and efficiently carry out procedures on them, or is it necessary to relate to them as person-to-person? Is this caring relationship in nursing itself a moral position? Does it mean that we must care first before we can be ethically good or right in our dealings with our patients? Contemplate these questions and reflect on your answers to them. They are among the most fundamental and important questions you may ever ask yourself in your nursing career.

Good as a call from the other

In the previous section we identified the possible source of good as being contained in relation, the way in which there is within us an urge to respond to others with care. Prior to that we considered the notion that good is within us, a feature of our humanness, and this indeed may be viewed as a prerequisite for caring in relation. A more existential view of this is to see good as something within the world into which we are thrown and within which we exist as persons.

This is all very different to the earlier view of ethics as being a social construction that we are obliged as part of a social contract to internalise. The fundamental premise here is that a part of this being thrown into the world involves being called to respond to it, and more specifically, to the persons within it.

The idea behind this premise emerges primarily from the writings of two philosophers whose work is remarkably similar, even though there is no evidence that they were aware of each other's positions. In a notable work, the French philosopher Emmanuel Levinas (1981) speaks of the way in which 'the Other' has a call on us, prior to even a face-to-face confrontation with that other. From a similar point of view, the Danish philosopher Knud Løgstrup (1997) proposes that in coming to meet the other they in a sense come into our care. By so doing they make an ethical demand upon us that is present and irrefutable. However, it is not suggested here that the person specifically and explicitly demands something of us (although this may sometimes be the case). It is simply by their mere presence that they constitute a demand. How we respond is, of course, the moral action that transpires. We can choose to take care of this other who is, so-to-speak and in terms of our ethical choices, delivered into our hands. Or we can choose to ignore or even destroy. For Løgstrup, using the terminology of Heidegger (1967), introduced earlier in this chapter, the authentic response is to respond with a caring disposition, the inauthentic response to ignore or even destroy.

Whether we see this as a call from 'the Other' (Levinas) or an 'ethical demand' (Løgstrup), the source of our ethic is the mere or even potential presence of another who has this call upon us. It is not some inner quality, some external social construction, or indeed some quality bestowed by a divine being. It is in effect a condition of how we exist in a world of self and others, a world within which such a demand exists, and where the next person we meet has this demand upon our resources. Dorothy Emmet (1979) illustrated this point when she put the question to

her pupils: 'Can we take moral holidays'. The response of one of her pupils, J. M. Brown (now a senior lecturer at the University of Ulster), was: 'We are not always (actively) on duty, but we are always on call' (Emmet, 1979, p. 143). In one sense this notion of the 'call' is significant. It is in line with the existential view of ethics that we considered in the section on ethical relativism. That is, that first we are called to a concern or care for the world we are thrust into, and second that in the final analysis we are alone in respect of our responsibility to choose.

While there is a fundamental difference between this and caring in relation as we discussed above, there is nevertheless a complementarity at play here. It might be argued that our openness to the ethical demand constituted by the mere presence of the other determines whether our relationship will reflect ethical caring. But the demand the other has upon us precedes our coming face-to-face. As nurses, we can determine how we will respond to those who are delivered into our hands, by calling upon consequentialist, deontological or relational approaches, or indeed by choosing an inauthentic position that *ignores* the ethical demand. But what we cannot do is deny the *existence* of this demand. In the sense meant here, the 'good' (or the call to respond ethically) is thrust upon us by the mere fact of our existence in the world with a free will to respond authentically or with sincere intent, to choose. Conversely, that which we might consider to be the bad, or at least the non-good, is when we choose not to respond with care, to in fact adopt an inauthentic response. At best, this may present as an uncaring nature. But at worst it may present in acts that are seen as of great evil, for if we have no concern for the other there is no block to treating them with indifference or even cruelty for our own pleasure or self-interest.

Good as an emerging discourse

Some of the previous sources of the good discussed above see this originating outside the person. This was the case in respect of the good as a social construct, as a Divine Command, as being in and of our relations with others, or as an existential Ethical Demand. There is a final sense in which we might argue that good emerges externally, from our discourse with others. This is not quite the same as good being a social construction or indeed being a facet of how we relate to others. It is, rather, a position arguing that good or right ethical choices cannot be internal and personal, nor can they be inflexible social constructs or rules. This is in fact a major shift from the premise that ethics can be monological (the idea that a rational and moral individual can arrive at sound ethical choices independently), to the premise that ethics must be collectivist (arrived at through rational discussion between community members, and agreement in each situation). In the case of health care, the community in question would be the major stakeholders, which may include health care professionals, managers, clients and their relations, and perhaps others who might contribute such as health lawyers, chaplains, or professional ethicists.

The main proponents of this perspective are Jurgen Habermas (1984, 1990) and Karl-Otto Apel (1980). They are jointly responsible for the perspective that is identified under labels such as 'discourse ethics' and 'communicative ethics'. The fundamental tenet in this approach is that ethical decisions emerge from discourse involving a group of co-equals capable of presenting their viewpoints in respect of any ethical dilemma. The basis of such discourse ethics includes the requirement that all involved have an equal right to be heard, and the belief that a concensus can and indeed must be reached in relation to what is the good or right choice. We therefore find that in this approach the source of the good is the consensus of a communication group. In this, we find the controversy. First, there is a doubt that some sort of consensus can indeed be reached, i.e. that the ideal communication community that Habermass proposes, committed to mutual respect and consensus, can ever exist. Second, there is the idea that the contract entered into by each individual is something like the following: they are not asked to

change or compromise their own values, but they are asked to accept that the final consensus position is accepted by all involved. This may cut across the idea, held strongly by many, that each person is responsible for their own moral choices and cannot relinquish this to others. One practical way around such difficulties is that suggested by the Woodstock Theological Center (1999). Applying discourse methods to health care ethics, the Woodstock participants developed a formula that aimed for consensus as a means of informing individual ethical choice.

FROM THEORY TO ACTION

Searching for frameworks

Thus far, we have presented various framings for understanding how we arrive at ethical choices. In general, we presented:

- A definition of ethics
- An overview of the main ethical theories
- The dimensions or distinctive features underpinning ethical theories (that essentially give such theories their *structure*)
- The source or essential nature of that which is adjudged good, or right, or virtuous (that essentially identifies the fundamental *content* of ethical theories).

It is useful at this stage to consider again the definition of ethics we proposed: ethics is the study of moral thinking, the values we attach to thoughts or actions; it is also the study of how we determine what we ought to do and what we actually do when we make moral choices.

The latter part of this definition draws attention to a vitally important matter. That is, how we move from ethical thinking to ethical doing; how we in fact put ethics into action in our practice. Broadly speaking, we can approach this in a minimalist or extended frame. Within the minimalist frame we can look to some ready-made system that allows us to deal with ethical decisions. This usually consists of some set of rules or maxims or principles, with or without additional advice on how they may be applied.

Usually rules specify exact prescriptions, maxims are more general statements that guide our conduct, and principles are even broader underlying laws or assumptions about the standards we should adhere to. In other words, all purport to guide our conduct, but at different levels of specificity. Ignoring controversy about the dividing lines, we will treat these all as within the more minimalist, prescriptive frame. The alternative, more extended, frame recognises that real-world ethical issues are by definition difficult and complex, presenting a range of conditions and conflicting calls on our moral choices. Because of this, there is a need for a more eclectic approach that allows for taking account of the variety of issues to be addressed. In addressing these two approaches, we are not presenting alternatives, because by definition an eclectic approach will encompass an ethic of principles. Also, because we are concerned with how nurses cope with their ethical choices, we present the more minimalist approach under the heading of professional ethics, which in most instances and certainly in nursing, have emerged as sets of ethical principles or rules.

Professional ethics

In the context of professional practice, therefore, practical ethics become professional ethics, a set of shared professional viewpoints pertaining to ethical standards. In most cases, these views are represented by a written code, which acts as guiding principles to the members of the profession.

One example of such a code is that of the International Council of Nurses, with membership being that of the nursing organisations of most countries in the world. The International Council of Nurses has an agreed Code of Ethics for Nurses. This presents general statements about how the nurse should behave in respect of people, practice, the profession, and co-workers. For example, the second of these, relating to practice, states:

> The nurse carries personal responsibility and accountability for nursing practice, and for

> maintaining competence by continual learning.
>
> The nurse maintains a standard of personal health such that the ability to provide care is not compromised.
>
> The nurse uses judgement regarding individual competence when accepting and delegating responsibility.
>
> The nurse at all times maintains standards of personal conduct which reflect well upon the profession and enhance public confidence.
>
> The nurse, in providing care, ensures that use of technology and scientific advances are compatible with the safety, dignity and rights of people.
>
> (International Council of Nurses, 2000)

Another such example is that of the Code of Professional Conduct issued by the Nursing and Midwifery Council in the UK (Nursing and Midwifery Council, 2002). Unlike the International Council of Nurses' code, this is the code issued by the UK regulatory body for nurses and midwives, and as such carries a statutory authority. Breaching the International Council of Nurses' code is breaking a professional undertaking given by a member body of the International Council of Nurses (which in the UK is the Royal College of Nursing). There is no legal imperative, and many nurses are not even in membership of these bodies. However, breaching the Code of Professional Conduct is breaching conditions of professional registration or licensure that have a legal obligation, and could lead to removal of the right to practise.

The Code of Professional Conduct (Nursing and Midwifery Council, 2002) covers clusters of principles that extend beyond the four areas identified by the International Council of Nurses. There are seven such areas:

> As a registered nurse or midwife, you are personally accountable for your practice. In caring for patients and clients, you must:
>
> • respect the patient or client as an individual;

- *obtain consent before you give any treatment or care;*
- *protect confidential information;*
- *co-operate with others in the team;*
- *maintain your professional knowledge and competence;*
- *be trustworthy;*
- *act to identify and minimise risk to patients and clients.*

These are the shared values of all the United Kingdom healthcare regulatory bodies.

(Nursing and Midwifery Council, 2002)

The one that is broadly equivalent to the International Council of Nurses' statements on practice is that requiring the nurse or midwife to maintain professional knowledge and competence. Under this heading come the following requirements:

You must keep your knowledge and skills up-to-date throughout your working life. In particular, you should take part regularly in learning activities that develop your competence and performance.

To practice competently, you must possess the knowledge, skills and abilities required for lawful, safe and effective practice without direct supervision. You must acknowledge the limits of your professional competence and only undertake practice and accept responsibilities for those activities in which you are competent.

If an aspect of practice is beyond your level of competence or outside your area of registration, you must obtain help and supervision from a competent practitioner until you and your employer consider that you have acquired the requisite knowledge and skill.

You have a duty to facilitate students of nursing and midwifery and others to develop their competence.

You have a responsibility to deliver care based on current evidence, best practice and,

where applicable, validated research when it is available.

(Nursing and Midwifery Council, 2002)

As will be noted, there are broad similarities between the two sets of practice requirements, but also some differences. This highlights one of the difficulties in identifying ethical demands in terms of rules or admonitions. That is, how to ensure that the rules are both comprehensive and practicable or workable. For example, in the final statement above, there is a responsibility to base care on evidence and validated research, and also best practice. First, in respect of comprehensiveness, it is clear that other forms of knowing are either assumed or not valued. It is vitally important that nursing as a complex caring activity draws on different ways of knowing, as highlighted in the work of Carper (1979), Chinn and Kramer (1999) and others (see Chapter 9). This is reflected in Flaming's (2001) statement that 'using the phrase "research-based practice" … whatever its power and appropriateness, limits practice because other ways of knowing that have already been adopted by the discipline are deemed inferior. This diminution is unfortunate'. On this basis, Flaming (2001) argues that 'practical wisdom' involves more than the application of empirical evidence in practice. Significant among such other ways of knowing is that which Carper and others term the ethical or moral. Nowhere, in this guidance on practice, or indeed elsewhere in the UK code, are requirements in respect of ethical competence and decision-making identified. While it may be argued that this is implicit, why then is it important to make other aspects explicit? Second, in respect of practicality, statements such as this provide insufficient specificity to genuinely guide practice: how, for example, is the nurse to determine what is the 'best practice' she is to be guided by?

Similar difficulties of comprehensiveness and practicality emerge in respect of other clusters of requirements, such as those presented under the heading concerning to 'be trustworthy'. This section of the UK code is devoted almost exclusively to issues such as the 'reputation' of the profession, not promoting or endorsing services or products, not accepting gifts for preferential treatment and not requesting or accepting loans. These are in themselves somewhat problematic. Does this allow nurses to participate in paid-for preferential provision of private health care within public National Health Service facilities, just because the profit is going to other professionals utilising the services to provide such care? Furthermore, are such admonitions sufficient if they are limited to negatives and exclude positives, such as ensuring that the nurse has adequate indemnity or insurance (through employers or otherwise), or protecting patients from others who would indulge in exploitative practices? However, even beyond these difficulties, there is the way in which being trustworthy is being interpreted here. It is interpreted as being almost exclusively pecuniary (i.e. concerning probity or correctness in respect of financial gain). But to be worthy of trust involves much more than matters pertaining to pecuniary gain. It is a matter of being worthy of (and maintaining) the patient's confidence, by virtue of such things as fiduciary practices (honesty and truth telling), assuring them of your ability, and conveying the clear confirmation that you will act in their best interests and in line with their wishes. This is in fact how the equivalent guidance to the medical profession (General Medical Council, 2001) addresses trustworthiness: it is treated predominantly as a relationship issue and sees its breach not exclusively in terms of pecuniary concerns, but in terms of poor relationships, including sexual or improper emotional relationships. There are, of course, other statements in the code that *do* address relational issues, but not explicitly from the perspective of promoting and meriting trust.

The aforementioned comments do not indicate a disaffection or argument against the Code of Professional Conduct (Nursing and Midwifery Council, 2002), or suggest that it is inferior to similar codes from other bodies. In so far as it goes, it is a valuable aid to ethical nursing. However, in keeping with all such sets of rules, maxims or principles, it suffers the weakness of being unable to identify rules or principles for all situations. Additionally, for those it *does* present, there are often contextual influences that make rules difficult to follow, or force the need for choice between rules. Therefore, such codes can be an aid to our ethical decision-making and choices, but they can never provide a comprehensive framework for coping with the complex moral world of health care.

Towards an eclectic framework for ethical practice

So far in this chapter we have addressed a wide range of ethical theories and ethical issues. It is certainly the case that reaching this point has been a long and arduous passage. However, if we are to recognise that all of this is relevant to our practice as not only competent but also moral agents, it is important that we can draw from any and all of these perspectives as appropriate, to ensure that we make the best moral choices. There are, of course, different ways that we can do this, and various frameworks that we can draw upon. For example, Seedhouse (1998), whose work has already been discussed, presents a most useful framework in the form of an ethical grid. However, we have already pointed out that this requires a particular rational approach that may not accommodate that aspect of moral thinking identified as non-rational (based upon such processes as intuition or emotions, or indeed the will of a supernatural being). We have also discussed the so-called Georgetown Mantra, the Four Principles Approach in biomedical ethics. This is perhaps the most commonly used of all frameworks in the health care field. But here also we recognised certain limitations, such as the difficulty of dealing with conflicts between the principles. Finally, we have also considered, in the previous section, the possibility of utilising a code of conduct or ethical code based upon definitive rules, but here also we recognised the limitations in terms of comprehensiveness and practicality within complex moral situations.

The alternative we propose here is a more

eclectic approach that attempts to draw on the best from the various positions we have addressed. This, of course, makes certain assumptions about how realistic it is to attempt to bring together disparate viewpoints that may in fact be incompatible. In this context we can, for example, recall our earlier consideration of Weber's (1991) view that ethics of responsibility (consequentialist ethics) and ethics of conviction (deontological ethics) are irreconcilable and Hare's (1993, 1997) opposing view that this reconciliation is indeed necessary. However, if we accept that we are, as persons in the world, open to all that is within us and all that is outside of us, there is already a unity to our existence as humans. We are not only influenced by our humanness and the call of our inner self, whether we see this as a conscience, or an intuitive knowing of what is right, or an emotional experience by which we *feel* what is the good thing to do. We are also influenced by others and by the consequences of what we do as moral agents and it would be futile to disregard this totally. Keegan and Keegan (1992) refer to this as a *holistic ethic*:

> ... *moral acts may be judged not solely in terms of their intrinsic nature nor solely in terms of their ends, but in both ways ... In addition, one can question the relationship of the act to the present and future of humanity. Through such a construct, holistic ethics is then both deontological and teleological.*
>
> (Keegan and Keegan, 1992, pp. 210–11)

Similarly, in the most recent edition of their seminal text on biomedical ethics, Beauchamp and Childress (2001) adopt a more pragmatic approach. They reject what they call top-down theories (that would include major consequentialist and deontological theories), which attempt the resolution of ethical issues exclusively by applying general rules, laws or principles. They similarly reject what they term bottom-up theories (that would include situation ethics and discourse ethics), which see such resolution as exclusively contextual and not subject to general principles. They argue instead for what they term a *coherence theory* of ethics that integrates these two orientations.

On similar arguments we propose an approach that does in fact draw on the best of the various viewpoints we have surveyed. This is presented here as a sequence or checklist that may aid the nurse in making the best ethical choices. Of course, in reality life is not so uniform and clear-cut: we would move backwards and forwards through the various elements within this sequence, and it is intended to be circular and reflexive rather than linear. In addition, it is a set of proposals that are *suggested* as a means of aiding in ethical decision-making. The approach may be modified to accommodate different ways of working in different situations. In the final analysis, the moral choices we make are our own and in this context it is essential that our framework is one that works for us. Beyond this, it will be noted that each of the elements has been discussed earlier in the chapter.

The eclectic sequence

Accepting the ethical demand
This requires that we recognise and embrace our being in the world as moral agents. In this context, the other has a call on our care, even before that other is present to us.

Committing ourselves to an authentic way of being
As a corollary to the latter orientation, there is a requirement for an intentional concern or care that involves a commitment to *caring about* the people and things in our world. Such intentionality requires an acceptance of the responsibility to attend to rather than ignore, and might be described as an orientation of authenticity or good faith.

Embracing the call to care
Where such an orientation confronts us with the needs of others, we must be prepared to respond

with an intention of *caring for* the other. This requires a decision to move beyond empathy or recognition of the needs and plights of others to a commitment to action.

Entering the relation as a moral agent

In so doing, there is a commitment to a caring relation that is person-to-person rather than contained by constraints of role and procedure. This involves the orientation of *informed moral passion* (Watson, 1990). It is established on the premise that if we really care *for* the other (with passion), we can do no other than consciously act in their best interests (with moral deportment). But it must be recognised that such caring in relation is depleted if it does not encompass the responsibility to bring best knowledge and competence to our intervention (as informed agents of that care).

Listening to the call from within

In making our ethical decisions, we must also attend to our tacit awareness of what we feel or know to be appropriate moral choices. Irrespective of the source of this moral wisdom (whether this is based in some intuitive or emotional sense that is uniquely human, a spiritual force that is within or acting upon us, or a conscience derived from our internalisation of cultural values), we must be sensitive to this call from within.

Attending to the consequences of actions

We must also recognise that all our actions have consequences, for our patients and for others. In considering ethical choices, it *is* important to attend to the possible consequences of our actions. This encompasses a responsibility to rationally seek the best or greatest good in each situation. However, in taking such account it is important that we do not work exclusively on the basis of the ends justifying the means. This requires a balancing of rational consideration of the merits and demerits of actions in terms of their outcomes, with the voice of our own conscience, in recognising that some actions cannot be justified irrespective of our ultimate

goals. That is, we must balance the recognition of valid means to achieve ends with the recognition of those we care for as ends in themselves.

Acquaintanceship with principles that may assist our decisions

In confronting the choices we make, we should make use of established principles that provide a framework for our decisions. Those such as the biomedical ethics framework known as the Four Principles Approach (incorporating beneficence, non-maleficence, respect for autonomy and justice) may provide particularly useful aids in this respect.

Adherence to our code of professional conduct

Similarly, as a member of the nursing profession, we have an obligation to adhere to the 'code of professional conduct' that establishes the regulatory basis for our practice.

Taking full account of the context of our choices

It is nevertheless important that we recognise that the choices we face occur in real-life situations, wherein the situation is more often complex and messy than clear and orderly. Within such contexts, it is often the case that we find principles in conflict, or that the rules of conduct we have depended upon are limited in respect of how they inform our choices. In such situations, we must give consideration to the particular context and how this impacts upon those involved. This involves taking account of the values and aspirations of those in the immediate situation and the wider environmental influences within which the specific situation is framed. We must be open to the need to balance a willingness to apply flexible use of the principles and maxims that inform our practice with the recognition that there are certain fundamental values to which we must hold.

Accepting that there can be no moral choice without moral discourse

The aforementioned contextual orientation draws attention not only to the complexity of the situations within which moral choices must be made, but also plurality of interests that are involved and the onerous responsibility this may place on one individual. It should, therefore, be taken as axiomatic that wherever possible, ethical choices are team choices. That is, the principles, outcomes and contextual features of the particular situation should be the subject of discourse involving the key stakeholders, including, where possible, the patients or clients involved. While the goal should be consensus, this must not be used as a mechanism for everyone relinquishing their personal moral responsibility or for later rejecting accountability for the decisions made. Such discourse must be viewed as a means of exploring the best possible choice and, where all are not clearly in agreement, the final responsibility rests with that individual who is the final moral agent. It is essential that this at least is agreed upon.

Seeking the counsel of our mentors
In such circumstances, it is important that where there are doubts the person with the final responsibility takes time to reflect on the moral choice being contemplated. This may be most usefully facilitated by the availability of a mentor or clinical supervisor. Such reflection and seeking of counsel should take place not only in those circumstances where you as the moral agent have expressed doubts, but also where they are the doubts of others.

Accepting responsibility
As indicated, even within the context of discourse, there is a need to establish moral agency. It must be recognised that there is someone who must accept the role of final moral agent. However, it is important that each of us accepts that there is no total relinquishing of moral responsibility. Each person is making *their* moral choice, even where this is being sought in discourse, and even when others are recognised as the final moral agents. These factors cannot be viewed as a veto on the individual's moral position; this is thrust upon us without the asking and its mere existence makes its relin-

quishment an impossibility. We can never apply a Pontius Pilate mentality that says this is a responsibility of the doctor, or the responsibility for that is in the hands of the administrator, and therefore beyond our control. We are responsible just by merit of association, and always at risk of being guilty by association. It follows from this that where ethical decisions are unacceptable to us, and in strong conflict with the call of our own rational assessment and/or call from conscience, we may be faced with the prospect of supererogatory action. That is, even where all others are in consensus, and even when a recognised final moral agent is involved, we may have to contemplate the possibility of our own individual concerned intervention as a moral agent. Here also, the counsel of a mentor or clinical supervisor may be vital.

Reviewing and reflecting
In the complex area of health care, it is inevitable that new moral challenges will emerge. In addition, the contexts within which ethical dilemmas emerge are paradoxically characterised by their uniqueness. The issues (ranging across such issues as rationing of resources, abortion, HIV/Aids, euthanasia, genetic engineering, etc.) may at one level have a sameness. However, in each instance the context invariably differs and this can have a significant influence on the moral choices that are made. By reflecting upon each instance of moral choice we can not only amass experiential moral wisdom, but also sensitise ourselves to functioning in a world within which contexts and relative values must be balanced with universal principles and core values.

Maintaining reflexivity throughout
This refers to the ways in which a number of influences are constantly at play throughout the ethical decision-making process. It can be seen to operate at a number of levels. First, there is the reflexivity or interplay between the nurse's reflections on the issues throughout the decision-making process, and her deeper reflection on how she is responding; in essence this is a critical reflection of self that questions how we

are interpreting the situation within which we are thrown and wherein we must make our decisions. Second, at another level, there is the reflexivity that is how ethical theory impacts upon the context, and how in turn that context impacts upon the theory. Rawls (1971) described this as a quest for reflective equilibrium, whereby judgements made in context are tested against ethical theories, and the ethical theories are in turn tested in respect of their relevance to the specific situation, until an equilibrium or best fit is achieved. We must be prepared to maintain a responsive critical orientation throughout the decision-making process that consciously calls us to not only fit best theory to circumstances, but also maintains a check on how *we* are responding to the various theoretical and contextual influences. This is not a stage of the ethical decision-making process; rather, it is an orientation that takes us back and forth through stages, and in and out between theory and context so that the process of arriving at our ethical choices is a spiral of discovery. Potentially, such reflexivity can lead us to consider wider contexts or to view specific contexts in different ways. It can also lead us to seek different ways of integrating theoretical perspectives, or indeed to seek and inject new theoretical perspectives that may have the potential to strengthen our ethical choices.

Study Activity 13.15

This final Study Activity may assist you in reviewing the eclectic framework presented above, and at the same time summarise important issues addressed throughout the chapter.

- First, re-read the eclectic framework. For each section make brief notes identifying what theoretical elements within the chapter underpin the proposed actions.
- Seek out the relevant passage in the chapter that you feel presents the underpinning features you have identified, and re-read this to confirm or modify your opinions.
- Finally, re-read the eclectic sequence again, this time in a more critical mode. Identify what you feel

are the main strengths and any weaknesses, and reflect upon how the weaknesses might be overcome.

SUMMARY

In this chapter, the fundamental importance of ethics to the practice of nursing was addressed in detail. Ethics was presented as a subject dealing with moral thinking and action that relates to decisions of good versus bad and right versus wrong. Major theories that purport to facilitate ethical thinking and action were addressed, and the dimensions, strengths and weaknesses of such theories were addressed. Attention was also given to the sources of that which we consider to be the good (or right, or virtuous).

In the final sections of the chapter we considered what might essentially be termed practical ethics. That is, how we move from ethical thinking and theorising to ethical doing or the making of moral choices. In this respect it became apparent that while each 'theoretical' perspective has its strengths, none would meet the test of guiding ethical decision-making in all circumstances. On this basis, an eclectic approach was proposed. This has three main features. First, it proposes an orientation within which elements of different theories may be brought to bear on our ethical practice. Second, it emphasises the importance of how context is important, and in particular recognises the influence of context on how theory is applied, and the influence of theory on how context is interpreted. Third, it encompasses a reflexive orientation that allows for critical appraisal across a number of dimensions, even to the extent that new sources of insight may be sought and inserted in the framework, in response to the specific nature of ethical demands.

In this extensive chapter, this book says almost all it has to say on the issue of ethics and nursing. It is indeed extensive, and in places complex. This is necessary. It is important that a composite statement can be made that shows not only the diverse positions but also how they can be brought together to inform our practice. To fragment this topic across chapters or attempt brevity at the cost of clarity would fail.

From this point, as a student or nurse you proceed into the field. In a highly charged and technological health care system, it may be easy in the day-to-day bustle to forget the moral dimension. However, this is constantly being thrust upon us, and at each moment we may be called to respond. In the most recent edition of their celebrated seminal text, Beauchamp and Childress (2001) end their book with this final sentence:

> *The more general (principles, rules, theories etc.) and the more particular (case judgments, feelings, perceptions, practices, parables, etc.) are integrally linked in our moral thinking, and neither should have pride of place.*
>
> (Beauchamp and Childress, 2001, p. 408)

We also have proposed an eclectic framework that advocates integrity and reflexivity, drawing on the strengths of a variety of theoretical perspectives. But we do, unlike Beauchamp and Childress, see a pride of place in all of this. This is encompassed in the commitment to care that is fundamental to our profession, and that is contained in the first four elements of our eclectic framework presented above. It claims that it is a part of our humanness that we are called to care. It is this call that is the core of our ethic. As Knud Løgstrup (1997) has stated:

> *The demand asks us to take care of whatever in the other person's life has been placed in our hands, regardless of whether he or she is one of our loved ones or a stranger, and regardless of the manner in which he or she has been placed in our hands.*
>
> (Løgstrup, 1997, p. 45)

If we respond authentically to this demand, with concern, compassion and commitment, with appropriate knowledge and skill to make our helping a genuine helping, and a willingness to harness other ethical perspectives to assist our deliberations, our moral choices will always be for the best interests of those in our care. This is what it means to be a nurse.

REFERENCES

Apel, K.-O. (1980) The *a priori* of the communication community and the foundations of ethics: the problem of the rational foundation of ethics in the scientific age. In: Apel, K.-O. (ed.) *Towards a Transformation of Philosophy* (trans. G. Adey and D. Frisby), Routledge and Kegan Paul, London

Argyris, M. and Schön, D. (1974) *Theory in Practice: Increasing professional effectiveness*, Jossey-Bass, London

Ayer, A.J. (1936) *Language, Truth and Logic*, Gollancz, London

Beauchamp, T. (1994) The 'Four Principles' approach. In: Gillon, R. (ed.) *Principles of Health Care Ethics*, John Wiley, Chichester

Beauchamp, T. and Childress, J. (1979) *Principles of Biomedical Ethics*, Oxford University Press, New York

Beauchamp, T. and Childress, J. (1983) *Principles of Biomedical Ethics* (2nd edn), Oxford University Press, New York

Beauchamp, T. and Childress, J. (1989) *Principles of Biomedical Ethics* (3rd edn), Oxford University Press, New York

Beauchamp, T. and Childress, J. (1994) *Principles of Biomedical Ethics* (4th edn), Oxford University Press, Oxford

Beauchamp, T. and Childress, J. (2001) *Principles of Biomedical Ethics* (5th edn), Oxford University Press, New York

Bellah, R., Madsen, R., Sullivan, W. *et al.* (1985) *Habits of the Heart: Individualism and commitment in American life*, University of California Press, Berkeley, CA

Bloom, A. (1987) *The Closing of the American Mind*, Simon and Schuster, New York

Carper, B.A. (1979) The ethics of caring. *Advances in Nursing Science* 1(3), 11–19

Cassell, J. (1998) Against medical ethics: opening the can of worms, *Journal of Medical Ethics* 24, 8–12

Chadwick, R. (1993) Justice in priority setting. In: *Rationing for Health*, BMJ Publishing, London

Childress, J. (2000) Bioethics on the brink of a new millennium. In: Kearon, K. and O'Ferrall, F. (eds) *Medical Ethics and the Future of Healthcare*, The Columba Press, Blackrock, Eire

Chinn, P.L. and Kramer, M.K. (1999) *Theory and Nursing: Integrated knowledge development* (5th edn), Mosby, St Louis, IL

Copleston, F.C. (1955) *Aquinas*, Pelican, London

Dickoff, J. and James, P. (1968) A theory of theories: a position paper. *Nursing Research* 1(1), 13–23

Dorkeno, E. (1994) *Cutting the Rose. Female genital mutilation: the practice and its prevention*, Minority Rights Publications, London

Dworkin, R. (1977) *Taking Rights Seriously*, Duckworth, London

Elhauge, E. (1994) Allocating health care morally. *California Law Review* 82, 1492–510

Emmet, D. (1966) *Rules, Roles and Relations*, Macmillan, New York

Emmet, D. (1979) *The Moral Prism*, Macmillan, London

EuroQol Group (1990) EuroQol – a new facility for the measurement of health-related quality of life. *Health Policy* 16(3), 199–208

Flaming, D. (2001) Using *phronesis* instead of 'research-based practice' as the guiding light for nursing practice. *Nursing Philosophy* 2, 251–8

Fletcher, J. (1966) *Situation Ethics*, SCM Press, London

Fox, M. (1990) *A Spirituality Named Compassion – and the healing of the global village, Humpty Dumpty and us*, Harper, San Francisco, CA

Gaita, R. (1991) *Good and Evil: An absolute conception*, Macmillan, Basingstoke

Gaylin, W. (1976) *Caring*, Alfred A. Knopf, New York

General Medical Council (2001) *Good Medical Practice* (3rd edn), General Medical Council, London

Gilligan, C. (1977) In a different voice: women's concepts of self and morality. *Harvard Educational Review* 47(4), 481–517

Gilligan, C. (1982) *In a Different Voice*, Harvard University Press, Cambridge, MA

Gillon, R. (1985) *Philosophical Medical Ethics*, John Wiley, Chichester (for *British Medical Journal*)

Gillon, R. (1994) Preface: medical ethics and the four principles. In: Gillon, R. (ed.) *Principles of Health Care Ethics*, John Wiley, Chichester

Green, F.L. (1945) *Odd Man Out*, Michael Joseph, London

Greene, M. (1990) The tensions and passions of caring. In: Leininger, M.M. and Watson, J. (ed.) *The Caring Imperative in Education*, National League for Nursing, New York

Habermas, J. (1984) *A Theory of Communicative Action*, Beacon Press, Boston, Mass

Habermas, J. (1990) Discourse ethics. In: Habermas, J. (ed.) *Moral Consciousness and Communicative Action*, MIT Press, Boston, Mass

Hanson, K. (1999) *Gender, Burden of Disease, and Priority Setting Techniques in the Health Sector*, Harvard Center for Population and Development Studies, Cambridge, Mass

Hare, R.M. (1993) Universal prescriptivism. In: Singer, P. (ed.) *A Companion to Ethics*, Blackwell, Oxford

Hare, R.M. (1997) *Sorting Out Ethics*, Clarendon Press, Oxford

Heidegger, M. (1967) *Being and Time*, Basil Blackwell, Oxford

Heller, J.G. (2002) Will public health survive QALYs? *Canadian Journal of Clinical Pharmacology* 9(1), 2–4

Hunt, G. (1992) Project 2000: ethics, ambivalence and ideology. In: Slevin, O. and Buckenham, M. (eds) *Project 2000: The teachers speak*, Macmillan, Edinburgh

International Council of Nurses (2000) *The ICN Code of Ethics for Nurses*, International Council of Nurses, Geneva

Johnstone, M.-J. (1994) *Bioethics: A nursing perspective* (2nd edn), W.B. Saunders, Sydney

Kant, I. ([1781] 1938) *The Fundamental Principles of the Metaphysic of Ethics*, Appleton-Century-Crofts, New York

Keegan, L. and Keegan, G.T. (1992) A concept of holistic ethics for the health professional. *Journal of Holistic Nursing* 10, 13

Kennedy, I. (Chairman) (2001) *Learning from Bristol: The report of the public inquiry into children's heart surgery at the Bristol Royal Infirmary 1984–1995*, Command Paper: CM 5207, HMSO, London

Kohlberg, L. (1973) *Collected Papers on Moral Development and Moral Education*, Harvard University, Cambridge, MA

Kohlberg, L. (1981) *The Philosophy of Moral Development*, Harper and Row, San Francisco, CA

Leininger, M.M. (1990) *Ethical and Moral Dimensions of Care*, Wayne State University Press, Detroit, IL

Levinas, E. (1981) *Otherwise than Being or Beyond Essence* (trans. A. Lingus), Nijhoff, The Hague

Løgstrup, K. (1997) *The Ethical Demand*, University of Indiana Press, Notre Dame, IN

MacIntyre, A. (1985) *After Virtue*, Duckworth, London

Mackie, J.L. (1977) *Ethics: Inventing right and wrong*, Penguin Books, New York

Mayeroff, M. (1971) *On Caring*, Harper and Row, New York

Midgley, M. (1983) *Heart and Mind: The varieties of moral experience*, Methuen, London

Mill, J.S. (1969) Utilitarianism (1863). In: Robson, J.M. (ed.) *J S Mill – Collected works*, Vol. 10, University of Toronto Press, Toronto

Moore, G.E. (1903) *Principia ethica*, Cambridge University Press, Cambridge

Murdoch, I. (1970) *The Sovereignty of Good*, Routledge and Kegan Paul, London

Noddings, N. (1984) *Caring: A feminine approach to ethics and moral education*, University of California Press, London

Nursing & Midwifery Council (2002) *Code of Professional Conduct*, Nursing and Midwifery Council, London

Rawls, J. (1971) *A Theory of Justice*, Harvard University Press, Cambridge, MA

Reed, C. (1947) *Odd Man Out*. Image Entertainment (UK).

Sartre, J.-P. (1993) The humanism of existentialism. In: Sartre, J.-P. (ed.) *Essays in Existentialism*, Citadel Press, New York

Seedhouse, D. (1998) *Ethics: The heart of health care*, John Wiley, Chichester

Seedhouse, D. (2000) *Practical Nursing Philosophy: The universal ethical code*, John Wiley, Chichester

Shaw, G.B. (1903) Maxims for revolutionists. In: Shaw, G.B. (ed.) *Man and Superman*, Constable, London

Smith, A.D. (1985) The self and the good. *Proceedings – The Aristotelian Society* LXXXV, 101–17

Taylor, C. (1991) *The Ethics of Authenticity*, Harvard University Press, Cambridge, MA

Thiroux, J.P. (1980) *Ethics, Theory and Practice*, Glencoe Press, Encino, CA

Tschudin, V. (1992) *Ethics in Nursing – The caring relationship*, Butterworth Heinemann, Oxford

Van Hooft, S. (1995) *Caring: An essay in the Philosophy of Ethics*, University Press of Colorado, CO

Watson, J. (1988) Introduction: an ethic of caring/curing/nursing qua nursing. In: Watson, J. and Ray, M. (eds) *The Ethics of Care and the Ethics of Cure*, National League for Nursing, New York

Watson, J. (1990) Caring knowledge and informed moral passion. *Nursing Science Quarterly* 13(1), 15–24

Weber, M. ([1919] 1991) Politics as a vocation or dead sociologists society. In: Weber, M. *From Max Weber*, Routledge, London

Weil, S. (1952) *Gravity and Grace* (trans. E. Crawford), Routlege and Kegan Paul, London

Weinstein, M.C. and Stason, W.B. (1977) Foundations of cost-effectiveness analysis for health and medical practices. *New England Journal of Medicine* 296, 716–21

Williams, A. (1985) The value of QALYs, *Health and Social Science Journal* 94, (4967) [Supplement]

Williams, A. (1995) *The Role of the EuroQol Instrument in QALY Calculations: Discussion paper 130*, Centre for Health Economics, University of York, York

Williams, A. (1997) *Being Reasonable about the Economics of Health*, Edward Elgar, Cheltenham

Wong, D. (1993) Relationism. In: Singer, P. (ed.) *A Comparison to Ethics*, Blackwell, Oxford

Woodstock Theological Center (1999) Ethical issues in managed health care organisations. *Woodstock Report, March 1999*, 57, Georgetown University Press, Washington DC

Yeo, M. and Ford, A. (1991) Integrity. In: Yeo, M. (ed.) *Concepts and Cases in Nursing Ethics*, Broadview Press, Ontario

14 Nursing models and theories: major contributions

Oliver Slevin

> *If the purpose of scientific method is to select from among a multitude of hypotheses, and if the number of hypotheses grows faster than the scientific method can handle, then it is clear that all hypotheses can never be tested. If all hypotheses cannot be tested, then the results of any experiment are inconclusive and the entire scientific method falls short of its goal of establishing proven knowledge.*
>
> *About this Einstein had said, 'Evolution has shown that at any given moment out of all conceivable constructions a single one has always proved itself absolutely superior to the rest', and let it go at that. But to Phaedrus that was an incredibly weak answer. The phrase 'at any given moment' really shook him. Did Einstein really mean to state that truth was a function of time? To state that would annihilate the most basic presumption of all science!*
>
> *But there it was, the whole history of science, a clear story of continuously new and changing explanations of old facts. The time spans of permanence seemed completely random, he could see no order in them. Some scientific truths seemed to last for centuries, others for less than a year.*
>
> (Pirsig, 1974)

LEARNING OUTCOMES

After studying this chapter you will be able to:

- Define the terms 'model' and 'theory', by highlighting claimed similarities and differences between the terms
- Discuss different views on the relationship between theory, science and research
- Explain the controversy surrounding the notions of a theory of and a theory for nursing
- Relate the debate on theory of-theory for nursing to the notions of simultaneity and totality theories of nursing
- Describe the structure of nursing knowledge and practice by demonstrating the linkages between different forms of knowledge and their relationship to practice
- Identify a theoretical framework that may provide a flexible and responsive approach to guiding practice in complex and rapidly changing health care systems.

INTRODUCTION

As we come to the final chapter in this module, we are approaching an important point of transition. In a rather simplified sense, this might be viewed as the point of linkage between theory and research. More specifically, it concerns thinking and action. It is often claimed that science (including *nursing science*) involves two processes: an internal, or thinking, or reflective, or theorising process whereby we attempt to make sense of the world, to explain the phenomena and processes we observe; and, an action or empirical process whereby we attempt to establish by observation, measurement, manipulation of variables, etc., whether or not our descriptions, explanations or predictions hold true in the real world. According to one argument, these are interrelated activities that together are necessary in helping us to make sense of the world.

This need to bring understanding and order to our knowledge of the world was well described by Carl Rogers (1961) when he stated that:

I have come to see both scientific research and the process of theory construction as being aimed toward the inward ordering of significant experience. Research is the persistent, disciplined effort to make sense and order out of the phenomena of subjective experience. It is justified because it is satisfying to perceive the world as having order, and because rewarding results often ensue when one understands the orderly relationships which appear in nature.

So I have come to recognise that the reason I devote myself to research, and to the building of theory, is to satisfy a need for perceiving order and meaning, a subjective need which exists in me.

(Rogers, 1961)

In nursing it is important that we construct valid and reliable knowledge which can be brought to bear on our work. In the earlier chapters of this module we considered the various types of knowing which we often utilise in arriving at the sound *knowledge* and *understanding* which guides our practice. In this final chapter we consider how this knowledge and understanding (or some of it) is built into theory and models that guide practice. This leads us naturally to the next module, within which in one sense we move from theorising to action – the empirical dimension that we considered under the chapter on empirical ways of knowing in this module.

ESTABLISHING THE PARAMETERS

In the opening quotation to this chapter, Pirsig speaks of the purpose of the scientific method as being to choose between a multitude of hypotheses. The term hypothesis means a tentative explanation for a phenomenon used as a basis for further investigation, or a statement that is assumed to be true for the sake of argument (at least until there is sufficient evidence to discount it). There are particular technical ways of working with hypotheses, and we return to these when we discuss research in the next module. However, if for now we stay with the level of

generality at which Pirsig speaks, we see that this term relates to how we attempt to make sense of the world. It concerns how we attempt to describe, explain or make predictions about what we see or experience. This is what Rogers (1961) also meant when he wrote about 'an effort to make sense and order out of the phenomena of subjective experience'.

Before proceeding it is useful to return to the opening quotation from Pirsig once again. He speaks about a 'multitude' of hypotheses, the rapid growth of these, and their transient nature (the speed with which they may be discounted and replaced). This is no less the case in nursing. Here also hypotheses (and theories and models) are introduced with great regularity and in constantly increasing numbers. Indeed, in the first edition of this book (Basford and Slevin, 1995) we devoted two chapters to North American and European nursing models or theories (presenting ten of the former and six of the latter). In the current edition, we do not do this for two main reasons, as outlined below.

First, the plethora of 'nursing' models and theories has increased to such an extent that even a whole book devoted to a presentation and critique of these could only address a fraction of the total. There are a number of brave attempts at doing this, but they are characterised by an excessive reliance on North American examples and by different choices in respect of what to include. Furthermore, it is often difficult to establish their real value or whether they have simply become 'known' through being spread by influential sources – what McKenna (1997) and others have described as 'the circle of contagiousness'. For background reading, you are referred to four influential texts (two from the UK and two from the USA), as detailed in Table 14.1.

Second, there are increasing concerns among nursing scholars and practitioners about the relevance and applicability of many of these models and theories to the complex modern world of nursing practice. In this respect, while there is an ever-increasing number of these, the results of research and the experience of practice have

Table 14.1 Seminal texts on theories and models

Authors	Country of publication	Total number of models/theories addressed	Number of UK models/theories included
McKenna (1997)	UK	19	1
Aggleton and Chalmers (2000)	UK	10	2
Fawcett (2000)	USA	7	0
Alligood and Marriner-Tomey (2002)	USA	16	1

failed to show an emerging and cohesive body of theory that is accepted within nursing and at the same time has been proven to be effective in sustaining high quality in nursing care. Meleis (1997) has pointed out that while a large number of these models or theories emerged in the last quarter of the twentieth century, nurses often chose to ignore them as largely irrelevant to their practice, even before they became licensed to practice and left the nursing colleges where such theories and models were being taught! Noak (2001) has expressed similar concerns in respect of the UK. Indeed, some nursing scholars (e.g. McCloskey and Bulechek, 2000) have suggested the need for a 'clearance' of these multifarious and inconsistent (if not indeed in some cases incompatible) attempts to establish a theoretical foundation. The argument put forward by such sources sometimes recommend alternative ways of organising nursing that is in fact *atheoretical,* proposing instead some managerialist categorisation of nursing work. We find here the vocabulary of nursing diagnosis (Carpenito, 1995; North American Nursing Diagnosis Association, 1999) and initiatives intent on developing local or international classifications of nursing practice activities (International Council of Nurses, 2002). The language moves away from terms such as model and theory, much favoured by nursing academics, to terms such as diagnosis and treatment, much favoured by medicine and those supportive of more standardised managed care orientations. Such positions have one strong argument in their favour. The state of nursing 'theory' is indeed to an extent in a state of disarray that requires serious attention. There is a need to address this

unsatisfactory state of affairs. However, to suggest a solution that moves away from a theory base may have at least three major disadvantages:

- In a modern health care system that increasingly demands evidence-based practice approaches, the suggestion that nursing turns away from science is a dangerous proposition. There is, of course, an assumption here that an evidence base implies a scientific approach, and that in turn theory is a part of this. This is a matter we return to below.

- As a corollary to the latter point, it is argued – most famously be Kuhn (1970) – that a discipline is characterised by a shared theoretical paradigm or worldview that guides its theoretical development. Rather than turning away from our theoretical problems, there is a need to welcome and explore the range of theoretical viewpoints. This may allow us to aim for a degree of synthesis that enhances our capacity to respond to complex health care systems, that in fact demands theories that are also complex and multifaceted.

- As an extension of the latter point, it might even be argued that in such a complex system, and within a complex occupation that requires its practitioners to respond at different levels and in different ways, the only sensible approach is that of eclecticism. That is, that nursing should be eclectic in developing and utilising *a range* of theoretical perspectives, fitting these to changing demands, as the occasion requires.

In this chapter we discuss major contributions to the *issue* of models and theories, *not* specific examples of such frameworks. The goal is not to help you in respect of understanding specific models or theories, thereby omitting many of these by necessity. Rather, it is intended that you will be armed with knowledge of major contributions in respect of the theory *issue*. In addressing issues *about* nursing theory, a process Meleis (1997) describes as *metatheory*, the aspiration is that you will be able to critically address theoretical approaches encountered in practice. We are aiming here for flexible and responsive tools for responding to the need for practice-guiding theory, not a commitment to any specific theoretical perspective.

THEORIES AND MODELS

Interchangeability or difference

The study of nursing, and indeed the practice of nursing itself, is increasingly influenced by what are termed nursing theories and models. Indeed, if you have already had practice placements or fieldwork experience you may have encountered nursing situations where practice is supposedly based on a particular theory or model of nursing. Therefore, it is important to define these two terms and to establish real or imagined differences between them. Rarely have any other two terms in the study of nursing led to more controversy or confusion.

The nursing literature is characterised by authors who adopt differing and often conflicting stances on this issue. Fawcett (1993, 2000) suggests that models, or what she terms conceptual models, are more abstract entities than theories. She suggests that knowledge occurs in the following sequence of abstraction, from the very abstract to the more concrete:

- metaparadigm (also discussed in the first chapter of this module)
- conceptual model
- theory
- empirical indicator (proposition or hypothesis – introduced above).

Others, such as Meleis (1997) and Chinn and

Kramer (1999), suggest that the terms theory and model are similar and overlapping if not indeed synonymous. Thus, Meleis (1997) states that:

> *The perspective of this text is to minimise the differences between conceptual models, frameworks, and theories and to relegate most of these differences to semantics and the confusion created by the many nursing scientists and theoreticians who have been educated in a multitude of fields. The rationale for taking this perspective is not to argue for a new position or to initiate a debate, but rather to cast some doubt on the significance of the differences between theories and conceptual models.*
>
> (Meleis, 1997, p. 139)

One can perhaps understand the stance taken by Meleis when it is noted that some (e.g. Kaplan, 1964, 1973) suggest (differently to Fawcett) that models are less abstract than theories in that they describe reality more fully. Indeed, the literature addressing the meanings of these terms is a quagmire of confusing and contradictory statements. It is important to recognise this fact in the first place and to cast a critical eye on those statements which attempt to clarify the situation in the sections which follow.

Study Activity 14.1

As a preparation for the next section, select one of the books in Table 14.1 (page 257). If you cannot find one of these in your library, search for a suitable alternative.

- Write a brief definition of the two terms 'model' and 'theory'.
- Select two models or theories – if possible one UK example and one North American example – and write a brief paragraph describing each. Do not spend too much time attempting to differentiate between 'model' and 'theory': we shall address this later. Retain your written notes, as we shall refer back to these later.

Models

Despite the confusion which reigns in this area, what almost everyone concedes is that a model is a reflection or a representation of reality rather than reality itself. Such representations are valuable for studying the real world, and in academic work this is their main function. They assist us in understanding reality. Thus, in what is probably the definitive academic treatise on the topic of models, Abraham Kaplan (1964, 1973) defines a model as follows:

> *Broadly speaking, we may say that any system A is a model of system B if the study of A is useful for the understanding of B without regard to any direct or indirect causal connection between A and B.*
>
> (Kaplan, 1973)

What Kaplan is suggesting is that while there must be similarities in form and structure between the model (A) and the reality (B), there does not have to be any direct connection between them, and they do not even have to resemble each other in content or in any physical sense. However, models do in fact sometimes resemble reality. Various types of model are described, but the most common among them are the following.

The physical or isomorphic model

Here the model represents the reality, not only in form and structure, but often in content. Because it is similar in appearance to the real-life object it represents, it is often also called an *empirical model*. Such models do, however, often differ in scale and are usually miniature forms of the real object. Typical examples are model resuscitation dolls, used to train nurses, doctors, and ambulance personnel in skills of cardiac and pulmonary resuscitation. Where such models are used for serious academic study, they are also often fully or partially working models.

The homomorphic model

This model is similar to the isomorphic one in that it is essentially a physical or empirical model. However, here the model builder deliberately leaves out some of the properties of the real object because they are not needed for the purpose for which the model was designed. Thus, scientists researching car accidents may design a model of a human being with a life-like skull but with the remainder of the body consisting of only a wire frame. In so doing, they have deliberately excluded all the complexities of the real object because they are only interested in one facet of reality at that particular time (namely head injuries in motor vehicle collisions).

The symbolic model

Here the model bears no physical resemblance to reality. Numbers or symbols such as shapes or words are used to map out the real situation. While the form and structure of the model follows or represents the original, the content or physical properties of the model do not. Because it does not resemble the real object in any physical sense, but only through words or symbols, this type of model is also sometimes referred to as a *theoretical model*. Fig. 14.1 presents a symbolic model of one version of what is known as the *nursing process method*, a topic which will be addressed in Module 6. It is in fact a model of the application of the

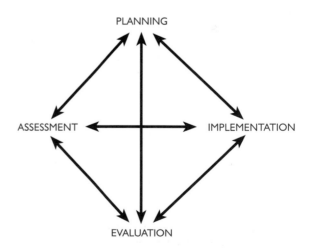

Figure 14.1 The nursing process: a symbolic model

problem-solving process in nursing and presents the interrelated stages of assessment, planning, implementation, and evaluation. It shows that the nurse must first assess the patient's needs, plan nursing action on the basis of this assessment, implement or carry out the planned nursing action, and then evaluate the outcome. By using arrows it also shows that the stages of the nursing process are interrelated, with each activity in the problem-solving process affecting the others.

Here the model is composed of symbols known as words, and arrows which denote a relationship or interactiveness between the words (or what they stand for). These words and arrows *represent* reality, but do not *resemble* nursing in action, and there is no portrayal of the actual nursing activity as it appears in reality. Sometimes the symbolic model is fairly concrete as in Fig. 14.2, which uses boxes, words, and interconnecting lines to present the sociological notion of the nuclear family, consisting of husband, wife, and children. Sometimes, however, as in Fig. 14.1, the elements within the model are more abstract.

The conceptual model

Where symbolic models *are* more abstract, the term conceptual model is used. Conceptual models represent reality through words or symbols but do not resemble it in any real sense. They, like symbolic models, may also be termed theoretical models. Here the words or symbols do not represent mere ideas or perceptions, but concepts. Concepts are constructs produced by abstracting or separating the characteristics of ideas, placing them together in classes or patterns. In so doing, we classify some things as cows, others as chairs, and others as beliefs. A conceptual model is one which reflects reality by placing words which are concepts into the model in the same way that the model aeroplane builder puts wings, a fuselage, and a cockpit together. The example of the nursing process in Fig. 14.1 is such a model; it is symbolic but also conceptual (consisting of concepts). A conceptual model is not just a list of the concepts which occur in some real situation. It must also include symbols (e.g. lines, arrows, or signs) which show how the concepts are interconnected or relate to each other. These lines and signs which link the concepts therefore represent *propositions*, which are claims about the relationships between the concepts. A conceptual model is thus best viewed in terms of the following formula:

Concepts + Propositions = Conceptual model.

There is immediately a definitional problem here. In Chapter 9 we defined a theory as a statement which describes and explains the relation-

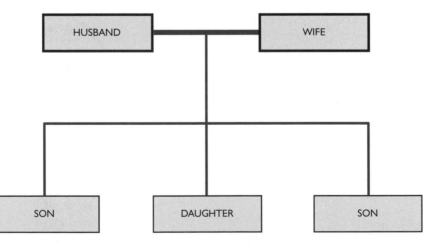

Figure 14.2   The nuclear family: a symbolic model

ships between concepts, and which may also predict how they interact and behave. It will be seen that this is exactly what is now being said in respect of a conceptual model. We have already considered the two main ways in which attempts are made to circumvent this difficulty. One is, for example, according to Fawcett (1993, 2000), to suggest that a conceptual model is at a higher level of abstraction than theory, which is expressed in more descriptive, concrete or real terms, such that it can be readily observed and indeed substantiated through research. The other, for example according to Meleis (1997) and Chinn and Kramer (1999), is to see the terms as essentially similar or inter-changeable. This is a matter we shall return to under theory below.

Nursing models

In the nursing literature it is common to find a specific meaning attached to the term *nursing model*. In one sense the conceptual model presented in Fig. 14.1 is a nursing model. It is a model in that in certain regards it represents or claims to represent aspects of the real situation. More specifically, it addresses aspects of the real situation of *nursing*. However, many do not consider such conceptualisations as true models of nursing. In such instances a very special meaning is attributed to the term *nursing model*.

Nursing models are within a type of conceptual model that applies a conceptual framework to the understanding of nursing and the guiding of nursing practice. It can be seen immediately that, while Fig. 14.1 is also cited as an example of a conceptual model, and while it is presented as an illustration of the nursing process, it is not a *nursing model* in the sense described above. It is simply a model of the problem-solving approach being applied to nursing. It does not physically, symbolically, or schematically represent the reality of nursing as it is or might be thought about and practised in reality.

The idea that a *nursing model* reflects nursing as it occurs in reality is central to the meaning of this term. Thus, drawing from Aggleton and Chalmers (2000), a *nursing* model may have several characteristics, including a representation of:

- the nature of the people receiving (or about to receive) nursing care
- the causes of problems likely to require nursing intervention
- the nature of the assessment process
- the nature of the planning and goal setting process
- the focus of nursing intervention during the implementation of the nursing care plan
- the nature of the process of evaluating the quality and effects of the care given.

Based on this focus on the practice of nursing, McFarlane (1986 p. 3) defines a nursing model as one which 'identifies and defines the factors or phenomena at work in a nursing situation and describes their relationship'.

This may again beg a question in regard to the difference between model, theory, and metaparadigm. As noted earlier in this module, a *metaparadigm* consists of the base elements to which nursing can be reduced. It is meant to be a brief but all-inclusive list of the phenomena that constitute nursing. It will be recalled that one such metaparadigm was that consisting of patient, environment, health, and nursing. Could this then be described as a nursing model in the sense defined by McFarlane? In the first instance, a metaparadigm simply identifies the areas of nursing concern at the *ultimate level* of abstraction. It does not present the relationships between these elements as they may exist in nursing practice. In the second instance, a nursing model, unlike a metaparadigm, is not presented as the total elements of nursing as agreed upon or accepted (or as should be accepted) by the majority of the profession. As Fawcett (1993) states:

> *Examination of the content of various conceptual models reveals that each model reflects the philosophical stance, cognitive orientation, research tradition, and practice modalities of a particular group of scholars within a discipline, rather than the beliefs,*

values, thoughts, research methods, and approaches to practice of all members of that discipline.

(Fawcett, 1993, p. 13)

Thus, while all nurses (or most nurses) *may* share a particular metaparadigm, they may subscribe to different nursing models. Some nurses have modelled nursing care by explaining it in terms of behavioural psychology or human need principles, which they propose should guide nursing action. Others explain it in terms of existential phenomenology. They claim that the complexity of human nature and nursing cannot be reduced to the simple processes of conditioned learning or response to biological, psychological and/or social needs, and that such an approach is a mechanistic and inadequate way of conceptualising what happens in nursing situations.

Thus, it is argued, a metaparadigm is different to a nursing model. The metaparadigm presents concepts or elements that are related to nursing. Indeed, by being stated at a high level of abstraction, it attempts to encompass the totality of nursing's concerns. However, in attaining this level of abstraction, it cannot provide the concrete and specific guidance necessary to guide nursing action. A nursing model is a framework that guides action; a nursing metaparadigm has a very different purpose, to provide a worldview of all that is contained within nursing. However, we *could* suggest that a metaparadigm is a *conceptual* model, in so far as it is a conceptual representation of nursing as a whole. In this sense, it is a second example of that type of conceptual model illustrated in Fig. 14.1, which presents the nursing process as a conceptual model. This begins to sound confusing: there are clearly some conceptual models that are more abstract than others!

It is similarly argued that a nursing model also differs from a theory in so far as a nursing model occupies a level of greater generality and abstraction. A nursing model reflects an attempt only to provide a general conceptual framework which will enhance our understanding of the nursing situation and guide our practice within that situation. In a theory (it is argued) the concepts are less abstract and more reflective of the real world. The links between them are intended to describe relational properties (i.e. to show that the concepts relate to and react to each other in certain ways), explain the nature of these relationships, and to, thus, enable us to predict how the concepts will work in similar situations. A nursing *model* based on behavioural principles may claim that nurse–patient relationships can be understood in terms of the nurse reinforcing patient behaviour, then suggest this as a basis for guiding nursing action, and not go beyond that. There is no attempt to make the concepts and relationships between them more precise or to prove that the relationships exist. The criterion is simply that the model provides a means of understanding nursing practice and that practice based on this understanding actually works. A behavioural *theory*, on the other hand, may state that:

$$\text{Random behaviour} + \text{reward (unconditioned behaviour)} = \text{Increase in that behaviour (conditioned behaviour)}$$

For the theory to be accepted, this relationship between concepts (random or unconditioned behaviour, reward, and conditioned behaviour) must be proven through empirical research.

It should not be assumed, however, that seeing nursing models as broad guiding frameworks is satisfactory to everyone in the world of nursing. Many nursing academics argue strongly that all practice should be based on sound research. They express concern that many nursing models being used in practice have not been tested empirically and that some are so general and abstract that in the form presented they could not be broken down into testable elements at all. The fundamental question is: should untested and untestable frameworks be used to guide nursing practice? There is a considerable degree of strength in this critical stance. It would seem to point to the need to develop models which are less abstract and more amenable to empirical testing. But would such entities be conceptual models of nursing, or would they become theories? We are again left with a difficulty of interpretation. Clearly, at least some people see theory as more concrete than a conceptual model, which (as noted above) is in turn less abstract than the metaparadigm. This is all, of course, a restatement of Fawcett's (1993) classification.

It can thus be seen, on the basis of the various statements above, that *nursing models* in fact possess the following general characteristics:

- They are a form of conceptual model.
- They represent or depict nursing situations in conceptual form.
- By virtue of being *conceptual,* they are at a level of abstraction that is removed from actual reality (for example, the conceptual units would include such notions as patient, homeostasis, human need, nursing problem, and nursing intervention, rather than more concrete and measurable units such as hunger, pain, and body temperature).
- By virtue of being abstract they provide a general framework of the nursing situation in each case rather than specific descriptions of actual nursing situations.
- Their primary function is to assist nurses in understanding the nursing situation and to guide their practice in that situation.

Study Activity 14.2

You may or may not find the above definition of 'nursing model' helpful. The clarity with which a definition is perceived often depends on the mental set of the individual and their style of thinking. Search the literature for three more definitions of the term 'nursing model'. Add these to your personal course notes and compare and contrast them with the definition proposed above.

Theory

We have already stated that a theory is a way of making sense of the world. It is about knowing that, or tentatively knowing that, things in the world are of a particular nature, and relate to each other in particular ways. In the first chapter of this module, we addressed Carper's (1978) patterns of knowing in nursing. Indeed, the subsequent four chapters of the module have each addressed one of Carper's patterns: the empirical, the personal, the aesthetic and the ethical patterns of knowing. In this context, theory is clearly within the cognitive or empirical domain (Chinn and Kramer, 1999). This implies a linkage to, or even containment of, theory within the scientific paradigm, although the term is often used in a much broader or less specialised sense. This is a matter of some controversy: not everyone outside of the sciences is happy about the suggestions that theory is exclusive to that domain and, as we shall see below, not everyone within the science paradigm accepts theory as a relevant scientific concept. By virtue of its complex nature, a brief and succinct definition of the term is difficult. This is witnessed by the plethora of such definitions, each one emphasising particular attributes and sometimes excluding elements considered essential in others. It is thus perhaps useful to consider a more inclusive explicatory statement that attempts to encompass at least most of the important features:

Theory is within the cognitive-empirical domain (Chinn and Kramer, 1999). It is the description or explanation of phenomena and the relationships between such phenomena
(Stevens, 1979)

In essence, our addressing of such phenomena (those things we observe or are conscious of) leads to the formulation of concepts, i.e. symbolic descriptions of how phenomena cluster or merge into meaningful notions. A theory occurs when these concepts are in turn linked by propositions which state relationships between them
(Kim, 1983)

Such statements may go beyond the purely descriptive or explanatory levels, to the level of prediction, where the propositions are of such a nature that they state cause–effect relationships between the concepts

(Alligood and Marriner-Tomey, 2002)

In some instances, it is further recognised that theory has a utility value in that it prescribes our actions

(Meleis, 1997)

A theory thus concerns concepts and the propositions that state relationships between them. In regard to these entities, a theory:

- describes
- explains
- predicts, and sometimes also
- prescribes.

The use of words here is of vital importance. Theory concerns phenomena, which are observable objects or happenings in the real world. In theory we do not just conceptualise phenomena, i.e. describe and categorise them, we also analyse how concepts behave in relation to each other. It can, therefore, be seen that the concepts used in theory are not as abstract as those presented in conceptual models. They have a much closer affinity with the real world. They cannot only be observed and sometimes even measured, but also manipulated so that their influence on other concepts can be observed and analysed. In scientific jargon, one entity (an *independent variable*) is manipulated in some way and the effect of this on another entity (a *dependent variable*) is observed. If changes in the former regularly cause changes in the latter, we can make statements about the relationship between them, and even predictions about how they will relate to each other in the future. Such statements are *predictive theories*, and if they can be made with a high degree of certainty, the theories become *scientific laws*. We consider this particular orientation to theory further when we address research in the next module. However, this linkage, between theory (thinking processes) and scientific activity (research), draws attention to the *process* of theory construction or theorising. Such theo-

rising, as indicated in Fig. 14.3, demonstrates the less abstract and more real world concerns involved. As will be seen, this is a process whereby through perceiving, conceptualising and theorising, we attempt to establish an understanding of the world. However, this is not a linear and closed sequential process. It is a reflexive cycle within which there is a constant moving backwards and forwards: posited theories are tested through theoretical analysis (Chinn and Kramer, 1999; Fawcett, 2000) or research (see next module); concepts are tested through specific concept analysis methods (such as those proposed by Walker and Avant, 1995); and, we constantly test our perception of phenomena by further perception, interobserver checks on reliability, and reflection upon what we are seeing and influences upon our perceptions. This production of cognitive, or propositional, or empirical knowledge is therefore a much more dynamic and ongoing cycle within which we are constantly subjecting our conjectures (theories) to the challenge of refutation (Popper, 1989).

Presenting this theorising process as in Fig. 14.3, with statements, lines and arrows, runs the risk of suggesting a rigid and mechanical process. Indeed, Fig. 14.3 could be taken as another example of that entity that we earlier described as a conceptual model: it is an abstract model of the 'theorising' process. By presenting such an abstraction, what goes on in the real world of theorising can be easily overlooked. However, the innovative and reflexive nature of this process must be emphasised. Good science involves good theory, and this is an insightful and creative process. David Bohm (1998) described this as *imaginative insight*. In the great 'discoveries' of science from Newton through to Einstein, and in the work of Crick and Watson in discovering the structure of DNA, the vital factor was this process of reflection and imagination, leading sometimes in an instant to an insight. The verification of the theory, the empirical testing of it, is almost in a sense an anticlimax. It is difficult to contemplate how anyone could suggest that such theorising is not an essential and vital part of the doing of

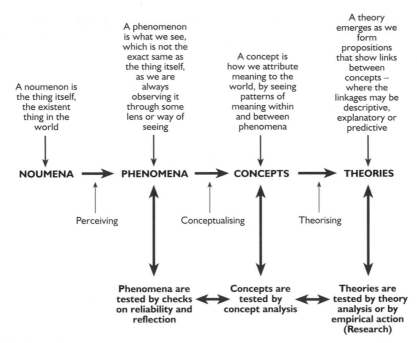

Figure 14.3 The theorising process

science. Yet, as we shall see below, even this has become a matter of dispute.

We have already noted an implied difference between what was earlier defined as a conceptual model and the explanation of theory presented above. Yet, when we consider how the various authorities define these terms, the differences are not immediately apparent and sometimes even confusing. This presents a problem. As we have already seen, one solution suggested by some nursing theorists involves accepting that there is no significant difference between them, or at least that it is not a worthwhile endeavour to nursing to be spending time endlessly debating this issue. Another solution is the suggestion that, as in the case of models, there are different types of theory, some of which *do* equate closely to models and others which are notably different. Merton's (1968) classification of theory is the most notable example. He suggested that theory can be divided into:

- *Grand theory* – a general macro-level theory, composed of abstract concepts in relationship,

which is at a level of abstraction which facilitates description but is not capable of research verification
- *Middle range theory* – composed of less abstract conceptual frameworks, closely aligned to observable reality and thus capable of research verification
- *Micro-theory* – composed of empirical concepts that are observable in reality and capable of research verification. This type of theory can be a research proposition or hypothesis drawn from middle range theory but usually not from grand theory.

While there is a clear difference between middle range theories and conceptual models based on the different levels of abstraction involved, the same cannot be said for grand theories. Here the level of conceptual abstraction is very similar to that involved in conceptual models. We can achieve a degree of clarity by considering the alignment between Merton's classification and that proposed by Fawcett (1993), as illustrated in Fig. 14.4, overleaf.

Fawcett (1993; 2000)   Merton (1968)

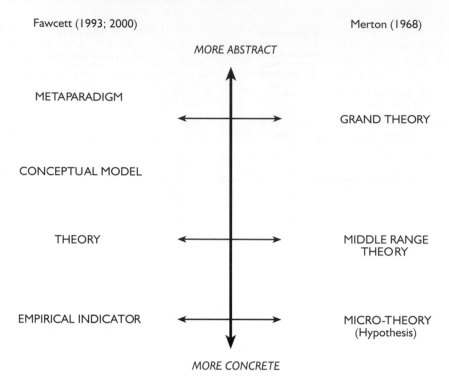

Figure 14.4   The levels of theoretical abstraction

Nursing theory

In line with Fig. 14.4, we can suggest that *nursing* theories can also be at different levels of abstraction. Those that are close to grand theories are similar to nursing models (or even a metaparadigm of nursing), while those which approximate middle range or micro-theory fall at a lower level of abstraction. This line of reasoning throws an entirely different perspective on the arguments surrounding theories and models. If, as suggested earlier, a nursing model is a special type of conceptual model, then such a model is only similar to theory if the theory being referred to is defined as the more abstract form.

It is unlikely, however, that such a rational argument will do much to remove the divisions that exist in the nursing literature regarding theories and models. Some nurses continue to argue against the value of model as a concept.

For example, Peplau (in Barker, 1993) states that:

> *According to my dictionary, a model is 'a facsimile, a miniature representation, a pattern of something to be made, a shape or mould'. I cannot see the vast complexities of a nursing science, or of a service and the people it serves, somehow being fitted into a model thus defined.*
>
> (Peplau, cited in Barker, 1993)

Yet others do subscribe to the notion of nursing models and in doing so do not necessarily subscribe to Peplau's limited definition. This argument in respect of the equivalence of models and theories is complicated by the differences of opinion pertaining to nursing theory. While most nursing academics now recognise the importance of theory *in* nursing, there is a divergence of opinion as to whether this should be theory *for* nursing or theory *of* nursing (*see*, for example, Barrett, 1991). Theory *of* nursing suggests that if nursing is to be an academic and professional discipline in its own right it must have a body of theory unique to itself and derived from its own education, practice, and research. This aspiration is particularly evident in the work of Martha Rogers and her 'science of unitary human beings' (Rogers, 1987). Theory *for* nursing implies that as nursing is an activity which shares broad orientations towards caring or helping with other professions, it is not a pure and unique science, or even a unique service in its own right. From this viewpoint, nursing is an applied science like these other professions. That is, it adapts theory from the various sciences to its own particular purposes. Such theory would be theory *for* nursing.

According to Reilly (1975) it is more important to strive for a synthesis of theory from other disciplines than to attempt to build a new and unique theory. Others have rejected such a viewpoint. For example, as far back as the 1960s authors such as Wald and Leonard (1964) have criticised attempts to apply other scientific disciplines, particularly those of the biological sciences, to nursing on the grounds that they only simplify the complexity of practice and fail to address fundamental nursing issues. However, even the most promising nursing theories presented to date, such as those of Rogers (1987) and Parse (1988, 1992) to some degree reflect creative adaptations of theories from other disciplines, in line with the notion of synthesis explicated by Reilly.

Study Activity 14.3 ──────────

There is a fundamental difference between adapting a theory to nursing and adopting a theory from another discipline. Write down your understanding of the difference between the terms ('adapting' and 'adopting') and list the advantages and disadvantages of each.

On the basis of the above comments, there are clearly areas of fundamental disagreement among nursing scholars, even when the notion of nursing theory is considered. Given this controversy, *nursing* theory should be defined according to its practical relevance, regardless of whether it is adapted or unique to the nursing field:

> *Nursing theory is any theory developed within or adapted to nursing which seeks to describe, explain, or predict relationships between concepts relevant to the practice of nursing, and which may also be used to prescribe or guide nursing actions.*

It should also be noted that there tends to be a fundamental divide in perspective wherever the terms model and theory are used. This relates to the approach being taken. If the aim is to explain how things are by identifying a set of components or elements that make up the situation, then the term 'model' is used. If the aim is to describe that which we are attending to in more holistic terms, as it exists in reality, then the term 'theory' is more appropriate. Kay and Connolly (1981), speaking of how the discipline of psychology studies people, refer to these as mechanistic and humanistic approaches, respectively. Parse (1987) defines this divide within nursing in terms of two opposing worldviews, the *totality paradigm* and the *simultaneity paradigm*.

The totality paradigm

Until recently this view has been the dominant paradigm. It is one which views man as a mechanistic organism who adapts to the environment and strives towards a state of well-being. It is grounded in a natural science perspective and to a lesser extent a social science perspective and has evolved from nursing's close affinity with medicine. Man is seen as a sum of parts which make up the totality and which can be acted upon as parts or a totality of parts. This paradigm is illustrated by the work of nursing scholars such as Orem (1995) and Roy (Roy and Andrews, 1999), who describe their frameworks as *models*.

The simultaneity paradigm

This paradigm operates from a completely different belief system. It sees man as more than the sum of his parts, changing simultaneously with his environment. Man is viewed as a holistic and integrated organism inextricably bound to the experience of his world. This worldview represents a break from the traditional natural and social sciences and often reflects an essentially phenomenological and existential perspective (in terms of how we experience being in the world as a person rather than a sum of parts). Examples of this are to be found in the frameworks of Watson (1997) and Parse (1998), where the terms '*science*' and '*theory*' rather than '*model*' are used.

These two paradigms represent fundamentally distinct worldviews which not only come from different origins but appear to develop along completely separate routes. Those within the totality paradigm continue to develop nursing models which are essentially adaptations of natural or social science theoretical frameworks. They attempt to advance nursing through objective logical-rational approaches. Those within the simultaneity paradigm continue to search for alternatives to what they see as mechanistic and reductionist models of practice. They seek a way forward through new paradigm approaches such as philosophical existentialism and phenomenological scientific perspectives, and they view such notions as *caring* and the *experience of health and illness* as central concepts in the nursing paradigm.

Some, such as Northrup (1992), view these two different worldviews as incompatible, potentially divisive influences in the development of nursing and argue for a unified perspective. Others, such as Barrett (1992), take a more pragmatic view by expressing the opinion that diversity is healthy. They believe that a new worldview of nursing will emerge from the interaction of these different paradigms which will reflect the best of all possible worlds by seeing the individual in his whole *and* in his parts. It is important that you are aware of each of these paradigms, how they are reflected in the various models and theories of nursing, and how each of them has something to say about the central concern of this book – how nursing can and should be practised.

Study Activity 14.4

In the preceding sections we considered the notions of model and theory, and the possible differences between them. This may all seem unclear and is highly unlikely to be any deficit on your part. The situation *is* unclear, and there *is* often little agreement in the writings of the various nursing theorists. It may help to reflect further on these issues:

- Re-read the sections on model and theory in the above sections of the chapter. It may be worthwhile making brief summary notes as you proceed. Compare these notes with those you made in Study Activity 14.1.
- Reflect upon this and re-read your notes; decide whether you see any advantages to nursing in differentiating between the terms.

THE THEORY–SCIENCE DEBATE

In our introduction to this chapter, an assumption is clearly being made about the complementary relationship between something we call theory and something we call research or empirical work. To a significant degree this relates to the understanding people have of the term *science*. To some, science encompasses theorising. It is only by first thinking about the world that we go out, in an empirical sense, to test our theory in the real world. This is the perspective reflected in Fig. 14.3. To others, theory is a highly subjective activity that only serves to compromise, if not indeed corrupt, what is the truth. The only true sense of science is thus an exclusively empirical activity.

The situation is more complicated when we consider the possibility that the theory part of this constellation is within a sequence. That is, that we *first* formulate a theory about how the world is, and we *then* test it out empirically in the real world. This, in its extreme form, states that theories always come from our internal thinking processes and are *never* informed by the empirical – that which is external to us. In essence, this assumes that we think up some theory in an *a priori* way, in isolation from any empirical experience of the real world. An alternative view is one that sees the relationship between theory and empirical activity or experience as much more reflexive, whereby there is a constant interplay between what we think and what we observe. Table 14.2 presents these three different and often opposing viewpoints.

Table 14.2 Theory and science

Position 1. The absolute empirical model

Premise I	Theory is conjecture and irrelevant in the quest for truth.
Premise II	Only research (empirical observation and analysis) establishes truth.
Premise III	Conjecture (theory) is therefore not an element of science.
Premise IV	The outcome is (claimed) empirical knowledge as absolute truth.

Position 2. The absolute theory-testing model

Premise I	Theory + Research = Science.
Premise II	Postulated theory → research → tested/validated theory (truth).
Premise III	Theory is therefore an element of science preceding research.
Premise IV	The outcome is proven theory as absolute truth.

Position 3. The relative integrated model

Premise I	Theorising (thinking) and empiricism (action) are integral elements of research.
Premise II	The thinking and action components are interactive and complementary.
Premise III	Theory thus informs the practice, but the practice also influences the theory.
Premise IV	The outcome is relative, not absolute truth – the strength of the theory is governed by the degree to which we fail to refute the conjecture.

It will be clear from Table 14.2 that the first position sees theory as having no place within science, while in the second and third positions theory is in effect an essential element of the

scientific endeavour; indeed, the third position is essentially that illustrated in Fig. 14.3. Furthermore, a vitally important difference in the third position is that it is usually accompanied by a less rigid faith in a quest for absolute truth. In this position, 'truth' is always in question and even when a theory has consistently withstood attempts to refute it, it is still only considered to be the best available knowledge at a particular time. It is the case that hardly anyone today would lay a claim to the narrow empirical position within which absolute truth is taken to be a realistic aspiration. This is an issue we have addressed earlier, in our chapter on empirical ways of knowing, and we return to this in the next module. However, the realistic recognition that all claims to knowledge must be relative or conditional presents a major scientific dilemma.

THE SCIENCE DILEMMA

This dilemma centres upon what Robert Pirsig asks in the opening quotation to this chapter. What if the body of knowledge is constantly being corrected or modified? What if it is not *sound* and *permanent* at all (or only *apparently* sound for a brief period), but fluid and changing, as is the case in health care? We are faced with what is in reality an explosive growth in medical and health science technology. Wider societal change is occurring with such velocity that we are forever being presented with new health and social problems, new diseases and the re-emergence of old diseases with new intensities and new presentations. As we attempt to respond to these changes, even the ways in which we organise our health care services – including our nursing services – are also being constantly modified and reformed. The social scientist Alvin Toffler (1971) coined the term *future shock* to describe the burgeoning speed of change in modern society, the problems of coping with this, and the disorientation, incapacitation, and powerlessness it causes for many people. When we reflect on the insights presented by commentators such as Pirsig and Toffler, we come to realise that the only permanent element of the modern social world *is* in fact change.

This situation has two significant implications for nursing. First, there is no such thing as a stable and permanent body of nursing knowledge. Our only valid concept of *sound* nursing knowledge must, therefore, be one which recognises the changing and progressive nature of our knowledge. Second, this is primarily, and indeed exclusively, a problem for nurses. We must accept the responsibility for constructing and constantly modifying our own body of knowledge. No-one else is going to do our thinking for us, carry out the research we need, or formulate the theory which gives us insights and guides our practice. Indeed, no-one else has either the motivation or the competence to embark on such undertakings.

The necessity of constantly building upon and modifying the body of knowledge requires a structuring of that knowledge, a task that involves building theories and models which map out and show interrelationships in the overall body of knowledge. What Pirsig (1974) says in the opening quotation of this chapter is true. Today's scientific 'truths' *are* undermined and cast aside in whole or in part by tomorrow's scientific 'truths'. But each new discovery requires a review of the body of knowledge and sometimes points to the need for new direction. In one sense we must be open minded, flexible, and change orientated, but in another we must also attempt to maintain consistency and order so that we can use the best and most sound knowledge available to bring order and clarity to our world. This issue is essentially a question of epistemology, as discussed in the first chapter of this module. It is a question of defining, structuring, and categorising knowledge, a question of how knowledge is developed and verified, and a question of utilising theories and models which show what Rogers (1961) describes as 'order and meaning'.

Our dilemma is one of establishing and building upon a sound body of nursing knowledge, while we in fact would appear to lack the agreed theoretical framework upon which such a

task would be founded. In this respect, Kuhn (1970) has suggested that a discipline is defined by having an agreed paradigm or way of perceiving and investigating the world; without this, he claims, it does not even merit the title discipline. Some, including Kuhn himself [and in nursing, Fawcett (2000)] prefer the term worldview. The situation is relatively straightforward for established disciplines, such as physics and biology. The fields of concern in such disciplines are fairly much circumscribed and suited to particular theoretical and research orientations. This is not to say that such disciplines are without problems. As Kuhn (1970) has pointed out, even in these disciplines the worldview can come under threat by some newly emerging knowledge that topples the dominant knowledge and beliefs, and what he termed a major *paradigm shift* occurs. However, in nursing the situation is very different. Such is the complexity of the health care system, such is the complexity of the human condition, and such are the complexities of the relationships between people (including nurses and their patients), that there can be little hope for a generally accepted single conceptual framework or theory that would guide all practice at the nurse–patient interface. We can, of course, look to a more abstract and all-encompassing metaparadigm that at least sets the parameters for our activities (although, as will be seen later, even this is not unproblematic). But for our work at the interface, we must recognise the value in seeking diversity rather than unity, and a more eclectic drawing upon a range of theoretical frameworks to guide our practice. And, where none has a goodness of fit for the particular practice situation, we must construct a suitable framework.

If such is the situation facing us, we clearly cannot proceed on the basis of some ready-made framework (be it called model, framework, or theory) that will adequately guide all of our practice. Using the science perspective, if we *do* accept theory as a science tool, then the traditional science model may not be a satisfactory template. According to one dominant version of this model, a theory is constructed, postulated and tested for its viability through established research methods (and we address these in the next module). However, we do not have such a generally accepted theory to test in the first place. The way out of this dilemma may lie in the recognition of a more eclectic approach to nursing science and practice, as suggested above. In such an approach we might turn instead to the human sciences and within them the qualitative scientific perspective as the source of our template. This perspective, as we will note in the next module, is not concerned with seeking objective knowledge of the world through a particular research process that involves the collection and analysis of measurable data. Rather, it is concerned with how people experience their world and attribute meanings to that which they experience. It is thus a much more subjective and interpretive enterprise within which measurable data are not available and the statistical means of analysing them therefore not so relevant.

Within this qualitative perspective it is increasingly recognised that situations can be so unique and so contextualised that a ready-made theoretical framework or model, or indeed a ready-made empirical method, is often inappropriate. Against this background the device known as *bricolage* has attained popularity (Denzin and Lincoln, 2000). This is taken from the French word *bricoleur,* which describes the handyman, or person who makes creative use of the limited tools available to him, or modifies his tools and methods to suit the task. The closest equivalent in the English language is the Jack-of-all-trades, the person who has a wide range of skills, and who then brings different configurations of these to the solving of particular context-bound problems. In doing so, he may even adapt or combine tools to make new tools, and invent new approaches to solving the problem. Within qualitative research, researchers similarly draw on a range of theoretical perspectives and/or methods to construct the approach best suited to the particular research topic or issue. Applying this approach to nursing, we would say that the particular patient or parti-

cular context determines the appropriate theory and/or nursing care approach. We would, therefore, draw from more than one theory or model, or perhaps even adapt or combine these to form a new theoretical perspective and method that best fits the nursing situation we are facing: we would in fact be constructing a *nursing bricolage.* This is what in fact expert and highly competent practitioners do in any case! There are no ready-made models or theories to suit all circumstances in this approach. The process of nursing therefore becomes a more reflexive and creative activity, driven by the demands represented by the patient, rather than any rigid adherence to a theory or method that may or may not be appropriate. This *does not* mean that we discount all nursing theories or models in existence, nor does it mean that we do not take account of the soundest knowledge made available to us through empirical research. Indeed, it is imperative that sound theoretical thinking and the best available evidence inform any framing of nursing interventions.

Study Activity 14.5 _____

Consider that you have a patient who has just been diagnosed as terminally ill. The person is clearly desolated by this information. He is also very weak and febrile at this time, as a consequence of the rapidly advancing illness pathology. Furthermore, he is clearly becoming more anxious about the thought of approaching death and the consequences for him, his wife and children.

- Using your library or Internet sources, seek out the following examples of nursing theories and models: Orem's self-care model (1995); Roper, Logan and Tierney's model of activities of living (1996); Watson's caring science (1997); and, Parse's science of human becoming (1992). List the key features of each model/theory.
- Given the brief outline of the patient, consider how you *might* construct a bricolage, drawing from each of these models/theories to construct a suitable framework that *might* guide the nursing interventions. Write up your bricolage as an eclectic

theoretical framework, in about 600 words. If fellow students have also undertaken the study, compare and discuss.

SCIENTIFIC AND NON-SCIENTIFIC KNOWLEDGE

The expanse of knowledge

Thus far we have, in general, been viewing theoretical constructs (models, theories, etc.) as being within the cognitive (empirical or factual knowledge) domain. On this basis, taking a narrow view of theory, it is not a concept of relevance outside of this propositional or factual knowledge construction parameter. However, it is important to recognise that there are different ways of knowing, and that not all of these fit within this perspective. We have already noted above, and in the first chapter of this module, the patterns of knowing proposed by Carper (1978). When the actual construction or production of knowledge as a whole is considered, two main types of knowledge can be discerned. One of these is knowledge derived from actual observation and experience, i.e. knowledge which is empirically derived. The other is knowledge which is derived without experience or prior to experience, i.e. knowledge which is derived through *a priorism*, through rational thinking processes, or perhaps even intuitive or tacit ways of knowing. The first of these is in fact, in its most systematic and methodical form, scientific knowledge. The second is often termed non-scientific knowledge. When it is the result of systematic and rational thinking processes, which give us insights or understanding and lead us towards beliefs and values about the world, the term philosophy is usually applied. Put in simple terms, science is about *facts*, the truth of which is established by agreed upon evidence in regard to observable phenomena. In similar simple terms, philosophy is about *values* and *beliefs*, the soundness of which is established by rational thinking and reflection in regard to particular objects or subjects of attention. Not

all of these are external observable phenomena at all (as in when philosophers may reason and reflect upon the nature of thinking).

It is useful to consider this differentiation by referring to statements made by notable nursing scholars.

On science

Afaf Ibrahim Meleis is Professor of Nursing at the Department of Mental Health, University of California. Her book, *Theoretical Nursing: Development and progress*, is internationally renowned as one of the major references on nursing knowledge. In this book Meleis (1997) states that:

> *Science is a unified body of knowledge about phenomena that is supported by agreed-upon evidence. Science includes disciplinary questions and it provides answers to questions that are central to the discipline. These answers represent wisdom based on the results of data that have been obtained through the different designs and methodological approaches. These answers are also the seeds from which science evolves and develops. There are different approaches to evaluating and judging scientific findings: support of truth through repeated findings; tentative consensus among a community of scholars supporting aspects of evidence; tentative consensus among other subcommunities attesting to descriptions of reality; and the use of objective criteria by members of the community.*
>
> (Meleis, 1997, pp. 10–11)

Meleis is particularly helpful here, in that she frames the *doing* of science – the empirical activity of observing, collecting, testing, and analysing data, in effect the research process – within the wider context of authenticating scientific knowledge.

On philosophy

Jacqueline Fawcett, Professor of Nursing at the University of Pennsylvania, is an internationally renowned nursing scholar, best known for her ideas on a metaparadigm of nursing. In one recent publication, Fawcett (2000) states that:

> A philosophy may be defined as a statement of beliefs and values about human beings and their world ... Philosophies encompass ontological claims about the nature of human beings and the goal of the discipline, epistemic claims regarding how knowledge is developed, and ethical claims about what members of a discipline should do.
>
> (Fawcett, 1993, p. 8)

Fawcett defines philosophy from the point of view of a discipline, and is obviously concerned with the discipline of nursing. But it is important to remember that while philosophy may inform all other disciplines, it is a knowledge perspective in its own right. Nevertheless, in her statement, Fawcett does capture the essential nature of philosophy. She includes recognition that philosophy is about beliefs and values.

It is important to recognise that while Fawcett frames her definition of philosophy within a particular perspective, philosophy itself recognises no limitations to its field of study other than that it concerns thought and knowledge. In essence, philosophy is knowledge about knowledge. It therefore informs all other disciplines.

Study Activity 14.6

Carry out a library-based study of the differences between science and philosophy. If your library has computerised cataloguing and CD-ROM or online search facilities, useful keywords may be philosophy, science, theory, humanities, arts, discipline, knowledge, research, ontology, epistemology, and ethics. Draw up a two-column table listing all the points of differentiation you can identify. If your fellow students also do this, discuss your tables with each other and refine and extend them as appropriate. You should spend no more than about an hour on this activity at this time. Retain your table to return to and expand upon throughout your programme.

However, the totality of knowledge which informs nursing is not encompassed by science and philosophy; philosophy is not the only form of non-scientific knowledge which is relevant. Donaldson and Crowley (1978) and Slevin (1992) have emphasised that human knowledge also includes insights from the humanities, from disciplines such as literature, history, and fine arts. Some, including Donaldson and Crowley, would include philosophy within the humanities. However, if it is accepted that science is generally empirical while philosophy is non-empirical, then the other humanities-based disciplines fall somewhere between these two. The humanities often draw from observation and experience of life, but do not apply rigorous methods of enquiry and the same burden of proof. Instead, their richness is often marked by a depth of understanding that is more philosophical than scientific. The value of such knowledge has been recognised to some extent by nurses. This is witnessed in Carper's (1978) aesthetic pattern of knowing, which we have already addressed in depth in an earlier chapter of this module. However, the contribution of the humanities is increasingly valued within the wider health care context. For example, there is already a growing interest in humanities in health care (Nuffield Trust, 1998), and there is a growing interest in a humanities-driven narrative-based medicine that is acting to counter the one-sidedness of evidence-based medicine (Greenhalgh and Hurwitz, 1998). The scope of human knowledge is thus perhaps best reflected by Fig. 14.5, overleaf.

We have already noted in this module how philosophy can inform our practice: the chapter on epistemology addressed how knowledge in nursing is constructed, and this was followed by a chapter on empirical knowing, which addressed factual or propositional knowledge; the chapter on personal knowing addressed ontological knowledge, our experiential way of being in the world and the meanings we ascribe to how we so exist; the chapter on aesthetic patterns of knowing provided a philosophical basis for recognising the contribution of the arts

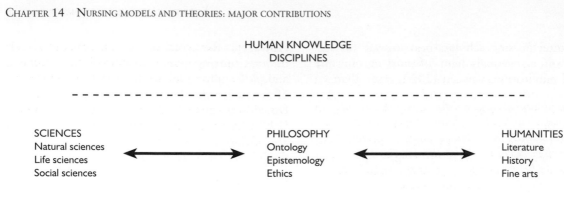

Figure 14.5 The scope of human knowledge

– both as a way of appreciating and thereby deepening understanding, and also in respect of the artistry that exists in nursing action itself; and the chapter on ethical ways of knowing addressed the moral aspects of nursing. This opened for us an understanding of the difference between cognitive, factual, propositional knowledge (knowing that) and practical wisdom (knowing how).

The structure of nursing knowledge

But where does theory fit into this general scheme? If the breadth of knowledge proposed above is accepted, and the views on theory are valid, then theory falls on the science side of this framework. How, then, do the humanities and philosophy fit in? And, more significantly, if theory is within the sciences, is it appropriate or even safe to have nursing actions guided by a framework or 'nursing model' that is exclusively

based upon this orientation? As indicated in Table 14.3, the orientation, content and even vocabulary of these three perspectives (science, philosophy and the humanities) can differ significantly. But, perhaps more importantly, the outcomes from the three areas of endeavour can also vary considerably. Clearly, the output from the scientific endeavour *is* of vital importance. We do need to 'know that', to have sound factual knowledge and theory that gives us confidence in how we see the world and operate within it. But, in the human relational context of nursing, we also need the output from the humanities endeavour. We do need to have insight into the meaning of health and illness and how these are being experienced by those we care for; and we do need to 'know how' to intervene in safe, skilful and competent ways.

Assuming it is accepted that all three sources of 'knowing' and in particular the 'outputs' we

Table 14.3 Knowledge orientations and their outputs

Science	Philosophy	Humanities
Factual	Rational	Experiential
Objective	Logical	Subjective
Detached	Transcending	Contextual
Source of verified knowledge	Source of wisdom and understanding	Source of shared experience
Accuracy	Exactitude	Meaningfulness
Outputs:	Outputs:	Outputs:
Factual knowledge/evidence	Sound arguments	Process of becoming
Verified/tested theory	Wisdom	Meaning and insight
'Knowing that'	'Knowing about knowing'	'Knowing how'

can expect from each them are equally important, we must establish some way of framing our world of nursing knowledge. A useful approach would be to view the interrelationships of each of these perspectives in terms of their level of abstraction, as presented in Fig. 14.6, overleaf. In this context, philosophy is the source of our values and beliefs about nursing. From these shared viewpoints, agreed areas of concern are identified and common problems to be solved are recognised. Kuhn (1970), as noted earlier, defined these as *paradigms*, emphasising that the crucial element was that these views or commitments were shared by a community of scholars, thus marking them off as a *discipline*. In essence, there is a shared interest in an area of knowledge, shared perspectives for thinking and speaking about it, and shared methods for studying or investigating it, such that the discipline and those who work within it are contained within a theoretical and methodological framework or paradigm.

At the most abstract level, paradigmatic outlooks can be specified as major areas of concern or attention, beyond which further reduction cannot be achieved. That is, the core elements which are the central concerns of a discipline can be identified. Such presentations are referred to as *metaparadigms,* a concept we have already met. As may be recalled, from the first chapter of the module and from our discussion above, Fawcett (1984) suggests that the metaparadigm of nursing includes:

- person
- environment
- health
- nursing.

Fawcett suggests that the total discipline is contained by a concern for these four elements. These elements must all be taken into consideration in the study of nursing and anything beyond them are of no concern. These four areas of concern mark the parameters of the discipline of nursing.

However, Meleis (1997) has suggested that to include nursing in the metaparadigm is a tautology, because as the metaparadigm is descriptive *of* nursing as a discipline, nursing cannot be a *part* of it; it is in fact *the whole*. Other theorists do not include nursing as an actual part of their metaparadigm. For example, in her *theory of human becoming,* Parse (1992) includes:

- person
- environment
- health.

In taking this stance she is clearly in line with the viewpoint expressed by Meleis. She is taking the discipline to *be* nursing, and the metaparadigm for it includes person, environment, and health. But nursing is not one of the elements, it is in fact the whole. Similarly, Newman *et al.* (1991) identify the following overriding metaparadigm elements:

- caring
- human health experience.

They argue that the concept of caring is fundamental to the discipline of nursing, but emphasise that this caring must occur in the health experience for it to be called nursing. They state that:

> *A body of knowledge that does not include caring and human health experience is not nursing knowledge. For example, knowledge about health without consideration of caring would be knowledge of a discipline of health. Nursing theories would link caring to the human health experience.*
>
> (Newman *et al.*, 1991)

This idea is similar to the views of Kirby and Slevin (1992). These authors do not set out to present a metaparadigm of nursing as such. Instead they are concerned with the essential nature of nursing work and the practice of nursing. In taking this stance they present nursing as a form of human activity involving certain elements which are essentially metaparadigmatic in that nursing is contained within them:

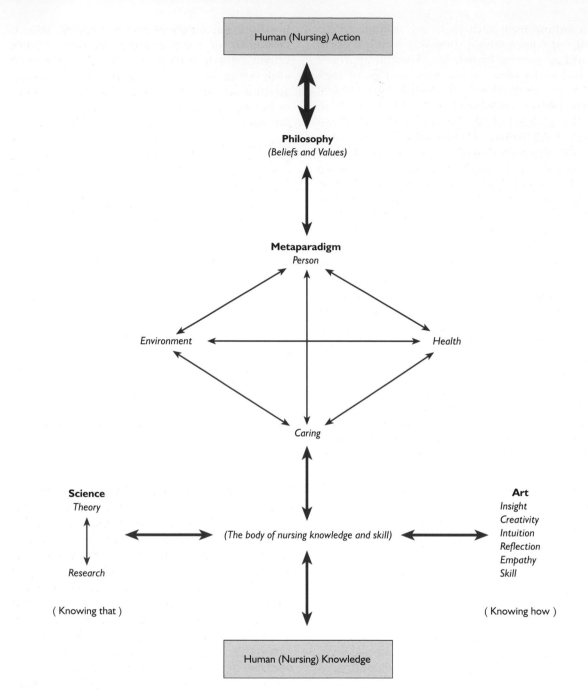

Figure 14.6   The structure of nursing knowledge and practice

- relationship
- caring
- health.

Here not only caring and health but also the nurse–patient relationship are viewed as major areas of concern. However, Kirby and Slevin are taking a narrower view than that of Parse in that by identifying relationship, they may appear to be restricting the environmental influence to an exclusively interpersonal dimension (i.e. considering only the human part of the environment). As we shall see in the final module of this book, the impact of the physical environment presents increased risk that is of a global nature, with many of these social and physical risks (global warming, flood, radiation, war and famine) being manmade to a greater or lesser extent.

It must be acknowledged that in responding to these criticisms, including nursing *within* the metaparadigm *of nursing* is a tautology, Fawcett has mounted a reasonable response. She points out that the term nursing as the title of the metaparadigm is meant to identify the discipline or profession, while the term nursing *within* the metaparadigm refers to the activity of *doing* nursing. Nevertheless, drawing on the views expressed by these different authors, a compromise metaparadigm for the profession (as suggested by Slevin, 1999) may be one which includes:

- person (the client or patient)
- environment (physical and social or interpersonal)
- health (ill-health and well-being)
- caring (helping, which is the core of nursing action).

On the basis of a philosophical foundation, and guided by such a metaparadigm, we can therefore proceed to establish frameworks for our nursing action for practice. As demonstrated in Fig. 14.6, this can be viewed broadly, in terms of science *and* art informing the practice, and in turn being informed by that practice. In Fig. 14.6 the items that occupy the space between nursing knowledge at the top and nursing action

at the bottom are connected by two-way arrows. They indicate that the interconnections are not linear and sequential; and by being presented from the top (nursing knowledge) to the bottom (nursing action), there is no hierarchical order suggested. It is true that philosophy may establish our beliefs and values, thus leading us to a metaparadigm of nursing which directs us towards knowledge construction, and which in turn guides our practice. But equally, the knowledge and skill gained from the practice of nursing influences our theories, our metaparadigm, and our philosophy.

Study Activity 14.7

The metaparadigm of nursing presented by Fawcett (1984) and briefly described above is very influential in nursing. Search the library for references to the concept of metaparadigm, particularly that presented by Fawcett, then write a brief 600-word critique of Fawcett's metaparadigm. If other students have also completed this activity, the group and tutor will find a discussion of the topic most valuable.

SUMMARY

In this chapter we have addressed the issues of theory and models from a particular perspective. We have considered how the terms are identified and to discuss the differences between them that are presented in the literature in an often unclear and conflicting manner. Throughout the chapter there have been constant references to these terms as reflecting means by which we attempt to understand our world, to make sense of it. We used the term theorising to describe this process, irrespective of whether terms such as conceptual model, conceptual framework or theory are the preferred terminology. Significantly, the chapter did not attempt to describe and critique the growing number of models and theories that continue to emerge on a regular basis, despite concerns about their relevance to nursing. The significant contributions addressed in this chapter were those that addressed the theory *issue*, rather than specific nursing theories. In this sense, it was suggested that the concerns of our discussion were those of metatheory. That is, we were concerned about the nature of theory (and models) in nursing rather than the explication of specific named theories.

In adopting the latter orientation, it was not intended that the importance of a theoretical underpinning to our practice be discounted. On the contrary, the position was taken that such an underpinning is of vital importance. However, against a backcloth of an ever-changing and complex health care system, it was proposed that a more reflexive and dynamic use of theoretical frameworks has become necessary. The devices of eclecticism, and more specifically the use of *bricolage*, were identified as useful means of proceeding in this manner. The position taken here was that, rather than holding rigidly to some given theory or model 'for all occasions', the demands presented by the particular patient or situation would determine the type of theoretical framework indicated. Such a framework could be adapted from current theory, or be derived from *parts* of current theories. In a sense, using this *bricolage* orientation we would construct from what is available, or what we might create from the parts of what is available, the 'theory' to suit the particular context.

This same orientation to a more open and flexible approach also led to an attempt to frame 'theory' within the wider context of a world of nursing knowledge and practice. Within this wider context, empirical or scientific knowledge, to which theory is aligned, was recognised as just one source that may inform our practice. Within the framing of an overall philosophy (beliefs and values), and within the parameters set by our nursing metaparadigm, we can also draw on the arts or humanities to establish a more holistic approach to our practice. We proceed from this point to the next module, within which much of the content is directed towards the empirical sources of nursing knowledge. This is, generally speaking, a movement into the area of research

and its impact on clinical effectiveness. That is, we are proceeding to consider science and how it is applied to nursing. However, in moving to this area it is hoped that this current chapter has demonstrated that good science is imaginative and creative, that it depends for its 'spark' and its leaps of insight and discovery on the quality of the theorising that is done. By a similar token, the chapter has also hopefully demonstrated that good nursing is not about the mindless application of some handed down model or theory, but about a similar process of theorising before, during and after practice. In such circumstances the theory we utilise is a dynamic and responsive process rather than a static framework growing steadily out of date and perhaps lacking relevance to the demands of practice as they change from day to day.

REFERENCES

Aggleton, P. and Chalmers, H. (2000) *Nursing Models and Nursing Practice* (2nd edn), Macmillan, Basingstoke

Alligood, M.R. and Marriner-Tomey, A. (2002) *Nursing Theory: Utilization and application* (2nd edn), Mosby, St. Louis

Barker, P. (1993) The Peplau legacy. *Nursing Times* 89(11), 48–51

Barrett, E.A.M. (1991) Theory: of or for nursing. *Nursing Science Quarterly* 4(2), 48–9

Barrett, E.A.M. (1992) Diversity reigns. *Nursing Science Quarterly* 5(4), 155–7

Bohm, D. (1998) *On Creativity*, Routledge, London

Carpenito, L.J. (1995) *Nursing Diagnosis: Application to clinical practice* (6th edn), J.B. Lippincott, Philadelphia, IL

Carper, B.A. (1978) Fundamental patterns of knowing in nursing. *Advances in Nursing Science* 1, 13–23

Chinn, P.L. and Kramer, M.K. (1999) *Theory and Nursing: A systematic approach*, Mosby Year Book, St. Louis, IL

Denzin, N. and Lincoln, Y. (2000) *The Handbook of Qualitative Research*, Sage, Thousand Oaks, CA

Donaldson, S.K. and Crowley, D.M. (1978) The discipline of nursing. *Nursing Outlook*, **February**, 113–20

Fawcett, J. (1984) The metaparadigm of nursing: present status and future refinements. *IMAGE: Journal of Nursing Scholarship* 16, 84–7

Fawcett, J. (1993) *Analysis and Evaluation of Nursing Theories*, F.A. Davis, Philadelphia, IL

Fawcett, J. (2000) *Analysis and Evaluation of Contemporary Nursing Knowledge: Nursing models and theories*, F.A. Davis, Philadelphia, IL

Greenhalgh, T. and Hurwitz, B. (1998) *Narrative-based Medicine*, BMJ Books, London

International Council of Nurses (2002) *International Classification for Nursing Practice*, International Council of Nurses, Geneva

Kaplan, A. (1964) *The Conduct of Inquiry*, Chandler, Scranton, PA

Kaplan, A. (1973) *The Conduct of Inquiry*, Intertext Books, Aylesbury

Kay, H. and Connolly, K.J. (1981) Foreward: reflections and recollections. In: Chapman, A. and Jones, D. (eds) *Models of Man*, The British Psychological Society, Leicester

Kim, H.S. (1983) *The Nature of Theoretical Thinking in Nursing*, Appleton Century Croft, Appleton, CA

Kirby, C. and Slevin, O. (1992) A new curriculum for care. In: Slevin, O. and Buckenham, M. (eds) *Project 2000: The teachers speak*, Campion Press, Edinburgh

Kuhn, T.S. (1970) *The Structure of Scientific Revolutions*, University of Chicago Press, Chicago, IL

McCloskey, J.C. and Bulechek, G.M. (2000) *Nursing Interventions Classification* (3rd edn), Mosby, St. Louis, IL

McFarlane, E.A. (1986) The value of models of care. In: Kershaw, B. and Salvage, J. (eds) *Models for Nursing*, John Wiley, Chichester

McKenna, H. (1997) *Nursing Models and Theories*, Routledge, London

Meleis, A.I. (1997) *Theoretical Nursing: Development and progress* (3rd edn), J.B. Lippincott, New York

Merton, R.K. (1968) *Social Theory and Social Structure*, Free Press, New York

Newman, M.A., Sime, A.M. and Corcoran-Perry, S.A. (1991) The focus of the discipline of nursing. *Advances in Nursing Science* 14(1), 1–6

Noak, J. (2001) Do we need another model for mental health care? *Nursing Standard* 16(8), 33–5

North American Nursing Diagnosis Association (1999) *Nursing Diagnoses: Definitions and classification 1999–2000*, North American Nursing Diagnosis Association, Philadelphia, IL

Northrup, D.T. (1992) A unified perspective within nursing, *Nursing Science Quarterly* 5(4), 154–5

Nuffield Trust (1998) *Humanities in Medicine: Beyond the millennium*, The Nuffield Trust, London

Orem, D. (1995) *Nursing: Concepts for practice* (5th edn), Mosby, St. Louis, IL

Parse, R.R. (1987) *Nursing Science: Major paradigms, theories and critiques*, Saunders, Philadelphia, IL

Parse, R.R. (1988) Man–living–health; a theory of nursing. In: Riehl-Sisca, L. (ed.) *Conceptual Models for Nursing Practice* (3rd edn), Appleton and Lange, Norwalk, CN

Parse, R.R. (1992) Human becoming: Parse's theory of nursing. *Nursing Science Quarterly* 5(1), 35–42

Parse, R.R. (1998) *The Human Becoming School of Thought: A perspective for nurses and other health professionals*, Sage, Thousand Oaks, CA

Pirsig, R.M. (1974) *Zen and the Art of Motorcycle Maintenance*, The Bodley Head, London

Popper, K. (1989) *Conjectures and Refutations*, Routledge, London

Reilly, D.E. (1975) Why a conceptual framework? *Nursing Outlook* 23, 566–9

Rogers, C. (1961) *On Becoming a Person*, Houghton Mifflin, Boston, Mass

Rogers, M. (1987) Rogers's science of unitary human beings. In: Parse, R.R. (ed.) *Nursing Science: Major paradigms, theories and critiques*, W B Saunders, Philadelphia, IL

Roper, N., Logan, W. and Tirney, A. (1996) *the Elements of Nursing* (4th edn), Churchill Livingston, Edinburgh

Roy, C. and Andrews, H. (1999) *The Roy Adaptation Model* (2nd edn), Appleton & Lange, Stamford

Slevin, O. (1992) Knowledgeable doing: the theoretical basis for practice. In: Slevin, O. and Buckenham, M. (eds) *Project 2000; The teachers speak*, Campion Press, Edinburgh

Slevin, O. (1999) The nurse–patient relationship: caring in a health context. In: Long, A. (ed.) *Interaction for Practice in Community Nursing*, Macmillan, Basingstoke

Stevens, B.J. (1979) *Nursing Theory: Analysis, application, evaluation*, Little, Brown & Co, Boston, Mass

Toffler, A. (1971) *Future Shock*, Pan Books, London

Wald, F.S. and Leonard, R.C. (1964) Toward development of nursing practice theory. *Nursing Research* 13, 309–13

Walker, L. and Avant, K. (1995) Strategies for Theory construction in Nursing (3rd edn) Appleton & Lange, Norwalk, CN

Watson, J. (1997) The theory of human caring: retrospective and prospective. *Nursing Science Quarterly* 10(1), 49–52

Reflections

In this module, we considered an epistemology of nursing as being the study of the knowledge of nursing: what it is, how it is constructed, the means by which it is validated, and ways of categorising or organising such knowledge. We then proceeded to consider one means of categorisation, which identified four patterns of knowing: empirical, personal, aesthetic and ethical.

Empirical knowing is concerned with knowledge that is cognitive, factual and derived from our observations of phenomena. It is derived primarily from research and consists of evidence that is in some way subjected to tests to establish its validity and reliability.

Personal knowing is concerned with knowledge that is experiential and embedded in our knowing of self and others. Such knowledge goes beyond the bounds of fact and cannot be directly observed, as it is founded upon the experience of being in the world and being with others. As such it is tacit and felt or at best described, and any attempt to *explain* detracts from the richness of what is experienced.

Aesthetic knowing is also an intensely personal pattern of knowing. It relates to how we value phenomena in terms of their shape and form, and how we see the beauty or patterns of meaning for us in such form. In a related sense, aesthetics is also about the artistry involved in how such aesthetic entities are created. Both senses are relevant to nursing: there is a grace and humanity in how nursing is performed in the service of others; but there is also an artistry in nursing that involves *knowing how* as opposed to *knowing that* which is characteristic of empirical knowing. Such *knowing how* is more than manual dexterity, it is a form of clinical wisdom emerging from experience and the intuition of knowing *what* to do as well as *how* to do it.

Ethical knowing is also concerned with values that we hold rather than any factual knowledge. However, the values involved are of a special form that we term moral. Ethical knowing addresses concerns about what is good or bad, right or wrong in such moral terms. But it is also about the ethical choices we make, so that ethics goes beyond ethical patterns of knowing to actions that may also be valued in moral terms.

We concluded the module by considering nursing models and theories. However, these were addressed at a level of principle: how do conceptual models and theories provide frameworks for making sense of the world or aspects of that world? In this specific sense, such cognitive entities are predominantly within the arena of empirical patterns of knowing. By recognising the importance of this and other ways of knowing, nursing is informed by both theoretical and philosophical insights.

You may wish to reflect on the relevance of these philosophical and theoretical insights to the practice of nursing. This might be best achieved by reflecting from within the practice situation itself. One way of doing this would be to consider within a forthcoming practice experience how the different patterns of knowing can be seen to inform the nursing choices that are made and the nursing actions that are taken.

MODULE 4: EVIDENCE-BASED PRACTICE

INTRODUCTION

Within the previous module, one important pattern of knowing was that identified as empirical knowing. This acknowledges an essentially human characteristic, that of attempting to make sense of the facts we are confronted with. The main means by which such factual knowledge is confirmed or validated is through the medium of research. Indeed, it was suggested in the final chapter of the previous module that the area we commonly describe as science is sometimes viewed as including the interrelated elements of theory and research.

The particular relevance of research to nursing (and indeed to health care in general) is contained in the premise that we should base our practice on the best available research findings. Because research is usually concerned with factual empirical knowledge, we view the product of such activity as being 'evidence'. It is now a widely held view that all practice or health care intervention should be established upon the best available evidence. On this basis, there is a constant demand for what we term evidence-based practice. All the chapters within this module centre on this concern to a greater or lesser extent.

15 THE RESEARCH PROCESS

Eamonn Slevin

LEARNING OUTCOMES

After studying this chapter you will be able to:

- Understand what research means
- Gain a rudimentary knowledge of the stages in the process of research
- Distinguish between the different stages in the research process
- Develop the necessary knowledge to be able to evaluate whether research you read has adhered to a logical research process.

INTRODUCTION

As a nurse you will need to have knowledge and skills of research at different levels. All nurses need to be able to understand research and to be able to interpret research findings. Some nurses will decide to develop a career in research and, therefore, they will need to become competent in undertaking research, while others may have to undertake an occasional research project or, as a student, undertake a research dissertation as part of a degree programme. Whatever level of knowledge and skills is required, there is little doubt that research knowledge is part of the nurse's knowledge base.

An important aspect for any nurse is to grasp an understanding of what research is. This chapter explains what research is, adhering to the traditional 'science' linear research process notion. There are, of course, different types of research and it is recognised that knowledge can develop from other methods, but these are not the focus of this chapter. The starting point of the chapter is to define what research is. Following this, a general overview of the research process is presented. In order to evaluate a research report, or for those who will undertake research, an essential requirement is knowledge of this process.

As this is not a nursing research book, this chapter presents only an introduction and overview to research and the research process. References to substantive nursing research texts are provided in Table 15.1 to allow you to access a more detailed account of research and research procedures.

WHAT IS RESEARCH?

Research is perceived by many to be a complex activity that can only be undertaken by professors and other academics. Yet Abbot and Sapsford (1998) maintain that doing research is really an extension of what many of us do in life. They assert that research is similar to the

Table 15.1 Useful research texts

Parahoo (1997)	A very useful all-round research book of particular value to those new to research
Polit and Hungler (1999)	A very useful book for the novice through to the more advanced researcher who leans towards quantitative research
Cormack (1996)	A useful all-round research book
Creswell (1994)	A concise book covering the research design
Crookes and Davis (1998)	Of particular value for sampling procedures and literature review
Hays (1994)	A comprehensive book covering most aspects of statistics
Holloway and Wheeler (1996)	A very useful text for qualitative research and methods

problem-solving common sense that many people use to discover answers to questions they encounter in life. This is undoubtedly true, but it is also true that our common sense is not always effective in guiding actions, if it were there would be fewer mistakes in life. Making mistakes is a trait of being human, hence the old saying 'anyone can make a mistake'.

While it is the case that anyone can make a mistake, in nursing, where the central concern is the care of people, mistakes need to be minimised. Therefore, nursing actions should be guided by knowledge that has a sound foundation. One approach to achieving this is the scientific method. In this chapter the term 'scientific method' is synonymous with 'research method'. A number of definitions of research have been suggested.

Burns and Grove (1987) define research as follows:

> *The root meaning of the word research is to search again or to examine carefully. More specifically, research is diligent, systematic inquiry or investigation to validate old knowledge and generate new knowledge.*
>
> (Burns and Grove, 1987)

Kerlinger's (1973) definition is one of the best known and most widely accepted. It was adopted by Polit and Hungler (1999) in their text on nursing research and by Cohen and Manion (1989) in a standard text on educational research. Kerlinger defines research as:

> *... a systematic, controlled, empirical, and critical investigation of hypothetical propositions about the presumed relationships among natural phenomena.*
>
> (Kerlinger, 1973)

Put in simple terms, these definitions indicate that research is a method involving searching for and investigating observable phenomena so that we can verify our tentative explanations about them and how they exist and relate to each other in the real world. The aims being that our tentative explanations become less tentative and

more certain. It is, therefore, an investigation of observable (or empirical) reality.

Stevens *et al.* (1993) define science as a coherent system of knowledge about the world (or part of it). They divide science into: science as an outcome – the body of knowledge acquired through scientific endeavour – and science as an activity, which is in fact research, the process of acquiring this knowledge.

Research is identified as involving:

- the perception of reality;
- induction (reasoning that draws general conclusions from specific instances); and,
- verification or falsification of facts.

These authors identify a scientific method that is empirical, but they also recognise research as a thinking activity involving reasoning.

Parahoo (1997) defines research as:

> *the study of phenomena by the rigorous and systematic collection and analysis of data [and it is] a private enterprise made public for the purpose of exposing it to others, to allow for replication, verification or falsification.*
>
> (Parahoo 1997)

Parahoo adds a new dimension in the assertion that not only must research be undertaken in a systematic rigorous manner, but that it should be laid open to the scrutiny of others to affirm or not the research outcomes.

The question is, what constitutes 'nursing research'? Hockey (1996) defines nursing research as 'research into those aspects of professional activity which are predominantly and appropriately the concern and responsibility of nurses'.

Drawing together the definitions of research as a scientific method as detailed in the various definitions above, and Hockey's view on nursing research, we can state the main component parts of *nursing research* as follows: it involves a systematic collection of empirical information through observing, measuring or otherwise evaluating, recording and analysing such information. Reflecting on the meanings that emerge from this analysis, and disseminating the research in order to:

- allow nurses and others in the scientific community to affirm or refute the research;
- gain new knowledge or verify current knowledge about aspects that are of significant concern to nursing;
- confirm hypotheses or propositions that illustrate relationships or justify predictions;
- describe or explain a situation with soundness.

Study Activity 15.1 ——————

- In the above section, research has been defined followed by an explanation of what 'nursing research' is. With a group of colleagues, debate whether or not you feel the idea of a 'nursing research' perspective is a useful one.
- A nurse working in a hospital was employed as a research nurse. Her role was to collect data in a drug trial experiment; a medical physician was directing the research. With your colleagues discuss whether or not you feel this nurse was undertaking 'nursing research'.

THE RESEARCH PROCESS

As a nurse you will be familiar with the idea of the nursing process, i.e. assessing, identifying a health need, planning care and evaluating that care (*see* Chapter 24). The research process has some parallels with this. It is also a process, i.e. a sequential series of actions that lead to an outcome. In both processes the aims are desirable outcomes. In the case of the nursing process the outcome planned for is health improvement, and in the research process the outcome is knowledge advancement. As it is nursing research that we are concerned with here, the knowledge developed is applied in that the overall aim is improvement to patients, community or society. This is so even if the research does not seem to have a direct application to patients, for example it might be research that helps improve nurse education, management systems or any other aspect that indirectly leads to improvements for those who require nursing care. An important point to remember is that research can improve care by identifying practices that develop and improve nursing care, and also by identifying practices that might be harmful and therefore should cease.

There are a number of sequential stages in the research process that customarily, but not invariably, follow each other. These stages can usually be found in any piece of research and should be discernible within the written research report, even when the sequence is not followed exactly. Thus, while there may be variations, the research process involves a number of elements:

- the research idea
- the research topic or problem
- the research proposal
- review of the literature
- refining the research topic into a specific question(s)
- methodology
- the research design/methods (incorporating ethical considerations and pilot work, or field trials, sample and sampling, data collection and data analysis – methods to enhance the robustness of the research)
- presentation of the findings from the analysis
- discussion of the findings of the research and overall conclusions that can be drawn
- a written report detailing the research and dissemination to the research/nursing community.

The research idea

The question is frequently posed – what is good research? Good research is no doubt identifiable in terms of the skilled manner, the rigour, and the adherence to the research cannons that a researcher follows. It would be quite difficult to argue that research was good if it was not undertaken rigorously. Rigorous research is research that is considered to be 'sound' from a scientific basis (McKenna and Mason, 1998). However, it is possible for research to be undertaken in a sound and rigorous manner and yet it might not really tell the nursing community anything new. In such instances the researcher/s may deserve credit for their skill in wading through the research process. Or, even if new knowledge is not an outcome, the researcher may be credited with verifying the findings of previous research. The worthiness of replicating previous research to confirm or refute its outcomes is a useful endeavour.

While not always recognised as part of the research process, it is suggested here that the first part of the process is the 'research idea'. In addition, it is asserted that good research begins with a good idea. Therefore, the research process begins in the researcher's mind. An idea for research may involve a leap of the imagination, a connection of observed phenomena, or in some of the best research, a chance encounter (or accidental discovery). Good research that will have an impact on the profession of nursing is research that is grounded in an 'idea' that forwards, expands and develops nursing knowledge.

Study Activity 15.2

Either individually or with colleagues search for some research (historical or modern) that began with a good idea, and try to identify how the idea emerged, e.g. through observations, by scientific endeavour, by chance or by a combination of these, or other means. You need not adhere to nursing or health care for this exercise. If you wish, you can look at the ideas of the following researchers and what led to the findings they are credited with: Albert Einstein, Alexander Fleming, Florence Nightingale, and Patricia Benner.

The research topic or research problem

A good research idea will lead to a research topic or problem. Or, indeed, the identification of a research problem may be the catalyst for a very good research idea. The purpose of any research is to discover new knowledge or verify knowledge that is currently judged to be true or sound.

Two examples of research purpose statements are as follows:

- The purpose of this research is to explore the life experiences of people living with a diagnosis of HIV.
- The purpose of this research is to test whether the provision of an education course on healthy living leads to weight reduction in obese people.

Both of the above statements represent potential health problems: the emotional effects of having a diagnosis of HIV and the potential physical problems of obesity.

The identification of a research problem and, within this, the statement of a research purpose, is a vitally important stage in the research process. From this the significance or insignificance of the research can be established. We can determine if the research has any real value or if it is merely done because it is easy or convenient. In addition, a well-formulated research purpose will guide the whole research project.

The aims and objectives for the research to be undertaken should be listed at this stage. An aim can be considered as a broad statement about what the research is going to achieve and the objectives are the various steps that lead to the achievement of the aims. The analogy of a set of stairs represents this well. At the top of the stairs is the wide landing, the aim or where we wish to reach. Each individual step might be considered an objective and we can walk up each step to eventually reach the landing. In research, then, the aim is the overall achievement one wishes to attain, and the objectives are succinct statements describing the stages the research will go through to achieve the aims.

Study Activity 15.3

Locate some research reports, either journals or dissertations, in the library. Examine these reports and see if you can find a list of aims and objectives. Do you feel that the aims and objectives provide you with a clear 'signposting' of the research?

The research proposal

Whenever a researcher discovers a good research idea, and he/she develops the idea into a feasible topic or research problem, there is a need to construct a research proposal. The reasons for preparing a research proposal are:

- to document what the researcher intends to undertake in the research
- to obtain permission to undertake the research – this may be from an academic institution as part of a course, a funding body in order to obtain funding to undertake a research study, or an ethics committee to obtain ethical approval to conduct research
- to obtain permission from the research site managers, the gatekeepers, to gain access to the research site and participants
- to obtain funding from a funding agency to carry out the research
- to clarify for the researcher what he/she intends to do and thus allow for any changes before undertaking the actual research.

A research proposal is, as the name suggests, a proposal to undertake research. Therefore, the stages in a written research proposal will mirror the subsequent study. It will, of course, be much briefer, and the length and content will vary depending on where the proposal is to be submitted. Some agencies will have guidance criteria for a research proposal (Polit and Hungler, 1999). Some organisations will require a succinct outline proposal, and others, like universities, may request a more detailed proposal. Whichever is the case, the main elements of most research proposals are as outlined in Table 15.2.

Literature review

Research is about advancing the frontiers of knowledge and should, therefore, be undertaken to discover something knew. However, it can also be conducted to confirm or verify current knowledge, in which case research can be repeated in order to strengthen or reject the claims for a particular body of knowledge.

Table 15.2 Outline for a research proposal

- An abstract or summary of the proposed research.
- Identification of the research problem.
- Rationale for addressing the problem, with particular emphasis on how the outcomes will improve nursing (care, management or education).
- Background literature – a limited review of the problem area that supports the proposal may identify gaps in current research knowledge related to the topic.
- A clear statement of the aims and objectives of the proposed research.
- A clear indication of the intended methods, to include: the research design, ethical aspects and how these will be addressed, the proposed sample and sampling methods, the data collection instruments to be used, the procedures for data collection, data analysis procedures.
- A time plan for undertaking the total study, as well as identification of periods when the various stages of the research will be completed, usually in weeks or months.
- Resource requirements – most often financial requirements, but might include the need for other resources.
- Skills and qualifications of the researcher/s that indicate their competence to undertake the research. (If you are undertaking research for the first time, e.g. perhaps for a dissertation, you may of course have no previous research experience; all researchers are at this point at some time in their careers.)

The method by which the state of the current body of knowledge is ascertained is through a literature review. Reviewing the literature is not done to create an impression of academic respectability. It is a vitally important element of the research process and is as much a part of doing research as any other aspect of the research process. While its primary function is to determine and present the current stage of knowledge in a particular area, there are also important ethical implications, which can be illustrated by the following assertions:

- Conducting research without determining what has already been done in a particular area is irresponsible and wasteful of resources.
- Failing to acknowledge that research is a replication of earlier research is misleading and

hinders the advancement of knowledge, rather than enhancing it. Presenting it as new research is dishonest and plagiaristic.

- Deliberately presenting literature that supports the researcher's propositions and claims introduces a bias in the research.

The literature review must be taken seriously as an essential part of the research process. The researcher must search out, read thoroughly and critically appraise all relevant literature, or at least as much as time, resources, and availability will allow. This step requires access to a good library with a comprehensive range of academic journals. There are efficient methods, such as searching under authors, abstracts, or subjects in indices to obtain the necessary information. Useful indices include:

- The International Nursing Index
- The Cumulative Index to Nursing and Allied Health Literature (CINAHL)
- Nursing Abstracts
- The Nursing Citation Index
- A Bibliography of Nursing Literature (Royal College of Nursing)
- *Index Medicus*
- Medical Literature Analysis and Retrieval System Online (Medline)
- Health Service Abstracts
- Cochrane Library (CD-Rom and Online)
- Psychological Abstracts
- Sociological Abstracts
- Dissertation Abstracts International.

Most large libraries will have all or some of these collections. A common and efficient method to conduct a literature search is to use a computer to search. Using online systems or CD-ROM, modern technology allows very sophisticated and extensive searches to be conducted. Computer searches for literature speed up the time it takes to conduct a search.

However, while obtaining literature via computer systems has greatly enhanced searching strategies, there is still the need for scrutiny and critical appraisal of the literature the researcher accesses. Sometimes research merely reports

literature (research published in journals might do this), but in more detailed research, literature needs to be 'reviewed'.

Reviewing entails reporting, analysing and critiquing literature. In addition, a review that omits significant contributions to the literature cannot be considered satisfactory. In general, the following principles should be followed:

Relevance
The principle of relevance is paramount. Only sources which are pertinent to the research project and which provide related knowledge should be used.

Depth
Works cited should be adequately described, analysed, and critiqued, particularly those that are significantly relevant to the research project.

Breadth
It is not necessary to include every relevant piece of literature; indeed, this would be an impossible task. However, the range of literature should be adequately sampled. It is also important to remember that research literature is not the only relevant literature. Theoretical and even non-scientific literature may be useful sources.

Honesty
As suggested earlier, there is an ethical obligation to present a comprehensive and balanced review. Particularly since the advent of computerised searching, it is possible to select works that are only supportive of the researcher's viewpoint. This biased approach to reviewing must be avoided.

Parahoo (1997) states that the functions of a literature review are to:

> *provide a rationale for the current study;*
> *put the current study into the context of what is known about the topic;*
> *review the relevant research carried out on the same or similar topics;*
> *discuss the conceptual/theoretical basis of the current study.*
>
> (Parahoo, 1997)

Study Activity 15.4 _____

Select a research paper from an academic journal such as the *Journal of Advanced Nursing*. Critique the literature review in the paper using the above principles and write a brief, approximately 250-word, account of it.

_____

Refining the research topic into a specific question(s)

Sometimes it is best to refine the research problem into specific questions, hypotheses or statements of purpose following the literature review. This is because following the review you may feel you have more knowledge and a clearer understanding of the research topic. There are three main ways that the research question may be stated.

A research hypothesis

A research hypothesis is used when you wish to test the relationship between two or more variables. The variables are referred to as the dependent variable – the variable that will change, be caused or in someway be affected by another variable – and the independent variable – the variable that causes the effect in the dependent variable. A simple explanation of this is: smoking (the independent variable) causes lung cancer (the dependent variable).

Parahoo (1997) defines a hypothesis as 'a tentative statement about the relationship, if any, between two or more variables'. There are a number of different types of hypothesis, but it is enough here to identify the two main types.

A directional hypothesis – in this type of hypothesis the researcher predicts there will be a relationship between the variables, and in addition, the direction of that relationship (Polit and Hungler, 1999). An example of a directional hypothesis is:

- Children aged 4 years who are given daily supplements of vitamins over a 5-year period will have higher IQ levels than children not given such supplements.

This is a directional hypothesis in that it not only states that there will be an effect, but also the direction of the effect, i.e. an increase in IQ.

A non-directional hypothesis – in this type of hypothesis a relationship between the variables is predicted, but no prediction is made regarding the direction of the relationship. An example of a non-directional hypothesis is:

- There is a difference in recovery rate between children who are nursed in individual side rooms in a hospital, and children who are nursed in an open ward with other children.

As you can see there is a stated relationship here between children nursed in side rooms and open wards, but there is no prediction regarding what direction this might take. Children in side rooms may recover faster, or slower, than those in an open ward.

A research question

This is the statement of a question that is more open than a hypothesis in that it queries rather than predicts. Examples of some research questions are:

- How many nurses drink eight units of alcohol or more in a week?
- What are the main reasons for patients attending accident and emergency departments at weekends?
- Where do children with learning disabilities spend most of their time when they come home from school?
- Do older people who live alone eat less well than other people?

Stated purpose

Sometimes it is difficult to formulate a clear research question or hypothesis. In such cases the researcher may describe statements that represent the purpose of the research:

- The purpose of this study is to identify how student nurses feel about being supernumerary.
- The main purpose is to ascertain how satisfied the patients were with the food they got in hospital.

- The purpose of the study is to discover why so many new mothers decide not to breast feed.

Study Activity 15.5 _____

- Look at the examples of directional and non-directional hypotheses above and decide which is the independent variable and which the dependent variable in each. Discuss with a few colleagues and see if you all agree.
- Think about and write down two examples of each of the types of research statements: hypotheses, research questions, statements of purpose.

Methodology

The term methodology is often used in research as an umbrella concept to describe the various stages or the methods used in a research study (Stevens *et al.*, 1993; Parahoo, 1997; Polit and Hungler, 1999). For example, sampling procedure, data collection, data analysis, and so on. In actual fact these are the methods, and they are different to the methodology. Methodology is the investigation, the evaluation and the theory that underpins the methods. The difference is succinctly stated by Mautner (1997): 'methodology is *about* method, and not the same as method'. It is suggested here that the researcher should at least write some sections, if not a full chapter, on the methodological underpinnings of the research.

Methodology, as discussed here, relates to the investigation of philosophical reasons why the particular design was chosen. There are three main factors influencing the selection of research methods. First, the philosophical underpinning of the research; second, the researcher's worldview educational and/or professional background, as well as his/her philosophical beliefs; and third, the purpose and aims of the study (Haase and Myers, 1988; Simmons, 1995).

1 If the philosophical underpinnings are detailed, this allows the reader to assess the fit between the approaches used and the method-

ological underpinnings. In some cases, mixed research methods are used and it is not always clear that doing this has not invalidated the methodological beliefs of one or more of the approaches used.

2 There is a consensus in literature that in qualitative research the researcher is in fact the data collection instrument (Field and Morse, 1985; Rew *et al.*, 1993; Sorrell and Redmond, 1995). This being the case, it seems appropriate that the researcher should make his/her worldviews known. It could also be argued that this should be the case in quantitative research also, as it would allow the reader to identify possible researcher bias in a study.

3 There is no doubt that the research methods should be seen to clearly 'fit' the study aims and objectives. However, it should be kept in mind that the link between research aims and methods is not an independent connection, but rather it occurs through the medium of the researcher. A circle then begins to form in that the researcher's 'worldview', as discussed above, is inextricably linked methodologically with the research approach used.

Many commentators and researchers believe that nurses often fail to explicate the methodologies that encapsulate the methods they use (Baker *et al.*, 1992; Walters, 1995). It is suggested that methodological issues are pivotal to the analytical vision of research and there is a 'requirement to go beyond a purely "cook book" version of research methods' (Silverman, 1997).

The research design/methods

The most essential aspect of research design is that it must be suited to the research purpose. It is imperative that the research purpose determines the research design and, within it, the research methods, rather than the other way around. An important factor in determining the design, and an important aspect of the research process in its own right, is that of establishing exactly what the research sets out to achieve. As indicated earlier, this involves identifying a research topic and narrowing it down to a research issue or problems, and then more specifically research questions. This should finally result in specific statements of intended outcome of the research which must be identified no later than the stage of determining the research design, because they influence that design. It is beyond the scope of this chapter to provide a detailed description of the various research designs that may be used. The texts identified in Table 15.1 can be referred to for details of the most common designs. Table 15.3 lists the main

Table 15.3   Outline examples of research designs

Design	Typical design/methods	Function	Reference
Quantitative research designs			
Experiment	True experiments must have three elements: (1) *manipulation* – the intervention that is applied to one group (the experimental group) and not the other (the control group); (2) *randomisation* – allocating participants to the control and experimental groups by random means (note: this is random allocation and not random selection); (3) control – this has two main components: (a) relates to having a control group, as in (2); (b) relates to control of all or as many variables as possible so that the researcher can state with as high a degree of probability as possible that the manipulation (the intervention) caused the hypothesised effect. The cause and effect are established on the basis of statistical measurements of the outcome on the dependent variable	To test a hypothesis that the independent variable will cause the dependent variable, therefore, the design aims to establish 'cause and effect'	Jocelyn *et al.* (1998)
Quasi-experiment	In all experiments, *manipulation* must be present or it cannot correctly be called an experiment. A quasi-experiment will, therefore, have manipulation, but it may not have one of the other two elements, randomisation or control. It is therefore a quasi-experiment and not a true experiment. In all other respects it is the same as an experiment	As for experiment	
Correlation	This involves the measurement of two variables (usually naturally occurring), perhaps from figures taken from records. There is no manipulation as there is in an experiment. An example might be that records seem to indicate that there is a high rate of teenage pregnancy among those living in lower class inner city areas. Statistical testing of these records may find that there is a statistical correlation between living in a lower class inner city area and teenage pregnancy. Note that this establishes only that there is a correlation, i.e. there is an association in the manifestation of both variables, but a correlation is not 'cause and effect' as can be established in experiments	Can establish that there is a correlation, but it cannot establish 'cause and effect' – living in a lower class inner city area may correlate with teenage pregnancy, but other factors such as education, health, drug or alcohol use, etc. are not considered in relation to their influence	
Survey	Most often (but not always) involves the administration of questionnaires or measurement scales to large, randomly selected samples of the overall population. An example is opinion polls at the time of elections. There may be 500 000 people in an election area, of which 10 000 are randomly selected. The 10 000 may be posted or given questionnaires asking how they will vote. When the questionnaires are analysed the result is that it indicates how the 500 000 will vote.	To establish opinions, perceptions or attitudes of large populations (need not always be very large)	

Table 15.3 Continued

Design	Typical design/methods	Function	Reference
Qualitative research designs			
Grounded theory	Also called 'constant comparative' method as it involves collecting data, analysing it and collecting further data based on the analysis. The sampling is based on the analysis and is thus called theoretical sampling. May involve various methods of data collection, such as interviews, observations, documentary and artefact collection, as well as traditional research literature. Data collection and analysis continues until concepts, categories and themes that emerge are verified over and over again and no new ones are emerging; this is referred to as saturation.	To generate a new theory or modify or extend an existing theory.	McCutcheon and Pincombe (2001)
Ethnography	Involves collecting data about a community or culture from within the studied group. The most common methods used are therefore observations of the group supplemented with other methods such as interviews. The two most common types of observation are: participant observation – the researcher lives/works among the group and collects data while doing so; non-participant observation – the researcher observes those in the group/community/culture and records and analyses data based on the observations but does not participate as a member of the group.	To describe and enlighten understanding of a culture – may be a group, subgroup, community, or a total culture. It is about learning from as well as describing the culture.	
Action research	Involves a number of methods: (1) researcher observes practice area; (2) problems are identified; (3) a plan of action is made to improve the problem; (4) the action plan is put into place; (5) observation, data collection, analysis and evaluation of the outcomes of the plan are undertaken; (6) the plan is revised and the process continues. Those who work in the practice area are seen as partners in the process and practitioners themselves are often the researchers who work in collaboration with a key researcher.	To generate knowledge about practice and through actions lead to practice developments/ improvements.	
Phenomenology	Most often, but certainly not always, involves interviewing participants about their lived experiences. Interviews will be in-depth, one-to-one and the same participants may be interviewed a number of times. There are different phenomenological approaches. The following apply to some but not all approaches: *essences* – the researcher identifies these as 'meaning units', e.g. in an interview with a nurse about how he/she feels about nursing, essences appear to be caring, holism, empathy, helping and presence; *intuiting* – this involves the researcher making connections between the essences and how and in what manner these essences are visualised in the world of the participant, e.g. how might the essences about what nursing is actually appear in the day-to-day nursing interactions with actual patients; *bracketing* – this involves the researcher bringing to a conscious level their beliefs, values, professional knowledge, etc. and suspending these. In simple terms, to put these out of mind so they will not bias, direct or influence the research (not all phenomenological types of research support the idea of bracketing).	To gain understanding of lived experiences, the intention being that such knowledge can sensitise nurses to the inner emotions, feelings, aspirations and needs of the patients and clients they care for.	Svedlund et al. (2001)

elements and functions of some research designs.

Whatever the research method, there are components that constitute a typical research design. Creswell (1994) suggests that the following research methods are aspects of a research design: pilot (field trial), sampling, data collection, analysis, and presentation of findings. Ethical issues and methods to enhance the validity and reliability of the research are also central areas of concern.

Ethical considerations

Ethical approval should be obtained to undertake the study at the preliminary planning stage of the research process. When the research proposal is completed is an appropriate time to do this. Many organisations, including the National Health Service in the UK and universities, have ethical committees for considering the ethical correctness of proposed research. It is usually necessary to obtain their approval before research can be performed.

There are a number of ethical considerations relevant to research. The Royal College of Nursing (1998) forward the following principles that need be adhered to in research.

- *Beneficence* – this principle states that an act should 'do good'. In relation to research, it implies that research should have benefit. This benefit may be direct in terms of improved patient/client care, or it may be at a more distance time, i.e. knowledge may develop that eventually will lead to betterment for patients.
- *Non-maleficence* – a maleficent act is a harmful act. Non-maleficence may be considered as the opposite to maleficence. Therefore, non-maleficence means that an act should not harm. Research should not harm the participants, or anyone else. If there is any degree of risk of harm to anyone, then this risk needs to be assessed by an ethics committee and if deemed necessary the research should not be undertaken.

- *Justice* – this principle has to do with equity and fairness. Considerations here might be:

   Is a participant in research at an advantage by receiving health care resources because of the research while someone else who may be in greater need is not receiving the health care resource in question?

   Is a nursing lecturer neglecting his/her responsibilities with regard to teaching and supporting students in favour of research (Royal College of Nursing, 1998)?

- *Respect for autonomy* – autonomy is about self-determination, being empowered and exercising choice in one's life. Informed consent is important here. It is, therefore, imperative that anyone who is a subject in a research project gives informed consent to participate. In other words, the subject must know what they are letting themselves in for. The dilemma is that telling subjects too much may change the research findings by affecting their behaviour. Telling them too little may be a serious breach of ethics.

Validity and reliability

The value of the data presented depends on the quality of the instruments or the methods used to collect it. If these are faulty, then the data are likely to be inaccurate, and the findings from them are called into question if not completely inauthenticated.

Validity – in research, validity is a technical term with a specific meaning. It refers to the extent to which a method or instrument actually measures or provides information about what it was used to measure or provide information about. For example, an instrument which purports to measure job satisfaction must really do this and not measure other variables or combinations of variables such as mood or intelligence.

Reliability – for a method or instrument to be reliable, it must produce the same result under the same conditions. In essence it must be accurate and stable as a measure. For example, a ruler must always accurately measure 20 cm.

If it expands or contracts with heat so that the measure varies each time according to the temperature of the environment, it is an unreliable tool. It is possible for an instrument to be reliable and yet invalid as an instrument. For an instrument to be valid it must measure exactly what it is supposed to measure. For example, estimating the weight of subjects from their shoe size may be totally reliable. A foot gauge which is highly accurate may have been used, but this is an invalid measure of body weight, because there is a very weak correlation between shoe size and weight. An entirely different instrument is needed for measuring body weight. Therefore, data must be obtained via methods which are both reliable and valid; they must accurately measure exactly what they are supposed to.

Study Activity 15.6

Reflect on some instruments that may be used in any aspect of everyday life to measure something.

- Consider how you might determine whether or not these instruments are valid and reliable.
- Also consider what the outcome might be if the instruments you have thought of are not valid or reliable in terms of their function.

Pilot study, or field trial

When a researcher develops a new research instrument, or when they modify an existing one, there is a requirement to pilot the instrument. A pilot study is a trial run of the actual main study and it is conducted in a different site than the main study. Participants for the main study should not be used in a pilot study. The reasons for carrying out a pilot study are:

- to identify any problems with the instrument, i.e. the language used in a scale or questionnaire
- to establish how long it takes to complete the questionnaire
- to conduct a trial of the analysis procedures to be undertaken in the main study

- as one means of facilitating the enhancement of the validity and the reliability of an instrument.

Some suggest that a pilot study should not be undertaken in qualitative research. However, it is suggested here that a field trial should be carried out in qualitative research. Some reasons for such a field trial are to:

- become familiar with the data collection method, e.g. interviewing
- gauge the value of questions in a semi-structured interview schedule
- practice use of the tape recorder
- time how long interviews will take
- identify a suitable area/environment to undertake interviews
- consider practical aspects of the research, such as typing transcripts from the tape-recorded data.

A field trial is also useful when other data collection methods such as observations are used.

Sample and sampling

Seldom can research be undertaken that involves the selection of all the people the researcher wishes to collect data from. It is therefore necessary to select a sample from the population to be studied. This is referred to as the 'sampling procedure'. The final group of people who are selected through this procedure to take part in the study are the 'research sample'. There are a number of principles to be followed in sampling:

1 Sampling by random means that it is more likely that a representative group of participants is identified. Random here does not mean haphazard. It means the systematic selection of participants from a population in such a manner that all of those selected have an equal chance of being selected (Polit and Hungler, 1999).

2 The larger the sample size the more probable the chances that data collected will be representative of the total population.

3 The more heterogeneous the population, the larger a sample must be to give a reliable reflection of all the various characteristics.

There are basically two broad types of sampling: random (also called probability) and non-random (non-probability) sampling. Within these two groups there are various sampling methods.

Simple random sampling – this utilises the principles that are followed in all the other types of random sampling:

- A 'sampling frame' is established. This is a list of all the people from which the sample will be drawn.
- All those on the list are numbered in sequential order.
- A table of random numbers (or computer-generated numbers) is then used to select the desired sample number from the sampling frame.

Suppose one wanted to select 100 people from a sampling frame of 1000. A good example of this is the analogy of the tombola draw for national lottery numbers. If 1000 balls are placed in the drum (each one numbered) and a random selection of 100 is required, then 100 balls are automatically selected and the numbers on these 100 are used to select 100 names in accordance with the sampling frame list. As there is a requirement that each person has an equal chance of being selected, i.e. in this case 1 in a 1000, each time a ball is selected the person's name is marked on the list and the ball is returned to the drum. If this is not done, by the time the last person is selected the chances of selection would have changed to 1 in 900. The selection continues until all 100 people are selected.

Study Activity 15.7

This is a full class activity. Arrange to do this as part of a research class with your lecturer. You and two or three other students should organise the activity. List all the names of everyone in your class and then number everyone consecutively on your class list. Write the numbers on pieces of paper and place them in a container. Next, select a number of variables from all the students in the class. These can be simple things that do not require anyone to provide private details, e.g. the numbers with long

hair and with short hair, the numbers wearing different colours of shoes, male to female, etc., and work out the percentage of these variables in your group. List these variables against each student's name and number. Then select numbers from the container as in the example of random sampling above, i.e. if there are 50 in your class, select 15. Finally, work out the percentages of the variables in the sample of 15 and compare these with the variables in the total in your class. If they are not similar, increase the number selected to 20 and continue increasing in fives to see how far you need to go before the percentage of the variables is the same as it is in the total 50.

In research, the researcher must make clear the sampling procedures followed to allow the reader to make a judgement about how representative of the population the sample is. Only random sampling is detailed here. For detailed descriptions of various random and non-random sampling procedures, refer to the texts listed in Table 15.1. Table 15.4 identifies the main types of sampling that can be used.

Table 15.4 The most common research sampling procedures

Random sampling types	Non-random sampling types
Simple	Convenience
Stratified	Purposive
Cluster (multistage)	Theoretical
Systematic	Snowball

Random sampling is used in quantitative research and non-random is used most often in qualitative research. However, for various reasons it is sometimes difficult to use random selection in quantitative research and, therefore, non-random sampling may be used on occasion.

Data collection

Two aspects of this phase may be distinguished:

1 the circumstances or context of data collection
2 the process of data collection.

The circumstances – the research should make clear answers to the following questions:

- What form does the contact with participants take?
- Is the communication oral or written, or both?

  Individual oral communication can be stimulating, but very time-consuming. Sometimes it is possible to find an intermediate method where the researcher makes personal contact with a group of respondents, for example to explain the intentions of the study. The research is followed up and carried out in writing afterwards.

- What is the frequency of the contact?
- How often is data collected?
- How will the respondents' confidentiality be protected? Is this carefully taken into account or hardly considered?

  The issue here is confidentiality during the course of the research and the impact of contact or confidentiality upon the process of data collection.

  The practical aspects of the research come under this heading as well. As conducting research is a human activity, a few practical and administrative matters, such as telephone calls, appointments, memos, visits, etc., will have to be taken care of.

All of these questions are related to the circumstances of the research and should be answered as part of the overall process.

The process of data collection – an important question here is how respondents can be motivated to optimum levels of co-operation? One major factor is respect for the individuality and independence of the participant. This respect and consideration should be made very apparent from the researcher's attitude towards keeping appointments, offering adequate explanations, and so on.

Second, it may be important to obtain the co-operation of key figures who have some influ-ence on the participants. These might be people from the institutions and organisations which co-ordinate the research and who can encourage respondents to participate.

Third, clear explanation of the intention of the research and the giving of straightforward instructions may contribute to the motivation of the participant.

Finally, the motivation of the researcher should be considered. If, for whatever reason, they do not appear interested or motivated, this attitude may be transferred to the participants and affect responses.

It is helpful as part of the process of data collection to record a diary of events. In this the course of events during the research is laid down. It is thus possible to account retrospectively for events such as a participant withdrawing from the study.

Data analysis

Before data are collected the researcher must have planned the analytical procedures that are to be used to analyse the information.

Because the raw material can be used more than once, it can be useful sometimes to apply different analytical techniques to meet specific purposes. Of course the researcher must be able to show how these choices fit within the total research plan. In the process of data analysis, at least two stages can be identified:

1 The processing of data – in the case of quantitative research, large databases are often used that are encoded, making it necessary to have a listing of the codes together with the given values of the variables. The manual entering of data in a computer file is very labour intensive and can sometimes be assisted by the use of an optical character reader.

2 The factual analysis – for simple analyses (frequency distribution and determination of average, median, mode and dispersion) and when the sample size is small, data are sometimes more easily processed without a computer. This certainly applies when one is relatively unfamiliar with statistical programs.

For more complicated analyses a computer is indispensable.

Statistical methods usually involve two types of procedure: descriptive statistics and inferential statistics. Descriptive analyses confine themselves to one variable only, such as frequency distribution, average, dispersion, etc. Typical would be the age ranges of the people in the sample, number of males to females, professional qualifications and so on. These may be presented as percentages, ratios or other descriptive representations. Inferential statistical methods, as the name suggests, are often applied for experimental research. Of these, the variance analysis and the t-test are commonly used. Inferential statistics usually involve testing for the differences or relationships between variables and whether this relationship is statistically significant. A statistical significance probability level is set, and this is tested for as a means of determining if differences are significant.

There is a wide variety of qualitative analysis techniques. Most involve transforming data into written transcripts, reading the total transcript, reading line-by-line or section-by-section and during this coding the data. The coding typically involves the identification of concepts, themes, subcategories, categories, and in some types of analysis (e.g. grounded theory) the identification of a core central category that captures conceptually all the other themes and categories. On occasion a process of 'content analysis' can be used to quantify qualitative narrative data.

Present the findings from the analysis

Following the data analysis, the findings are presented. In some types of quantitative research, this is a pure descriptive presentation with no discussion or interpretation of what these mean. Presentation of the results is accomplished by two means, a descriptive account and by visual portrayal. These are presented separately here, but in reality both means of presenting support and accompany each other.

Descriptive accounts

Written descriptive details of findings are presented with a mix of narrative and numeric symbols. For example, one might write that the sample group consisted of 177 (87%) females and 27 (13%) males. The presentation of inferential statistical tests involves the results of significance probability tests. The most common probability level is 0.05, represented as p (probability) (meaning equal to or less than). Therefore, $p \leq 0.05$ would indicate that if a cause results it is probable that this same result will occur 95 times out of 100, or on only five times in 100 would the result not occur.

Visual portrayal

The visual portrayal of findings will be in the form of some of the following: graphs, pie charts, scatter plots, or tables. These should be clear and easy to follow. They should be well labelled and the reader should be able to tell at a glance what is represented.

Qualitative presentation

Qualitative presentation usually involves the telling of a 'story line' and this is supported by direct narrative accounts from the data. Figures and diagrams may also be used, but these tend to be more in the form of theoretical or conceptual maps.

Discussion of the findings

In this part of the research process the researcher interprets the findings and what they mean in terms of implications, limitations, and recommendations. This is the aspect of the research process where most problems can arise. To avoid problems the researcher should:

- make no claims that cannot be founded on the findings of the research
- avoid 'sweeping statements'– statements that are not based on the evidence in the research.
- generalise to well beyond that warranted by the findings or have otherwise no sound foundation

- not attempt to highlight findings that are insignificant, as some are tempted to do due to personal bias
- maintain an objective perspective.

Implications

Most nursing research will have implications for one or more of four aspects: nursing education, nursing care, management or future research. The researcher should objectively interpret what the findings mean for one or all of these aspects.

Recommendations

Following on from the implications of the research will be the recommendations that can be made based on the findings. Generally speaking one of three recommendations can be made:

1 There is evidence from the findings to support a recommended course of action and thus it is recommended that change be introduced.
2 The study provides evidence that no change should be made in respect of the topic under investigation.
3 The results from the research are inconclusive and thus a recommendation is made to conduct further research in relation to the topic. Such a recommendation may suggest an alternative research approach, a different or larger sample group, or that the research is repeated in a different location(s).

Limitations

It is vitally important, and an ethical obligation, that any limitations to the research are identified. This takes courage and openness in the researcher, but it should be remembered that nursing research inevitably involves investigations related to the care of ill and vulnerable people. It is therefore a moral imperative that readers of research are fully aware of any limitations, particularly significant ones that may call the results of the research into question.

Conclusion to the study

The final part of the discussion should be a section in which the researcher draws together the overall findings. This is a succinct detail of the most relevant findings of the research and what can be drawn from these. A good conclusion of such an extensive piece of work is difficult to conceptualise and then write. The researcher may need to read the report a number of times, leave it for periods and come back to it before he/she can write an appropriate conclusion.

The written report and dissemination

This is the final part of the research process. Undertaking research is difficult to justify if it is not disseminated to the nursing academic and professional community. This is achieved by a number of means:

- There is an onus on the researcher to present the research to those who agreed to participate in the study. In addition, those who facilitated access to the research site should be given access to the completed research.
- If the research is undertaken in fulfilment of an academic degree, then it will need to be presented in accordance with the guidance for this.
- The findings may be presented through a research colloquium or conference.
- The study may be published in an academic or professional journal.
- Increasingly, researchers are publishing via online journals.

If the research is to be submitted to a journal or as a dissertation, the researcher will be able to obtain guidance on how the written report should be presented. In general, as far as layout is concerned, the research account should meet the general conditions for written reports. To present the research as well as possible, the following should receive particular attention:

- title, and subtitle if any
- author(s)
- summary or abstract
- introduction and context for the research
- an exposition of the relevant literature
- the formulated question(s) or issue(s)

- theoretical basis
- the methodological approach – identified at least
- type of research and research design (the sample and sampling; instruments used; data collection and analysis; ethical considerations; validity and reliability)
- results
- conclusions, recommendations, points of discussion
- bibliography or list of references cited.

SUMMARY

In this chapter, the meaning of research has been identified as a scientific method involving a systematic collection of empirical information through an analytical linear process. This process is referred to as the 'research process'. It is suggested here that nursing has reached a stage of professional and academic maturity where it is reasonable to forward the perspective of 'nursing research'. Nursing research is research undertaken with the ultimate goal of benefiting all aspects of nursing, most importantly the patients/clients that nurses care for. The idea of 'nursing research' may seem an insular and isolationist approach, but there is no suggestion here that nurses should refrain from participation in multidisciplinary research. Nurses can contribute to and gain from collaborate research with other professionals.

Good research will have two main characteristics. One is a good research idea. This will occur when a nurse makes an imaginative conceptual connection. The idea may be triggered by an unanticipated occurrence, personal study or questions from clients. This idea will become the seed from which research and ultimately practice knowledge advancement shall grow.

The second characteristic of good research is the competence, skill and methodological grasp of the various stages of the research process that the nurse researcher demonstrates. This chapter has identified these stages as signposts to follow. It is asserted here that like nursing care, expertise in research requires practice, and in a similar vein to nursing care, nursing research requires a reflective process to draw theory and knowledge together in the doing of research.

REFERENCES

Abbot, P. and Sapsford, R. (1998) *Research Methods for Nurses and the Caring Professions* (2nd edn), Open University Press, Buckingham

Baker, C., Wuest, J. and Stern, P.N. (1992) Method slurring: the grounded theory phenomenology example. *Journal of Advanced Nursing* 17, 1355–60

Burns, N. and Grove, S.K. (1987) *The Practice of Nursing Research – Conduct, critique and utilization*, W.B. Saunders, Philadelphia, IL

Cohen, L. and Manion, L. (1989) *Research Methods in Education*, Routledge, London

Cormack, D.F.S. (1996) *The Research Process in Nursing*, Blackwell, Oxford

Creswell, J.W. (1994) *Research Design: Qualitative and quantitative approaches*, Sage, London

Crookes, P. and Davis, S. (eds) (1998) *Research into Practice*, Baillière Tindall, Edinburgh

Field, P.A. and Morse, J.M. (1985) *Nursing Research: The application of qualitative approaches*, Croom Helm, London

Haase, J.E. and Myers, S.T. (1988) Reconciling paradigm assumptions of qualitative and quantitative research. *Western Journal of Nursing Research* 10(2), 128–37

Hays, W.L. (1994) *Statistics* (5th edn), Holt, Rinehart and Winston, New York

Hockey, L. (1996) The nature and purpose of research. In: Cormack, D.F.S. (ed.) *The Research Process in Nursing*, Blackwell, Oxford

Holloway, I. and Wheeler, S. (1996) *Qualitative Research for Nurses*, Blackwell Science, London

Jocelyn, L.J., Casiro, O.G., Beattie, M.S.W., Bow, J. and Kneisz, J. (1998) Treatment of children with autism: a randomized controlled trial to evaluate a caregiver-based intervention program in community day-care centers. *Developmental and Behavioral Pediatrics* 19(5), 326–33

Kerlinger, F.N. (1973) *Foundations of Behavioral Research*, Holt, Rinehart and Winston, New York

Mautner, T. (ed.) (1997) *Dictionary of Philosophy*, Penguin Books, London

McCutcheon, H.I. and Pincombe, J. (2001) Intuition: an important tool in the practice of nursing. *Journal of Advanced Nursing* 35(3), 342–8

McKenna, H. and Mason, C. (1998) Nursing and the wider R&D agenda: influence and contribution. *NT Research* 3(2), 108–15

Parahoo, K. (1997) *Nursing Research Principles, Process and Issues*, Macmillan, London

Polit, D.F. and Hungler, B.P. (1999) *Nursing Research Principles and Methods* (6th edn), J.B. Lippincott, New York

Rew, L., Bechtel, D. and Sapp, A. (1993) Self-as-instrument in qualitative research. *Nursing Research* 42(5), 300–1

Royal College of Nursing (1998) *Research Ethics: Guidance for nurses involved in research or any investigative project involving human subjects. Standards of care*, Royal College of Nursing, London

Silverman, D. (1997) Introducing qualitative research. In: Silverman, D. (ed.) *Qualitative Research Theory, Method and Practice*, Sage, London, pp. 1–7.

Simmons, S. (1995) From paradigm to method in interpretive action research. *Journal of Advanced Nursing* 21(5), 837–44

Sorrell, J.M. and Redmond, G.M. (1995) Interviews in qualitative nursing research: differing approaches for ethnographic and phenomenological studies. *Journal of Advanced Nursing* 21(6), 1117–22

Stevens, P.J.M., Schade, A.L., Chalk, B. and Slevin, O. (1993) *Understanding Research: A scientific approach for health care professionals*, Campion Press, Edinburgh

Svedlund, M., Danielson, E. and Norberg, A. (2001) Women's narratives during the acute phase of their myocardial infarction. *Journal of Advanced Nursing* 35(2), 197–204

Walters, A.J. (1995) The phenomenological movement: implications for nursing research. *Journal of Advanced Nursing* 22, 791–9

16 RESEARCH PARADIGMS

Eamonn Slevin

LEARNING OUTCOMES

After studying this chapter you will be able to:

- Understand the term 'research paradigm'
- Gain knowledge about research paradigms that will allow you to compare and contrast these
- Recognise the main values and limitations of the most common research paradigms
- Develop the necessary knowledge to be able to evaluate the appropriateness of the use of particular paradigms within research
- Recognise why and how paradigms change.

INTRODUCTION

The purpose of research is to produce the 'best available evidence' (or knowledge) to inform practice (an issue addressed later in the module, in the chapters concerning evidence-based practice). It is therefore important to recognise the values, methods, strengths and limitations of a particular approach (or paradigm). In order to be able to systematically review and critique a piece of research, the dominant discourse reflected by the 'paradigm' used within the study must be considered critically. As a student, and in your future role as a nurse, you need to develop a suitable degree of scepticism about the appropriateness of any paradigm for addressing particular health care/nursing issues.

Elsewhere in this book the term paradigm has been discussed in relation to nursing theory. A paradigm is generally taken to mean a set of beliefs, principles, values, rules and ideas that form the *'worldview'* held by a group or discipline (Kuhn, 1970; Fawcett, 1992; Stevens

Barnum, 1994). It also means the methods and philosophical underpinnings used to investigate phenomena of interest to a discipline. Theories can be grouped together according to paradigmatic worldviews and such theories may then be used to guide or frame practice (McKenna, 1997; Thompson, 2000). Just as there are paradigms or worldviews (the terms worldview and paradigm are used interchangeably in this chapter, both terms having similar meaning) that provide the basis of theory, there are also research paradigms. In the previous chapter, research was defined and the stages in a typical research process were detailed. However, it is important to remember that there are different types of research. These different types of research can be grouped together in a number of ways, but the most common way of grouping is according to which paradigm the research approach used is considered to belong to. Therefore, research undertaken will be underpinned by a particular worldview, although in some cases mixed research methods (drawing on more than one worldview) may be used within a single study.

Some researchers have strong beliefs in adhering to particular research paradigms and argue that the research methods used are influenced significantly by the researcher's personal worldview (Simmons, 1995). Parahoo (1997), commenting on the influence of research paradigms, states 'a paradigm creates it own cultural environment that regulates the behaviours of its followers and favours research conforming to its own rules'.

THE MAIN RESEARCH PARADIGMS

It is important to recognise the paradigm assumptions that underpin different research

---

303

methods, as the approaches used differ significantly. According to this notion of different research paradigms, methods can be broadly divided into the following:

- *Quantitative research* – essentially modelled on the traditional natural sciences (physics, chemistry, biology, etc.), and is sometimes termed positivistic science (although some see the term positivism as archaic now) because of the emphasis on measurement, experimentation and objectivity.
- *Qualitative research* – more concerned with description, meaning, and subjective experience, and which some describe as humanistic science (although some see this term as disparaging because of the suggestion of it being an art rather than true scientific endeavour).
- *New paradigm research* – a term that has been used to describe research that does not fit neatly into the above paradigms. It attempts to establish new approaches that are seen to be more appropriate for researching complex human situations. However, whether these approaches are 'new' or merely alternative ways of using and combining existing research methods is open to debate. Perhaps the term 'alternative' or 'critical' paradigm may be more appropriate.

Quantitative perspectives

Because of its positivistic roots, quantitative research has the longest tradition, both in nursing and in the social and life sciences as a whole. A positivist viewpoint suggests that only empirical knowledge is valid and that all knowledge must be based on observing phenomena and establishing facts. This approach usually means basing knowledge on objective observation and measurement and refuting interpretation and conjecture as irrelevant. While positivism is not a strong disciplinary force today, the tradition of relying on observable behaviour and rejecting interpretation other than on the basis of what can be seen (or measured) is still at the core of quantitative methods. Because

of its apparent scientific respectability, nursing espoused this perspective for many years as the only legitimate form of research. But in recent years this has changed. There is now a greater recognition within nursing for the need to use other paradigms to research practice (Hicks and Hennessy, 1997).

The vocabulary that appears in the literature on quantitative research methodology is markedly different. Here words such as 'experiment', 'quasi-experiment', 'hypothesis', 'generalisation', 'measurement', 'cause', and 'statistical significance' abound. This approach originates in the positivistic tradition, modelled on the natural sciences and relegating the humanistic approach to the arts. Subjectivity is a failing, while objectivity is the goal. In this case the medium for advancing scientific truths is the experiment or at the very least a descriptive survey. Analysis is conducted on the basis of measured data obtained by direct observation and structured closed-question interviews or questionnaires, almost always requiring large data sets and statistical numerical analysis.

The classical, purist example of a quantitative approach is the experiment. An experiment by its very nature involves a controlled situation, variables which are measurable in quantitative terms, and a goal of establishing a highly probable cause–effect relationship. In order to establish causality, there must be a strong relationship between the proposed cause and the effect. The cause must precede the effect and should always be present prior to the effect occurring. In its simplest form, a variable (a phenomenon, person, or object which is capable of change) is measured, a second variable is brought to bear on it, and it is again measured to see if the second variable caused it to change in any way. The more often this effect can be replicated, the stronger the claim for a cause–effect relationship. Statistical tests can be applied to establish the strength of this claim, as opposed to the changes having occurred by chance.

However, in the social sciences, as well as nursing, such experimental opportunities are rare. A scientist could place a piece of metal in a vacuum container and apply heat to it and then record at what exact heat the metal bends. This could be repeated and if the size, shape and chemical elements of the metal remain the same, the vacuum container maintains the same pressure and the heat is applied in exactly the same way the metal will bend at the same degree of heat. Such an experiment could be repeated and time after time the metal will bend at the same degree of heat. This might be a very useful experiment in terms of the fire safety of buildings, or constructing fireproof safes.

However, isolating variables and subjecting them to single influences is very difficult in real situations involving complex human beings. More often when social phenomena change in some way there is a complex interaction of difficult-to-control causal influences at play. No two people are exactly the same in the way that one piece of metal is the same as another which has the same chemical elements. Nor can placing the person in any can of vacuum control that person's environment, life experiences and other aspects. The best that can be hoped for is a relative rather than absolute claim to causality, that there is a degree of probability that a cause–effect relationship exists and thus, by definition, a degree of possibility that the relationship only appears to exist by chance.

Study Activity 16.1 _____

Happiness, success, and sound relationships depend on letting go of controlling things that are beyond your control. Examples of things that you cannot control are the feelings of others, the future, the past and whether or not other people like you.

(Hendricks, 1998)

- Reflect on the above citation. Do you agree that these are things that one cannot control in life?
- Think about things in life that might need to be controlled (kept constant) if you were to undertake experimental research that compared two or more groups of people. Make a list of the things you identified (in research these are called variables)

and discuss them with a group of your colleagues. Questions you might wish to debate are:

– How can all the variables that may affect the outcome of an experiment be kept constant in human beings?
– Can experiments be undertaken on human beings at all?

- Having undertaken the above exercises, go to the library and search for some research papers in journals that use experimental, or other quantitative methods. Read one or two and then reflect again on your views above.
- With a group of your colleagues make a list of possible practice problems (or areas of interest) that you feel could be researched using quantitative methods. To begin, include anything at all that you and your colleagues identify. Use brainstorming techniques and do not worry about how you would go about researching the problems you identify.
- Go over your list a second time and consider whether there are any research problems on it that you feel would be too difficult, or even impossible to study using human beings as subjects.

Qualitative perspectives

Qualitative research, sometimes referred to as 'interpretive', is a more recent approach that sees human beings as complex entities, not susceptible to measurement and manipulation as are minerals, metals, plants, or even lower order animals. Because of their complexity, humans need to be studied in their subjective contexts by describing how they experience and find meaning in their world. The approach essentially finds its roots in the social sciences, particularly in sociology, anthropology, ethnography, psychology and philosophy (Maggs-Rapport, 2001).

Qualitative methods – variously described as fieldwork, naturalistic methods, interpretive research, phenomenological methods, ethnography (all with similar qualitative perspectives but variations in approach) – emphasise the real world and the particular personal or social situation of the subjects. The primary purpose is to describe and evaluate this world. Agar (1986) stresses that the issue is not what the hypothesis is, or whether the findings can be generalised. Rather, it is about what is taking place and the meanings people assign to their lived actions or experiences. The approach is essentially humanistic in that it attends to subjects as persons in their social contexts.

Qualitative research is defined here as an approach to researching human beings that centres on unique experiences, is holistic and in-depth, and utilises various methods to collect rich narrative (non-numerical) data in natural settings with the aim of identifying meanings that people ascribe to a phenomenon (or phenomena).

Key words in the literature on qualitative methodology convey the perspective: 'humanistic', 'naturalistic', 'descriptive', 'introspection', 'understanding', and 'holistic explanation'. Advocates of the approach stress accuracy and scientific endeavour, in the sense of a science of understanding the real world as others experience it. And the medium for conveying scientific truths is via description and analysis of the world on the basis of information gained from such methods as participant observation (where the researcher becomes an active participant in the social situation, perhaps becoming a member of staff or a group member, while at the same time observing and recording what is happening), in-depth open-ended unstructured interviews, and research of personal documents, diaries, and life histories.

The main criticism offered by opponents of qualitative research methods is that there is an over-reliance on the use of subjectivity, intuition, human senses and expressed views that are not 'tested' by rigorous scientific means. On the other hand, Parahoo (1997) suggests that the practice of nursing shares characteristics such as 'patient centred, holistic and humanistic' with qualitative research and therefore these approaches are suitable for researching nursing phenomena.

Study Activity 16.2

For this activity, you can actually undertake some very limited data collection.

- *Observation* – the next time you are in the clinical area, observe one or more patients' behaviours and see if you can identify anything that you feel may have more significance to the person than your initial view of the behaviour, i.e. the behaviour may have a function but is there anything else going on that tells you something else? Perhaps the behaviour has another hidden function?
- *Interview* – until you are skilled at interviewing it might be better to undertake this with a colleague or close friend. If you are aware of any experience/s that your friend has had that is interesting, ask them if they would let you interview them about this. Make it a short interview, 20 minutes or so. Before you interview your friend, think of questions you would like to ask. Use some of the words in italics in the following lines by Rudyard Kipling (cited in Hargie et al., 1991) to guide you in the interview:

    I keep six honest serving men (they taught me all I know);
    Their names are *What* and *Why* and *When*,
    And *How* and *Where* and *Who*.

- Record the interview if you can (if not make notes) and afterwards listen to it a number of times and ascertain if you can understand how your friend perceives the experience he/she had. Discuss your findings with your friend – does he/she agree with your interpretation of what was said in the interview?
- With a group of colleagues, make a list of possible practice problems (or areas of interest) that you feel could be researched using qualitative methods.
- Use the library to search for some research papers in journals that use qualitative methods. Read these and discuss with your lecturer and colleagues what value you feel these offer to nursing practice.

QUANTITATIVE AND QUALITATIVE PERSPECTIVES – COMPARISON OF MAIN ASPECTS

The above overviews of quantitative and qualitative perspectives can be further explained by considering some of the differences between the two approaches. It must be recognised that the opposing pictures are more in the nature of ideal types or extreme pictures than realities. However, the differences are notable enough to allow differences to be tabulated (*see* Table 16.1 for a comparison of the two paradigms).

The issue can be simplified to the level of a debate about words and numbers, which perhaps highlights the potential weaknesses in both perspectives. Numbers without words, or with very few of them, as in the extreme quantitative perspective, dooms research to the position of presenting an incomplete picture, one weak in depth and meaning. This risk is high where data collection has emphasised measurement and the collection of numerical data, while ignoring descriptive information and analysis. Later, at the usually separate stage of analysis when such verbal information may be vital, it is too late. And to attempt to introduce descriptive or interpretive information at this stage – after the event, so to speak – would be to introduce information liable to all the subjectivity that the natural scientists attempt to avoid.

However, the qualitative perspective with an emphasis on words and an absence or lack of numerical data at its most extreme is also incomplete. Some supporters of the perspective argue that this position is justified, indeed suggesting that it is the definitive and essential characteristic of their approach. To them, their role is to explore, discover, and describe the world humans occupy, and by so doing to give it meaning (Field and Morse, 1985; Holloway and Wheeler, 1996). There is little concern with establishing laws of human behaviour here.

Theory testing and theory generating research

The two paradigms are sometimes presented within the perspectives of 'theory testing' or 'theory generating' research. In the former,

Table 16.1 Some of the main differences in the quantitative and qualitative paradigms

Quantitative	Qualitative
Numerical measurable data	Narrative interpretative data
Objective	Subjective
Belief in single truth about a phenomenon	Belief in multiple truths about a phenomenon
Associated with *inductive* processes	Associated with *deductive* processes
Mistrust of human senses in data collection – use of structured instruments	Human senses acknowledged in data collection – researcher is instrument
Singular elements of a phenomenon are the focus of study (parts make the *person*)	Total person as an integrated whole is the focus of study (*person* is greater than the parts and parts cannot be researched in isolation from the total person)
People researched are *subjects* and are selected by random means	People are research *respondents* – selection is intentional/ purposive and/or because of theoretical richness
Person can be isolated – environment, context, life influences and other variables can be controlled (*value free*)	Person is integrated with environment, context, life influences and other variables – these influence people individually and cannot be controlled (*value dependent*)
Robustness measures – validity, reliability	Robustness criteria – truth value, consistency and confirmability
Findings stem from large random samples (or random allocated experimental groups) and usual aims are to:	Small purposive sample and usual aims are to:
– generalise to total population	identify unique experiences
– identify cause and effect	– give voice to hidden phenomena
– identify collective views, opinions or behaviours	– sensitise others to the experiences, culture, roles or symbolic importance of life events of research respondents

'theory testing', a hypothesis is established and this is tested in practice, usually using experimental research. An important point to remember about this term is that seldom if ever is a total theoretical perspective tested. In fact, Moody (1990) states with regard to nursing, or other theories, that 'the theory or model is never tested directly itself, but the propositions or hypotheses derived from it are submitted to empirical testing'.

In the latter of these two perspectives, 'theory generating research', theoretical perspectives arise from the data, and are developed from information unfolding in the course of carrying out fieldwork. The work of Glaser and Strauss (1967) on 'grounded theory' (so-called because of the emphasis on theory emerging 'from the ground' in the course of fieldwork rather than elsewhere) is the most often quoted example of this perspective. For an up-to-date account of the approach, you may find it helpful to consult Strauss and Corbin (1990, 1998).

Research robustness

Perhaps the major weakness in qualitative research is its emphasis on a descriptive, situation-specific and non-measurement-orientated approach. It is usually not possible to establish the reliability of such work. In research, *reliability* is a technical term with a very specific meaning. It refers to the capacity for a test, instrument, or measure to present the same results each time it is carried out under the exact same conditions. Thus, a thermometer should record 100°C each time it is immersed in boiling water, and each observer who uses the thermometer should be able to come up with the exact same result. If, however, the thermometer is immersed in 10 different containers of boiling water and records grossly different temperatures each time, we conclude that it is an unreliable instrument. The research methods employed in qualitative research, e.g. participant observation by a single researcher who makes non-quantitative descriptive records, and dyadic, in-depth unstructured interviews, do not allow for the usual checks on reliability, such as test–retest

schedules. The value of the research, irrespective of how well written and colourful, is therefore open to some doubt.

Indeed, the tendency for researchers in this field is to occasionally select colourful or controversial topics [*see*, e.g. the classical studies by Becker (1955) on marihuana users and Punch (1986) on public schooling]. This tendency increases the sense of doubt in cynical critics of the qualitative approach; they see such studies as attempts to dramatise rather than as serious scientific works. As a justification for their viewpoint, they often point not only to the dubious subject matter of qualitative research, but also to what they see as dubious and unscientific methodology; such work, they claim, does not even meet one of the basic tenets of science, that of reliability.

However, it should be recognised that qualitative researchers often do not make claims for reliability in their work; indeed many reject reliability as a concept that has any relevance to their area of science. They would argue that they strive only to give valid and meaningful insights into little known corners of the social world. But there is an expanding body of knowledge, evident in rigorous publications, that nurse researchers are using varied and appropriate methods to enhance the robustness of their research (*see*, for example, Hinds *et al.*, 1990; Beck, 1994; Appleton, 1995; Cutcliffe and McKenna, 1999; Slevin and Sines, 2000).

In research, validity is also a technical term with a specific meaning. It refers to the extent to which a method or instrument actually measures or provides information about what it was used to measure or provide information about. For example, an instrument which purports to measure job satisfaction must really do this and not measure other variables or combinations of variables such as mood or intelligence. Essentially, qualitative researchers attempt to establish validity by use of a number of techniques, such as presenting an audit trail of how their findings emerged; undertaking member checks (taking data back to respondents to ascertain their agreement, or not, with the findings); collecting data until saturation is reached; or using various different methods together to research the phenomenon of interest, e.g. interviews, observations, and document analysis. Using more than one research method to study the same situation in this way is a technique known as the *mixed methods* approach, or *triangulation*. The assumption in this approach is that bias that is a specific risk of one method can be overcome if more than one method is used. This approach is addressed again in the next section of this chapter.

Paradigm terms

To conclude this section, some of the terminology you might come across as you read about research is presented. Table 16.2 lists various terms that are used by different nurse theorists and others when referring to the two main paradigms. In each case the terms used are associated with either the quantitative or the qualitative perspectives.

Use of varied complex terminology can be quite off-putting to a student who is beginning to study research paradigms. However, the terms used in Table 16.2 are really only different semantic labels for the two main research paradigms, although the authors who use these may not agree with this assertion.

Table 16.2 Terminology associated with the quantitative and the qualitative paradigms

Associated with the quantitative paradigm	Associated with the qualitative paradigm
Logical positivism	Interpretivism
Natural science	Human science
Received view	Perceived view (Meleis, 1997)
Realism	Conceptualism (Stevens Barnum, 1994)
Totality	Simultaneity (Parse *et al.*, 1985; Cody, 1995)

Study Activity 16.3 ———

Organise a class debate with the agreement of your lecturer. The debate statement is: 'The use of varied terminology to describe research paradigms is not useful, creates confusion and does little to promote research in nursing.'

HOW AND WHY PARADIGMS CHANGE

Before moving on to new paradigms in research, it is necessary to consider how and why paradigms might change. There are a number of reasons for the change in research methods.

The reasons for change

In some disciplines, nursing being one, there is a recognition that qualitative or quantitative perspectives are not always the best means to research the many and varied phenomena that are of concern. As a result there has been an emergence of new paradigms (or perspectives) that are seen as being more relevant to addressing problems or issues in the particular field of inquiry. This is not only so in nursing, there have been calls for new research paradigms that address 'human' as opposed to 'mechanistic medical' issues in medicine (Underwood *et al.*, 1986; McWhinney, 1991).

The problem is that, as suggested earlier, the mainstream quantitative approach is limited in the extent to which it can answer some of the questions being asked, particularly in nursing, an activity which is essentially humanistic, concerned with intimate caring and deeply subjective interpersonal relationships. It is argued by some that, by virtue of its essentially objective and neutral perspective, the quantitative approach, dominated by randomised controlled experiments, frequently overshadows the use of alternative methods of research (Hicks and Hennessy, 1997). The need for a different scientific paradigm is thus particularly important.

We can, of course, answer some of our questions through the quantitative approach. Indeed, where the variables (phenomena under study) are easily identified, measured, controlled and manipulated, these are the methods of choice. Rogers (1985) suggested that:

> *The Newtonian, mechanistic, reductionist, linear cause–effect, behaviorist view of science is not thrown out but is seen as simply one aspect of science, a perfectly good way of investigating some problems, but decidedly inappropriate for others.*
>
> (Rogers, 1985)

We can, for example, identify the types of back injury most common among nurses and investigate the influence of training in lifting techniques on the incidence of such injury. Similarly, we can use observational time sampling studies to measure the levels of activity among the elderly residents of a nursing home. But in reality it is not that simple. There may be other variables that we cannot control and which corrupt our findings or introduce margins of error that question the results. For example, back injury is notoriously difficult to diagnose and classify, and there may be malingering or psychosomatic influences at play.

There are means of overcoming such problems by controlling their influence or by statistically estimating the degree of potential error they bring to the findings. But what if, for example, we are interested not simply in levels of activity among elderly residents, but in the meaningfulness of life in nursing homes or the nature of the nurse–patient relationship and how it may be therapeutically constructed? In these cases the straightforward quantitative approach is of little value.

In some instances the qualitative approach is the alternative of choice which provides the depth and meaning we require. But sometimes even this is inadequate. The challenging questions, and those we sometimes tend to avoid because of their difficult and often emotive nature, are more problematic. Here are questions concerning the nature of caring, coping with death and dying, or emotional aspects of the nurse–patient relationship. Of these, Schön (1987) has stated:

> *In the varied topography of professional practice, there is a high, hard ground overlooking a swamp. On the high ground, manageable problems lend themselves to solution through the application of research-based theory and technique. In the swampy lowland, messy confusing problems defy technical solution. The practitioner must choose. Should he remain on the high ground where he can solve relatively unimportant problems according to the prevailing standards of rigour or shall he descend to the swamp of important problems and nonrigorous inquiry?*
>
> (Schön, 1987)

The argument presented by Schön is important. Is he really suggesting that the most important questions we must answer should not be approached rigorously? This position would surely not be acceptable; there is in no sense a justification for basing the most crucial aspects of practice on subjective thinking. However, if what Schön means by 'rigorous inquiry' is, as he words it, the *prevailing* approach, i.e. the standard natural scientific quantitative methods, or even the standard qualitative approaches that have developed as an alternative perspective in the social sciences, he is fundamentally correct. Such approaches may indeed not be the most appropriate means of informing our practice in these areas. But the solution is not non-rigorous inquiry, it is rather to search out and use alternative methods of rigorous inquiry. These alternative methods have been called *new paradigm research* because they break away from the traditional exclusively quantitative and qualitative paradigms.

How change takes place

Generally, paradigm changes occur by three means. The first of these is revolution, which is synonymous with Kuhn's (1970) perspective of 'paradigm shift'. This suggests that one dominant paradigm prevails in a discipline until it is replaced by an alternative one. The new paradigm then prevails in the discipline and the old one is rejected, thus the theory of revolution.

This perspective also suggests there is a period of chaos when paradigms compete, a pre-paradigmatic state from which the dominant paradigm emerges. Coppa (1993) suggested that nursing may be at a pre-paradigm juncture, where old theories are beginning to yield to a new paradigm.

The second theory of change is evolution. An evolutionary theory based on Darwinian thinking suggests that development occurs over time. Old perspectives are not rejected, as in Kuhn's revolutionary ideation, but rather there is slow building, developing and adaptation, which culminates in a higher level of knowledge (Meleis, 1997). The process is considered to be incessant and previous paradigms may not be rejected, merely modified.

In the third perspective, Meleis (1997) suggests that neither of the above two explanations fully describes the path nursing has taken. She rejects a monistic explanation in the epistemology of nursing. If revolution is the epistemological basis, then nursing could not be considered a discipline, as it would be in a pre-paradigmatic state. Likewise, an evolutionary view would fail to show that nursing had succeeded in evolving to disciplinary status. Meleis (1997) maintains that nursing is a specific discipline and she describes a third perspective that she refers to as integration or convolution to justify this. Nursing, she says, has taken a divergent pathway which is unique in that it has drawn on evolution and revolution to guide its pathway:

> *The discipline of nursing evolved through peaks, valleys, detours, circular paths, retracing of steps, and series of crises as well as through an evolutionary process.*
>
> (Meleis, 1991)

According to Meleis, this integrative process explains and even justifies the divergent views within nursing. It also explains why there is a need for divergent research paradigms. Figure 16.1 illustrates how paradigms change.

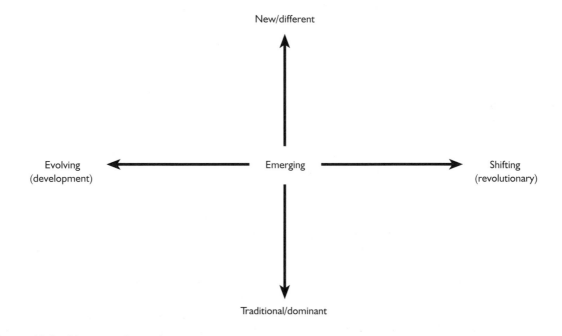

Figure 16.1 How paradigms change

Study Activity 16.4 _____

- Reflect on what you have read so far in this section. Focus on the reasons why paradigms change – do you agree with these? Can you think of any other reasons for change?
- In relation to how paradigms change, which one of the three processes – revolution, evolution or convolution – do you feel offers the soundest explanation for how change takes place?

NEW PARADIGM RESEARCH

There is difficulty in defining what new paradigm methods are, other than by recognising that they are methods that represent significant breaks from the current dominant paradigms. Not unexpectedly, this difficulty has caused a certain degree of confusion and lack of clarity. For example, some see new paradigm research as essentially synonymous with qualitative research, a view understandable when in fact qualitative methods tend to predominate in new paradigm approaches. Indeed, in the previous chapter, this common link is recognised. However, this need not always be the case. Holloway (1997), in referring to one form commonly recognised as 'new paradigm' (action research), states:

> *Action research generally involves small-scale intervention in a process or treatment in a work situation, and an evaluation of the impact of this process. Because it is small-scale, the research is generally, though not always, qualitative.*
>
> (Holloway, 1997)

This is a position further clarified by John Heron (a significant scholar within new paradigm and action research circles). Heron, together with Peter Reason and John Rowan, established the New Paradigm Research Group in the late 1970s/early 1980s, and their book (Reason and Rowan, 1981), discussed below, was a major influence in this orientation. Heron uses the term co-operative inquiry while others use terms

such as participatory research, action research, and even participatory action research. All share a common commitment to a paradigm that involves a removal of the barrier between the researcher and the researched, whereby they both become 'co-researchers'. Heron (1997) states that:

> *Qualitative research, using multiple methodologies, is about other people studied in their own social settings and understood in terms of the meanings those people themselves bring to their situation. To say that it is about other people in their own setting is to say one central thing: the researcher in mainline qualitative research does not involve informants in decisions about research methodology, about the design of operational procedures. He or she only seeks to negotiate, with the people being studied, (1) access to their setting, (2) issues involved in ongoing management of the research, and (3) the interpretations arrived at. Co-operative inquiry by contrast does research with other people, who are invited to be full co-inquirers with the initiating researcher and become actively involved in operational decision-making, and are committed to this kind of participative research design in principle, both politically and epistemologically.*
>
> (Heron, 1997)

It would appear that while so-called 'new paradigm' research, including action research (and the approaches closely aligned to it), are usually of a qualitative nature, this is not always so. Furthermore, while the approaches may usually be qualitative, they differ from most (mainline) qualitative research in their use of new ways of thinking about and doing research, including the participation of 'subjects' as co-researchers.

Clamp and Gough (1999) state that:

> *new paradigm research is another way of doing research. It puts forward alternatives to*

"orthodox" research methods and capitalises on the contribution of those who are normally just subjects.

(Clamp and Gough, 1999)

In general, we can state that new paradigm methods are those which:

- differ significantly from the standard quantitative and qualitative methods
- are essentially approaches involving new perspectives and methods, or new ways of combining and using established approaches
- tend to be less inflexible, not based on the commonly accepted research conventions and are designed to deal with specific research problems.

As you may have noted from the list above, there is in fact no single new paradigm approach, but rather a shared perspective which is characterised by a willingness to be creative in the application of the research approach to the subject or problem.

There are a number of such new paradigm perspectives; only three examples are identified here.

New paradigm research as collaboration

The term 'new paradigm research' was first made popular by Reason and Rowan (1981) and later refined by Reason (1988). Indeed, the term is often reserved specifically for the approach advocated by these researchers. The basis of their perspective is essentially established on the assertion that traditional research methods are inadequate for a science of persons. Clamp and Gough's (1999, pp. 50–1) definition of new paradigm research: 'research which is done with people rather than on people. It involves working with people so that they may discover some truth about themselves' is synonymous with that of Reason.

The idea is to conduct inquiries by breaking down barriers between the researcher and the researched. All those involved collaborate in the particular quest for knowledge as both researchers and subjects. The term 'research

participants' is most appropriate as it indicates the perspective of co-researchers. Thus, this approach is not only research, but also a form of education, personal development, and social action. In essence, research participants work together to:

- discuss the research problem
- decide on the method of research or inquiry
- self-observe, as they (or a number of them) are researchers and subjects
- reflect on experience
- decide together on problem resolution and
- take action on the basis of findings.

Reinharz (1981) suggested that new paradigm methods fall within the general rubric of qualitative research. However, they are characterised by the researcher and his reflections being included in the data. In more traditional natural science research, it is a cardinal rule that the researcher does not intrude into the field in any way, and great effort is devoted to avoid the subjective influence of the researcher. This stance is also taken in most qualitative research.

Study Activity 16.5 _____

Undertake a library search to find a research paper that uses a method/s involving true participation, i.e. researcher and those being researched working in collaboration to achieve the research aims.

New paradigm research as triangulation

Earlier in this chapter, weaknesses in both quantitative and qualitative methods were identified. One solution to addressing the weaknesses in these paradigms is to mix methods, so that both quantitative breadth and qualitative depth can be presented, thus resulting in more holistic and meaningful findings. The mixing can technically speaking involve mixing quantitative methods, or mixing qualitative methods. However, it often involves mixing quantitative and qualitative methods together. It may also involve mixing not only methods but theoretical perspectives and forms of analysis. This mixing of perspectives and methods is a relatively recent approach and as such is recognised by many as an essentially new paradigm in the human sciences.

By using more than one method, the problems of bias, which are inherent weaknesses of single methods, may be overcome. However, the notion that using different methods can cancel out biases intrinsic to individual methods used alone is not necessarily sound. Fielding and Fielding (1986) suggest that if bias-checking procedures are not incorporated into methodology, the net result may be a multiplication of error rather than a cancelling-out process.

Cautions do need to be kept in mind when mixing research methods. The assumption that quantitative and qualitative approaches can be integrated in a single research project is often rejected. Quantitative research gives broad descriptions of population characteristics; for example, it may claim to measure the incidence of depression and depressive symptoms in a group of patients. Qualitative research, on the other hand, may involve studying depression by giving an in-depth description of the subjective experience of living through this type of illness. The sum total of both pieces of research certainly adds up to the total knowledge of this illness. But there are limited situations where the qualitative research from its phenomenological theoretical base of understanding experience enhances the quantitative research from its epidemiological theoretical base of statistical analysis in a population of patients, or vice versa.

While the notion that mixing methods or triangulation may in itself cancel out biases should indeed be viewed with caution, the argument that mixing quantitative and qualitative methods is not possible should perhaps be viewed as a purist's position. In the above example it is not sufficient to simply know the incidence of depression in a group of patients. We need to know what the depression actually is and what it is like to experience it to get the full picture. In this sense we should not get hung up

on differences in theoretical perspective and be prepared to take a more pragmatic view. Carey (1993) argues that rather than adopting entrenched theoretical positions, researchers should be prepared to allow the research topic or problem to determine the methods and, where this is justified, to mix methods. The increasing popularity of this new paradigm in nursing can be attributed to the fact that as the research issues or problems are often complex human issues, triangulation of qualitative and quantitative methods is often the method of choice. In this context, Fielding and Fielding (1986) suggest that:

> It is impractical and unwise to list all the available means of data collection and analysis and use as many as possible. What is important is to choose at least one method which is specifically suited to exploring the structural aspects of the problem and at least one which can capture the essential elements of its meaning to those involved.
>
> (Fielding and Fielding, 1986)

Creswell (1994) refers to three types of combined study that may be used:

Two-phase design – this involves two separate methods. For example, first a phase is undertaken involving a qualitative approach such as grounded theory, and then a second phase is undertaken; this could involve testing the theory that has been generated using a quantitative approach (or vice versa – quantitative followed by qualitative). This has the advantage of the underpinning philosophies of both approaches being used to guide the research without any contamination from the other. However, a disadvantage is that in some research the link between the two phases is not clear.

The dominant–less dominant design – this involves utilising a small aspect of one paradigm within a single study that is dominated by the alternative paradigm.

Mixed methodology design – this involves mixing the paradigms throughout the research, in all or many of the methods of a study. The advantage of this is that both approaches contribute to and support each other. A disadvantage to using a total mixed methodology design is that the researcher needs to have in-depth knowledge of both paradigms. In fact Peterson and Martin (2000) suggest in their discussion on transdisciplinary approaches (research undertaken by researchers from cross-disciplines) that such researchers should hold at least two or more disciplinary qualifications, e.g. anthropology, sociology and a health-related qualification. Additionally, some see mixing paradigms in this manner as unacceptable as they feel both of the main paradigms (quantitative and qualitative) are incompatible.

Mixed methods have a number of advantages:

- They can be used to study practice phenomenon for which one approach may not be suitable
- They can add to the validity of the findings if findings from one approach converge with the other (Mitchell, 1986; Neuman, 1991)
- They have the potential to enhance links with practice, e.g. they could generate theory and then also test the theory in practice.

Study Activity 16.6

Organise a class debate with the agreement of your lecturer. The debate statement is: 'Mixed research methods should not be used as the two main paradigms (quantitative and qualitative) are not compatible'.

New paradigm research as action

An essential notion within the original concept of new paradigm research as expounded by Reason and Rowan (1981) is that of taking action on the basis of findings. The new paradigm for many researchers is essentially applied rather than pure research. It is this action orientation that is seen as the main innovative feature of the new paradigm (*see*, for example,

Cohen and Manion, 1989). This approach is often presented under the title action research. While there are some variations in definition, action research is usually defined as being:

- a small-scale study of the real world, in the field rather than in the laboratory, and concerned with day-to-day issues
- situational and interventionist, i.e. action-orientated and aimed at developing practices, policies, and procedures
- collaborative, with researchers and subjects working together and
- aimed at organisational development and change.

The approach draws much from the seminal work of Lewin (1946) who emphasised the importance of joint studies involving social scientists and practitioners working together to bring about social change through joint planning, action, observation, and reflection. The notion has gained recent popularity through a disaffection with traditional quantitative research as a means of researching complex human problems and a view that in both the quantitative and qualitative traditions the distancing of the professional researcher from the field and the subjects not only compromises the findings but is less likely to result in their successful implementation.

Action research has in some cases moved away from the original notion of professional researchers and staff collaborating as co-researchers to the idea that staff or practitioners should regularly undertake action research themselves. In this context, Carr and Kemmis (1986) define action research as:

A form of self-reflective enquiry undertaken by participants in a social situation in order to improve the rationality and justice of their own practices, their understanding of these practices, and the situations in which those practices are carried out.

(Carr and Kemmis, 1986)

In nursing, the introduction of action research is closely aligned with another innovation known as nursing development units. Here, clinicians, educators, and sometimes researchers, work together to identify nursing problems. They agree on methods of research designed to suit the problem rather than making the problem suit a dominant research method, and then develop and introduce new and improved methods of practice as a result of these activities.

Study Activity 16.7

Action research is considered to be a good approach to use in the study of new situations or roles. For example, 'nurse consultants' are a new type of nurse in the UK: an action research project could be established involving these nurses, researching their role as they forge new positions within nursing and health care.

- With a group of colleagues, construct a list of research ideas that you feel could be appropriately investigated using an action research approach.

It will be evident from this discussion of new paradigm research that there are different approaches and not a single perspective. However, there are some assumptions underpinning new paradigm research that allow broad principles to be compared with the two traditional approaches. Table 16.3 presents the

Table 16.3   Differences and similarities between the main research paradigms

Quantitative	Qualitative	New paradigm
Numerical measurable data	Narrative interpretative data	May combine narrative and numeric
Objective	Subjective	May combine objectivity and subjectivity
Belief in single truth about a phenomenon	Belief in multiple truths about a phenomenon	Open to critical inquiry and constructivism
Associated with *inductive* processes	Associated with *deductive* processes	May use induction and deduction within same study
Mistrust of human senses in data collection – use of structured instruments	Human senses acknowledged in data collection – researcher is instrument	Context driven – research problem dictates and any methods may be used
Singular elements of a phenomenon are the focus of study (parts make the *person*)	Total person as an integrated whole is the focus of study (*person* is greater than the parts and parts cannot be researched in isolation from the total person)	Similar to qualitative
People researched are *subjects* and are selected by random means	People are research *respondents* – selection is intentional/purposive and/or because of theoretical richness	Participants – researcher and researched are co-researchers. Selection is liable to be problem focused.
Person can be isolated – environment, context, life influences and other variables can be controlled (*value free*)	Person is integrated with environment, context, life influences and other variables – these influence people individually and cannot be controlled (*value dependent*)	Similar to qualitative
Robustness measures – validity, reliability	Robustness criteria – truth value, consistency and confirmability	Use of quantitative and qualitative methods as well as mixed approaches to validate

Findings stem from large, random samples (or random allocated experimental groups) and usual aims are to:
  – generalise to total population
  – identify cause and effect
  – identify collective views, opinions or behaviours
	Small purposive sample and usual aims are to:
	  – identify unique experiences
	  – give voice to hidden phenomena
	  – sensitise others to the experiences, culture, roles or symbolic importance of life events of research respondents
		Usually small sample purposive or self-selection (e.g. action research) and aims are to:
		  – answer complex questions that other approaches do not
		  – study new phenomena
		  – create change as part of the process of the research
		  – question traditional worldviews

comparisons of quantitative and qualitative research (as presented in Table 16.1) with that of the new paradigms.

SUMMARY

It is important to nursing as a discipline, and more so on moral grounds to the patients who receive nursing care, that research undertaken generates and establishes the 'best' possible knowledge. There are a number of ways to discover knowledge to underpin nursing practice, but few would argue that research leads the way in this endeavour. However, it is not enough to say that research has found something so it must be useful; there is flawed research just as there is valuable and useful research. One of the criteria in making a decision about how valuable research findings are is that which is most fundamental to all research – the paradigm or approach that is most suitable to answer the research question. It is suggested here that if the paradigm selected is not appropriate to address the research problem or question under study, then the findings of such research are at best dubious, if not completely useless in terms of knowledge advancement.

This chapter provides the necessary information to allow an informed choice to be made about the appropriateness of using specific research paradigms. Each of the three perspectives detailed is valuable.

If a research investigation aims to establish a cause and effect relationship between variables then an experimental approach, whenever this is possible, is the approach of choice. Or, if a researcher wishes to collect demographic detail related to health aspects from a large population, then a survey may be most appropriate. In either case, the quantitative paradigm is best suited to address the research aims.

Should the aim of a research study be to elucidate life experiences, e.g. what it is like to live with a chronic illness, a phenomenological approach philosophically and methodologically rooted within the qualitative paradigm is the approach of choice.

However, for research problems that are not amenable to the rubrics of either of the two main paradigms, there is a need to look for alternative research canons. Such canons are to be found by looking beyond the two main paradigms to what have been referred to here as new paradigm approaches. Only three new paradigm perspectives have been presented in this chapter. There are others, and innovative researchers will continue to develop these. Various new approaches are being used now and more will develop in the future. It will be those researchers who wade into the 'swampy lowlands' to which Schön refers who will lead the way in the development of new research paradigms.

REFERENCES

Agar, M.H. (1986) *Speaking of Ethnography*, Sage, Beverley Hills, CA

Appleton, J.V. (1995) Analysing qualitative data: addressing issues of validity and reliability. *Journal of Advanced Nursing* **22**, 993–7

Beck, C.T. (1994) Reliability and validity issues in phenomenological research. *Western Journal of Nursing Research* **13**(3), 254–67

Becker, H.S. (1955) Marihuana use and social control. *Social Problems* **3**, 35–44

Carey, J.W. (1993) Linking qualitative and quantitative methods: integrating cultural factors into public health, *Qualitative Health Research* **3**(3), 289–318

Carr, W. and Kemmis, S. (1986) *Becoming Critical: Education, knowledge and action research*, Falmer Press, London

Clamp, C. and Gough, S. (1999) *Resources for Nursing Research* (3rd edn), Sage, Thousand Oaks, CA

Cody, W.K. (1995) About all those paradigms: many in the universe, two in nursing. *Nursing Science Quarterly* **7**(4), 144–7

Cohen, L. and Manion, L. (1989) *Research Methods in Education*, Routledge, London

Coppa, F.D. (1993) Chaos theory suggests a new paradigm for nursing science. *Journal of Advanced Nursing* **18**(6), 985–91

Creswell, J.W. (1994) *Research Design Qualitative and Quantitative Approaches*, Sage, London

Cutcliffe, J.R. and McKenna, H. (1999) Establishing the credibility of qualitative research findings: the plot thickens. *Journal of Advanced Nursing* 30(2), 374–80

Fawcett, J. (1992) Contemporary conceptualisations of nursing: philosophy or science? In: Kikuchi, J.F. and Simmons, H. (eds) *Philosophic Inquiry in Nursing*, Sage, Newbury Park, CA

Field, P.A. and Morse, J.M. (1985) *Nursing Research: The application of qualitative approaches,* Croom Helm, London

Fielding, M.G. and Fielding, J.L. (1986) *Linking Data,* Sage, Beverley Hills, CA

Glaser, B.G. and Strauss, A.L. (1967) *The Discovery of Grounded Theory: Strategies for qualitative research*, Aldine, New York

Hargie, O., Saunders, C. and Dickson, D. (1991) *Social Skills in Interpersonal Communication* (2nd edn), Routledge, London

Hendricks, G. (1998) *A Year of Living Consciously*, Harper Collins, New York

Heron, J. (1997) *Co-operative Inquiry: Research into the human condition*, Sage, London

Hicks, C. and Hennessy, D. (1997) Mixed messages in nursing research: their contribution to the persisting hiatus between evidence and practice. *Journal of Advanced Nursing* 3(25), 595–601

Hinds, P.S., Scandrett-Hibden, S. and McAulay, L.S. (1990) Further assessment of a method to estimate reliability and validity of qualitative research findings. *Journal of Advanced Nursing* 15, 430–5

Holloway, I. (1997) *Basic Concepts for Qualitative Research*, Blackwell Science, Oxford

Holloway, I. and Wheeler, S. (1996) *Qualitative Research for Nurses*, Blackwell Science, London

Kuhn, T. (1970) *The Structure of the Scientific Revolutions* (2nd edn), University of Chicago Press, Chicago, IL

Lewin, K. (1946) Action research and minority problems, *Journal of Social Issues* 2, 34–46

Maggs-Rapport, M. (2001) Best research practice: in pursuit of methodological rigour. *Journal of Advanced Nursing* 35(3), 373–83

McKenna, H. (1997) *Nursing Theories and Models*, Routledge, London

McWhinney, I.R. (1991) Primary care research in the next twenty years. In: Norton, P.G., Stewart, M., Tudiver, F. *et al.* (eds) *Primary Care Research: Traditional and innovative approaches*, Sage, Newbury Park, CA

Meleis, A.I. (1991) *Theoretical Nursing Development and Progress*, J.B. Lippincott, Philadelphia, IL

Meleis, A.I. (1997) *Theoretical Nursing Development and Progress* (2nd edn), J.B. Lippincott, Philadelphia, IL

Mitchell, E.S. (1986) Multiple triangulation: a methodology for nursing science. *Advances in Nursing Science* 8(3), 18–26

Moody, L.E. (1990) *Advancing Nursing Science through Research*, Vol. 1, Sage, London

Neuman, W.L. (1991) *Social Science Research Methods: Qualitative and quantitative approaches*, Allyn and Bacon, Needleham Heights

Parahoo, K. (1997) *Nursing Research Principles, Process and Issues*, Macmillan, London

Parse, R.R., Coyne, A.B. and Smith, M.J. (1985) *Nursing Research: Qualitative methods*, Brady, Bowie, MD

Peterson, C. and Martin, C. (2000) A new paradigm in general practice research – towards transdisciplinary approaches. The utilisation of multiple research methodologies in general practice research. *Online Journal: Priory Lodge Education*

Punch, M. (1986) *The Politics and Ethics of Fieldwork*, Sage, London

Reason, P. (1988) *Human Inquiry in Action – Developments in new paradigm research*, Sage, London

Reason, P. and Rowan, J. (1981) *Human Inquiry: A sourcebook of new paradigm research*, John Wiley, New York

Reinharz, S. (1981) Implementing new paradigm research. In: Reason, P. and Rowan, J. (eds) *Human Inquiry: A sourcebook of new paradigm research*, John Wiley, New York

Rogers, C. (1985) Toward a more human science of the person. *Journal of Humanistic Psychology* 25(4), 7–24

Schön, D. (1987) *Educating the Reflective Practitioner*, Jossy Bass, San Francisco, CA

Simmons, S. (1995) From paradigm to method in interpretive action research. *Journal of Advanced Nursing* 21(5), 837–44

Slevin, E. and Sines, D. (2000) Enhancing the truthfulness, consistency and transferability of a qualitative study, *Nurse Researcher* 7(2), 79–97

Stevens Barnum, B.J. (1994) *Nursing Theory Analysis Application Evaluation* (4th edn), J.B. Lippincott, Philadelphia, IL

Strauss, A. and Corbin, J. (1998) *Basics of Qualitative Research Grounded Theory Procedures and Techniques*. Sage, London

Strauss, A. and Corbin, J. (1994) Grounded theory methodology – an overview. In: Denzin, N.K. and Lincoln, Y.S. (eds) *Handbook of Qualitative Research*, Sage, London, pp. 273–85

Thompson, N. (2000) *Theory and Practice in Human Services*, Open University Press, Buckingham

Underwood,P., Owen, A. and Winkler, R. (1986) Replacing the clockwork model of medicine. *Community Health Studies* 10(3), 275–83

17 CLINICAL EFFECTIVENESS: AN EVIDENCE BASE FOR PRACTICE?

Alan Pearson

LEARNING OUTCOMES

After studying this chapter you will be able to:

- Define and explain evidence-based practice as a basis for nursing practice
- Identify major criticisms of evidence-based practice from within nursing
- Recognise the importance of the best available evidence for effective practice
- Discuss the values and limitations of an approach that sees evidence as primarily a tool to enhance clinical effectiveness
- Argue for a more holistic approach that combines evidence and judgement in the best nursing practice.

INTRODUCTION

All areas of the health care system in the industrialised world are currently facing increasing demands for health care and an escalation in the costs associated with this demand. Governments and health care professionals have responded to these realities in a variety of ways. Some responses focus on cost cutting by rationing services, introducing measures to increase productivity and imposing cost-shifting exercises. Some responses are grounded in serious ethical discussions focusing on what can be afforded and what cannot and in developing processes to provide essential health services to those who most need them. Some promote a user-pays approach and some just simply blame others (in the case of politicians, other politicians; in the case of health professionals, health professions or specialist groups other than their own).

Yet another response (and, in my view, the most acceptable) is that of the evidence-based practice movement. The emergence of evidence-based practice has led to a focus on best practice based on the best available evidence in most Westernised countries.

In this chapter, I intend to overview the development of evidence-based nursing, consider the major criticisms of evidence-based practice, and then focus on the limitations of focusing only on evidence of clinical effectiveness in nursing. Needless to say, it is my view that clinical performance and professional judgement in this, the information age, must increasingly be based on our exposure to summarised evidence and that, in the not-to-distant future, practice that is not based on a consideration of the evidence will be difficult to justify. What counts as evidence in nursing is, though, the critical question; but more on that later.

HEALTH CARE PRACTICES AND EVIDENCE-BASED GUIDELINES

Most health professions are increasingly embracing the use of evidence-based guidelines to inform (rather than direct) practice and this is in response to high profile initiatives of governments and provider agencies. In the US, considerable resources have been invested in high-quality, high-cost research and development programmes to develop clinical guidelines. The National Institutes of Health now has a well-established strategy to review international literature and conduct meta-analyses to generate clinical guidelines based on the best available evidence.

In the UK, recent policy initiatives have directed health care provider agencies to develop research and development strategies, to establish research and development units, and to promote practices based on the best available knowledge. At the same time, the British Government has established a number of centres for evidence-based practice and health research centres such as the Kings Fund support these.

At an international level, the Cochrane Collaboration has linked research and development sites across the world to review and analyse randomised clinical trials from an international perspective and to generate reports to inform practitioners, to influence practice, and to be a resource in the development of consensus guidelines.

The practical application of rigorously reviewed evidence is now promoted through the development and dissemination of practice guidelines in most developed health care systems. Clinical practice guidelines consist of statements to assist practitioner and patient decisions about appropriate health care for specific clinical circumstances which are systematically developed on the basis of consensus within expert groups. An increasing number of well-constructed, practical and evidence-based guidelines are being developed, largely within the US.

Sackett and Rosenberg (1995) suggested that evidence-based medicine is concerned with five linked ideas:

1 Clinical and other health care decisions should be based on the best patient-, population- and laboratory-based evidence.
2 The nature and source of the evidence to be sought depends on the particular clinical question.
3 The identification of the best available evidence requires the application of epidemiological, economic and biostatistical principles plus pathophysiology and personal experience.
4 This identification and appraisal of the evidence must be acted upon.
5 There should be continuous evaluation of performance.

Bearing the above in mind, there is little sense in rejecting this process designed to assist practitioners rather than control them.

Study Activity 17.1

In this chapter we note that evidence-based practice is not simply about applying evidence as it is presented in a thoughtless way, irrespective of context and taking no account of practitioners' judgement.

- Carry out a literature search in your library on the issue of clinical judgement in evidence-based practice.
- Write a brief statement (approximately 250 words) on the meaning of clinical judgement and the activities it involves.

Evidence-based practice is now almost institutionalised in most industrialised countries, especially in Europe, the UK, North America and Australasia. Many of these countries have established centres for evidence-based health care, evidence-based medicine and evidence-based nursing. For example, there are Cochrane Centres in all of these countries and centres for evidence-based nursing in the UK and North America. The Joanna Briggs Institute for Evidence-Based Nursing, based in Australia, has collaborating centres in China and New Zealand and is seeking to establish collaborating centres in Singapore and Thailand.

Simply defined, evidence-based practice is the combination of individual clinical or professional expertise with the best available external evidence to produce practice that is most likely to lead to a positive outcome for a client or patient. Evidence-based nursing is therefore nursing that is characterised by these attributes. Needless to say, such definitions are simplistic, and need to be subjected to close scrutiny by nurses.

Although medicine and nursing are the health care occupations most advanced in the evidence-based practice movement, the ideas and arguments are common to all professionals who work in health care. These concepts are not without controversy and I will examine the debates that surround their adoption and the implications of these debates for nursing later.

EVIDENCE-BASED MEDICINE

Evidence-based medicine can be defined as medical practice that is characterised by the attributes of evidence-based practice. Sackett *et al.* (1996) contend that evidence-based medicine had its philosophical origins in the mid-nineteenth century in Paris. They define it as being 'the conscientious, explicit and judicious use of current best evidence in making decisions about the care of individual patients' (p. 71).

EVIDENCE-BASED NURSING

Nursing is a relatively recent recruit to the evidence-based practice movement and its involvement in multidisciplinary centres, such as Cochrane Centres, is minimal. Furthermore, there is considerable evidence to suggest that nurses still do not find it appropriate to apply research findings in their practice. Pearson *et al.* (1997, p. 4) have cited quite a number of examples of this. As to why this is so, it has been suggested that:

- a nurse may be unaware of the research findings
- a nurse may not understand the findings
- a nurse may not believe the findings
- a nurse may not know how to apply them
- a nurse may not be permitted to apply the findings.

It is important to look behind these possible explanations. For instance, to blandly state that nurses may be unaware of some important research implies that they are remiss by failing to keep up to date. However, it is important to recognise that the demands of work and family often leave little time for ensuring the currency of one's knowledge. Even if a person has time to devote to this purpose, the information explosion ensures that it is not possible to keep up with all of the developments. Similarly, a nurse

might not understand the findings of a given piece of research. Many nurses have had little or no exposure to research training and therefore lack the knowledge necessary to understand some areas of research. Just as importantly, if they have had limited experience of research methods, how are they to assess the reliability and validity of the research they are reading? How will they know what weight to attach to a given piece of research?

It is in these areas that the evidence-based practice movement is able to afford considerable assistance. It recognises that it is unrealistic to expect busy health professionals to have the time to stay abreast of all the latest research. Hence, one of its key strategies is the meta-analysis of research. This involves having a trained researcher or team of researchers gathering all the available research on a given question and systematically reviewing it for reliability and validity; that is, assessing its quality. Systematic reviews can provide the raw materials for establishing clinical guidelines and assist in identifying gaps in existing research, often discovering that there has been no research (or none of sufficient quality) on a given question.

It should be clear that I am of the view that evidence-based practice has much to offer nursing. The problem of frequently being unable to identify why we do what we do in practice has undermined the potential of nurses to influence the management of our clients. One might ask why this should be so when the medical profession seems not to have been so afflicted, notwithstanding that it has declared itself to be in no better position with respect to the evidence. The reality is that the availability of evidence has to be taken in the context of the many other factors that contribute to the uniqueness of a given profession. The traditional situation of nursing as a relatively less powerful field of practice, ensures that the impact will be more pronounced. The corollary of this is, of course, that generating evidence is likely to be relatively more beneficial in nursing.

There is a small but growing literature on evidence-based practice in nursing. Much of the work has originated in the UK, but there is a growing awareness in the USA too. In Australia, there has been considerable development of the infrastructure underpinning evidence-based nursing and there is an increasing amount of work on evidence-based practice in nursing, emanating largely from the Joanna Briggs Institute and its 10 collaborating centres in Adelaide, Perth, Darwin, Toowoomba, Brisbane, Sydney, Melbourne (where there are two centres), Auckland (New Zealand) and Hong Kong.

The development of evidence-based nursing has not been uncontroversial. It is relatively easy to find papers espousing the benefits of evidence-based nursing, but there is a growing literature opposing this development. Much of this criticism is relatively defensive and not at all well justified, but nursing does have a substantive objection to evidence-based health care as it is presently construed. So, just what are the major criticisms of evidence-based practice?

1 *Nurses are already doing it* – there is a good deal of truth in this. Many nurses do engage in evidence-based practice to the extent that this is possible given the constraints of time and the availability of quality evidence. However, there is substantial and compelling evidence against the existence of widespread evidence-based practice. First, in all health care sectors there is widespread and extensive variability in practice. This indicates that the one best way of doing something (if there is 'one') has yet to be determined for many of the services nurses provide.

2 *Evidence-based nursing is 'cookbook' care* – aims to coalesce the individual professional's clinical expertise with the best available evidence in order to produce the best possible outcome for a particular patient or client. This necessarily involves taking into account the circumstances of the recipient of care. Thus, it is ideally a client-centred approach which, when properly practised, is highly individualised. The other side of this coin is, however, that it has the potential (if not properly applied) to give rise to 'cookbook'

care. The same pressures that produced the impetus for evidence-based care could be responsible for mechanisms of evidence-based practice, such as practice guidelines being used simply as a recipe for care delivered without due consideration of the individual patient or client. This is then arguably not evidence-based practice.

3 *Evidence-based practice relies on randomised clinical trials and meta-analyses* – this is the nub of nursing's difficulty with the current style of evidence-based health care, focusing as it generally does on effectiveness. At the heart of the issue lies the critique of traditional science and the emergence of new paradigms for knowledge. While the randomised clinical trial is probably the 'best' approach to generating evidence of effectiveness, nurses are concerned with more than cause and effect questions, and this is reflected in the wide range of research approaches utilised by nurses to generate knowledge for practising nurses.

Although its proponents would argue that evidence-based nursing is not limited to traditional research, there has been considerable emphasis on randomised clinical trials and meta-analyses, especially in medicine and by the Cochrane Collaboration. This has drawn criticism from those professions who regard qualitative research methods as equally valid forms of research and, thus, generators of legitimate evidence for nursing practice. It is, of course, stating the obvious to note that nursing has been one of the more prominent advocates of qualitative research, and much of the research that has been done in and on nursing has been qualitative in nature. Qualitative research fares rather poorly in systematic reviews. These are a key tool for the evidence-based practice movement. The question here becomes one of what is acceptable research in terms of generating knowledge that amounts to evidence for the purpose of informing practice. There are currently different views on the subject and these generally align with the various positions that characterise the longstanding debate between qualitative and quantitative researchers. This is clearly not an easily resolved argument, but it is vitally important in terms of ascertaining the value of research-generated 'evidence' to the practice of nursing.

4 *There is no evidence* – for largely historical reasons, this criticism is even more applicable to nursing than to medicine, but the gist of the complaint is that if we wish to engage in evidence-based practice, then there needs to be a body of research to provide the evidence on which to base that practice. However, in the great majority of systematic reviews that have been conducted on nursing questions, the result has been that the research is either non-existent or inconclusive. That is to say, there is no evidence one way or the other. For example, in a systematic review of research on the effectiveness of support for carers of people with Alzheimer's type dementia, the main result was that the research was inconclusive. The authors said that with '... the limited nature of the research evidence in mind, it is not possible to recommend either wholesale investment in caregiver support programs or withdrawal of the same ...' (Thompson and Thompson, 1999).

While the lack of evidence could be perceived as a barrier to evidence-based practice, it should be recognised that the need to base practice on evidence has only relatively recently penetrated the consciousness of the nursing profession. Thus, identifying the lack of evidence is an important first step in developing the evidence base.

5 *Theory is more important than evidence in guiding practice* – flowing from the previous criticism is the argument that it is much more important that practice be well grounded in theory than in research. One of the main reasons for this is the rapidity with which 'evidence' – and especially technical evidence – becomes obsolete.

Thus, the term evidence-based practice begs the question – evidence of what; and what constitutes evidence when one is interested in how people feel or how practical an action or intervention is in a specific setting or culture.

Study Activity 17.2 _____

Here we have considered five major criticisms of evidence-based practice that are frequently presented by nurses. Re-read the sections on each of these criticisms.

- Identify an experienced qualified nursing colleague and ask her/him to discuss the value of evidence-based practice and any weaknesses or limitations she/he sees in this approach. Use the five criticisms as a checklist and establish how many of these (and also any additional criticisms) the practitioner identifies.
- Identify an experienced registered medical practitioner within a secondary care/hospital environment and ask her/him to discuss the value of evidence-based practice and any weaknesses or limitations she/he sees in such an approach. Again, use the checklist to establish how many of the five items (and any additional criticisms) the practitioner identifies.
- Look for any differences in the two responses and reflect on the possible reasons for these, considering in particular the professional orientations of the two practitioners.

EFFECTIVENESS, APPROPRIATENESS AND FEASIBILITY

To date, the evidence-based practice movement has focused on *evidence of effectiveness*. Pearson (1998), in arguing that evidence-based practice includes an interest in research into clinical effectiveness but is not confined to this interest, says:

> ... *randomised trials are the gold standard for phenomena that we are interested in studying from a cause and effect perspective, but clearly they are not the gold standard if*

> *we are interested in how patients and nurses relate to each other, or if we are interested in how patients live through the experience of radiotherapy when they have a life threatening illness. We have yet to work out how to assess the quality of alternative approaches to research other than the RCT.*
>
> (Pearson, 1998)

He goes on to suggest that '... evidence-based practice is not exclusively about effectiveness; it is about basing practice on the best available evidence'.

The diverse origins of problems in nursing practice require a diversity of research methodologies. Thus, methodological approaches in this area need to be eclectic enough to incorporate classical, medical and scientific designs and the emerging qualitative and action-orientated approaches from the humanities and the social and behavioural sciences. The development of interdisciplinary research and a greater understanding of the relationship between medical, nursing and allied health interventions are also fundamental to the emergence of research methodologies which are relevant and sensitive to the health needs of consumers.

There is a small, although growing, literature on the role of qualitative research in evidence-based practice and recognition of a need to move beyond the effectiveness of interventions to consider their appropriateness and practical feasibility.

Lemmer *et al.* (1999), in attempting to conduct a systematic review in an area of health visiting focusing on the randomised clinical trial as the 'gold standard', report on a paucity of trials in this field and argue that clinical complexity demands a need to integrate qualitative methods into systematic reviews. They argue that:

> ... *[t]he comprehensiveness and synthesis of a systematic review are more important to emphasise than whether the literature is outside the clinical remit of an RCT.*
>
> (Lemmer *et al.*, 1999, p. 323)

The need to more fully integrate the results of qualitative research into the systematic process is well argued for by Popay *et al.* (1998), who suggests that:

> ... *there are many proponents of evidence-based decision making within health care who cannot and/or will not accept that qualitative research has an important part to play* ...
>
> (Popay and Williams, 1998)

She asserts that the results of qualitative research do more than simply enhance those of quantitative studies and suggests that qualitative research is capable of generating evidence that:

- explores taken-for-granted practices
- increases understanding of consumer and clinical behaviour
- develops interventions
- illuminates patient's perceptions on quality/appropriateness
- gives guidance to understanding organisational culture and change management
- evaluates complex policy initiatives.

Green and Britten (1998) state that:

> [q]*ualitative research may seem unscientific and anecdotal to many medical scientists. However, as the critics of evidence-based medicine are quick to point out, medicine is more than the application of scientific rules.*
>
> (Green and Britten, 1998)

They go on to argue that qualitative research findings provide rigorous accounts of treatment regimens in everyday contexts and that there is an increasing need within the evidence-based practice arena for an awareness that different research questions require different kinds of research. They are unequivocal in asserting that '... "good" evidence goes further than the results of meta-analyses of randomised controlled trials'.

The Cochrane Qualitative Methods Network, established in 1998, is currently exploring the scope for incorporating qualitative research into Cochrane reviews and a number of protocols and checklists have been developed by the group (see *Qualitative Methods Network: Report on Rome Workshop*, November 1999 on *http://www.salford.ac.uk/jhr/cochrane/homepage.htm* and *Draft Methods Group Module*). There are still no internationally reviewed approaches to assessing the quality of specific qualitative methods and no accepted way to rank or rate qualitative research findings reported in the literature. There have been, however, a number of attempts to synthesise (as a form of meta-analysis) the results of similar qualitative studies, and these are well described by Sandelowski *et al.* (1997); these authors have also developed an in-depth theoretical approach to the systematic meta-synthesis of qualitative findings that maintains the integrity of individual studies. Drawing on the work of Sandelowski *et al.*, the Cochrane Qualitative Methods Network, Popay *et al.* (1998), and Lemmer *et al.* (1999), an approach to qualitative meta-analysis, quality assessment and the development of a quality rating scale for qualitative research results could be used to add appropriateness and feasibility dimensions to the currently effectiveness-orientated systematic review process.

Study Activity 17.3

A question has been raised about evidence being primarily to establish effectiveness.

- Carry out a literature review to identify definitions of clinical effectiveness. On this basis write a brief statement (approximately 250 words) that defines and describes the main attributes of the concept 'clinical effectiveness'.
- Re-read the section on effectiveness and identify other goals of nursing care that may not fit easily into a clinical effectiveness frame.
- Reflect upon the evidence or other forms of knowledge that may be needed to underpin these additional goals, and the ways in which such evidence may differ from that required to underpin clinical effectiveness.

SUMMARY

There are signs that the evidence-based practice movement is beginning to develop a more comprehensive view of evidence and there are research initiatives attempting to construct approaches to assess and synthesise the results of interpretive and critical research so that these forms of evidence can become an integral part of systematic reviews and, thus, inform practice. Such an approach to evidence-based practice will help us, as practitioners, to perform well in our practice, using our professional judgement and appropriate evidence.

The rejection of evidence-based practice by practitioners or researchers because of its current obsession with effectiveness is not, in my view, in the best interests of our clients or of the health care professions. Our role is to constructively critique the over-emphasis on effectiveness and develop approaches to systematically review other forms of evidence.

REFERENCES

Green, J. and Britten, N. (1998) Qualitative research and evidence-based medicine. *British Medical Journal* **316**, 1230–2

Lemmer, B., Grellier, R. and Steven, J. (1999) Systematic review of nonrandom and qualitative research literature: exploring and uncovering an evidence base for health visiting and decision making. *Qualitative Health Research* **9**, 315–28

Pearson, A. (1998) Excellence in care: future dimensions for effective nursing. *NT Research* **3**(1), 25–7

Pearson, A., Borbasi, S., Fitzgerald, M. *et al.* (1997) Evidence-based nursing: an examination of nursing within the international evidence-based health care practice movement. RCNA Discussion Paper no. 1, *Nursing Review*, Sydney

Popay, J., Rogers, A. and Williams, G. (1998) Rationale and standards for the systematic review of qualitative literature in health services research. *Qualitative Health Research* **8**(3) 341–51

Sackett, D.L. and Rosenberg, W.M.C. (1995) On the need for evidence-based medicine. *Health Economics* **4**, 249–54

Sackett, D.L., Rosenberg, W.M.C., Gray, J.A.M. *et al.* (1996) Evidence-based medicine: what it is and what it is not. *British Medical Journal* **312**, 71–2

Sandelowski, M., Docherty, S. and Emden, C. (1997) Qualitative metasynthesis: issues and techniques. *Research in Nursing and Health* **20**, 365–71

Thompson, C. and Thompson, G. (1999) Support for carers of people with Alzheimer's type dementia. *The Cochrane Library*, issue 4

18 THEORY, PRACTICE AND RESEARCH

Oliver Slevin

> *Living theory is encountered in praxis, a dance wherein ideas, concepts and theories may arise in the intellect from reading, discussion, lectures, classroom learning activities, or in practice. Practice both tests and enhances theory, and theory both tests and enhances practice. Each enlightens the other, provoking insights, altering and changing the form, shape, and meaning of each. As the theory evolves, so the practice evolves. In this way, in the truly professional curriculum, each informs the other in the magical whole of praxis.*
>
> (Bevis, 1988)

LEARNING OUTCOMES

After studying this chapter you will be able to:

- Explain the term praxis in the context of theory–practice, research–practice and theory–research relationships
- Describe the dyadic relationship between research and practice
- Provide definitive statements in respect of the various perspectives on evidence-based practice and service delivery
- Provide a comprehensive case supporting the relevance and importance of research to practice
- Describe the dyadic relationship between theory and research
- Provide a comprehensive case supporting the relevance and importance of theory to research
- Describe the dyadic relationship between theory and practice
- Provide a comprehensive case supporting the

relevance and importance of theory to practice
- Identify and explicate the interactions and interconnections in the theory–research–practice triad, and the implications these have for the profession of nursing.

INTRODUCTION

In any new edition of a book such as this there is a desire to not only update but to make changes that improve the reading and learning experience for the student. This would include searching for more relevant and contemporary opening quotations, where these are used. However, we commence this chapter, as we did its equivalent in the first edition, with the same quotation. In the intervening period, Olivia Em Bevis, the author of that quotation, sadly passed away. She will be a great loss to nursing, and her seminal work on the relationship between practice and theory set the scene for reflections upon such matters for decades after she introduced them.

The relationship between theory and practice is indeed very complex. Bevis spoke, in our opening quotation, of a 'living theory', and 'praxis' or integration of theory with practice. Theory, she argued, influences practice, and practice influences theory. In effect, theory and practice constantly interact with each other. Bevis spoke particularly of a dance between theory and practice in the curriculum, but it is nowhere less evident than in the actual practice of nursing. In essence, behind this seminal work there is a recognition that the influence of knowledge upon practice ultimately occurs in those moments when nursing actions are carried out. It is there, in those moments, that the nurse brings all her knowledge and skill to bear upon the matter that is immediately at hand. This is, in the truest sense, knowledge-in-action, and it is what praxis is all about. It is in such contexts that people speak of this knowledge for and in practice in terms of theory *and* research.

In simple terms it might be said: research produces sound theory, and this theory informs our practice. But this is indeed a simplification. It fails to recognise, for example, that the theory that best fits is often that which emerges from the experience of practice, and that the means of procuring or generating *this* sort of theory differ significantly from the traditional methods of formulating and then testing the theory in practice or real-world settings. It also fails to recognise that the theory–research relationship is a matter of some controversy. Not everyone accepts that the purpose of research is to generate or test theory. And, it fails to recognise that in those moments within which practice takes place, the clinical wisdom that comes to bear is often informed by tacit knowledge derived from extensive experience and expertise in discerning what needs to be done (Benner *et al.*, 1999; Cimino, 1999). In such contexts, there may even be *no* explicit theory or research evidence to call upon and the nurse must seek the information she utilises in here-and-now situations that are often highly dynamic and rapidly changing. In reality we are confronted with a situation in which the theory–research–practice interface is a complex configuration of relationships.

It will be recalled that in the final chapter of the previous module we referred to how 'theory' fits within science and the relationship between theory and research. This set the scene for the current module, within which we have discussed research and how it contributes to our clinical and nursing effectiveness. In this final chapter of the current module we conclude by considering the complex relationships that exist between theory, practice *and* research.

THE ISSUE OF A THEORY–PRACTICE GAP

You may be aware of an ongoing debate in the nursing profession about the theory–practice gap. Some have argued that there is no clear relationship between the theory taught in college and the practice carried out in the practice areas. However, irrespective of such 'gaps', some form of theory is always involved. It may not be the same theory that is taught in college, and the nurses may not even be conscious of applying the theory to which they subscribe, but it is there just the same. This 'gap' has become a major concern within nursing. Much attention is given to means by which the gap may be narrowed or even closed altogether, so that all practice is explicitly informed by a clearly stated theory for nursing. This in effect amounts to a naive assumption, which fails to recognise that:

- this pattern of knowing that we call theoretical or propositional knowing may not be the only form of knowledge that informs our practice
- theory is never a static state but a dynamic process whereby theory is constantly being refined, not least by changes in the practice environment
- practice is also a dynamic and changing process, and in health care settings the rate of change may be so rapid that at some times practice runs in advance of theory (requiring it to be refined to explain the new circumstances), while at other times the theory (or new research-generated knowledge) guides or even prescribes the practice, thus running in front of it.

According to the notion of *theory-of-action* versus *theory-in-use*, explained by Argyris and Schön (1974), the actual theory-in-use professionals apply in their practice may be quite different from the particular theory to which they publicly subscribe (the *theory-of-action*). Of course, there are problems if the theory taught in the college is different from the *theory-in-use*. Why are nurses not using the *theory-of-action* taught in the curriculum? Is there something wrong with the theory, if nurses are ignoring or actively rejecting it? Is the *theory-in-use* a better theory, and are nurses right to adopt it and reject the *theory-of-action* being promoted by others? Is it a waste of time to persist in teaching one theory if another is being utilised in practice? Regardless of the answers to these difficult questions, practice is always praxis in the reality of day-to-day practice: wherever there is practice, there is always theory.

Gary Rolfe has elsewhere reflected upon this situation. In an enlightening statement whose ending is remarkably similar to that by Bevis (1988) in the opening quotation to this chapter, Rolfe (1996) argues that:

> *Nursing theorists tell us that the theory–practice gap is between what research and theory says ought ideally to be happening, and what actually happens in the 'imperfect' clinical area. From this perspective, the problem is that nurses fail, for a variety of reasons, to make use of research findings, and the gap will only be bridged if practice moves closer to the ideals of nursing theory by nurses reading and implementing research reports. On the other hand, practitioners tell us that the gap is between what actually works in real life and the unrealistic textbook ideals. From this perspective, the gap will be bridged by nursing theory more closely reflecting the realities of clinical life … The fact that the gap is still very much with us suggests that neither view is an accurate representation of the actual situation … the refusal of the gap to go away is actually a symptom of a serious underlying problem resulting from outdated theoretical concepts and a misconception about the relationship of theory to practice. The gap is a consequence of the way in which theory has failed to keep pace with changes in the concept and practice of nursing. It is an illusion, created by a way of conceptualising theory which can never fully account for what happens in clinical practice, and as such, the theory–practice gap cannot be bridged either by practice moving closer to theory, or by theory conforming to the constraints and limitations of real-life practice. It is a problem which must be dis-*

> *solved rather than solved, by developing a new concept of nursing theory and a new relationship between theory and practice, in which each informs and is responsive to the other.*
>
> (Rolfe, 1996, pp. 2–3)

But how does research fit into this scheme? In the relationship between theory and research discussed in the previous module, we suggested that the process of thinking about phenomena, issues, and problems leads to theories being proposed as we attempt to establish meaning in the phenomena we perceive. These untested theories then have to be tested and confirmed through research in a process known as the *theory-testing model* of theory building. However, an alternative model, known as the *grounded theory model* of theory construction, shows that theories can arise 'from the ground' so to speak, from experience and insights gained in the practice situation.

We return to this issue of the theory–research relationship below. But for now it is important to note that in the complex relationship between theory and research we come upon another praxis. Here the 'magical whole' is one encompassing theory (or thinking) and research (or doing), as knowledge is tested and enhanced. The idea presented by Bevis in the opening quotation can in fact be paraphrased as follows:

> *Research both tests and enhances theory, and theory both tests and enhances research. Each enlightens the other, provoking insights, altering and changing the form, shape and meaning of each. As the theory evolves, so the research evolves.*

Thus far we have introduced the issue of the relationship between theory and practice and between theory and research. But what is the relationship between research and practice? It may seem clear that as research influences or confirms theory construction, and as theory in turn influences practice, this is an indirect relationship mediated by theory, as illustrated by the following sequence:

Research → Theory → Practice

However, we have already seen that in at least one approach, that of grounded theory, observation and empirical evidence in the practice field lead to theory, as in the following sequence:

Practice → Research → Theory

These are just two examples of how research and practice are in direct, or alternatively indirect, relationships. But even here there are assumptions about the relationship or relevance of research to theory, and about whether research influences practice, or is influenced by it. There are also issues of the extent to which research and theory impact upon the real world of practice at all!

It will be clear by now that the matter we are addressing is indeed one of complex relationships. We can separate these out in terms of dyadic relationships as follows:

- the relationship between research and practice
- the relationship between theory and research
- the relationship between theory and practice.

However, in the real world of health care there is also an overriding triadic relationship between all three:

- the relationship between research, theory *and* practice.

It will assist us in moving towards this triadic relationship if we first address the three dyads.

Study Activity 18.1 ⎯⎯⎯⎯⎯⎯

The issues we shall address in this chapter are theory, research, and practice, addressing each of these primarily in a health context and with specific reference to the practice of nursing. The concepts are, therefore, research, theory, practice, health and nursing. You have engaged each of these concepts in this book already, to a greater or lesser extent. However, the purpose of this first Study Activity is to make the subsequent discussions easier to follow, by

undertaking a mini-concept analysis of each term. As may be recalled from Chapter 14, a concept is a term that describes a discrete entity in terms of its specific characteristics, and in general all examples of the entity would possess these characteristics. Thus, a chair normally has four legs, a flat surface to sit on, and a back to lean upon. In a *concept analysis* the concept is subjected to critical analysis to help us clarify the concept. This may be achieved by means of an analysis involving: reviewing the literature and the practice situation/environment to establish a definitive statement of the concept; through such reviewing, identifying the characteristics of the concept and stating these as an *exemplar case* (one that describes the ideal presentation of the concept); identifying alternative cases that help to distinguish the defining properties of the concept, such as a *contrary case*, where the other concept is entirely different (for example, 'intelligence' is entirely different to 'theory'), or a *borderline case*, where the other concept is very similar (for example, 'well-being' is very similar to 'health', but there are fundamental differences allowing us to have well-being even when we are in poor health). Concept analysis can be a complex and extensive undertaking, involving a number of analytical stages (see, for example, McKenna, 1997; Walker and Avant, 1999). However, for the purpose of this Study Activity:

- Carry out a brief concept analysis of each of the five concepts, using a brief review of the literature to identify the main characteristics, expressing the exemplar case and identifying just one contrary and one borderline case.
- Write a brief concept analysis report of approximately 200 words (half an A4 page) for each concept.
- Retain these statements for reference as you proceed through the remainder of the chapter.

RESEARCH AND PRACTICE

Evidence-based health care

In recent times, the most dominant discourse by far in almost all modern health care systems relates to this particular dyad: the relationship between research and practice. More specifically, the discourse pertains to the phenomenon that has become known variously as evidence-based health care, evidence-based practice, evidence-based medicine (and variations such as evidence-based nursing, evidence-based physiotherapy, etc.). Evidence-based medicine (and the variations) simply refers to the commitment to base the particular profession's practice on an evidential basis. Evidence-based practice is a broader term that relates to all the professions and their practices. Evidence-based health care is broader still, and pertains to the establishment of the total health care system on an evidence basis.

The terms find their origins in medicine, from which the variations are derived. In its most simple form, evidence-based medicine seems to be stating that medical interventions of whatever form should be based exclusively on evidence, in effect the *best available evidence*. This would seem to be indicating that medicine should be exclusively 'scientific' and that there is no place within it for that phenomenon we describe as 'clinical judgement' that is largely derived from experience as a form of intuitive or tacit knowing. Such assumptions have led to various modifications of the term, in efforts to avoid this restrictive interpretation. Therefore, various other terms such as 'evidence-informed medicine' and 'evidence-informed nursing' (McSherry *et al.*, 2002) have come into use, intended to indicate that the practice is central and that evidence informs this rather than dictating the practice.

This all draws attention to a subtle yet fundamental point. It is sometimes assumed that because there may be an unreasoned and unrealistic faith in empirical ways of knowing as the only legitimate source of real knowledge or absolute truth, the same accusation can be levelled at evidence-based medicine, or indeed the other variations in the evidence-based perspective referred to above. However, in all these variations there tends to be two significant positions that allow us to refute such claims.

- First, it is almost universally the case that the evidence-based movement adopts a modern post-positivistic approach to empirical evidence. That is, the post-positivistic position that recognises that empirical evidence can only ever produce a degree of probability that the knowledge claims hold and that such claims are always subject to possible refutation by further research. Therefore, the carefully worded phrase 'best *available* evidence' is almost always used.
- Second, the evidence is always taken as an aid to clinical decision-making. It is again an almost universal principle that the application of clinical wisdom taking into account context and the individual patient, is an important final arbiter (*see also* Chapters 17 and 27).

It is indeed fair to state that the most influential advocates of evidence-based medicine do not suggest a narrow understanding of the term. This is eloquently demonstrated in the work of Sackett *et al.* (2000), who have been perhaps the most important champions of this approach. It is worth considering their definition of evidence-based medicine, even though it is a little lengthy:

Evidence-based medicine (EBM) is the integration of best research evidence with clinical expertise and patient values.

- *By best research evidence we mean clinically relevant research, often from the basic sciences of medicine, but especially from patient-centered clinical research into the accuracy and precision of diagnostic tests (including the clinical examination), the power of prognostic markers, and the efficacy and safety of therapeutic, rehabilitative, and preventive regimes. New evidence from clinical research both invalidates previously accepted diagnostic tests and treatments and replaces them with new ones that are more powerful, more accurate, more efficacious, and safer.*
- *By clinical expertise we mean the ability to use our clinical skills and past expertise to rapidly identify each patient's unique*

> *health state and diagnosis, their individual risks and benefits of potential interventions, and their personal values and expectations.*
>
> • *By patient values we mean the unique preferences, concerns and expectations each patient brings to a clinical encounter and which must be integrated into clinical decisions if they are to serve the patient.*
>
> *When these three elements are integrated, clinicians and patients form a diagnostic and therapeutic alliance which optimizes clinical outcomes and quality of life.*
>
> (Sackett *et al.*, 2000, p. 1)

The contribution by Sackett *et al.* (2000) is particularly important in promoting a more holistic approach to evidence-based practice. However, it is important to recognise subtle differences in the various aforementioned terms. The following, while not necessarily universally accepted, may be useful rules-of-thumb:

• When the term *evidence-based medicine* is used, the emphasis tends to be on the safety and efficacy of *medical* interventions such as diagnosis, prognosis, and treatment interventions. The evidence sought is usually of an objective form and almost universally of that type derived from *randomised controlled trials* (where at least one randomly assigned group is given an intervention and outcomes are compared with at least one control group that has not received the intervention), or *experimental research* (laboratory research under controlled conditions).

• When the term *evidence-based nursing* is used, the emphasis is again on the safety and efficacy of interventions. However, nursing as a caring practice sees itself as operating within a wider context than that designated by diagnosis and treatment (Watson, 1997). The range of 'evidence' therefore tends to be broader – including caring as well as treatment knowledge. Also, because some nursing concerns are more subjective and relational, the means of procuring the best knowledge can extend beyond more objective and quantitative research into more qualitative domains. This is not to say that medicine ignores such domains of knowledge, and the growth of *narrative-based medicine* (Greenhalgh and Hurwitz, 1998) bears witnesses to this. However, this broader orientation is the norm rather than the exception in nursing, whereas in medicine it is very much a recently emerging perspective.

• When the term *evidence-based practice* is used, it is sometimes indicative of an attempt to avoid the *nature* of the evidence being determined by the bias of a particular professional grouping. The emphasis is on *practice*, and this determines the nature of the evidence that would be sought. In its most flexible and responsive form, the assumption is that practice is multidisciplinary and determined by the patients'/clients' needs. This in turn will determine the nature of the evidence that is sought, which by definition will be contextual and targeted towards particular needs.

• When the term *evidence-based health care* is used, it can in fact denote two different perspectives that do not in effect share all that much in their orientation. In the first sense, the orientation is essentially holistic. Evidence is sought that will respond to the total health care needs of the patients or clients partaking of the service. In this sense, there is a certain affinity with evidence-based practice. However, this may imply a certain degree of narrowness, while the hallmark of this first sense of the meaning is its breadth of concern. It encompasses evidence-based practice and indeed evidence-based medicine, evidence-based nursing, etc. But it extends beyond this to a concern with ensuring that policy development and health care management are also established on a sound evidence base (Hicks, 1997). Furthermore, it encompasses a more inclusive approach whereby patients or clients participate. Here patients or clients are presented with evidence in understandable form and involved in the decisions arising (an aspect within evidence-based health care that is sometimes labelled *evidence-based patient choice*). In the second sense, the term evidence-based health care has a more specific meaning. It refers to the evidence base for making decisions about the management and administration of health care systems as a whole (Muir Gray, 1997). As such, the decisions, and therefore the evidence needed to support them, are at a higher or different level to that concerned with clinical decision-making at the patient–professional interface. The nature of the evidence sought also tends to be notably different, being derived from such activities as epidemiological surveys or programme evaluation research. As will be noted, this is a much narrower perspective, including only one of the elements identified in the first meaning of evidence-based health care (that of an evidence base for the management of health care systems).

Irrespective of the perspective adopted, all of these share a common set of values to a greater or lesser extent. This includes attaching a premium to empirically derived knowledge, in the sense in which this was described in Chapter 10. This is totally justified and indeed essential if safe and effective service provision is to be assured. However, where all other forms of knowledge are rejected or disvalued, there is a real risk that services and individualised care may suffer as a result.

The burgeoning research and development agenda

Following on from the advancing influence of evidence-based approaches to practice, the development of research and development strategies across the UK heralded a commitment to basing best services on a research and development footing. The increasing emphasis on high standards within the health services in response to public demands and the need for more cost-effective services in the face of escalating costs, has led to an increasing emphasis on research. This emphasis was reflected in Great Britain by the introduction of a new research and develop-

ment strategy within the National Health Service in England (National Health Service Management Executive, 1991). The approach here is one that stresses the need to link research with the development of services to prevent it from becoming an isolated function. As it is reflected in slightly different ways in the four home countries within the UK, for ease of reference we concentrate primarily on the situation in England.

The research and development strategy has been co-ordinated by a research and development directorate within the National Health Service and the emphasis is on multidisciplinary and service-orientated approaches. Similar initiatives have been carried forward in the other three UK countries. Although there has been a change of Government in latter years, this is one area of commitment that Labour carried forward from the previous Conservative Government. It is important to note that the research and development strategies are part of a wider drive towards quality in the National Health Service, which preceded the change in UK Government in 1997 but has continued with increasing force since that year. The general thrust has been that of a commitment to improving quality and enhancing standards, modernising health services to meet new and changing demands, and providing the infrastructures necessary to achieve these ends. This began with three significant Department of Health policy documents issued during the first 2 years of the current Labour Government's coming to power: *The New NHS: Modern, dependable* (Department of Health, 1997), *A First Class Service: Quality in the new NHS* (Department of Health, 1998a), and *Our Healthier Nation – Saving lives* (Department of Health, 1999). The emphasis within these documents was that of a commitment to modernisation (interpreted as making the National Health Service more up-to-date and responsive to the modern world) and means of establishing higher quality (interpreted in terms of efficiency, cost-effectiveness and greater responsiveness to and involvement of the public).

It was recognised that to achieve these aspirations there was a need to ensure that adequate infrastructures were in place. These were interpreted as including: a general programme of modernisation, extending across resources, structures and processes; an effective workforce, adequately trained and constantly updated through effective continuing professional development, as part of an education and training thrust; an adequate evidence foundation carried forward as a research and development thrust; extension of and recognition of responsibility for clinical as well as corporate standards (not only for clinicians but to include those responsible for managing services), as reflected in new clinical governance initiatives; a more direct involvement of the professional regulatory bodies to the quality agenda and greater responsiveness of these bodies to the public, and a greater involvement of, and responsiveness to, this same public within the services in general.

In a sense, these initiatives created a 'no hiding place' scenario. Clinicians are now being driven towards accepting responsibility for wider quality issues and cost-effectiveness, and their regulatory bodies are being challenged to respond to policy and public demands. Similarly, health service managers are no longer able to say that clinical matters are outside of their sphere of concern: under clinical governance they carry responsibility and accountability for ensuring that clinical effectiveness would be achieved. To ensure that there is adequate support for clinical governance, the Department of Health has established within the English National Health Service a National Clinical Governance Support Team. The good practice advice emanating from this body, and its availability to provide support, would make it difficult to claim inability to meet the clinical governance challenge.

Of course, the success of these policy initiatives would depend on adequate infrastructures being in place. In respect of education and training, two significant Department of Health publications, *Working Together: Securing a quality workforce* (Department of Health, 1998b) and *A Health Service of All the Talents:*

Developing the National Health Service workforce (Department of Health, 2000a), established a commitment to providing adequate training and continuing development for staff. As an extension of this, there is a further commitment to establishing National Health Service organisations as learning organisations. This places an emphasis on moving away from a blame culture that tends to result in covering up mistakes and various other blame-avoidance strategies, to a more open environment within which there is a commitment to learning from mistakes (Department of Health, 2000b). To support this cultural change, the Department of Health has established a National Health Service National Patient Safety Agency whose task it is to receive reports of errors without risk of reprimand and disseminate such information so that adverse events threatening patient safety can be avoided.

Alongside the latter education and training (E&T) thrust, the equally forceful research and development (R&D) thrust aims at improving the evidence base essential to clinical effectiveness and a safe, high-quality service. This commitment is reflected in the support of Government for centres that facilitate the development of evidence-based approaches. Significant among these are the support for the Cochrane Collaboration Centre connected to which is the Cochrane Library, a database of research evidence that is available as a CD-ROM and online source, and the establishment of the National Health Service Centre for Reviews and Disseminations based at the University of York. The latter body carries out systematic reviews (see below) of health-related research and disseminates this throughout the services. This commitment is further reflected in a comprehensive approach to the future support of research and development within the health services. In carrying this forward, the Department of Health (2000c, 2001) proposes to fund research development on two fronts:

- National Health Service priorities and needs research and development funding
- National Health Service support for science.

335

The first of these relates to research and development activities directly targeted at modernising services and quality improvement, while the second relates to supporting scientific research necessary to underpin the evidence base of health care (and in this respect the Department of Health clearly defines evidence-based health care in terms of the broader of the two senses of this term, as presented earlier in this chapter).

In carrying these initiatives forward, the Department of Health is also cognisant of the need not only to create quality but to audit its achievement. Two additional mechanisms, proposed first in *A First Class Service: Quality in the new NHS* (Department of Health, 1998a), as referred to earlier, have been established as organisational entities to further this cause. The first of these is the National Institute for Clinical Excellence; the other is the Commission for Health Improvement.

National Institute for Clinical Excellence (NICE)

This is a special health authority established by the Department of Health in 1999. Its function is to appraise new evidence and new health care technologies, and on the basis of this, to facilitate the production and dissemination of evidence-based guidelines and standards for care delivery. Such standards are issued by the Department of Health as national service frameworks pertaining to particular client groups or areas of service delivery.

Commission for Health Improvement (CHI)

The Commission was established by the Department of Health in 2000 as an independent inspection body. Its role (across England, Wales and – by invitation – Northern Ireland) is to monitor the implementation of standards (as, for example, specified in the national service frameworks) and to carry out inspections where there are major systems failure (for example, in 'failing hospitals').

The push towards increasing standards and enhancing quality is a continuing and rapidly changing process. The demands of a more informed and increasingly critical public constantly grow. The very advances in technology and therapeutics occasioned by research and development which improve the public's lot have the paradoxical effect of increasing demand and dissatisfaction. At the same time, the scarcity of resources makes responding an increasingly difficult challenge. As a consequence, new strategies are constantly emerging, each with its own organisational structures and processes. These sometimes replace other approaches and sometimes add to the range of initiatives being carried forward.

The consideration of these various elements is by necessity brief within this chapter. However, it can be clearly seen from Fig. 18.1 (which for clarity presents only some of the main initiatives) that the UK Government is taking a serious and aggressive stance in respect of improving quality. It will also be clear that within this, research and development and in particular evidence-based practice and health care, are important underpinning strands. This indicates most decisively the point made earlier, that the relationship between research and practice has intensified in its importance to levels never previously encountered.

Study Activity 18.2

In the preceding sections we have by necessity concentrated on developments within the English National Health Service that relate directly or indirectly to the issue of research and practice. Using an Internet search engine, explore your own country's Health Department/Ministry web site to identify its research and development strategy. Write a brief overview of around 400 words (one A4 page) that highlights the arrangements and any differences to the English system. Keep these notes within your course notes for future reference. If England is in fact your own home country, search the English Department of Health web site and do a similar overview, in particular identifying any recent developments of the research and development strategy.

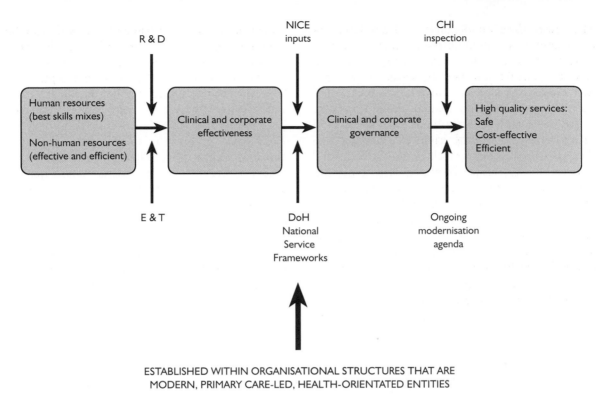

Figure 18.1 The National Health Service quality infrastructures

CHI, Commission for Health Improvement; DoH, Department of Health; E&T, education and training; NICE, National Institute for Clinical Excellence; R&D, research and development

Scientism

It is important to note that within the above developments there is a risk that a profound faith in research may exist. That is, it may be believed that science or research, by providing the requisite evidence, may be sufficient to provide the total knowledge foundations necessary for 'good' health care. It is not the case that such aspects are unimportant. It has already been argued that research and development is vital to the provision of safe and effective care. The danger is that such a blind faith may fail to appreciate limitations of scientific knowledge in health care. A claim is often made (not entirely with justification in all circumstances) that the medical profession in particular espouses a traditional positivistic scientific paradigm that mainly values quantitative information derived from experimental research and randomised controlled trials. Given the exceptional political power of the medical lobby within health, it may hardly be surprising that primacy is given to this particular source of knowledge.

What is witnessed here is the phenomenon of *scientism* which has become dominant in modern society in general, and thus also in health care settings. Scientism relates to the situation in which there is an almost blind faith in what is viewed as hard science. It is the view that the characteristic inductive methods of the natural sciences are the only valid sources of genuine factual knowledge about man and society (Williams, 1983). It is the further view that knowledge produced by any other method is invalid and unreliable.

It is a fact of life that the managers and senior executives who manage modern health services may not have a detailed understanding of nursing theory. Their interests tend to be predominantly in measurable performance indicators, health care statistical indices, and quantitative research designed to prove the efficacy and cost-effectiveness of particular health interventions. It is also a fact of life, well known to researchers in the health care field, that Government departments are much more likely to fund quantitative research which may lead to savings or cost-effectiveness than they are to fund qualitative research which may address apparently more nebulous issues such as the promotion of caring relationships or the refinement of nursing theory. In short, the reality of the situation is that those in the health services, including many of those in the nursing profession, view the knowledge domain of practice mainly from a particular research perspective that excludes both a theory perspective *and* the possibility of alternative ways of knowing. A number of influences, professional, social, and policy related, are important in the development of this situation.

Professional influences

The professional influence is perhaps the most important because it arises from within nursing itself. The result is an aspiration towards excellence and a desire to ensure that practice is safe and effective. In the UK an example of this influence was witnessed in the introduction of a new and revolutionary restructuring of nurse education at the end of the 1980s (United Kingdom Central Council for Nursing, Midwifery and Health Visiting, 1986). The new education, entitled Project 2000, aimed to educate a single level of nurse practitioner known as the 'knowledgeable doer'. It had been recognised that there was a gap between the theory or knowledge of nursing (itself underdeveloped) and the practice of nursing (largely based on tradition and subjective judgement). The new education would ensure that practice would be based on a sound body of knowledge, and that this knowledge would, by definition, have to be science and research based.

This emphasis on science (and research) as an exclusive basis for best practice has also been present in the field of nursing academia. In an attempt to achieve full professional status and academic respectability, nursing academics have a particular interest in espousing a scientific perspective. To a large extent, this has been realised as a bias in favour of quantitative research approaches. These trends have only recently yielded to some extent towards qualitative, humanistic approaches. While in North America there are a number of influential nurse theorists, Great Britain currently has a relatively small cadre of nurse theorists. As a result, the main knowledge base available to nursing practice (other than that imported from North America or elsewhere) is that of research-derived knowledge, most of which is not theory linked and not set within a framework of theory enhancement and development.

Social–legal influences

With major advances in health care and a better educated and more sophisticated public, society is becoming more demanding and more critical of health care provision. Professions such as nursing are under scrutiny more than ever before. This significant shift in societal attitudes puts the social contract between nursing and society in high profile. Its sharpest edge, particularly in North America but now also in the UK and other Western societies, is the threat of litigation. This emphasises the imposition on nurses to be able to show that what they do is based on sound up-to-date knowledge. In this regard, over 15 years ago Hockey (1987) stated that:

> *Legally, a professional nurse in the UK is held responsible for his or her actions and has to be able to defend them on the basis of the latest knowledge. The latest available knowledge must be based on research because this is the only way by which the body of knowledge can be changed or extended.*
>
> (Hockey, 1987)

Given this societal challenge and the legal imperative that hangs over nursing, it is hardly surprising that many are now preoccupied with research findings. Such research findings will not only establish the safety and effectiveness of practice, but provide a concrete defence for that practice should it be questioned in the courts or in the course of other forms of investigation.

Policy influences

We have already considered the significant policy developments that are focused upon in the quest for quality within UK health services. There are perhaps two major threads within this drive that lead towards a scientific- or research-orientated perspective, and perhaps also drive this further into unrealistic expectations that we might see as an example of scientism. These influences can be identified by considering the subtle yet fundamental nature of the aspirations. Most of the policy documentation is stated as supporting research to promote *clinical effectiveness* and *cost-effectiveness*.

In respect of the first of these aspirations (clinical effectiveness), the tendency is to emphasise evidence that makes specific statements about the efficacy of clinical work, extending from diagnostic and prognostic techniques through to the therapeutic efficacy of particular therapeutic interventions and health technologies. However, this tends to be interpreted as being research findings or 'evidence' of a particular nature. That is, research that is derived from randomised controlled trials or experimental research is given priority. Nevertheless, the quest remains that of evidence that directs health care interventions towards best practices. In respect of the second of these aspirations, it is expected that research will also provide evidence on the relative costs of interventions. In effect, the research is expected not only to provide evidence of the most effective health interventions, but also the cheapest that are still effective to some given standard (which itself may be stated so as to direct choices towards cheaper options rather than best practices). Evidence in this context is not only a clinical issue but also a highly political one.

Study Activity 18.3

Using your library and online resources, carry out a literature and subject review using the terms 'clinical effectiveness' and 'cost-effectiveness'.

- Present brief definitions of what the two terms mean. In doing this you may wish to review Chapter 17 on clinical effectiveness within this module.
- List all the ways you can identify in which the two terms and their goals differ or concur, drawing particular attention to any circumstances in which they might actually be in conflict.

The relationship in reality

While much lip service is paid to the application of research to practice, the extent to which research findings are actually applied is open to question. In fact, we are not yet in a position where we can claim that research is significantly guiding practice in its totality. In this regard, it is interesting to note this comment by Chalmers (1993), which relates to midwives but could equally be applied to nurses:

> *Midwives are using pregnant women and babies as guinea pigs in uncontrolled experiments in their everyday practice. For example, how many midwives have recommended that women use 'Epifoam' or 'Rotersept', or hairdryers for drying the perineum; and what unbiased evidence would they point to as justification for promoting these forms of care? Can midwives point to evidence that weighing women routinely during pregnancy is likely to do more good than harm?*
>
> (Chalmers, 1993)

This statement, albeit now of only historical interest, carries an element of truth in it, as practice is often based on tradition and convention rather than research. In effect, despite the imperatives discussed above, the relationship between research and practice is often more an aspiration than a reality.

There are a number of reasons that can explain this state of affairs. These can be generally considered under the headings of amassing, evaluating, disseminating, and implementing.

Amassing

The one thing that is clear is that the volume of health-related research is massive in proportions. On an international level, there are in excess of 20 000 biomedical journals publishing more than 8000 scholarly papers per week. There are literally millions of individual research reports and the likelihood of collecting and collating all that exists is an almost impossible task. The advances in information and communication technology have, of course, made such activities more manageable. However, there are difficulties in respect of converting the mountain of 'evidence' into clusters that make it possible to proceed to the next stage of establishing usefulness. One problem is not only the sheer volume of published work, but the rapidity with which it is added to. Another relates to the amount of research that is not actually published as yet, some of which may be of vital importance.

Yet another problem relates to the nature of the material available, i.e. what is included and what is excluded. The great majority of published research papers are directed towards illness-orientated medicine and therapeutics, and consist mainly of randomised controlled trials. For example, Oakley (1999) suggests that the Cochrane Collaborations (the source of the Cochrane Library of Evidence) is based on a model that embodies the three assumptions of: an illness focus; a greater emphasis on treatment than prevention; and a prioritisation of systematic reviews (see under 'Evaluating' below) above other kinds of research activity. There is indeed evidence to suggest that, while there is a massive volume of health-related research, some areas such as primary care (National Health Service Executive, 1997; McKenna and Ashton, 2000) and mental health (Department of Health, 2002) are under-researched.

It is also the case that research that is most likely to be funded is of the aforementioned randomised controlled trials type. While there is some indication of an increasing acceptance of qualitative research and other sources of knowledge, the so-called 'gold standard' in respect of clinical evidence remains randomised controlled trials, evaluated through 'systematic reviews' (see under 'Evaluating' below). This is reflected in the means by which evidence is classified, in terms of 'strength'. The most commonly used classification is that developed within the Cochrane Collaboration, as illustrated in Table 18.1. As will be seen, qualitative research does not appear until at least type IV: it is classified as non-experimental research (only accepted if it emanates from more than one centre or research group), or possibly even as descriptive studies, where it drops to type V, the very lowest valued 'evidence'. Of course, the crux of this matter lies in the notion of evidence. Most qualitative research does not aspire to the production of evidence of a propositional cause–effect nature. However, as noted in the earlier chapters of this module, and in Module 3, the knowledge obtained from such qualitative approaches is vitally important to a deeper understanding of health issues and any system of 'evidence' that excludes it (or places it at so low a level that it is disvalued and seldom funded) would create a bias and a vacuum in the knowledge needed to inform our practice.

Evaluating

The next and equally daunting challenge is that of evaluating the available evidence. It is again the case that with advances in information and communication technology, published research is more widely available. Databases, both online and in CD-ROM format, are increasingly accessible to nurses. These include the Medline database of medical and health science research, and the equivalent nursing database known as CINAHL (Cumulative Index to Nursing and Allied Health Literature). However, the problem

Table 18.1 Assessment criteria: type and strength of evidence

Type	Strength
I	Strong evidence from at least one published systematic review of multiple, well-designed, randomised controlled trials.
II	Strong evidence from at least one published properly designed randomised controlled trial of appropriate size and in an appropriate clinical setting.
III	Evidence from published, well-designed trials without randomisation, single group pre–post, cohort, time series or matched case-controlled studies.
IV	Evidence from well-designed, non-experimental studies from more than one centre or research group.
V	Opinions of respected authorities, based on clinical evidence, descriptive studies or reports of expert consensus committees.

(*Source*: Bandolier, 1994)

of interpreting the findings of specific research papers, particularly where these are complex, must be surmounted. The National Health Service Centre for Reviews and Dissemination and the Cochrane Library (both referred to earlier) provide a helpful service by undertaking or reporting reviews. There are essentially two approaches employed:

- *Systematic reviews* – reviews that are undertaken of key research reports on a particular topic. An attempt is made, at the most comprehensive level of a systematic review, to scan the world literature and identify all important contributions. The individual research reports are critiqued and a report includes an overview of consistent findings across these reports. Of course, there need to be criteria for establishing the acceptability of research included in the review, and this may include the clarity of the research goals, the research method (if randomised controlled trials or controlled experiments were used), how issues of reliability and validity were addressed, and the consistency of analysis of findings. It is important when considering such systematic reviews to consider *their* methods, and in particular the criteria they

used to value the research that was reviewed. Systematic reviews that exclude certain research (e.g. qualitative research that does not meet a review criterion of only including randomised controlled trials) may exclude important information that would inform practice.

- *Meta-analyses* – data that are taken from a number of completed research projects on the same topic, and then analysed as if they were data from one massive study. Such a meta-analysis involves synthesising the data from a number of studies, or sometimes attempting to synthesise the findings. This can, of course, present a number of methodological difficulties. Not only are the data increased, but so also are the risks of bias or confounding variables in the various studies that are clumped together. For this reason, systematic reviewing tends to be the preferred option.

Disseminating

There is clearly a wide range of techniques that can be utilised. These include the primary resources themselves (i.e. research journals such as the *Journal of Advanced Nursing*, the *International Journal of Nursing Studies*, *Advances in Nursing Science*, *Nursing Science Quarterly*, and similar journals), and evidence-based practice bulletins and research reports or research monographs (individually published or circulated research reports). Many of these resources are also available in online electronic journal form. In addition, research information is distributed electronically, by agencies such as those referred to earlier (Medline, CINAHL and, as systematic reviews, through the Cochrane Library and the National Health Service Centre for Reviews and Dissemination). Unfortunately, there are often major barriers between the source of this information and the actual practice setting. As indicated above, such research may be complex and difficult to interpret and staff may lack the educational preparation to interpret research findings or reviews. But even if this obstacle is overcome, it is often the case that, despite the UK Government's commitment to modernisation, many health care facilities do not have the infrastructures in place to access disseminated information (McDaid, 2000; Slevin, 2002). There is often a lack of library facilities, poor access to research publications, and/or absence of computers with access to online databases.

Implementing

Despite the amount of research that is increasingly being made available, there are concerns about the extent to which this is implemented in actual practice situations. For example, Smith (1992) estimated that as little as 15% of medical activity is scientifically validated, and Roberts (1995) estimated that around 20% of therapeutic interventions within the National Health Service were inappropriate. It has been crudely estimated that if the National Health Service Centre for Reviews and Dissemination had a 10 year all-freeze period it could not review all the research literature currently available and, of course, by the end of that period most of it would be out of date anyway. Indeed, it is also crudely estimated that only around 1–5% of the research available is reliable enough to inform practice with confidence. Baker (1998), one of the leading figures in setting up the English research and development strategy, has indicated that the most successful research and development strategy would be unlikely to ensure that more than 50% of health care practice is based on the best evidence that is available.

Undoubtedly, some practitioners are resistant to change, including change which originates from research. It is also the case that overstretched practitioners may not have sufficient time or opportunity to evaluate the applicability of research findings or, alternatively, where they are negatively disposed towards the very concept of evidence-based practice, they claim that this is the case. Such attitudinal barriers may be increased in circumstances where managers do not emphasise the importance of evidence, and where the culture within a health care agency does not promote an evidence-based ethos. Professionals cannot, however, avoid the increasing imposition placed upon them to develop the skills to search literature, critique and understand research reports and systematic reviews, and apply research findings where appropriate. Similarly, as the scrutiny of agencies such as the Commission for Health Improvement extends across the health services, those responsible for managing the quality of services will be unable to avoid this imposition.

The research–practice link: a basis for best practice or mass confusion?

In this section we have considered the direct link between research and practice, and in particular the impact of the evidence-based health care movement that has attempted to strengthen this link. It must be recognised that such developments have led to real and significant improvements in quality of care. Dangerous medicines are now much more unlikely to reach the patient, mass hysterectomies and tonsillectomies, for which there was no real supporting evidence, are a thing of the past, and new life-saving technologies enter our health care systems at an ever-increasing rate. These achievements alone justify the commitment to the link between research and practice.

However, as noted above, it is still the case that only a fraction of what is done for or to the users of our services can genuinely be claimed to be on the basis of best available evidence. There are, of course, reasons for this that are intrinsic to the systems for promoting evidence-based practice. We have noted these above, from the point of amassing evidence, through its evaluation and dissemination, to issues of implementation at the practice interface. However, there are other issues that impact upon this situation. We noted above Baker's (1998) assertion that only 50% at most of what we practice would be evidence based. To a certain extent this is attributable to the barriers to implementation we referred to above. But it must also be recognised that not all of the knowledge that informs our practice can be empirical, in the sense conveyed by evidence-based practice. In Module 3 we considered the various forms or patterns of knowing that may inform our practice. These included not only the empirical, but also the personal, aesthetic and ethical modes of knowing (Carper, 1978). We do, of course, need the best empirical evidence to inform our practice, but other forms of knowledge – such as that related to ethical decision-making – are no less vitally important. Sometimes practitioners turn away from the empirical knowledge because they know, intuitively and from their clinical wisdom, that other knowledge must inform their actions.

However, there may also be a more fundamental process at play here. If you have just read the earlier sections on research and practice you will not have failed to note the increasingly complex array of arrangements, strategies, information sources, and Government and independent organisations involved in the evidence-based health care movement. In such circumstances, even those directly involved find the system unclear and confusing. Practitioners need clear and transparent systems that are accessible at the point of care delivery and easy to utilise on a day-to-day basis. It is questionable whether the confusing array of strategies and agencies meet this requirement. Furthermore, despite the efforts of Government and health service agencies to relate research to practice realities, it is not always clear that this has been successful. Almost 40 years ago Raulin (1963) presented this confusing array in a fable, in which bricks were used as an analogy for research:

> And so it happened that the land became flooded with bricks. It became necessary to organise more and more storage places, called journals, and more and more elaborate systems of bookkeeping to record the inventory. In all of this the brickmakers retained their pride and skill and the bricks were of the very best quality. But production was ahead of demand and bricks were no longer made to order. The size and shape was now dictated by changing trends in fashion. In order to compete successfully, production emphasised those types of brick that were easy to make and only rarely did an adventuresome brickmaker attempt a

> difficult or unusual design. The influence of tradition in production and in types of product became a dominating factor. Unfortunately, the builders were almost destroyed. It became difficult to find the proper bricks for a task because one had to hunt among so many. It became difficult to find a suitable plot for construction of an edifice because the ground was covered with loose bricks. It became difficult to complete a useful edifice because, as soon as the foundations were discernible, they were buried under an avalanche of random bricks. And, saddest of all, sometimes no effort was made to maintain the distinction between a pile of bricks and a true edifice.
>
> (Raulin, 1963)

Raulin could only have guessed that the flood of bricks (or research) he referred to would increase to oceanic proportions over the next four decades. The moral of this tale is clear. There is a need for the brickmakers (or researchers) to manufacture bricks (research) that allow the builders (managers and practitioners) to construct an edifice (of safe and effective health care practices). This can be put another way. Unless research helps us develop a meaningful way of understanding the health care world and how practice must work within it, it becomes a disjointed body of information that is of limited use. Rather than helping us to make sense of the situation, it may indeed serve to confuse and paralyse effective practice. In short, to inform our practice in an ordered and structured way, research must be applied within a theoretical framework. If the relationship between theory and research is not addressed, the relationship between research and practice may lapse easily into the world of Raulin's fable.

THEORY AND RESEARCH

Constructing knowledge

The empirical act of research produces factual knowledge and structures and analyses this knowledge. In comparing the theory–research relationship with the theory–practice relationship of praxis that we discussed in the introduction to this chapter, research is the practice analogue, the action part of the process. Theory is the non-empirical process of thinking about knowledge. The product of this thinking or 'theorising' is the organisation of associated concepts into useful frameworks or worldviews that we describe as theories. The motivating force behind theory building is to provide meaningful constructions of our world, constructions that not only explain the world but help us to live and work in it (an issue raised consistently in Chapter 14). Together these two closely related research and theory functions create knowledge, in this case nursing knowledge. Through the complementary interaction of these two entities in a scientific praxis, knowledge is born. But can each of these entities separately and alone produce sound knowledge? Or can research only produce sound knowledge when it is theory linked? These are fundamental questions, which must be addressed.

Study Activity 18.4 ⎯⎯⎯⎯⎯

A nurse carried out research into back injury among nurses. She claimed to be interested in this area because of the high rate of absenteeism related to back injuries. The nurse administered a questionnaire to a sample of nurses, asking about the nature of the back injury, the cause of it (in the subject's opinion), the extent of sick leave taken, the treatment, and any residual disability. Her analysis was presented with excellent descriptive and inferential statistics (see Chapter 15). One of her main findings was that a large majority of nurses declared that their injury was due to excessive lifting of patients in staff shortage situations. However, a colleague asked the researcher about the theoretical basis of her research: What was the theory she had attempted to verify? What was the contribution of her research to theory development? The researcher responded that she had no such theoretical viewpoints; her research was empirical not theoretical.

- The nurse in the above example apparently felt that research and theory have little to do with each other. Write down some personal thoughts on this viewpoint. You may find it helpful to review the discussion on theory as science presented in Chapter 14. State whether you agree or disagree with the nurse and justify your position.
- Look up the subject 'attribution theory' in your college library's psychology section and write a brief and simple explanation of this theory. Explain the nurse's finding in the above example in terms of attribution theory. Write a brief account of how her finding could be used to apply attribution theory to the issue of back injury in nursing.

Theory as science

To many scientists, including nurse-scientists, theory and research are closely related. Thus, nursing scholars such as Fawcett (1999) and Meleis (1997) see research as the vehicle for theory development. Both authors see theory and research as being closely related aspects of science. In fact, from this point of view:

Science = theory + research.

This concept is clearly described by Burns and Grove (1987), who define science as:

> ... a coherent organisation of research findings and tested theories related to a specific field of knowledge. Science is both a product and a process. For example, within physics is Newton's Law of Gravity, which was developed through extensive research. The knowledge of gravity (product) is a part of the science of physics that evolved through formulating and testing theoretical ideas (process). The science of a field determines the accepted process for obtaining knowledge within that field. Research is an accepted process for obtaining scientific knowledge.
>
> (Burns and Grove, 1987, pp. 10–11)

Yet it is true that many professional scientists, as for the nurse in the Study Activity above, do not see theory as an important aspect of scientific work. She merely collected information about back injury and was puzzled when asked about the relationship between her research and theory. To her, theory was irrelevant, a belief shared by many researchers. For example, according to Burns and Grove (1987) one view (clearly different to the alternative view they state above) is that:

> *Science and theory are different yet very dependent on one another. They both require the use of abstract thought processes. The object of each is to promote understanding or 'knowing' of the empirical world. Science is seen as being closer to 'truth,' whereas theory is associated with conjectures or possibilities. Science is thought of as being more certain than theory. People who favor a strong science tend to discount the value of theories, whereas those who stress the greater importance of theories tend to discount the wisdom of using scientific knowledge alone for adequate explanation of the empirical world.*
>
> (Burns and Grove, 1987, p. 16)

Such thinking clearly suggests a separation of theory from research and supports the view that theory is in some way unscientific, that it is not even a part of science at all. This idea is tantamount to saying that the formula presented above, that science = theory + research, is unsound, and that the following is actually correct:

Research = science

and

Theory = conjecture.

This view is not shared by Fawcett and Meleis, as indicated above, and in fairness in subsequent editions of their book, Burns and Grove (1993, 1997, 2000), while still speaking of science *and* theory, recognise the close affinity between theory and research and the importance of research as a source of emerging theory. It is

also not the view presented in Chapter 14 of this book. There theory in its most orthodox sense is taken to be knowledge which is exclusively scientific knowledge, arrived at through scientific rigour, and closely aligned with research from which, in its final confirmed form, it is derived. As such, theory is clearly and unequivocally within the scientific domain. Indeed, Kuhn (1970), in a classical study of the nature of science, argues that a discipline characterised by research that simply addresses problems that come to attention in a haphazard manner, must be viewed as pre-paradigmatic. That is, such disciplines are not fully developed scientific disciplines with a shared knowledge or theoretical framework.

Such an overall lack of consensus about where theory stands in regard to science in general and research in particular does little to bring clarity to the mind of the student. But the situation is not entirely hopeless. To a large extent the problem is associated with the meaning people ascribe to the term theory. For some, theory is simply thinking as opposed to doing; thus, in nursing we talk about theory and practice. In other contexts people use the term theory to mean simply their propositional statements which attempt to explain ideas or phenomena in the real world. Clearly, theory in this sense is largely conjectural, and as such less rigorous than scientific thinking and enquiry. However, in Chapter 14 we gave a more specific definition of theory in its scientific context:

> *Theory is the description or explanation of phenomena and the relationship between such phenomena. In essence concepts, i.e. symbolic descriptions of phenomena, are linked by propositions which state relationships between them. Such statements may go beyond the purely descriptive or explanatory levels to the level of prediction.*

Making such statements on the basis of empirical findings or, conversely, confirming them through empirical investigation, places theory well within science. But only if theory is defined and under-

345

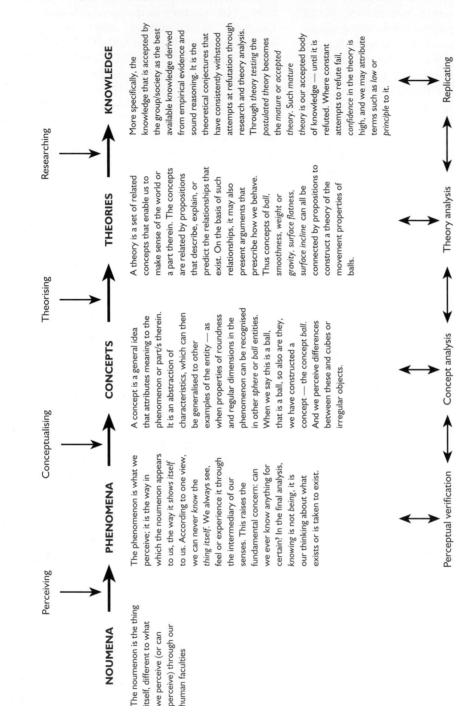

NOUMENA

The noumenon is the thing itself, different to what we perceive (or can perceive) through our human faculties

Perceiving

PHENOMENA

The phenomenon is what we perceive; it is the way in which the noumenon appears to us, the way it *shows itself* to us. According to one view, we can never *know the thing itself*. We always see, feel or experience it through the intermediary of our senses. This raises the fundamental concern: can we ever know anything for certain? In the final analysis, *knowing is not being*, it is our thinking about what exists or is taken to exist.

Conceptualising

CONCEPTS

A concept is a general idea that attributes meaning to the phenomenon or part/s therein. It is an abstraction of characteristics, which can then be generalised to other examples of the entity — as when properties of roundness and regular dimensions in the phenomenon can be recognised in other *sphere* or *ball* entities. When we say this is a ball, that is a ball, so also are they, we have constructed a concept — the concept *ball*. And we perceive differences between these and cubes or irregular objects.

Theorising

THEORIES

A theory is a set of related concepts that enable us to make sense of the world or a part therein. The concepts are related by propositions that describe, explain, or predict the relationships that exist. On the basis of such relationships, it may also present arguments that prescribe how we behave. Thus concepts of *ball*, *smoothness*, *weight* or *gravity*, *surface flatness*, *surface incline* can all be connected by propositions to construct a theory of the movement properties of balls.

Researching

KNOWLEDGE

More specifically, the knowledge that is accepted by the group/society as the best available knowledge derived from empirical evidence and sound reasoning. It is the theoretical conjectures that have consistently withstood attempts at refutation through research and theory analysis. Through *theory testing* the *postulated theory* becomes the *mature* or *accepted theory*. Such *mature theory* is our accepted body of knowledge — until it is refuted. Where constant attempts to refute fail, *confidence* in the theory is high, and we may attribute terms such as *law* or *principle* to it.

Perceptual verification
Reflection

Concept analysis

Theory analysis
Theory testing
Theory construction/
reconstruction

Replicating
Critiquing
Systematic reviewing

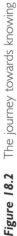

Figure 18.2 The journey towards knowing

stood in this way. This perspective clearly establishes a close relationship between theory and research. They are, as suggested in the introduction to this chapter, inextricable: one is informed and enhanced by the other, and vice versa. We can visualise the situation, as in Fig. 18.2 (an elaboration of the similar Fig. 14.3 in Chapter 14), as being a process of knowledge construction within a particular theoretical frame. Thus, we move from the initial perception of noumena (things in our world) that we experience as phenomena, which we would attempt to understand, through processes of conceptualisation and theorising. We then test these theories in the real world (by research) and this in turn further informs our theory and the concepts and propositions that make it up.

The theory–research relationship

The relationship between theory as outlined above and research (what is commonly described as the theory-testing approach) is not as simple as it may at first seem. There are in fact a number of different relationships which can exist here. Considered in the context of nursing (although the same applies in regard to most professional disciplines), the main types of relationship that may be found are as follows.

Theory testing

Theory testing is the most orthodox approach to the theory–research relationship, which sees the primary function of research as theory construction. It is characteristic of the traditional empirical-positivistic scientific approach. Here ideas, explanations, and predictions may be posited about specific problems or areas of concern within a discipline. These are then researched and – when the data are analysed – descriptions, explanations, causal relationships, and predictable generalisations emerge which are formulated as a theory. Thus, an explanation of reality comes out of the research in the following relationship:

intradisciplinary problems or concerns (with propositions or hypotheses that *may* explain

or predict relationships, and causes) → research → confirmed theory.

In some circumstances, initial thinking about the problem or area of concern is advanced to the stage where an untested theory is actually proposed. In this situation the individuals involved have a notional view of how phenomena relate to each other and behave. They formulate a conceptual framework which describes the situation, and explains the relationships, causal and otherwise, between the concepts. Theory may also predict how these concepts will interact and generalise such predictions into other similar situations. But what they have to do is formulate their theoretical propositions in empirical terms and test their validity and reliability through research. The relationship between theory and research which exists here is as follows:

Unconfirmed or untested theory (with a fully stated theory being proposed)	→	Research (tested or confirmed theory

In both of the above situations the primary function of research is to test and confirm a theory. There are still few major examples of a theory developed within nursing and tested and confirmed through nursing research, which was not in some way derivative of a theory in some other discipline. However, this situation is not unusual in a discipline that in terms of scientific and professional development is still quite young. Indeed, even in the pure sciences such as physics and chemistry, the discovery of a major new theory is a rare and momentous achievement.

Theory adoption

Here a theory which has been developed in another discipline is identified as being useful for the resolution of nursing problems or the guiding of nursing practice. One example is operant and classical conditioning theories, which are learning theories developed within the discipline of behavioural psychology. These theories have been adopted by nurse therapists as the theoretical underpinning of psychotherapeutic practice. In theory adoption, the theory is taken in its totality and applied in an unmodified form. In this case the relationship between theory and research is of a confirmatory nature. That is, the research function is to confirm the appropriateness of the theory to nursing by evaluating the extent to which the adoption of the theory has been successful.

Theory adaptation

Here the theory is again taken from another discipline. However, it is not borrowed in its entirety. Indeed, Barnum (1990) disagrees with the notion of 'borrowing', stating that:

> Borrowed theories remain borrowed as long as they are not adapted to the nursing milieu and the nursing image of man. Once such theories have been adapted to the nursing milieu, it is logical to refer to these boundary overlaps as shared knowledge rather than as borrowed theories.
>
> (Barnum, 1990)

The essential difference between adopted (or 'borrowed') and adapted theory is that in the former the theory is taken in its entirety and not modified in any substantive way to accommodate the nursing situation, while in the latter case the theory is modified and refined to suit the new situation. Here again research is used to evaluate and confirm the appropriateness of the application of the adapted theory to the nursing situation. However, in essence, research goes a step further. An adapted theory is a modified theory, and indeed, it may have been changed in quite substantive ways from its original form. In addition, it may not have been adapted from just a single theory, but from two or more theories, possibly originating from more than one discipline. This process often involves much work of an original and creative nature in terms of amalgamating, synthesising, and reforming theoretical knowledge. What emerges may be a new theoretical formulation in which it may even be quite

difficult to identify or trace the theories from which it was originally derived. In this instance, the function of research is to test the validity of the new theory, as well as confirm its relevance or applicability to nursing. The theory–research relationship here therefore not only shares the evaluative aspects of research in theory adoption as referred to above, but also aspects of the theory-testing approach.

Examples of such adaptive theories can be found in the work of a number of nurse-scientists. One example is the work of Virginia Henderson (1966), who integrated a psychological 'needs' theory and biological homeostasis or 'physiological balance' theory in her definition and theory of nursing.

Study Activity 18.5

- Using references in your college library, conduct brief reviews of the following:

  – Parse's *Theory of Human Becoming*
  – Rogers' *Science of Unitary Human Beings*
  – Roper et al.'s *Activities of Living Model*

- In each case identify how the authors have adapted theories from other disciplines or academic fields. You are expected to seek out the above authors as primary sources, but useful starting points may be McKenna (1997) and Alligood and Marriner-Tomey (2002). Each statement should be 150–200 words. It may be useful to share ideas with other students who have also undertaken this exercise.

Grounded theory

Part of the problem of derivativeness in nursing theory lies in the fact that nurses have until fairly recently looked to other disciplines for the solutions to their problems. This situation has led to the development or introduction of theory which is either adopted or adapted from other disciplines. However, as nursing is a unique activity, involving close and usually complex caring relationships, the source of true nursing theory can only be found within the nursing practice situation. In this sense, theory adopted or adapted from other disciplines may be less than adequate for describing and explaining nursing, predicting nursing events, or guiding nursing practice.

Nursing theory that is derived from practice is likely to be more relevant to that practice. In this approach, nursing problems and concerns are known in practical nursing situations. From investigating these problems in the field within their own contexts, the theory arises from the ground, so to speak; thus, the term 'grounded theory'. Such theory is completely context bound and therefore has complete relevance; there is no adaptation of theories from different contexts which have been constructed for understanding different situations. There is no need to manipulate or distort a theory to make it explain situations for which it was never constructed and for which it may not be ideally suited. Even fairly straightforward theories, such as the operant conditioning theory given as an example of adopted theory, may not be very helpful in the complex interpersonal environment of nursing. In this setting there are many variables, and the controls of reinforcement and reward that are usually so simple in the animal psychology laboratory become exceedingly problematic. Indeed, critics of that theory claim that it is of limited relevance in any human situation, given the capacity of human beings for rational thought and the complex nature of determining what exactly is reinforcing or rewarding to any individual human being.

While the idea of grounded theory comes from sociology (*see*, for example, the work of Glaser and Strauss, 1967), nursing theory developed through this method would arguably be true nursing theory. In this approach the relationship of research and practice to theory is vital. Theory is in fact developed from observation and analysis of practice 'on the ground'. It is derived directly from research in the field, without any presuppositions about theory and without any pre-empirical formulation of untested theory. The sequence is therefore different from the classical theory-testing approach where propositions, hypotheses, or even full-blown untested theories are formulated to explain phenomena and then tested or verified through research. It can be illustrated as follows:

Practice	→	Research	→	Theory
(problems or concerns are 'known' about, but no prior explanations or theories are formulated for testing.)		(the research follows and is guided by the practice issues.)		(the theory emerges from the research 'on the ground'.)

Research without theory

In Study Activity 18.4 we encountered research which, it would appear, was not related to theory. We then proceeded to demonstrate the relationship between theory (in the context of its specific scientific meaning) and research. However, the frequency of research work which seems to bear no relationship to theory continues to be problematic in debates such as that presented in this chapter. This is particularly so when many researchers continue to take the view that theory is not science, but something less precise and more conjectural than research.

This position has led to a recognition of two types of research: theory-linked research, where, as described above, there is a close interactive relationship between theory and research; and, isolated research, which is not consciously linked to theory in any way. Chinn and Kramer (1999) recognised such research as addressing specific problems or questions that face nursing. In regard to such issues, researchers formulate research questions or hypotheses and proceed to confirm or reject these on the basis of empirical evidence. These authors go on to state that such isolated research can be of excellent quality. However, according to them, 'Isolated research, which often focuses on particulars of a specific problem, offers little potential for speculating about the significance of the research beyond that which can be justified by the method, design, and analysis of study results'. When this view is considered in relation to the one expressed by Kuhn (1990) that when research is conducted in a haphazard manner without paradigmatic parameters, it is reflective of a lack of scientific maturity, the preponderance of isolated research may be viewed as less than satisfactory. Such research may indeed answer specific problems in isolation. But if not considered in the context of nursing theory and the development of nursing knowledge, its value may be greatly curtailed.

This risk of a haphazard and uncoordinated development of nursing knowledge is a matter of some concern. By working within a theoretical framework we can map out the world of nursing knowledge, identify the gaps in that world, and carry forward theory-linked research to fill in these vacuums. Of course the map will never be finished because the world in general and the world of nursing in particular is always changing. However, we would at least be moving forward in a planned and co-ordinated manner to the best of our ability, and building up a body of research-based theoretical knowledge which would both explain and guide nursing practice. Should isolated research predominate, nursing may move forward as an incompletely understood and fragmented world because isolated research has no theoretical quest, no commitment to mapping out the world of nursing knowledge. It is guided only by expediency, the demands of the moment, the particular fads of researchers or the dominant interests in any particular period.

This view is illustrated to some extent by the developments in nursing research in recent years. In the 1960s and 1970s, quantitative research, primarily utilising survey and questionnaire methods, was dominant. The choice of research topics was more often determined by the dominant research method than by the specific areas of nursing knowledge that were most in need of researching. Of course, the profession was also striving for professional and academic recognition and espoused the most

respectable research approaches. By the 1980s, nursing academics were increasingly discovering qualitative approaches, particularly ethnographic methods of describing the world from the point of view of those living within it (nurses, doctors, patients, etc.). Again, areas that fit well with this particular approach were much more likely to get researched. By the 1990s, nursing had discovered phenomenological approaches which looked more deeply at meanings attributed to those living in the world by interpreting the lived experiences of those 'thrust into' the world of health and disease. The pattern again started to shift. It seemed from these various 'shifts' that to a significant extent nursing research was more determined by infatuation with method (or the new and exciting method currently in vogue) than the actual concerns or problems facing nursing. Of course, the methods were not always new, but merely newly encountered by nursing scholars. The danger here was that method would determine how 'truth' or 'sound knowledge' in respect of nursing issues would be constructed, rather than the issues themselves determining the method, a danger recognised by the philosopher Gadamer (1989).

When the topics for research are considered, similar biases can be discerned. In one review, Smith (1994) found that the most common research papers in nursing journals were those which reported research studies on nurses rather than on nursing or clinical practice, in contrast to medical journal papers which emphasised clinical research or management of care. This preoccupation with 'navel gazing' is possibly a direct consequence of an isolated research orientation and a lack of theoretical direction.

The purpose here is not to convey a total rejection of all research which is not related to theory and is thus described as isolated research. However, if research is generally theory linked it is much more likely that it will be attuned to addressing the development of a co-ordinated body of knowledge, and attending to that which should be the main concern of research, i.e. the practice of nursing.

Study Activity 18.6

Browse through the nursing journals of the past 12 months in the journals section of your library. Select and scan 20 research papers. You should not attempt to read them in detail. However, scan them closely enough so that you can answer the following questions:

- How many of the papers specifically address the practice of nursing as opposed to some other aspect, such as nurses' roles or educational topics?
- How many of the papers are clearly linked to theory and profess to advance a particular theory or theoretical perspective, and how many are examples of isolated research as described above?
- If other students are also doing this activity, agree to scan different journals, so that you can combine the results.
- Write a brief commentary of about 500 words that relates to the biases in reported nursing research presented in this section of the chapter.

Theory without research

On the basis of the previous discussions, it could be argued that theory which is not linked to research is by definition untested theory. Does this mean that it falls into the category of conjecture, as described by Burns and Grove (1987)? Or, to put it another way, if the orthodox scientific definition of theory presented earlier and in Chapter 14 is adhered to, is such untested theory – in the context of that definition – best described as non-theory?

In essence, the answers to these questions depend on the definition of theory. The definitions referred to above attach a very specific meaning to the term. It is in fact the type of theory described in Chapter 14, which Merton (1968) described as the theory of the middle range. Remember that such a theory falls somewhere between general or grand theory, which is at a very high level of abstraction, and operational terms such as hypotheses, which are the least abstract and closest aligned to the actual empirical situation. Such statements are sometimes called micro-theories.

Micro-theory is already stated in operational terms and can be readily subjected to empirical scrutiny through research. Middle range theory is not so abstract that it cannot be reduced to similar operational terms (i.e. micro-theory or hypotheses) and then tested by research. However, grand theory is generally so abstract as to be irreducible in this way. It provides an abstract macro-worldview and as such lacks the precision needed to operationalise theory into researchable terms. Such a theory is extremely difficult if not impossible to reduce. But grand theories are not put forward as statements for researching in any case. As stated earlier, their purpose is to give an overview of the particular world they describe.

When these different definitions of various theories are considered, the situation becomes much clearer. Some theories, those described as micro-theory and middle range theory, can be validated through research and must, it may be argued, be linked to research. Grand theory usually cannot be researched in the same way and, therefore, cannot be directly linked to research in the sense that the research can 'test' the authenticity of the theory or that the theory presents propositions or hypotheses that can be empirically tested. However, such theory can provide the overall worldview of our discipline, the theoretical framework that will guide our practice. Indeed, it is perhaps better to term such overviews as theoretical frameworks to avoid the controversy that seems to constantly beset similar abstract terms such as grand theory, macro-theory or metaparadigm. When viewed as a guiding framework for our middle range and micro-theory, and thus for the general thrust towards building up a body of nursing knowledge through research, such theoretical frameworks are highly important. They too have an important relationship with research, albeit in an indirect way. The relationship is, of course, not one that permits the research to test the theory, and for this reason there must be alternative means of testing or establishing the relevance and viability of such theory.

THEORY AND PRACTICE

Relevance of theory to practice

The introduction to this chapter suggested that theory and practice are inextricably linked in the action of praxis. In this situation, theory is enacted in practice, where theory enhances practice, and practice in turn enhances theory. If this notion is accepted, then the relationship between theory and practice, indeed the idea that they cannot and should not be separated in the real-life situation, must be taken as irrefutable.

However, the theory contained in praxis must by definition be sound and relevant theory. The good fit of theory to practice is paramount. If a theory *describes* or *explains* practice, it must do so accurately. However, of even greater importance, particularly with regard to professional practice, is the utilisation of theory to *guide* practice. It must never be forgotten that in the practice of nursing, interventions can have life or death outcomes. In this context, the guiding of practice by theory can never be taken lightly. It is imperative that in such situations the theory which guides practice is both relevant and sound. In this context, 'sound' implies that the theory must promote and guide practice which is effective and safe. There are a number of ways in which the soundness of theory as a guide to practice can be established. In general, these can be divided into empirical and non-empirical approaches.

Empirical theory testing

In the previous section, the importance of research, specifically research that is sometimes referred to as theory-linked research, in verifying or testing theory and establishing its applicability in practice, was emphasised. Theory is normally tested and its relevance to practice verified via this research-orientated approach. However, there can sometimes be a time-lag between

theory implementation and theory testing through research. The research process is usually a highly structured method and the time taken to design a research project, execute it, and produce results can extend over many months. One way around this situation is to remove the boundaries between theory, research and practice, so that they can occur in unison, each interacting with and influencing the other as practice is advanced on a theory–research base. An increasingly common way of achieving this is through the approach known as action research (which was considered in more depth in Chapter 16). In this approach, the barriers between practice and research are effectively removed: practice is research and research is incorporated in practice. Researchers cease to be external agents but work with the subjects, and the subjects themselves (in this case nurses) become co-researchers (*see*, for example, Heron, 1996). This approach is characterised by:

- small-scale studies of real-world practical situations
- being situational and interventionist, i.e. action orientated and aimed at developing practices, policies, and procedures
- being collaborative, with researchers and subjects working together as co-researchers
- aiming at solving organisational or practice problems and actively promoting organisational or practice change.

A second approach, specific to nursing, is the innovation of nursing development units. These specialist units are aimed at improving and enhancing practice through research and development activities. While various research orientated and non-research-orientated approaches may be utilised, the close alignment of these to practice, the direct application to practice and the almost immediate if not concurrent evaluation of innovation, means that the normal time-lag between theory implementation and theory testing can effectively be removed. There are some similarities between the principles underlying action research and nursing development units, and indeed, action research is an approach often (although not exclusively) adopted in such units.

Non-empirical theory testing

It is often assumed that only empirical methods are valid for testing theory. However, this perception is reflective of a tendency to undervalue non-scientific approaches towards knowledge. It also fails to recognise that some theories, especially grand theories, are essentially formulated at a very abstract level. Such theories are aimed at providing broad frameworks or worldviews and are so formulated as to be incapable of operationalising and testing through research.

There are in fact some effective non-empirical methods for theory testing. Examples of such approaches are provided here. For a more comprehensive consideration of such theory-testing approaches, *see* Silva and Sorrell (1992), two of whose approaches are included here.

Critical reasoning

Critical reasoning implies a detailed critique of the theory based on reasoning rather than empirical evidence. It involves a detailed description and critical analysis of the various aspects of the theory. Questions which may be addressed are:

- *Claims* – What is the theory actually claiming in terms of description, explanation, relationships between concepts, predictable nature of concept relationships, and generalisability in terms of application in different settings? Are these aspects of the theory clearly stated and logically consistent? This point relates to what is known as the internal consistency of the theory.
- *Parsimony* – Is the theory stated clearly and concisely? This question concerns the extent to which the theory is comprehensive and fully encompasses the phenomena and their relationships, yet does so with brevity and clarity so that redundant or irrelevant information is excluded.

- *Philosophy* – Is the philosophy underpinning the theory sound and consistent with the content of the theory?
- *Biases and influences* – Has the theorist made clear his biases and influences on his theory, particularly if it is adapted from other theoretical works?
- *Conceptual integrity and cohesiveness* – Are the concepts which are incorporated in the theory clearly explicated and discrete conceptual entities? Concept analysis, as this process is named, involves a description of the concepts and the establishment of boundaries between them, particularly in terms of concepts that are antecedent and consequent to them. For example, the concept of loss may have an antecedent concept of bereavement and a consequent concept of depression in relation to it. Are the concepts clearly explained, presented as discrete concepts and in apposition and connectedness? *See*, for example, Meleis (1997) and Walker and Avant (1999) for useful discussions of concept analysis.
- Does the theory have value in terms of guiding practice, and is it applicable in this regard across separate but similar situations? *See*, for example, Chinn and Kramer (1999), who discuss this property of theory in terms of empirical applicability.

Problem-solving

Via the problem-solving approach the theory is tested in terms of its outcomes or applicability in practice. The main relevance of theory to nursing is the extent to which it is useful in informing and guiding practice. In this regard, Dickoff and James (1968) described such theory as situation-producing theory, because it was specifically designed to facilitate a profession's practice and 'to guide the shaping of reality to that profession's purpose'.

Implicit in the problem-solving approach to theory testing is a view that to be relevant and successful as a nursing theory, a theory must by definition prove itself to be effective in practice. The approach here is thus similar to the critical reasoning approach in that it applies rigorous reasoning to establish the success of the theory. However, it does involve an element of empirical input, in that those testing the theory draw from experience in the use of the theory. It is by definition exclusively concerned with how the theory helps in the problem-solving process that is nursing practice.

Tacit knowing

Earlier in this chapter it was noted that in some instances practitioners choose not to apply a particular theory in practice, even when it is officially accepted or openly espoused. This situation is often explained as resistance to change, to a 'flat Earth' mentality, whereby practitioners reject anything new out-of-hand, particularly if it is being promoted by management or educators. This explanation is undoubtedly true in some circumstances, and such negative attitudes present real problems for those who manage services, particularly where these attitudes have a detrimental influence on the quality of care provision.

However, in some circumstances practitioners reject a theory simply because they believe it will not work. And often they are right, although in such circumstances these practitioners cannot articulate their reasoning. They may say, 'I don't know why it will not work, I just do'. This intuitive type of knowing what to do and what not to do is born out of extensive experience and developed to the stage where there is deep know-how. These practitioners have the capacity to implicitly know without having to or being able to explain a situation. It is characteristic of the expert practitioner described by Benner (1984) and Benner *et al.* (1999) and the notion of tacit or personal knowing described by Polanyi (1967). Such intuitive judgement has its empirical counterparts in the concepts of face validity and expert validity utilised in research. The importance of such tacit knowing to skills mastery is also referred to by Slevin (in Chapter 12) and is addressed by Benner later (in Chapter 27). However, as Slevin and Kirby have indicated (see Chapter 11), there are subtle differ-

ences between personal knowing as the fact that *all* our knowledge is viewed through the lens of the person, a tacit knowledge *of* things that is closely related to implicit knowledge or know-how *in* practice, and a knowledge that is embedded in the experience of self and other. To the practitioner, these differences and shades of meaning are seldom considered, she/he just knows.

It is important that the experience and expertise of practitioners is not discounted in theory testing. While such forms of knowing are increasingly being recognised in nursing, many view them with a degree of cynicism. Our profession has courted the models of natural sciences for many years, and it is difficult to replace the measurement tool, the survey, and the statistical analysis with something we may variously describe as intuition, implicit knowledge, or personal knowing. The solution to such dilemmas is to avoid dependence on a single approach to theory testing. If the validity of a particular theory in practice is at issue, the use of empirical and non-empirical methods of theory testing can be readily justified and should be utilised wherever possible. In such circumstances, where nurses intuitively have doubts about the applicability of a particular theory in practice, it is likely that other theory-testing approaches will reflect this tacit understanding of the situation.

SUMMARY

This chapter addressed a number of important relationships, including the relationships between research and practice, theory and research, and theory and practice. The first relationship, between research and practice, is dominant in modern health care situations. An increasing emphasis is being given to the importance of research as a sound basis for practice, even to the exclusion of a consideration of theory. Across all corners of health care systems and increasingly across all corners of the Earth, the dominant concern is to establish health care on an evidence base. In this chapter the variations of this orientation – evidence-based medicine and its equivalents (including evidence-based nursing), the less discipline-specific notion of evidence-based practice, the wider notion of evidence-based health, and even the more radical notion of evidence-based patient choice – were all considered as variants of the research–practice relationship. In the second relationship, between theory and research, it was noted that research is important in confirming and testing postulated theory (the 'theory-testing' orientation), but that theory can also emerge from research in the field (the 'grounded theory' orientation). There is potential conflict between a perspective that sees research as the tool for establishing a sound body of nursing knowledge (that we may term theory), and a perspective that sees theory as being of little relevance to the real world, and sees research as being essentially to provide factual information to directly guide practice (isolated research). In the third relationship, between theory and practice, theory guides practice and within nursing there are attempts to adopt theory from other disciplines, sometimes also adapting that theory to best fit the nursing situation. There is an ideal of constructing theory, either by postulating a theory and then testing it in nursing practice situations, or by theory that emerges from the practice field through grounded theory approaches. However, examples of such theory that are truly original, uniquely nursing, and non-derivative are rare. Nevertheless, the professional aspiration is to establish a close interactive relationship between theory and practice, so that theory not only informs and is integrated within practice, but also is in turn informed and refined by that practice.

As was noted, there is the capacity for gaps or breaches in the relationships in each of these situations. It is often found that no recognised or explicit theory seems to be informing practice. Similarly, research often takes place as isolated research, not within any theoretical framework, and not with the intention of developing or enhancing theory. While much lip service is paid to basing practice on research, there are indications that much of current practice has not been validated through research. This raises the possibility that practice may not be informed by theory, or research, or any integrated theory–research orientation. Of course, it was also noted that while practitioners may not support any explicit theory-of-action, there is often an implicit theory-in-use that appears to be tacitly operated in the practice situation. It may be reasonable to be concerned about whether such theory is based on the best possible knowledge or evidence. However, it was also recognised that such tacit or implicit theory-in-use most often develops and achieves currency because practitioners find that it works for them and their patients/clients in their real-world situations. As also noted in the chapter, there is the issue of aspects of nursing practice that would not in any case be best informed by empirical knowledge or 'evidence' of that form derived from research. By the same token, if we see theory as a part of science, constructed through research, these aspects of nursing would not be best informed by theory so construed. In these circumstances we must look to other patterns of knowing that also inform our practice, and such alternative patterns of knowing were considered in depth within Module 3.

Underlying the possibility of gaps in each of these three relationships there is the risk of an even more dangerous disintegration, a lack of integration within the overall theory, research, and practice triad. If the three areas of endeavour in nursing – theory, research and practice – were not in any way related to each other and did not influence and enhance each other, then each would, like severed limbs, wither and die.

To preserve the integrity of nursing and ensure that practice – which is the core of nursing – is developed and enhanced to levels of ever-increasing excellence, the notion of praxis (where knowledge and practice, or thinking and doing, become one) must be extended to encompass all three elements, as indicated in Fig. 18.3. However, in considering this relationship, it is important to place it in a wider context. In this chapter, we have been viewing theory as essentially a way of stating propositional knowledge about how things are in the world. While such things may be actual external objects that we perceive, they may also be in the nature of abstract ideas or concepts or experiences that are not directly visible in any way. One example, important to nursing, might be the experience of pain. This is not something we can directly observe, although we can observe some of its manifestations. But for all such phenomena, those we can directly observe and those we can feel or experience, we can say that they are empirical in that we can directly or indirectly observe them. The means of doing this, in an orderly and systematic way, comes within the sphere of research. Therefore, theory, construed as part of the scientific or empirical domain, is linked in various ways to research, and both have an impact on practice. However, as stated above, if we *do* view theory in this way (essentially as a part of science, as discussed earlier), a

degree of caution is required. We must be wary that the praxis we describe as an integration of knowledge and practice is not confined to integrating only the theory–research or empirical dimension of knowledge. Within this praxis, as also illustrated in Fig. 18.3, we find influences of: ethical or moral thinking; personal knowledge that is of an experiential, meaningful nature that includes knowing self and other, and being-in-the-world and being in relation with others; and, aesthetic knowledge that includes a dimension of know-how or skilful mastery.

Within this conceptualisation:

- Research informs practice and is informed by that practice.
- Research informs theory and is informed by that theory.
- Theory informs practice and is informed by that practice.

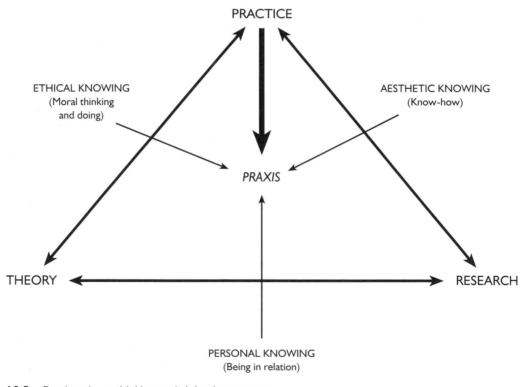

Figure 18.3 Praxis: where thinking and doing become one

- Where theory informs practice directly, that theory has often already been informed (or tested) by research.
- Where research informs practice directly, that research has already been guided in most cases by a theoretical framework.
- In some instances the research that guides practice has no links with theory (being termed isolated research), and in these instances the research does not contribute to an evolving body of nursing knowledge.
- The knowledge that informs practice is not exclusively propositional knowledge (which we might also term evidence or 'knowing that' knowledge), but also includes ethical, personal and aesthetic knowing (which includes within aesthetic knowledge that form of artistry or skilful knowledge that we term 'know-how').
- At the moment of doing, within the nursing act, these various ways of knowing and doing become a knowledgeable doing, within which the knowing and doing become one: practice in this moment becomes praxis.

Through such a framework, each nurse would approach practice with fundamental questions, such as: What theory will best guide my practice? To what extent is this theory validated by sound theory-linked research? What other research is available to guide my practice? To what extent is this research sound and applicable to the care of my patients? To what extent can my colleagues and I ensure that our experiences in applying these theories and research findings are utilised to strengthen and enhance the knowledge base? If research-based knowledge is unavailable or inappropriate, what other forms of knowledge are available to me and how might I best apply this in my practice?

The capacity to ask such questions, to seek out the correct answers to them and respond appropriately, is fundamental to the future of nursing. This fact implies that for each individual nurse and the profession as a whole, and in the course of continuous appraisal of nursing practice, there would be a holistic orientation.

This perspective not only brings together theory, research, and practice (which come within that domain that we have identified as propositional, or factual, or empirical knowledge), but also other forms of knowledge (which in Fig. 18.3 are referred to as ethical, aesthetic and personal forms of knowledge). As Pearson has already suggested in Chapter 17, there is more to nursing than a clinical effectiveness based exclusively on a narrow interpretation of evidence-based practice. It is this capacity to bring all to bear, in the moment of doing, and in full harmony with the context, that is important. We have described it here as a nursing praxis (as does Rolfe, later, in Chapter 26). Others have termed it differently. Benner *et al.* (1999) speak of a 'thinking-in-action' approach that they describe as clinical wisdom (see also Benner's contribution later, in Chapter 27). Schön (1987) speaks of a form of reflection-in-action, which is different to the preparatory reflection or thinking about action prior to that action, and different also to the evaluative reflection that occurs after that action. This notion has been taken up enthusiastically within nursing, as the idea of 'reflective practice'. Johns (2000), perhaps one of the most lucid proponents of this approach, comes closest to the position presented in this chapter by speaking of 'reflection-within-the-moment'. Such reflection in action involves a constant intercourse between thinking and doing, each dynamically informing the other in a reflexive cycle.

When this ethos of reflexive praxis and the ability to actualise it is the norm, nursing will have truly achieved a level of professional excellence. But in the current chapter we have discussed the theory–research–practice triad and how it (and other patterns of knowing) informs our praxis. In so doing, we have not extended our discussion further into the practice situation. This, as we have emphasised elsewhere (e.g. in Chapters 2 and 29), is a situation of relation. Within that *context* of practice that we refer to above is the patient or client, and our informed practice or praxis must in the final analysis be played out within the relationship between nurse and patient. We see here the insightfulness of the definition of evidence-based medicine proposed by Sackett *et al.* (2000) presented earlier in this chapter, where the third element of that definition, that of patient involvement and patient choice, is an important and essential element. In praxis, the circle is never fully closed until the patient is fully empowered to participate, because this is the source of the final element of knowledge that informs our praxis. We may bring to this encounter all the explicit evidence and theory, and all the implicit and tacit ways of personal, ethical and aesthetic knowing we have developed for responding to the context. But just as each patient differs from all others, each moment of praxis is different to everything that came before. It is, as Bevis so rightly stated in the opening quotation to this chapter, a living theory.

REFERENCES

Alligood, R. and Mariner-Tomey, A. (2002) *Nursing Theory: Utilization and application* (2nd edn), Radcliffe Medical Press, Oxford

Argyris, C. and Schön, D. (1974) *Theory in Practice: Increasing professional effectiveness*. Jossey-Bass, London

Baker, M. (1998) Challenging ignorance. In: Baker, M. and Kirk, S. (eds) *Research and Development for the NHS* (2nd edn), Radcliffe Medical Press, Oxford

Bandolier (1994) Assessment criteria. *Bandolier* **July**, 6–5

Barnum, B.J. (1990) *Nursing Theory: Analysis, application and evaluation*, Little, Brown & Co, Boston, Mass

Benner, P. (1984) *From Novice to Expert: Excellence and power in clinical practice*, Addison-Wesley, Menlo Park, CA

Benner, P., Hooper-Kyriakidis, P. and Stannard, D. (1999) *Clinical Wisdom and Interventions in Critical Care: A thinking in action approach*, W.B. Saunders, Philadelphia, IL

Bevis, E.M. (1988) New directions for a new age. In: National League for Nursing (ed.) *Curriculum Revolution: Mandate for change*, National League for Nursing, New York

Burns, N. and Grove, S.K. (1987) *The Practice of Nursing Research: Conduct, critique and utilization*, W.B. Saunders, Philadelphia, IL

Burns, N. and Grove, S.K. (1993) *The Practice of Nursing Research: Conduct, critique and utilization* (2nd edn), W.B. Saunders, Philadelphia, IL

Burns, N. and Grove, S.K. (1997) *The Practice of Nursing Research: Conduct, critique and utilization* (3rd edn), W.B. Saunders, Philadelphia, IL

Burns, N. and Grove, S.K. (2000) *The Practice of Nursing Research: Conduct, critique and utilization* (4th edn), W.B. Saunders, Philadelphia, IL

Carper, B.A. (1978) Fundamental patterns of knowing in nursing. *Advances in Nursing Science* **1**(1), 13–23

Chalmers, I. (1993) Effective care in midwifery – research, the professions and the public. *Midwives Chronicle* **106**(1), 3–13

Chinn, P.L. and Kramer, M.K. (1999) *Theory and Nursing: Integrated knowledge development* (5th edn) Mosby, St Louis, IL

Cimino, J. (1999) Development of expertise in medical practice. In: Sternberg, R. and Horvath, J. (eds) *Tacit Knowledge in Professional Practice*, Lawrence Erlbaum, Mahwah, NJ

Department of Health (1997) *The New NHS: Modern, dependable*, HMSO, London

Department of Health (1998a) *A First Class Service: Quality in the new NHS*, Leeds NHS Executive, Leeds

Department of Health (1998b) *Working Together: Securing a quality workforce for the NHS*, Department of Health, London

Department of Health (1999) *Saving Lives: Our healthier nation*, The Stationery Office, London

Department of Health (2000a) *A Health Service of All the Talents: Developing the National Health Service workforce*, Leeds NHS Executive, Leeds

Department of Health (2000b) *An Organisation with a Memory – Report of an expert group on learning from adverse events in the NHS*, The Stationery Office, London

Department of Health (2000c) *Research and Development for a First Class Service – R&D funding in the new NHS*, NHS Executive, Leeds

Department of Health (2001) *NHS Priorities and Needs R&D Funding – A position paper*, NHS Executive, Leeds

Department of Health (2002) *Strategic Reviews of Research and Development – Mental health main report*, Department of Health, London

Dickoff, J. and James, P. (1968) A theory of theories: a position paper. *Nursing Research* **17**, 197–203

Fawcett, J. (1999) *The Relationship of Theory and Research* (3rd edn), F.A. Davis, Philadelphia, IL

Gadamer, H.-G. (1989) *Truth and Method* (2nd edn), Sheed and Ward, London

Glaser, B. and Strauss, A. (1967) *The Discovery of Grounded Theory*, Aldine, Chicago, IL

Greenhalgh, T. and Hurwitz, B. (1998) *Narrative-based Medicine*, BMJ Books, London

Henderson, V. (1966) *The Nature of Nursing: A definition and its implications for practice, research and education*, Macmillan, New York

Heron, J. (1996) *Co-operative Inquiry: Research into the human condition*, Sage, London

Hicks, N. (1997) Evidence-based health care, *Bandolier* **May**, 39–49

Hockey, E. (1987) Issues in the communication of nursing research. In: Hockey, E. (ed.) *Recent Advances in Nursing – Current issues, 18*, Churchill Livingstone, Edinburgh

Johns, C. (2000) *Becoming a Reflective Practitioner*, Blackwell Science, Oxford

Kuhn, T.S. (1970) *The Structure of Scientific Revolutions*, Chicago University Press, Chicago

McDaid, C. (2000) *Clinical Effectiveness and Evidence-based Nursing, Midwifery and Health Visiting: Barriers, resources and practical implications*, NBNI, Belfast

McKenna, H. (1997) *Nursing Models and Theories*, Routledge, London

McKenna, H. and Ashton, S. (2000) *Evidence-based Practice in Primary-led Health Care: Barriers and strategies for clinical effectiveness*, University of Ulster/NBNI, Belfast

McSherry, R., Simmons, M. and Abbott, P. (2002) *Evidence-informed Nursing: A guide for clinical nurses*, Routledge, London

Meleis, A.I. (1997) *Theoretical Nursing: Development and progress* (3rd edn), J.B. Lippincott, New York

Merton, R.K. (1968) *Social Theory and Social Structure*, Free Press, New York

Muir Grey, J.A. (1997) *Evidence-based Healthcare: How to make health policy and management decisions*, Churchill Livingstone, Edinburgh

National Health Service Management Executive (1991) *Research for Health: A research and development strategy for the NHS*, National Health Service Management Executive, London

National Health Service Executive (1997) *R&D in Primary Care: Report of a working group (Chair: D. Mant)*, Department of Health, London

Oakley, A. (1999) *An Infrastructure for Assessing Social and Educational Interventions: The same difference?* University of London, Institute of Education, London

Polanyi, M. (1967) *The Tacit Dimension*, Doubleday, London

Raulin, M. (1963) The importance of scientific theory, *Science* **142**, 3590–2

Roberts, C. (1995) Rationing is a desperate measure, *Health Services Journal* **12**, 15

Rolfe, G. (1996) *Closing the Theory–Practice Gap: A new paradigm for nursing*, Butterworth-Heinemann, Oxford

Sackett, D.L., Straus, S.E., Richardson, W.S., *et al.* (2000) *Evidence-based Medicine: How to practice and teach EBM*, Churchill Livingstone, Edinburgh

Schön, D. (1987) *Educating the Reflective Practitioner*, Jossey Bass, San Francisco, CA

Silva, M.C. and Sorrell, J.M. (1992) Testing of nursing theory: critique and philosophical expansion. *Advances in Nursing Science* **14**(4), 12–23

Slevin, O. (2002) Valuing the past, embracing the future. In: McDaid, C. (ed.) *From Past to Future*, NBNI, Belfast

Smith, L.N. (1994) An analysis and reflections on the quality of nursing research in 1992. *Journal of Advanced Nursing* **19**(2), 385–93

Smith, R. (1992) Where is the wisdom? *British Medical Journal* **303**, 798–9

United Kingdom Central Council for Nursing, Midwifery and Health Visiting (1986) *Project 2000: A new preparation for practice*, United Kingdom Central Council, London

Walker, L.O. and Avant, K.C. (1999) *Strategies for Theory Construction in Nursing* (3rd edn), Appleton and Lange, Norwalk, CN

Watson, J. (1997) The theory of human caring: retrospective and prospective. *Nursing Science Quarterly* **10**(1), 49–52

Williams, R. (1983) *Keywords* (2nd edn), Fontana, London

MODULE 4: EVIDENCE-BASED PRACTICE

REFLECTIONS

In this module we considered in greater depth one of the patterns of knowing from the previous module, the empirical pattern of knowing. We recognised that empirical knowing, with its production of evidence to substantiate knowledge claims, is vitally important in a modern health service where interventions involve risk of harm, and where the availability of the best evidence to justify such interventions is essential.

The first two chapters addressed research as the process by which empirical evidence is produced. We examined the traditional research process (collecting and analysing data to propose new knowledge or validate current knowledge claims) in some detail in the first chapter. We recognised, however (in the second chapter), that this is only one paradigm (way of viewing the world) for contributing to our knowledge. On this basis, an alternative qualitative paradigm was considered, and finally 'new' paradigms were suggested that seek to establish modes of inquiry into issues not readily researched through the established quantitative and qualitative paradigms.

The second two chapters addressed the practical aspects of knowledge obtained from research. First, we noted that research is the source of best evidence that informs clinical effectiveness. However, we also acknowledged that as an interpersonal caring activity, nursing goes beyond aspects that are exclusively clinical. On this basis, the evidence required to inform *nursing* practice includes but extends beyond that which is exclusively clinical in its orienta-

tion. Second, given that the product of science includes technology, the issue of harnessing such technology to practice was considered. In respect of this, the importance of health technology assessment as a particular form of empirical inquiry that establishes the efficacy and safety of new technologies was explored.

The final chapter had the specific goal of demonstrating the interrelationships and indeed interdependence of theory, practice and research. There is first the dyadic (two-way) relationship between research and practice, as exemplified by the push towards evidence-based health care in all modern health care systems. There is second the complex dyadic relationship between theory and research, wherein theory can guide research and research in turn can test and validate theory. Third, there is the dyadic relationship between theory and practice, wherein theory may guide practice, but so also relevant theory may emerge from practice. In considering these separate dyadic relationships it becomes apparent that they are part of a wider triadic (three-way) relationship that culminates in an integration of practice and knowledge within the nursing act itself. We call this practice knowledge-in-action *praxis*.

Using your personal experience, you may find it useful at this stage to reflect upon the extent to which practice that is guided by evidence and theory is realised in real day-to-day practice settings. However, reflecting with other colleagues might also be useful in identifying areas of practice where empirical evidence is absent or perhaps not even relevant. In doing so, you might consider *what does* inform practice in such circumstances?

MODULE 5:   THE SOCIAL AND HUMAN CONTEXT OF NURSING CARE

INTRODUCTION

The social and human context of nursing is covered in Module 5. Here the concepts of care in a political context are explored, which enables you to focus on nursing in conflict and conflict resolution. We describe nursing within a multicultural and multiracial society which requires an understanding of religion and the broader remit of spirituality in a nursing context.

In engaging with broader issues that relate to nursing practice, we cannot ignore the very nature of gender and how nursing has evolved synonymously with the emancipation of women and a greater awareness of the oppression of women, and as such, nursing, throughout the world of health care. As women have struggled for political recognition from social exclusion, nursing has also struggled to forge its way as an equal partner in care.

In addition, the module recognises that we have become an ageing society whose health care needs are very different from those of children and younger adults. However, there has been a particular problem with discrimination, with exclusion from health care based on age. In the chapter on older people we cover the problems of ageism as it relates to a nursing context.

Exploring these domains enables you to gain a knowledge and understanding of issues that are contemporary and those that require a solution to old problems. Hopefully this will provoke a social conscience on the world of nursing. Awakening your conscience on these issues will enhance your ability to cope better with these central core issues as you go about your everyday practice.

19 THE POLITICS OF CARE

Oliver Slevin

> *The margin is where nursing's embedded practices are being uncovered and where they differ from the medical text.*
>
> (Watson, 1999)

LEARNING OUTCOMES

After studying this chapter you will be able to:

- Explain the term 'politics' and demonstrate insight into its origins and their relevance in the modern age
- Present an argument for politics as a phenomenon founded upon power
- Identify the sources of power or influence in politics
- Explain how political influence is established on the basis of social discourses, using a social constructionist perspective
- Identify the various political influences that impact upon health care and upon nursing
- Consider the sociopolitical domain as an additional pattern of knowing that is relevant to nursing
- Discuss how nursing may respond to the politics of the future.

INTRODUCTION

In this module, all the chapters address the social or human context within which nursing takes place. It has been suggested (e.g. White, 1995) that there is a tendency for nursing to look inwardly to the issues that seem to be of immediate concern, without a counterpointing gaze that also looks outwardly to the context within which nursing takes place. This is dangerous. It is dangerous not only to nursing itself, but more importantly to those for whom we care.

We have spoken of this notion of care before in this book. There are chapters within Module 1 and subsequently that indeed consider the caring element that is at the core of the nursing spirit, and it would be superfluous to review all this in detail at this point. But you will recall that, in all our previous discussions of this notion, there are common features that have emerged. We have said that in being caring we exhibit a sense of compassion that goes beyond an empathy or understanding of the other, or even a sympathy or feeling for the other, to a commitment to help. This commitment we have identified as a moral imperative, upon which basis we have spoken of an ethic of care. That is, we have suggested an argument that states if we really care for the other, we cannot knowingly do them harm. In this respect we drew on the suggestion by Noddings (1984) that to care is by definition 'ethical', that we may need no more than care as the fundamental basis upon which to base our ethic. Furthermore, such a moral stand by definition requires that our helping is an informed and competent helping. Care, and indeed an ethic based upon care, is empty if we cannot meet that extension of our understanding of compassion as helping, and if we lack the competence to help. On this basis, Watson (1992a) suggested her insightful phrase describing the essence of nursing as 'informed moral passion', bringing together this triad of knowledge and skill, ethical comportment, and compassionate concern.

Of course, where we have presented these ideas previously, we have attempted to adopt a critical approach that adequately considers such notions against challenges to their validity.

Where appropriate, we have presented alternative perspectives. However, an honest critique would admit to an orientation within the book that argues *for* this caring orientation. Indeed, that argues for the important role of nursing in maintaining a human and caring dimension within modern health care systems that might otherwise be impersonal, dispassionate and perhaps even alienating to those such systems exist to help. But this is not a one-way process. We do not deliver care, in the nursing context, in the same way the postman delivers our mail. Caring, even when it relates to one other, is a relation: there is *always* the one caring and the one cared for. And this relation may extend in different directions: it may include the care of families, groups, communities, the wider society, or even caring on a global scale.

Nursing must, therefore, always relate to the other, even when that other is not, for the moment, in our presence. This in itself demonstrates that nursing must involve looking outward. But, more specifically, it also draws to our attention how these wider considerations may impact upon our caring even at its more intimate interpersonal levels. The very time we have available to care may be limited by the resources that are put at our disposal, and the decisions about such matters (so it is often said) are taken elsewhere. And here we find the base cause of the danger to which we alluded earlier: this notion of the 'elsewhere'. It implies an 'otherwise-than-us' orientation, an idea that suggests such things are not matters for us; they are in essence outwith our concern and beyond our control. Such matters, which relate to the power to make decisions, are what politics is about. In so far as such matters impact upon our commitment to care, the call for nursing to involve itself is not a matter of choice. It is in fact a moral imperative, and indeed an aspect of that ethic of care to which we referred earlier. Of course, this is not to suggest that such involvement is a simple matter. The agencies that wield such power and (as some may claim) disenfranchise nursing from the decision-making processes, are extremely potent. We will see this later in this chapter, and elsewhere (e.g. in the chapter on gender later in this module). In this chapter we concentrate on this issue of social power and influence that we call politics, how it impacts upon health care and nursing, and how we might respond now and in the future.

POLITICS IN A NUTSHELL

Politics concerns organising, influencing, controlling. Here, as is so often the case, we must thank the Greeks. In the centuries before Christ, Greece moved from a disorganised region of rival kingdoms and nomadic tribes to residential and commercial centres of population. These centres became city-states in their own right – and each city-state (*polis*, in ancient Greek) was faced with how it should organise itself. From the ancient Greek *polis* or city-state comes *politics*, how such an entity can best be organised, according to which values, applying what rules, governed by whom.

The story is not as simple as this. Part of the greatness of Greece in this era was the creativity and innovativeness of the quest for an ideal politic, an ideal way of organising and governing the state (even the word 'govern' is taken from the Greek word meaning 'to steer' or 'to direct'). We find from this era almost all the forms of political structure that we know of in the modern world. Aristotle (a Greek scholar of this era) spoke of three fundamental forms of government and their alternatives.

- *Monarchy and tyranny* – in monarchy the state was governed by a single head or king, who usually ascended to this position through heredity (the word monarch coming from the Greek term *monos* meaning one or one-ness, and the term *arche* meaning origin or basis of). The expectation is that the monarch's primary concern is the well-being of his subjects, who come under his protection. In instances of tyranny, self-interested individuals or groups would overthrow the monarch to further their own interests rather than those of the people.

- *Aristocracy and oligarchy* – in aristocracy a small group of people who were adjudged to be the best equipped to rule or govern ascended to this task (the Greek word *aristos* means 'best'). The view here was that by being the best or most able, these few would be most able to know what to do in the best interests of the whole. This is not to be confused with different views of aristocracy that emerged in subsequent centuries (such as hereditary peerage in Great Britain). The notion of oligarchy (as Aristotle conceived it) identified a similar governing by a few (the Greek term *oligos* alluding to 'few'). But this was not necessarily a few selected on merit as being the best able to govern, and in modern-day politics we see the cabinets (group of senior ministers within a governing political party) extending from able groups to oligarchies of weak members.

- *Timocracy and democracy* – in timocracy the right to rule was determined by the possession of property. Part of the logic here was that *all* those with a lot invested in the state (and thus a lot to lose) would share in governing the state, and be particularly diligent in looking to the best interests of the state and its people. The Greek root of this form (*timos*, meaning 'valued' or 'of value', but also 'to be valued' or 'honoured') meant that while Aristotle viewed it as a system based upon property or valuables, Plato (another ancient Greek scholar) saw it as a system based upon people of value or of honour. A risk would of course exist, that some members of such a group or class might look only to their own interests (but this would be tyranny rather than timocracy). The alternative form here, termed democracy, would (in its pure form) allow for all citizens to share in the government of the state. According to Aristotle, this was less desirable than its alternative as the commitment to state well-being could not be guaranteed by such a diversity of opinion, which lacked the strength of being governed by a few who were the best able (the aristocracy).

Of course, around these systems, various other types evolved, each with terms (again often of Greek origin) intended to explain their chief characteristics. Thus, we hear of political (or indeed any group) leadership that is *autocratic* (based upon a single leader or dictator), *democratic* (shared by the group), or *laisez faire* (undirected and open). Also, with the passage of time, these ideas changed within cultures. Thus, in France, the view of the monarchy and aristocracy as tyrants led to the French Revolution. Similarly, the idea of a timocracy that allowed only those with property to participate in government has been viewed as a corrupt system in the modern era. Such is the difficulty surrounding terminology, that while we view democracy as the most common and most desirable form of political system, it is difficult to ascertain what the term actually means in the modern context. The following statements demonstrate a number of shades of meaning that are often taken to be included in the term:

- It involves all the people who are recognised as citizens participating, but usually only by exercising a vote (and even this right is dependent on certain conditions in various countries). However, the voting relates specifically to electing who will represent the people and make choices on their behalf (and presumably in their interests). It is thus also often termed representative democracy, as opposed to participatory or direct democracy (see below).

- It involves the election of a few to represent the many, and to govern with their consent. In terms of the people's judgement about who is best able to do this, the government in power is an aristocracy (in the original Greek sense).

- However, because people are often not in a position to judge 'accurately', or because they are influenced by election campaigns, those elected may not necessarily be 'the best', and may most closely resemble the ancient Greek form defined as oligarchy.

- Because many feel that they have no real say, they feel powerless and disenfranchised, and become alienated from the political process and the governmental oligarchy; many even choose not to exercise their vote (Taylor, 1991).

- In more recent times, people have tended to react against the disempowering and exclusionary nature of modern democracies, and begun to demand a more active involvement (Putnam, 2000). This is most evident in such phenomena as the modern referendum, where the electorate vote on an important issue rather than for individuals who will make their choices for them. This in fact indicates a more recent shift from representative government (where we vote on who will make our choices for us) to participatory government (where we vote directly on the specific issues of choice). Some see this shift as a movement towards what is often termed 'direct democracy', something more akin to the original Greek meaning of the term.

Fundamentally, politics is about *power* and its distribution on the basis of:

- *wealth* or capital (Marx, [1907] 1999)
- *might* of the 'chosen few' (Mosca, [1934] 1980) or
- *knowledge* or control of information (Foucault, 1970, 1976).

This highlights the hard, but in fact realistic, face of politics. It is about how issues are addressed and, in the final analysis, how one argument or position is sustained and carried through against others. Thus, according to the Marxist argument, those who have control of 'wealth' or capital have the most power and capability to carry through their position. The relationship of social groups to wealth is of course complex. Juxtaposed with capital is labour. The capacity to determine or negotiate working conditions and pay, and indeed to give or withhold labour is a powerful influence on how capital is realised and distributed. The term 'might' refers to the premise that some people are more able than others and emerge naturally

as superior and thus are naturally destined to lead the party, or country, or even the world. This is not dissimilar to the ancient Greek notion of an aristocracy (those best able), but the emphasis here is on the natural superiority of a particular group. This is essentially the position adopted within the Fascist perspective (and indeed Mosca's work as cited above was influential in the thinking of Hitler and Mussolini). Particularly pertinent in the modern age is the idea that power resides in 'knowledge'. Michel Foucault (1970) argued that the control of knowledge and, in particular, the dominant knowledge discourses, determine our values and which views become normative and accepted. While his arguments were controversial in the 1960s and 1970s, today in what we now call the information age, it is much easier to appreciate his position.

It would be wrong, however, to assume that there are either/or choices, or indeed that they reflect any sequential or historical progression. It would be tempting to suggest that in our modern egalitarian age, wealth is no longer a great social divider. However, the gap between rich and poor continues to widen and increasingly multinational corporations influence our environments and even our governments. We may also confidently comment that Fascism is a thing of the past, but it would be naive to believe that political elites do not exist, and that these do not have the features of exclusive clubs to which only some gain entry. Similarly, while we may believe that in the modern information age knowledge is accessible to all, and just a keyboard move away on our Internet screens, this may not be the case. Not all have access, what is available to be accessed is increasingly controlled and sanctioned and, perhaps more importantly, some groups (governments, multinational corporations) have the capacity to withhold or manipulate information. There is a modern-day paradox in which it is increasingly possible for knowledge to be withheld *from us*, while the agencies that would do this are increasingly able to accumulate knowledge *about us*. The reality is that political power tends to be a more subtle mix of these various influences, and that in fact they are interplaying variables: wealth pays for knowledge, 'insider' knowledge is often restricted to elite groups, elite groups are predominantly the wealthy. We see, therefore, that not only is knowledge a powerful political force, but there is the potential for it to be used for good or evil.

Study Activity 19.1

Assume that the above three dimensions (wealth, might and knowledge) *are* the main indices upon which political power is based.

- How does nursing fair in respect of each of these three dimensions?
- On the basis of your considerations, *should* nursing be a powerful group in modern society?
- If the latter *is not* the case, what factors in your opinion act to limit nursing's full political potential?

In its usual sense, politics is the *activity* of government, but it can also be to do with organised social activity in any social context. Thus, people speak of politics with a small 'p': institutional politics, professional politics, etc. In this context, any social grouping, such as the profession of nursing, is exposed to politics in two senses. There is exposure to external politics, politics with a capital 'P': the influence of government and the policies and legislation emanating from it. And, there is also exposure to internal politics: the politics with a small 'p', which are the organised social influences within the profession itself or within other groupings which influence the profession. It is this often powerful sense of politics that occurs in the margin [as suggested by Watson (1999) in the opening quotation to this chapter], often beneath the surface or disguised in some other more wholesome 'text'. And this is the space within which, for example, whistleblowers such as nurse Graham Pink or Dr Stephen Bolsin (whose cases were addressed in Chapter 13) suffered greatly for speaking against the dominant 'discourse'.

In another sense, the term politics implies the *study* of politics or what today is termed political science. As a discipline, political philosophy has existed since at least the ancient Greeks, but as political science it commenced in the seventeenth century and extended into the latter half of the twentieth century as an essentially *descriptive* discipline. Its main influences were the disciplines of moral philosophy, history and law. The concerns were to describe the machinery of government and the workings of the state (Easton, 1953). In more recent times, as the discipline has matured it has become recognised that various social institutions such as business agencies, trades unions and international organisations influence government, state and national politics, and vice versa. As a consequence, the parameters of the discipline have extended to include: the study of such bodies as political entities in their own right, as influences on government and state; and, in turn, the influence of government and state on these institutions.

More recently, like so many of the softer disciplines, political science has invested in developing itself as a *science* in the sense of being an *empirical* activity aimed at producing theories and predictive knowledge (Blondel, 1963). Much of the activity of political scientists nowadays draws on the social and behavioural sciences, concerned with political beliefs and attitudes, voting patterns, etc. The discipline thus encompasses not only descriptive but empirical dimensions. As such, it is as informative to nursing as to any other walk of modern life. The external political systems are significant influences on how nursing as a discipline evolves and there are, of course, political influences within the health care system and within the profession itself.

Study Activity 19.2

Above we identified the possibility of a more robust approach to *studying* political structures and processes: the discipline of political science (sometimes confusingly just called 'politics'). Earlier, we recognised the potential for knowledge to be a powerful political force. It is sometimes argued that political science cannot only be used to increase our insight into politics but also to manipulate political situations by manipulating how knowledge is used. A term that is increasingly met is that of 'spin' or the 'political spin', and those adept at this activity are termed 'spin doctors'. Look up the meanings of these terms (spin and spin doctor) and relate them to our discussions on political power and how it may be constructed and manipulated.

Study Activity 19.3

In the USA there is a political activity known as 'lobbying' and there is even an emerging occupation or profession whose practitioners are called 'lobbyists'. This area of activity is concerned with not only determining the political 'climate' or emerging views about particular issues, but also with influencing politicians or procuring their support for particular political positions or initiatives.

- Look up the terms 'lobbying' and 'lobbyist', and write brief definitive statements of each.
- Compare and contrast the concept of lobbying with that of political spin introduced in Study Activity 19.2.
- Within the UK, which groups within the health professions have the most highly developed lobbying skills?
- Is nursing successful in this activity, and if not, why not?

POLITICS AND POWER

The power of knowledge

As suggested above, to a very large extent the survival of that which is political (state, government, legislature, etc.) depends on a *shared and accepted knowledge*, which is a social construction. Within this shared knowledge resides almost all of the power that underpins modern politics. It is, of course, true that to a certain extent politics, or political systems, are sustained

by authoritarian and coercive influences. If we breach certain norms, mores, laws, etc., we may be punished, or we may be coerced into certain ways of behaving, particularly in some totalitarian states. But in general, these are instances when the fundamental power, the power of shared knowledge and belief, has failed.

The perspective presented here is postmodern or deconstructionist social constructionism [for a good general introduction see Burr (1995)]. This draws much from the work of the French scholar Michel Foucault (1970, 1976), as referred to above. According to Foucault we derive knowledge from a socially constructed *discourse*. Those who control or impose the dominant discourse hold power. This may include the total populace (at least theoretically) in a democracy, of a few in a totalitarian state. The knowledge or discourse is shared and accepted as the norm, because it is ours, because we all sign up to it, because we feel obliged or coerced into complying. The device known as the *discourse* is a narrative about phenomena, persons, groups, institutions, etc. It is a language which paints a picture, describes phenomena, in effect gives such phenomena structure and meaning. For those who benefit from such a discourse and who can nurture its growth within society, the advantages are extreme and powerful. Their view, that which is to their benefit, has become the dominant accepted knowledge. It has become reified as unquestioned truth and all members of society to greater or lesser extent are subordinated to it. In this perspective, the power behind social action is not to be found within the individual and internal characteristics of people: ideas such as 'attitude', 'belief', 'prejudice', etc., even as shared constructs, are not recognised as being of relevance. The relevant source of social action is the discourse or discourses which are shared and which exist as a societal level. Even when we are not subordinated to them, when we do not accept their legitimacy, we are aware that we are going against the social order, that we are subscribing to a conflicting discourse and may be subject to ridicule or worse as a result.

The power to influence

For any 'object', e.g. family, medicine, nursing, Christianity, etc., there is a discourse, indeed a number of subdiscourses, which give it a shared meaning. The discourse presents a way of seeing things, of objectivising them so that they are viewed as 'common sense', are in effect recognised by the social group as the truth of the matter as regards this object or that. This is not only true of the dominant members who benefit from this interpretation of reality; it is a 'common sense' which is shared and accepted as the natural order by the remaining members who are in fact subordinated to it. Thus, in the era of Conservative dominance in the UK, the words of the discourse were individualism, competition, privatisation, law and order, family values, etc. We know now that not only did the Conservative Party itself subscribe to this discourse, but through public relations consultants and the medium of the Conservative press it promoted this discourse to such an extent that opposing discourses, such as that of the Labour Party, were swept aside for more than a generation. Those who spoke against, such as the National Union of Mineworkers, were sanctioned, almost to the point of being criminalised. The New Labour era is now unfolding its *discourse*, and already we see its phrases: one nation, family values, no-one excluded, education, welfare, responsibility, a 'third way', etc. But behind this apparently softer politics, the power of sanction is no less present, as the British politician Ken Livingstone would no doubt testify! In his election campaign to become Mayor of London he became the subject of a number of demonising discourses and indeed was expelled from the Labour Party. Who his protagonists were, and the justice or otherwise of their viewpoints, are not a matter for judgement here. What is important is that, had he been a less robust individual, who was held in less respect by his constituents, his proverbial goose would have been well and truly cooked.

In describing the power of the discourse, Foucault referred to the nineteenth century prison device known as the *Panopticon*. In this invention, French prison cells were arranged around a central watch tower from which the supervisor could directly observe all the prisoners. As prisoners could not be certain whether or not they were being watched, and possibly as a consequence be disciplined, they started to police their own behaviour, to exercise a self-discipline predicated by the prison's disciplinary discourse of 'don't do this' and 'do do that'. It has been suggested that an equivalent form exists in modern society today (Sarup, 1988). We all know we are increasingly visible, and there are modern-day Panopticon equivalents – computer, telephonic and satellite surveillance. And also, in the case of nursing, the monitoring through health service managers, the statutory bodies and so the suspicious would claim devices such as clinical supervision (*see* Chapter 7).

All this influences us to subscribe to the dominant discourses. We get married because the dominant discourse is true love, the family and caring for our spouse and children. We do not reject marriage on an alternative discourse, such as the Marxist discourse which claims that the family is a device to allow men to be available to work to maximum output through the exploitation of women to provide free services such as housekeeping, child minding and sexual favours, all of which would have to be paid for otherwise (Illich, 1980).

Discourses are not of course permanent entities to be mindlessly followed. There are, there always will be, conflicting discourses and if such obtain a foothold they may in turn become the dominant discourse; we have recently observed the replacement of one dominant political party with its very different discourses by another, both in the UK and the USA. But at any one time, there are dominant discourses which represent shared knowledge, which gives power. The power derives from the acceptance of the truth of that knowledge and this power resides in the principal purveyors and benefactors of the discourse. For example, the increasing emphasis on an evidence-based health care system has its discourse. This discourse is one which draws on a particular scientific perspective which is the language of traditional empirical science – experimental research, randomised controlled trials, statistical measurement, meta-analyses, etc. It is a discourse common to the traditions of medicine and health service managers. Against this backcloth power resides with managers, doctors, and biological/natural scientists. If nurses want to share in the power and decision-making, obtain a share of the resources, they must participate in and sign up to this discourse, take part in this dance. However, their voice is excluded (Davies, 1995) from this male domain and their caring work is devalued (James, 1989). Frankly, if in the recent past nurses had presented a different discourse – a discourse encompassing a feminist interpretation of health care and a philosophical-humanistic source of health care knowledge – they would have been on the proverbial 'hiding to nothing'! The discourse would either have been merely tolerated or openly attacked [see, e.g. the attack by Barker *et al.* (1995) on Kirby and Slevin (1992) and Watson (1985, 1992b)].

POLITICAL DISCOURSES AND NURSING

The external political influences on nurses: discourses that stereotype and devalue

In society, stereotypes of the nurse are dominant social discourses, as evidenced in the work of Muff (1982), Salvage (1985), Savage (1987) and Davies (1995). Such imagery emerges as the result of social psychological processes, deriving from prejudice, stigmatising processes, etc. Thus, all nurses (or most female nurses who make up the majority) are young handmaidens who are also sex objects until they age into battle-axes or leave; male nurses are quite eccentric to enter such an occupation, and quite possibly gay. To the person in the street, images of nursing as a highly complex occupation, with a substantial body of empirical and theoretical knowledge, tend to be absent or partial.

The problem with the analyses of Muff, Salvage and Savage is that they present imagery which is viewed as examples of antisocial stereotyping: something which is recognised as negative and which must be fought against. The position proposed by the social constructionist perspective is that, contrary to being a recognised negative aspect of social life, these images are in fact part of the dominant discourse. That this is in fact how society, to a greater or lesser extent, views nursing. The political implications for nursing arise when even government, as suggested by Salvage (1985), use such discourse in recruitment drives, with terms such as 'nurses are born not made' and photography depicting soft, caring womanhood. The implications are exponentially driven when health service managers, doctors and even patients sustain this discourse, as often we nurses do ourselves.

The political and professional outcome of this discourse is that nursing continues to be relegated to a secondary position. As a group, nurses have always been viewed as secondary to, and indeed subservient to, doctors. But they are held in a similar subservient position to social workers, professions allied to medicine and health service managers. Even the new-from-college health service trainee manager occupies a higher status than the nurse. The discourse holds nursing in this position, and holds the power elsewhere. The counter-discourse involves confronting powerful elements: medicine, health service management, society at large, and even government itself. This may seem a formidable task, and indeed it would be wrong to underestimate the challenges. It is of course the case that society in general values nursing and this to some extent counters the devaluing influences. However, this is a valuing of the nurse as a handmaiden or ministering angel, and such stereotypes are no less difficult to overcome, as was noted in our earlier chapter on 'nursing as a profession'.

The internal political influences on nurses: discourses that oppress and obstruct

Even within the profession and its immediate sphere of activity there are discourses which determine power and direction. Some of these are the internalisation of the external discourses referred to above. We still find within the profession a strong sense of the handmaiden role. This has been sustained since the political machinations of Florence Nightingale, who stressed the vocational and 'religious calling' nature of nursing, accepted a subservient role for women entering the occupation and opposed any moves towards professionalisation such as registration (*see*, for example, Skretkowicz, 1992; van der Peet, 1995).

This subservient model continued to some extent in the UK until recently and is only now beginning to change, but only within the profession itself. The emphasis, within nurse education and within wider professionalisation processes, towards rule-following, task-orientated working and highly structured and hierarchical bureaucracy – still reflective of Nightingale's militaristic model of nursing – has not only been sustained by the wider social discourse but to an extent has continued to be sustained within the profession.

There has, however, been a subtle yet definite shifting of perspectives within the profession within the last third of a century. This is well documented elsewhere (e.g. Kirby and Slevin, 1992; Slevin, 1995, 1999; Meleis, 1997; Burns and Grove, 2001). The significant developments began with the pioneering work into nursing research commencing in the mid-1950s and extending to the present. The dominant influence here was the aspiration to a science of nursing, drawing largely from the natural or quantitative sciences. Schulman (1958, 1972), whose work was also discussed in an earlier chapter, spoke of this as a move from a 'mother-surrogate' to a 'healer' role (where 'healer' had a narrow meaning of technical/specialist/medical role). The natural progression of this was the early work on nursing theory which commenced mainly in the 1960s but gathered momentum in the 1970s and 1980s. This represented a commitment to adopt or adapt theories from other disciplines and attempt to establish their relevance to nursing through empirical endeavour. This led to a plethora of nursing theories

and models which were essentially derivative, established from the traditional, positivistic natural sciences and to a large degree particulate rather than holistic.

The discourse here is characteristic of nursing's natural science aspirations. The language of this discourse will be familiar. It is replete with words such as research, experiment, observation, measurement, empirical, data, quantitative, theory, hypothesis, causation, validity, reliability, evidence-based practice, etc. This discourse is still active, fuelled by the development within the UK health services of service-wide research and development strategies and a call for evidence-based practice, since the publication of Government proposals in this area (National Health Service Executive, 1991). While in reality to date there has been no real investment in nursing as a research-based profession, and the handmaiden discourse is still very much alive, the scientific research paradigm is its strongest adversary. The problem here is that the research-based models are increasingly being recognised as limited in the nursing context. This is not to say that evidence-based approaches are of no value; indeed, there is a great and growing need for sound empirical underpinning as a basis for the best available evidence to inform practice.

However, given that nursing is by definition a deeply subjective and intensely human relational activity, there are significant aspects of nursing which are not amenable to verification through traditional, natural scientific, empirical approaches. This is not a situation exclusive to nursing. Even in the wider health care context, Baker (1998), a leading figure within the UK health services research and development scene, has acknowledged that realistically the best that could be hoped for in a highly successful research and development strategy would be around 50% of care being delivered on a sound evidence base.

The limitations of this discourse led to another discourse, arising mainly in the 1970s in the USA but reaching these shores mainly from the mid-1980s on. This took a number of forms, arose from a number of different perspectives, but in total represented a move away from a natural science, *particulate* perspective, to a broader, *holistic* perspective. The significant aspect of this discourse is that it is not narrowly confined to an evidence-based, research-derived knowledge. It is *eclectic* in that it moves beyond this to a broader knowledge base and indeed to sources of nursing action and wisdom which do not easily fit into a knowledge categorisation at all. This was perhaps well reflected in two significant publications. Carper's (1978) seminal work on different ways of knowing, which recognised not only the empirical but also personal, ethical and aesthetic ways of knowing, is the first of these (*see* also Chapter 9). Of equal seminal influence was the work of Belenky *et al.* (1986) which drew attention to the imposition of male ways of thinking and knowing as reflected, for example, in the traditional models of science and medicine, and which proposed alternative modes of thinking and addressing issues which are characteristic of a more human, but no less effective, perspective.

The significant differences between this holistic discourse and the more scientifically orientated discourse can be identified as follows:

- Here there is a more eclectic approach, and a willingness to draw on a wider range of sources. Method and paradigm do not determine the pathway to knowing; it is nursing as a way of being and relating which determines and calls upon the sources. The breadth of sources extends well beyond the parameters of traditional science, to areas ranging from empirics to aesthetics, from theology to biology.
- Here these diverse sources facilitate more holistic as opposed to more particulate understandings of nursing reality. Where theoretical knowledge is the product, Parse (1987) refers to such theories as being within the simultaneity paradigm (where all that is the client and his environment is considered at once, as one) as opposed to the totality paradigm (where all are parts, and the whole merely a total of parts).

There is a conflict between the latter two discourses (holistic-caring and scientific-technical) and between each of them and the still more or less dominant traditional subservient-handmaiden discourse. The scientific, evidence-based discourse continues to gain strength from the rising importance of research and the quest for an evidence-based service, and a professionalism established on the model of professions as monopolistic, specialised, highly technical occupations entered via advanced discipline-specific education. However, the increasing recognition of the limits of such a discourse and recognition of the strength of a broader, more holistic, discourse also gain momentum. This aspires to a professionalism established on a *new* professional model, based on a relationship and a partnership with clients, and upon an outward rather than an inward seeking of knowledge to guide practice (Slevin, 1999). The politics within nursing, as represented by these three opposing discourses, will determine the future of nursing as we proceed into the new millennium.

Study Activity 19.4

Select at least three of the mainstream scholarly journals in the discipline of nursing. By scanning the contents lists and, where available, the brief abstracts of the published papers for the past 3-year period, note the topics and list these under the two headings – scientific/empirical and humanistic/holistic. Note any differences in the sizes of your two lists. Reflect upon the discourses that underlie the two perspectives and the differences between them.

The politics of difference

In this section we have so far concentrated on the direct impact of political influences on nursing. However, one aspect impacting upon all members of society might be broadly termed the politics of difference. Particularly as the influences of globalisation and global migration advance, there is an increasing tendency for societies to become multicultural. The situation within a multicultural society can take a number of different forms. In an attempt to model this situation, Gordon (1978) proposed three possible models:

- *Assimilation* – where the immigrant group is expected to abandon its own culture in favour of the dominant culture of the host society.
- *The melting pot* – where, as a society becomes increasingly 'mixed', all its groups change and a new culture emerges.
- *Cultural pluralism* – where cultural differences are tolerated, or even promoted, and a richness of cultural diversity exists alongside common commitment to the society as a whole.

It is often the case that, particularly where there is a lack of assimilation, prejudice towards the immigrant group emerges. They are first labelled as undesirable, or a threat, or inferior in some way. Such prejudice can then become overt in the form of persecution and discrimination. Prime examples of this have included discrimination against black people in the USA and South Africa, and Jewish people in Nazi Germany. It is also seen in the UK, where discrimination is said to be widely present in respect of black and Asian peoples, and where its most overt expression is in movements such as the National Front and the British National Party. Such reactions are often termed racism (*see* Back and Solomos, 2000; Fredrickson, 2002). This is defined in the *Collins English Dictionary* (2000) as:

> *the belief that races have distinctive cultural characteristics determined by hereditary factors and that this endows some races with an intrinsic superiority over others . . .*
> (whereby there is) . . . *abusive or aggressive behaviour towards members of another race on the basis of such a belief.*
> (Collins English Dictionary, 2000)

Other groups within society can also be disadvantaged, and later in this module we consider some of these, such as women, older people, and ethnic groups (sometimes coterminous with race, but not always so). There are two aspects of these phenomena that are of importance to nurses:

1 Discrimination against such groups can emerge as inequalities in health, even though there is extensive race relations legislation within the UK (*see* Townsend *et al.*, 1992). This has led to the need for Government action, such as the commitment to reducing inequalities in the *NHS Plan* (Department of Health, 2000).
2 Within an increasingly multicultural society, nurses must develop transcultural knowledge and skills to meet the needs of people from different racial, ethnic and cultural backgrounds (Leininger, 2002).

Study Activity 19.5

Using your library sources, review the topic 'transcultural nursing' and consider how it might inform your practice.

SUMMARY

We have spoken of powers (political forces) that may stereotype and devalue, and those that may oppress and obstruct. We have furthermore spoken of the various discourses that are the 'vehicles' for these 'forces'. At the same time we have suggested that, albeit within a particular stereotype of the nurse as a handmaiden and ministering angel, society holds nursing in high regard. And we have identified nursing consciousness as essentially of these three forms:

- *Traditionalists* – who subscribe to the mother-surrogate or handmaiden role.
- *Scientists–technicians* – who subscribe to the rational-technical role.
- *Radical carers* – who subscribe to new ways of knowing and being, empowerment and a feminist ethic of care.

373

The latter consciousness tends to subscribe to different patterns of knowing (empirical, personal, ethical and aesthetic) as explicated by Carper (1978). In a more recent critique of Carper's patterns, White (1995) proposed a fifth pattern of knowing, which she termed sociopolitical knowing. That is a pattern characterised by:

- a questioning of taken-for-granted assumptions about practice, the profession, health care
- awareness of the sociopolitical context of persons (including nurses and their patients)
- awareness of how nursing is influenced by the wider political world (nationally, internationally, globally), and how nursing can influence that world and indeed its own future.

This highlights the need to address how we must cope with 'forces' that would stereotype and devalue us, or oppress and obstruct us. But it also highlights politics as a 'vehicle' for opportunity and emancipation. We must not only be more politically aware, but we must be more politically competent and more politically active. Or, as Watson (1999) suggests, we must deconstruct and then reconstruct *our own* futures. This may seem a difficult undertaking. But there is about the world in this post-modern age, that some describe as the new modernity, an openness to dialogue and negotiated solutions.

Groups are no longer held to restricted and confined ways of looking at the world and responding to its problems. Now, and in the future, we can expect to be confronted by new problems and new risks for which there are no old solutions. Some, such as Etzioni (1997), see this as a new paradigm situation, a new approach that is communitarian or dependent on dialogue and agreement rather than conflict and imposition. Etzioni (1997) describes this communitarian outlook, characterised by dialogue and negotiation, as 'the new Golden Rule', the new way of determining how we should live. This presents to nursing a new opportunity, an opportunity to participate in determining how it will emerge as a helping profession in the future. It requires of us a consciousness of our own political power, based upon our value to society as vitally important workers, thinkers and skilful practitioners. It also requires of us a development of the political skills necessary to be effective participants in determining our future. But, importantly, it requires that we negotiate how we will be as nurses with those who will be nursed. We must say to the people: this is how we can be for you; recognise in us the capacity to respond to your needs in sickness and in health.

REFERENCES

Back, L. and Solomos, J. (eds) (2000) *Theories of Race and Racism: A reader*, Routledge, New York

Baker, M.E. (1998) Challenging ignorance. In: Baker, M. and Kirk, S. (eds) *Research and Development for the NHS – Evidence, evaluation and effectiveness* (2nd edn), Radcliffe Medical Press, Oxford

Barker, P.J., Reynolds, W. and Ward, T. (1995) The proper focus of nursing: a critique of the 'caring' ideology, *International Journal of Nursing Studies* **12**(4), 386–97

Belenky, M.F., Clinchy, B.M., Goldberger, N.R. *et al.* (1986) *Women's Ways of Knowing*, Basic Books, New York

Blondel, J. (1963) *Voters, Parties, Leaders*, Penguin, Harmondsworth

Burns, N. and Grove, S.K. (2001) *The Practice of Nursing Research* (4th edn), W.B. Saunders, Philadelphia, IL

Burr, V. (1995) *An Introduction to Social Constructionism*, Routledge, London

Carper, B.A. (1978) Fundamental patterns of knowing in nursing. *Advances in Nursing Science* **1**, 13–23

Davies, C. (1995) *Gender and the Professional Predicament in Nursing*, Open University Press, Buckingham

Department of Health (2000) *The NHS Plan: A plan for investment – a plan for reform*, The Stationery Office, London

Easton, D. (1953) *The Political System*, Doubleday, New York

Etzioni, A. (1997) *The New Golden Rule*, Profile Books, London

Foucault, M. (1970) *The Order of Things: An archaeology of the human sciences*, Tavistock, London

Foucault, M. (1976) *The Birth of the Clinic*, Tavistock, London

Fredrickson, G. (2002) *Racism: A short history*, Princeton University Press, Princeton, NJ

Gordon, M. (1978) *Human Nature, Class and Ethnicity*, Oxford University Press, Oxford

Harper Collins (2000) *The Collins English Dictionary*, Harper Collins, Glasgow

Illich, I. (1980) *Shadow-work*, University of Capetown, Capetown

James, V. (1989) Emotional labour: skill and work in the social regulation of feelings. *Sociological Review* 37(1), 18–35

Kirby, C. and Slevin, O. (1992) A new curriculum for care. In: Slevin, O. and Buckenham, M. (eds) *Project 2000: The teachers speak*, Campion Press, Edinburgh

Leininger, M. (2002) *Transcultural Nursing: Concepts, theories, research and practice* (3rd edn), McGraw-Hill, New York

Marx, K. ([1907] 1999) *Capital*, Oxford University Press, Oxford

Meleis, A.I. (1997) *Theoretical Nursing: Development and progress* (3rd edn), J.B. Lippincott, Philadelphia, IL

Mosca, G. ([1934] 1980) *The Ruling Class*, Greenwood Press, Westport, CT

Muff, J. (1982) Handmaiden, battle-axe, whore: an exploration into the fantasies, myths and stereotypes about nurses. In: Muff, J. (ed.) *Socialisation, Sexism and Stereotyping*, C.V. Mosby, St Louis, IL

National Health Service Executive (1991) *Research for Health: A research and development strategy for the NHS*, National Health Service Executive, London

Noddings, N. (1984) *Caring: A feminine approach to ethics and moral education*, University of California Press, London

Parse, R.R. (1987) *Nursing Science*, W.B. Saunders, Philadelphia, IL

Putnam, R.D. (2000) *Bowling Alone: The collapse and revival of American civic community*, Simon and Schuster, New York

Salvage, J. (1985) *The Politics of Nursing*, Heinemann, London

Sarup, M. (1988) *An Introductory Guide to Post-structuralism and Postmodernism*, Harvester Wheatsheaf, Hemel Hempstead

Savage, J. (1987) *Nurses, Gender and Sexuality*, Heinemann, London

Schulman, S. (1958) Basic functional roles in nursing: mother surrogate and healer. In: Jaco, E. (ed.) *Patients, Physicians and Illness*, Free Press, New York

Schulman, S. (1972) Mother-surrogate – after a decade. In: Jaco, E. (ed.) *Patients, Physicians and Illness*, Collier-Macmillan, London

Skretkowicz, V. (1992) *Florence Nightingale's Notes on Nursing*, Scutari, London

Slevin, O. (1995) Theories and models. In: Basford, L. and Slevin, O. (eds) *Theory and Practice of Nursing*, Campion Press, Edinburgh

Slevin, O. (1999) The nurse–patient relationship: caring in a health context. In: Long, A. (ed.) *Interaction for Practice in Community Nursing*, Macmillan, London

Taylor, C. (1991) *The Ethics of Authenticity: The malaise of modernity*, Harvard University Press, Cambridge, MA

Townsend, P., Whitehead, M. and Davidson, N. (1992) *Inequalities in Health: The Black report and the health divide*, Penguin Books, London

van der Peet, R. (1995) *The Nightingale Model of Nursing*, Campion Press, Edinburgh

Watson, J. (1985) *Nursing: Human science and human care*, Appleton-Century-Croft, Norwalk, CT

Watson, J. (1992a) Caring knowledge and informed moral passion. *Nursing Science Quarterly* 13(1), 15–24

Watson, J. (1992b) Window on theory of human caring. In: O'Toole, M. (ed.) *Miller-Keane Encyclopedia and Dictionary of Medicine, Nursing and Allied Health* (5th edn), W.B. Saunders, Philadelphia, IL

Watson, J. (1999) *Postmodern Nursing and Beyond*, Churchill Livingstone, Edinburgh

White, J. (1995) Patterns of knowing: review, critique and update. *Advances in Nursing Science* 17(4), 73–86

20 RELIGION, ETHNICITY AND THE DEVELOPMENT OF MORE INCLUSIVE HEALTH CARE

Paul Weller

LEARNING OUTCOMES

After studying this chapter you will be able to:

- Outline some of the forms of believing and belonging that shape the contemporary context of health care
- Identify at least one way in which religious prejudice may affect your nursing practice
- Identify at least one way in which those for whom you are providing health care may be affected by indirect religious discrimination or religious disadvantage
- Evaluate the extent to which a religion or religions may inform or pose questions to your professional identity and practice as a nurse
- Identify at least one issue around health care where consultation with a religious group may result in the development of more inclusive health care.

INTRODUCTION

This chapter explores the role, diversity and significance of religion in the lives of population groups, patients and their families, together with the importance of taking account of religion for the development of a more inclusive health care practice and policy.

The contemporary context and variety of religion in British society is outlined. A number of approaches to understanding the nature of religion as a form of 'believing' and 'belonging' are explored. Consideration is also given to the significance of religion in the lives of population groups, patients and their families.

The relevance of existing legislation to unfair treatment on the basis of religion is explained, and the results of research into the nature and extent of religious discrimination are reported, with special reference to unfair treatment in health care settings. Some examples are set out of what people of various religions perceive as unfair treatment, along with a number of initiatives for addressing these issues.

A framework is offered for understanding and locating the various experiences that are reported by people of various religions as unfair and discriminatory treatment. Finally, ways forward are suggested towards the development of a more inclusive health care policy and practice.

The issues relating to religion and health care are wide-ranging and complex and the constraints of this chapter do not allow for a fully adequate overview. The reader is therefore directed towards a number of key resources, which will enable them to gain a wider knowledge of a range of religions and of the key issues that arise at the interfaces between the religions and the policies and practice of health care. Throughout the chapter, students are encouraged to draw upon their own experience to consider the relevance of religion to their professional identity and practice, their attitudes and behaviour, and for the policies and practices of the health care organisations within which they work.

Study Activity 20.1 _____

- Before reading this chapter, reflect upon, and make a note about, any role that religion has played in your life.
- Note down any example that may come to mind from your nursing practice in which a patient and/

or their family seemed to be either helped or distressed by an aspect of their religion.

THE RELIGIOUS CONTEXT OF CONTEMPORARY HEALTH CARE

As health care and the nursing profession have been changing and developing, so too has the nature of the society (Abrams *et al.*, 1985; Jones, 1993; Mason, 1995) in which health care is exercised. If health care is to be as effective as possible, it needs to find ways of avoiding discrimination and to take account of diversity in ways that facilitate and develop the inclusivity of the health care provided (Department of Health, 1991, 1992a, b).

The UK has a strong heritage from Christianity and this remains the predominant religious tradition, particularly in Northern Ireland, Scotland and Wales (Davie, 1994; Bruce, 1995). In the 1960s, it was often popularly assumed that the processes of secularisation would lead to a diminishing of the significance of religion, at least in the public sphere. However, in the last decades of the twentieth century, religion has again more generally been recognised to be a significant – sometimes the determining – factor in the lives of individuals, families and communities. This has been particularly (although not exclusively) the case in respect of those who are also members of minority ethnic groups (Ballard, 1994; Modood *et al.*, 1994). The UK is now more religiously diverse (Parsons, 1993, 1994; Weller, 2001) than any other country of the European Union and the religions found within it continue to exhibit a considerable degree of vigour despite the effects of secularisation.

There are, of course, a whole range of socio-economic factors (Davey Smith *et al.*, 1990; Benzeval *et al.*, 1995) that have a bearing upon the care both of individual patients and particular population groups. Social class, wealth, employment status and gender all affect the perceptions, experiences and access to health care of individuals and groups in society. The relationship between ethnicity, health and treatment (Henley, 1982a; Hopkins and Bahl, 1993), and the impact of racial discrimination and disadvantage upon both health itself and the provision of health care, has received increasing attention in research studies (Donovan, 1984; Ahmad, 1993; Balarajam and Soni Raleigh, 1995; Smaje, 1995; Modood *et al.*, 1997; Nazroo, 1997a, b), as well as in nurse training and professional development (Dobson, 1991; Beishon *et al.*, 1995).

Other chapters in this book highlight and explore these continuing issues. Although some attention has been paid to issues related to the religious identifications of individual patients, their families, and population groups (Henley, 1982, 1983a, b; Henley and Schott, 1999) in health care, as in other areas of policy, practice and service delivery, this has often not been done in a focused or systematic way in relation to issues of religion considered in their own right.

At the time of writing, there is no agreed and reliable information on the religious composition of the population, with only estimated figures being available (Barley *et al.*, 1987; Anwar, 1993; Brierley, 2000).

For discussion of the figures and the issues involved in estimating them, *see* Weller, P. (ed.) (2001), also Table 20.1).

Alongside those who belong to the major world religions in the UK are groups often popularly referred to as 'sects' or 'cults'. In academic usage (Barker, 1990), these groups have more normally come to be described as 'New Religious Movements' (NRMs). Those who understand themselves as Pagans have also begun to emerge into the wider public consciousness, as have 'New Age' spiritualists (York, 1995), whose beliefs are characterised by a concern for personal growth and draw upon spiritual practices and traditions from a variety of sources.

There continue to be many humanists and atheists who uphold strong ethical and moral values but do not profess any form of religious self-identification, as well as large numbers of people who are indifferent to organised religion, but who may have a concern with spirituality. Nevertheless, the fact that religion is increasingly being recognised as a factor to take into account in policy, practice and service delivery is evidenced by the inclusion of a question on religion in the decennial Census. New Census questions are only added after a protracted process of debate (Weller and Andrews, 1998), which both justifies and demonstrates the requirements of national and local government, business and academia for the information to be derived from any new question. While a religion question has traditionally been asked in the Census as conducted in Northern Ireland, 2001 is the first time that such a question has been asked in England and Wales, and in Scotland. With some additional variations for Scotland, respondents to the 2001 Census in England, Wales and Scotland were asked to choose from the options of 'None', Christian, Buddhist, Hindu, Jewish, Muslim or Sikh, or to write in the name of any other religion.

Table 20.1 2001 estimates of the numbers in various religious groupings in the UK

Baha'i	6000
Buddhist	30 000–100 000
Christian	38 100 000
Hindu	400 000–550 000
Jain	25 000–30 000
Jewish	283 000
Muslim	1 000 000–1 500 000
Sikh	350 000–500 000
Zoroastrian	5000–10 000

(From Weller, 2001)
(Estimates prior to the publication of results of the 2001 decennial Census question on religion.)

The publication of the 2001 Census results will ensure – as did the inclusion of an ethnic question (Ballard and Kalra, 1994; Peach, 1996) in the 1991 Census – more accurate demographic information than is currently available based on estimates. Regional and local datasets derived from the Census will enable more inclusive planning at regional and local levels of service delivery, including health care.

DEFINITIONS OF RELIGION

As with 'ethnicity' (Barth, 1969; Bacal, 1991) there is no simple definition of 'religion'. In both popular usage and some legal usage in connection with charity law, religion has often been considered to be something to do with belief in a God or divine being. Such an understanding is, however, problematic, since it does not take account of the world religions of Buddhism or Jainism, which are non-theistic. In addition, such definitions locate the significance of belief more centrally than would be the case in some traditions. As Grace Davie (1994) has argued, there is a phenomenon of 'believing without belonging', which means that religious belief is likely to be considerably wider than either active involvement in, or even passive identification with, a religious tradition or community.

At the same time, the relationship between religion, culture and ethnicity is not straightforward, either in terms of the self-understanding of groups of people described by these terms, or in terms of the factors affecting the composition of these groups in particular social and historical contexts. 'Culture' and 'religion' are clearly often connected in interdependent ways even if they are, in principle, distinguishable. However, the nature of their relationship is evaluated differently both among and between the different religious traditions and within varied approaches to the study of religions.

Etymologically, the English word 'religion' derives from the Latin word *religio*, which has a root meaning related to the idea of a 'binding' together and which contains the sense of an organised culture. In terms of contemporary definitions of religion, the best that exist are various 'working definitions', which also tend to reflect the various disciplinary traditions within which the definitions are made.

The sociologist Emile Durkheim's definition of religion ([1915] 1947) is that of 'a unified system of beliefs and practices relative to sacred things'. Anthropologist Clifford Geertz defined religion as:

... a (1) system of symbols which acts to (2) establish powerful, pervasive and long-lasting moods and motivations in men [sic] by (3) formulating conceptions of a general order of existence and (4) clothing these conceptions with such an aura of factuality that (5) the moods and motivations seem uniquely realistic.

(Geertz [1996], 1996, p. 90)

By contrast, it has been argued that what are today described as distinct 'religions' are, in fact, historical constructions superimposed upon what are actually the very diverse experiences of people of 'personal faith' who live within what Cantwell Smith prefers to call 'cumulative traditions'.

Perhaps religious identification is best understood in terms of different combinations of a 'believing' (in certain values, ideals and doctrines) that often goes closely together with a 'belonging' (to certain organisations, movements and communities) and is expressed through 'practice' (that is, related to shared symbols, rituals, observances and ethical orientations).

Study Activity 20.2

- Note down the variety of religions that you have come across in your nursing practice.
- Identify one example that you have come across in your nursing practice where religion and culture seem to go hand in hand.
- Identify one example that you have come across in your nursing practice where an aspect of religion seems as though it might be separate from the cultural norms of a patient or their family.

RELIGION AND DISCRIMINATION

Parallel to the re-emergence of the recognition of the significance of religion has been a growing concern with the possibility that individuals, families and communities may experience discrimination and unfair treatment, not only in respect of race and ethnicity, but also on the grounds of religion (Department for the Environment, Transport and the Regions, 1996; Commission for Racial Equality, 1997). In the UK, legislation on religious discrimination currently exists only in the jurisdiction of Northern Ireland, under the terms of the Northern Ireland Act 1998. This prohibits discrimination by government or public bodies on grounds of religious belief or political opinion, while the Fair Employment and Treatment (Northern Ireland) Order 1998 covers religious discrimination in employment and extends protection to cover the provision of goods, services and facilities. The possibility of legislation on religious discrimination in the rest of the UK is under active debate (Hepple and Choudhary, 2001). In particular, by December 2003, the government will need to implement the Directive of the Council of the European Union (2000/78/EC) on equal treatment and discrimination in employment, including discrimination on the grounds of religion or belief.

There are, however, aspects of current legislation that are relevant to equitable treatment in respect of people of various religions. Although the House of Lords' decision in the 1983 case of *Mandela v. Dowell Lee* made clear that the Race Relations Act could not apply to religious groups in their own right, the case did establish that, within the Act, 'ethnic' is judged to have a meaning wider than simply 'racial'. The principle was also established that a 'common religion' should be taken into account as one of the contributing factors of shared ethnicity found among 'racial groups' as defined in the terms of the Act.

Sikhs were therefore judged to be an ethnic group in the meaning of the Act. Jews are also covered, as an ethno-religious group, but Buddhists, Christians and Muslims are not covered, since they are part of universal, global religious traditions and communities. Thus, a white person who embraces Islam is not covered by the Act although a Muslim who is also a member of a minority ethnic group might be covered under the Act's provisions relating to 'indirect discrimination'.

The incorporation into domestic law of the European Convention on Human Rights, through the Human Rights Act 1998, has introduced into UK law new obligations with respect to religion. The Convention upholds the unqualified right to freedom of thought, conscience and religion, together with the qualified right, either alone or in community with others, in public or in private, to manifest one's religion or belief. Under the 1998 Human Rights Act the government and all bodies acting as 'public authorities' must examine the degree to which their current policies and practices, as well as their future proposals, are in conformity with the rights upheld by the Convention. The Human Rights Act thus already creates a significantly new legal context that requires fresh and systematic consideration of issues of how public policy impacts upon religion across a wide range of areas, including health care policy and practice.

RESEARCH ON RELIGIOUS DISCRIMINATION AND HEALTH CARE

While much work has been undertaken in relation to discrimination on the grounds of ethnicity, until recently there has been no systematic research undertaken into unfair treatment specifically on the ground of religion. However, in 1999 the Home Office commissioned the University of Derby to undertake a research project on religious discrimination in England and Wales. The project published an interim report and the Home Office published the project's final report, *Religious Discrimination in England and Wales* (Weller *et al.*, 2001). The section that follows is based on this research project's findings with regard to health care (*see* note at end of the chapter).

The findings of the research were based upon the results of a postal questionnaire survey distributed to a total of 1830 (643 national, 66 regional and 1121 local) religious organisations throughout England and Wales, asking about the reported experience of their members. Of the 628 questionnaires returned, 154 were from national organisations, 16 from regional, and 458 from local. For a variety of reasons, the results of the survey need to be treated with caution; for a discussion of the issues involved, see the project's technical report in Weller *et al.*, 2001 (pp. 147–72). Nevertheless, the survey results do tally reasonably well with the findings from the project's qualitative research and therefore give a reasonable insight into the areas that are of particular concern for specific religious groups.

The project's qualitative findings are based on the results of 156 meetings for fieldwork interviews and discussions involving 318 individuals from religious organisations and secular agencies in four localities (Leicester, the London Borough of Newham, Blackburn and Cardiff) for approximately six weeks in each area during 1999–2000. Interviewees were not taken systematically through the same list of topics but were asked to volunteer their own experiences as a member of a faith community or as a representative of a secular agency, together with their observations about policy and practice in this area, their awareness of ongoing problems, and their views on how discrimination can be avoided or tackled.

Unfair treatment on the basis of religion in health care settings

In general terms, ignorance and indifference towards religion were of widespread concern among research participants from all religious groups. Ignorance and indifference do not themselves constitute discrimination, but in organisational settings they can contribute towards an environment in which discrimination of all kinds (including 'unwitting' and institutional discrimination) are able to thrive. In the local interviews, those who actively practised their religion often said that they were made to feel awkward and that they experienced pressure to conform. They claimed that other people based their views on pre-conceived ideas and stereotypes and seemed neither to know nor to care about the things that are central to the experience of those for whom religious identity constitutes an important, or the key, aspect of their life.

In relation to health care in particular, the questionnaire included specific questions about the policies and practices of NHS surgeries and health centres, NHS hospitals, and private health care, as well as questions about the attitudes and behaviour of staff and patients in these settings. As with other sections of the postal survey, where organisations and their members had experience of unfair treatment they were asked to indicate if this was 'frequent' or 'occasional'. The respondents were asked to give specific examples of any unfair treatment and to suggest possible ways of tackling the problems experienced in the health care sector.

If responding organisations had no experience of the question asked, their responses were excluded from analysis of the questionnaire findings.

Unfair treatment on the basis of religion in NHS hospitals

Asked about NHS hospital staff, patients, policies and practices (see Tables 20.2, 20.3 and 20.4), organisations from the Sikh, Muslim, Hindu and Christian traditions responding to the postal survey were most likely to indicate that staff were the main source of unfair treatment. Around two-thirds of Sikh organisations

Table 20.2 Unfair treatment from NHS hospital medical staff attitudes and behaviour

Religion	Some unfair treatment	Frequent unfair treatment	Occasional unfair treatment	Total respondents
Baha'i	1	1	0	21
Buddhist	0	0	0	25
Christian	37	5	32	234
Hindu	14	2	12	30
Jain	2	1	1	4
Jewish	2	0	2	20
Muslim	28	10	18	53
NRM/Pagan	9	1	8	17
Sikh	14	2	12	30
Zoroastrian	2	1	1	4

(From Weller et al., 2001)

Table 20.3 Unfair treament from NHS hospital policies

Religion	Some unfair treatment	Frequent unfair treatment	Occasional unfair treatment	Total respondents
Baha'i	2	1	1	20
Buddhist	0	0	0	24
Christian	19	4	15	217
Hindu	6	2	4	23
Jain	2	1	1	4
Jewish	0	0	0	19
Muslim	20	9	11	47
NRM/Pagan	8	1	7	14
Sikh	9	0	9	25
Zoroastrian	3	2	1	4

(From Weller et al., 2001)

Table 20.4 Unfair treatment from NHS hospital practices

Religion	Some unfair treatment	Frequent unfair treatment	Occasional unfair treatment	Total respondents
Baha'i	2	1	1	20
Buddhist	0	0	0	24
Christian	19	4	15	217
Hindu	6	2	4	23
Jain	2	1	1	4
Jewish	0	0	0	19
Muslim	24	9	15	46
NRM/Pagan	8	1	7	14
Sikh	9	0	9	25
Zoroastrian	2	0	2	4

(From Weller et al., 2001)

and over half of Muslim organisations reported that their members experienced unfair treatment from the attitudes and behaviour of NHS staff. A majority of the small number of responses from New Religious Movement and Pagan organisations did the same. Muslims were the most likely to say that the unfairness was 'frequent' rather than 'occasional'. No unfair treatment in any aspect of health care within the NHS was reported by Buddhist organisations.

Unfair treatment on the basis of religion in NHS surgeries and health centres

In respect of NHS surgeries and health centres (*see* Tables 20.5 and 20.6), Sikh organisations were the most likely to identify unfair treatment, with around two out of three reporting unfair treatment of their members by medical and non-medical staff. At the same time, nearly all of these organisations said the unfair treatment was 'occasional' rather than 'frequent'. This figure of two out three compares with a much smaller proportion of Christian organisations, although the proportion was higher for organisations belonging to the black-led and 'other Christian' categories than for the majority Christian traditions. In nearly all religious traditions, fewer organisations recorded unfair treatment from the policies and practices of health centres and surgeries than from the attitudes and behaviour of staff.

Unfair treatment on the basis of religion in private health care

Fewer organisations were in a position to answer questions about private health care (*see* Tables 20.7 and 20.8) but the patterns of unfair treatment experienced were similar to those in NHS settings.

The nature of unfair treatment on the basis of religion in health care

The raw data in Tables 20.2–20.8 gives a broad indication of the relative experience of unfair treatment among different religious groups in relation to the various sectors of health care, and among the various groups of health care personnel. Detailed analysis of the survey findings yields a number of indications about the specific areas in which concern was concentrated.

In relation to unfair treatment in health care, a number of areas of concern were cited in the postal survey, including:

- admissions (Muslims)
- attitudes and behaviour of medical staff (Muslims, new religious movements/Pagans, Sikhs)
- attitudes and behaviour of patients (new religious movements/Pagans)
- attitudes and behaviour of administrative staff (Muslims)

Table 20.5 Unfair treatment from NHS surgery and health centre staff attitudes and behaviour

Religion	Some unfair treatment	Frequent unfair treatment	Occasional unfair treatment	Total respondents
Baha'i	2	1	1	23
Buddhist	0	0	0	24
Christian	41	2	39	237
Hindu	10	3	7	29
Jain	2	1	1	4
Jewish	1	0	1	21
Muslim	23	5	18	50
NRM/Pagan	7	2	5	16
Sikh	19	1	18	30
Zoroastrian	3	0	3	4

(From Weller et al., 2001)

Table 20.6 Unfair treatment from NHS surgery and medical centre policies/practices

Religion	Some unfair treatment	Frequent unfair treatment	Occasional unfair treatment	Total respondents
Baha'i	1	1	0	23
Buddhist	0	0	0	24
Christian	23	3	20	231
Hindu	6	0	6	23
Jain	1	1	0	3
Jewish	1	0	1	21
Muslim	20	8	12	48
NRM/Pagan	6	1	5	15
Sikh	15	1	14	28
Zoroastrian	2	0	2	5

(From Weller et al., 2001)

Table 20.7 Unfair treatment from private health care staff

Religion	Some unfair treatment	Frequent unfair treatment	Occasional unfair treatment	Total respondents
Baha'i	2	1	1	17
Buddhist	0	0	0	18
Christian	13	2	11	177
Hindu	3	0	3	19
Jain	2	1	1	3
Jewish	1	0	1	20
Muslim	15	2	13	34
NRM/Pagan	1	0	1	5
Sikh	9	1	8	21
Zoroastrian	1	0	1	3

(From Weller et al., 2001)

Table 20.8 Unfair treatment from private health care policies/practices

Religion	Some unfair treatment	Frequent unfair treatment	Occasional unfair treatment	Total respondents
Baha'i	2	1	1	17
Buddhist	0	0	0	17
Christian	9	1	8	175
Hindu	2	1	1	3
Jain	1	0	1	20
Jewish	1	0	1	20
Muslim	14	3	11	34
NRM/Pagan	1	1	0	4
Sikh	7	1	6	20
Zoroastrian	1	0	1	3

(From Weller et al., 2001)

- chaplaincy and facilities for worship (Muslims, new religious movements/Pagans)
- dietary needs (Jains, Muslims, Sikhs)
- general ignorance towards culture and beliefs (Muslims, Sikhs)
- language interpretation barriers (Sikhs)
- medical policies (new religious movements/Pagans)
- medical practices/techniques (Jains, Muslims).

The questionnaires also provided the opportunity to add brief written examples of unfair treatment on the basis of religion being experienced within health care. Table 20.9 shows quotes from the postal survey, giving a little more insight into the nature of the unfair treatment perceived and reported by respondents.

Study Activity 20.3

- Make a preliminary assessment of why some religious groups may feel more than others that they experience unfair treatment within health care settings.
- In relation to your nursing experience, identify an attitude or behaviour that may be an expression of religious prejudice.
- Based on your nursing practice, identify a policy or practice in your health care organisation which, in relation to religion, may cause indirect discrimination.

Table 20.9 The nature of unfair treatment in healthcare, as perceived by patients

Religion	Comment
Jains	'Medication tested on animals'.
Muslims	'Elderly overlooked', 'unsuitable medicines', 'no female doctor for women patients', 'lack of attention', 'proper care not given by GPs', 'doctor not responsive to needs', 'circumcision not available', 'no Muslims at higher levels', 'stereotyping female mental patient', 'Muslims ignored', 'impolite staff', 'post-death and female requirements'
New religious movements/Pagans	'Pagan not listed on forms', 'categorised as C of E', 'verbal abuse', 'hospital refuses donations from our religion', 'medical staff are suspicious and biased'
Sikhs	'Hair removal', 'will not remove 5 K's', 'GPs don't care for elderly'

Issues and dilemmas and innovations in religion and health care

Health care was not a major focus of the project's local fieldwork, but interviewees sometimes referred to health care issues, and a number of discussions took place with hospital chaplains. From these interviews and discussions, the following clusters of issues emerged. These are briefly described, together, in a number of instances, with the initiatives that have been taken to try to address them.

Food and clothing in hospitals

In one location Hindus experienced difficulties when family members were not allowed to bring their own food into the hospital. For the more elderly and devout patients, the hospital's standard vegetarian meals were not felt to be adequately appropriate to their religious dietary requirements. It was also noted that, for reasons of modesty connected with culture and religion, many women did not feel comfortable wearing the standard hospital nightdress during the daytime and preferred to wear their saris. The local religious community had been very active in contacting the hospital to explain these concerns and, as a result, it was reported that the need for specific interventions had gradually decreased.

The deceased

A number of concerns were reported around procedures and practices in relation to the deceased. These included instances when Muslims were not allowed access to prepare the body in traditional ways for burial, despite provisions of the Coroners Act that allow for exemptions. A group of Buddhists also noted difficulties in connection with arrangements for the deceased and felt that there should be a co-ordinator in hospitals who can contact community members to provide the appropriate rites.

Circumcision

For Jews and Muslims, issues connected with circumcision of male children can sometimes give rise to problems. It was noted that the availability of the operation on the NHS varies from one area to another. Interviewees also noted that 'in England, there is a black economy' of unlicensed GPs who perform the procedure without proper insurance or authority.

Blood-based treatments

For Jehovah's Witnesses significant difficulties often arise in relation to their refusal, on religious grounds, to accept blood-based treatments. They were concerned that, because of this, they are stigmatised as 'martyrs' and 'child murderers', or are sometimes seen as 'having a death wish'. An interviewee from this tradition explained that he understood concerns about possible legal liability if blood-based treatments are not provided, and also the feeling among many health care staff that not giving blood hinders the possibility of helping a patient. At the local level, Jehovah's Witnesses have often taken the initiative in establishing hospital liaison committees in order to encourage consideration of available alternatives, including the provision of lists of surgeons who perform bloodless surgery. In one locality, Jehovah's Witnesses had donated cell salvage machines to the local hospital.

Chaplaincy services

A number of issues were identified in respect of organised support for religious and spiritual needs in hospitals. The provisions for chaplaincy and spiritual needs vary considerably from hospital to hospital, depending upon a variety of factors such as demographics, the size of hospital, and the resources available. Religious minorities have not had the tradition of privileged access that has more traditionally been available to Christian chaplains, although a number of hospitals had tried to accommodate the changing religious profile of the local populations (Beckford and Gilliat, 1996a, b). In this context, one chaplain drew attention to the complex problems connected with representation of minority religions on the regulatory bodies responsible for hospital chaplaincy. A Christian chaplain said he felt hospitals should be proactive and that they should apply for outside funding to develop their services. His hospital had set up various partnerships with lay religious organisations.

Study Activity 20.4 _____

- Taking each of the following issues in turn:

    - food in hospitals
    - clothing in hospitals
    - preparation of the deceased

– circumcision
– blood-based treatments
– chaplaincy services,

consider each one from the perspective of both the nurse and health care organisations.

Varieties of unfair treatment on the basis of religion

The project's interim report identified a framework for understanding the range of different experiences and dynamics that the overall phrase of 'religious discrimination' or 'unfair treatment on the basis of religion' can cover. A number of categories were identified, as follows.

Religious prejudice

'Religious prejudice' involves the stereotyping of particular religious groups such as that observed in the phenomenon described by Muslims as 'Islamophobia' (Runnymede Trust, 1997). Such religious prejudice does not necessarily of itself lead to discriminatory actions but it is possible for it to translate into directly discriminatory behaviour through decisions taken by individuals holding positions of power within the health care system. It can also result in indirect discrimination through the exclusivity of recruitment policies, employment practice and service provision.

Religious hatred

Attitudes of religious prejudice, when intense, can spill over into manifestations of 'religious hatred', which can result in intimidatory or violent behaviour towards religious minorities.

Religious disadvantage

Christianity, especially in its Established forms, has a privileged presence, sometimes as of right, and sometimes as a consequence of tradition, which is not available to other non-Established traditions. An example of 'religious disadvantage' can be found in respect of the provisions made for religious chaplaincy services in public institutions, including the health care organisations.

Direct religious discrimination

'Direct religious discrimination' occurs where there is deliberate exclusion of people from opportunities or services on grounds related to their religious belief, identity or practice.

Indirect religious discrimination

'Indirect religious discrimination' can be understood in terms of the exclusionary effects of historical decisions, contemporary structures or patterns of behaviour and organisation that have not been examined in the light of a current wider religious plurality. This can lead to culturally exclusive requirements and provisions in terms of diet, clothing, religious festivals and a range of other matters, which can, in turn, result in unintentional or unwitting discrimination against people of various religious traditions.

Institutional religionism

The neologism 'institutional religionism', understood by analogy with the Stephen Lawrence Inquiry (Macpherson, 1999) report's analysis of 'institutional racism', is an attempt to describe the endemic and structurally embedded forms of discrimination that can occur within organisations. This is the product of a combination of several factors into a mutually reinforcing environment and ethos. It thus occurs in a context in which 'religious prejudice', 'direct' and 'indirect' religious discrimination combine in the collective failure of an organisation to provide an adequate and professional environment and service.

Study Activity 20.5 ───────────

● From your own nursing experience, note down a specific example of each of the following dimensions of unfair treatment on the basis of religion:

  – religious prejudice
  – religious hatred

- religious disadvantage
- direct religious discrimination
- indirect religious discrimination
- institutional religionism.

GOING FORWARD: RELIGION AND THE DEVELOPMENT OF MORE INCLUSIVE HEALTH CARE

At the heart of any development of more inclusive health care must be the quality and the appropriateness of the service that is delivered to individual people who have entrusted themselves, or have been entrusted by others, to health care systems and organisations, and to the health care professionals working within them. Good care for people of varied religious backgrounds means that that care should be equitable. In order to achieve this equity, care needs to be offered from a perspective that takes seriously the distinctiveness of the whole person to whom care is offered. This includes key aspects of their cultural and religious identity, some of the implications of which can also be challenging to the identity, role and practice of professional carers. Some of these may be more immediately obvious than others – for example, issues related to dress, diet, gender traditions, hygiene and familial norms and the like. Other aspects may be less immediately obvious, but are often no less significant for the individuals being cared for; indeed, they are sometimes more significant. These aspects include their beliefs, values and spiritualities.

Study Activity 20.6

For a more detailed view of the very complex and varied religious traditions and practices, and the ways in which these interact with issues of inclusivity in health care, you should refer to the following resources:

- for short overviews and introductions to the major world religious traditions, their key beliefs, main traditions and movements, consult the website produced by the Multi-Faith Centre at the University of Derby, at *www.multifaithnet.org.*
- For information – written with the general professional reader in mind – on the world religious traditions and their community structures and organisations in the UK (including contact details for their organisations at national, regional and local levels), consult the directory of religions in the UK (Weller, 2001).
- For key background materials and a range of more detailed examples of how religions interface with issues in health care organisations and for health care professionals consult Henley and Schott, (1999).

Having a basic knowledge about a range of religions can lead to more effective care. Professionals are better able to avoid cultural and religious mistakes that can cause distress and offence and thus impede the healing process. Even small tokens of understanding and recognition can promote well-being. At the same time, a little knowledge can be a dangerous thing, especially when this leads to stereotyping (all Muslims believe 'x'), or when assumptions are made about an individual's degree of orthodoxy or observance within the religion with which they appear to be identified. Such assumptions, although often well-motivated, can lead to awkwardness and difficulty for the individuals about whom they are made.

As well as people who have an active involvement in the corporate life of their religious communities, the UK also has a significant proportion of people whose religious belief and practice is often described as 'folk religion' or 'residual Christianity'. Such people may turn to an active involvement in Christian religious life only, or mainly, at times of crisis or personal significance such as birth, marriage and death, or at religious festivals. Other religions also have followers whose religious observances are relatively limited. In relation to all communities there are in addition some individuals and groups who acknowledge their connection with a particular tradition but find themselves in conflict with its official representatives over one or other single issue, or across a whole range of ways of understanding the significance of their inherited or adopted tradition.

Compensation can be made, to some extent, for lack of information about religions, or aspects of their tradition and practice, by appropriately attentive listening and receptivity to the needs of those being cared for. Such listening and receptivity can also enable sensitivity to an individual's personal and unique positioning in relation to a specific religion and/or tradition within it. One of the best ways to learn what needs to be considered with regard to religion is to ask people from within the religious traditions to articulate the needs and concerns that they have. At the same time, because of their vulnerability, those who are within health care settings are not always in the best position to express their real needs and feelings. Responding sensitively and appropriately to individual needs often represents a starting point in engaging with the implications, for health care, of a religiously plural society. However, while the response of individual professionals to individual care issues in an ethnically and religiously diverse context is necessary, it is not sufficient. Sometimes it is necessary to go beyond those for whom one is already providing health care in order to consult with leaders and representatives of religious communities and organisations in order to discover what, from their perspective, appropriate and religiously inclusive care might entail.

Alongside the professional's development of individually responsive care, it is also important to examine the written policies and unwritten practices of professions, health care systems, institutions and organisations, and for such examination to lead to active consideration of planning issues in health care.

Alongside these structural and professional challenges and responses, it would also be wise to consider how the religious contexts and contents of health care either inform the nurse's professional identity and practice and/or impact upon it. Through the communities that transmit religious traditions, significant numbers of individuals have experienced religions as a constraint on their life opportunities and personal freedoms and/or as something that has been responsible for great hurt in their life. At the same time, religious traditions contain resources of practical wisdom, tried and tested on the anvil of experience throughout thousands of years, amidst great diversities of culture, place and time. They are a repository of experience from which millions of people find motivation, challenge, inspiration and a contribution to their well-being.

For both of these reasons, as well as for matters related to public policy, religion is an important factor to take account of in the provision of care for individual patients and their families. For health care professionals, the realities of sickness, the uncertainties of health – and particularly the inevitability of one's own death – cannot be avoided. Dealing with life, illness and death can pose profound questions and challenges (Hinnells and Porter, 1999). Some of these challenges – and especially those concerned with care of those who are dying – are challenging not only organisationally and professionally (Green, 1991a, b; Firth, 1993; Neuberger, 1994), but also personally (McGilloway and Myco, 1985). Therefore, alongside the *questions that are posed to religions* through the experience of health care practitioners in dealing with human suffering and death, and their impact upon both those who suffer this and their carers, and the *questions that are posed to professional practice* in terms of taking proper account of the place of religion in the lives of patients, their families and their communities, there are also *questions that the religions pose to both those experiencing these things and those who care for them.*

Study Activity 20.7

- In what ways might your professional practice as a nurse pose questions to religion?
- In what ways might religion inform your professional identity and practice as a nurse?

- In what ways might religion pose questions to your professional identity and practice as a nurse?
- Identify one health care issue where consultation with a religious group may result in the development of more inclusive health care.

REFERENCES

Abrams, M., Gerard, D. and Timms, N. (eds.) (1985) *Values and Social Change in Britain*, Macmillan, London

Ahmad, W. (1993) *'Race' and Health in Contemporary Britain*, Open University Press, Buckingham

Anwar, M. (1993) *Muslims in Britain: 1991 Census and other statistical sources*, Centre for the Study of Islam and Christian-Muslim Relations Papers, Birmingham

Bacal, A. (1991) *Ethnicity in the Social Sciences: A view and review of the literature on ethnicity*, Reprint Paper on Ethnic Relations, No.3, Centre for Research in Ethnic Relations, University of Warwick, Coventry

Balarajam, R. and Soni Raleigh, V. (1995) *Ethnicity and Health in England*, HMSO, London

Ballard, R. (ed.) (1994) *Desh Pardesh: The South Asian presence in Britain*, Hurst

Ballard, R. and Kalra, V. (1994) *The Ethnic Dimensions of the 1991 Census: A preliminary report*, Manchester Census Group, University of Manchester, Manchester

Barley, C., Field, C., Kosmin, B. *et al.* (1987) *Religion: Reviews of United Kingdom statistical sources*, Volume XX, Pergamon Press, Oxford

Barker, E. (1990) *New Religious Movements: A practical introduction*, HMSO, London

Barth, F. (1969) *Ethnic Groups and Boundaries*, Allen and Unwin, London

Beckford, J. and Gilliat, S. (1996a) *The Church of England and Other Faiths in a Multi-Faith Society, Volume I and Volume II*, Department of Sociology, University of Warwick, Coventry

Beckford, J. and Gilliat, S. (1996b) *The Church of England and Other Faiths in a Multi-Faith Society: Summary report*, Department of Sociology, University of Warwick, Coventry

Beishon, S., Virdee, S. and Hagall, A. (1995) *Nursing in a Multi-Ethnic NHS*, Policy Studies Institute, London

Benzeval, M., Judge, K. and Whitehead, M. (1995) *Tackling Inequalities in Health: An agenda for action*, The King's Fund, London

Brierley, P. (2000) *Religious Trends No. 2, 2000/01 Millennium edition*, Christian Research Association, London

Bruce, S. (1995) *Religion in Modern Britain*, Oxford University Press, Oxford

Commission for Racial Equality (1997) *Religious Discrimination: Your rights*, Commission for Racial Equality, London

Davie, G. (1994) *Religion in Britain since 1945: Believing without belonging*, Blackwell, London

Davey Smith, G., Bartley, M. and Blane, D. (1990) The Black Report on socioeconomic inequalities in health 10 years on. *British Medical Journal* **301**, 373–7

Department of Health (1991) *The Patients' Charter*, HMSO, London

Department of Health (1992a) *A Strategy for Health in England. The health of the nation*, HMSO, London

Department of Health (1992b) *Ethnicity and Health. A guide for the NHS*, HMSO, London

Department for the Environment, Transport and the Regions (1996) *Challenging Religious Discrimination: A guide for faith communities and their advisers*, Department for the Environment, Transport and the Regions, London

Dobson, S. (1991) *Transcultural Nursing*, Scutari Press, London

Donovan, J. (1984) Ethnicity and health: a research review, *Social Science and Medicine* **19**(7), 663–70

Durkheim, E. ([1915] 1947) *The Elementary Forms of Religious Life*, The Free Press, New York

Firth, S. (1993) Cross-cultural perspectives on bereavement. In: Dickenson, D. and Johnson, M. (eds.) *Death, Dying and Bereavement*, Sage, London, pp. 254–61

Geertz, C. ([1966] 1990) Religion as a cultural system. In: Bainton, M. (ed.) (1990) *Anthropological Approaches to the Study of Religion*, Tavistock, London, pp. 1–46

Green, J. (1991a) *Death with Dignity: Meeting the spiritual needs of patients in a multi-cultural society, Volume I*, Nursing Times, London

Green, J. (1991b) *Death with Dignity: Meeting the spiritual needs of patients in a multi-cultural society, Volume II*, Nursing Times, London

Henley, A. (1982) *The Asian Patient in Hospital and at Home*, DHSS/King's Hospital Fund for London, London

Henley, A. (1983a) *Caring for Hindus and their Families: Religious aspects of care*, DHSS/King's Hospital Fund for London, London

Henley, A. (1983b) *Caring for Sikhs and their Families: Religious aspects of care*, DHSS/King's Hospital Fund for London, London

Henley, A. and Schott, J. (1999) *Culture, Religion and Patient Care in a Multi-Ethnic Society: A handbook for professionals*, Age Concern Books, London

Hepple, B. and Choudhary, T. (2001) *Tackling Religious Discrimination: Practical implications for policy makers and legislators*, Home Office Research Study 221, Home Office Research, Development and Statistics Directorate, London (*www.homeoffice.gov.uk/rds/pdfs/hors221.pdf*)

Hinnells, J. and Porter, R. (eds.) (1999) *Religion, Health and Suffering*, Kegan Paul International, Kegan Paul, London

Hopkins, A. and Bahl, V. (eds.) (1993) *Access to Health Care for People from Black and Ethnic Minorities*, Royal College of Physicians, London

Jones, T. (1993) *Britain's Ethnic Minorities*, Policy Studies Institute, London

Macpherson, Sir W. (1999) *Stephen Lawrence Inquiry: Report, Sir William Macpherson's Inquiry into matters arising from the death of Stephen Lawrence on 22nd April 1993 to date, in order particularly to identify the lessons to be learned for the investigation and prosecution of racially motivated crimes*, 24th February, Cm 4262-I, The Stationery Office, London

Mason, D. (1995) *Race and Ethnicity in Modern Britain*, Oxford University Press, Oxford

Modood, T., Beishon, S. and Virdee, S. (1994) *Changing Ethnic Identities*, Policy Studies Institute, London

Modood, T., Berthoud, R. *et al.* (1997) *Ethnic Minorities in Britain: Diversity and disadvantage*, Policy Studies Institute, London

McGilloway, O. and Myco, F. (eds.) (1985) *Nursing and Spiritual Care*, Harper and Row, London

Nazroo, J. (1997a) *The Health of Britain's Ethnic Minorities: Findings from a national survey*, Policy Studies Institute, London

Nazroo, J. (1997b) *Ethnicity and Mental Health*, Policy Studies Institute, London

Neuberger, J. (1994) *Caring for Dying People of Different Faiths* (2nd edition), Mosby, London

Parsons, G. (ed.) (1993) *The Growth of Religious Diversity: Britain from 1945. Volume I: Traditions*, Routledge, London

Parsons, G. (ed.) (1994) *The Growth of Religious Diversity: Britain from 1945. Volume II: Issues*, Routledge, London

Peach, C. (ed.) (1996) *Ethnicity in the 1991 Census. Volume 2: The ethnic minority populations of Great Britain*, Office for National Statistics, London

Runnymede Trust (1997) *Islamophobia: A challenge for us all*, Runnymede Trust, London

Smaje, C. (1995) *Health, 'Race' and Ethnicity: Making sense of the evidence*, King's Hospital Fund for London, London

Weller, P. (ed.) (2001) *Religions in the UK: Directory, 2001-3*, Multi-Faith Centre at the University of Derby, Derby

Weller, P. and Andrews, A. (1998) Counting religion: religion, statistics and the 2001 census. *World Faiths Encounter* **21**, November, 23–34

Weller, P., Feldman, A. and Purdam, K. *et al.* (2001) *Religious Discrimination in England and Wales*, Home office Research Study 200, Research, Development, Statistics Directorate, The Home Office, London. (*www.homeoffice.gov.uk/rds/pdfs/hors220.pdf*)

York, M. (1995) *The Emerging Network: A sociology of new age and neo-pagan movements*, Rowman and Littlewood, London

FURTHER READING

Abrams, M., Gerard, D., and Timms, N. (eds.) (1985) *Values and Social Change in Britain*, MacMillan, London

Note

This section draws on text in the Home Office Research Study 220, *Religious Discrimination in England and Wales*, Research Development Statistics Directorate, the Home Office, London, by Paul Weller, Alice Feldman, Kingsley Purdam *et al.*, which is Crown Copyright, 2001, as well as on other research materials gathered in the course of the Religious Discrimination in England and Wales Research Project. Contributions to the publication were also made by Ahmed Andrews, Anna Doswell, John Hinnells, Marie Parker-Jenkins, Sima Parmar and Michele Wolfe. The authors and contributors also express their acknowledgements to the fieldwork informants and questionnaire respondents, whose experiences and views form the basis of the research findings. The views expressed in this section and the chapter as a whole are those of the author, and not necessarily those of the Home Office; nor do they reflect government policy.

21 GENDER ISSUES IN A NURSING CONTEXT

Lynn Basford

LEARNING OUTCOMES

After studying this chapter you will be able to:

- Explain the term 'gender' and itentify the main gender characteristics in humans
- Understand gender issues as they relate to work, and in particular, nursing work, drawing on sociological and feminist theories
- Discuss female gender identity and differences, as prescribed in psychological, sociological and feminist literature
- Identify and critique the concept of ways of knowing characteristic of a feminine perspective
- Discuss issues pertaining to nursing as a predoninantly female occupation and the implications of these issues for the work and professional status of nurses
- Identify issues of quality pertaining to gender and discuss the impact of such issues on nursing and health

INTRODUCTION

Throughout history the division of labour between men and women has been polarised, with women often undertaking work that is unpaid or badly paid and undervalued by men and by society at large. Inherent within the division of labour between men and women is the notion that men are strong and women weak; men are rational thinkers while women are subjected to emotional outbursts that are directly linked to their hormones and child-bearing biological capacity.

To assume there are no gender issues in any work environment is both naïve and false, given the evolution of social systems and divisions of labour. Acker (1989) made this point pungently clear when he stated that all social relations are indeed gendered and impact on every aspect of social phenomena. This includes the world of nursing. The profession of nursing is undeniably predominantly female; the role of the nurse is perceived socially and culturally to be a feminine one, intrinsically linked to the notion of human (feminine) caring values, and the domestic and nurturing role of women.

Militating against the recognition of nursing as a profession is the idea that it is a 'calling', that is, service-orientated and subordinated to male (medical) dominance (Chinn and Wheeler, 1985). The male dominance perspective in health care reflects a wider representation of women in all aspects of societal life – women are constructed around a system of social hierarchy and a political arena of male dominance and female subordination.

Feminist commentators assert that the link between women and the domestic environment is indisputably related to their sex. The social construction of femininity is an all-pervading aspect of women's lives, behaviour, attitudes, achievements, abilities and skills. They are usually defined in terms of marriage and the family. This condition reflects a patriarchal value system based on sex and gender, whereby the male is perceived as inherently superior to the female. Feminists contend that this position is reinforced by the fact that women's biological and physical differences are used to legitimate male dominance and female subordination.

Attempts to eradicate male dominance and provide gender equality have been a feature of British governments throughout the last four decades of the twentieth century. Nonetheless, the success of such aspirations has fallen significantly short; statistical information continues to demonstrate the gender imbalance at executive and management level in numerous domains.

BIOLOGICAL DIFFERENCE

Scientists adopting a naturalistic stance would argue that men and women have a very different biological make-up and therefore their place in society should be different. Others contend that this is a spurious argument, which overrides the nurture debates and the fact that all individuals, regardless of gender, have individual characteristics and personal attributes (Davies, 1995). Whilst the individualistic phenomenon is well recognised, both in the domains of psychology and sociology, it has not served to de-myth the stereotypical images that reinforce the positive value of men and the negative value of women.

The biological account of male dominance is based on the assumption that women are physically smaller and weaker, and therefore physically inferior, and dependent on men. The supposedly debilitating effects of menstruation, pregnancy and menopause reinforce this. The male biological traits became the yardstick by which to measure all humanity. As a result, women are not defined by their individuality, but in direct comparison to men. Firestone (cited in Eisenstein, 1988) makes the point that women's innate ability for pregnancy and lactation creates 'an inherently unequal power distribution' within what she terms the 'biological family'. For example, a child's dependence on the mother, initially created by lactation, is extended beyond the period of necessity and confines women to the domestic environment. It is a position that identifies women as closer to nature and, as a result, more suited to the private domestic world.

Men, on the other hand, are identified and described in the context of public life, where the culture of law, religion and politics prevails. The distinction between culture and nature is one of control; culture is an expression of the need to regulate whereby the male exerts his control over nature and, therefore, the female.

The nature versus nurture debate is a long-standing one. What is evident is the interdependent nature of both strands of the argument. The importance of women's 'natural' ability to bear children cannot be ignored. As Rich (cited in Day, 1985) points out, a woman's capacity for motherhood under-employs the female consciousness, femininity demanding instinct rather than logic and intelligence, selflessness rather than self-realisation. This idea suggests that breeding is a fatalistic and unquestioning attitude, and that the only awareness women possess is a sense of duty as wife and mother; in turn, this is believed to lead to a sense of guilt if they do not fulfil this natural role. Marriage is then considered to be a woman's true role in society, forming the legal, social, economic, emotional and sexual basis of male-female relationships. A woman's 'true' femininity may only be attained through child-bearing within marriage.

Any feelings of sympathy with the difference debate are problematic for feminists, both in theory and practice, given the fact that the acknowledgement of a distinct sexual difference has led to accusations of 'biologism' and 'essentialism' (Davies, 1995, p. 20). Nonetheless, it should be acknowledged that women have gained political ground based on their sexual differences and roles based on their reproductive capacity. Recognising gender difference is not so much wrong in itself, but the emphasis has been placed on the difference between men and women and not on the notion of masculinity and femininity. These are concepts which are identified as being 'non-gender specific', given that either sex can have a predominance of masculine or feminine attributes.

GENDER

The phenomenological process of gendering describes the ways in which humans engage with each other, and the social structures and organisations through which they live. Social structures exist within the private domain of family life and in the public world of work and politics. It is this separation of the private versus the public world of work that has allowed gender divisions to occur. Women, as child-bearers and child-rearers, are firmly positioned within the private world, while men have cemented a role that allows them to operate in the public domain. So far, the focus of attention has been the notion of gender difference, with a view that men and women are polar opposites and separately defined.

Such separation models exist within the context of western ideologies, but it could be argued that in the East a more complementary position is upheld. The Chinese philosophy of Yin and Yang, for example, projects the inter-relationship of the sexes, which are intertwined and exist because of each other, not independently of each other. This philosophy celebrates the diversity of the sexes, and promotes the rich tapestry of human life and human existence.

However, despite the romantic image, for most societies the division of labour reflects the powerful domineering male that is superior in all human functioning to the female. The complementary model is something to which sympathetic governments and societies can only seek to aspire.

FEMINIST THEORISTS

Feminists have attempted to explain the phenomenon of gendering through cultural and societal evolution as separate and distinctive paradigms of male and female identity. Davies (1998) cites three such women:

1 Nancy Chodorow, a sociologist, who provides an explanation from the position of feminist psychoanalysis
2 Carol Gilligan, a psychologist whose research identified different ways of thinking, acting and making moral choices characteristic of a feminine perspective
3 Rosalyn Bologh, a political scientist, who provides an understanding of the dynamic inter-relationship between the masculine and feminine and the way in which this serves to deny and malign the feminine attributes of

human functioning. Bologh also highlights the the masculinity of organisational develop-ment, a precursor of organisation construc-tions that exist today.

Nancy Chodorow

The work of psychoanalyst Sigmund Freud was pivotal to Chodorow's articulation and develop-ment of gendered personalities (1978, 1989). She calls into question the biological arguments and social psychological views and her theoretical framework debates the position from a sexual role valorisation, to one that acknowledges the complex relationships both at the individual and the organisational level of development.

From the individualistic perspective, Chodorow suggests that gender identity relates to the notion of self within the familial roles of family life and the nurturing (mothering) role. Drawing on psychoanalytical theories, she proffers the notion that all children begin their life through attachment and unity with the mother, gradually moving from this dependent position in stages, until the individual self emerges as a separate identity.

The process of moving from dependence to independence is a complex phenomenon and defies a simple explanation. It requires the process of disengagement that has an appropriate response at each stage. Should inadequacies be affirmed at any stage, this could have a disas-trous effect on the child's ability to mature into full adulthood. The process of disengagement is fundamental to the science and practice of thera-peutic psychoanalysis.

Pivotal to Chodorow's theory is the notion that the division of labour is indicative of the parenting process predominantly undertaken by women, which means that the period of attach-ment of girls is longer than that of boys. The logical outcome of this is the assumption that, because of the longer period of attachment, girls are much slower to complete their separation and development than boys. Chodorow does not uphold this view and offers the suggestion that, because the mother nurtures both girls and boys, the relationship patterns are fundamentally different, providing a distinctive development route. For example, girls model the mother's feminine roles in the innate knowledge that they are alike. In this sense the relationship remains principally a primary dyadic mother-child relationship, which allows the girl to experience merging and separation in the context of attachment, characterised by 'primary identification and object choice' (pp. 166–7). In contrast, sons are viewed by their mothers as male opposites and are encouraged to disengage from the pre-Oedipal relationship, thus reducing their 'primary love and empathetic tie with their mother' (pp. 166–7). The different engagement that the boy has with his mother formulates a defensive reaction that consolidates the ego (gendered) boundaries.

The daughter's experience with her mother is clearly very different from that of the son. The girl has a strong sense of affinity and empathy with the mother, which provides an opportunity to experience another's needs as if they were the girl's own. This experience provides a foundation through which the internalisation of unconscious sets of meanings, fantasies and image of herself can occur. The whole process becomes a framework of continuity, both with the girl's internal and external worlds. When she attempts to form a relationship with the father, the girl does this through seeking approval with the mother at each step of the way. The severing of the connection is therefore reduced, which also impacts on the development of the psyche. That psyche is more complex than that of the boy, since the boy has a much cleaner disengagement from his attachment to his mother.

Chodorow views the whole gendered process in terms of the ways in which girls and boys obtain their personality and psychological development from the process of attachment and disengagement in the formulation of a self identity. Others support her arguments, suggesting that infants acquire a sense of self through the process that provides a basis of differentiating girls from boys.

The theoretical discourse based on personality and mothering provided by Chodorow has its critics. Nonetheless, it provides a framework for others to develop and is useful in attempting to understand the nature of femininity and the position of women in society as a whole.

Carol Gilligan

Carol Gilligan (1982) moves the debate from the work of Chodorow to moral reasoning among men and women. Gilligan does not find a sympathetic resonance with Chodorow's psychoanalytical discourse, viewing the process as a negative account. Gilligan critiqued ten years of research and challenged the prevailing assumptions that female children were less equipped to have rational deductive abstract thoughts than boys were. The experiments used to support these assumptions suggested that, when given an ethical dilemma, 11-year-old boys would apply the kind of deductive reasoning that might be used to solve a mathematical problem. Girls, on the other hand, would appear less confident, and would articulate uncertainty, as if the answer could not be given in absolute terms. Instead of deducing that the experimental results supported girls' inferior and limiting ability to apply moral reasoning, Gilligan argued that the difference was based on two perspectives:

- 'the perspective of maturation as a process of developing the integrity of the autonomous self' and
- the 'connectedness and inter-subjectivity', which is based on a totally different world view (p. 26).

Boys and girls, according to Gilligan, formulate opinions that are different and of equal value and, as such, their views should not be judged in a hierarchical framework.

Study Activity 21.1 _____

Consider the following dilemma. Discuss it with a male and a female colleague for their solutions, then compare their responses.

John is married to Mary. They live in the USA, where social medicine is not the norm. Mary is dying from terminal cancer and desperately needs certain drugs, which would ease her pain and offer her a quality of life before her death. John has used all their financial assets for experimental treatment and has no further reserves. He ponders on whether he should steal the drugs from the local pharmacy, or just allow Mary to die in great discomfort.

- In your discussions, did both genders offer solutions that were similar?
- Did they rationalise their choice?
- Was there remarkable difference between the male and female maturity in thinking?
- Did your results strike a chord with Gilligan's theory?

Rosalyn Bologh

Sociologist Rosalyn Bologh (1990) shares a perspective that draws from the seminal works of Max Weber. During her process of awakening and understanding she moves away from his treatise, perceiving that his work is too limiting, but she does continue to share Weber's view that the public world is masculine.

Bologh goes on to raise the debate by claiming that children express two desires:

1 the desire for love, protection and consolation; and
2 the desire for power, action and ability to make a difference in the world.

The first desire is feminine while the desire for action is masculine, based on the notion of controlling one's life independent of others. The problem with having two options is that a choice has to be made. The choice of 'masculine' action embraces the public world but is empty of expectation, and a caring, nurturing environment. It commands independence, and rational deductive thought full of self-interest. In this context, the masculine public life contains ethical guilt. Bologh acknowledges that Weber ruminated this point but also recognised that men can engage with brotherly love and, in the pursuit of a common cause, can unite. In such instances, Weber claimed that one man stands above the other – the hero or leader who achieves greatness. However, the leader does not always operate from an altruistic position or with any deference to moral reasoning.

Weber argued that the choice of love and protection is an illusion and can only be acknowledged in the private world, where men protect women. In this world, femininity can thrive with unrepressed emotion. For men, femininity is undisciplined and should not contaminate the public world of order and structure.

From these positions, masculinity and femininity remain dichotomously opposed, with only the masculine characteristics displayed in the public arena. Conversely, feminine characteristics are repressed and can only be acknowledged through a veil of secrecy that is seductive and disreputable. Masculinity examined in the private world operates on different levels, from the dominant position of erotic love to a portrayal of 'manliness' that strives to gain affection and respect from women. The woman in turn offers the man devotion while he is affectionate to the cause.

Weber exemplifies the loneliness of the male world, which is often isolated, and highlights the difference of the public world of masculinity versus the private world of femininity. In the final analysis, masculinity is given meaning through the repression of femininity. From this position, the contempt, disrespect and fear of women can be explained from the evolution of societal and public life.

WOMEN IN EMPLOYMENT

Gender in organisational life

The bias relationship within the fabric and structures of organisational life has evolved over time, cementing the dominance of men at the very heart of organisations. From this position, men have been able to use their powers and influence, which has served to ensure the continuity of that dominance of men over women in the public world of work. Sometimes the process has been planned, using the biological arguments to support decisions that are made. On other occasions, the male 'genderisation' process has evolved in an insidious fashion, but it has nonetheless been effective. The implications of a gender-biased organisation are far-reaching, in that women are prevented from having equal opportunities, equal access and equal recognition within pay structures.

In the West, governments have persistently attempted to eradicate male dominance within organisations (including the National Health Service, which is a predominantly female workforce), to combat discrimination practices and provide a more balanced, egalitarian organisational framework. Frameworks have been introduced to enable women to have equal opportunities and to function on an equal basis at all levels of organisational life. Unfortunately, such policies and legislation have so far failed to have any major sustained effect. It is a circular discourse that is a travesty of justice towards women.

Any real changes in organisational gendered frameworks require detailed reflection, both on the theory and practice, to inform the present and provide a vision for the needs of the future – politically, organisationally and professionally.

Capitalism and industrialisation

Long before capitalism, a culture of femininity was already established within the fabric of society. The fulcrum of capitalism, however, rested on the separation of society by function. That is to say, the general signifier of productive work and labour became the wage, which distinguished between production for use and production for exchange, the latter being awarded higher status and financial reward. Furthermore, the introduction of a factory system, where production and waged labour became focused in one building or area, contributed to the separation between home and work, and, more significantly, between men's work and women's work. After the destruction of women's craft industry, women were encouraged to join the ranks of paid workers as a source of cheap and unskilled labour, usually on a casual basis. This situation required women to juggle the two worlds of home and work, and engage in the contradictions of both of them.

The nature of capitalism encouraged the sexual division of labour and increased male dominance in both economic and social relations, directing family and social needs, and, in so doing, subordinating them to the market economy (Braverman, cited in Beechey, 1991). Men controlled production, labour and wages. Domesticity confined women to an existence as unwaged, unproductive and undervalued members of society, financially dependent upon men. This created a financial contract based on moral obligation and duty, not law. Women's labour power (in the capitalist sense) no longer existed as a separate commodity; it was a duty that women were expected to perform out of love for their family.

Women were further disadvantaged in terms of gaining permanent access to paid employment through the 'marriage bar', which meant that women were required to leave any employment after taking their marriage vows. The operation of a marriage bar reflected the notion that a woman's primary role centred on child-rearing and domestic management. No consideration was ever given to the fact that many women supported their families and, as a result, were often compelled to take ill-paid, arduous jobs as home-workers, which had a detrimental effect on their health and well-being. Attitudes towards a married woman working were often hostile, because work outside the home was believed to be harmful to her natural primary role as wife and mother. The fact that constant pregnancies and heavy domestic work in ill-equipped homes had dire consequences for the health and well-being of women was never really considered (Hunt, 1988).

Study Activity 21.2 ────────

Read about Karl Marx's theories on capitalism.
- What is a capitalist society?
- How did capitalism change the nature of both women's and men's work?

The influence of two world wars

The two world wars of the twentieth century were instrumental in changing the status quo for women's employment opportunities. There was an overriding need for women to join the war effort, particularly in occupations that were previously classified as men's work. These were either in engineering and munitions industries, or in occupations that were newly created during the conflict. Furthermore, work opportunities were not solely for single women; married women were also invited to join the ranks of the employed. To enable this to happen, the government encouraged and facilitated workplace nurseries. There were no altruistic reasons for this action, nor any change in societal beliefs and attitudes; the motivation behind it was the simple fact that all women were needed to contribute to the war effort (Yeandle, 1984; Hunt, 1988).

At the end of the First World War, pressure was exerted both socially and politically for women to return to previous occupations, including employment in domestic work. Political pressure was exerted via benefits regulations and the enactment of the Restoration of Pre-war Practices Act. As Yeandle (1984) succinctly states, there was no acknowledgement of women's newly acquired skills, or recognition that there was any necessity for women recently widowed during the war to work and receive a reasonable wage. With hindsight it is easy to recognise that the government showed little consideration for the needs of women due to their changed situation. This lack of insight contributed to the extensive female unemployment that occurred after the First World War. Married women were encouraged back into the home while single women were directed either into domestic service, or caring and clerical occupations.

During the Second World War, the situation was similar, although the ideological climate had changed significantly. Professional and psychological reasons reinforced the idea that the woman's primary role was in the home,

nurturing the family. Women therefore retreated into family and domestic life, supported by rising affluence during the 1950s and almost full employment for men (Yeandle, 1984).

Study Activity 21.3

- Visit your library and find out about the types of occupations women were engaged in during the war years. In your opinion, did some of these occupations require heavy manual labour? If so, does this contradict the biological theories that women are the weaker sex?

- In the clinical areas, are there any tasks that are considered to be heavy? If so, can you list them? What do you know of height–weight ratios when moving and handling patients?

The post-war period

The post-war period was to see very significant changes and further developments in women's employment. First and foremost, demographic trends facilitated the return of more married women to paid employment, together with the decline in numbers of school-leavers and an economic survey that indicated that the prospective labour force fell substantially short of that required to reach national production objectives (Lewis, 1992). The demand for women's labour increased, but the prevailing ideology relating to the woman's primary role still existed, creating a potential conflict.

The important decision came from policy-makers, who perceived that women would be able to combine marriage and motherhood with a limited amount of paid work (Summerfield, 1984), without their home responsibilities being seriously undermined. Employers in a wide range of industries increasingly viewed the extension of part-time work as an ideal means of upholding this situation. Within this framework, feminist writing unquestioningly accepted the association of women with maternal and domestic responsibilities. Myrdal and Klein (1957) quoted domestic work, catering, social services and child-rearing as suitable part-time employment for women.

The trend towards part-time employment continued to increase: in 1951, the number rose by 12 per cent; in 1961 by 26 per cent; in 1971 by 35 per cent; in 1981 by 42 per cent; and in 1987 by 44 per cent (Lewis, 1992). Female part-time employment statistics in the UK demonstrate this shift, from 4006 in 1984 to 5124 in 2001 (Department of Employment, 2001).

The phenomenon of part-time employment was largely centred on the expansion of the service sectors, resulting in low rates of pay, poor conditions of service, and lack of promotion opportunities. Through this process, women and men were segregated in the workplace. It is this situation, according to Bruegel (1979) and Walby (1985), that has protected women from unemployment in times of recession.

Study Activity 21.4 ━━━━━━━━

Read the works of John Bowlby and write down your own analysis of how his ideas reinforced the role of women within the private sphere.

━━━━━━━━━━━━━━━━

Feminist perspectives

It is evident from reading the current literature that an analysis of women's position in paid employment defies a simple explanation. Evidence does conclusively identify the position of women within paid employment and their responsibilities for child-rearing and domestic management as mutually determined. This feature requires further examination of the biological and social aspects of the role of women in reproduction and their position in the labour market (Harris and Young, 1981). Feminist analysis from this period focused on the above concepts, but provided no more than a limited explanation.

Contemporary analyses have featured women's participation in paid employment and their representation within it. These studies are said to have been useful in explaining inequalities and for shedding light on the ways in which women's subordinate position in the workforce is reinforced or, as feminists claim, can be challenged (Redclift and Sinclair, 1991).

Throughout the 1960s, feminists focused attention largely on two theories that were derived from a sociological perspective: 'the dual labour market theory' and 'a reserve army of labour' (Hunt, 1988; Lewis, 1992).

Dual labour market theory

The dual labour market theory suggests that there are two labour markets. The primary labour market is characterised by high pay, job security, good working conditions, and favourable promotion prospects. The secondary labour market consists of lower-paid jobs with less job security, inferior working conditions, and few opportunities for promotion. Primary and secondary labour markets often exist side by side within an organisation, but transfer from the secondary to the primary is seen to be difficult (Yeandle, 1984; Beechey, 1987; Redclift and Sinclair, 1991). Both men and women can be found in the secondary sector, but research indicates that women are more likely to be employed in it.

Employers tend to ascribe characteristics to women that make them particularly suited to jobs in the secondary labour market. They are seen as easy to replace, as having less interest in gaining additional skills, and as being less concerned than men with the size of their wage packet, since men are expected to be the main breadwinners within families (Beechey, 1987; Hunt, 1988). The relatively low status of women in society, and their tendency not to belong to unions, weakens their position further and makes it especially difficult for them to transfer to primary sector employment. Once they have been recruited to the secondary sector, women are likely to remain in it (Beechey, 1987; Redclift and Sinclair, 1991).

The dual labour market theory moves away from looking at family life to explain the position of women in the labour market. It avoids concentrating on individual cases of discrimination, and stresses the structures limiting female employment opportunities. However, Beechey (1987) makes the point that this explanation focuses attention on the manufacturing model, which is inadequate for analysing the majority of women's work, particularly work in the state sector. She maintains that the theory fails to explain why women gain promotion less often than men, and why some women, for instance, in the textile industry, do skilled manual work and still receive low pay even though the work is similar to work done in the primary sector. Marxists and Marxist feminists criticise the model on the basis that it does not address the position of women in the workings of the capitalist economy as a whole.

Beechey (1987) maintains that monopoly capitalism has resulted in a progressive decrease in the skills required for clerical and service sector work, and retailing. According to Braverman, women have been drawn into these areas of work as the service sector has expanded, while the mainly male manufacturing sector has declined. The weakness in this explanation is the over-emphasis on decreasing skills, as not all women are in unskilled jobs (Beechey, 1987; Hunt, 1988).

Reserve army of labour

Beechey (1987) has developed a second strand of Marxist thought in order to explain the position of women in the labour market. Marx argued that capitalism required a 'reserve army of labour', that is, a spare pool of potential recruits to the labour force. According to Marx, because of their built-in contradictions, capitalist economies went through cycles of slump and boom; it was essential to be able to hire workers during the booms and to fire them during the slumps. Furthermore, in their pursuit of surplus value, capitalists tried constantly to improve the efficiency of their machinery. This condition reduced the workforce needed to produce existing products, but new ones were constantly being introduced. A reserve army provided the necessary flexibility to deal with these changes (Armstrong and Armstrong, 1988).

One of the main features of this framework is that a reduced level of wages is maintained, not only for the reserve army but also for all workers. This provides opportunities for employers to exploit the workforce (Beechey, 1987; Armstrong and Armstrong, 1988).

Occupational segregation

The theory of the reserve army of labour is a useful way of explaining some of the changes that have taken place in the twentieth century in the proportion of women in employment in Britain. For example, it would appear to account for the increased employment of women during the two world wars. The theory, however, cannot explain horizontal segregation in the labour market. It serves capitalism in times of recession and rising unemployment because women are cheap substitutes for male workers (Gardiner, cited in Beechey, 1987). According to the Equal Opportunities Commission Report of 1983, in the period of recession from 1971 to 1983 male employment declined from 13 million to 11.5 million, but female employment actually increased from 8.2 to 8.8 million. This increase was largely due to more women working part-time, supporting the notion that women do form a relatively flexible workforce.

These early studies have often been criticised for their subjectivity. Recent studies have engaged in a degree of empirical research to provide a more substantive analysis of the position of women in paid work. Some feminists have centred attention on theories of economics and argue that inequality in the position of men and women in work is perpetuated by a complex combination of factors. Cockburn (1985) and Game and Pringle (1984) suggest that the complexity of these factors arises because the labour market is not gender-neutral. It has inherent ideological features that are activated through the practices of male managers, unions, workers and women themselves. Consequently, economic theories concentrate on the changes in quantifiable variables such as wages, family circumstances, including age and number of children, pay bargaining procedure, the career ladder for the male worker, and the role of the worker within the primary sector.

Critics point out that this approach fails adequately to address the effects of the non-quantifiable causes of choices that people make – choices that, according to Redclift and Sinclair (1991), are made within the context of inequality. Women participate with men in the labour markets on an unequal basis because of persistent gender assumptions and an unequal distribution of power. In addition, it is suggested that economists fail to analyse ways in which labour markets are structured in terms of horizontal and vertical segregation. Cockburn (1985) supports this notion and claims that 'there is a never-ending articulation of work into new horizontal and vertical sub-divisions'.

It remains clear from reading feminist literature that no single theory is sufficient to explain women's position in the sphere of paid employment. Inequalities within paid work evidently continue to exist, with women predominantly occupying subordinate and low-status positions. From a historical perspective, men have shaped female history. The culture that surrounds them is masculine. The patterns of women's behaviour are influenced by values that assign them a subordinate place in public life. For women to ascend to public prominence in an equal power relationship with men, women have to believe that it is proper to participate in public life. Studies conducted by social scientists have indicated that women are less interested than men in politics or public life. Some claim it is a natural phenomenon and is congruent with the different roles played by men and women in society. On the other hand, feminists who say that this claim lacks foundation on serious biological research, reject the notion that there are natural differences between the interests of men and women. They prefer the construct that women's lack of interest in public life is rooted more firmly within the domains of the socialisation process, and is firmly entrenched within capitalist society.

EQUAL OPPORTUNITIES LEGISLATION

The Impact of Legislation

Over 100 years ago, John Stuart Mill wrote the following:

> *I believe that women's disabilities elsewhere are only clung to in order to maintain their subjection in domestic life, because the generality of the male sex cannot yet tolerate the idea of living with an equal. Were it not for that, I think that almost everyone ... would admit the injustice of excluding half the human race from the greater number of lucrative occupations.*
>
> (Cited in Hunt, 1988)

In the year 2003, governments, policy-makers, sociologists, feminists, psychologists and human rights activists continue to draw attention to the position of women in the labour market. It is poignantly clear that the position remains unequal and discriminatory. Davies (1995) points out that it is useless to focus attention solely on equal opportunities and equal access if the fabric of the organisation is left 'unexamined' (p. 44). She goes on to stress that women who do succeed in traversing the hierarchical ladder do so at tremendous expense to their personal well-being, doing things that no male colleague is expected to do (for example, the constant juggling of home, family and work pressures).

Equal opportunities legislation has had a limited impact on the unequal position of men and women in large organisations. For example, in the NHS, some 90 per cent of the workforce is female but the key positions are held by men. Legislation such as the Sex Discrimination Act has offered opportunities for men to access midwifery programmes within the context of equal opportunities between the sexes, however, Davies (1995) contends that this has had a limited value in balancing out equal opportunities for female nurses.

Problems with the legislation

Lewis (1992) draws attention to the fact that feminists have vociferously attempted to gain equal treatment and equal opportunities for women in the labour market, public service, tax and security laws. While there is evidence that legislation has attempted to address these issues, there is still a long way to go. In the 1960s and 1970s, great strides were made in this domain, marking the most significant of advancements for women since the 1920s (Carter, 1988). The changes in social attitudes were instrumental in bringing about such legislative reforms underpinned by the philosophy of social justice between all men and women (Benjamin, 1988). Nonetheless, the political rhetoric and government policy was not always for the benefit of women per se, but as a token gesture to gain useful political votes (Carter, 1988; Lewis, 1992). For example, the Equal Pay Act 1970 outlawed the explicit discrimination against women in terms of conditions of their employment. While there were some obvious benefits – narrowing of the pay differentials between men and women, sick pay, holidays and hours of work – the main obstacle in the way of true equality of pay was the fact that the woman had to demonstrate that she was doing work of a similar nature or equivalent to that of a man. With the segregation of work activities this was problematic in itself and woman were therefore unable to claim discriminatory practice.

The Sex Discrimination Act 1975, while a milestone achievement in terms of appointments, dismissal, promotion, redundancy, and access to training and education, was still ineffective in bringing about real, sustained change in employment practice. Carter (1988) suggests that one of the major factors in the ineffectiveness of the legislation was in the wide range of its scope, which made it difficult to enforce or monitor. Women also had difficulty in proving that discrimination had occurred, for example, that they had been overlooked for promotion. In addition, the woman was required to take a case against her employer, and this was untenable for most, who would fear reprisal or even loss of their job.

For the most part, discriminatory legislation against women has been ineffectual and, according to some feminists, has served to entrench the patriarchal power and dominance of men (Bottomley, cited in Atkins, 1986). Carter (1988) points out that the legislations were largely inadequate and full of loopholes, which successive governments attempted to redress with the Social Security Act 1975 and the Employment Protection Act 1975. According to Atkins (1986), these Acts did not really address the inadequacies of the earlier laws and remained in form only.

With hindsight, it is easy to understand that legislation can only be implemented if the attitude of society corresponds with government thinking. Lack of interest on the part of the public is rooted more firmly within the domains of the socialisation process of men and women, and can be seen to be a product of capitalist societies. The male commentary relating to equal rights for women is eloquently depicted by Secretary of State Patrick Jenkin (1979):

> *If the good Lord had intended us all to have equal rights to go out to work and behave equally, you know he really wouldn't have created men and women.*
>
> (Cited in Cooke and Campbell, 1982)

In recent years, changes in public attitudes have emerged in favour of promoting equality in the workplace. There is a greater representation of women in occupations that were previously male-dominated. Equality laws can only be an instrument of change and not a panacea, but they do add weight to raise debate and apply pressure to organisations to make changes that are more women-centred. Thornton's view of equality (1986) is as follows:

> *Only 'equal freedom' or 'equal consideration of interests' will empower the gender, but*

thus far no workable means has been found to achieve equality for women qua *women.*

(Cited in Lewis, 1992)

ANALYSING THE NOTION OF GENDER

Davies (1995, p. 44) suggests that a different approach is now required that challenges the ways in which masculinity and femininity are understood as cultural phenomena that are transferred to organisational life. Organisations should not be seen as 'gender-neutral spaces' that are occupied by specific genders, but as a 'social construction' of patriarchal values that verifies and affirms organisations. In Davies's view, gender is pivotal in explaining and understanding organisations, and, in order to do this, 'gender' should be seen as a verb. In this way, it is possible to speak of the 'gendering' of organisations and the 'gendered' character that is embraced within policies. Davies goes on to analyse the notion of gender from the following standpoints:

- gender on the surface
- gender and the logic of organisations
- the gendering of bureaucracy, and
- the gendering of profession.

Discussing gender in this way provides good opportunities for clarity of understanding.

Study Activity 21.5

Consider the work experiences of the women in your family – mother, grandmothers, aunts – and reflect upon them. Identify any barriers that inhibited their progression or career development. Consider, if appropriate, any roles that they took on during the war. Finally, compare their work experiences with your own.

Gender on the surface

The visibility of gender is all around – in speech, dress codes and physical appearances – so that it is possible to differentiate quite easily between the two sexes. This differentiation is reinforced through social norms and expectations, and has been transferred to the workplace, with job positions, roles and responsibilities that reflect a specific gender. The influence of gender at every level of public life is so pervasive that it often goes unnoticed, and organisations have been constructed to differentiate and separate women's roles from those of their male counterparts. The dominance of men has secured their position as rulers of the workforce, often occupying senior or high-status positions. For example, in the NHS, where 75 per cent of employees are women, the vast majority of senior positions are occupied by men. In 1991, the Equal Opportunities Commission identified that only one per cent of female doctors held consultant positions, while in nursing 10 per cent of employees were men, but that 10 per cent held a disproportionate share of senior positions.

The representation of gender throughout every fabric of societal activity serves to reinforce the gender divide. At the surface level, gender interactions both in the private and public worlds of work require closer examination and, according to Gherardi (1994), the continuous polarisation of the concept of masculinity and femininity needs blending.

Gender and the logic of organisations

The logic of organisational structures defies simple analysis, and, there has been critical thought on the subject, with the belief that gender is fundamentally a principle through which organisational logic is manifest. It is covert rather than overt and provides a medium of abstract thinking, which is gender-neutral.

Acker analyses the notion of the 'job' as a series of jobs, subsets and hierarchical frameworks. The overriding assumption is that the higher the hierarchy the greater the skill mastery and responsibility held. Organisations are structured in this fashion and great energy is expended with regard to recruitment, training and promotional activities, rather than assessing the composite skills of the workforce and realigning the organisational structures to correspond. The job, from this position, is abstract and yet it is this sense of abstraction and adherence to masculine construction of organisations and jobs that reinforces the gender roles and responsibilities. For example, a secretary (female) may have the skills, knowledge, experience and understanding to fulfil the role of her manager (male), but that would usurp his dominant position.

Jobs are modelled on men and their ability to be employed on a continuous full-time basis, supported in their domestic life by women. On the contrary, women are viewed negatively when it comes to the job acquisition, often perceived as operating transient behaviours that are subjected to the vagaries of child-bearing, child-rearing and the domestic world. In addition, the career woman does not usually have a supporting 'wife' to allow her to have undistracted time in periods of study, or to move jobs every couple of years for a decade or more, thus gaining a varied experience. Such male-centred organisational philosophies prevent women from accessing a career or job promotion. Even organisations that are largely female also operate from these assumptions, and there is ample evidence of this within the NHS.

Organisational (masculine) logic brings out and reinforces the notion of gendered identities. Hierarchical structures and career progressions are based on male values and male visions relating to how the workplace should be constructed. Fortunately for women, but unfortunately for men, the shortage of skilled manpower and the collapse of the traditionally male-dominated organisations (for example, the steel, mining and shipping industries), along with technological advances, have led to an increased demand for a flexible workforce with transferable skills. Women since the post-war period have excelled at flexibility, and can capitalise on the changes that are currently challenging the logic of male organisational structures that remain inflexible and are not women-friendly.

The gendering of bureaucracy

Organisations are synonymous with the notion of bureaucracy. The bigger the organisation, the more bureaucratic it is. The bureaucratic process can lead to delays, absurd decisions, ineffective communication and obstructive rules. The problems associated with bureaucratic empires are all too familiar and are experienced on a daily basis within the NHS.

The principal factor used within bureaucratic structures is based on the theories offered by social scientist Max Weber. Weber considered a past based on familial authority and patrimonial authority that assumed a personal allegiance to a master (with a man as master of the household and in public life). The dominance of the master could be capricious and volatile. Thus, a move to a framework that embraced rationality within a legal structure was considered to represent an advance in effectiveness, efficiency and in continuity (Pringle, 1989).

Within the bureaucratic organisation the posts of officers were structured hierarchically and rules were rigidly adhered to. In this sense, bureaucratic decisions were based on personal judgement of the officers and the application of the rules. Rules were said to enforce order and predictability, and this forms the basis of Weber's criteria, through which an analysis of organisations and management thinking may be undertaken (Davies, 1995).

The bureaucratic framework is based on commands from an authority figure. It is described as being non-compassionate and rigid, and following male logic in its execution. By contrast, feminists such as Jones (1993) suggest there should be a move towards a more user-friendly, compassionate and caring bureaucratic system, with the capacity to nurture. This would change the emphasis and encourage a system that would apply moral reasoning and moral judgement, based on the perceived needs of individuals operating within a climax of assistance and help.

Bureaucratic organisations are gendered in that they afford and reinforce male values, clouded by the idea that men have constructed ordered and rational frameworks from which organisations can operate. A cursory study of this premise reveals that it is merely another form of masculine rationale that excludes feminine values and thinking.

The gendering of profession

Bureaucracy and professional practice are often portrayed as being polar opposites, given the fact that a professional can and does operate autonomously without account of the bureaucratic machinery – for example, doctors working within the constructs of the NHS. However, a consideration of the evolution of the professions and organisational bureaucracy shows that there may be more of an affinity than is perceived, given the fact that professional groups, values and belief systems are constructed from cultural norms of masculinity (Glazer and Slater, 1987). In support of this, Gamarnikow (1978) found that professional identities were based on masculine values, with women seen in a supporting role; this construct is exemplified in health care, with the nursing profession (mostly female) by and large supporting the activities of (male) doctors. Witz (1992) identified the division of labour in health care as evolving from historical beginnings, where women have continued to be excluded. Women who did break through the 'glass ceiling', and managed to enter the male-dominated professions, did so on recognition they would have to relate to that gendering and gendered values.

Professions claim their professional status as a result of holding a body of knowledge and having mastery of a set of skills. Following this line of logic, it is clear that extending that body of knowledge and skills within the domains of specialism gains credibility and recognition. Medicine has followed this route in a reductionistic manner that does not serve the interest of the patient, who is more than the sum of his parts, but does enable the specialist to protect his empire through erosion of his knowledge (power) base by others.

Displaying emotion within the professional context is not approved as suitable professional conduct. Maintaining a professional detachment to the client or patient is accepted and encouraged, and commonly practised by the hospital consultant. Stivers (1993) suggest this is a subversive ploy to reflect the male characteristic and suppress female characteristics within the professional world.

Study Activity 21.6

- How many men are there in your study set? Within your organisation, how many senior managers are men?
- How many women study at university and what is the percentage compared to men?
- In your opinion, is there still a power relationship between doctors and nurses?

GENDER AND NURSING

Nursing is a predominantly female profession, operating within the 'masculine' organisational structures, values, bureaucracy and professional (male) dominance of the medical profession. Over the years, nursing's aspiration to be a profession has been a difficult challenge that has been complicated by its subservient behaviour towards its medical colleagues. Nurses have continued to play the 'doctor-nurse' game, acting in a subservient role to the doctor and, as a consequence, their knowledge and skill are less valued. The suggestion is that nursing is not a profession but merely an adjunct to medicine. Nursing, by definition and practice, is the feminine role that allows medicine to represent the forms of masculinity and male rational thought, which supports its power base of authority. Until recently, health and healing were reflected as the principle domain of medicine and nurses were instrumental only in implementing the doctor's instructions that would assure restoration of health.

Davies (1995, p. 61) contends that nursing's pursuance of a professional identity should reconsider its position and 'challenge the gendered basis of the concept'. She believes this is not so sacrilegious, recognising that nursing is striving to secure its own body of knowledge through research and evidence-based practice. Nursing has become more specialised, and has developed a level of competence at mastery level that is different from that of the male medical colleague.

Notwithstanding the above, there is a wind of change, both politically and professionally. Through the legal frameworks, nurses can employ a doctor, they can prescribe medicines (previously the sole domain of medical colleagues), and they can operate independently of doctors in new roles such as consultant nurses, triage, Nurse Direct, and in walk-in centres. These developments offer opportunities for the profession of nursing to change the balance of power, to influence organisational structures and values, and create a bureaucracy that is more women-centred, compassionate and caring. This can only be achieved if nurses rise to the challenge, deconstruct the gender stereotypes and provide frameworks for gender equality.

SUMMARY

The issue of gender pervades all aspects of human functioning and, as such, remains a complex phenomenon that is difficult to unravel. Sociologists, psychologists, anthropologists, politicians and feminists have all attempted to explain it, moving from the biological deterministic perspective of the sexes to the socialisation of the roles men and women occupy, both in the private world of the home and within the public arena.

Separation and segregation of men and women has become such a strong feature within the workplace that it has served to maintain, and, in some instances, increase the masculine dominance. On examination, organisations are constructed around male values, needs, language and role representations. Women, by contrast, occupy a supporting role, or, as in the traditional doctor-nurse relationship, a subservient one. Women who have attained a powerful position within an organisation have historically modelled themselves on masculine attributes and characteristics.

Changing this imbalance of power within the workplace has been a source of concern for several governments. Attempts to redress the balance through discriminatory Acts have raised a social conscience in relation to the plight of women, but the Acts themselves have been largely ineffective in changing organisational structures and attitudes.

Organisations and working practices are increasingly under scrutiny and many have to consider their structures, policies and value systems, moving from a male-centred domination to an approach that is women-friendly and in tune with the values that are associated with femininity. To achieve this, radical changes are required, with a workforce that is prepared to be flexible – as women have been in their work practices throughout the period of modernity.

The roles and responsibilities of professional groups working within the NHS are undergoing significant changes, with challenges to traditional working practices and the structure of the organisation. Time will tell if gender perspectives have changed sufficiently to allow true gender equality to exist.

REFERENCES

Acker, J. (1989) Making gender visible. In: Wallace, R. (ed.) *Feminism and Sociological Theory*, Sage, London

Armstrong, D. and Armstrong, D. (1988) *Political Anatomy of the Body: Medical knowledge in Britain in the 20th century*, Cambridge Press, London

Atkins, S. (1986) The Sex Discrimination Act: the end of a decade. *Feminist Review* **24**, October

Beechey, V. (1987) *Unequal Work*, Verso, London

Benjamin, J. (1988) *The Bonds of Love*, Pantheon, New York

Bologh, R.W. (1990) *Love or Greatness: Max Weber and masculine thinking, a feminist enquiry*, Unwin Hyman, London

Bruegel, I. (1979) Women as a reserve army of labour, a note on recent British experience. Cited in

Evans, M. (ed.) *Women's Question*, Fontana, London

Carter, A. (1988) *The Politics of Women's Rights*, Longman, London

Chinn, P. and Wheeler, C.E. (1985) Feminism and nursing: can nursing afford to remain aloof from the women's movement? *Nursing Outlook* 33, 74–7

Chodorow, N. (1978) *The Reproduction of Motherhood: Psychoanalysis and the sociology of gender*, University of California Press, London. Cited in Davies, C. (1998) *Gender and the Professional Predicament of Nursing*, Open University Press, Buckingham

Chodorow, N. (1989) *Feminism and Psychoanalytical Theory*, Yale University Press, London. Cited in Davies, C. (1998) *Gender and the Professional Predicament of Nursing*, Open University Press, Buckingham

Cockburn, C. (1985), *Machinery of Dominance: Women, men and technical knowledge*, Pluto Press, London

Cooke and Campbell (1982) *Sweet Freedom: The struggle for women's liberation*, Picador, London

Davies, C. (1995) *Gender and the Professional Predicament of Nursing*, Open University Press, Buckingham

Day, R. (1985) *The Changing Experience of Women*, The open University, Milton Keynes

Department of Employment (2001) *National Statistics*, DoE, London

Eisenstein, H. (1988) *Contemporary Feminist Thought*, Unwin, London

Equal Opportunity Commission (1983) *Women and Trade Unions: A survey*, HMSO, London

Gamarnikow, E. (1978) Sexual division of labour: the case of nursing. In: Kun, A. and Wolfe, A.M. (eds.) *Feminism and Materialism*, Routledge and Kegan Paul, London

Game, A. and Pringle, S. (1984) *Gender at Work*, Pluto Press, London

Gherardi, S. (1994) The gender we think, the gender we do in our everyday organisational lives. In: Rothschild and Davies, C. (eds.) Gender and organisational Life. *Human Relations* (special issue) 47(6)

Gilligan, C. (1982) *In a Different Voice: Psychological theory and women's development*, Harvard University Press, London. Cited in Davies, C. (1998) *Gender and the Professional Predicament in Nursing*, Open University Press

Glazer, N.Y. and Slater, M. (1987) *Unequal Colleagues: The entrance of women into the professions, 1890–1940*, Rutgers University Press, New Brunswick

Harris, B. and Young, S. (1981) *The Anthropology of Pre-Capitalist Society*, Macmillan, London

Hunt, A. (1988) *Women and Paid Work*, Macmillan Press, London

Jones, K.B. (1993) *Compassionate Authority: Democracy and the representation of women*, Routledge, London

Lewis, J. (1992) *Women in Britain Since 1945*, Blackwell, Oxford

Miles, R. (1998) *The Women's History of the World*, Paladin, London

Mitchell, J. (1974) *Psychoanalysis and Feminism*, Penguin, London

Myrdal, V. and Klein, R. (1957) *Women's Two Roles*, Routledge and Kegan Paul, London

Pringle, R. (1989) *Secretaries Talk: Sexuality, power and work*, Verso, London

Redclift, N. and Sinclair, T. (1991) *Working Women*, Routledge, London

Stivers, C. (1993) *Gender Images in Public Administration*, Sage, London

Summerfield, P. (1984) *Women Workers in the Second World War: Productive patriarchy in conflict*, Croom Helm, London

Walby, S. (1985) *Patriarchy at Work*, Polity Press, Cambridge

Witz, A. (1992) *Professions and Patriarchy*, Routledge, London

Yeandle, S. (1984) *Women at Work*, Tavistock, London

FURTHER READING

Acker, J. (1990) Hierarchies, jobs, bodies: a theory of gendered organisations. *Gender and Society* **4**(2), 139–58

Evens, M. (ed.) (1982) *Women's Question*, Fontana, London

Miles, R. (1989) *The Women's History of the World*, Paladin Books, London

Rosser, J. and Davies, C. (1987) What would we do without her? Invisible women in the NHS administration. In: Spencer, A. and Podmore, D. (eds.) *In a Man's World: Essays on women in male-dominated professions*, Tavistock, London

22 A NURSING PERSPECTIVE ON OLDER PEOPLE: THE PROBLEM OF AGEISM

Oliver Slevin

> *If an old man sees that you are really interested in his personal life, you will see a wonderful transformation take place in him. His eyes that seemed dull will light up with a new fire; his face will come alive with unexpected emotion. He felt that he had been thrown on the scrap-heap, and all at once he comes to life again, becomes a person once more. Just like the child, the old man needs to be spoken to and listened to in order to become a person, to become aware of himself, to live and grow. You will have brought about something that no social service can ever do of itself: you will have promoted him to the rank of person.*
>
> (Tournier, 1972)

LEARNING OUTCOMES

After studying this chapter you will be able to:

- Describe the concept of old age
- Define the terms 'labelling' and 'stigma'
- Discuss the concept of 'blaming the victim'
- Explain the concept of ageism
- Identify societal attitudes towards older people
- Discuss the attitudes of nurses towards older people
- Discuss the implications of ageism in health care and nursing practice
- Present strategies for combating ageist influences in caring settings.

INTRODUCTION

The above quotation is both enlightening and frightening. Tournier, a Swiss doctor, was the founder of what he called 'the medicine of the person', in which medical knowledge, psychological humanism and spiritual enlightenment were combined. Although he never trained as a psychiatrist and considered himself a general practitioner, he had a profound influence in the fields of psychiatry and psychotherapy.

At the time Tournier wrote *Learning to Grow Old,* the book from which the opening quotation is taken, he was in his mid-70s. He was speaking from the lived experience of being what we term in our society 'old'. His statement opens up to us a wealth of insight. There is a question of the older person actually having true personhood in the fullest sense. There is a comparison of the older person with a child. There is a suggestion that, as with a child, the older person needs to be sustained and thus – by definition – treated differently to other adults if his personal identity is to be protected. And there is a plea against the alienation and depersonalisation of older people.

In Tournier's statement there is both a strength and a weakness. Its strength is its claim for a recognition of older people as persons. Its weakness is in the need for such a claim in the first place. There is a suggestion that simply by being old an individual is at risk of not being a full person, of being 'thrown on the scrap-heap'. It is this risk, and indeed its reality, which is the concern of this chapter.

The chapter is also relevant to Chapter 41 which addresses gerontological nursing. The word 'gerontology' derives from the Greek root *geras,* meaning 'old', *geront,* meaning 'old man/person', and *logos,* referring to study or science. It therefore means, in its most precise sense, the science or study of old age. By such association, gerontological nursing is the nursing care of older people. The present chapter is concerned with a particular aspect of this study, the position of older people in society and the negative aspects of this position. It therefore more specifically addresses the topic of *social gerontology*.

To emphasise the concerns in this chapter, it is worth reflecting upon another term commonly met, the word 'geriatric' or 'geriatrics'. Here again the Greek term *geras* is combined with another Greek word *iatros* associated with doctor or medical. Geriatrics is thus the medicine of old age, and by association, geriatric nursing is another term for the nursing care of older people. However, because of all the negative associations of 'oldness', which we will address later in this chapter, the term geriatric has attained strong negative connotations. It is even sometimes used as a term of derision to describe an older person (with implications of physical deterioration, lack of mental competence and/or unhygienic habits). To avoid such stigmatisation, we have arrived at the more common usage of the term gerontology. Geriatricians (doctors specialising in the medicine of old age) now often prefer to describe themselves as gerontologists or gerontological specialists, and so too – as indicated above – we have gerontological nursing.

However, it is important to recognise that underlying the terms gerontologist and gerontological nursing there is a dual purpose. The first purpose, as we indicated above, is to escape the negative connotations associated with terms such as geriatrics. The second purpose is associated with a recognition that the problems of old age are not exclusively physical or medical but extend into wider concerns (physical, psychological and social). Furthermore, as older people are a discrete group with their own particular characteristics, the ways in which various phenomena (health, illness, social problems, etc.) present in this group differ to how they present in other groups. The perspective extends the traditional geriatric (medical–illness orientation) to the wider gerontological (study of old age) orientation.

At first glance, such an approach appears laudable. It does after all take a more holistic approach to old age and its problems. This is a necessary and positive development. But herein lies a problem. Illich (1976) has described how medicine has extended beyond dealing with illness (or lack of health) into other aspects of life. As a consequence issues that are seen to be (or claimed to be) in some way deviant or problematic are redefined as *medical* problems. As Illich (1976) termed it, medicine *expropriated* such phenomena. In this context we might argue that medicine and its sister professions and institutions have expropriated gerontology (which is specifically the *study* of old age and older persons), and under the guise of an apparently honourable and well-intentioned endeavour to be 'holistic', have claimed old age as a medical concern or a medical problem. The point here is not intended to undermine the use of 'gerontological' terminology in medicine and nursing, but rather to sensitise the reader to cast a critical eye on the medical and nursing discourses that adopt such terminology. It is important that a more holistic approach is taken to how health is defined and actualised in old age. It is also important that a more holistic approach is taken in situations where ill-health exists in members of this age group. But it is vitally important that simply being an older person does not become defined as a medical, or health, or social welfare problem in and of itself. This, unfortunately, is often the case.

OLD AGE

The age criterion

There are various problems in identifying who older people actually are and in defining old age. People speak of old age, the elderly, the aged, and – in the context of health care situations – geriatric patients. There is also a problem when such terminology acquires negative and stigmatising connotations. The term 'older people' has been adopted in this chapter, as it is a term currently popular, in an attempt to avoid such stigma. However, all these terms are to some extent problematic in that they do not clearly identify older people or define old age.

One common approach is that which defines this population as being all those who are eligible to receive a state retirement pension. In the UK, this is women who have reached their 60th birthday and men who have reached their 65th birthday. In Great Britain this totalled 9.82 million persons (18.1%) of the resident population at the 1991 decennial census. However, another more universally accepted benchmark is that of *all* people (male and female) who have reached their 65th birthday, i.e. the 65 years plus population, of whom there were 9.03 million in the UK as a whole at the time of the 1991 census. By the most recent UK Government statistics, updated in 2002, these figures remain confirmed. Therefore, using the age criterion, an elderly or older person is generally taken as being someone who is 65 years of age or older.

Biological theories of old age

Chronological age is, of course, a very crude way of defining old age. For others, old age is defined in biological, psychological or sociological terms. The biological viewpoint sees the essential changes of ageing as occurring at the cellular or subcellular level. For example, Curtis (1965) proposed a *somatic mutation theory* of ageing. This theory proposes molecular changes within body cells as a result of spontaneous mutations which are irreversible and which accumulate with age. In essence, the theory claims that after a period, cells wear out and die, with a consequent fate for the organism as a whole.

An alternative *immunological theory* of ageing was proposed by Walford (1965). This postulates that an undifferentiated immune response increases with age. In effect, with advanced years, the body fails to recognise its own cells and attacks them, producing the typical picture of physical and mental decline in old age. In this context, old age is viewed as an autoimmune reaction. That is, at a particular age the body starts to attack itself.

These theories are, of course, broadly in line with a chronological age definition of old age, as it is recognised that such biological changes usually occur or accelerate beyond the commencement of the sixth decade of life. Their general thrust is towards recognising that when we reach this age range there are bodily and mental changes which present a typical picture of old age as the individual reaches the final stages of life. As a consequence of cell level changes there are macroscopic bodily changes (dry wrinkled skin, lack of mobility, cataracts, teeth loss, etc.) and perhaps also a decline in mental functioning.

Study Activity 22.1

- List 10 visible body changes that, in your view, are characteristic of old age.
- Consider each of your 10 items and decide whether they are in fact exclusive to older people.

Social and psychological theories of old age

In contrast to exclusively biological theories, there are psychological and sociological theories of ageing which emphasise environmental and psychic as well as biological influences. The most controversial of these is probably that known as *disengagement theory* proposed by Cumming and Henry (1961). This theory states that society and the individual always seek to maintain themselves in equilibrium to avoid disruption. The older person thus prepares for the ultimate disengagement of death by a mutual and accepted disengagement from society. In simple terms, the individual wishes to withdraw from society, society wishes him to withdraw, so he does so gracefully and with minimum disruption to the social order. This in essence involves a relinquishing of social roles, a reduction in social activity and the severing of actual and affective (emotional) ties with other members of society. According to this theory, old age is a state of social withdrawal in preparation for the ultimate withdrawal of death.

Study Activity 22.2 _____

- Using a library search and the above comments, write up a brief 200-word description of the disengagement theory.
- Carry out a similar library search on the topic 'medical model' and write up a brief 200-word description of this.
- Assume that the nurses on an elderly care ward subscribe to the disengagement theory and the medical model as opposed to an alternative nursing model of care. In a further 200 words describe how you think these nurses would approach the care of their patients.

A major criticism of disengagement is presented in the antithetical activity theory of old age as proposed by Havighurst (1963). This theory assumes that the natural success of old age is to remain active and to replace previous centres of activity, such as work and politics, with new forms of activity which compensate for such losses. According to those who subscribe to this view, high morale and life satisfaction are correlated with social integration. The argument here is that social disengagement is not the natural career in old age. Indeed, it is suggested that disengagement is both undesirable and unhealthy. According to this theory, old people are not, and indeed should not be, socially isolated and inactive. Instead, they are characterised as people who occupy active but alternative lifestyles to the young. They usually do not still work, but they may be active in leisure pursuits or community work. While they may be less active physically, they do indulge in recreational, religious and family life. In brief, older people are not those who disengage, but are people in the latter years who indulge in an active, albeit more sedentary, daily life.

A question can be begged here as to why older people should even find themselves occupying such sedentary lifestyles. Why should older people who are healthy and active retire from work? Why is it assumed that their leisure time is taken up with less physical recreational activities – bowls rather than football, watching television rather than dancing, walking the dog rather than hunting and fishing? This can, in part, be explained by socialisation processes and what has become known as the *role theory* of old age proposed by Rosow (1974).

According to role theory, in more primitive societies property, strategic knowledge and productivity accumulated to the old who thus held power. The young depended on the old as the holders of wealth and wisdom, while older people increasingly depended on the young for physical support and sustenance as they became increasingly frail. There was thus mutual dependency. It was also often the case that in such societies religion, tradition and kinship retained older people in a venerated social position. However, in modern Western societies these situations are to a large extent reversed. There is often a diffusion of property ownership across the population, and ownership and management are largely separated. Such is the speed of change that traditional knowledge becomes obsolete and new knowledge is held by the young rather than the old. With advances in new knowledge and new skills, the older person becomes obsolete in the workplace. With the separation of work from home, mobility becomes more important and advantages the physically more mobile younger person. Religion and tradition are no longer major forces in what has increasingly become a 'youth' culture. There is in fact a shift in institutional power from the old to the young.

Role theorists suggest that in modern societies these changes impose a marginalised position on the elderly. Rosow (1974) suggested that these trends are characterised by the following:

- *Devaluation* – the status of the older person as a non-worker, non-vital member of the social group, whose knowledge, values and general abilities are largely redundant, comes to the fore. This is reflected in the wider social group's negative attitudes, relative indifference towards, or even overt rejection of older people.

- *Stereotyping* – predominantly negative characteristics are often attributed to older people as a group. Such opinions are usually strongly held and seldom questioned, even though they are largely unsubstantiated.
- *Exclusion* – older people are often actively excluded from equal opportunity for participation in many areas of social life, e.g. work, politics, community and recreational activities.
- *Role loss and role ambiguity* – while previous roles such as worker, community leader, union official, etc. are removed, there is little activity prescribed or acknowledged for old age, other than inactivity. This lack of a prescribed, required or recognised social role can generate as much ambiguity, anxiety and strain as can the conflicting role pressures (e.g. between work and family commitments) of younger life. Indeed, most younger people probably cannot even visualise what it would be like to have no recognised role in society whatsoever.
- *Youthful self-image* – in the absence of a clearly prescribed role and in the face of devaluation, exclusion and negative stereotyping, the older person sometimes rejects the older person reality for a more tolerable self-image, which sees himself as a younger person. This aspiration to youthful status indicates a discrepancy between the older person's perspective and those of younger people and even many other older people. This can lead to strained relationships and to such older people being subjected to ridicule and rejection.

Old age is thus characterised as a situation in which strong social pressures direct the older person towards a marginalised peripheral position in society. As Cavan (1962) states, 'we have a man still motivated by his old self-conception, but separated from his previous roles and many of his previous evaluative groups. He is a true social isolate'. He is, in terms used by Cavan, in a situation which can best be described as 'rolelessness'.

Overview

It may be hoped that the outcome of the above comments would be a clear-cut definition of what old age – and thus elderly or 'older people' – actually means. This, regrettably, cannot be the case. There is no generally accepted definition of old age. There is instead a lack of consensus and a variety of often conflicting views. However, on the basis of the above comments, it is possible to suggest a listing of descriptive statements which at least give a general notion of the characteristics generally or often contained in our conceptualisations about this phenomenon. On this basis, old age is:

- membership of that section of the population who are 65 years of age or older
- the stage in the lifecycle, usually commencing in the mid-60s or later, when the effects of biological decline become apparent in terms of physical and possibly also mental frailty
- a state in which, as a result of the above two conditions, there is a mutual disengagement of the older person from society, and society from the older person – or, in opposition to this – a state in which the older person retains an active and full lifestyle, albeit involving different activities to those of the younger adult population
- a stage at the latter part of the lifecycle when a person is denuded of former social roles and exists in a state of relative rolelessness, sometimes made anxious by a lack of any recognised or prescribed role within the wider social group.

Study Activity 22.3

- Ask six of your fellow students or colleagues to write down their definition of old age.
- Determine the common elements in the six definitions and analyse how each of the six definitions fit in with the above descriptive statements.

LABELLING

In the role theory perspective above it is suggested that as a result of devaluation, stereotyping and exclusion, older people are forced into roleless positions. It is important to understand the processes by which this state of affairs can come about. This can be approached through a consideration of the process of social labelling postulated within the perspective known as the sociology of deviance (*see*, for example, Rock and McIntosh, 1974). *Labelling theory* describes how a number of factors in sequence and in combination lead to negative labelling of a group or individual. This tends to run as follows.

First, there is the dominant social group which by virtue of numbers and/or power controls the norms and values or moral position of a society.

Second, the dominant group has concerns or anxieties in various areas. Sometimes these achieve the level of what Cohen (1972) described as *moral panics*. In Cohen's study, people viewed what in essence were petty skirmishes between rival youth cultures in the 1960s as a major threat to the social order. These skirmishes occurred between 'mods' – young people who dressed in suits and duffel coats and rode motor scooters – and 'rockers' – young people who wore black leathers and rode motor cycles. Both groups and their skirmishes were built up into major social problems, the groups being viewed as evil devils by many (Cohen's book is entitled *Folk Devils and Moral Panics*). In more recent years, moral panics have developed in regard to social problems such as Aids. In regard to older people, the moral panic is that the older population will become more numerous and will impose intolerable burdens on society and its health and social care systems.

Third, the social or moral concerns become associated with or attached to certain individuals or a social group. They are the cause of the social problem; they *are*, in effect, the social problem. This requires that the social group is easily identifiable. That is, they may dress and act similarly (as in the case of mods and rockers), they may have a specific health disposition (such as Aids or mental illness), they may be of a particular ethnic background (be Jewish or black), or they may have some other clearly discernible social characteristics (such as being Protestant, Catholic, poor, female, or elderly).

Fourth, the identified group is not only discernible from, and thus different in some ways to, the dominant group, but is smaller in terms of numbers and/or power. In this sense it is by definition a *minority group* and thus susceptible to the influence of the larger group. Often this setting apart occurs in actuality, in that the group is socially and perhaps also physically set apart from the majority group or society as a whole. In sociological terms it is described as an *outgroup*. Its members interact more with each other than with people outside the group and gradually develop their own internal social networks, social life, values and beliefs, codes of behaviour, etc. They in fact develop their own culture or, as it is described by sociologists, their own *subculture*.

Fifth, the minority group is blamed for the social problem. In some circumstances this is relatively straightforward, as in situations where the moral panic relates to crime waves. The individuals are criminals, to be caught and punished. However, even when blame cannot be applied in a straightforward way, as may be the case with the mentally ill or older people, a *form* of blame is still attributed. Ryan (1971) describes this phenomenon as *blaming the victim*. Here, while liberal thinking refuses to sanction the individual or minority group in any punitive manner, those affected are seen to be victims of misfortune. The misfortune is still centred in them and as such they are still viewed as inferior and must be treated in some way. Ryan (1971) states:

> *Victim-blaming is cloaked in kindness and concern, and bears all the trappings and statistical furbelows of scientism; it is obscured by a perfumed haze of humanitarianism . . . . In this way, the new ideology is very different from the open*

prejudice and reactionary tactics of the old days. Its adherents include sympathetic social scientists with social consciences in good working order, and liberal politicians with a genuine commitment to reform. They are very careful to dissociate themselves from vulgar Calvinism or crude racism; they indignantly condemn any notions of innate wickedness or genetic defect. 'The Negro is not born inferior,' they shout apoplectically. 'Force of circumstance,' they explain in reasonable tones, 'has made him inferior.'

(Ryan, 1971, pp. 6–7)

Sixth, once the problem is identified and linked or attributed to the minority group, they are labelled accordingly. They are criminals (evil and destructive), or Aids sufferers (contagious, unclean and degenerate), or mentally ill (dangerous and unpredictable), or elderly (a social burden, lacking in competence, mentally and physically infirm). This label normally has two characteristics:

- It possesses *stigma*. That is, the person or group is viewed as being in a position of negative characteristic or disgrace. In this regard Goffman (1970) speaks of blemishes of character (e.g. criminal behaviour), abominations of the body (e.g. deformities or contagions such as Aids) and tribal stigma (e.g. regarding race, nationality, religion).
- It is characterised by *stereotyping*. This is the application of rigid, biased and inaccurate beliefs to the individual or their minority group. Such beliefs are usually not based on accurate perception and factual evidence, and indeed do not stand up to rational scrutiny. Yet they are held to be true by a significant proportion of the majority group. It is possible to apply stereotypes to people that are positive and valuing. For example, clergymen may be stereotyped as saintly people of high moral standing (even though this is often not the case). However, where such a belief is not only inaccurate and illogical, but also of a clearly negative,

devaluing and hostile nature, the term 'prejudice' is used. Thus, older people may be viewed as dirty, undependable, incompetent, slow, mentally infirm, etc.

Seventh, labelling is more than the attributing of a label, it is a process. This process can be explained in terms of the sociological–social psychological discipline known as symbolic interactionism. This is largely based on the work of George Herbert Mead (1934) and his concept of *taking the role of the other*. The suggestion here is that a person's role grows out of his interaction with *significant others*. The individual observes what these significant (influential or powerful) others expect of him, how they expect him to behave, and this exerts a powerful influence upon him to act accordingly. He in effect *takes* his role *from* the significant others. While this interactive influence is involved in all role development, it also applies in regard to deviant roles or roles expected of people who are labelled as members of minority groups. Using the example of disengagement theory discussed earlier, it could be argued that if the dominant group adopts this perspective and expects older people to disengage, there are powerful social pressures on older people to conform, even if this is not their personal choice.

Eighth, in labelling situations, the simple process of accepting the prescribed position, the role designated by the significant other (which in this case may be the dominant social group) operates as a vicious circle. The person adopts the role expected of him. As an older person he retires from work and politics, becomes less active in community and social life, accepts a dependent rather than independent social role. He may actually initially be capable of continuing in work and a more active life. However, by accepting the prescriptions and living according to them, he soon starts to 'fit the bill' in these regards. He actually *does* become dependent, incapable of work, less able to be active in community and social life. Within the vicious circle, this confirms society's stereotypes of older people and places even greater pressures on them to conform to the dependent role; it becomes virtually impossible to do anything else. In effect, the stereotype starts to become a reality. This conversion of socially constructed expectations into reality is known as the *self-fulfilling prophecy*.

AGEISM

Ageism defined

Ageism is the direct result of negative labelling. It cannot occur unless this negative labelling occurs first. That is, there must be stereotyped, prejudiced views held by the majority group (the society) or a major part of it, towards the minority group (the elderly). But stereotyping and prejudice are about negative beliefs; thinking, not doing. Robert Butler (1969), who coined the word ageism, emphasised that it is also about *negative action*. That is, it is a tendency to *discriminate* against older people and the actual realisation of this discrimination within the particular social system. As suggested by Levin and Levin (1980) and Blythway (1995), the realisation of this discrimination may take various forms of victimisation, from social isolation and segregation, through to legal or moral sanctions, and even direct injury.

On the basis of the above comments, ageism is defined by the following statements:

- It is directed towards a target minority group – older people.
- It is shared by the majority or is institutionalised.
- It is characterised by negative stereotypes – prejudice.
- It involves negative punitive action – discrimination.

It is not enough simply to define a term such as ageism. Defining something does not necessarily prove that it exists! The concept depends on whether older people are a clearly defined homogeneous group who are seen to present social problems for the majority and who through a process of labelling can be subjected to stereo-

typing, prejudice and discrimination. Some argue that this is indeed the case. Others question the claim. For example, Victor (1994), referring to the claim that older people are an identified subculture with ascribed negative characteristics, states:

> *The obvious weakness of this view is that the theory does not apply universally for the elderly are a highly diverse group. Some older people are ascribed considerable power and prestige in areas such as the law and politics. Additionally, though poverty is common in old age, not all the elderly are poor (Walker, 1980; Falkingham and Victor, 1991). Neither are the elderly characterized by residence in age-segregated communities, or by patterns of social interaction confined within their own social groups. Thus, given the heterogeneous nature of the elderly population, this perspective is of only limited utility as a conceptual framework.*
>
> (Victor, 1994, p. 39)

However, it is important to note here that Victor is stating that the perspective is of 'only limited utility'. She is not disclaiming its existence to a greater or lesser extent. In stating that 'though poverty is *common* (author's italics) in old age, not all the elderly are poor', she is recognising some degree of inequality and disadvantage. This is almost like saying that because not all women or black people are disadvantaged the notion of discrimination in regard to these groups is of limited utility.

The limited utility suggested by Victor is perhaps better understood in terms of the nature of the social processes at play in regard to minority groups such as women, ethnic groups or older people. These processes are often subtle or even covert in their manifestations. For example, women or older people are not small groups numerically. But they are often minorities in terms of the limited power they hold and the social pressures placed upon them to conform to stereotypes. Women may, like Victor's older people, appear to be a heterogeneous group;

there are, after all, female barristers as well as housewives and office cleaners. But when women aspire to be company directors rather than secretaries, or to break the male mould by being the bricklayer rather than the tea-lady, the social influences become less subtle. And, while we *do* have female barristers and judges within our legal professions, the prospect of the first female Law Lord (the highest echelon of the UK legal professions) is only emerging in 2003.

There are indeed older people who are still active in areas such as the law – High Court judges in their late 60s. But what of the butcher, the baker, the candlestick maker who wishes to continue working at 66 or even 76 years of age, and is quite capable of doing so? For the majority of older people, the right to continue working has in fact been taken away in Western society (although this is not so in other societies, such as Japan). In accordance with the stereotype and the dominant social order, the work role is removed at age 65 years, if indeed not well before this time. This is not, or at least seldom, done forcibly. It does not need to be so overt. Through the process of labelling and conformity to social expectations, the older person, like the proverbial criminal caught red-handed, accepts that it is 'a fair cop' and goes quietly! He is essentially in a no-win situation. If he goes quietly, he accepts the label of retired, inactive older person and enters the inactive or alternative activity world of the aged. If he refuses to go, he is labelled differently, as a social misfit and a disruptive social influence. He runs the risk of being forcibly evicted from his workplace, perhaps even of being labelled as mentally unstable.

The sources and abuses of ageism

Ageism as an issue in modern society arises from the sources of the phenomenon and the abuses it leads to. As has been explained in the discussion of labelling theory and the definition of ageism above, these elements are inextricably connected. First a problem is identified, second beliefs and attitudes arise in relation to it, and third action is taken in an attempt to address or solve the problem. The sources of the phenomenon – the

problem identification, beliefs and attitudes – determine the action. If the problem is seen as one of threat to the well-being or survival of society, and if the beliefs and attitudes are negative in their orientation and in fact amount to prejudice, the action is in turn inclined to be negative and to emerge as abuse or discrimination. It is useful in this context to address the problem, the beliefs or attitudes, and the abuses which arise.

The problem

Older people have not always been considered a problem. In earlier times there were fewer older people and they were essentially integrated with and a part of the wider society. Indeed, within the community and the family group they played a central and important role. They continued to work until they were less able. They were a source of wisdom and guidance to the young. They cared for the children when the younger adults engaged in more strenuous labour.

However, by the twentieth century, older people began to present as a problem in modern society. There has, of course, been a sustained increase in the population of over-65s since the turn of the twentieth century. The increases, with projections carried through to the year 2031, are presented in Table 22.1.

Table 22.1 Increases in the 65 years plus population in the UK

Year	Population (millions)
1901	1.8
1931	3.4
1951	5.5
1971	8.5
1991	9.0
2001	9.2
2011	9.7
2021	11.0
2031	12.6

(From Department of Health, 2001)

In effect, after the population of older people (those at 65 years plus) remaining constant at 6 or 7% of the total population since the middle ages, it soared to approximately 14% by the 1990s. However, the concern has not just been with the overall increase, but with the increase in what has been described as the older elderly within this age group, i.e. those in the 85 years plus age range. This particular increase reflects improvements in living standards and health care. But it also is taken to represent a significant problem for the health and social care services, as there are many more frail older people in this age range. For example, Carstairs (1981) has estimated that over two-thirds of those in this age group would suffer some degree of disability with approximately one-fifth being severely disabled or bed-fast.

With an increasing proportion of the population not involved in production, the demands on the economy in terms of state pensions and welfare services, and the demands on health and personal social services particularly from the 85 years plus age group, major problems are anticipated. This situation has in some cases reached the proportions of moral panic, as described earlier. Some people even suggest that the demands placed on society by older people will seriously undermine the wealth and living standards of the remainder of the population, and bring the National Health Service and personal social services to their knees. Thus, a social problem – older people – has become recognised and perhaps even amplified by moral panic and scare-mongering.

The attitudes

Attitudes are primary sources of social action. As defined by psychologists, attitudes consist of cognitive, affective and behavioural elements. Each attitude comprises:

- *cognitions* or *beliefs* about persons, objects, institutions or issues
- *affects* or *feelings* about these persons, objects, institutions or issues
- *behavioural tendencies* that are in line with the attitude's cognitive and affective elements.

Thus, an individual may believe that older people are dirty and unhygienic (cognition), may feel that they are smelly and unpleasant (affect), and may avoid drinking from utensils used by them (behaviour).

It is thus not surprising that if negative beliefs about older people arise out of seeing them as a social problem, societal attitudes towards them may also be negative. There is in fact research evidence to support this. In what has become the classical study in this area, Tuckman and Lorge (1953) administered an attitude inventory to university students and found a significant presence of negative stereotyped attitudes towards older people. Subsequent studies by Drake (1957), Kogan (1961), Campbell (1971), Harris (1975), Baker (1978) and Slevin (1991), all point to negative attitudes and stereotyping. The studies by Campbell, Baker and Slevin are of particular interest as the subjects were nurses. Campbell (1971) utilised the Tuckman and Lorge attitude inventory and found similar negative attitudes among nurses as those discovered among other adults and – through the use of a Nurses Preference Scale – identified a significant preference among nurses for working with younger adults. Slevin (1991), using a purpose-designed inventory, also found that nurses exhibited negative attitudes. However, it was found here that as young women entered nurse training, proceeded through this training and subsequently gained experience in working with older people, their attitudes became progressively more negative. This would seem to suggest that exposure to and socialisation into elderly care situations strengthens negative attitudes and stereotyping.

Study Activity 22.4 _____

You will need five to six fellow students or colleagues to assist you with this activity. You will also need a pencil and paper. Seat your colleagues in a circle. Tell them you are going to present a phrase and then go around the group asking each person to utter a word in response to this phrase. They are not to think about it, just utter the word that comes immediately to mind. State the phrase 'old people' and go around the group clockwise. Allow no-one time to think; if an individual has a block, go immediately to the next person. Go around the group several times, writing down each word uttered, and do not stop until the group is starting to dry up. This technique is known as 'brainstorming'. When you have finished you should have between 30 and 50 words. List these words under three columns headed 'Positive', 'Neutral' and 'Negative'. Are there more negative words such as dirty, frail, deranged, undependable than positive words such as good, loving, wise, understanding? Even if there are as few as 10–20% of the total words in the negative category you should reflect on the extent of negative attitudinal viewpoints this may reflect in your group.

The discrimination and abuse

The argument, thus far, runs as follows. Older people are a social problem, society in general holds negative attitudes towards them, there is thus a tendency to *behave* negatively towards older people. This is in fact the *prejudice* component of ageism, as defined earlier. The question is, does the action component of ageism, the *discrimination*, then become a reality? Are older people discriminated against, are they abused in any way?

The possibility of older people actually being abused came to notoriety in the 1960s with the publication of the controversial book entitled *Sans Everything* by Robb (1968). This work presented a virtual litany of examples of actual physical and mental abuse of older people by staff in elderly care institutions. The resulting furore was heightened by a number of public enquiries into abuse in hospitals and elderly care institutions throughout the 1960s and 1970s. There is no indication that today such problems are disappearing (Decalmer and Glendenning, 1997). This is clearly acknowledged in a courageous publication from the UK's Royal College of Psychiatrists (Garner and Evans, 2000), which not only recognises and analyses the possible

causes of such abuse, but also proposes guidelines for its eradication.

The non-institutional population of older people is not necessarily free from such concerns. Child abuse and the abuse of younger adults (particularly that form sometimes referred to as 'wife-battering') have a long history as significant social problems. However, the abuse of older people outside institutions has only been recognised since the 1970s, when attention to the phenomenon of 'granny-battering' first came to attention in the media. Information on the incidence of such abuse is imprecise, as is the case with most forms of personal abuse. In the USA, a Government report estimated the prevalence of elder abuse as being 4% of the elderly population (US House of Representatives, 1981). In a separate study in the USA, Pillemer and Finkelhor (1988), in a random study of 2000 older people in Boston, found reports of abuse in 32 older people per 1000 (i.e. approximately 3.2% of the sample). The common pattern in such abuse is victims who are in the older groups, in the 75–84 and 85 years plus age ranges, who are more frail and highly dependent and who live with younger relatives; male relatives being more frequent perpetrators than females.

It is often the case, of course, that elder abusers have great love and affection for their older relatives and are themselves guilt-ridden as a consequence of their abuse. The abuse is at least as much the result of exhaustion and frustration as any negative attitudes or prejudices. However, it might be argued that the placing of these older people and their relatives in these most difficult of circumstances is the result of discriminatory practices at society-wide or national level. The lack of community support, the lack of residential places, the poor provision of or absence of respite care, all contribute to making both the older person and their informal carers victims.

The possibility of discrimination against older people by virtue of failure to respond to their needs is in itself extremely worrying. However, the possibility of deliberate discrimination, particularly if this is contained in government policy, is a more sinister possibility. One must, of course, question the motives of a society which knows about its older members being disadvantaged and yet does nothing about it. It is now over 20 years since the publication of the Black Report (Department of Health and Social Security, 1980) on inequalities in health (*see* Townsend and Davidson, 1982). In this controversial report it was noted that malnutrition among the elderly was estimated at 7%. In 1980, the year the Black Report was first published, the Government's own estimate was that 23% of older people had incomes below the supplementary pension rate (the accepted baseline below which poverty was taken to exist at that time). A further 33% were on incomes just above this, thus indicating that over 50% of older people were living at or almost at poverty levels. Arber and Ginn (1991) reported that 10 years later estimates of older people in poverty were still of the order of 17%. This does not suggest a strong Government commitment to positive action in favour of older people. For a society to be aware that approximately one-fifth of its older population is living in poverty and to do nothing about it is a most terrible indictment in our affluent world. This cannot be explained away by claims to ignorance or incompetence on the part of governments. This is the real face of ageism, and it encompasses the possibility of abuse through neglect (Action on Elder Abuse, 2000).

A more worrying recent development is the suggestion that, because they represent an intolerable strain on the health services, older people may be excluded from certain forms of treatment and care. Against this trend, in an increasingly economics-driven National Health Service, the Royal College of Physicians (1994) published a most outspoken report for such a conservative body. This insists that there must be equity of care for elderly people and stresses that in regard to acute emergency medical care there should be 'no distinction or negative discrimination on grounds of age'. Linda Thomas (1994), the Editor of the journal *Elderly Care*, addressed this trend with courage and conviction in an editorial

for that journal. She stated:

> *Age is a state of mind: if you don't mind, it doesn't matter.... But age, it seems, matters quite a lot when it comes to the health service. In fact your age could be quite crucial in dictating the type of treatment you receive. Over the past few weeks, a number of allegations have been made suggesting that elderly people are being denied access to NHS treatment. There is nothing hysterical about the claims, which have come from widely respected sources, including the Royal College of Physicians and the British Geriatrics Society.*
>
> *In an emphatic statement with anger barely concealed, the British Geriatrics Society cites a particular case study, that of thrombolytic therapy, to support its claim that there is age-related discrimination in access to treatment. The effectiveness of 'clot-busting' thrombolytic therapy for elderly patients with myocardial infarction is proven. In fact, says the Society, in patients over 70 years of age, the number of lives saved per thousand treated was 80. In patients under 60 it was only 25.*
>
> *Yet 40 per cent of British coronary care units operate an upper age limit for offering thrombolytic therapy. The illogicality of withholding treatment from those who, it appears, are likely to benefit most is quite breathtaking.*
>
> *It really is nonsensical, isn't it, to think that lying about your age could end up becoming a matter of life and death instead of a silly vanity. The irritation at being asked how old you are when you present for any kind of treatment is likely to be replaced by paranoia. Before we know where we are, there will be an upsurge of break-ins to GPs' surgeries as pensioners fight to falsify the birthdates on their medical records.*
>
> (Thomas, 1994)

This intrusion of the question of ageism into the health care setting has implications for nursing.

Study Activity 22.5 —————

It is suggested by some that older people should have equal access to all health services and treatment by right. Others say that if there are insufficient resources to go around, priority should always be given to younger people, who can still lead a full and productive life.

- Discuss the arguments for and against each of these viewpoints. Write up your analysis in about 500 words. If possible discuss your arguments with fellow students who have also completed this exercise.

AGEISM AND NURSING

Attitudes

Does ageism exist in nursing? This is undoubtedly an uncomfortable question to be raising in a textbook for nurses. As with all caring professions, nursing aspires to the highest standards of excellence and proclaims a commitment not only to treatment but also to meeting the personal and social needs of patients and clients. Yet nurses are members of the social majority. If ageism exists in society, the possibility of it being reflected to some extent in nursing must be accepted.

This possibility raises the most serious implications for the care of older people. Nurses play a major part in the care of older people in the community. In the institutional setting – in hospitals and nursing homes – the situation is even more critical. Here nurses are the group who have more contact than any other group with older patients. In this regard one thinks first of specialist units for older people, including nursing homes, medical geriatric units and units for the elderly mentally infirm. However, many older people are treated and cared for in other settings. Approximately 50% of beds in general medical wards and 33% of beds in surgical wards are occupied by patients in the 65 years plus age group. The prospect of prejudice

towards and discrimination of older people by nurses is thus very serious.

Unfortunately there is some evidence to suggest that this may be so to some extent. As noted above, some research (Campbell, 1971; Baker, 1978; Slevin, 1991) suggests that nurses do in fact hold negative attitudes towards older people, in common with other younger adults. Slevin (1991) claimed that with entry into and progression through the profession these attitudes may in fact become more negative in orientation. In addition, in the research carried out by Campbell (1971) it was found that the majority of nurses stated a preference for working with younger adults and children.

An important factor here may be the lack of attention and even the lack of prestige which nursing itself assigns to the nursing of older people. This is reflected in the commitment to this area of care in the nursing curriculum. In 1977, the General Nursing Council, then one of the statutory bodies governing nurse education in the UK, issued a significant policy statement on nurse education. In opening statements the document highlighted the dramatic demographic changes already anticipated at that time. This included recognition of a significant increase in the elderly population and changes in the population profile for this group, particularly as regards the older elderly. The document called for nursing curricula which would reflect these demographic changes. Surprisingly, in the same document, the General Nursing Council recommended only a minimum of 3 months' care of the elderly experience in 3 years' training.

Some 10 years later, an even more significant change in the nursing curriculum took place. The United Kingdom Central Council for Nursing, Midwifery and Health Visiting (UKCC), by this time the statutory body responsible for setting nurse education standards on a UK-wide basis, published proposals for a major review of nurse education known as *Project 2000* (UKCC, 1986). There would now be just one level of nurse, but four branches of nursing – adult, mental health, mental handicap and children's nursing.

In view of the anticipated demographic changes discussed earlier, the high numbers of older people in the in-patient population and the anticipated increased demands on the geriatric services, it may seem surprising that increased emphasis was again not given to this specialty. Indeed, during consultation on Project 2000 there was a strong lobby for the introduction of a care of the elderly branch. However, this was not included in the final proposals (UKCC, 1987). Various arguments were put forward for the final decision not to have an elderly branch. One was that an integrated approach to all adult nursing, including that of the elderly, is a more economical and educationally sound approach, given the similarities across the age ranges. Another argument had an affinity with the anti-segregation lobby in medicine. This argument decries the segregation of elderly people, suggesting that this may lead to a 'ghettoising' effect. It also submits that less resources would be made available to geriatric units, given the demand for more high technology care for younger adults (see, for example, Leonard, 1976; Laurence, 1979).

The above arguments, while possessing some strengths, particularly in regard to an increased sensitivity to the dangers of segregation, also contain fundamental weaknesses. They would limit the extension of specialist knowledge and skill which is characteristic of all specialisation. They also fail to recognise that older people have special needs which are significantly different to younger adults. In regard to the ill older person, these have been identified as:

- multiple pathology
- non-specific or atypical presentation of disease
- rapid deterioration of illness if untreated
- high incidence of complications
- importance of environmental factors – housing, income, social support, etc.

These arguments, which in fact are among the major influences which have sustained a flourishing and vitally important *medical* specialty, would be equally important in nursing. Against such arguments, it may be difficult to see how the previous arguments held sway in the major Project 2000 reforms. But perhaps a more fundamental and less overt argument was the deciding factor at the end of the day. Even in the latter half of the 1980s, recruitment into nursing was a major problem. There was a real fear that if a separate branch was introduced for this essentially unpopular area of nursing, it would be impossible to recruit the numbers needed.

It is interesting to compare the situation in the UK with that in the USA. There, in the predominantly generic nurse training curriculum, it has also been argued by Edel (1986) and Hirst and Metcalf (1988) that there is inadequate preparation for care of the elderly. However, care of the elderly or gerontological nursing is a growing postgraduate specialty in the USA. There are approximately 2000 geriatric and gerontological nurse specialists educated to master's level. There are, in addition, 40 chairs (professorships) in geriatric gerontological nursing in universities throughout the USA. No such trends are apparent in the UK.

Study Activity 22.6

As indicated above, it has been suggested by some that there should be an elderly care branch of nursing in addition to adult, mental health, mental handicap and children's nursing. Identify the arguments for and against such a proposal. Incorporate in your analysis a consideration of the implications for ageism in such a proposal.

Practice

Earlier in this chapter it was emphasised that the existence of a social problem in regard to an identifiable minority group together with negative attitudes towards that group were essential springboards to ageist action or discrimination. It has been suggested above that nurses, in addition to possibly sharing negative attitudes towards older people in common with the wider social group, are also subjected to intraprofessional and intrahealth service influences. The low profile given to the care of older people in the curriculum may not only serve to confirm the low prestige and unpopularity of this area, it may also serve to perpetuate ignorance in regard to this client or patient group. Such circumstances may well set the scene for discriminatory nursing action.

Such discriminatory action would be at its most visible in in-patient settings devoted to the care of older people – specifically geriatric units and nursing homes. In these settings, nurses are the most constant and most influential presence; it is they who in fact set the scene. A large body of literature presents a picture of the institutionalised older person as being passive, withdrawn, disengaged, dehumanised, apathetic, despairing and – together with or as a consequence of these conditions – deteriorating (Townsend, 1962; Henry, 1963; Robb, 1968; Gubrium, 1975; Fontana, 1977; Bowker, 1982; Baltes and Skinner, 1983; Slevin, 1989; Wall, 1997). The overall picture in these institutional settings was one of what Henry described as 'tombs for the living' within which the majority of the activity was, in Gubrium's words 'bed-and-body work' carried out by the nursing staff – washing, cleaning, feeding, dressing, etc.

Such pictures are substantiated by studies into levels of interaction between nurses and their older patients. Most of these studies (e.g. Norton *et al.*, 1962; Wells, 1980; Wade *et al.*, 1983; Slevin, 1989) have illustrated that nurses interact with patients for only a small proportion of their on-duty time and that this interaction is indeed mainly concerned with physical care or what Gubrium termed 'bed-and-body work'. The lack of more holistic care, addressing social and psychological as well as physical needs, and the limiting of the nurse–patient relationship to that of physical maintenance contacts, could be viewed from one perspective as being dehumanising.

It is a fact that nurses in Great Britain aspire to the highest standards and that actual physical or mental abuse of older patients is a rare occurrence. Nurses would indeed be horrified to contemplate the possibility that they treated their patients with anything other than kindness and this is to a large extent true. However, in the practices which have existed in the past, and which today continue to be perpetuated in some care settings, there remains a vestige of ageism. It is ageism by default rather than any overt punitive action. It is an ageism of depersonalisation, that which Tournier (1972) refers to in the opening quotation to this chapter when he speaks of the ultimate injury, the failure to regard another as a person in the fullest sense.

Strategy

Protesting innocence is not a strategy. The real danger of ageism in nursing is that of not recognising it as a threat and taking positive action to limit and indeed remove ageist influences. We can take our cue from Tournier (1967) here. The key is in the value we place on persons, irrespective of their age. If we acknowledge the older person as a person in the fullest sense, if we value and honour him, accept his right to a full and meaningful life within his own wishes and capabilities, and commit ourselves to the primacy of care and equity of access to our resources, ageism has been dispelled. This requires the existence of real commitment and an overt expression of intent.

The commitment to such care in practice is dependent on an equal commitment in terms of management, leadership, research and education. Practitioners cannot embrace this commitment if it is not first embraced by our managers and leaders. Fundamental to success is the provision of adequate education, founded on a sound theoretical and research base. This has been emphasised in a report by the UKCC in which concern is expressed about nursing standards and the increase in professional misconduct in nursing homes (UKCC, 1994). In this report the Council stated:

> *The lack of induction courses, readily available written procedures, poorly defined responsibilities of staff, almost non-existent in-service training and staff not being released to attend courses emerge as key problems. A*

> *combination of these factors contributes to the poor standards of care and unsafe practices in some homes. The most significant deficit is the lack of any kind of induction for new staff. Registered nursing staff, new to the home, find themselves to be the only nurse on duty and have to become familiar with procedures from untrained staff. In some nursing homes this appeared to be acceptable practice.*
>
> (UKCC, 1994, p. 8)

Quality education is in itself an assault on ageism in nursing. However, it must also be a direct and overt assault. Today it would be inconceivable that our nursing curriculum would not have child abuse in its syllabus content. In our increasingly multiracial society, racism and transcultural nursing are increasingly essential aspects of the curriculum (Leininger, 2002). Now we also recognise gender issues as important aspects of health and health care delivery. So too must it be with ageism. It must be placed firmly and overtly on the agenda, in both our nursing curricula and in our nursing practice. By talking about our ghosts we are well on the way to exorcising them. There is such a commitment in nursing. However, the prospect of this having a real and lasting effect is influenced by the wider social system. While on a UK-wide level there is a commitment to introduce equality legislation in respect of the older population over the next few years, in line with European Union developments, as yet there is no such protective legislation for the elderly (unlike the situation in respect of race, gender and disability). A notable exception is in Northern Ireland where, under devolved government, the Northern Ireland Act 1998 does provide the same protection against discrimination to older people as in other instances (such as gender, race, religion, disability, etc.).

SUMMARY

In this chapter the issue of ageism and its relevance to nursing was considered. The labelling theory perspective was adopted as a vehicle for understanding the development of ageism. The phenomenon of ageism was defined in terms of perceived social problems (age-related threats), a target group (older people), prejudice (negative attitudes and stereotypes) and discrimination (abuse and victimisation).

The sources and abuses of ageism in society were then discussed in terms of the specific social problems underpinning its construction, the attitudes or prejudices upon which it is based, and the discrimination and abuses which then arise as a consequence of these precedents. In the final sections of the chapter, the issue of ageism and nursing was discussed, once again in terms of problems, attitudes and discriminatory action. The issue of a strategy for addressing ageism in nursing was then briefly outlined.

This chapter commenced with a quotation from the work of Paul Tournier. So too should it end. In that same work Tournier (1972) states:

> *The problem of old age does not concern only the old. It calls in question the whole of our society, and exposes its faults. That it is inhuman is veritable at any age. But this is felt more especially in childhood, when we begin to discover the world and its injustices, and when we are too weak to defend ourselves. Later on, in the full strength of active life, we can at least fight, stand up to injustice, contend with fate. But when old age comes, we find ourselves powerless once again, and feel once more the pain of the faults in our civilization.*
>
> (Tournier, 1972, p. 36)

Elsewhere, Tournier (1967) speaks of this humanity in terms of personhood. He suggests that we live in two worlds, the world of persons and the world of things. To live primarily in the world of objects, to relate to both ourselves and others in this world in terms of things and concepts, is to exhibit our inhumanity. Alternatively, Tournier suggests, 'one can lay oneself open to the world of persons, awaken to the sense of person. By becoming oneself a person one discovers other persons round about, and one seeks to establish a bond with them' (Tournier, 1967, p. 179). This is the world of humanity.

It is certainly true that in caring for our children we are demonstrating our humanity. But there is also instinct here, as witnessed by the fact that most animals exhibit this need to support their young. However, in caring for its older people, a society demonstrates its true humanity. It is this one attribute which more than all others is the true test of our humanity or – in its absence – our inhumanity. The view from here does not see older people as a social problem, as a burden which leads us down the pathway to that prejudice and discrimination we have come to know as ageism. The view from here sees our older people as the ultimate gift, the opportunity for a society to answer the call to humanity. And it is we as nurses, more than all others, who receive this gift from the older members of our society. In caring for the old, in relating to them as persons, in committing ourselves to their empowerment and fullness of life, we as nurses can bear witness to the humanity of our society.

REFERENCES

Action in Elder Abuse (2002) *Without Due Care and Attention – The abuse of older people by neglect (including self-neglect)*, Action on Elder Abuse, London

Arber, S. and Ginn, J. (1991) *Gender and Later Life*, Sage, London

Baker, D.E. (1978) Attitudes of nurses to care of the elderly, PhD thesis, University of Manchester

Baltes, M.M. and Skinner, E.H. (1983) Cognitive performance deficits and hospitalisation: learned helplessness, instrumental passivity, or what? *Journal of Personality and Social Psychology*

Bowker, L.H. (1982) *Humanizing Institutions for the Aged*, Lexington Books, New York

Butler, R.N. (1969) Age-ism: another form of bigotry. *Gerontologist* **9**, 243–6

Blytheway, B. (1995) *Ageism*, Open University Press, Buckingham

Campbell, M.L. (1971) Study of attitudes of nursing personnel toward the geriatric patient. *Nursing Research* **20**, 147–51

Carstairs, V. (1981) *Our Elders*, Oxford University Press, Oxford

Cavan, R. (1962) Self and role in adjustment during old age. In: Rose, A. (ed.) *Human Behaviour and Social Processes*, Routledge and Kegan Paul, London

Cohen, S. (1972) *Folk Devils and Moral Panics: The creation of the mods and rockers*, Routledge and Kegan Paul, London

Cumming, E. and Henry, W.E. (1961) *Growing Old*, Basic Books, New York

Curtis, H.J. (1965) The somatic mutation theory of aging. In: Kastenbaum, R. (ed.) *Contributions to the Psychobiology of Aging*, Springer, New York

Decalmer, P. and Glendenning, S. (1997) *The Mistreatment of Elderly People* (2nd edn), Sage, London

Department of Health (2001) *The National Service Framework for Older People*, Department of Health, London

Department of Health and Social Security (1980) *Report of the Working Group on Inequalities in Health (The Black Report)*, Department of Health and Social Security, London

Drake, J. (1957) Some factors influencing students' attitudes toward older people. *Social Forces* **35**, 266–71

Edel, M. (1986) Recognizing gerontological content, *Journal of Geriatric Nursing* **12**(10), 28–32

Falkingham, J. and Victor, C.R. (1991) The myth of the woopie. *Ageing and Society* **11**(4), 471–93

Fontana, A. (1977) *The Last Frontier*, Sage, Beverley Hills, CA

Garner, J. and Evans, S. (2000) *Institutional Abuse of Older Adults*, Royal College of Psychiatrists, London

General Nursing Council for England and Wales (1977) *Educational Policy Statement*, General Nursing Council, London

Goffman, E. (1970) *Stigma: Notes on the management of spoiled identity*, Penguin, Harmondsworth

Grimley Evans, J. (1981) *Hospital Care for the Elderly*, Oxford University Press, Oxford

Gubrium, J. (1975) *Living and Dying at Murray Manor*, St. Martins Press, New York

Harris, L. (1975) *The Myths and Reality of Aging in America*, National Council on Aging, New York

Havighurst, R. (1963) *Successful Ageing*, University of Chicago Press, Chicago, IL

Henry, J. (1963) *Culture Against Man*, Random House, New York

Hirst, S.P. and Metcalf, B.J. (1988) *Selective Issues in Gerontic Nursing Education*, Churchill Livingstone, Edinburgh

Illich, I. (1976) *Limits to Medicine – Medical nemesis: the expropriation of health*, Penguin Books, New York

Kogan, N. (1961) Attitudes toward old people: the development of a scale and an examination of correlates, *Journal of Abnormal and Social Psychology* **62**(1), 44–54

Laurence, M. (1979) Geriatric cuckoo. *World Medicine* **14**(23), 19–20

Leininger, M. (2002) *Transcultural Nursing: Concepts, theories, research and practice* (3rd edn), McGraw-Hill, New York

Leonard, J.C. (1976) Can geriatrics survive? *British Medical Journal* **1**, 1335–6

Levin, J. and Levin, W.C. (1980) *Ageism: Prejudice and discrimination against the elderly*, Wadsworth, Belmont, CA

Mead, G.H. (1934) *Mind, Self and Society*, University of Chicago Press, Chicago, IL

Norton, D., McLaren, R. and Exton-Smyth, A.M. (1962) *An Investigation of Geriatric Nursing Problems in Hospital*, Churchill Livingstone, Edinburgh

Pillemer, K. and Finkelhor, D. (1988) The prevalence of elder abuse: a random sample survey. *The Gerontologist* **28**, 51–7

Robb, B. (1968) *Sans Everything*, Nelson, London

Rock, P. and McIntosh, M. (1974) *Deviance and Social Control*, Tavistock, London

Rosow, I. (1974) *Socialization to Old Age*, University of California Press, Berkeley, CA

Royal College of Physicians (1994) *Ensuring Equity and Quality of Care for Elderly People: The interface between geriatric medicine and general (internal) medicine*, Royal College of Physicians, London

Ryan, W. (1971) *Blaming the Victim*, Vintage Books, New York

Slevin, O.D. (1989) Communicating with the elderly: social and educational influences in nurse–patient interactions, PhD thesis, The Queen's University of Belfast

Slevin, O.D. (1991) Ageist attitudes among young adults: implications for a caring profession. *Journal of Advanced Nursing* **16**, 1197–1205

Thomas, L. (1994) Age-related matter of care. *Elderly Care* **6**(3), 5

Tournier, P. (1967) *The Meaning of Persons*, SCM Press, London

Tournier, P. (1972) *Learning to Grow Old*, SCM Press, London

Townsend, P. (1962) *The Last Refuge*, Routledge and Kegan Paul, London

Townsend, P. and Davidson, N. (1982) *Inequalities in Health – The Black Report*, Penguin, Harmondsworth

Tuckman, J. and Lorge, I. (1953) Attitudes toward old people. *Journal of Social Psychology* **37**, 249–60

United Kingdom Central Council for Nursing, Midwifery and Health Visiting (1986) *Project 2000: A new preparation for practice*, UKCC, London

United Kingdom Central Council for Nursing, Midwifery and Health Visiting (1987) *Project 2000: The final proposals (Project Paper 9)*, UKCC, London

United Kingdom Central Council for Nursing, Midwifery and Health Visiting (1994) *Professional Conduct – Occasional report on standards of nursing in nursing homes*, UKCC, London

US House of Representatives (1981) *Elder Abuse: An examination of a hidden problem*, Government Printing Office, Washington, DC

Victor, C.R. (1994) *Old Age in Modern Society* (2nd edn), Chapman and Hall, London

Wade, B., Sawyer, L. and Bell, J. (1983) *Dependency with Dignity: Different care provision for the elderly*, Bedford Square Press, London

Walford, R.L. (1965) *Immunology and Aging*, Springer, New York

Walker, A. (1980) The social creation of poverty and dependency in old age, *Journal of Social Policy* **9**, 49–75

Wall, R. (1997) The living arrangements of the elderly in contemporary Europe. Annual Conference of the British Sociological Association. University of Loughborough, Loughborough

Wells, T.J. (1980) *Problems in Geriatric Nursing Care*, Churchill Livingstone, Edinburgh

23 SPIRITUALITY AND NURSING

Oliver Slevin

> *He who has a why to live for can bear with almost any how.*
>
> Friedrich Nietzsche

LEARNING OUTCOMES

After studying this chapter you will be able to:

- Define and reflect upon the different meanings attached to the terms 'spirit' and 'spiritual'
- Describe how notions of the spiritual and the secular are often juxtaposed, or even seen as being in opposition
- Relate this to a wider societal tendency towards two different outlooks or worldviews
- Reflect upon deeper meanings of the spiritual dimension
- Consider ways in which the spiritual dimension may impact upon health and well-being
- Identify ways in which nurses may address such a spiritual dimension in their work.

INTRODUCTION

In this chapter we embark upon a quest for the meaning of a term and its relevance to nursing. The Latin word *spiritus* relates to breath, life, soul, or mind. It suggests a quality or presence that is the living characteristic or life force. When it leaves, the being becomes lifeless, breath is gone, mind ceases to function. Within our legal systems, we so define death as a cessation of breathing and/or brain function. In resuscitation, the nurse quite literally breathes life into the victim again. But the situation is more complex than this. We can choose to explain such things in purely biological–physiological terms, or we can consider whether there is something else in each of us that is spiritual or life-giving. In effect, we can consider whether there is a dimension that can be termed 'spiritual' (relating to the spirit) that we must take into account in our caring practices.

Had the student of today been commencing education 10 years ago, she or he would have been confronted with a frequently heard call to 'the holistic approach to care'. It was argued that we should address not only the physical, psychological and social, but also the spiritual dimensions of care. Various neologisms or jargon terms were invented to emphasise this orientation, such as 'bio-psycho-social care', with the spiritual dimension thrown in for good measure, or as an afterthought.

In one sense, this trend marked a significant advance. There was at least an overt recognition that when we care for others it is not sufficient to attend only to their physical disorders or biological needs. However, it also presented some risks. First, there was the risk of assuming that what 'holism' implies is simply taking account of everything. As the American nursing academic Rosemarie Parse (1995) noted, such stringing together of different dimensions actually represents a fragmentary approach to nursing. Thus she described nursing theories that simply attempt to encompass all that must be contained in caring as *totality theories*, wherein the totality of care is simply the sum of the parts. Conversely, she described those theories that consider the person as a whole being, irreducible to different dimensions, as *simultaneity theories*, wherein the whole is more than the sum of its parts. Second, there was the risk that by tagging the spiritual dimension onto a cluster of other concerns, this rather difficult and uncomfortable notion could be dealt with easily and without too much dwelling on what – in the era of science and technology – was an uncomfortable and even embarrassing concept. There would appear to be some justification for the view that we often leaned towards ignoring or rejecting the spiritual dimension or, alternatively, paying it a lip service that failed to address the issue in any meaningful way.

The notion of spirituality as a caring dimension is no less difficult in our present time. Earlier in this module (i.e. in Chapter 20) we have already addressed religion and its impact upon health care, and this was no less difficult a topic to broach. In today's secular age, within which we look to science for the solving of our remaining mysteries, and where organised religion is said to be in decline, it is understandable that the student may reflect seriously upon the relevance of such topics to modern nursing. Before we proceed to consider the spiritual aspect of nursing, or even attempt to define spirituality, it may help to consider your own initial reaction to this dimension.

Study Activity 23.1 _____

- Without resorting to literature or seeking advice (or reading forward), reflect upon the term 'spiritual' and what it means to you personally. It may help to consider any experiences you have had that you feel were spiritual. Or you may wish to consider someone whom you feel to be a spiritual person, and why you feel this to be so. Avoid any attempt to censor your thoughts: write down your reflections as they come to you.

- When you have done this, read your notes and make an objective judgment about how well you have encapsulated some of the essential meaning of the term. You may wish to compare notes with a fellow student. At this stage you may feel that you are in no position to judge, if you have not even looked up the term! However, the important thing is that you have moved from an intuitive, subjective account in your own words to a more objective and reasoned way of thinking about the concept. As you will see later, spiritual issues are of

an intensely personal nature, and this first serious consideration of the phenomenon by looking to your own internal self will be of much value.

- Retain your notes, as they will be needed in a subsequent Study Activity.

At this early stage in the chapter, you may still be begging a question about the relevance of spirituality to modern health care. This should neither worry nor frustrate you. Throughout this book, there is a constant call to be sceptical and questioning, to think critically about the knowledge that must inform practice. The same is the case here. The purpose of this chapter is to facilitate you in such a sceptical and critical consideration of spiritual dimensions of health care and nursing. You will be able to approach the dimension in three different, though interrelated, ways.

1 You will be able to recognise within your own persona a spiritual dimension that has a direct influence on your capacity as a carer of persons.
2 You will be able to relate to your patients on the level of their spirituality, as person-to-person or spiritual being to spiritual being.
3 You will be able to frame such knowledge of self and others within a sound knowledge of the spiritual and its dynamic (i.e. its ways of acting upon people and relationships).

OPENING ARGUMENT

Throughout your career there will be times when you will stand beside the most eminent medical consultants, whose work is guided by the most complex science and technology, and hear them say to colleagues or relatives, 'She has lost the will to live, her spirit has gone.' More importantly, the day will come when you will yourself recognise this phenomenon in your patients. This begs a most fundamental and intriguing question. How can it be that people whose very core of being is contextualised in a hard scientific perspective not only recognise but also seem to place such blind faith in a concept that is so nebulous? In a sense, this is almost a question that answers itself. By definition, that which is spiritual is an invisible essence. Its existence cannot be proved or disproved on the basis of observation and analysis. There is, after all, nothing there that can be directly perceived, measured or analysed. It may appear to be – quite literally – a matter of blind faith. Yet, these people of great knowledge and extensive experience do recognise some element or spirit within people that can have a profound effect upon their health and well-being. We are not speaking here of religious maniacs or latter-day mystics. These experienced clinicians are exceptionally rational people – some would say they are rational to a fault. They are not given to easily accepting surmise instead of evidence, or practising according to metaphor rather than theory. In fact, they are operating on the basis of the evidence of their own experience. They know that there is something within each person that is akin to a life force – a will to be. And they know that when this is weakened, when this inner strength gives up, there can be significant consequences.

This lack of spirit is as dangerous as the most virulent micro-organism. In the account of his experience in Nazi concentration camps, written in 1959, we find this passage from the distinguished psychoanalyst, Viktor Frankl ([1959] 1984):

> The prisoner who had lost faith in the future – his future – was doomed. With his loss of belief in the future, he also lost his spiritual hold: he let himself decline and became subject to mental and physical decay . . . We all feared this moment – not for ourselves, which would have been pointless, but for our friends. Usually it began with the prisoner refusing one morning to get dressed and wash and go out on the parade grounds. No entreaties, no blows, no threats had any effect. He just lay there, hardly moving. If this crisis was brought about by an illness, he refused to be taken to the sick-bay or to do anything to help himself. He simply gave up. There he remained, lying in his own excreta, and nothing bothered him any more.
>
> (Frankl, 1984, pp. 95–6)

In this, Frankl was recognising a link between spirit and life. He was himself able to avoid the decline into oblivion by clinging to his memory of and hope for being reunited with his wife, and by his calling as a doctor to help his fellow inmates. In this work, he recognised repeatedly the impact of loss of hope upon the survival of his fellow prisoners. Of course, to the rational mind there are various explanations that provide grounds for rejecting Frankl's premises. These prisoners were malnourished and dehydrated. Typhus was endemic in the camps. The prisoners were subjected to the terrors of torture, brutality and mass extermination. In such circumstances the physical body is highly at risk of deterioration. The mental state may understandably revert to a catatonic stupor. All of this is readily explained by medical science, and (so the argument runs) it is unhelpful to interject with unsubstantiated mumbo-jumbo that belongs to a bygone age. Yet, Frankl shows that even the hard statistics of the camps flew in the face of such rational argument. When rumours that prisoners were to be liberated failed to materialise at the anticipated time, this simple fact led to a massive increase in mortality without any discernable worsening of camp conditions. Clearly, any dampening of 'spirits' in such precarious circumstances had the most lethal consequences.

The impact of a weakening of the spirit on health and even survival is well documented elsewhere. However, the seminal work in this area is probably the important research carried out by Rees and Lutkins (1967). This research had such a profound and shocking effect upon the medical establishment that it caused a whole reappraisal of the impact of life events on the health and psyche of the person. The report of their research was entitled 'The mortality of bereavement' but is now commonly referred to as 'Dying of a broken heart'. In this research, the

429

mortality at one year in a group of close relatives of deceased persons was compared with a control group living in the same area who had not suffered bereavement. There was a sevenfold increase of risk of death in the group of bereaved persons, with no discernable variation in the control group. It is interesting that, in summarising their findings, Rees and Lutkins (1967) quoted from the poetry of Sir Henry Wotton. This quotation admirably summarised the point emerging from their findings. The original seventeenth-century wording, rather than their modernisation of it, is presented here:

> *He first deceas'd; she for a little tri'd*
> *To live without him: lik'd it not, and di'd.*
> Death of Sir Albertus Moreton's Wife

While this work had a significant impact on medical attitudes, the dominant view within the scientific medical community tended to be sceptical (*see*, for example, Archer, 1999). However, the danger in failing to recognise the importance of a spiritual dimension is not exclusively related to its rejection on a rational–scientific argument. As is often the case in such matters, the real danger lies in the arena of prejudice, wherein extremes to either side of a balanced view are equally threatening. The spiritual well-being of the individual may be threatened by an extreme rejection of such matters as being unscientific and irrelevant to the care and treatment of the patient. This might be termed a form of medical terrorism. Alternatively, spiritual viewpoints may be imposed upon the patient, or attempts may be made to encourage spiritual reflection against his will. This may in turn be viewed as a form of spiritual terrorism.

Keizer (2001), himself a physician, describes his own father's final days within a health care system. He commences by describing the death of Lord Byron in the nineteenth century, and how this was speeded – if not indeed caused – by the relentless bleeding and leeching carried out by his physicians. Keizer then describes how, at the end of the twentieth century, his father was similarly subjected to an increasing barrage of surgical and investigatory procedures by his medical attendants, so that finally his relatives sought the intervention of the family doctor. At this stage, the elderly patient had lost all powers of resistance and wished for nothing more than to be left to die in peace. This he did, approximately one week later, following transfer to an elderly care facility. On autopsy, it was found that the 'growth' that led to the intense series of interventions was nothing more than a benign tumour.

There is perhaps an important message in such narratives, which suggests that there is a need to avoid extremes on the basis of the viewpoints of others and look instead to the wishes and values that are fundamental to the individual affected by such decisions. At the core of this respecting of the person as an individual there is a respecting of self that indeed moves us towards spiritual concerns.

Study Activity 23.2

- While it may be painful to do so, try to recall an elderly relative or acquaintance who was ill and declining. Reflecting on their apparent attitude, place them somewhere on the following set of dimensions in Figure 23.1: copy the dimensions out and place an X on each line as appropriate.

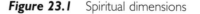

Hope-ful	Hope-less
Enlivened	Deadened
Vital	Lethargic
Alert	Listless
Energetic	Weakened
Inspirited	Despirited

Figure 23.1   Spiritual dimensions

- Consider how there may have been a lack of a will to live, and how this may have influenced well-being and recovery, or indeed led to a decline or even death.

Some undertaking this above exercise may have found it particularly difficult, having lived through this scene with a loved one within their own life. For them, living through this experience of the spirit touched them also; they were not merely observers but participants in the drama. Henri Nouwen, a distinguished theologian who spent much of his life working within a community of people with learning disabilities, recounts a poignant memory of his own mother's death. In this, Nouwen (1980) presents his own understanding of his mother's delirious and painful progress towards the final moments:

> *What am I talking about? Am I making an existential drama out of the death of a woman who lived a good life but died a painful death? The doctors and nurses in the hospital, who surrounded my mother with competent care, neither could nor would speak with the words and concepts that I have been using. They referred to a growing lack of oxygen, a hard-to-explain restlessness and a difficult-to-understand groaning. But is that all there is to say? No doubt lack of oxygen creates anxiety, but not all anxiety is experienced as a struggle of faith in the moment of encounter with God himself. What am I saying when I speak about a sharing in Christ's agony? Some, mostly the medical staff, interpreted her struggle primarily as a physical response to a very radical operation. Others, who had known her piety, perceived it as the emergence of old memories and deeply embedded routine phrases repeated during a state of semi-consciousness. But I saw something else. I saw my own mother entering into that moment in which we are totally alone with God, in which the final decision of life must be made: the decision of faith.*
>
> (Nouwen, 1980, pp. 31–2)

Around every deathbed or sickbed there is arrayed a range of positions on the spiritual question, and Nouwen draws attention to these.

For him and the other members of his family, who were devout Dutch Catholics, there was an intense spiritual awareness. This reached from them to the mother and beyond her to their God. In different circumstances, those who have no profession of faith in any god may experience no less a heightened sense of existential awareness of finality and loss in the departure of a loved one.

For nurses, there is no call to adopt these various positions as our own. However, irrespective of our own beliefs, there is a call to accept and respond to them. Somehow, when this spiritual or essential state of being calls from our patients and their relatives, we must respond to their need. We must create the responsive and supporting space within which their search for meaning and coping can be facilitated. This is not simply an option. There is no sense in which we can argue that we treat only the body and the symptoms of the mind, or that this marks the limits of our professional responsibility. There is an ethical imperative to enter this space and to care for the spirit as well as the body and mind.

MEANINGS

It should be clear from the comments above that there is at least one sense in which the spiritual is relevant to health care and to nursing: that is the sense in which spirit is a will to live. However, there are various albeit interconnecting meanings that can be applied to the notions of spirit and spirituality. In the first sense, discussed above, 'spirit' is something akin to the life force within a person, and 'spirituality' is the adjective describing the presence of this phenomenon. Indeed, the Latin origin of spirit – to breathe – with its associated terms of inspiring and expiring quite literally means to take on life or to live. As we noted at the beginning of this chapter, the word *spiritus* in Latin can mean breath, life, soul, or mind, depending on the context.

The terms 'spirit' and 'spiritual' are used in various ways and in each instance there may be a relevance to nursing and health care. For

431

Table 23.1 The meaning of the terms 'spirit' and 'spiritual'

'Spirit'	'Spiritual'
A vital force that characterises a living being as being alive	Any matter concerning the spirit
A person's will or enthusiasm for living	A way of connectedness with the experience of being alive – a zest for living
A sense of self, or consciousness of being a living entity – the meaning of such being	Having an affinity with the mind or spirit of self and others (other people, other living things, etc.), a transcendence that is characterised by a heightened sense of consciousness
The inner being or soul that characterises our essential human quality (seen by some to be an immaterial being that survives the human body)	Being attuned to the inner being within self and others (as in the experience of being a 'soul-mate')
A divine (God-like) being or presence, that may be visible, invisible, felt or assumed – by being divine it is different to the natural, i.e. supernatural	Relating to religious or sacred things rather than worldly or secular matters, concerning the supernatural rather than natural world
A liquid produced by distillation, so that particular essences are extracted	A religious song associated with some ethnic groups, notable for its arousing capacity

example, a brief scan of several dictionaries reveals the range of meanings given in Table 23.1, not all of which are mutually exclusive.

Some of these meanings may seem to have little relevance to nursing in the modern world. Nurses who aspire to a particularly narrow scientific perspective may argue that there is no empirical evidence to justify notions that people may have some life-engendering inner force, the lack of which may remove a will to live and even lead to death. Similarly, nurses who are of an essentially secular orientation, with no particular commitment to or interest in religious belief, may view spiritual matters as out-of-date and irrelevant. This is particularly likely where these include the idea of an inner self, spirit or soul, or indeed the notion that there is some higher spiritual being or creator who determines our destiny.

A central problem in all this is the fact that, by most of their definitions, the spirit and things spiritual are not visible in the normal sense of being phenomena or objects within our world that can be perceived (seen, heard, touched), and as such subjected to measurement and analysis. If these spiritual dimensions exist, they can only be confronted on their own plane, through

sensing, intuition or tacit knowing of their presence. However, the existence of such things, while ever the source of controversy, is notable by the allusions to spirit and things spiritual across cultures and across time. James Hillman (1997), the renowned Jungian psychoanalyst, is informative in this respect:

> The concept of this individualized soul-image has a long and complicated history; its appearance in cultures is diverse and widespread and the names for it are legion . . . I will use many terms for this acorn – image, character, fate, genius, calling, daimon, soul, destiny – rather interchangeably, preferring one or another depending on the context . . . We should not be afraid of these big nouns; they are not hollow . . . These many words do not tell us what 'it' is, but they do confirm that it is. They also point to its mysteriousness. We cannot know what exactly we refer to because its nature remains shadowy, revealing itself mainly in hints, intuitions, whispers, and the sudden urges and oddities that disturb your life . . .
>
> Consider this event. Amateur Night at the Harlem Opera House. A skinny, awkward

sixteen-year-old goes fearfully on stage. She is announced to the crowd: 'The next contestant is a young lady named Ella Fitzgerald . . . Miss Fitzgerald here is gonna dance for us . . . Hold it, hold it. Now what's your problem honey? . . . Correction, folks. Miss Fitzgerald has changed her mind. She's not gonna dance, she's gonna sing.'

Ella Fitzgerald gave three encores and won first prize. However, 'she had meant to dance'.

Was it chance that suddenly changed her mind? Did a singing gene suddenly kick in? Or might that moment have been an annunciation, calling Ella Fitzgerald to her particular fate?

(Hillman, 1997, pp. 10–11)

There is little doubt that Hillman, a trained scientific psychologist and psychoanalyst, recognised the lack of a scientific foundation for these views. For him, and indeed for Frankl and the other experienced physicians and nurses referred to above, there is undoubtedly a sense of unease. However, there is also a recognition emerging from wisdom and experience that there are things that cannot be left to the psychology laboratory or the scientific experiment. Beyond all the attempts to measure what is human in us, there is a recognition – even in that most human of the sciences, psychology – that the very root of its name, the ancient Greek term psyche, most accurately translates to 'soul' or 'self'.

It must by now be clear that there is no way in which a concrete and patently obvious designation of meaning to the terms 'spirit' and 'spiritual' can be attained, in the same way that we can say without serious equivocation that this is a shoe or that is a table. If it is something that is unseen, can only be felt intuitively, or described by metaphor rather than physical attributes, who can confirm or contest it? Yet, even should we as nurses be inclined to disregard or reject such ideas, we cannot ignore the central meaning they have for others. In Chapter 20 of this book, Paul Weller draws attention to the degree to which religion (which to some extent encapsulates organised spiritual movements) is a central and meaningful aspect of many people's lives. Indeed, in their influential and extensive study of changes in American life, Bellah *et al.* (1985) found that while many Americans had turned away from organised religion, the great majority of people held to either some public (church-linked) or private sense of spirituality. While not always a central aspect of life, this was nevertheless held to be a vital foundation for how they lived and the meaning they attributed to their world. Given the importance to their very existence that our clients and patients may attribute to this spiritual dimension, it becomes an important consideration in terms of how we provide care.

Study Activity 23.3

Within the past 20 years there have been four seminal books on spiritual aspects of nursing published in the UK. These are:

1 McGilloway, O. and Myco, F. (1985) *Nursing and Spiritual Care*, Harper and Row, London
2 Narayanasamy, A. (1991) *Spiritual Care: A resource guide*, Quay Books, Lancaster
3 Bradshaw, A. (1994) *Lighting the Lamp: The spiritual dimension of nursing care*, Scutari, London
4 McSherry, W. (2000) *Making Sense of Spirituality in Nursing Practice: An interactive approach*, Churchill Livingstone, Edinburgh.

You may find it useful to consult these texts in extending your study of spirituality in nursing. However, for the purpose of this exercise, carry out the following activities:

- Undertake a literature search in your library to see if you can identify any additional books published in the UK within the past 20 years that are dedicated exclusively to the study of spirituality in nursing. If you find any, add them to the list above.
- Extend your literature search by identifying books published in the UK that are dedicated exclusively to nursing science, i.e. books on theory and research. Do a simple count of those you find.

433

- Consult textbooks published within the UK within the past 10 years on nursing practice and search their index sections for the topics 'spirit', 'spirituality' and 'spiritual care'. Again, do a simple count of those you have found.
- On the basis of your investigations are there some grounds for arguing that the spiritual dimension of care is under-represented in our literature? If so, suggest reasons for this state of affairs.

After considering all of this, we must commit ourselves to some statement of meaning for the spiritual dimension. At best this will serve as a basis for considering how we can address the spiritual dimension in our practice. At worst, it at least provides a set of statements that can be tested and rejected or refined. On this basis, we can attempt to describe and explain the spiritual dimension with the following statements:

- It refers to an inner essence of life or being alive, which we may term a life force or source of psychic energy.
- It is intangible in that it cannot be seen or observed, and is not locatable in terms of bodily organs, etc.
- It is therefore not subject to scientific investigation, or to the verifications or (importantly) the refutations of science.
- Our descriptions must therefore fall largely within the realm of metaphor, using terms such as 'self', 'soul', 'spirit', 'life force', etc.
- While there are major difficulties in describing what it is, there are attestations across cultures and ages confirming that the spiritual exists as a human dimension.
- While issues of the spirit may not be directly observable and subject to scientific investigation, there is a substantial body of statistical and expert experiential evidence to indicate that a weakening or loss of a life force or will to live, which we may label 'spirit', is a threat to health and well-being, and even to survival.
- As a life force, the spiritual dimension calls us to strive for meaning and purpose in terms of

our sense of self, our relations with others and the wider cosmic universe.
- This striving for meaning encompasses a concern or caring for what and who we are, and by definition, extends from ourselves to others. Thus, as we have this care and concern for our own existence and survival, we face the other with an equal concern for their existence and survival.
- It can thus be suggested that good spirit is by definition compassionate and caring.
- Where such striving extends into a more cosmic domain of understanding, for some the source of meaning and destiny is located in a deity or creator, and this emerges in various cultures as religious affiliations.
- The calling to an intentional and authentic concern for a sense of meaning in respect of the internal spirit or psyche is not an everyday way of being and (except for those following a religious contemplative life) heightened awareness is usually triggered by some major life event that calls into question our existence. This would include illness or impending death.
- By virtue of the call to care for persons confronted by their destiny in this way, issues of a spiritual nature become an important dimension in nursing.

Study Activity 23.4

- Consider these three readings. They are presented in chronological order, and each presents the author's view on the inner self or spiritual dimension.
- William James is recognised as the father of modern psychology. This reading is taken from his book entitled *Principles of Psychology*, and the section entitled 'The self'.

> *The more active-feeling states of consciousness are thus the more central portions of the spiritual Me. The very core and nucleus of our self, as we know it, the very sanctuary of our life, is the sense of activity which certain inner states possess. This sense of activity is often held to be a direct revelation of the*

living substance of our Soul. Whether this be so or not is an ulterior question. I wish now only to lay down the peculiar internality of whatever states possess this quality of seeming to be active. It is as if they went out to meet all the other elements of our experience. In thus feeling about them probably all men agree.

(James, 1892, pub. 1954, pp. 267–9)

- Thomas Moore was a Catholic monk who later became a therapist. He enjoys considerable success as an author on spiritual matters, particularly in America. This reading is taken from his book entitled *Care of the Soul*:

'Soul' is not a thing, but a quality or a dimension of experiencing life and ourselves. It has to do with depth, value, relatedness, heart and personal substance. I do not use the word here as an object of religious belief or as something to do with immortality. When we say someone or something has soul, we know what we mean, but it is difficult to specify exactly what that meaning is.

(Moore, 1992, p. 5)

- Susan Greenfield is a distinguished neurophysiologist, who has worked at the forefront of neuroscience and pharmacology developments, primarily at Oxford. This reading is taken from her paper entitled 'Soul, brain and mind':

I suggest there is no magic ingredient for consciousness: the critical factor in the brain is not some special qualitative magic bullet that some lucky neuroscientist is going to eventually unearth. Rather, the issue is a quantitative one, depending on the degree of recruitment of neurones: the extent of recruitment will determine your consciousness at any one time from one moment to the next . . . Once we can obtain a high resolution in human brain imaging, similar to that with invasive techniques in animals, we will be able to test out this idea and develop it. It is only a matter of time, for imaging techniques are improving at an awesome rate. It is a big step for scientists to start to theorise about the modern

soul, the mortal soul, consciousness and mind. Hard experimental data may be just around the corner.

(Greenfield, 1999, p. 124)

- Each of these readings has a different view on what the spiritual dimension actually is. For James it is an inner force or energy; for Moore it is a way of experiencing and being; while for Greenfield the interest is in the quest for a neurophysiological explanation for what she describes as 'consciousness'.
- Reflect on these different viewpoints in the context of the discussion of meanings we have considered in this section of the chapter. Then take a blank sheet of paper and on it provide a definitive statement that describes in your own words the spiritual dimension of human existence, as you now understand it. You must do this in a brief paragraph of approximately 150 words.
- Now revisit the notes you made at the end of Study Activity 23.1. Compare those with the statement you have just written. Note any significant ways in which the two statements differ.

DISCOURSES

Dilemmas

So far, we have considered the argument for a spiritual dimension and attempted to gain a sense of its meaning. The student reader may still be experiencing difficulties with all that has been said. Indeed, the topics of this chapter are commonly defined as a mystery, and as such will forever present such difficulties. Some religious authorities, who see spirit as a divine entity, define a mystery in this sense as by definition beyond human understanding. Acceptance of the spiritual then becomes purely a matter of faith, and in such circumstances the responsibility of the nurse may extend only to respecting the values and beliefs of those in her care. However, in moving beyond this to a more detailed consideration of the issue, we should recognise that we are influenced by various discourses.

Between science and humanity

One significant discourse is that which we may term the 'scientific discourse'. In the 'modern' era, there has been a turning to science as the main or only source of truth. This has been accompanied by a decline in traditional ways of life, which looked much to religion and its spiritual directors for the source of solutions to problems of living. As a consequence, two major and opposing discourses have emerged. These were usefully described by C.P. Snow (1959) in his highly influential publication entitled *The Two Cultures*. On the science side of this controversy, there is a claim that the only valid source of truth is that derived from empirical evidence, as procured through the scientific method (*see* Chapter 10). At its extreme, this has been described as scientism – the irrational faith in the capacity of science as the source of all knowledge (Williams, 1983).

On the opposing side – the humanities – there is a claim that not all sources of knowledge and understanding can be achieved through the sciences. In their different ways, the arts, philosophy and religion have much to contribute to our knowledge, particularly as this relates to how we should live. The positions taken by Greenfield and Moore (*see* Study Activity 23.4) reflect opposing positions on each side of this science-humanities divide.

In considering the spiritual dimension, it is important that the nurse is aware of these opposing views. These different discourses, between science and humanities, reason and belief, objective and subjective reality, are of particular concern to those working in health care systems. There is at once a call to use the best available evidence and the most effective technology to advance the well-being of the patients and clients. At the same time, there is, more than in most other situations, recognition of the complexities of the human condition, the importance of people's beliefs, and the capacity for the human condition to defy science and reason. In determining your position on the spiritual dimension you should be aware of these discourses and how they may influence your choices and actions.

The politics of meaning

Michael Lerner was a conscientious objector in the 1960s and 1970s, jailed for his views on American foreign policy. He later became a psychoanalyst and is now an influential Rabbi. J. Edgar Hoover, the past Director of the FBI, once described him as one of the most dangerous men in America. However, while Hoover is remembered with notoriety, Lerner has become one of the most influential and respected figures in modern America. His quest is for a more just and caring society, and he condemns the lack of meaning within modern politics. He was influential in Hilary Clinton's call for 'a new politics of meaning' and his book entitled *The Politics of Meaning: Restoring hope and possibility in an age of cynicism* (Lerner, 1997) is now viewed as an influential masterpiece. His argument is as follows. Both the econo-marxist politics of the Left and the Market-ist politics of the Right hold things and not meaning to be of fundamental importance. Their concerns are with power and material things and not with that fundamental meaning, which Lerner describes as a sense of purpose in existence and a reaching out to others in a spirit of togetherness. He states:

> A politics of meaning aims to shift the bottom line from a focus on profit or other material values to a focus on ethical, spiritual, social, and ecological values. Accordingly, the productivity or efficiency or rationality of any given program is to be judged by these criteria.
>
> (Lerner, 1997, p. 216)

This discourse – essentially a discourse on politics and authenticity versus inauthenticity in the context of our relations with each other – is also important to nursing. There are insights here into the political and social world from which those in need come into our care, within health care facilities where vulnerability and loneliness may be increased. There are also insights into the wider technological, depersonalised and mechanised world, which are accentuated in the centres of modern medicine, and which add to this vulnerability by creating a sense of powerlessness and alienation. Here, in this intensified microcosm of the wider political world, there is a crying out from the patient for acceptance as a person and for understanding and meaning in the face of their own vulnerability. As carers we are called upon to respond in a way that counterbalances these alienating and depersonalising influences. If we give any credence to the evidence of the impact of a weakened spirit upon health and well-being outcomes, this call to sustain the spirit in a health-giving and healing way becomes justified on moral as well as professional effectiveness grounds. Indeed, we might argue that in a health care world of material politics, depersonalising technologies, and impersonal people-processing, the nurse occupies a vital position as the human and humanising face of health care.

Between surface and depth

The final discourse we deal with here is that of the pull between the superficial and the deep. In all those meanings we ascribed to the spiritual above, there is a recognition that spirit is something deep, something personal and something that must be sensed and responded to intuitively. The premise emerging from this is that there is a superficial or surface mode of being that is the normal mode, which is characterised by routine, reasoning and objectivity, and dealing with matters of a concrete and predictable nature. Opposed to this there is an alternative, deeper mode of being, which draws us into more fundamental concerns about the nature of our existence, the knowledge of our own vulnerability and eventual death or non-existence, and the meanings we can seek that will assist us in coming to terms with such insights. This is a highly subjective mode of being, full of mystery and unpredictability, which can only be fathomed through intuitive insight. It is here that matters of the spirit reign. If we exclude the mystic or those involved in drug-assisted transcendence, this is not the normal mode of being but one that is thrust upon us at certain times, by major life events, including illness or

bereavement. In essence, it is when our existence is in question that we are drawn to these depths.

One aspect of this discourse draws on ideas from existential philosophy. In 1943, Sartre spoke of opposing attitudes of 'authenticity' and 'bad faith' (Sartre, 1969). In the authentic mode of being we confront the nature of our existence with courage. But, as is often the case, we avoid this confrontation and live safely in bad faith behind barriers of role and convention. Another philosopher, Martin Heidegger, whose ideas in fact preceded those of Sartre by many years, described similar modes of being in 1927, but used the terms 'authenticity' and 'inauthenticity' rather than bad faith (Heidegger, 1962). However, Heidegger adopted a less negative view of the inauthentic way of being. For him, this is the normal mode of being, and living permanently in the intense angst created by authentic confrontation with our existence would be intolerable.

For carers such as nurses and doctors, living in day-to-day contact with suffering and death, there are real problems in confronting these realities. Indeed, there are well-documented accounts of how professionals cope in these situations. The psychoanalyst Sister Mary Wolff-Salin (1989) describes how intellectualisation and rationalisation are used to avoid painful personal involvement. It is on this basis that within the traditional medical model there is a tendency to address problems and cases rather than people and feelings. In nursing also, Isobel Menzies (1960) has described what she termed 'social defence mechanisms'. In her study, nurses used rituals and routines, and preferred task-centred rather than person-centred approaches, which would require them to relate person-to-person with their patients. Robin Downie (1989) similarly described how social workers preferred to adopt professional roles with their prescribed behaviours, rather than entering into more personal relationships, which may have been appropriate to the needs of their clients. In an insightful comment on the resistance of professionals to entering the deeper areas of activity, including personal relations and spiritual distress, Donald Schön (1987) states:

> *In the varied topography of professional practice, there is a high, hard ground overlooking a swamp. On the high ground, manageable problems lend themselves to solution through the application of research-based theory and technique. In the swampy lowland, messy confusing problems defy technical solution. The practitioner must choose. Should he remain on the high ground where he can solve relatively unimportant problems according to prevailing standards of rigour or shall he descend to the swamp of important problems and non-rigorous inquiry?*
>
> (Schön, 1987, p. 187)

Sister Mary Wolff-Salin (1989), refers more specifically to the matter of relating on a deep, spiritual level, when she states:

> *What all this is about is alienation. It seems that in the spiritual as in the psychological life there is no happy ground of mediocrity. Refusal to choose the depths, the centre, the heart condemns one to wander forever in a domain of superficiality where both one's life with God and one's human relationships become only a fraction of what they could be. And perhaps this is a case where indeed 'the last shall be first', for it is often those simple and poor in what our culture and world value who find it easier to live on the level of the heart – often, or more often at least, than those who seem more gifted by fortune.*
>
> (Wolff-Salin, 1989, p. 67)

It is apparent in all this that the major discourse here relates to the choice between remaining within the superficial – the 'high, hard ground' described above by Schön – or descending to the depths or 'swampy ground' of the patient's troubled spirit. However, this would be not only short-sighted but dangerous. There is a vital

need to address the issues at the surface. It is here that science draws us to practice based upon the best available evidence; and, it is here that clinical effectiveness and the need for safe use of technology are issues of importance. But there is an equally vital need to recognise the point beyond which science and technology will not help, and an equally vital need to recognise that if we are to respond to the spiritual needs of our patients we must follow into this domain. One or the other will not do. We must be constant in our movement between the surface and the deep, between the rational and objective observation of the physical and mental state of those in our care and the appropriate response to these, and the subjective and existential response to the deeper search for meaning and peace in those whose very existence is in question.

A FRAMEWORK FOR SPIRITUAL CARE

Limits

It is not the intention to present a detailed description of the elements of spiritual care, particularly regarding how we may relate to those in our care. Where such attempts have been made, it is invariably the case that the interventions suggested cannot easily be distinguished from interventions that may be prescribed or proposed under labels other than the spiritual. For example, we may very well identify such elements as presence, availability, compassion, empowerment, etc. But Carol Kirby addresses these same issues as elements of the therapeutic relationship in Chapter 29. Similarly, we may consider means by which we can move beyond treatment of disease as encapsulated within the mainstream medical model, to a healing of the whole person. But Lynn Basford addresses these same issues in Chapter 31, where she considers approaches to complementary therapy.

What we can do here is to speak of the spiritual orientation and how we may encompass this in our care of the whole person. This means how we can reach out to and help those who are in spiritual need or pain in situations such as where there is a sense of loss or hopelessness that may even extend to a loss of the will or psychic energy to continue; where the other feels a sense of existential loneliness and alienation within a new, strange and threatening environment; where the intrusion of illness or disability is leading the other to seek meanings behind their very existence; where the other feels so threatened by the emergence of serious illness that they are filled with an existential dread of the approaching end of life; or, where a crisis of faith is occurring in someone who previously had held to this lifeline.

Working in contexts

In moving forward we must have some acceptance of the concept of spirit and how this will inform a spiritual dimension in our caring practices. In this chapter we have attempted to address meanings and how these may relate to the health and well-being of those in our care. You should not feel obliged to accept the meanings put forward. Indeed, your capacity to respond on this spiritual level would be bound to failure if you embarked on such a project without true acceptance and commitment. In this most personal of dimensions you must make you own mind up about these matters. It is sufficient that you bring to those in your care what spiritual support your conscience permits. But included in this must be an acceptance of the beliefs of those in your care and a capacity to provide them with the space to confront their own spiritual dilemmas.

Also of importance are those other contexts or discourses that we discussed above. There is no call here to accept or reject these various orientations, one in favour of another. From the discourse between the sciences and humanities we must draw insights into the contribution that science brings to what we called surface care and the equally important insights the humanities bring to that which we described as deep care. From our awareness of the political discourses, we must bring insights into how the modern technological world, with its valuing of individualism and material things, threatens and alienates the person, and how those who are ill or damaged are particularly vulnerable and in need of spiritual support.

Framing the spiritual dimension

Some quarter of a century ago Henri Nouwen (1975) presented a framework for reaching out spiritually. He presented this in terms of three polarities:

1 The polarity of self and relation to self, with its polarity of loneliness as opposed to solitude and meaningful knowing of the inner self or being.
2 The polarity of self in relation to others, with its polarity of hostility as opposed to hospitality or making a space available for the other to find meaning and peace.
3 The polarity of self in relation to the wider cosmos or a creator, in which the polarity is between illusion and faith or true reality.

Many years later, in a nursing context, Reed (1992) presented a similar emerging paradigm for addressing the spiritual dimension in nursing. Reed viewed the spiritual dimension as a propensity to make meaning through relatedness. This may be experienced:

- *Intrapersonally* – as a connectedness within oneself
- *Interpersonally* – as a connectedness with others
- *Transpersonally* – as a connectedness with an unseen God or greater cosmic force.

From a medical perspective, Robert Twycross (1999), a distinguished palliative care physician, more recently presents a very similar framework, in which he suggests that spiritual dimension must address:

- the meaning and purpose of life for the individual
- interconnectedness and harmony with others
- relationship with God/ultimate reality.

The similarity between these different frameworks is notable, which is perhaps not surprising. Each author speaks from a wealth of experience concerning the spiritual dimension of care – one in the field of caring ministry, one in the field of nursing practice, and one in the field of palliative medicine. In proceeding to confront the spiritual dimension we can use such framings to give direction to our way forward. In essence, they provide an approach that extends from the necessary beginning of self-knowledge, the journey out from self to connection with the other, the supportive presence with and for that other and, finally, the helping of that other in the journey towards facing his or her own destiny.

Commitment of self

This relates in part to the relation to self, referred to by Nouwen (1975), Reed (1992) and Twycross (1999) above. In proceeding on this basis, we are recognising that there are no tried and tested formulae that will tell us how we may address spiritual needs, in the same way that we may have a formula for the making up and application of a plaster to a fractured limb. The make-up of each person's psyche or spiritual being is different and the challenges confronted are unique to each person. Furthermore, if we are to respond to the other at this deep and intuitive level, we are calling upon our own psyche, our own spiritual dimension, and this we cannot construct to order. As Wolff-Salin states:

> . . . the issue is one of personal being and personal becoming. No techniques, no learning on a superficial or intellectual level prepare one for this work, but only a certain choice of how to live, and the gift to live it. In other words, the first requirement is the depth, seriousness, and perseverance of one's own journey.
>
> (Wolff-Salin, 1989, p. 137)

In the words expressed by Schön (1987), we must have a willingness to enter into the swampy ground that is the troubled and painful presence of the other. This calls us to move beyond the surface or superficial, to a willingness to live authentically. It is in fact an intentional choice: the choice to shed the protections of intellectualism and role behaviour and offer the self to the other.

Connection

The most difficult step after this choice is to enter into the spiritual presence of another person. As we have noted, many and varied are the defences constructed by professionals to avoid personal entanglements with patients or clients. In a review of spiritual phenomena in nursing, Golberg (1998) identified a number of such phenomena that were found to cluster in two groupings. The first of these was labelled emotional phenomena and included meaning, empathy/compassion, hope, love, and religion/transcendence. The second was labelled physical phenomena and included presencing, touch and healing. Because the spiritual is embodied in the person and the separation of physical, psychological, social and spiritual belies the integration and interdependence of these elements, the two categories were further collapsed to a single encompassing category labelled 'connection'.

The latter study was limited as it drew its data from nursing literature and failed to present a sound argument for connection being a discrete element that can be shown to relate specifically to the spiritual dimension and as such differentiate it from other caring dimensions. For example, someone who completely rejects the value or even existence of a spiritual dimension, might undertake the same study and present the same case for connection being the fundamental underlying element within a psychotherapeutic relationship. Nevertheless, the study does justify a case for recognising that connection is at least an important element within the spiritual dimension. However, what is important here is the nature of the connection. It demands that we connect on a spiritual level and while touch may assist the communication between beings and compassion may merge in the contact, the connection itself is beyond words of description and is an allusion to the coming together of spirit-being with spirit-being. It is vitally important that this lack of explanation of the connection is not rejected as being esoteric or meaninglessly abstract. It is quite simply true that when such spiritual connection occurs there is an experiencing of contact that is instantly more intimate, more whole, more alive, and characterised by an insightful realisation of coming into the presence of the other that is akin to an awakening or an epiphany. If it could be described in more objective terms, it would be something other than spiritual.

Creating a spiritual space and responding appropriately

This relates to that element that Nouwen (1975) referred to as the polarity of relationship with others and Reed (1992) referred to as interpersonal relating. In line with Nouwen's perspective, the challenge here is to create a hospitable space within which the patient feels both accepted and received and in which he or she feels at liberty to express their concerns and to unfold their deepest anxieties and inner suffering. The techniques involved – listening, reflecting together, responding with compassion – will be addressed elsewhere and are not detailed here. What is important is the willingness to be the host, the receptacle of the patient's fears and concerns, and going beyond this to being the servant of compassion.

Transcending the immediate

For Nouwen (1975), Reed (1992) and Twycross (1999) there was a third dimension, which related to the idea of a higher power or creator, and as such transcended the immediate situation. It is a relation that is above, beyond or in the hereafter. Where it exists, it calls the patient and those loved ones close to him to an act of faith. Such faith is a personal thing and as such it is a place to which the individual must journey alone. The call here is to demonstrate acceptance and respect, and to ensure that this space accommodates this journey, the choices it involves and the leaps of faith it entails.

Study Activity 23.5

At the end of a lengthy chapter on the most difficult and complex of issues, you are probably asking the question 'Where do I go from here?'. In his excellent account of a history of humanity through the eyes of women, Theodore Zeldon (1998) ends his book with these words:

> It is in the power of everybody, with a little courage, to hold out a hand to someone different, to listen, and to attempt to increase, even by a tiny amount, the quantity of kindness and humanity in the world . . . (History) has so far been largely a chronicle of ability gone to waste. But next time two people meet, the result could be different.
>
> (Zeldon, 1998, pp. 471–2)

● This Study Activity invites you to take up Zeldon's challenge. Using the above guidelines on responding to the spiritual call, for the next week go out with intentionality to seek spiritual connections in your clinical area or even in your day-to-day life. It is of course essential that you do this unobtrusively, with sensitivity and in an ethical and responsible manner. Keep a journal or diary of these contacts. It is important that you make a record of each contact as soon afterwards as possible. After each contact reflect upon what took place and use these reflections to 'inform' your subsequent contacts. At the end of the week, re-read this section of the chapter and consider how well you addressed the key elements and what you might do to improve this dimension of your caring practice. It may be particularly useful if you carry out this activity under the advice and supervision of your mentor.

SUMMARY

In this chapter we have attempted to address one of the most difficult areas in nursing. That is, responding to the spiritual dimension within our caring practices. The difficulties begin with establishing some clarity in what we mean by the spiritual dimension. This has always been a troublesome undertaking. By accepting that there is such a dimension, we are in effect acknowledging the existence of something we might call the spirit. This has been variously described within the chapter as spirit, soul, self, consciousness and heart. One understanding of this term, the idea of a deep/internal life force or enlivening core was identified, and on this basis we proceeded to identify a number of elements that were presented as reflecting the spiritual domain.

However, there was also recognition of lack of clarity and consensus about what spirit and the spiritual domain consist of. In this respect, we acknowledged the need for a sceptical and critical approach to arriving at some understanding of these phenomena. As an aid to this journey of discovery, particular attention was paid to various discourses that influence how people think about these concepts. These included the science–humanities discourse, including the opposing positions of what might be termed the secular and the sacred; the political discourse and the influences of a modern materialistic and depersonalising society on the oppression of the spirit; and the discourse in respect of deep and superficial ways of living and relating. In each instance, the implications of these various discourses for nursing were briefly addressed.

A framework for spiritual care was then suggested. Although not exhaustive, it is hoped that the ideas presented at least form the basis for proceeding to develop appropriate approaches to the spiritual dimension in the practice setting, and that they provide the foundation for more extensive reading. In carrying this project forward, the student may find it helpful to return to the framework for spiritual care presented in the chapter, and refine and adapt it to best suit their particular ways of working. In doing so, it is important to keep in mind that the purpose of this chapter is to recognise a spiritual dimension of need in those people we call patients, and to establish how we can best respond to their soulful call. In ending, we might recall the powerful reference to such

responding in the writing of Paul Solomon (1991):

> *If I want to know what you're thinking right now, all I have to do is care more about what you're thinking than what I'm thinking . . . As soon as I care more about what you're thinking than what I'm thinking I will give up my thoughts and I will absorb yours, and I will understand you.*
>
> (Solomon, 1991)

REFERENCES

Archer, J. (1999) *The Nature of Grief*, Routledge, London

Bellah, R., Madsen, R., Sullivan, W. *et al.* (1985) *Habits of the Heart: Individualism and commitment in American life*, University of California Press, Berkeley, CA

Bradshaw, A. (1994) *Lighting the Lamp: The spiritual dimension of nursing care*, Scutari, London

Downie, R.S. (1989) *Roles and Values*, Methuen, London

Frankl, V. ([1954] 1984) *Man's Search for Meaning* (revised and updated edition), Simon and Schuster, New York

Golberg, B. (1998) Connection: an exploration of spirituality in nursing care. *Journal of Advanced Nursing* 27(4), 836–42

Greenfield, S. (1999) Soul, brain and mind. In: Crabbe, M.J.C. (ed.) *From Soul to Self*, Routledge, London

Heidegger, M. (1962) *Being and Time*, Blackwell, Oxford

Hillman, J. (1997) *The Soul's Code: In search of character and calling*, Bantam, London

James, W. (1954) *Principles of Psychology*, World Publishing, Cleveland, OH

Keizer, B. (2001). Living well, dying well (1). In: Marinker, M. (ed.). *Medicine and Humanity*, King's Fund, London

Lerner, M. (1997) *The Politics of Meaning: Restoring hope and possibility in an age of cynicism*, Addison-Wesley, New York

McGilloway, O. and Myco, F. (1985) *Nursing and Spiritual Care*, Harper and Row, London

McSherry, W. (2000) *Making Sense of Spirituality in Nursing Practice*, Churchill Livingstone, Edinburgh

Menzies, I. (1960) *The Functioning of Social Systems as a Defence Against Anxiety*, Tavistock, London

Moore, T. (1992) *Care of the Soul*, Piatkus, London

Narayanasamy, A. (1991) *Spiritual Care: A resource guide*, Quay Books, Lancaster

Nouwen, H. (1975) *Reaching Out*, Collins, London

Nouwen, H. (1980) *In Memorium*, Ave Maria Press, Notre Dame, IA

Parse, R.R. (1995) *Illuminations: The human becoming theory in practice and research*, National League for Nursing, New York

Reed, P. (1992) An emerging paradigm for the investigation of spirituality in nursing. *Research in Nursing and Health* **15**, 349–57

Rees, W. and Lutkins, S. (1967) The mortality of bereavement. *British Medical Journal* **4**, 13–16

Sartre, J-P. (1969) *Being and Nothingness*, Routledge, London

Schön, D. (1987) *Educating the Reflective Practitioner*, Jossey-Bass, San Francisco, CA

Snow, C.P. (1959) *The Two Cultures and the Scientific Revolution*, Cambridge University Press, Cambridge

Solomon, P. (1991) Paul Solomon speaks on spiritual roots and the journey to wholeness. *Human Potential Magazine*, **16**(3), 28–32

Twycross, R. (1999) *Introducing Palliative Care* (3rd edition), Radcliffe Medical Press, Oxford

Williams, R. (1983) *Keywords*, Flamingo, London

Wolff-Salin, M. (1989) *No Other Light: Points of convergence in psychology and spirituality*, Crossroad, New York

Zeldon, T. (1998) *An Intimate History of Humanity*, Vintage, London

MODULE 5: THE SOCIAL AND HUMAN CONTEXT OF NURSING CARE

REFLECTIONS

On reading this module you will have become very aware of the politics that impinge on the world of nursing and that nursing does not operate in a political vacuum. As the world becomes a 'global health community' where we have become increasingly interdependent and interrelated, we are made aware of the issues of social injustice, social economics and the lack of moral and ethical integrity that influence health care. Working on the premise that nursing work is within multicultural and multiracial societies, you need to have a broader understanding of religion and spirituality to ensure holistic care is given to all. To have augmented your knowledge you will have examined the literature and related it to your practice arena.

Religion and spiritual care are often misunderstood and largely overlooked when giving care. Sometimes they are considered to be one and the same. However, having explored these chapters you will have gained useful insights as to the differences. It may be useful at this juncture for you to write in your portfolio your understanding of the terms and how they are used in your practice arenas.

Spirituality and religious beliefs are of paramount importance to the dying person. When we have lived the fabled, 'three score years and ten', we can assume death is on the horizon. While this philosophy is congruent with people's beliefs, we have collectively failed to recognise people's individuality and their physical and psychological wellness that provides a framework to recover from illness and achieve longevity. The facts are that increasingly more people are reaching advanced age but their experience with health assessment and therapeutic interventions has for the most part been discriminatory. The National Service Framework for Older People clearly highlights this situation and plans to eradicate any discrimination based on a person's age.

We would advise you to continue to be politically aware, be conscious of discriminatory practice, social exclusion and equality based on age, gender, racism, and religion. As a bonus we would hope you become a true advocate of the needs of all your patients and thus enhance the political position of nursing.

MODULE 6:   FRAMEWORKS FOR PRACTICE

INTRODUCTION

The movement from Module 5 to Module 6 is something of a watershed. The first five modules of the book concentrated, to a large extent, upon the knowledge aspect of nursing. From Module 6 we concentrate primarily on the practice of nursing. That is not to say that Modules 1–5 excluded any concern for practice. Indeed, the link between the knowledge being considered and the practice of nursing has been a feature of every chapter so far.

However, it is common within nursing to speak of the theory and practice of nursing. This, of course, implies a difference between the knowledge of nursing and the doing of it, and indeed is often, in a more extreme way, a term used to differentiate the academic study of nursing and the real world of nursing practice. In this context, it is common also to hear of the 'theory–practice' gap, a thesis that argues that

there is a problem within nursing, whereby there is a failure to apply the theories that would enhance care to the practice of nursing. There are dangers implicit in such positions.

Obviously there is the risk that by seeing theory and practice as different and perhaps lacking in relevance to each other, the risk of a gap between theory and practice may be increased. Indeed you may think that we are adding to this ourselves through the structure of this book. However, every project must commence somewhere and there is a certain logic in addressing the knowledge (or theory) that is relevant to practice and then attending to that practice. In doing so, we have attempted in the first five modules to relate the knowledge issues to practice at each point and in the same way, in the next four modules, the issues of practice will be linked to their knowledge or theory underpinnings.

24

PROBLEM-SOLVING FRAMEWORKS: THE NURSING PROCESS APPROACH

Oliver Slevin

> *Too much discussion of critical thinking focuses either on the discipline of logic or on general skills in problem solving. As long as critical thinking is conceived of exclusively as a form of logic or some watered-down version of the scientific method, the focus will remain purely instrumental, objective and impersonal.*
>
> (Meyers, 1986, p. 117)

LEARNING OUTCOMES

After studying this chapter you will be able to:

- Present an argument for utilising frameworks that may guide practice
- Identify and critique common approaches to solving problems
- Describe the framework known as the problem-solving approach
- Compare and contrast the problem-solving process and the research process
- Demonstrate an awareness of critical thinking and the capacity to develop critical thinking skills in practice
- Present the nursing process method as an application of the problem-solving approach that is cyclical, iterative and dynamic
- Describe the stages or elements of the nursing process method
- Discuss the controversy surrounding the notion of nursing diagnosis, including the advantages and disadvantages of this concept and alternatives to its use
- Demonstrate the capacity to develop skills in using the nursing process method.

INTRODUCTION

How can we develop an approach for dealing with nursing problems that is systematic and effective, yet does not make nursing an impersonal and excessively objective endeavour? Is it possible to have a problem-solving framework, established upon a high degree of critical and analytical thinking, that still fits with the highly personal, relational and caring orientations that are characteristic of nursing? These are the questions raised by the above opening quotation from Meyers (1986). These are the questions this chapter attempts to address.

Thus far in this book we have proceeded along a logical course that endeavours to bring together the knowledge and theoretical basis of nursing with the practice or doing of nursing. In Module 1 we outlined the emergence of nursing as a caring occupation and Module 2 explored the movement of this occupation towards its present-day orientation as a professional discipline. A characteristic of such professional disciplines is the possession of a specific and sophisticated body of knowledge that underpins practice. Module 3 detailed the philosophical and theoretical basis upon which the discipline of nursing may be based. In that module it was recognised that nursing is a complex relational activity involving nurses as carers and those being cared for (patients or clients, their families, communities). Such work requires different patterns of knowing: not only empirical or scientific knowledge, but also ethical, aesthetic and personal ways of knowing (Carper, 1978). While this emphasised the need for a balanced approach, it was nevertheless recognised that in complex, high-risk health care situations there is an imperative to ensure that practice draws on the best available knowledge.

This is increasingly recognised as health care systems embrace approaches to evidence-based health and as the health care disciplines (including nursing) are increasingly expected to establish evidence-based practice approaches. This particular emphasis was explored in Module 4.

In essence, the first four modules of the book established a knowledge or theoretical foundation for the study and practice of nursing. However, throughout these modules the emphasis was on how this knowledge base relates to practice. This was framed within a view that the nurse is involved in a relationship of *caring* for *others* in the *context* of *health*. These four terms were identified within Chapter 9 as encompassing the *metaparadigm* of nursing: those elements which together establish the totality of nursing's concerns. Both the original and most influential metaparadigm presented by Fawcett (1993, 2000), consisting of person, health, environment and nursing, and a variation (Slevin, 1999), consisting of person, health, environment and caring, were presented. In both instances, it will be noted that *environment* is a significant element of the paradigm. This recognises that nursing always occurs within some context or other, and that this context is highly significant in shaping nursing activities. At a broad level, environment can be recognised as both physical and social. The physical environment can impact significantly on health and on how health care is delivered. Later, in Module 8, we consider public health and the extent to which issues such as water, sewage, and pollution can impact upon the health of communities. In Module 10 we consider the global dimensions of risk which include the impact of major disasters that (whether natural or manmade) impact upon health and safety.

However, the environment is also a social setting: we are greatly influenced by others in our environment at all stages, from the cradle to the grave. We note above that even within the micro social system that is the nurse–patient interface, we are involved in social relationships; nursing, as we have claimed, is primarily a relational activity. Indeed, Module 7 of this book is devoted exclusively to therapeutic modes of intervention established primarily upon the nurse–patient relationship. But it was in the previous module, Module 5, that we concentrated primarily upon the social and human context. Each individual in our society is influenced by political forces, and by social phenomena such as race, ethnicity, culture, gender, and age. At a more personal level, there is also a spiritual dimension that greatly influences our life and responses to illness, loss, death, etc. While this has an internal aspect, it also has a social aspect, discussed in the context of religion.

As indicated in the Introduction to this module, the end of Module 5 marked a watershed. This represents a movement from knowledge and scientific theory and other forms of cognitive, moral, personal and aesthetic awareness that underpin our work as nurses, to a more specific concern with the *practice* of nursing. It is important to recognise that it is this, the *practice* of nursing, that is our primary concern. All those dimensions of knowledge that we considered in the first five modules are important only in so far as they inform this practice, and are in turn informed by it. We might indeed claim with justification that knowledge that does not *inform* nursing practice and/or *emerge* from that practice is of no importance to nursing and should be excluded from this book and indeed from our attention as practitioners of nursing.

The main problem we face in nursing is, however, of a rather different order. Nursing is about the delivery of care, often within complex high technology situations. It has the aim of promoting, enhancing and sometimes restoring health, which itself is a complex phenomenon. It occurs within a range of physical and social contexts, each in turn with *their* complexities, both individually and in terms of how they interact. The problem facing nursing is not so much the seeking of relevant knowledge, but the realisation that by its very nature nursing must call upon an exceptionally broad range of knowledge and *ways* of knowing.

The claim being made here is fairly straightforward. The knowledge and ways of knowing that we draw to nursing are useful in that they can be harnessed to a particular purpose. That is, the forming of frameworks that will inform and guide our practice. In nursing, as noted in Module 3, the important theory is a practice-guiding theory – what Dickoff and James (1968) defined in their ground-breaking paper as *situation-producing theory*, and what Argyris and Schön (1974) explored in their study of theories-of-action and theories-in-use. Indeed, we also noted in Module 3 that one particular facet of theorising is the establishment of theoretical statements as conceptual models – broad frameworks that can provide a general direction to our nursing activities. In this module we carry this further by considering particular ways in which we frame and guide our practice at the point of delivery of nursing care. Subsequent chapters in the module address how we frame our practice on the basis of such constructs as nursing competencies, or on reflective and clinical reasoning processes. In this first chapter we concentrate particularly upon that rational-logical perspective that is commonly described as the problem-solving method, and its particular implementation in what has become known as the nursing process method.

THINKING AND ACTION

Problem-solving

At many points in each day the working nurse approaches her patient. She is confronted with particular phenomena. There is a situation or context within which a patient exists, and into which the nurse now enters. The context is within a *health* parameter; the nurse is not entering here to carry out the legal conveyance of a property sale, or to undertake the cooking of a meal. It must be assumed that there will be some health-related matter or problem to be dealt with, and that it is the nurse's duty to respond to this matter. As the nurse carefully observes and interacts with the patient, she iden-

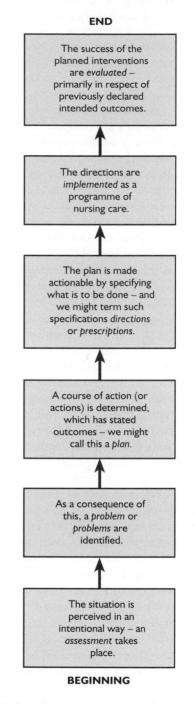

END

The success of the planned interventions are *evaluated* – primarily in respect of previously declared intended outcomes.

The directions are *implemented* as a programme of nursing care.

The plan is made actionable by specifying what is to be done – and we might term such specifications *directions* or *prescriptions*.

A course of action (or actions) is determined, which has stated outcomes – we might call this a *plan*.

As a consequence of this, a *problem* or *problems* are identified.

The situation is perceived in an intentional way – an *assessment* takes place.

BEGINNING

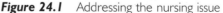

Figure 24.1 Addressing the nursing issue

tifies nursing 'problems' or 'issues' that *she* must respond to. The patient may appear flushed, a clinical thermometer reading may demonstrate an elevated body temperature, and the patient may complain of feeling hot, or weak, or unable to think straight. The nurse identifies the patient as febrile. Or, the patient may appear pale and frightened, and be bent over; when asked he may complain of abdominal pain. Further queries may identify characteristics of this pain, and palpation of the abdomen may isolate tenderness in a particular area. The nurse is faced with a problem in each case, and each of these problems presents risks to the patient's comfort, health and well-being, or even survival. She must determine how she will move forward, how she will *solve* this problem.

Much of the seminal work on what is today referred to as the *nursing process* derives from the work of Ida Orlando (1961, 1972), on what she termed 'the process of nursing'. This centred upon the three interactive elements of patient behaviour, nurse reaction (to this), and nurse action (the response to the call or need for help). Within this triadic sequence there is something going on: the nurse is thinking about the patient's problems and how she can help to resolve them. In a simplified form, the process we refer to (problem-solving) involves something like the process identified in Fig. 24.1 overleaf.

It will be noted that there is about this course of action a certain degree of tidiness, a logical movement from an initial point to a conclusion, a beginning to an end. Of course, in reality things are seldom as tidy as this: various influences may emerge that make the linear progression no longer feasible, or the planned actions are found on evaluation to have been unsuccessful or only partly successful. In real-life practice situations, there tends to be a more cyclical and interactive process at play, whereby not only is the process influenced by intervening variables (such as changes in the patient's condition, or environmental influences), but the evaluation leads to further assessment and subsequent planned interventions. This is indicated in Fig. 24.2, overleaf.

This more dynamic presentation of the process involved is in fact a *problem-solving* process. It is similar to that which we shall present below as *the nursing process method*. It *is* a process, and as such presents in clear and logical stages what may be happening when nursing care is countenanced, planned and then delivered. But it still has about it a degree of linearity, and it is still an essentially rational and instrumental approach.

It has been claimed that such a process is *scientific*, and it indeed resembles the dominant research process of the natural sciences, as described in Chapter 15. In that process, a research problem or issue is considered. This is primarily a problem associated with issues of knowledge of the world, or of understanding or establishing how phenomena in the world act or interact. The problem is, therefore, one of describing, or explaining or predicting. In identifying such a problem, preliminary consideration endeavours to clarify it and an exhaustive review of the literature establishes what is known about the particular area of knowledge. This establishes whether there are gaps in this knowledge that justify the research project. Tentative hypotheses that might explain the knowledge (in terms of how phenomena act and interact) are formulated, and the viability of these claims is then established through various methods of data collection and analysis. The robustness of the data collection and analysis is appraised using various tests of validity and reliability. The outcome of the study is evaluated: first by considering the extent to which hypotheses have been confirmed; then by the judgement of peers in the scientific community; and, finally by the extent to which the research and its findings are replicable. In the similar problem-solving method, a problem is also identified. This is not to do specifically or exclusively with establishing knowledge. Although this is important, the concern is usually with some practical real-world problem. Possible solutions are considered that will achieve the outcome (resolution of the problem), there is a plan for carrying forward the tentative best solution, and an evaluation

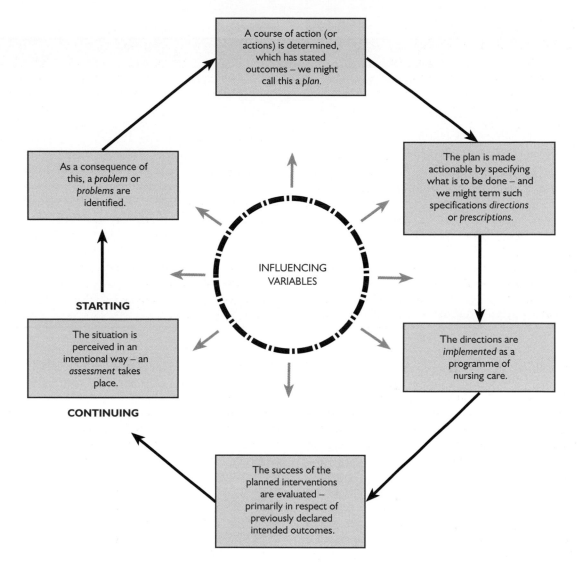

Figure 24.2 A cyclical progression

(that establishes if the outcome has been achieved). In both processes (research and problem-solving) there is an element of what is known as *trial and error*. If one hypothesis or solution is unsuccessful then others are tried, until one that most adequately describes, explains or predicts knowledge (in research) or resolves the difficulty (in problem-solving) is identified. This then holds as the best fit until it is found to be inadequate or something better (in terms of validating the knowledge or solving the problem) comes along. Table 24.1 (overleaf) shows the similarities and differences between the two processes.

It is important to differentiate the above use of *trial and error* from that commonly presented in cognitive psychology. Cognitive-behavioural psychologists often describe *trial and error* as a process whereby various solutions are attempted without any real endeavour to understand the

Table 24.1   The research and problem-solving processes

Research process	Problem-solving process
Addresses knowledge (in natural science/traditional research)	Addresses issues or problems that emerge in the world within which we live and work
Aims to construct knowledge and theory	Aims to resolve practical problems
A knowledge deficit is identified	Practical problem/s identified and explicated
Hypotheses or propositions for testing are formulated	Resolutions are formulated and prioritised in terms of anticipated fit
A research project is designed and methods of collecting and/or manipulating data are constructed	A plan to implement resolution/s is formulated, including identification of anticipated outcomes and prescriptions or directions for actions to be taken to achieve these ends
There is an emphasis on unbiased observation, precision of measurement, and validity and reliability of methods	While there is also a commitment to high standards in terms of method, in general the rigour demanded does not equal that of the formal research process
Data are collected and analysed	The plan of action is implemented
Findings are presented and subjected to critical appraisal, including that of peers within the particular scientific discipline	The process and achievement of desired outcomes are evaluated

relationships and meanings, and this is simply continued in an almost random way, until after a series of not thought-out *trials and errors,* one trial results in success. This is then accepted and carried forward as the normal way of responding to that situation, again without any real concern to understand *why* it is successful. Without such real understanding of how and why the solution works, it is unlikely that the individual will be able to adapt it to different circumstances or cope with situations where the solution fails. In research *and* problem-solving, real attempts are made to think critically about the problem, and tentative solutions (or hypotheses) are constructed in an informed and thoughtful way.

Study Activity 24.1

- Identify some problem you may have had in your own personal life. Reflect upon each of the following, writing short summary notes of your response in each case:
  - How you became aware that you had a problem.
  - How you defined the problem at the time.

- The various solutions to the problem that crossed your mind, and why you chose one rather than the others.
- Whether you sought anyone else's advice, why you chose this person, and how helpful they were.
- How successful your chosen way forward was in resolving the problem.

- Re-read your notes and then compare your strategy with the problem-solving approach described above. Was it broadly similar or different to the problem-solving approach? If it was different, do you think the problem-solving approach as outlined above would have been more effective in resolving your particular problem?

Critical thinking

It is important to recognise that the problem-solving method is essentially a *process* in the sense that this means a series of stages gone through to achieve certain goals. It tells us little of the actual *thinking* processes that are happening as this method progresses. This point can be clarified by referring again to the work of Orlando (1961, 1972) cited above. As will be recalled, she proposed a nursing process approach with the following elements: patient behaviour; nursing reaction; nursing action.

The reaction phase involves the following three components:

- *Perception* – the phenomena that the nurse observes, including the problems the patient presents;
- *Thinking* – the nurse's thoughts and reflections about her perceptions of these phenomena or problems, including reflections upon how she may assist the patient in their resolution;
- *Feeling* – the feelings these engender in the nurse.

Orlando emphasised the vital importance for these three components of dialogue with the patient. Through interacting with the patient, the nurse can validate her perceptions and thinking (the meanings she attributes to these perceptions), or where appropriate correct these through dialogue. By sharing her feelings, the nurse conveys to the patient the extent to which she understands and empathises.

It is important to note what is happening here, and the impact it has upon subsequent nursing actions. The nurse is in fact thinking *about* her perceptions, her thinking about the patient's problems, and her emotional or affective reaction to these. Within cognitive science, a process of *metacognition* has been identified in recent years (Paris and Winograd, 1990; Paul, 1993). This is in essence the process of thinking about thinking that Orlando referred to over 40 years ago, and it demonstrates the originality and importance of her work, which was not derivative of other scientific or nursing theories. This metacognitive process involves being critical and evaluative about our own thinking, and it is an essential part of what has become known as 'critical thinking'.

Unfortunately, as is the case with most technical terms, there are problems of interpretation and definition to cope with here also. Some use the term critical thinking as a synonym for any rational thinking process; as such it is often also used as a synonym for the problem-solving method. However, the problem-solving approach, as it is outlined above, is primarily a sequence of events leading to the solution of a problem, and as such does not necessarily incorporate the specific critical thinking perspective (Bevis, 1993; Boychuk Duchscher, 1999). Indeed, at its most instrumental and mechanistic level, it might even be antithetical to a critical orientation, often depending instead on an unquestioning allegiance to logical-deductive processes and laid-down protocols.

In appreciating this term, it is useful to start at a simple level of tautology: critical thinking is thinking that is critical. That is, a process whereby we approach the objects of our thinking with a sceptical and questioning orientation, taking none of it for granted but instead demanding grounds for its acceptance. In his famous treatise on this topic, the pioneering educator John Dewey ([1909] 1982) described critical thinking as 'suspended judgement' or 'healthy scepticism'. He defined such thinking as:

> *Active, persistent, and careful consideration of a belief or supposed form of knowledge in the light of the grounds which support it and the further conclusions to which it tends.*
>
> (Dewey, [1909] 1982, p. 9)

In a more recent definitive text, Fisher and Scriven (1997) similarly define such thinking as:

> *. . . a skilled and active interpretation and evaluation of observations and communications, information, and argumentation.*
>
> (Scriven, 1997, p. 20)

Putting such definitive statements with the earlier notion of thinking *about* our thinking, we might therefore recognise that critical thinking involves two related processes:

- a cognitive process of healthy sceptical questioning of claims or statements about the object of our thinking
- a metacognitive sceptical appraisal *of* this questioning, and reflection about how sound and balanced *it* is.

The claims or statements about the object of our thinking may of course be based upon our own observations (whether informal and qualitative or formal and quantitative), or upon our critical appraisal of the accounts of others (including our patients and professional colleagues). The claims may also be derived from apparently more robust sources, as in the case of research evidence. In each case, it is important that a critical eye is cast upon the information that presents itself to us. Where this is the case, there is an active and dynamic consideration of the situations and problems that are presented, and an equally active and dynamic consideration of the solutions. Orlando (1972) differentiated between an approach she described as the 'automatic nursing process' dimension and one she termed the 'deliberative nursing process' dimension. In the former, nurses carry out activities *on* the patient automatically, without any degree of critical appraisal, as in following doctors' orders or task-orientated routines. In the latter, there is a more deliberative approach wherein the nurse contemplates the patient's problems (through the processes of perception, reaction and action, as referred to above), discusses them with him, and arrives at an agreed course of action that is carried forward *with* the patient. Orlando later referred to the former automatic process as 'the nursing process without discipline' and the latter deliberative process as 'the nursing process with discipline' (Orlando Pelletier, 1990).

It is clear from the above deliberations that while the problem-solving approach is not necessarily synonymous with critical thinking, problem-solving that does not incorporate such critical orientation is a much more automatic and less effective process. A process of nursing that is automatic and without the discipline of such a critical orientation is more likely to present as a process whereby the nurse jumps to conclusions without adequate examination of the data. This is close to the trial and error situation described above, and returned to briefly below. The contrasting positions may be summarised as in Table 24.2.

Study Activity 24.2

One of the processes we identified with critical thinking was metacognition (thinking critically *about* our thinking).

- Re-read the explanation of metacognition in the above section.
- Carry out a review (using your library and the Internet) using the search term metacognition and the similar terms reflection and self-examination.
- Write your own summary (approximately two pages/500 words) of the processes involved in

Table 24.2 Critical and uncritical thinking

Critical thinking	Uncritical thinking
Careful consideration across the breadth and depth of all data available	Little or no attention to data
Healthy scepticism in approaching data	Low levels of scepticism extending to unquestioning acceptance of facts
Judgement suspended until a case for acceptance is justified	Tendency to jump to conclusions
Highly reflective orientation	Highly unreflective orientation
Solutions to problems carefully thought out and prioritised	Single solutions carried forward on a trial-and-error basis
Metacognition (thinking critically about one's own thinking) present	Metacognition absent

metacognition that also compares it with the other two terms. In particular, identify how each may differ in terms of the processes involved and in terms of their goals.

- Ask your personal tutor or a colleague/fellow student to comment on your summary.

ALTERNATIVES TO THE PROBLEM-SOLVING APPROACH

Orientations

We return to the use of the problem-solving framework in nursing presently. However, in the reality of day-to-day practice, there is a variety of ways in which nurses approach their work. Some of the more important of these in the context of modern nursing are addressed in the subsequent chapters of this module. However, it is useful to note the existence of these and other approaches at this stage. This is important in a complex human and relational activity such as nursing, where it must be recognised that different circumstances may call for different approaches. However, this is not to say that all such approaches are valid. This is why it is so important that nurses adopt a critical thinking orientation such as that discussed above. This enables them to question the validity of different approaches rather than mindlessly continuing with practices that are ineffective and perhaps even dangerous.

Trial and error

We have already considered this approach in the previous section of the chapter. Of course, it was recognised that in the problem-solving approach, and even in the course of formal research, there is an element of trial and error. However, what we are concerned with here is that other meaning of the term, where there is a thought-less and uninformed approach to problems. Here, the problem is approached by trying out solutions that are not thought-out. The success of such an approach is largely down to luck and

coincidence. Furthermore, as noted earlier, the nurse has given no thought to *why* or *how* the solution works. As a consequence, when the 'solution' runs into trouble there is no way in which the nurse can identify what is happening and how to respond to it. It will also be clear that such an approach has major ethical implications. These not thought-out solutions are after all being tried out on real people, in circumstances where the nurse has no knowledge of how the intervention will affect the patient. Not only does the nurse have no idea whatsoever about whether the trial will solve the problem; by the same token she can have no real knowledge of possible detrimental or harmful consequences. Such 'trial and error' approaches are by definition not only generally ineffective but also morally reprehensible.

Traditional approaches

When problems are being addressed on the basis of tradition, historical values are the determining factors. In nursing there is a long history of nursing practice based upon tradition. For example:

- Daily washing takes place in some hospital wards very early in the morning, irrespective of the patients' wishes.
- Such activities as the latter, and other activities such as medicine administration or wound dressings, are carried out as tasks at particular times and according to particular protocols, often by particular nurses being allocated tasks for the day.
- In wards for older persons, patients are sometimes put to bed in the early evening, sometimes with no-one still being up and dressed as early as 7 p.m.

It is, of course, possible that some of these activities were originally based upon sound thinking and if addressed through active, problem-solving approaches they may still be the best way of doing things. However, the situation is that the practices have been passed on from generation to generation of nurses, so that they are practised in an automatic and unthinking way. Not only does no-one question them, but such questioning tends to be strongly resisted. It may be recalled that in Chapter 9 we noted that Kerlinger (1987) drew attention to the high degree of tenacity with which such traditional practices are held once they become embedded in a culture.

It does not automatically follow that such traditional approaches are harmful. Indeed, it is usually the case that no overt harm can be readily perceived, because if this was the case the practices would have long since been discarded. The fact that they have been retained and become part of the culture of nursing testifies to the fact that such overt perceived harm is absent. This does not mean that they are *harmless* or that they are best practices. Referring to the third example in the previous paragraph (concerning wards for older persons), there is ample research evidence to indicate that prolonged bed rest and enforced inactivity are detrimental to the health of older people. However, such detrimental influences tend to be more insidious and for many years their consequences may not be readily attributable. Approaches that adopt critical thinking, including a critical and judicious application of evidence to practice, have increasingly called into question traditional methods of practice.

Research

In some instances the nature of the problem/s may justify proceeding to a full-blown research project, as referred to in the previous section and as detailed in Module 4 of this book. This approach is at the opposite end of a continuum to the trial and error and traditional approaches outlined above, and of course exceeds the problem-solving approach in terms of rigour. It is generally the case that the day-to-day problems we face do not justify such a more formal approach. In addition, the more rigorous research process, sometimes requiring special instruments or technology and the involvement of professional researchers, would normally involve costs that are prohibitive. However, in some instances the problem may be of such a

nature, or the consequences of inappropriate solutions may be so extreme, that such an approach is justified. This is particularly the case where the issue is one of establishing the best available evidence upon which to base practice. Where such evidence is not already available to inform the resolution of a particular problem, a decision may be taken to commission a piece of research to inform our decisions.

Intuitive approaches

The issue of using intuition to resolve problems is one of considerable controversy. This centres upon the meaning that we attach to this term. In some instances, when the word intuition is used, it refers to some sixth sense and attributes almost magical powers to those who are said to possess it. Such an orientation would, of course, be totally unjustifiable in circumstances where the health, well-being or perhaps even survival of those in our care is at risk. However, it will be recalled that in Chapter 11 we also explored another sense in which this term is used. There it was recognised as a form of personal or tacit knowing that emerges from extensive experience in a particular field. By virtue of such experience, the expert practitioner is able to perceive patterns and rapidly respond to these without having to go through a mechanical process of assessment, problem explication and planning as involved in the problem-solving process. Indeed, often such practitioners cannot even explicate how they arrived at their insights and decisions, sometimes almost instantly. This tacit or intuitive dimension is identified in the work of Polanyi (1958, 1966) and (within nursing) Benner (1984), and is essential to that form of clinical reasoning discussed by Benner in her chapter within this module.

There is a danger in seeing such approaches as tradition, problem-solving, research and intuition as alternative approaches that are mutually discrete. In the reality of best practice, problem-solving requires drawing upon the best evidence available, and where this is not available there may be due recognition of traditional approaches that through years of practice have been found to be successful. By the same token, critical thinking about the *practical* problems nurses encounter is always within a health context and is informed by a clinical wisdom that is tacit or intuitive. In such best practice situations, plans of action are not formulated to exclude tacit experiential knowledge, but allow for its use in the course of the implementation of care.

Authoritarian approaches

Authority is associated with power. Such power may be acquired through:

- a position in the hierarchy of an organisation, such as in the case of the chief executive of a health services trust or a director of nursing services
- a position of acknowledged expertise, such as in the case of a medical or nursing consultant.

If the decision-making is attributed to the source of authority or power, the individuals subjected to such authority accept no responsibility; indeed, the individuals do not even have to participate in the problem-solving or agreed solutions. The actions to be taken are prescribed by others, and any actions to the contrary may often be proscribed.

Such an approach in fact says nothing about the *means* of arriving at solutions to problems. It is a statement rather of the *locus* of the problem-solving or indeed any alternative approach. Those in authority may impose resolution of problems on the basis of trial and error, tradition, research, intuitive, or particular problem-solving approaches. The method used may indeed be a mix of any or all of these, and may be of varying degrees of effectiveness. However, by virtue of being distanced from the actual situation within which the problems may occur, it is likely that the decisions being imposed suffer from a lack of consideration of the specific situational context. Meyers (1986), in his classical study of critical thinking, points to evidence that general principles of logic and reasoning carry us only so far. The importance of having experience of the situation within which

problems occur is vital to forming insights into emerging and recurring patterns (as identified also in the tacit knowledge contained in the intuitive approach above). In general, it can be expected that being distanced from the problem, having no first hand experience of how it affects those directly experiencing it, and attempting to propose solutions in line with abstract principles, are unlikely to result in truly effective measures being adopted. Nouwen (1994) is insightful in his reference to leaders of authority who might try to resolve difficulties in this way when he states that 'The great illusion of leadership is to think that man can be led out of the desert by someone who has never been there'. The role of those in authority in promoting effective approaches to practice cannot be underestimated. However, this is most effective where those in authority adopt leadership roles within which they acquaint themselves fully with the practice situation and where they adopt flexible and facilitative approaches rather than attempting to impose specific solutions from a distance.

Study Activity 24.3 ━━━━━━

Each of the above methods of framing our practice has its advantages and disadvantages, and in some cases it is hard to see how the limited advantages could justify the use of the approach when the major disadvantages are considered. In this Study Activity you should concentrate on one of these, described as tradition above.

- Re-read the section on tradition and extend your consideration of this by further library study of the concept.
- Select from within your current or previous clinical area an example of practice that fits this model (i.e. is based primarily on tradition).
- Using the skills or attributes of critical thinking presented in the first column of Table 24.2, critique the practice you have identified. Your critical thinking should result in a balanced appraisal of the practice that includes a case for or against continuing the practice.

THE NURSING PROCESS METHOD

Background

It is important to appreciate that the nursing process method, as it is understood today, is a nursing implementation of that approach described earlier as the problem-solving approach. The term may thus be defined as:

> *a rational, logical, purposive, goal-orientated, systematic and planned approach to the resolution of problems within nursing contexts. It is to a large extent linear and sequential in its orientation, usually involving stages that follow a general progression from the assessment of a situation, through the identification of problems and tentative solutions, resulting in a plan of action that following implementation is evaluated. There is recognition of the interactivity of the elements and the cyclical and progressive nature of the method: evaluative information leads to further modification of the assessment, the problem and the plan as implementation proceeds. The method is nevertheless characterised by adherence to a systematic logic that extends from the assessment through to the evaluation of outcomes.*

Two provisos may be considered here. The first proviso is that not everyone agrees that the nursing process method is an application of the problem-solving approach. For example, Barnum (1998) suggests that there are fundamental differences between the two, sufficient to justify an alternative approach of *problem-orientated nursing* that is more closely modelled on the problem-solving approach. She presents some justifications for this. In problem-solving a problem must first exist, while the nursing process is carried forward when a person is identified as a patient or client, irrespective or prior to problems emerging. For example, in health promotional nursing activities, no specific health problem may be apparent. Also, the problem-

orientated approach may be adopted to solve problems for nurses that are not directly related to care (such as staff absence rates), while the nursing process is always centred upon care delivery. While such arguments may have certain academic interest, to all intents and purposes the nursing process follows the broad problem-solving approach discussed earlier.

The second proviso is that it is also important to recognise the subtlety at play in the term *nursing process*. The specific nursing process method, as it is described in the nursing literature and practised in clinical settings, is different to the process of nursing that occurs at the point of delivery of care. The latter process is highly relational and reflective, and involves the helping relationship between nurse and patient. Such a caring process may of course be provided within a nursing process method framework, but it may also occur in circumstances where such a systematic method is not in use at all.

The idea of a nursing process method finds its origins in American nursing during the 1950s. Lydia Hall (1955) and, later, Dorothy Johnson (1959) were speaking of such a method based upon researching or assessing the situation, arriving at decisions, and implementing these in nursing action. Orlando's work (1961, 1972, 1990), referred to earlier, placed this process within a nurse–patient relational frame, again using a three-stage process but describing the process in terms of patient behaviour, nurse reaction to this, and the nursing action ensuing from this reaction. By the 1980s the nursing process was being referred to as a four-stage process of research, planning, implementation and evaluation proposed by Yura and Walsh (1988). Not everyone was comfortable with the first stage being described as research. In line with the discussion earlier in this chapter, it was felt that research is not only a particularly rigorous approach, usually directed at the verification or validation of knowledge or building of theory, but is in fact a whole process in its own right, as illustrated in Table 24.1. It became more popular, particularly in the UK, to replace the term 'research' with 'assessment' and to identify the four phases or components of the nursing process method as:

- assessment
- planning
- implementation
- evaluation.

Study Activity 24.4 ⎯⎯⎯⎯⎯⎯

The above paragraphs provide a brief overview of the development of the nursing process method. As a critical thinker, you will be aware that often such historical accounts are selective and tell their story from a particular perspective. Given its prominence as a method of framing our practice, it is important that *you* have a sound understanding of this process and how it emerged as an important aspect of modern nursing. Write your own brief (two page/500 word) review of the emergence of the nursing process method, with particular reference to its development in the UK.

The diagnosis versus problem controversy

By the end of the 1980s it was becoming common to find the nursing process method presented as a five-stage rather than four-stage process. The variations to the five-stage process (of which there are at least two) primarily involve the splitting of the first 'assessment' stage into assessment and diagnosis, or assessment and problem identification. The controversy surrounds not the splitting of this first stage, but the use of the term diagnosis. The meaning of the term is not in itself problematic. Diagnosis is identifying a problem or fault, together with its nature or causes. The word derives from the Greek terms *gnosis* (knowing) and *dia* (through), thus meaning 'knowing through'. In its most common usage, i.e. medicine, it involves *knowing* a medical problem or disease *through* such means as touch (palpation), hearing (auscultation), sight (signs), recounted experiences of the patient (symptoms), and many more ways of searching

through and into the body or (in the case of psychiatric medicine) mind of the individual. While there is an artistry in diagnosis born out of extensive experience, it is also a scientific process. This is increasingly so in the world of modern technology and medicine, as means of exploring the body to microscopic levels and beyond come within our grasp. The difficulty with diagnosis derives mainly from its association with the medical profession and with certain characteristics some critics associate with that profession. In essence, the perceived difficulties include:

- The particular scientific orientation of medicine (primarily rooted in the natural and biological sciences) is seen to be a core value within diagnosis, and this is particularly the case in modern, high-technology health care systems. Nursing claims an approach that draws on a wider range of patterns of knowing (as demonstrated in Module 3 of this book), only one of which (the empirical pattern) fits with the diagnostic process. One illustration of this is the claim that doctors touch primarily to investigate or treat, while nurses also touch in a caring and healing manner. This is a point very aptly demonstrated by van Manen (1999), where he speaks of two forms of touch. The first of these is the *gnostic* probing touch, which is directed towards obtaining information (and as will be recalled, we draw attention to this etymological root of the term 'diagnosis'). The second of these is the *pathic* touch (the term 'pathic' derives from suffering and passion, and from the pity engendered by suffering). Such touch is a reaching out to the other, to comfort, to share in and ease suffering, to communicate togetherness in adversity, a message to the other that one is there, with them. The difficulty for nursing is that the diagnostic orientation (so the argument runs) tends to be primarily scientific and as such excludes other forms of knowledge that are important in nursing. In this respect, the restriction of 'touch' to a 'gnostic' purpose accentuates the objectification of the patient.

- It has been argued, most notably by Barnum (1987), that diagnosis is by definition a fragmentary approach, concentrating on specific issues (such as anatomical parts, body organs and systems, and their dysfunctions), and as such is antithetical to the holistic (whole-person) orientation of nursing. Stated in rather biased (and not always reasonable) terms, medicine treats cases, nursing cares for persons.

- It is recognised that many in the medical profession (and in other professional and social groups) display a degree of antagonism towards the nursing process method. It is understandable that where elaborate systems for planning care are being developed, other groups may feel their 'turf' is being threatened. In such circumstances, the inclusion of the term 'diagnosis' has been seen as a possible source of additional antagonism, sufficient to lead some nurses to seek alternative terms.

- The nursing diagnosis movement incorporates attempts to identify extensive data sets (lists of diagnoses) that are not necessarily shown to be effective or manageable (because of the increasing number of such diagnoses), or fully comprehensive (given that contextual influences upon nurse and patient often result in problems that are to an extent unique and situational). This has led some critics to suggest that this movement may be more about standardising care into forms suitable for managers and health economists whose aim is to cost care, rather than being about improving the quality of care.

In the face of such difficulties, nurses have sought alternatives to the 'diagnosis' terminology. One such alternative is to use the term 'nursing problem'. But here also difficulties arise. As noted above, all issues to be addressed in practice are not necessarily 'problems'. Notwithstanding the latter difficulties, the term *nursing*

diagnosis has increased massively in popularity. As a term it has existed as long as the nursing process method (back as far as the 1950s), but in more recent years it has become a major concern in nursing. The term is generally differentiated from medical diagnosis by emphasising that the intention here is to identify a specific human response (of a patient/client/family/group/community) to an actual or potential health problem that requires a nursing intervention. In general, these tend to be framed in terms of a stated nursing diagnosis, a corresponding nursing intervention, and an anticipated outcome. There are a number of developments within the nursing diagnosis and nursing problem movements, but the two most influential are identified here.

North American Nursing Diagnosis Association (NANDA)

For a number of years, this body has been developing a data set of nursing diagnoses that has been updated on a number of occasions. The body defined nursing diagnosis as:

> . . . *a clinical judgment about individual, family, or community responses to actual and potential health problems/life processes. Nursing diagnoses provide the basis for selection of nursing interventions to achieve outcomes for which the nurse is accountable.*
>
> (NANDA, 1990, p. 5)

Essentially, the NANDA classification consists of an extremely long list of diagnoses that has been updated regularly through NANDA conferences and publications. As an illustration, the following is the recent entry in respect of diagnoses for incontinence:

> *Incontinence, functional*
> *Incontinence, reflex*
> *Incontinence, stress*
> *Incontinence, total*
> *Incontinence, urge*
>
> (NANDA, 2001)

The NANDA organisation has actively promoted acceptance of its system at an international level, and there was even a little-publicised unsuccessful attempt to have the classification included in the World Health Organisation's International Classification of Diseases (*see* Hogston, 1997). There can be real advantages in identifying a taxonomy of diagnoses that may inform nursing practice. However, where this extends into very large lists (the most recent list includes 155 diagnoses) that are not always easy to interpret, the practicality of such an undertaking may be questioned. This is further complicated by the fact that the diagnoses are accompanied by nursing interventions and outcomes. In this respect, Barnum (1998) has stated:

> *Although the nursing process steps are easily learned and used by inexperienced nurses, the nursing diagnoses are so numerous as to make application a trial. The same can be said for the taxonomies of nursing interventions. The question is whether such a complex system can have a major impact upon practice.*
>
> (Barnum, 1998, p. 152)

International Classification for Nursing Practice (ICNP)

This is a project carried forward by the International Council of Nurses. It bears similarities to the NANDA approach. However, there has been a view that NANDA reflects the purpose for which it was constructed, within US culture and health care systems (Clark, 1998). In a sense, ICNP attempts to overcome such cultural limitations by moving towards a truly international classification. The ICNP uses the terms *nursing phenomena* (equivalent to NANDA's nursing diagnoses), and *nursing interventions,* again aimed towards achievement of specific nursing outcomes (as in the case of NANDA).

Like NANDA, the ICNP has developed through revisions from an alpha set to a more recent beta set (International Council of Nurses,

2002). However, as with the NANDA approach, questions may be begged about the practicality of large complex lists. In a recent study, Ruland (2001) carried out research into the ICNP beta set in Norway. This research scrutinised nursing records to identify terms that corresponded to ICNP terms relating to circulation of blood and elimination of body waste in a cardiac intensive care unit and a nursing home. For nursing phenomena (the equivalent of nursing diagnoses), 47% of the circulation terms found in records were similar to ICNP nursing phenomena, while 69% of elimination terms were similar. These figures may be deemed worrying. After all, for something like elimination of body waste, there should not be a great variation in terms. When considering nursing interventions, the figures were significantly lower. Only 27% of circulation terms (describing nursing interventions) corresponded with the ICNP intervention terms, with only a marginally higher 35% in respect of elimination. It is possible that this may demonstrate ambiguities in intervention terminology that may be resolved by further refinement of the ICNP taxonomy. However, the more likely case may be that interventions tend to be so situation and patient specific (and thus varying from situation to situation) that the formulation of such 'lists' of standard interventions is of limited value.

The difficulties in respect of nursing diagnosis are clearly considerable, and the practicality of such complex systems is still in question. That is not to say, however, that the alternative of using the term nursing *problem* is without difficulties. We have already noted Barnum's (1998) suggestion that in nursing it may not always be the case that the issues the nurse must address are suitably labelled as *problems*. There is of course an opportunity to seek an alternative term. The ICNP term *nursing phenomenon* referred to above might be one such alternative. The difficulty here is that it is to a large extent a synonym for diagnosis, but further to this the term phenomenon is so broad as to be of limited value. We noted in Module 3 that a phenomenon is simply some fact, or occurrence, or entity that we perceive. If we accept this, everything we observe or perceive that is to do with nursing is a nursing phenomenon – even a nurse's uniform! Another alternative is to backtrack to a four-stage nursing process of assessment, planning, implementation and evaluation. For the purpose of the final subsection we use the term 'problem identification'. While it is recognised that most modern texts (e.g. Meleis, 1997; Aggleton and Chalmers, 2000) now use the term nursing diagnosis, the argument here is that 'problem identification' is less controversial and fits more appropriately with what is intended to be a simple, practical and useful framework for everyday nursing practice.

Study Activity 24.5 ─────────

This Study Activity assumes access to a computer and the Internet. Using your browser, locate the websites for NANDA International and ICNP (the latter can also be accessed through the International Council of Nurses' website).

- Explore the list of nursing diagnoses in the current NANDA database, and the equivalent listing of nursing phenomena in the current ICNP version. Compare how these are worded and grouped into a taxonomy in each case.
- Explore how NANDA and ICNP state nursing interventions.
- Reflect upon how such extensive lists might assist you in carrying forward your own nursing practice.

The nursing process in action

The process as presented here consists of five elements or stages:

1 Assessment
2 Problem identification
3 Planning
4 Implementation
5 Evaluation.

It will be noted that, in line with the earlier arguments, the term 'problem identification' is

used rather than 'nursing diagnosis'. However, you may prefer the latter term. It is important to recognise that using this term does not necessarily imply an acceptance of either NANDA or ICNP philosophies. The important thing is that the activity involved identifies a *nursing* issue or problem that must be addressed, rather than the identification of a medical disorder. Of course, in some instances where nurses are involved in advanced practice roles (e.g. nurse therapists), they *may* be involved in the medical diagnosis process. In addition, all nurses collect data that may be used by medical practitioners in making medical diagnoses. It is important to make a clear distinction between those situations in which nurses are participating in medical diagnoses, and those situations where the diagnosis is seeking to uncover nursing problems or issues that must be addressed. It will be recalled that while there is a sequential aspect to this problem-solving process, there is also an interactivity that is dynamic and ongoing across and between the elements making up the stages of the process. This is demonstrated in Fig. 24.3.

While each stage impacts upon the others, each also has its particular function in contributing to the integrity of the overall process. These functions are outlined below. It should be noted that so far little has been said about *who* carries this process forward. In most situations there is a ward or facility manager, team leader or primary nurse with overall responsibility (and these are terms we return to in the final chapter of this module). However, in best practice situations the care team as a whole is involved at each stage of the process. This is particularly important where team members collaborate on the assessment, and where the team takes a group approach to problem identification and planning. In the latter situation in particular, the group can brainstorm possible solutions, and different areas of expertise of individual group members can be brought to bear on the problem/s. Where care is being implemented, it is again important that good teamworking takes place, so that care is adequately co-ordinated. Similarly, at the stage of evaluation, the experi-

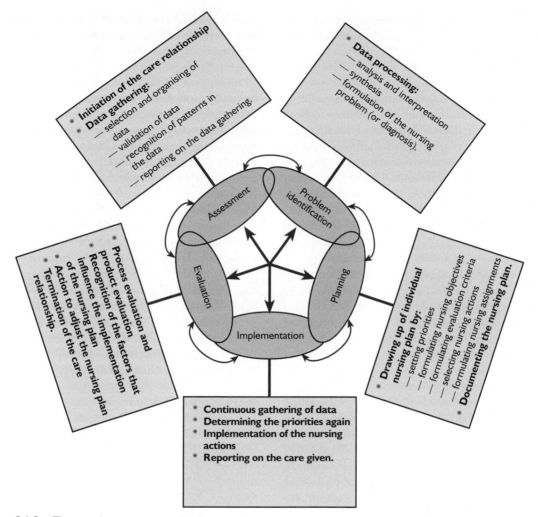

Figure 24.3 The nursing process method

ences of the whole group can contribute to the appraisal. It is important to recognise, however, that this approach is named the *nursing* process method. There is a danger here that, irrespective of how efficient the nursing team is, the care may be divorced from and not co-ordinated with the contribution of the other members of the health care team. It is therefore important that the nursing process is not carried forward in isolation, but is part of the overall programme of care. This is again a matter to which we return in the final chapter of this module. For now, we

give some further consideration to the stages or elements that make up the nursing process method.

Assessment

- Initiation of the caring relationship
- Data gathering:
  - selection and organising of data
  - validation of data
  - recognition of patterns in the data
  - reporting on the data gathering.

Traditionally, this is the equivalent of the nursing history, wherein quantitative information (height, weight, bodily characteristics, temperature, pulse, blood pressure, etc.) and qualitative information (mental state, social background, family status, etc.) are accumulated. However, while in the past this tended to be a routine and automatic procedure, carried out without much thought, in the nursing process the nurse should make attempts to validate the data and actively look for patterns emerging from that data. This does not mean that assessment protocols (identifying the assessment areas to be covered) or instruments (such as mental status questionnaires or coma scales) should not be used. Such protocols and instruments are useful aids to assessment, and in some health care settings particular protocols may be required within policy. However, it is important that data collected are examined in an analytical and careful way. It will be clear from this that the critical thinking orientation described earlier is vitally important within the nursing process. One useful device here is the concept of *triangulation* sometimes used in the human and qualitative sciences. This term is borrowed from mathematics and navigation, and involves examining the same phenomena from different perspectives (Denzin, 1989; Leininger, 1992). Such triangulation may be theoretical (involving using different theories that may explain the situation), or methodological triangulation (where the phenomenon is examined using different methods). Methodological triangulation may be particularly useful in assessment, where, for example, two or more measures for determining short-term memory may be employed.

It is also important to note the importance of the patient's contribution to the assessment process. It will be recalled that Orlando (1961, 1990) emphasised the dialogical nature of the nursing process, and the need to involve the patient in establishing the health care issues to be addressed. This is an important principle also recognised in more recent approaches to nursing, such as the *theory of human becoming* developed by Parse (1995). One useful orienta-

tion is that of the emic–etic perspectives identified within qualitative research (*see*, for example, Headland *et al.*, 1990). The *etic* perspective is essentially the scientific, detached, outsider view. It involves a dispassionate consideration of the situation and at its most extreme even views any subjective information as of limited or no value. The *emic* perspective is the alternative more humanistic, involved, insider view. It involves a more passionate and interested commitment to attempting to view the situation from the point of view of the subject (or in this case, patient). This is the orientation adopted in participant observation, for example, where the researcher attempts to observe the situation from the subject's perspective, and even uses the subject's language to describe those situations. An etic orientation is highly important in assessment: there is a need to accurately record important health indicators such as temperature, blood haemoglobin levels, etc. However, it is also important to obtain information about health from the emic (or patient's) view.

Problem identification

- Data processing:
  - analysis and interpretation
  - synthesis
  - formulation of the nursing problem (or diagnosis).

At this stage it becomes clear that the nurse must be even more critical and analytical in her thinking. It is often the case that there must be synthesis of information emerging from the assessment that leads to the formulation of a problem (or diagnosis, if this term is preferred). For example, taking together such data as pallor, cold sweating, rapid pulse, low blood pressure, and expressions of anxiety from the patient, a pattern reflective of circulatory shock may emerge. In so far as this is a situation to which the nurse must respond, it becomes a nursing *problem* and it must be clearly stated as such. All such problems must be similarly clearly identified.

It will be noted that in Fig. 24.3 the terms

problem identification and nursing diagnosis are identified as being interchangeable. As indicated above, this can be a matter of choice. However, even where there is no commitment to adopt a nursing diagnosis approach, taxonomies of nursing diagnoses and corresponding nursing interventions such as those presented by NANDA or in the ICNP can be a useful source to browse when attempting to formulate and state nursing problems.

It is important when attempting to discern nursing problems to constantly return to the data from the assessment phase. This may even involve the need to return and obtain further data. This constant movement between the data and the nurse's thinking about it is termed the *iterative* process (*see* Coffey and Atkinson, 1996), or *tacking* (*see* Geertz, 1996), where tacking is a metaphor for how sailing ships turn one way and then another to maximise wind energy. It will be clear from how Fig. 24.3 is presented that this iterative process is not exclusive to the assessment–problem identification interface, but occurs between each stage and all the others.

Planning

- Drawing up an individual nursing plan by:
  - setting priorities
  - formulating nursing objectives
  - formulating evaluation criteria
  - selecting the nursing actions
  - formulating nursing assignments.
- Documenting the nursing plan.

It is important to note that the planning process is not simply identifying a set of nursing problems and listing these. The process of prioritising the problems is vitally important. This must first of all rank the problems in terms of immediacy of the action needed: some problems may actually be life-threatening, while others are of less importance or urgency and can be left for attention at a later date. Of particular interest here is the method of *triage,* which involves the prioritisation of patients according to their problems within accident and emergency depart-

ments (Manchester Triage Group, 1997). Here, patients may be categorised into priority groups, as follows:

- Group 1 patients will be seen immediately by medical staff, and have absolute priority.
- Group 2 patients will be seen as soon as possible, preferably within 10 minutes of arrival, but not until all Group 1 patients have been seen.
- Group 3 patients will be seen as soon as possible, usually within 1 hour, but not until all Group 2 patients have been seen.
- Group 4 patients will be seen, if possible, within 3 hours, but not until all Group 3 patients have been seen.
- Group 5 patients will not be seen until all Group 1, 2, 3, and 4 patients have been seen.

Triage is, of course, a dynamic process that develops and can change literally from moment to moment, as sudden changes in patients' conditions and stability occur. It takes place in emergency care and also primary care settings. However, it demonstrates the fact that nurses must prioritise and that sometimes this must happen within relatively short time spans.

Also of significance here is how the goals to be achieved (variously defined as objectives or intended outcomes) must be stated. This requires a capacity to verbalise a solution to the problems in terms of the optimal or at least adequate outcomes that must be achieved. On the basis of these intended outcomes, those activities referred to as selecting nursing actions and formulating nursing assignments in Fig. 24.3 are carried forward. In terms of documenting the nursing plan, these are of particular importance. It is sometimes the case that these particular statements are referred to as *nursing prescriptions,* although (as with the term diagnosis) many nurses are reluctant to use this term because of its medical connotations. As a consequence, alternative terms such as nursing orders, nursing instructions or nursing directions are sometimes used. It must be realised that these statements are part of a formal record, and that the nurse who formulates them is professionally and legally accountable. It is therefore important that on the planning document or nursing orders sheet, the name of the nurse making the instructions is clearly stated, dated and accompanied by a signature. The importance of stating such required nursing actions or nursing prescriptions cannot be overemphasised. They must be presented clearly and succinctly and state clearly *what* actions are to be taken, *when* they are to be taken, *how* they are to be carried out and by *whom*.

Implementation

- Continuous gathering of data
- Determining the priorities again
- Implementation of the nursing actions
- Reporting on the care given.

The emphasis within this stage on continuous data collection (assessment) and ongoing determining of priorities (problem identification and review of same) highlights the iterative nature of the nursing process as discussed earlier. It should also be noted that there is a commitment not only to carry out the agreed nursing actions, but also to report the care given. As in the case of nursing instructions, such reporting is part of a formal official record. Staff carrying out the actions must therefore again record what was done in clear and succinct terms, and such records must be dated and have the name and signature of the person reporting clearly entered.

Evaluation

- Process evaluation and product evaluation
- Recognition of the factors that influence the implementation of the nursing plan
- Action to adjust the nursing plan
- Termination of the care relationship.

It is again useful to remind ourselves that the nursing process is an iterative process, and this is reflected to some extent in the commitment to process and product evaluation. In one sense, both of these can take place at an endpoint, at which time the team may review not only the process and how effective it was, but also the outcomes achieved. However, in a more fundamental sense, this also refers to the timing and nature of the evaluative processes. It is sometimes useful to separate evaluation into what is known as *formative* and *summative* evaluation. The latter, summative evaluation, is that which takes place at the endpoint, and usually involves seeking information on how efficiently the process worked and if and to what extent the identified outcomes were achieved. In some cases this may take place at the end of the particular patient's period of care, when it is also important to terminate the caring relationship appropriately. Formative evaluation is different. It is that ongoing process of evaluation that takes place throughout the period of care delivery, commencing at the stage of assessment and continuing on an ongoing basis. It is thus evaluation *during* the process rather than evaluation *of* the process. This is vitally important, as difficulties encountered must be identified and dealt with as and when they occur; but it also provides a growing body of evaluative information that can be incorporated in the summative stage later.

Study Activity 24.6

This is an extensive Study Activity that requires adequate preparation and would be completed over several days within a clinical situation.

The purpose of the Study Activity is to produce a simulated nursing process plan within a real-life situation. You will need to obtain the approval of your facility manager, the agreement of your mentor/facilitator, and the informed consent of a patient. In doing so, you must make it clear that this is a simulation (mock care plan) and will not be used to guide the actual care of the patient, and that full confidentiality will be maintained.

- Conduct an assessment of the patient, using the normal range of assessment protocols in use within the facility. Ensure that the assessment includes quantitative data in respect of the patient's general physical and mental health. Ensure that it also includes qualitative data obtained from the patient. Remember to apply both the emic and etic processes discussed earlier, so that you are accurately representing the patient's viewpoint.

- Review the data to identify any problems or nursing diagnoses that appear to be emerging. In doing so, ensure that you conduct this as an iterative process, returning to the data as necessary, but importantly (in line with Orlando's approach discussed earlier) also discussing the problems/diagnoses with the patient so that there is agreement on those identified. This should end with a set of problems/diagnoses that are clearly stated, and you might wish to consult the NANDA or ICNP databases for useful ways of expressing these statements.

- Draw up a plan that reflects the following properties:

  - a prioritising of the problems/diagnoses (which must reflect the health or life-threatening nature of each problem).

  - outcomes that need to be achieved to resolve each problem (including the identification of success criteria and the timeframe for achievement).

  - nursing instructions/directions/prescriptions that are to be implemented in order to achieve the outcomes (including details of *who* does it, *when* they do it, and *how* they do it).

- Arrange a session with your mentor to go through the documentation of your assessment, problem identification/diagnoses, and plan in detail. This will allow you to reflect on how well you conducted each of the three clusters of activities that are in fact the first three stages of the nursing process method.

(It may be the case that at the time you are studying this material you have no access to clinical facilities. But remember everyone has 'health' and health-related concerns or interests. Ask a friend or fellow student to be your proxy patient and conduct the exercise with that person as the subject.)

SUMMARY

In this chapter we have outlined that approach known as the nursing process method. You will have noted that this was presented as a special application of the problem-solving approach. While the chapter identified a number of variations to the nursing process method, the most common modern form consisting of a five-stage process of assessment, problem identification or diagnosis, planning, implementation and evaluation was considered in detail. It is sometimes suggested that such an approach provides a relatively simple yet systematic and organised way of managing nursing care. But it is also suggested that it may impose a highly instrumental and rigid approach that fails to take account of the specific contextual features and the needs of the individual patient. It is hoped, however, that the particular approach presented in this chapter would overcome such dangers. This approach emphasises the importance of critical thinking in problem-solving. It also aims to balance the need for a staged and manageable approach to care delivery with a more iterative approach that recognises the ways in which the different components or stages interact with each other. It furthermore takes account of the particular situation and the involvement of the patient, by suggesting an emic as well as an etic approach.

It must nevertheless be recognised that the nursing process is just one means by which we can organise our approaches to nursing care. We must also recognise that there are other ways of framing care that do not involve attempts to sequence or organise it into stages or to place it within highly structured taxonomies. Such approaches concentrate instead on such issues as the competency of the nurse, or the nature of the clinical reasoning that takes place within caring relationships. The subsequent chapters of this module address some of the more important of these different ways of viewing and framing nursing work. These are presented as *other* ways that nursing care may be structured and managed within the process of nursing, rather than as *alternatives* to the nursing process method. Indeed, where the nursing process method is grounded in practice, and responsive to the needs of individuals and the contexts within which care occurs, it can be a creative and reflexive vehicle within which other ways of organising the delivery of care can be sustained and indeed flourish.

REFERENCES

Aggleton, P. and Chalmers, H. (2000) *Nursing Models and Nursing Practice* (2nd edn), Macmillan, London

Argyris, C. and Schön, D. (1974) *Theory in Practice: Increasing professional effectiveness*, Jossey-Bass, London

Barnum, B.K. (1987) Holistic nursing and nursing process. *Nursing Practice* 1(3), 27–35

Barnum, B. (1998) *Nursing Theory: Analysis application evaluation* (5th edn), J.B. Lippincott, Philadelphia, IL

Benner, P. (1984) *From Novice to Expert: Excellence and power in clinical nursing practice*, Addison-Wesley, Menlo Park, CA

Bevis, E.O. (1993) All in all, it was a pretty good funeral, *Journal of Nursing Education* 32, 101–5

Boychuk Duchscher, J.E. (1999) Catching the wave: understanding the concept of critical thinking. *Journal of Advanced Nursing* 29(3), 577–83

Carper, B.A. (1978) Fundamental patterns of knowing in nursing, *Advances in Nursing Science* 1, 13–23

Clark, J. (1998) The International Classification for Nursing Practice project. *Online Journal of Issues in Nursing* 30 September 1998

Coffey, A. and Atkinson, P. (1996) *Making Sense of Qualitative Data: Complementary research strategies*, Sage, Thousand Oaks, CA

Denzin, N.K. (1989) *The Research Act: A theoretical introduction to sociological methods*, Prentice-Hall, Englewood Cliffs, NJ

Dewey, J. ([1909] 1982) *How we Think*, Heath, Lexington, MA

Dickoff, J. and James, P. (1968) A theory of theories: a position paper. *Nursing Research* 17, 197–203

Fawcett, J. (1993) *Analysis and Evaluation of Nursing Theories*, F.A. Davis, Philadelphia, IL

Fawcett, J. (2000) *Analysis and Evaluation of Contemporary Nursing Knowledge: Nursing models and theories*, F.A. Davis, Philadelphia, IL

Fisher, A. and Scriven, M. (1997) *Critical Thinking: Its definition and assessment*, University of East Anglia, Centre for Research in Critical Thinking, Norwich

Geertz, C. (1996) From the native's point of view: on the nature of anthropological understanding. In: Basso, K. and Selby, H. (eds) *Meaning in Anthropology*, University of New Mexico Press, Albuquerque

Hall, L. (1955) Quality of nursing care. *Public Health News* 36(6), 212–5

Headland, T.N., Pike, K.L. and Harris, M. (1990) *Emics and Etics: The insider/outsider debate*, Sage, Newbury Park, CA

Hogston, R. (1997) Nursing diagnoses and classification systems: a position paper, *Journal of Advanced Nursing* 26, 496–500

International Council of Nurses (2002) *ICNP Beta 2 – International Classification for Nursing Practice*, International Council of Nurses, Geneva

Johnson, D.E. (1959) A philosophy of nursing. *Nursing Outlook* 7, 198–200

Kerlinger, F.N. (1987) *Foundations of Behavioural Research*, Holt, Rinehart and Winston, New York

Leininger, M. (1992) Current issues, problems, and trends to advance qualitative paradigmatic research methods for the future. *Qualitative Health Research* 2(4), 392–415

Manchester Triage Group (1997) *Emergency Triage*, BMJ Publishing, London

Meleis, A.I. (1997) *Theoretical Nursing: Development and progress* (3rd edn), J.B. Lippincott, Philadelphia, IL

Meyers, C. (1986) *Teaching Students to Think Critically: A guide for faculty in all disciplines*, Jossey Bass, San Francisco, CA

North American Nursing Diagnosis Association (NANDA) (1990) *Taxonomy I – Revised 1990*, NANDA, St Louis, IL

North American Nursing Diagnosis Association (NANDA) (2001) *Nursing Diagnoses: Definitions and classification 2001–2002*, NANDA International, Philadelphia, IL

Nouwen, H. (1994) *The Wounded Healer*, Darton, Longman and Todd, London

Orlando, I.J. (1961) *The Dynamic Nurse–Patient Relationship: Function, process, and principles*, G.P. Putnam, New York

Orlando, I.J. (1972) *The Discipline of Teaching of Nursing Process: an evaluative study*, G.P. Putnam, New York

Orlando Pelletier, I.J. (1990) Preface. In: Orlando Pelletier, I.J. (ed.) *The Dynamic Nurse–Patient Relationship: Function, process, and principles* (new NLN edition), National League for Nursing, New York

Paris, W. and Winograd, T. (1990) How metacognition can promote academic learning and instruction. In: James, B. and Idol, L. (eds) *Dimensions of Thinking and Cognition Instruction*, Lawrence Erlbaum, Hillsdale, NJ

Parse, R.R. (1995) *Illuminations – The human becoming theory in practice and research*, National League for Nursing, New York

Paul, R. (1993) *Critical Thinking: How to prepare students for a rapidly changing world*, Foundation for Critical Thinking, Santa Rosa, CA

Polanyi, M. (1958) *Personal Knowledge: Towards a post critical philosophy*, Routledge and Kegan Paul, London

Polanyi, M. (1966) *The Tacit Dimension*, Doubleday and Company, New York

Ruland, C.M. (2001) Evaluating the beta version of the International Classification for Nursing Practice for domain completeness, applicability of its axial structure and utility in clinical practice: a Norwegian project. *International Nursing Review* **48**, 1–8

Slevin, O. (1999) The nurse–patient relationship: caring in a health context. In: Long, A. (ed.) *Interaction for Practice in Community Nursing*, Macmillan, Basingstoke

van Manen, M. (1999) The pathic nature of inquiry and nursing. In: Madjar, I. and Walton, J. (eds) *Nursing and the Experience of Illness: Phenomenology in practice*, Routledge, London

Yura, H. and Walsh, M. (1988) *The Nursing Process: Assessing, planning, implementing, evaluating*, Appleton and Lange, Norwalk, CN

25

COMPETENCE-BASED APPROACHES

Lynn Basford

LEARNING OUTCOMES

After reading this chapter you will be able to:

- Describe pre-registration outcomes and competencies
- Reflect upon the ways in which these competencies are gained through the development of theory and practice
- Describe the different aspects of being a totally competent practitioner
- Understand the professional and legal requirements of being competent to practice
- Define National Occupational Standards
- Discuss the notion of fitness for practice, fitness for purpose and fitness for academic award
- Describe a competence-driven curriculum.

INTRODUCTION

The notion of having a competent health care workforce has been a driving factor behind the government's modernisation agenda to assure the public that all professional health care workers are competent and fit for practice, and underpinned and suitably monitored by a regulatory framework. For the nursing profession, this means ensuring that continuing competence and fitness to practice is addressed and monitored at 'the point of entry to pre-registration education and continues throughout the working life of the practitioner' (UKCC, 1999). It is therefore acknowledged that individual practitioners must be accountable and responsible for maintaining their competence to practice, which is audited through the regulation process (UKCC, 2001).

Having said this, the issue of how to determine and define competence to ensure that the practitioner is not only 'fit to practice', but is also 'fit for purpose' and 'fit for academic award' has been hotly debated. The debates commenced with the evolution of the National Occupational Standards movement, which provided a template for occupational standards and performance indicators to provide a framework for measuring occupational competence that was agreed and clearly understood by all. In the beginning, professional groups perceived that such routes for determining competence were for workers who would undertake national vocational qualifications and were not a suitable mechanism for measuring competence within the professional workforce. Nonetheless, service failure and the growing lack of public confidence in the ability and competence of professional health care workers have continued to increase in profile. This has drawn to the attention of government agents and others the need for clear indicators and benchmark standards to determine professional competence at all levels of practice.

DEFINING COMPETENCE

A glance at the *Oxford English Dictionary* defines competence as 'an attribute of someone who is adequately qualified or capable and who is fit and proper'. From a nursing perspective being suitably qualified refers to the fact that you have undertaken a programme of study that meets the outcomes required by the Nursing and Midwifery Council (NMC). While these outcomes may be met, this does not necessarily prove competence to practise in the contemporary arena, or that you are of *proper* standing. Competence defined within the occupational standards framework means that you have the relevant knowledge that underpins the clinical task, which you clearly understand and have internally synthesised, and for which you have gained the dexterity of skill and the necessary experience. This definition has become widely accepted as a useful framework for a common understanding.

NATIONAL OCCUPATIONAL STANDARDS

National Occupational Standards (NOS) were introduced in the 1980s as a conceptual framework to describe and measure occupational performance, in response to the growing recognition that many workers did not hold the relevant qualifications to undertake their job. Each performance is broken down into the knowledge required to underpin the task or skill, the determination of the range of skills and the understanding and experience to perform the task unsupervised (*see* Fig 25.1). Upon achieving all these elements the student or worker is deemed competent and fit to practise (Healthwork UK, 2001).

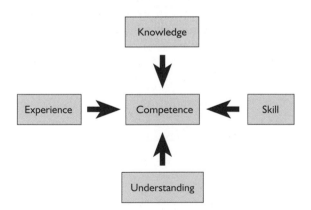

Figure 25.1 Components of National Occupational Standards

In essence, NOS are focused on the needs and scope of practice within the organisation and the identification of good practice that can be emulated and standardised. This is to ensure that all workers can demonstrate consistency of application and occupational competence across the field of practice. Having identified the components required for each field of practice, the structure and content of education and training can be designed for the various qualifications. Curricula models based on this framework can assist organisations to establish a positive link between the aims and objectives of the organisation and can empower individuals to become independent learners, who are able to identify and develop their own knowledge base to underpin their practice. This model of learning requires close relationships between the learner, the organisation and the trainer.

The process of developing NOS is rigorous and involves a National Training Organisation recognised by the government, which will oversee the process, including the following stages:

1 *Production of an occupational map* – essentially a report describing the nature and characteristics of a sector.
2 *Production of a functional map* – used to chart the type of work activities across the sector.
3 *Standards development* – undertaken by technical/professional consultants.
4 *Approval of the standards*.

The process is labour intensive and takes considerable time. However, it does enable appropriate accreditation of National Vocational Qualifications (NVQs) and Scottish Vocational Qualifications (SVQs), and associated funding.

Since their early days NOS have defied their critics in that most vocational industries, including care organisations, have recognised their value both to the organisation and to the individual. Quality and consistency have been achieved through the workforce gaining these qualifications, which have been a catalyst for professional bodies to review their own standards and competencies. This has included the nursing professional body, which was originally opposed to the development of NVQs in care, perceiving that these standards in care compromised professional competence and practice. This created an unnecessary tension between what was considered to be professional nursing care and care given by health care assistants.

FITNESS FOR PURPOSE AND PRACTICE

The concept of ensuring fitness for purpose and practice was endorsed by the UKCC's Commission report (1999), which identified 33 recommendations constructed around three areas:

1 Increasing flexibility
2 Achieving fitness for practice
3 Working in partnerships.

Increasing flexibility

This is a necessary concept when considering fitness for purpose and practice to enable a workforce with the relevant knowledge, skill, understanding and experience to work in any care setting, given the changing dimensions and focus of health care. For example, the advancements in health care technology and therapeutic interventions will allow current hospital services to be delivered in a broader range of care settings and acute hospitals will deliver specialist forms of care only (Hayes, 2001). As a consequence, the demarcation between hospital and community-based care will become increasingly integrated, using 'seamless' organisational structures and a flexible, competent workforce.

By definition, competence described within a changing kaleidoscopic framework is clearly not a static entity and requires a total rethink when defining competence for practice and purpose. Practitioners will require the ability to transfer their knowledge and skill when organisational boundaries change and when external factors generate a need for change due to technological innovations, therapeutic advancements, epidemiological and demographic changes, genetic engineering, evidence of practice and the health needs of an increasing diverse population.

Achieving fitness for practice

The process of achieving 'fitness for practice' begins at the pre-registration stage, through which the standard, type and content of such programmes are determined by the professional body and is endorsed through legislation. Currently, there is debate as to whether these regulations and standards adequately prepare the new nurse practitioner to be fit and 'competent' to practice at the point of registration. Scotland's Nursing for Health document (The Scottish Executive, 2001) has identified the need to review pre-registration programmes so that they enable and empower the new practitioner to work with communities and develop public health competencies. Other debates suggest that competence should be gained in the arena of complementary therapies, chronic disease management, telemedicine, genetic screening and triaging (UKCC, 2001). All acknowledge the need for the new practitioner to have the skills to take an increasingly autonomous role within the frameworks of multidisciplinary and multi-agency teams. Tables 25.1 and 25.2 show key areas to be considered here.

Table 25.1   Points of emphasis in achieving fitness for practise

- Care is delivered in the community, rather than the hospital.
- Health promotion is emphasised by all health care professionals.
- There is continuity of care within and between specialist settings.
- There is holistic care, linking health and social care.
- Chronic disease, both mental and physical, is tackled.
- The determinants of health, including poverty and social inclusion, are addressed.

(Adapted from UKCC, 2001, p. 30)

Table 25.2   Requirements of practitioners

- Work in partnerships with patients, families and communities.
- Assess complex needs and refer appropriately.
- Manage and deliver care in a range of settings.
- Work within and across care teams.
- Take responsibility for their continuing professional development needs in order to delivery quality patient-centred care

(Adapted from UKCC, 2001, p. 30)

There is a growing belief that if nurse education prepared nurses to work within these competency frameworks they would be able to 'make a major contribution to reducing diseases as well as promoting health and improving the quality of life' (World Health Organisation, 2000; UKCC, 2001, p. 30). Based on these recommendations, the new Nursing and Midwifery Council (established in 2002) will be responsible for ensuring that nurse education programmes that enable new practitioners to achieve competence to practice. Six models had been given by the UKCC to raise the debates around pre-registration programmes. In the main, they considered amending the common foundation, retaining four branch programmes, models that embrace a generalist practitioner and approaches that engage with inter-professional education (UKCC, 2001).

Working in partnerships

Working together in multidisciplinary and multiagency settings is a topical and much explored phenomenon. Over the past four decades this issue has been debated to address the issue of service failures, the lack of clinical effectiveness and efficiency and the growing economic burden on governments. The medium to enhance working more effectively in partnerships has been thought to be inter-professional education. However, to date there has been a fragmented approach towards inter-professional education particularly at the undergraduate pre-qualifying level. The reasons have been well documented, centring on professional 'territorialism', professional regulation, curricula design and length, large groups of students with minor groups feeling disadvantaged in the educational setting, lack of fundamental resources and the lack of preparation of teachers to be able to teach effectively using multidisciplinary models. Nonetheless, current policy indicates a growing need for professional bodies and curricula designers to address these issues. There is evidence of growing support from professional bodies, such as the Nursing and Midwifery Council, the General Medical Council, the Council for Professions Supplementary to Medicine and the Central Council for Education and Training in Social Work. Representatives from each of these groups are cooperating to explore the way forward and to identify core competencies that transcend all professional groups. The Scottish Qualifications Authority has developed 'qualifications frameworks that assist in broadening the entry gates to professional education and in determining academic equivalencies', (UKCC, 2001, p. 31). In addition, the Quality Assurance Agency has developed statements for benchmarking and standards for professional health workers to enable a framework and philosophical foundation for inter-professional education and competence to be developed.

Study Activity 25.1

- Read the following policy documents and identify references to competence, benchmarking, fitness for practice and purpose and working and learning together.

  - *The National Health Service Ten-year Plan* (Department of Health, 2000a)
  - *Our Healthier Nation* (The Scottish Executive, 2000)
  - *Creating the Potential: A plan for education* (The National Assembly for Wales, 2001)
  - *Valuing Diversity: A way forward* (The Northern Ireland Executive, 1998)
  - *Fitness for Practice* (UKCC, 1999)
  - *Making a Difference: Strengthening the nursing, midwifery and health visiting contribution to health and health care* (Department of Health, 1999)
  - *Towards a New Way of Working* (The Scottish Executive, 1998)
  - *Rebuilding our National Health Service* (The Scottish Executive, 2001)
  - *A Health Service for All the Talents: Developing the NHS workforce* (Department of Health, 2000)
  - *Delivering for Patients* (The National Assembly for Wales, 2000)
- Identify the key knowledge and skills required for you to learn in your pre-registration programme.

> Reflect on how the learning outcomes identified in your curriculum for you to achieve enable you to become competent to practise.

Shared professional competencies have been under-explored with regard to their efficacy to change practice and enable effective team working. However, a study by Barr *et al.* (2000) has drawn conclusions that inter-professional education can have differing outcomes. But there is evidence that work-based inter-professional education can be more effective than university-shared learning, which results directly in changes to practice and the quality of care. Miller *et al.* (1999) enlarge the explanation by identifying that the quality of care can be enhanced through the increased development of team knowledge and skills used more effectively when working in cooperation and collaboration with each other. Tope (1999) concluded that patient-focused care can be used effectively for inter-professional education and states that cross-training and multiskilling are key factors.

On a much wider framework, the notion of supporting inter-professional learning through common competency frameworks has been considered around the clinical governance agenda with the view that better clinical outcomes will be more effective. To enable this to occur, common practices, shared competencies, common learning opportunities, and suitable resources must be identified. The mapping of common practices, professional roles and responsibilities should provide a mechanism through which shared competencies relevant to practice and integrated care pathways can be developed.

NURSING COMPETENCE

Training and educating the nursing profession came under much scrutiny during the 1990s, and the conclusion commonly held was that '... students completing their training have not been equipped at the point of qualification with the full range of clinical skills they need' (Department of Health, 1999). While it was recognised that they did have the ability to rectify deficits in skills relatively quickly, this was not an acceptable situation in the demanding environment of a modern service. The Department of Health (1999) made strong recommendations that the profession should change the structures and standards of nurse training and education to embrace a stronger focus on clinical skills development with the relevant underpinning knowledge. Curriculum designers were encouraged to review curricula to meet these recommendations and to enable the nurse to be 'fit for practice, fit for purpose and fit for academic award' (UKCC, 2001).

The Department of Health stated that there should be stronger links between vocational training and pre-registration education, allowing flexible routes through the programme within the notion of 'stepping on' and 'stepping off'. In this sense, health care assistants with appropriate vocational qualifications will be able to fast track to nurse training. In addition, an individual on the traditional educational programme will be able to step off with occupational credits. To illustrate this, an HCA with an NVQ in Care at level three will gain access into nurse training, while an HCA with an NVQ in Care at level four may gain exemption from the common foundation programme. Similarly, on successful completion of care competencies, a learner entering nurse training through traditional access routes will be able to gain credits within the NVQ system, should they wish to leave nurse training (*see* Table 25.3, overleaf).

Marrying the frameworks of occupational standards and professional competence is a complex procedure, but it has been shown to be an effective model if detailed curriculum planning has been undertaken with all key stakeholders involved in the process (Day and Basford, 1995; *see* Fig. 25.2). Key stakeholders are considered to be educationalists, clinicians (both from the NHS and private sector), user representatives, The Workforce Confederation, vocational training organisations, further education establishments who run access to nursing programmes and NVQ in care and cadetship schemes.

Table 25.3 Making a difference

Typically, people here will, at a minimum, be competent . . .	Typically, posts will include . . .	Typically, people here will have been educated and trained to . . .
I ... to provide basic and routine personal care to patients/clients and a limited range of clinical interventions routine to the care setting under the supervision of a registered nurse, midwife or health visitor.	... cadets and health care assistants and other clinical support workers.	... National Vocational Qualification levels 1, 2 or 3.
II ... to do the above and exercise clinical judgement and assume professional responsibility and accountability for the assessment of health needs, planning, delivery and evaluation of routine direct care, for both individuals and groups of patients/clients; to direct and supervise the work of support workers and mentor students.	... both newly registered nurses and midwives and established registered practitioners in a variety of jobs and specialties in both hospital and community and primary care settings.	... higher education diploma or first degree level, hold professional registration and in some cases additional specialist-specific professional qualifications.
III ... to do the above and assume significant clinical or public health leadership of registered practitioners and others, and/or clinical management and/or specialist care.	... experienced senior registered practitioners in a diverse range of posts, including ward sisters/charge nurses, community nurses, midwives, health visitors and clinical nurse specialists.	... first or masters degree level, hold professional registration and, in many cases, additional specialist-specific professional qualifications.
IV ... to do the above and provide expert care, to provide clinical or public health leadership and consultancy to senior registered practitioners and others and initiate and lead significant practice, education and service development.	... experienced and expert practitioners holding nurse, midwife or health visitor consultant posts.	... masters or doctorate level, hold professional registration and additional specialist-specific professional qualifications commensurate with standards proposed for recognition of a 'higher level of practice'.

(From Department of Health, 1999, p. 35)

THEORY VERSUS PRACTICE GAP

The purpose of Project 2000 (UKCC, 1986) was to prepare 'knowledgeable doers' – nurses who were to be competent practitioners with the academic skills needed to understand and develop their practice. Unfortunately, after more than a decade, the perception is that while the intellectual dimension of nursing has been addressed, the practical acquisition of students has been diluted. It was hoped that the inclusion of an integrated assessment system would have resulted in nurses who were 'fit for practice, fit for purpose and fit for academic award'. The fitness for practice report (UKCC, 1999)

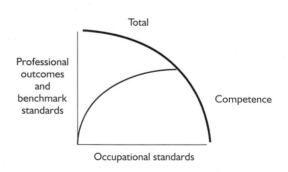

Figure 25.2 Professional outcomes versus occupational standards (Adapted from Day and Basford, 1995)

recommends 'competence–outcomes based curricula' in an attempt to redress the balance. This is consistent with the direction in which higher education is moving through outcomes-based learning curricula models. Jackson (2000) illustrates the benefits of such approaches in relation to professional education such as nursing by claiming that the integration of occupational standards and professional outcomes facilitates a clear access and progression route through the learning process in ways that more compartmentalised systems are unable to achieve.

In 2001, the UKCC provided a list of outcomes and competencies that a student nurse must achieve prior to registration (*see* Table 25.4). These are developed around four domains of practice:

1 Professional and ethical practice
2 Care delivery
3 Care management
4 Personal and professional development.

This framework provides a clear focus on what is to be learned, as the domains are broken down into two major levels: (i) outcomes; and (ii) competencies. Progression occurs when the

Table 25.4 Pre-registration nursing: course outcomes and competencies

Domain	Outcomes to be achieved for entry to the branch programme
	Professional and ethical practice: discuss in an informed manner the implications of professional regulation for nursing practice:
	• demonstrate a basic knowledge of professional and self-regulation
	• recognise and acknowledge the limitation of one's own abilities
	• recognise situations that require referral to a registered practitioner.
	Demonstrate an awareness of the UKCC's Code of Professional Conduct:
	• commit to the principle that the primary purpose of the registered nurse is to protect and serve society
	• accept responsibility for one's own actions and decisions.
Professional and ethical practice	*Demonstrate an awareness of, and apply ethical principles to, nursing practice:*
	• demonstrate respect for patient and client confidentiality
	• identify ethical issues in day-to-day practice.
	Demonstrate an awareness of legislation relevant to nursing practice:
	• identify key issues in relevant legislation relating to mental health, children, data protection, manual handling, and health and safety, etc.
Professional and ethical practice	*Demonstrate the importance of promoting equity in patient and client care by contributing to nursing care in a fair and anti-discriminatory way:*
	• demonstrate fairness and sensitivity when responding to patients, clients and groups from diverse circumstances
	• recognise the needs of patients and clients whose lives are affected by disability, however manifest.
	Manage oneself, one's practice, and that of others, in accordance with the UKCC's Code of Professional Conduct, recognising one's own abilities and limitations:
	• practise in accordance with the UKCC's *Code of Professional Conduct*
	• use professional standards of practice to self-assess performance
	• consult with a registered nurse when nursing care requires expertise beyond one's own current scope of competence
	• consult other health care professionals when individual or group needs fall outside the scope of nursing practice
	• identify unsafe practice and respond appropriately to ensure a safe outcome
	• manage the delivery of care services within the sphere of one's own accountability.
	Practise in accordance with an ethical and legal framework that ensures the primacy of patient and client interest and well-being and respects confidentiality:
	• demonstrate knowledge of legislation and health and social policy relevant to nursing practice
	• ensure the confidentiality and security of written and verbal information acquired in a professional capacity
	• demonstrate knowledge of contemporary ethical issues and their impact on nursing and health care

(cont.)

Table 25.4   Pre-registration nursing: course outcomes and competencies (cont.)

Professional and ethical practice	• manage the complexities arising from ethical and legal dilemmas • act appropriately when seeking access to caring for patients and clients in their own homes. *Practise in a fair and anti-discriminatory way, acknowledging the differences in beliefs and cultural practices of individuals or groups:* • maintain, support and acknowledge the rights of individuals or groups in the health care setting • act to ensure that the rights of individuals and groups are not compromised • respect the values, customs and beliefs of individuals and groups • provide care that demonstrates sensitivity to the diversity of patients and clients.
Care delivery	*Discuss methods of, barriers to and the boundaries of effective communications and interpersonal relationships:* • recognise the effect of one's own values on interactions with patients and clients and the carers, families and friends • utilise appropriate communication skills with patients and clients • acknowledge the boundaries of a professional caring relationship. *Demonstrate sensitivity when interacting with and providing information to patients and clients*
Care delivery	*Contribute to enhancing the health and social well-being of patients and clients by understanding how, under the supervision of a registered practitioner, to:* • contribute to the assessment of health needs • identify opportunities for health promotion • identify networks of health and social services.
Care delivery	*Contribute to the development and document nursing assessments by participation in comprehensive and systematic nursing assessment of the physical, psychological, social and spiritual needs of patients and clients:* • be aware of assessment strategies to guide the collection of data for assessing patients and clients, and use assessment tools under guidance • discuss the prioritisation of care needs • be aware of the need to reassess patients and clients as to their needs for nursing care. *Engage in, develop, and disengage from therapeutic relationships through the use of appropriate communication and interpersonal skills:* • utilise a range of effective and appropriate communication and engagement skills • maintain and, where appropriate, disengage from, professional caring relationships that focus on meeting the patient's or client's needs within professional therapeutic boundaries. *Create and utilise opportunities to promote the health and well-being of patients, clients and groups:* • consult with patients, clients and groups to identify their need and desire for health promotion advice • provide relevant and current health information to patients, clients and groups in a form that facilitates their understanding and acknowledges choice/individual preference • provide support and education in the development and/or maintenance of independent living skills • seek specialist/expert advice, as appropriate. *Undertake and document a comprehensive, systematic and accurate nursing assessment of the physical, psychological, social and spiritual needs of patients, clients and communities:* • select valid and reliable assessment tools for the required purpose • systematically collect data regarding the health and functional status of individuals, clients and communities through appropriate interaction, observation and measurement • analyse and interpret data accurately to inform nursing care and take appropriate action.
Care delivery	*Contribute to the planning of nursing care, involving patients and clients and, where possible, their carers, demonstrating an understanding of helping patients and clients to make informed decisions:* • identify care needs based on the assessment of a patient or client • participate in the negotiation and agreement of the care plan with the patient or client and with their carer, family or friends, as appropriate, under supervision of a registered nurse • inform patients and clients about intended nursing actions, respecting their right to participate in decisions about their care.

(cont.)

Table 25.4   Pre-registration nursing: course outcomes and competencies (cont.)

Care delivery	*Contribute to the implementation of a programme of nursing care, designed and supervised by registered practitioners:* ● undertake activities that are consistent with the care plan and within the limits of one's own abilities. *Demonstrate evidence of a developing knowledge base, which underpins safe nursing practice:* ● access and discuss research and other evidence in nursing and related disciplines ● identify examples of the use of evidence in planning nursing interventions. *Demonstrate a range of essential nursing skills, under the supervision of a registered nurse, to meet individuals' needs, including:* ● maintaining dignity, privacy and confidentiality; effective communication and observational skills, including listening and taking physiological measurements; safety and health, including moving and handling and infection control; essential first aid and emergency procedures; administration of medicines; emotional, physical and personal care, including meeting the need for comfort, nutrition and personal hygiene. *Formulate and document a plan of nursing care, where possible in partnership with patients, clients, carers and family and friends, within a framework of informed consent:* ● establish priorities for care based on individual or group needs ● develop and document a care plan to achieve optimal health, habilitation and rehabilitation based on assessment and current nursing knowledge ● identify expected outcomes, including a time frame for achievements and/or review in consultation with patients, members of the family and friends and with members of the health and social care team. *Based on the best evidence, apply knowledge and an appropriate repertoire of skills indicative of safe nursing practice:* ● ensure that current research finding and other evidence are incorporated in practice ● identify relevant changes in practice or new information and disseminate it to colleagues ● contribute to the application of a range of interventions to support patients and clients and which optimise their health and well-being ● demonstrate the safe application of the skills required to meet the needs of patients and clients within the current sphere of practice ● identify and respond to patients' and clients' continuing learning and care needs ● engage with, and evaluate, the evidence base, which underpins safe nursing practice.
Care management	*Contribute to the evaluation of the appropriateness of nursing care delivered:* ● demonstrate an awareness of the need to assess regularly a patient's or client's response to nursing interventions ● provide for a supervising registered practitioner, evaluative commentary and information on nursing care based on personal observation and actions ● contribute to the documentation of the outcomes of nursing interventions.
Care mamagement	*Recognise situations in which agreed plans of nursing care no longer appear appropriate and refer these to an appropriate accountable practitioner:* ● demonstrate the ability to discuss and accept care decisions ● accurately record observations made and communicate these to the relevant members of the health and social care team. *Provide a rationale for the nursing care delivered, which takes account of social, cultural, spiritual, legal, political and economic influences:* ● identify, collect and evaluate information to justify the effective utilisation of resources to achieve planned outcomes of nursing care. *Evaluate and document the outcomes of nursing and other interventions:* ● collaborate with patients and clients, and, when appropriate, additional carers to review and monitor the progress of individuals or groups towards planned outcomes ● analyse and revise expected outcomes, nursing interventions and priorities in accordance with changes in the individual's condition, needs or circumstances. *Demonstrate sound clinical judgement across a range of differing professional and care delivery contexts:* ● use evidence-based knowledge from nursing and related disciplines to select and individualise nursing interventions

(cont.)

Table 25.4 Pre-registration nursing: course outcomes and competencies (cont.)

Care management	• demonstrate the ability to transfer skills and knowledge to a variety of circumstances and settings
	• recognise the need for adaptation and adapt nursing practice to meet varying and unpredictable circumstances
	• ensure that practice does not compromise the nurse's duty of care to individuals or the safety of the public.
	Contribute to the identification of actual and potential risks to patients, clients and their carers, to oneself and to others, and participate in measures to promote and ensure health and safety:
	• understand and implement health and safety principles and policies
	• recognise and report situations that are kpotentially unsafe for patients, clients, oneself and others.
	Demonstrate an understanding of the role of others by participating in inter-professional working practice.
	• identify the roles of the members of the health and social care teams
	• work within the health and social care team to maintain and enhance integrated care.
	Demonstrate literacy, numeracy and computer skills needed to record, enter, store, retrieve and organise data essential for care delivery.
	Contribute to public protection by creating and maintaining a safe environment of care through the use of quality assurance and risk management strategies:
	• apply relevant principles to ensure the safe administration of therapeutic substances
	• use appropriate risk assessment tools to identify actual and potential risks
	• identify environmental hazards and eliminate and/or prevent them where possible
	• communicate safety concerns to a relevant authority
	• manage risk to provide care that best meets the needs and interests of patients, clients and the public.
	Demonstrate knowledge of effective inter-professional working practices, which respect and utilise the contributions of members of the health and social care team:
	• establish and maintain collaborative working relationships with members of the health and social care team and others
	• participate with members of the health and social care team in decision-making concerning patients and clients
	• review and evaluate care with members of the health and social care team and others.
	Delegate duties to others, as appropriate, ensuring that they are supervised and monitored:
	• take into account the role and competence of staff when delegating work
	• maintain one's own accountability and responsibility when delegating aspects of care to others
	• demonstrate the ability to coordinate the delivery of nursing and health care.
	Demonstrate key skills:
	• literacy – interpret and present information in a comprehensible manner
	• numeracy – accurately interpret numerical data and their significance for the safe delivery of care
	• information technology and management – interpret and utilise data and technology, taking account of legal, ethical and safety considerations, in the delivery and enhancement of care
	• problem-solving – demonstrate sound clinical decision-making, which can be justified even when on the basis of limited information.
Care management	*Demonstrate responsibility for one's own learning through the development of a portfolio of practice and recognise when further learning is required:*
	• identify specific learning needs and objectives
	• begin to engage with, and interpret, the evidence base that underpins nursing practice.
	Acknowledge the importance of seeking supervision to develop safe nursing practice.
	Demonstrate a commitment to the need for continuing professional development and personal supervision activities in order to enhance knowledge, skills, values and attitudes needed for safe and effective nursing practice:
	• identify one's own professional development needs by engaging in activities such as reflection in, and on, practice and lifelong learning
	• develop a personal development plan, which takes into account personal, professional and organisational needs
	• share experiences with colleagues, patients and clients in order to identify the additional knowledge and skills needed to manage unfamiliar or professionally challenging situations

(cont.)

Table 25.4 Pre-registration nursing: course outcomes and competencies (cont.)

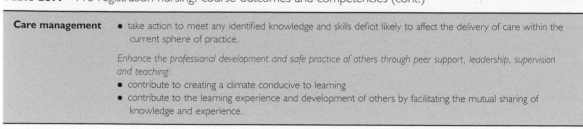

Care management	• take action to meet any identified knowledge and skills deficit likely to affect the delivery of care within the current sphere of practice. *Enhance the professional development and safe practice of others through peer support, leadership, supervision and teaching:* • contribute to creating a climate conducive to learning • contribute to the learning experience and development of others by facilitating the mutual sharing of knowledge and experience.

(From UKCC, 2001)

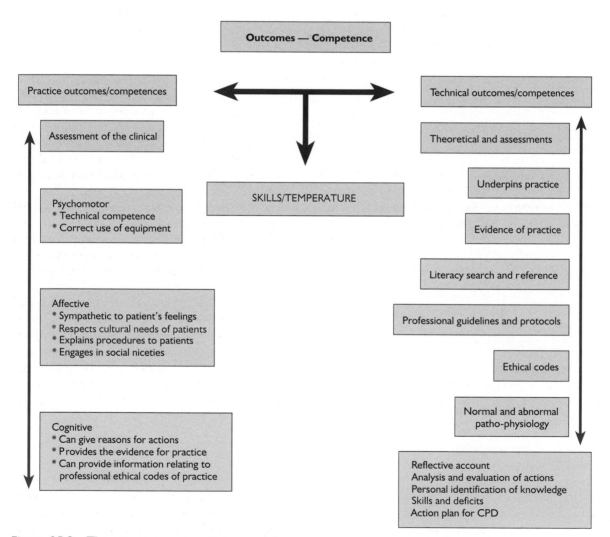

Figure 25.3 The outcomes–competence model

student achieves the outcomes required for successful completion of the foundation programme and moves into the branch programme (i.e. adult, child, learning disability or mental health). Competencies and outcomes for the branches are also determined in this manner and upon successful completion of these, the student can apply for registration.

To achieve total competence the student is required to demonstrate the knowledge, skill and understanding of each component of clinical practice that develops into a comprehensive portfolio. For example, if we take a nursing task such as temperature recording, the student would explore the pathophysiological aspects of heat homeostasis, the psychological determinants and the social external factors that may hinder normal homeostasis. Assessment would be by a collection of evidence contained within a portfolio of learning, demonstrating competence through clinical and academic achievement (see Fig. 25.3).

The repertoire of skills acquisition continues with the student developing higher level skills and competencies, which enable them to undertake comprehensive health assessments, implementing care and evaluating the outcomes of the care that is given within a framework of professional and ethical practice. Thus, it is clearly demonstrated that each of the four UKCC domains have been achieved.

GAINING COMPETENCE IN THE CLINICAL SETTING

Clinical skills development is of pivotal concern. If the learner is to gain competence and confidence to practise, exposure in the clinical environment under supportive supervision is of paramount importance. The clinical learning environment must meet the learning outcomes of the learner and it is recognised that the quality of the environment must meet the standards set by clinical governance. In addition, clinical placements should be long enough for the learner to develop clinical competence and

gain the necessary experience. Clinical education should be gained from an expert practitioner who has the relevant competence to practice within a particular domain.

FITNESS FOR ACADEMIC AWARD

So far the discussion has centred around competence from a professional perspective; however, the relevant knowledge that underpins practice must also be considered. While a nurse may develop the skill component of the competence without having the knowledge and understanding, then total competence is not achieved and the student would not be able to register as a nurse.

In the UK, the current minimum academic level of attainment is at Higher Education Diploma level (Dip HE). However, each of the four countries is in the process of identifying its own minimum academic level. England will maintain the Dip HE as a minimum outcome, while Scotland, Wales and Northern Ireland will consider a full degree as a minimum academic level.

Such changes have evoked emotional outbursts from both within and outside the profession. There are proponents who claim that nursing should have parity of academic standards with all other health care professional groups, while opponents state that nursing is fundamentally a vocation, and academic attainment is of secondary consideration to practice competence. Others believe, more cynically, that blocks are put on England, given that England has the greatest number of nurses and the economic burden would increase beyond sustainable levels should the minimum academic level of attainment be increased.

SUMMARY

These debates can be circular and do not get to the heart of the core competencies that would enable a professional to be 'fit for practice, fit for purpose and fit for academic award'. What is clearly demonstrated is that professional bodies need to examine the standards that measure professional competence, and how these standards can meet contemporary practice within a climate of changing roles, organisational structures and health care policy. The nurse of the future needs to develop a range of competencies that can be adopted and used in any care setting. In addition, competencies will be shared with other professional groups in the growing emphasis of working and learning together to enhance clinical governance and quality of life for patients.

Study Activity 25.2

Examine your clinical assessments to date and re-evaluate the depth of your knowledge, confidence and competence to undertake the clinical task. Measure your opinions on a scale of 1 to 10. Repeat this test in six months' time and identify any differences.

REFERENCES

Barr, H., Freethe, D., Hammick, M. *et al.* (2000) *Establishing the Evidence Base for Inter-professional Education: Outcomes from three reviews by the Joint Evaluation Team*. Centre for the Advancement of Inter-Professional Education, London

Day, M. and Basford, L. (1995) Fit for care. *Nursing Times*, **91**(14), 42–3.

Department of Health (1999) *Making a Difference: Strengthening the nursing, midwifery and health visiting contribution to health and health care*, The Stationery Office, London

Department of Health (2000) *A Health Service for All the Talents: Developing the NHS workforce*. DoH, London

Department of Health (2000) *The National Health Service Ten-year Plan*, DoH, London

Hayes, M. (2001) *Acute Hospital Review Group*. The Stationery Office, London

Healthwork UK (2001) *National Occupational Standards*, Healthworks UK, London, www.healthwork.co.uk/standards.htm

Jackson, N. (2000) Programme specification and its role in promoting an outcomes model of learning. *Active Learning in Higher Education* **1**(2), Sage, London

Miller C., Ross, N. and Freeman, M. (1999) Researching professional education – shared learning and clinical teamwork: new directions in education for multiprofessional practice. *ENB Research Reports*, Series no. 14, English National Board For Nurses and Midwives and Health Visitors, London

The National Assembly for Wales (2000) *Delivering for Patients*, The National Assembly for Wales, Cardiff

The National Assembly for Wales (2001) *Creating the Potential: A plan for education*, The National Assembly for Wales, Cardiff

The Northern Ireland Executive (1998) *Valuing Diversity: A way forward*, Northern Ireland Executive, Dublin

The Scottish Executive (1998) *Towards a New Way of Working*, The Scottish Executive Department, Edinburgh

The Scottish Executive (2000) *Our Healthier Nation*, The Scottish Executive Department, Edinburgh

The Scottish Executive (2001) *Rebuilding our National Health Service*, The Scottish Executive Department, Edinburgh

Tope, R. (1999) *Inter-professional Education – A literature review*. NHS Executive South West Region, London

UKCC (1999) *Fitness for Practice*, UKCC, London

UKCC (2001) *Requirements for Pre-registration Nursing Programmes*, UKCC, London

World Health Organisation (2000) Second WHO Ministerial Conference on Nursing and Midwifery, Munich, Germany, 15–17 June. *The Family Health Nurse: Context, conceptual frameworks and curricula*. WHO, Geneva

26 REFLECTIVE PRACTICE

Gary Rolfe

LEARNING OUTCOMES

After studying this chapter you will be able to:

- Identify the processes that are at play when an act of reflection takes place
- Recognise that propositional knowledge drawn from research is insufficient to fully inform our practice in complex caring situations
- Draw a distinction between research-based practice (where factual knowledge is simply adopted in practice) and a more sophisticated view of *evidence*-based practice that includes integration of the best available evidence with clinical expertise and judgement
- Discuss four different forms of reflection relevant to practice, extending from reflection *about* knowledge or evidence, through reflection *on* practice (where we reflect on how we acted or performed), and emancipatory reflection (where there is a deep and critical reflection on the forces or assumptions that influence our practice), to reflection *in* practice (where we reflect while we act, and in fact our knowledge or theory and practice become one in the act of praxis).

INTRODUCTION

A great deal has been written about reflection over the years, and it has been heralded by some as a radical new approach to nurse education and practice. In fact, reflection as a form of education dates back at least as far as Socrates, who facilitated his pupils to find the answers to philosophical problems within themselves, and

for whom 'the unexamined life is not worth living'. In modern times, its educational use can be traced to John Dewey (1938), who claimed that 'we learn by doing and realising what came of what we did'.

Despite all the theorising around reflection, it is seen by many as a perfectly natural and common-place learning mechanism in which most of us engage on a regular basis without prompting and without even realising it. It can happen, for example, during informal discussions with colleagues, friends and family, in the 'internal conversations' we hold with ourselves while walking home from work, or even while we are asleep as part of our dreams. In nursing, we use the term 'reflective practice' to refer to the *application* of this reflective tool to an exploration of our thoughts, feelings and beliefs about our own practice. Thus, Taylor (2000) describes reflective practice as:

> *The throwing back of thoughts and memories, in cognitive acts such as thinking, contemplation, meditation and any other form of attentive consideration, in order to make sense of them, and to make contextually appropriate changes if they are required.*
>
> (Taylor, 2000, p. 3)

If reflective practice is a cognitive act by which we make sense of our thoughts and memories, then it clearly has implications for learning, and particularly what Gibbs (1992) calls 'deep learning'. Deep learning takes the student beyond the memorisation of information, and involves 'thinking, seeking integration between components and between tasks, and "playing" with ideas' (Gibbs, 1992). Deep learning, therefore, requires a form of critical reflection, an introspective exploration of our current conceptual view of the world with the aim of adjusting it to accommodate new information. Critical reflection of this kind involves more than passive thought; it is an active and at times painful process of transforming information into knowledge in order to improve practice.

Andrews (1996) refers to this 'deep learning' view of reflective practice as 'conceptual modification', and extends it from reflection on knowledge and theories *about* practice to reflection on practice itself. For Andrews, reflective practice goes beyond merely thinking about what we do, and 'is not to be confused with thinking about practice, which may only involve recalling what has occurred rather than learning from it'. This notion of reflective practice as a form of 'deep learning' from and about practice is echoed in the definition offered by Fitzgerald (1994) of reflection as 'the retrospective contemplation of practice undertaken in order to uncover the knowledge used in a particular situation, by analysing and interpreting the information recalled'.

As well as focusing on knowledge from and about practice, reflection can also provide access to knowledge about ourselves. For example, Taylor (2000) encourages us to reflect on our own personal histories as 'it may help to "fill in some gaps" in your appreciation of who you have become and why you think and act the way you do in your home and work life'. More radically, Wright (1998) sees reflective practice as 'an instrument of inner work', and suggests that 'reflective practice may not only concern the transformation of practice, but also the transformation of the nurse, and the nurse as a person ...'. We can see, then, that reflective practice can be used not only to critique research-based theory and knowledge, but also to create experiential knowledge and theory out of our own experiences and to uncover and explore personal knowledge about ourselves.

However, many writers would consider that these definitions of reflective practice as essentially a cognitive learning process do not go far enough, and we can see in Wright's statement that he considers reflection not only as a way of generating knowledge, but as a way of transforming the world. As Jasper (1998) has pointed out, what nurses usually refer to as reflective *practice* is, in fact, merely reflective *process*. In other words, we only complete the reflective cycle when reflective knowledge is applied back to the practice from which it was generated. Of course, the difficulty is that if we take Fitzgerald's definition of reflection as the *retrospective* contemplation of practice, then by the time we come to reflect on a particular issue it is often too late to employ our insights to change it. Certainly, some models of reflection ask 'could I handle this better in similar situations?' (Johns, 1998), or even 'if it arose again, what would I do?' (Gibbs, 1988), but in many cases it is already too late to influence the current situation, which has probably moved on and even resolved itself by the time we come to reflect on it. All that reflection-on-action allows us to do, then, is to avoid making the same mistakes a second time, and it cannot usually help us to bring about change in the actual situation that is being reflected on. In order to move from *reflective* practice to *reflexive* practice, it is therefore necessary to reflect *in* rather than *on* action, that is, actually in the clinical setting while the action is underway. For Schön, this reflection-in-action is the hallmark of expert practice, although it is rarely discussed and almost never formally practised in nursing.

We can see, then, that reflective practice in nursing has a number of different meanings and foci. First, it is an essential component of scholarly practice, a deep intellectual consideration of propositional knowledge and theory and its application to practice. Second, it is a method for generating a complementary or alternative form of knowledge and theory that is embedded in practice itself, that is, knowledge derived from practice rather than from research and grand theory. Third, it is a method of generating personal knowledge and theory about ourselves, that is, a way of coming to understand ourselves and our practice more deeply. And fourth, it is a method of directly influencing practice in ways that scientific research and traditional forms of reflection-on-action simply cannot manage to do. Each of these concepts of reflective practice will be considered in this chapter.

REFLECTIVE PRACTICE AND EVIDENCE-BASED PRACTICE

If we look back over the short history of reflective practice in nursing, we might be forgiven for thinking that it is already in decline. Certainly, it appeared to reach a peak in the early 1990s, particularly in the UK, when it found its way into most nursing curricula and was seen as an essential component of clinical supervision and portfolio writing. However, the growth of the evidence-based practice movement in the second half of the 1990s initially appeared to reject not only reflective practice, but also the personal and experiential knowledge that it produced. For example, early advocates of evidence-based practice claimed that 'evidence-based medicine de-emphasizes intuition [and] unsystematic clinical experience … and stresses the examination of evidence from clinical research' (Evidence-based Medicine Working Group, 1992). More recently, French (1998) has defined evidence-based practice in nursing as 'the process of systematic identification, rigorous evaluation and the subsequent dissemination and use of the findings of research to influence clinical practice', with the gold standard of research being the randomised controlled trial. These definitions are clearly aimed at marginalising reflective practice, which is neither a rigorous process (in the scientific sense) of generating knowledge, nor, as some critics have pointed out, has it been rigorously evaluated itself (Mackintosh, 1998).

Fortunately for reflective practice, this rather simplistic concept of evidence-based practice is beginning to be challenged from within. On the one hand, the role of intuition and experience is now accepted not only as a source of evidence, but as the glue that holds the various types of evidence together. Evidence-based practice is now more usually considered to be a process of

'integrating *individual clinical expertise* with the best available external clinical evidence from systematic research' (Sackett *et al.*, 1996, my emphasis). If we take clinical expertise to include the knowledge and wisdom gained from experience (Benner, 1984), then access to our expertise can only come about through introspection, that is, through reflecting on our store of experiential knowledge. Furthermore, if evidence-based practice entails an *integration* of these internal and external sources of knowledge, then it is reasonable to suppose that the process of integration itself requires a deep critical reflection on knowledge and theory and the ways in which it might best be applied to practice. Seen in this light, expertise has almost replaced external research evidence as the 'gold standard', because, as Sackett *et al.* (1996) point out:

> *external clinical evidence can inform, but can never replace, individual clinical expertise, and it is this expertise that decides whether the external evidence applies to the individual patient at all and, if so, how it should be integrated into a clinical decision.*
>
> (Sackett *et al.*, 1996, p. 72)

This apparent sea-change has possibly been brought about by the recognition that, in its original form of practice based on the findings of randomised controlled trials, evidence-based practice is little more than what Benner (1984) refers to as 'novice practice', that is, practice done 'by the book'. Not only is such practice rigid, inflexible and impersonal, but evidence-based decisions could be made by anyone who can read and digest a meta-analysis of recent studies. As Gadamer (1996) has observed:

> *Once science has provided doctors [and, we might add, nurses] with the general laws, causal mechanisms and principles, they must still discover what is the right thing to do in each particular case, and this seems to be something which hardly seems predictable or knowable in advance.*
>
> (Gadamer, 1996, p. 95)

485

A note of caution is required, however, as despite the rhetoric of a much broader approach to evidence-based practice, the reality for nursing is that it is still equated in the minds of many with research-based practice. Reflective practice is beginning to appear on the evidence-based practice agenda, but there remains a long way to go before it is fully accepted and integrated.

REFLECTIVE PRACTICE AS A NEW PARADIGM

There are a number of reasons why reflection has not been fully integrated into the paradigm of evidence-based practice. First, there is still a high degree of ambivalence surrounding its status, and while the expert knowledge derived from reflection is seen as a necessary component of any evidence-based clinical decision, such that 'clinical expertise ... may override [research evidence] for a given decision' (DiCenso *et al.*, 1998), it rarely features even at the bottom end of most hierarchies of evidence (Muir Gray, 1998). Second, there is a real danger for reflective practice that even if it did become accepted as part of a broader evidence-based paradigm, it would continue to be judged according to the narrower, research-based criteria of evidence-based practice. We can see this bias in many of the critiques of reflective practice:

> *Much of the published evidence regarding the [reflective] model's impact on clinical practice appears to be based on personal anecdote, and again, evidence in support of its impact on patient care is of a mainly qualitative and descriptive nature.*
>
> (Mackintosh, 1998, p. 556)

Mackintosh is clearly judging reflective practice against the gold standard of the randomised controlled trial, in which qualitative and descriptive research and personal knowledge are low down in the hierarchy of evidence, rather than according to the criteria of reflective practice itself, where knowledge obtained from personal anecdote and narrative would be considered

good reflective evidence. Unfortunately, even advocates of reflective practice feel the need to apologise for its lack of compliance to the gold standard. Thus, Atkins and Murphy (1994), while acknowledging that reflection 'does seem to have real potential for nursing practice', temper their praise by adding, however, that 'there is as yet little research to support the use of reflection'. Similarly, Andrews (1996) adds that what little research evidence does exist 'is not always fully validated by the findings'. Clearly, if reflective practice is ever to be seen as of equal worth to the randomised controlled trial, it cannot do so from within a paradigm that continues to privilege 'hard' research evidence above 'soft' evidence from introspection. Reflective practitioners therefore need to re-situate themselves in a paradigm where introspective knowledge and narrative generated from practice by the practitioner herself is valued above (or at least equal to) the evidence from large-scale, generalisable research studies.

Such a practice-based paradigm has a number of far-reaching implications. It suggests, for example, that curriculum writing teams, journal editorships and research grant committees might come under the control of practitioners rather than academics, that education might be ward based rather than classroom based, that journals might be full of reflective diary entries rather than research reports, and that basic-grade staff nurses might obtain large grants to carry out reflective research into their own practice.

Although such a practice-based paradigm might be difficult for many nurses to imagine, much of the groundwork has already taken place in other disciplines such as education. For example, there is a long tradition of teachers valuing and learning from their own practice, initiated by the work of Lawrence Stenhouse (1975) and his 'teacher as researcher' movement which encouraged school teachers to work in partnership with trained researchers to explore their own practice. Other educationalists later dispensed with the outside researcher and developed an action research methodology in which the teachers explored their own practice through reflection. Ebbutt (1985) describes this as:

> ... *the systematic study of attempts to change and improve ... practice by groups of participants by means of their own practical actions and by means of their own reflections upon the effects of those actions.*
>
> (Ebbutt, 1985, p. 156)

This reflective research did not aim to produce generalisable findings in the tradition of scientific research, but rather to initiate a new paradigm in which concrete knowledge about individual teachers and pupils in specific situations is considered more useful than abstract decontextualised knowledge about large populations. As van Manen (1990) points out:

> *Pedagogic situations are always unique. And so, what we need more of is theory not consisting of generalizations, which we then have difficulty applying to concrete and ever-changing circumstances, but theory of the unique; that is, theory eminently suitable to deal with this particular pedagogic situation, this school, that child, or this class of youngsters.*
>
> (van Manen, 1990, p. 155)

Clearly, such theory of the unique will be different for every new situation, whether it is an encounter between teacher and pupil or nurse and patient. Such theory cannot be generated by traditional scientific research methods that subsume individual experience into a greater decontextualised whole, nor even by qualitative research that concerns itself with small groups of specific individuals. Theory of the unique is embedded in practice, and can only emerge through critical reflection on that practice. Thus:

> *A 'practice', then, is not some kind of thoughtless behaviour which exists separately from 'theory' and to which theory can be 'applied'. Furthermore, all practices, like all observations, have 'theory' embedded in them.*
>
> (Carr and Kemmis, 1986, p. 113)

Schön (1987) referred to these personal, practice-based theories as theories in use, 'implicit in our patterns of spontaneous behaviour', while Usher and Bryant (1989) coined the term 'informal theory', and added:

> *Since without such a 'theory' practice would be random and purposeless, we can say that it 'forms' practice. It enables practitioners to make sense of what they are doing and thus appears to have an enabling function.*
>
> (Schön, 1987, p. 80)

Although nursing continues to lag behind the discipline of education in respect of reflective practice, the importance of individual 'theory of the unique' is beginning to be recognised and valued as an important component of clinical decision-making (Radwin, 1995; Clarke *et al.*, 1996; Rolfe, 1998; Benner *et al.*, 1999).

REFLECTIVE PRACTICE AND CRITICAL THEORY

We can see, then, that this new practice-focused paradigm turns the traditional hierarchy of evidence on its head by valuing informal 'theory of the unique' over generalisable research-based theory, and reflection-on-action over scientific research as the principal method of generating such knowledge and theory. However, some reflective practitioners would wish to extend the focus of reflection beyond either research-based knowledge or knowledge generated from practice, to the 'self'. Thus, Boyd and Fales (1983) describe reflective practice as 'the process of creating and clarifying the meaning of experience in terms of self in relation to both self and the world'. There is a suggestion here that self-reflection has a direct impact on the outside world, and this implication is made explicit by Atkins and Murphy (1994):

> *For reflection to make a real difference to practice, it is important that the outcome includes a commitment to action. This may not necessarily involve acts which can be observed by others, but it is important that*

> *the individual makes a commitment of some*
> *kind on the basis of that learning. Action is*
> *the final stage of the reflective cycle.*
>
> (Atkins and Murphy, 1994, p. 51)

However, it is the critical theorists who have done the most to link inward-looking reflection with outward-looking action. Thus, in addition to the *technical* reflection on formal theory which is employed as part of evidence-based nursing, and the *practical* reflection on informal theory which helps us to explore and understand our own practice, Taylor (2000) also advocates *emancipatory* reflection which 'seeks to free nurses and midwives from taken-for-granted assumptions and oppressive forces which limit them and their practice'.

This emancipatory reflection borrows heavily from the work of Kim (1999), for whom the critical/emancipatory phase of reflection flowed naturally from the descriptive phase and the reflective phase. Thus, whereas Taylor's three types of reflection are independent of one another, and 'each has its own value for different purposes', Kim's three phases follow in a natural progression, each building on its predecessor. However, for both writers, the focus of emancipatory reflection is not practice *per se*, but rather the self, and in particular, our potential for self-deception. Thus, emancipatory reflection:

> *... involves discourses about the nature and*
> *sources of distortions, inconsistencies and*
> *incongruence between (a) values/beliefs and*
> *practice, (b) intentions and actions, and (c)*
> *clients' needs and nurses' actions.*
>
> (Kim, 1999, p. 1209)

We can see, however, that self and practice are inextricably linked, and that the process of exploring these sources of distortions, inconsistencies and incongruities entails a radical focus back on practice that Taylor (2000) refers to as 'transformative action'. For Taylor, this is a deep and searching form of reflection that 'requires practitioners to make a deep, systematic and direct analysis of their work to locate the features which constrain effective practice'.

There is a suggestion in these accounts that emancipatory reflection is based on a more objective footing than other forms of reflection, and that it is able to refute the criticism sometimes levelled against reflective practice that it is purely subjective and, in particular, that retrospective reflection is open to distortion and self-delusion (Newell, 1992). Indeed, emancipatory reflection regards itself as a method of correcting these distortions as it promises self-emancipation through 'raised awareness and a new sense of informed consciousness to bring about positive social and political change' (Taylor, 2000). Emancipatory reflection offers to raise awareness beyond the possibility of self-deception and thereby to bring about not just change, but *positive* change. Taylor (2000) continues:

> *Emancipatory reflection also offers nurses*
> *and midwives the potential to identify their*
> *own misguided and firmly held perceptions of*
> *themselves and their roles, to bring about*
> *change for the better. The process of*
> *emancipatory reflection for change is praxis.*
>
> (Taylor, 2000, p. 148)

For the critical theorists, then, the product of emancipatory reflection is 'praxis', which is concerned with exploring the true nature of the self in order to improve practice through social and political action.

PRAXIS AND REFLECTION-IN-ACTION

Other writers have taken a broader view of praxis. For example, Gadamer (1996) describes it simply as the interrelationship between practice and research. Thus, 'praxis ... is not merely an application of scientific knowledge. Rather, aspects of praxis react back on research, and the results of research must consistently prove and confirm themselves in turn with reference to praxis'. However, whereas most writers describe praxis in terms of action, Carr and

Kemmis (1986) identify it as a form of knowledge 'which "resides in" the knowledgeable actor or knowing subject'. Rolfe (1996) combines Gadamer's notion of an interplay between research and practice with Carr and Kemmis's concept of a kind of practical knowledge personal to the practitioner, to arrive at a definition of nursing praxis as 'the coming together of theory and practice involving a process of hypothesising and testing out informal theory, and modifying practice according to the results'. Rolfe is using Usher and Bryant's (1989) term 'informal theory' to mean the theories that practitioners employ to make sense of their practice *in the midst of practice itself*. Praxis, then, is a process of reflection-in-action (Schön, 1983, 1987), whereby the practitioner constructs an informal 'theory of the unique' to explain the specific clinical situation they are faced with, formulates hypotheses from that theory, tests the hypotheses by acting on them, and modifies their theory in the light of the outcome. Clarke *et al.* (1996) describe a very similar process, which they refer to as professional judgement, while Andrews (1996) refers to it as intuition, which she describes as 'a complex critical skill that is the result of modification of personal theory through reflecting in action'.

Study Activity 26.1

In this chapter a case is made for an approach to reflection in practice that is encompassed within the notion of praxis. The term has its roots in Aristotelian philosophy, subsequently in Marxist theory, and more recently in professional practice disciplines.

- Do a library and Internet search for meanings of the term 'praxis' (and you may wish to include the final sections of Chapter 18).
- Make brief notes as you work, and then write a brief statement (citing and referencing your sources) explaining the term in no more than 300 words.

For Rolfe, as for Schön, this process of reflection-in-action is the key to advanced practice, as it offers a way out of Benner's (1984) dilemma of the expert nurse who is unaware of the tacit knowledge base on which her practice is based. Reflection-*in*-action provides the practitioner with a running commentary on her practice that she can later reflect *on* and articulate in order to 'open up inquiry', to share her *modus operandus* with her colleagues, and more importantly, to offer as evidence for her clinical decisions.

Nursing praxis and the method of reflection-in-action fully unites reflection with practice as two aspects of the same act. It provides a constant interplay between looking outwards, gazing inwards, interpreting, sharing and transforming in action, and fully integrates the roles of practitioner, researcher and educator in a single person. Unfortunately, it is largely overlooked in nursing, and generally when we talk about reflective practice, we are referring to reflection *on* action rather than *in* action. The problem might simply be that, as Clarke *et al.* (1996) maintain, 'we just do not know enough about the process of reflection in action'. However, it is possible that we have inherited a notion of expert practice as essentially tacit and unknowable, such that 'if experts are made to attend to the particulars [while they are practising] ... their performance actually deteriorates' (Benner, 1984). However, against Benner's suggestion that expertise is an intuitive and unknowable art, Schön (1983) observed that 'when people use terms such as "art" and "intuition", they usually intend to terminate discussion rather than to open up inquiry', and that ultimately such a strategy served only to widen the theory–practice gap. Certainly, Benner's book, *From Novice to Expert*, provided an articulate argument against the possibility of reflection-in-action that influenced an entire generation of nurses, but the work of Schön (1983) makes an equally strong case, not only that reflection-in-action is possible, but that it is necessary if practitioners are to avoid selective inattention, repetitive patterns of error and ultimately, burnout.

Study Activity 26.2 _____

Carry out a meta-reflection (a reflection *on* reflection) of your own reflective practice:

- Do you consciously reflect in an anticipatory way before your practice, and what form does this take?
- Do you ever reflect introspectively upon your own assumptions about practice?
- Do you reflect *in* practice, by integrating ongoing reflection within your practice in a reflexive way?
- Do you consciously reflect in an evaluative way *after* practice has occurred?

It may be that you do some or all of these things constantly, without consciously thinking about them. However, intentionally attending to how you reflect may help you transform your own practice development. Re-reading the section on emancipatory reflection may help you consider such possibilities of becoming a more reflective practitioner.

SUMMARY

In the course of this chapter I have outlined and discussed four different foci for reflective practice. First, I explored reflection on empirical research-based knowledge and theory. This is an important component of evidence-based practice, and resembles Gibbs' (1992) concept of deep learning. This approach to reflection explores propositional knowledge from the perspective of its application and relevance to the individual practitioner, who integrates it into their own knowledge base and, in a sense, makes it their own. Second, I looked at practice experiences as a focus for reflection, what Schön (1983) referred to as reflection-on-action. This approach to reflection challenges the paradigm of evidence-based practice, in which knowledge and theory are applied to practice in a one-way process, and argues instead that the most important knowledge for practitioners is that which emerges *from* practice. Third, I looked at the self as a focus for emancipatory reflection, and demonstrated how a deep and critical introspec-

tive exploration of self leads ultimately to practical changes in the outside world through praxis. And finally, I argued for a broader view of praxis as the integration of theory and practice in a single act that Schön referred to as reflection-in-action. I ended with the observation that reflection-in-action is yet to be widely adopted in nursing, largely because of the belief that expert or advanced practice has no underpinning rationale on which we might reflect, and that focusing on our practice while we are doing it leads to a deterioration and a regression back to novice practice. However, if nursing is to become truly reflective and (more importantly) reflexive, then the move to reflection-in-action has to be the next challenge for the profession.

Study Activity 26.3 _____

At one level, this chapter draws a distinction between reflection *on* practice (which may occur before or after that practice) and reflection *in* practice (where thinking and doing become one). These are fundamentally important distinctions:

- Undertake a library search, including sources cited in the chapter, to identify further statements about these distinctions.
- Make your own brief notes on each form of reflection identified.

REFERENCES

Andrews, M. (1996) Using reflection to develop clinical expertise. *British Journal of Nursing* 5(8), 508–13

Atkins, S. and Murphy, K. (1994) Reflective practice. *Nursing Standard* 8(39), 49–54

Benner, P. (1984) *From Novice to Expert*, Addison-Wesley, Memlo Park, CA

Benner, P., Hooper-Kyriakidis, P. and Stannard, D. (1999) *Clinical Wisdom and Interventions in Critical Care*, W.B. Saunders, Philadelphia, IL

Boyd, E. and Fales, A. (1983) Reflective learning: the key to learning from experience. *Journal of Humanistic Psychology* 23(2), 99–117

Carr, W. and Kemmis, S. (1986) *Becoming Critical*, Falmer Press, London

Clarke, B., James, C. and Kelly, J. (1996) Reflective practice: reviewing the issues and refocusing the debate. *International Journal of Nursing Studies* 33(2), 171–80

Dewey, J. (1938) *Experience and Education*, Macmillan, New York

DiCenso, A., Cullum, N. and Ciliska, D. (1998) Implementing evidence-based nursing: some misconceptions. *Evidence-Based Nursing* 1(2), 38–40

Ebbutt, D. (1985) Educational action research: some general concerns and specific quibbles. In: Burgess, R.G. (ed.) *Issues in Educational Research: Qualitative methods*, Falmer Press, Lewes

Evidence-Based Medicine Working Group (1992) Evidence-based nursing: a new approach to teaching the practice of medicine. *JAMA* 268(17), 2420–5

Fitzgerald, M. (1994) Theories of reflection for learning. In: Palmer, A., Burns, S. and Bulman, C. (eds) *Reflective Practice in Nursing*, Blackwell Scientific, Oxford

French, B. (1998) Developing the skills required for evidence-based practice. *Nurse Education Today* 18, 46–51

Gadamer, H-G. (1996) *The Enigma of Health*, Polity Press, Cambridge

Gibbs, G. (1988) *Learning by Doing: A guide to teaching and learning methods*, Further Education Unit, Oxford Polytechnic, Oxford

Gibbs, G. (1992) *Improving the Quality of Student Learning*, Technical and Education Services, Plymouth

Jasper, M. (1998) Using portfolios to advance practice. In: Rolfe, G. and Fulbrook, P. (eds) *Advanced Nursing Practice*, Butterworth Heinemann, Oxford

Johns, C. (1998) Opening the doors of perception. In: Johns, C. and Freshwater, D. (eds) *Transforming Nursing through Reflective Practice*, Blackwell Science, Oxford

Kim, H.S. (1999) Critical reflective inquiry for knowledge development in nursing practice. *Journal of Advanced Nursing* 29(5), 1205–12

Mackintosh, C. (1998) Reflection: a flawed strategy for the nursing profession? *Nurse Education Today* 18, 553–7

Muir Gray, J. (1998) *Evidence-based Healthcare*, Churchill Livingstone, Edinburgh

Newell, R. (1992) Anxiety, accuracy and reflection: the limits of professional development. *Journal of Advanced Nursing* 17, 1326–33

Radwin, L. (1995) Knowing the patient: a process model for individualized interventions. *Nursing Research* 44(6), 364–70

Rolfe, G. (1996) *Closing the Theory–Practice Gap: A new paradigm for nursing*, Butterworth-Heinemann, Oxford

Rolfe, G. (1998) *Expanding Nursing Knowledge: Understanding and researching your own practice*, Butterworth Heinemann, Oxford

Sackett, D.L., Rosenberg, W.M.C., Muir Gray, J.A. *et al.* (1996) Evidence-based medicine: what it is and what it isn't, *British Medical Journal* 312, 71–2

Schön, D.A. (1983) *The Reflective Practitioner*, Temple Smith, London

Schön, D.A. (1987) *Educating the Reflective Practitioner*, Jossey-Bass, San Francisco

Stenhouse, L. (1975) *An Introduction to Curriculum Research and Development*, Heinemann Educational, Oxford

Taylor, B.J. (2000) *Reflective Practice: A guide for nurses and midwives*, Open University Press, Buckingham

Usher, R. and Bryant, I. (1989) *Adult Education as Theory, Practice and Research*, Routledge, London

van Manen, M. (1990) *Researching Lived Experience*, The Althouse Press, Ontario

Wright, S. (1998) The reflective journey begins a spiritual journey. In: Johns, C. and Freshwater, D. (eds) *Transforming Nursing through Reflective Practice*, Blackwell Science, Oxford

27 CLINICAL REASONING: ARTICULATING EXPERIENTIAL LEARNING IN NURSING PRACTICE

Patricia Benner

Nursing, like medicine, involves a rich, socially embedded clinical know-how that encompasses perceptual skills, transitional understandings across time, and understanding of the particular in relation to the general. Clinical knowledge is a form of engaged reasoning that follows modus operandi *thinking, in relation to patients' and clinical populations' particular manifestations of disease, dysfunction, response to treatment and recovery trajectories. Clinical knowledge is necessarily configurational, historical (by historical, I mean the immediate and long-term histories of particular patients and clinical populations), contextual, perceptual, and based upon knowledge gained in transitions ... Through articulation, clinical understanding becomes increasingly articulate and translatable at least by clinical examples, narratives and puzzles encountered in practice.*

(Benner, 1994)

LEARNING OUTCOMES

After studying this chapter you will be able to:

- Recognise clinical judgement as an essential aspect of practice
- Appreciate that while such clinical judgement is informed by the technical and scientific, in real-world practice clinical reasoning extends beyond the point at which such information alone is sufficient
- Explain the difference between technical knowledge and 'knowing that' (or propositional knowledge) and the tacit and intuitional knowledge embedded in practice that draws also on practical knowledge or 'know-how'
- Describe the process of clinical reasoning as an embedded and contextual form of clinical judgement, different but complementary to rational forms of problem-solving
- Identify the clinical and moral aspects of clinical reasoning as it is enacted in practice settings, where narrative unfolding, experiential tacit knowing, and technical knowledge come together in informed ethical caring
- Recognise the developmental nature of clinical reasoning, whereby through experiential learning the practitioner progresses from novice to expert.

INTRODUCTION

The nurse–patient relationship sets up the conditions of possibility for the patient to disclose their concerns, fears and discomforts. If the nurse is too hurried, or too task oriented to notice the patient's and families' experience, then the level of disclosure on the part of the patient/family will be constrained. Likewise, the nurse's attunement and engagement with the patient allows the nurse to notice subtle changes. Clinical judgement requires engaged reasoning across time about the particular changes in the patient's condition and changes in the clinician's understanding of the patient's situation (Benner *et al.*, 1999). In addition to the narrower 'rational technical' account of rationality handed down in the Cartesian tradition, and captured in early Greek thought by Plato as 'techne' or technique, Aristotle called attention to practice or *praxis* that requires *phronesis*, something qualitatively distinct from techne. A practice is a socially embedded form of knowledge that has notions of the good internal to the practice (MacIntyre, 1981). Aristotle's example was that of a statesman who had to develop character, skilled know-how, practical reasoning and comportment that included appropriate emotional responses, and relationships. This contrast form of rationality and skill-based character called *phronesis* is similar to clinical judgement. A rational technical mode (techne, the know-how and skill of producing things), sometimes called rational technicality, separates means and ends and focuses on achieving pre-specified outcomes. Rational technical thought is a powerful strategy for those areas of science and technology that can be standardised and routinised. But where clinical judgement, relationship, perception (or noticing), timing and skilled know-how are involved, more than techne or rational calculation is required. Guignon (1983) points out that separating means and outcomes often devalues or does violence to the means, especially where means and ends are closely interwoven. For example, it is not sensible to separate means and ends in birth, comfort, health promotion, or end-of-life care. In each of these caring practices, means and ends are in many ways not separable, as most often there are multiple means and ends at stake in any clinical encounter.

Care-giving relationships may open up possibilities, or close them down. But even with the best intentions and comportment, the one cared for may not be able to respond to care. 'Outcomes' in care-giving relationships are necessarily interdependent and mutual. Some types of influence are morally unacceptable. Manipulation, coercion, or misuse of professional influence in persuading a patient to accept a treatment are unethical. When things go well and the patient/family is able to respond to caring practices, the practitioner cannot attribute the good outcome solely to the efficacy of some technique they may have used. The current focus on 'pre-specified outcomes' and identifying and

evaluating nursing outcomes in case management is based on the premise that only technique is involved in health care, that one knows the outcomes to expect, and that all things can be 'fixed'. The problem is further complicated by institutional constraints to good care-giving. Meeting and responding to the other, may clash with the bureaucratic goals of care for the many in the most cost-efficient manner. For all these reasons, developing moral agency and the skills of involvement present ongoing demands for experiential learning and character development. Viewing nursing as a basic human encounter and as a practice that requires phronesis, has major implications for nursing education and the moral development of practitioners.

Technical cure and restorative care must not become mutually exclusive for the nurse. One way to create more equal dialogical partners between technical medicine and lifeworlds is to understand medicine, nursing and other health care practices as *practices* that encompass more than the science and technologies that they use to effect cures.

THE NATURE OF PRACTICE: A SOCIALLY EMBEDDED FORM OF KNOWLEDGE

A socially organised practice such as nursing has notions of good internal to the practice (MacIntyre, 1981). For example, attentiveness, not neglect, recognition practices, not depersonalisation, are notions of good internal to the practice of nursing. A nurse educated to be an excellent nurse can recognise, in most instances, good and poor nursing care, even though it would be impossible to formally list all the precise behaviours and comportments of excellent nursing care. In philosophy, the inability to make explicit or formal all elements of a social practice is called the 'limits of formalisation' (Dreyfus, 1992). Likewise, the practical knowledge embedded in the traditions of science cannot be made completely formal and explicit (Lave and Wenger, 1991; Benner *et al.*, 1996). Every complex social practice has a foreground of focused attention and a background of comportment, practical skills and understanding of the social practice. Science and technology have extensive traditions of formalising the reasoning and knowledge associated with scientific experiments. Consequently, it can appear to the naive scientific practitioner that thinking within a particular scientific discipline is restricted to what can be made formalisable. However, as Thomas Kuhn (1970) demonstrated through historical examples, every science has non-rational (not *irrational*) aspects of thinking such as the use of metaphors; understandings about constitutes an interesting scientific problem, skilful know-how in conducting experiments etc. The practice of a particular discipline such as nursing or a science such as crystal growing, or genomics, contains the *ethos* or notions of what counts as good nursing or good scientific practice. In practice disciplines such as nursing and medicine, the ethos of the practice shapes and is shaped by relevant science. Knowledge development occurs in science, and in experiential learning directly from practice. Practice is a way of knowing in its own right, in this non-technological understanding of what constitutes a practice (Kuhn, 1970; Dunne, 1993).

In order to make good clinical judgements, the nurse must be skilful in moral and clinical perception (Benner and Wrubel, 1982; Blum, 1994; Vetleson, 1994). While conceptual knowledge is essential, it is not sufficient to ensure that the nurse will form relationships with patients that lead to salient disclosures, or that the nurse will notice and correctly identify an instance of pulmonary oedema, despair, or pain when he or she sees it, even though the nurse may know conceptually what the formal characteristics of these patient conditions are in principle.

In the practice of medicine and nursing, science and technology are used to increase certainty about the measurement of signs and symptoms. The practice of the objective measurement of signs and symptoms reduces errors and improves clinical judgement. No one would recommend going back to guessing body temperatures by palpation alone. However, even the most formal measurements cannot replace the perceptual skill of the clinician in recognising when a measurement is relevant, or the meaning of a particular measurement. Also following the course of the patient's development of signs and symptoms (the trajectory or evolution of signs and symptoms) informs the clinician's understanding of the meaning of the signs and symptoms. This may seem patently obvious to any practising clinician, yet current strategies for applying algorithms or making particular clinical judgements based upon aggregate outcomes data alone, ignore the clinical know-how, relational skills, and need for clinical judgement as reasoning across time (Halpern, 2001).

Study Activity 27.1

A significant aspect of the ideas presented in this chapter is that while technical knowledge and 'know-how', and scientific evidence can help inform and enhance our practice, beyond this we must make clinical judgements that draw upon our experience and tacit knowledge of the unique clinical situations we encounter. Ask an experienced nursing practitioner in your next (or current) practice placement how she/he arrives at clinical judgements, and compare her/his response with the insights presented in this chapter.

Technique is defined here as pre-specified outcomes that can be reduced to routine, predictable, standardised care. A more robust understanding of practice needs to be developed in an era when science and technology have become the dominant public legitimised discourses for modern practices.

Good nursing practice requires ongoing clinical knowledge development through experiential learning. Experiential learning is not automatic. It requires openness, attentiveness and responsible engaged learning on the part of the practitioner. Reflection on practice and active engaged thinking are required. Here a distinction is being made between detached, disengaged reflection and engaged thinking-in-action (Benner *et al.*, 1999). Standing outside the situation and reflecting back on it is a powerful critical thinking strategy for improving practice, especially in situations of breakdown and error (Schön, 1987) (see Chapter 26, Reflective practice). However, being emotionally attuned to the patient/family and the demands of the situation in the immediate moment is required for well-timed expert performance.

The Dreyfus Model of Skill Acquisition (Dreyfus, 1979; Benner, 1984) is based upon determining the level of practice evident in particular situations. It elucidates strengths as well as problems. Situated practice capacities are described rather than traits or talents of the practitioners. At each stage of experiential learning (novice, advanced beginner, competent, proficient, expert), clinicians can perform at their best. For example, one can be the best advanced beginner possible, typically the first year of practice. However, no practitioner can be beyond experience regardless of the level of skill acquisition in most clinical situations and despite the necessary attempts to make practice as clear and explicit as possible. If the nurse has never encountered a particular clinical situation, experiential learning is required. For example, referring to critical pathways is not the same as recognising when and how these pathways are relevant or must be adapted to particular patients. Experiential learning that leads to individualisation and clinical discernment is required to render critical pathways sensible and safe. Such individualisation requires clinical discernment based upon experience with past whole concrete clinical situations. This ability to make clinical comparisons between whole concrete clinical cases without decomposing the whole situation into its analytical components is a hallmark of expert clinical nursing practice (Kuhn, 1970; Ruddick, 1989). A renewing, coherent, recognisable identity requires that practitioners develop notions of good that are constantly being worked out and extended through experiential learning in local and larger practice communities. Practice is a way of

knowing, as well as a way of being in the world (Ruddick, 1989; Dunne, 1993; Taylor, 1993, 1994). A self-renewing practice directs the development, implementation and evaluation of science and technology. Clinical judgement requires moral agency (defined as the ability to effect and influence situations), relationship, perceptual acuity, skilled know-how, and narrative reasoning across time about particular patient transitions (Kuhn, 1970; Benner *et al.*, 1999). As Joseph Dunne (1993) notes:

> *A practice is not just a surface on which one can display instant virtuosity. It grounds one in a tradition that has been formed through an elaborate development and that exists at any juncture only in the dispositions (slowly and perhaps painfully acquired) of its recognized practitioners.*
>
> (Dunne, 1993, pp. 378–80)

Study Activity 27.2

Using the authorities cited in the text and through a wider library and Internet search (using search terms such as novice, expert, expertise, competence, proficiency), outline the Dreyfus Model of Skills Acquisition by making brief descriptive notes (each approximately 150 words) of each stage of the model.

THE ROLE OF NARRATIVE IN CLINICAL JUDGEMENT AND ARTICULATION OF CLINICAL KNOWLEDGE

One way to extend and evaluate clinical practice is through the study of narratives about actual practice. Narratives can capture what is universal in a particular clinical or human situation. The person telling a story about their practice experience may reveal more than they intend, or even have direct access to. For example, why the nurse had the concerns described, or took the action taken, may not be immediately apparent even to the storyteller. Telling a story of experiential learning can reveal new understandings or taken-for-granted meanings even for the storyteller.

A narrative mode of description and memory best captures clinical judgement and experiential learning because a narrative can capture chronology, the concerns of the actor, and even the ambiguities and puzzles as the story unfolds (Ruddick, 1989; Hunter, 1991). Jane Rubin (1996) points out that the agent/actor's concerns organise how the story is told, what is included, left out and even where the story begins and ends. Nurses' clinical narratives can reveal their taken-for-granted clinical understandings. Articulating those understandings publicly and in writing can assist in making innovations and experiential learning in practice accessible to others, thus opening the possibility of making clinical knowledge cumulative and collective, as well as generating new questions and topics for research. Practising nurses develop clinical knowledge and their own moral agency as they learn from their patients and families. Experiential learning in high-risk environments requires courage and supportive learning environments. Nurses' stories can reveal agent-centred experiential learning. Local practice communities develop distinct clinical knowledge and skills. A lack of public recognition of the nature of nurses' knowledge of work causes nurses' clinical learning to be neglected in local practice settings. Collecting narratives and doing interpretive reflection on these narratives uncovers new knowledge and skills; identifies impediments to good practice as well as areas of excellence. Teaching reflective thinking about first-person, experience narrative allows clinicians to identify concerns that organise the story, identify notions of good embedded in the story, identify relational, communicative and collaborative skills, and articulate newly developing clinical knowledge. The goal is to articulate new clinical knowledge. The forming of the story, what concerns shape the story and how the story ends are revealed in the dialogue and perceptions of the storyteller. Narratives reveal contexts, process and content of practical moral reasoning. Thus, stories create moral imagination even as they expose knowledge gaps and paradoxes. The following interview excerpt is taken from a naturalistic study of actual clinical situations in intensive care units (ICUs) (Benner *et al.*, 1999). The interview is taken from an advanced practice nurse (APN) and illustrates clinical grasp and clinical forethought, as well as experiential learning:

> APN: *A man had been admitted to the ICU on a mechanical ventilator with a status post cardiac arrest. The patient had been intubated, on full ventilatory support for less than a day ... He did not appear to have any problems initially, at least in terms of ventilation and oxygenation, with ruling in for an MI. He was basically in a stabilization period of support. He was not instrumented with a PA catheter, was awake, cognitively aware, at least as best as we could tell ... I remember getting a call late in the afternoon and the staff nurse thought that the patient seemed to be working a little bit harder on the ventilator, and she had approached the intern and the resident. I work in a teaching facility, and they looked at the patient, didn't really notice, particularly, that the patient was struggling with his breathing, or that there was a slight increase in the respiratory rate that seemed to be sustained. The nurse also had reported to me that the heart rate had been elevated, but he didn't appear to be hemodynamically compromised, so she wasn't too worried about it, but she was wondering if the ventilator settings were appropriate ... One of the first things that I noticed when I went in the room, was that the patient wasn't breathing very rapidly, but was using a lot more respiratory effort on each breath, using more accessory muscles, and this patient was actively exhaling. The breathing appeared paradoxical, meaning, he wasn't using the diaphragm, he*

was using accessory muscles. But there really wasn't a marked tachypnea pattern. And, again, I looked at the ventilator sheets to see again how long the patient had been on the ventilator and just wondering if it was just maybe an agitation situation, and maybe they needed some sedation, or [to figure out] what was going on. The nurse also remarked that in the last 20 minutes, the patient's mentation had deteriorated, where he had been a little more responsive, he was now less responsive, and so she was even more nervous. So the three us – I believe it was either the senior resident or the junior assistant resident, myself, and the staff nurse, talking in the patient's room, or looking at the ventilatory parameters, and clearly the patient's mentation had deteriorated, breathing appeared to be more labored. So, I had asked them if they had taken a recent chest X-ray, or if there was anything else new going on with the patient that was important, and they said, 'No, the patient had a chest X-ray in the morning as part of a routine check, but there hadn't been any follow up.' I asked the nurse if there had been any change in breath sounds, and she said, 'No.' And the junior resident who was in the room said he had noticed no differences as well. So I took a listen, and the chest was really noisy, but I, I thought that the breath sounds appeared to me to be a little more diminished on the right side as opposed to the left side. So I asked whether or not if there was any indication to repeat the chest X-ray, or if that was their finding as well. Now with breath sounds often, there isn't symmetry necessarily and, but there wasn't anything outward in terms of chest excursion, and by visual inspection it looked like it would be symmetric. But nevertheless, I went ahead and looked at the ventilator parameters. The ventilatory support settings appeared to be appropriate. Possibly the back-up rate could have been a little higher, but the patient wasn't really assisting much over the control rate. The patient had a pulse oximeter. Those settings were fairly stable, in the low 90s, as I recall, and the patient was not hypotensive, was a little more tachycardiac though than what the nurse had led me to believe over the 'phone, during our telephone conversation … somewhere around 120s, 130s, something like that. But the patient wasn't exhibiting signs of, you know, EKG changes or hypotension associated with that. He was on no vasoactive drugs at the time. There was a slight increase in the airway pressures, ah, but it wasn't high enough that would really warn me that I felt that there was a marked change in compliance at that time. The patient appeared to be returning most of the tidal volume that was being delivered by the ventilator.

… So I stayed in with the nurse, and we were talking and going over what the plan was and, things we might be looking for in the evening, because it was late afternoon, and I was going to be getting ready to go home. So, right before I left – the nurse had temporarily left the room, I noticed, and at first I wasn't sure if it was just the room lighting, or, if there was a true color change, subsequently there was a color change in the patient. But I noticed that the patient's upper torso looked a little duskier to me, especially the head and neck area. And I pulled his gown down. And I noticed there was a clear demarcation and color, and this was sort of in the mid-chest area, up to the neck and to the head. I took a look at breath sounds again and noticed that the breath sounds appeared even more diminished on the right side, as opposed to the left side. So I was thinking that this was maybe a pneumothorax. Again, the patient's mentation had not improved, When I brought this up to the junior resident, and actually the cardiology fellow was up there as well, in the latter part of the afternoon, they didn't think it was a pneumothorax because the patient was returning most of the exhaled volume. And they thought that under positive pressure, this would be a tension

pneumothorax, and we should see a decrease in exhaled volumes, or marked increase in airway pressures. And I know from the literature and at least my own experience, it isn't always so clear-cut like that. So the chest X-ray was ordered, and not – probably 10 or 15 minutes from the time that I get this curb side consult with the fellow and even before Radiology came up, this patient dropped his blood pressure, his heart rate went up, when we listened to his breath sounds, it was clear the patient's breath sounds had decreased even more.

Int.: Oh. . .

APN: And, here happened to be a doctor attending over on the MICU in the Coronary Care Unit attending a post arrest, who came over, and emergently inserted a chest tube and clearly it was a big pneumothorax. And I guess what sort of stood out in my mind, was that people were really looking at a lot of the classic parameters that they're taught that you should see. And I don't know if it was necessarily because of what I've read, or I think a lot of it has to do with what I've seen clinically, and I try to incorporate at least what I know, from knowledge, and what I've seen in practice, is that, it isn't always so clear cut. I mean, it just isn't. And sometimes you really have to kind of go on physical exam findings, and not necessarily – it's important to pay attention to the things you anticipate, but sometimes the things that aren't so obvious can be very clinically significant.

(Benner *et al.*, 1999)

This narrative account of experiential learning about clinical manifestations of a tension pneumothorax contains much practical knowledge about interpreting ambiguous clinical signs and symptoms, advocating for a needed diagnostic test (chest X-ray), negotiating

different interpretations by getting different opinions, and finally responding quickly to a dramatic change in the patient's rapidly changing condition. It is a good example of the kind of *modus operandi* thinking involved in clinical judgement. The patient's trajectory matters in interpreting clinical signs and symptoms. This story also illustrates two pervasive habits of thought and action in clinical practice: clinical grasp and clinical forethought (Benner *et al.*, 1999).

Clinical grasp

Clinical grasp describes clinical inquiry in action. Clinical grasp includes problem identification and clinical judgement across time about the particular transitions of particular patients/ families. Four aspects of clinical grasp include: (1) making qualitative distinctions; (2) engaging in detective work; (3) recognising changing relevance; (4) developing clinical knowledge in specific patient populations.

Making qualitative distinctions

Qualitative distinctions refer to those distinctions that can only be made in a particular, contextual, or historical situation. In the clinical example above, the nurse was listening for qualitative changes in the breath sounds, and changes in the patient's colour, also changes in the patient's mental alertness. The context and sequence of events are essential for making qualitative distinctions. Therefore, they require paying attention to transitions and judgement (Kuhn, 1970; Benner *et al.*, 1999). Many qualitative distinctions can only be made by observing differences through touch, sound or sight, as in skin turgor, colour, and capillary refill (Hopper, 1995).

Engaging in detective work: *modus operandi* thinking and clinical puzzle solving

Clinical situations are open-ended and under-determined. *Modus operandi* thinking keeps track of the particular patient, the way the illness unfolds, the meanings of the patient's responses as they have occurred in the particular time sequence. *Modus operandi* thinking requires keeping track of what has been tried, and what has or has not worked with the patient. In this kind of reasoning-in-transition, gains and losses in understanding that are error reducing are evaluated for their significance (Taylor, 1994; Dreyfus *et al.*, 1996). However, the clinician also thinks of a possibility of pneumothorax. A second comparative chest X-ray is needed. Later in the interview he states:

APN: *I guess it could have been a pulmonary embolus. But I was really sort of focused on the differences, and the fact that it was fairly similar appearance, which can happen with pulmonary emboli. The heart rhythm pattern had not changed, although it, it was elevated. There was some tachycardia. Uhm, but, it sort of was leading me to believe that this was more sort of a pulmonary problem, as opposed to a pulmonary circulation problem, you know.*

(Benner *et al.*, 1999)

The clinician is guessing that this is a problem of physically moving air in and out rather than obstructions to pulmonary circulation. The evidence is subtle, so the clinician stays open to disconfirmation, but proceeds with trying to get the chest X-ray and is prepared to recognise the sudden change in the patient's respiratory status when that occurs. Another qualitative distinction was the judgement of whether the patient's change in mental status and agitation was due primarily to anxiety or to hypoxia.

Recognising changing clinical relevance

Recognising changes in clinical relevance is an experientially learned skill that enables clinicians to distinguish what is relevant in situations. The meanings of signs and symptoms are changed by sequencing and history. The patient's mental status and colour continued to deteriorate, as did the diminishment of his breath sounds. Once the chest tubes were in place there was a dramatic change in the patient's colour. Each of these changes in the patient's signs and symptoms are made by examining the transitions as they occur.

Developing clinical knowledge in specific patient populations

Because this clinician has had the opportunity to observe both pulmonary circulation problems and mechanical breathing problems he is able to recognise a kind of 'family resemblance' with other mechanical breathing problems (as opposed to pulmonary circulation problems) that he has noticed with other patients.

Refinement of clinical judgement is possible when nurses have the opportunity to work with specific patient populations. The comparisons between many specific patients create a matrix of comparisons for clinicians, as well as a tacit, background set of expectations that create active detective work if a patient does not meet the usual predictable transitions in recovery. What is in the background and foreground of the clinician's attention needs to shift with changes in the patient's condition. Understanding a particular patient population well can assist with recognising these shifts.

Clinical forethought

Clinical forethought is another pervasive habit of thought and action in nursing practice evident in this narrative example (Kuhn, 1970; Benner *et al.*, 1999). Clinical forethought plays a role in clinical grasp because it structures the practical logic of clinicians. Clinical forethought refers to at least four habits of thought and action: (1) future think; (2) clinical forethought about specific diagnoses; (3) anticipation of risks for particular patients; (4) seeing the unexpected.

Future think

Future think is the broadest category of this logic of practice. In the example, the APN states 'So I stayed in with the nurse, and we were talking and going over what the plan was and, things we might be looking for in the evening'.

Anticipating likely immediate futures assist with making good clinical judgements and with preparing the environment so that the nurse can respond to the patient's immediate needs in a timely manner. Without the 'lead time' developing a sense of salience for anticipated signs and symptoms and preparing the environment, essential clinical judgements and timely interventions would be impossible in rapidly changing clinical situations. Future think governs the style and content of the nurse's attentiveness to the patient. Whether in a fast paced or slower paced rehabilitation setting, thinking and acting with anticipated futures guide clinical thinking and judgement. Future think captures the way judgement is suspended in a predictive net of thoughtful planning ahead and preparing the environment for likely eventualities.

Clinical forethought about specific diagnoses and injuries

This habit of thought and action is so second nature to the experienced nurse that he or she may neglect to tell the newcomer, the 'obvious'. Clinical forethought involves much local specific knowledge, such as who is a good resource, how to marshal support services and equipment for particular patients. The staff nurse used good judgement in calling the APN to assist in solving the puzzle when she was unable to convince the less clinically experienced junior resident. The APN made use of all available physicians in the area. Part of what made a timely response possible was actually planning that the situation might change rapidly.

Examples of preparing for specific patient populations abound in all settings. For example, anticipating the need for a pacemaker during surgery and having the equipment assembled ready for use saves essential time. Forecasting an accident victim's potential injuries, for example, when intubation might be needed for the accident victim.

Anticipation of crises, risks and vulnerabilities for particular patients

The narrative example is shaped by the fore-boding sense of an impending crisis for this particular patient. The staff nurse uses her sense of nervousness or uneasiness about the changes in the patient's breathing to initiate her problem search. This aspect of clinical forethought is central to knowing the particular patient, family or community. Nurses situate the patient's problems almost like a topography of possibilities. This vital clinical knowledge needs to be communicated to other caregivers, and across care borders. Clinical teaching could be improved by enriching curricula with narratives from actual practice, and by helping students recognise commonly occurring clinical situations. For example, if a patient is haemodynamically unstable, then managing life-sustaining physiological functions will be a main orienting goal. If the patient is agitated and uncomfortable, then attending to comfort needs in relation to haemodynamics will be a priority (Dreyfus *et al.*, 1996). Providing comfort measures turns out to be a central background practice for making clinical judgements, and contains within it much judgement and experiential learning. When clinical teaching is too removed from typical contingencies and strong clinical situations in practice, students will lack practice in active thinking-in-action in ambiguous clinical situations. With the rapid advance of knowledge and technology, students need to be good clinical learners and clinical knowledge developers. One way nurse educators can enhance clinical inquiry is by increasing experiential learning in the curriculum. Experiential learning requires open learning climates where students can discuss and examine transitions in understanding, including their false starts or their misconceptions in actual clinical situations. Focusing *only* on performance and on 'being correct' and not on learning from breakdown or error dampens students' curiosity and courage to learn experientially.

One's *sense* of moral agency as well as *actual* moral agency in particular situations change with level of skill acquisition (Kuhn, 1970). Furthermore, experiential learning is facilitated or hampered by learning skills of involvement with patients/families and engagement with clinical problems at hand. Those nurses who do not go on to become expert clinicians have some learning difficulty associated with skills of involvement and consequently with making clinical judgements, particularly making qualitative distinctions (Hopper, 1995). Experienced, non-expert nurses saw clinical problem-solving as a simple weighing of facts, or rational calculation. They did not experience their own agency in making clinical judgements. They failed to see qualitative distinctions linked to the patient's well-being.

Seeing the unexpected

One of the keys to becoming an expert practitioner lies in how the person holds past experiential learning and background habitual skills and practices. If nothing is routinised as a habitual response pattern, then practitioners cannot function in emergencies attending to the unexpected. However, if expectations are held rigidly, then subtle changes from the usual will be missed and habitual, rote responses will rule. The clinician must be flexible in shifting between what is in the background and the foreground. This is accomplished by staying curious and open. The clinical 'certainty' associated with perceptual grasp is distinct from the kind of 'certainty' achievable in scientific experiments and through measurements. It is similar to 'face recognition' or recognition of 'family resemblances'. It is subject to faulty memory, false associative memories, and mistaken identities. Therefore, such perceptual grasp is the beginning of curiosity and inquiry and not the end. In rapidly moving clinical situations, perceptual grasp is the starting point for clarification, confirmation and action. The relationship between the foreground and background of attention needs to be fluid, so that missed expectations allow the nurse to *see* the unexpected. For example, when the background rhythm of a cardiac monitor changes, the nurse notices, and what had been background tacit awareness becomes the foreground of attention. A hallmark of expertise is the ability to notice the unexpected (Kuhn, 1970). Background expectations of usual patient trajectories form with experience. These background experiences form tacit expectations that enable the nurse to notice subtle failed expectations and pay attention to early signs of unexpected changes in the patient's condition. Clinical expectations gained from caring for similar patient populations form a tacit *clinical forethought* that enables the exper-ienced clinician to notice missed expectations. Alterations from implicit or explicit expectations set the stage for experiential learning depending on the openness of the learner.

Study Activity 27.3 ⎯⎯⎯⎯

This chapter is a rich repository of reflection about the importance of clinical reasoning in practice. Read it again more closely, with particular attention to the distinctions drawn between 'techne' and 'phronesis'.

● Make notes on this second journey through the text, so that you can reflect upon these later.
● Return to Chapter 26 (Reflective practice). Note the slight difference in emphasis and in particular the incorporation in the present chapter of a moral dimension to praxis.

SUMMARY

Learning to be a good nurse requires not only technical expertise but also the ability to form helping relationships and engage in practical ethical and clinical reasoning (Dreyfus *et al.*, 1996). Aristotle linked experiential learning to the development of character and the moral sensitivities of a person learning a practice (Benner and Wrubel, 1982). No doubt rational calculations available to techne – population trends and statistics, algorithms – created as decision support structures, can improve accuracy when used as a stance of inquiry in making clinical judgements about particular patients. But in the end, the skills of phronesis (clinical judgement that reasons across time, taking into account the transitions of the particular patient/family/community and transitions in the clinician's understanding of the clinical situation), will be required for nursing, medicine or any helping professional (Benner *et al.*, 1999).

Experiential learning in clinical practice is expensive because the stakes are so high for patients and clinicians. Therefore, making experiential learning public, accessible to others, so that clinical wisdom can become cumulative and collective, is crucial to clinical knowledge development. Health care settings have not begun to tap the clinician's wealth of experiential learning.

REFERENCES

Benner, P. (1984) *From Novice to Expert: Excellence and power in clinical nursing practice*, Addison-Wesley, Menlo Park, CA

Benner, P. (1994) The role of articulation in understanding practice and experience as sources of knowledge in clinical nursing. In: Tully, J. (ed.) *Philosophy in an Age of Pluralism: The philosophy of Charles Taylor in question*, Cambridge University Press, New York

Benner, P. and Wrubel, J. (1982) Clinical knowledge development: the value of perceptual awareness. *Nurse Educator* 7, 11–17

Benner, P., Tanner, C.A. and Chesla, C.A. (1996) *Expertise in Nursing Practice: Caring, clinical judgment, and ethics*, Springer, New York

Benner, P., Hooper-Kyriakidis, P. and Stannard, D. (1999) *Clinical Wisdom and Interventions in Critical Care. A thinking-in-action approach*, W.B. Saunders, Philadelphia, IL

Blum, L. (1994) *Moral Perception and Particularity*, Cambridge University Press, Cambridge

Dreyfus, H.L. (1979) *What Computers Can't Do: The limits of artificial intelligence* (rev. edn), Harper and Row, New York

Dreyfus, H.L. (1992) *What Computers Still Can't Do: A critique of artificial reason*, MIT, Cambridge, MA

Dreyfus, H., Dreyfus, S. and Benner, P. (1996) Implications of the phenomenology of expertise for teaching and learning everyday skilful ethical comportment. In: Benner, P., Tanner, C.A. and Chesla, C. (eds) *Expertise in Nursing Practice: Caring, clinical judgment, and ethics*, Springer, New York

Dunne, J. (1993) *Back to the Rough Ground, Practical Judgment and the Lure of Technique,* Indiana University Press, Notre Dame, IN

Guignon, C.B. (1983) *Heidegger and the Problem of Knowledge*, Hackett, Indianapolis, IN

Halpern, J. (2001) *From Detached Concern to Empathy. Humanizing medical care*, Oxford University Press, Oxford

Hopper, P.L. (1995) Expert titration of multiple vasoactive drugs in post-cardiac surgical patients: an interpretive study of clinical judgment and perceptual acuity, Doctoral Dissertation, University of California, San Francisco, CA

Hunter, K.M. (1991) *Doctors' Stories: The narrative structure of medical knowledge*, Princeton University Press, Princeton

Kuhn, T.S. (1970) *The Structure of Scientific Revolutions* (2nd edn), University of Chicago, Chicago, IL

Lave, J. and Wenger, E. (1991) *Situated Learning: Legitimate peripheral perspectives (Learning in doing: Social, cognitive and computational perspectives)*, Cambridge University Press, Cambridge

MacIntyre, A. (1981) *After Virtue: A study in moral theory*, University of Indiana Press, Notre Dame, IN

Rubin, J. (1996) Impediments to the development of clinical knowledge and ethical judgment in critical care nursing. In: Benner, P., Tanner, C.A. and Chesla, C.A. (eds) *Expertise in Nursing Practice: Caring, clinical judgment, and ethics*, Springer, New York

Ruddick, S. (1989) *Maternal Thinking: Toward a politic of peace*, Ballantine, New York

Schön, D. (1987) *The Reflective Practitioner: How professionals think in action*, Basic Books, New York

Taylor, C. (1993) Explanation and practical reason. In: Nussbaum, M. and Sen, A. (eds) *The Quality of Life*, Clarendon Press, Oxford

Taylor, C. (1994) Philosophical reflections on caring

practices. In: Phillips, S.S. and Benner, P. (eds) *The Crisis of Care: Affirming and restoring caring practices in the helping professions*, Georgetown University Press, Washington, DC

Vetleson, A.J. (1994) *Perception, Empathy, and Judgment: An inquiry into the preconditions of moral performance*, Pennsylvania State University, University Park, PA

28 NURSING IN THE WIDER CONTEXT: ORGANISATIONAL FRAMEWORKS

Oliver Slevin

> The culture of managed care is different from the culture of the society around it, and it makes people nervous.
>
> (Friedman, 1999)

LEARNING OUTCOMES

After studying this chapter you will be able to:

- Recognise that nursing takes place within and as a part of the endeavours of wider health care organisations
- Define the concept of organisation, as an orderly social structure with specific social functions
- Explain the complex nature of organisations and the various internal and external influences that may impact upon them
- Discuss the principles of complexity and chaos that impact upon modern society and organisations within it, including health care organisations
- Present a case for modern health care organisations being established upon an overriding framework described as the adaptive learning organisation
- Present examples of organisational frameworks that are adaptive at both point of care and national levels
- Recognise that specific frameworks that may guide nursing need not conflict with organisational frameworks, but can in fact enhance the nursing contribution within such frameworks.

INTRODUCTION

In this module we have concentrated upon frameworks that may guide practice. It is impor-
tant to understand what such a framework *is*, and what its primary purpose is. A 'frame' is a concept taken primarily from the physical world, and is most often encountered in areas of interest such as engineering and architecture. The most common conceptualisation is that of interconnecting structures with their interstitial spaces. Such structures are essentially manmade for a specific purpose, which is usually to provide some form of support. Thus, a framework of steel girders or a wooden frame forms support for a building, or a wire frame provides a frame for spectacles. It is the use of materials *and* space that is of particular interest. The girder framework does not become a building until some of the space becomes filled with concrete or other building materials, and until services such as electricity, water, gas, etc. are installed; similarly the wire frame does not become a pair of spectacles until the lenses are inserted. The frame is the *infrastructure* upon which the *structure* is built. It not only provides the support for the structure but acts as a guide to its construction.

This physical concept may, however, become a metaphor for a *thinking* framework. Here, a set of principles, guidelines or rules (the equivalent to the steel or wood in a physical frame) becomes the frame or infrastructure for how we think and act in respect of particular phenomena. It in fact becomes a guide to how activities can be carried forward. The framework presented in the first chapter of this module was of course such a framework. There, we noted how the principles and rules making up the problem-solving approach might be utilised as a framework for guiding nursing work. We described that particular application of the problem-solving approach as the nursing process method. In the subsequent chapters of the module we also considered other conceptual frames that might guide nursing practice. In this respect we considered how conceptual frames such as competence, reflection, and clinical reasoning (including its tacit or intuitive dimensions) may also be helpful frameworks for guiding our nursing practice.

It is important to reiterate, once again, that these do not have to be alternative frameworks for practice. While the nursing process is a highly structured, problem-solving approach it does not by definition have to impose inflexible methods of delivering care. Indeed, an effective use of the framework would demand reflexive approaches to practice that allow care to be modified to respond to specific situations, effective use of tacit knowledge derived from experience, and the development of competence in the delivery of care identified in care plans. However, all of these orientations are by definition nursing specific. The delivery of health care is a wider undertaking, and at an organisational level involves a number of occupational groups across a range of health care settings. The need for frameworks at this organisational level is the primary focus of this final chapter of the module.

There is one final consideration that can inform our analysis of such frameworks. It is important to recognise that the basic elements of these thinking frameworks are ideas, constructed into concepts through language. In a significant and important sense, how we think about issues is determined by the language we use, and this is what, to a significant extent, determines how we think and act. We speak, therefore, of 'frames of reference' and in so doing allude to the particular paradigm or worldview that informs our thinking. Another way of seeing this is to recognise that how we deal with health care issues is 'framed' or contained within particular social discourses, and the dominant social discourse determines how health care will be delivered. A good example of this is the current Labour Government's discourse on care provision (Poole, 2000). This uses as one of its frames of reference a dual commitment that combines 'best practices' and effectiveness with 'best value'

and efficiency. On one hand this aims, primarily through establishing evidence-based health care, to implement what works best. On the other hand, it also aims at efficient use of resources through the redistribution and containment of costs. What is really being stated in this discourse is not that the very best will be provided, but that the very best *that can be afforded* will be provided. In turn, what can be afforded is determined by the overall funding made available for health care, and this part of the discourse relates to how health is valued against how other activities such as, for example, education and defence are valued. It is beyond the remit of this chapter to delve further into the complex political and economic considerations that underlie such social discourses, as indeed the fact that the UK spends less on health than other Western countries such as the USA, Germany and France. But it is important to recognise three important points:

- The framework within which health care as a whole is delivered is always determined by some social discourse that has underpinning values.
- Within the modern health care context, this discourse involves a balancing of best practices and best value.
- Nursing care is always delivered within such discourses and the frameworks they construct, such that in the modern world of health care it is essential that we are cognisant of these constraints within which we must maximise our contribution to care.

Study Activity 28.1

Consider the following two statements:

'My philosophy of care is one that is determined by my individual patient's needs. I must always do the very best that I can, basing my interventions on the best available evidence and ensuring that the medicines and technology I use are the most up-to-date and effective available'.

'I feel a responsibility to ensure that I can do the best I can for all my patients. This often means I must make hard choices about devoting resources to those who will benefit most, and I sometimes will elect to use cheaper interventions even where they are not as effective so that I can spread my resources wisely'.

● Reflect on each of these statements, then write brief summaries (about one A4 page/400 words each) of the discourses you feel are informing the two viewpoints.

THE ORGANISATIONAL ORIENTATION

Organisations

If we are to understand how frameworks at an organisational level impact upon care, we must first have some view on what organisations are. In the sense intended here, an organisation is a social structure, consisting of people, and a social process, consisting of certain rule-governed activities. It is essentially a construction of modern cultures, particularly in more highly developed societies. Jary and Jary (1995) define such an organisation as:

> A type of collectivity established for the pursuit of specific aims or goals, characterized by a formal structure of rules, authority relations, a division of labour and limited membership or admission. The term is used mainly to refer to large-scale or 'complex organizations' which pervade all aspects of social life in modern society, e.g. business enterprises, schools, hospitals, churches, prisons, the military, political parties, trades unions, etc. Such organizations involve patterns of relationships which differ from other social groups such as the family, peer groups, and neighbourhoods which are largely spontaneous, unplanned or informal . . .
> Forms of association in organizations tend to occupy only a segment of a person's life (with the notable exception of Total Organizations).
>
> (Jary and Jary, 1995, p. 464)

It may help our later understanding of frameworks at the organisational level if we give further brief consideration to this term. The term seems to emerge from a range of word usages that have a particularly confusing history. The Latin word *organum* related to an instrument (thus the particular musical instrument we today know as an organ). However, extending back into antiquity, the Greek work *organon* also referred to an instrument, but this might have various usages. It could refer to a musical instrument, but also to any instrument or machine or mechanism that had a purpose. This included social organs or instruments such as a rule or law (thus today we speak of statutory *instruments,* such as Nurses Rules that are laid in Parliament). In those early times mechanical was a synonym for organic. By the eighteenth and nineteenth centuries, the term 'organic' emerged as having biological significance. It was recognised that living organisms are composed of interacting mechanisms or organs that each have a function within the living being. However, the interdependence of organs in the body set it aside from crude machines that tend to be isolated and free-standing mechanisms with specific invariable functions. Within the living 'organism' the bodily systems and their organs are sophisticated and complex systems that are ordered in highly effective ways to sustain each other in a common purpose – the process of living and growing. To this end, the organs making up the living body have the capacity to respond to changes within the systems, to adapt to change and to self-correct in response to such change – to in fact maintain a balance of living that we might describe as a stable living organism capable of continuing its purpose of living. This capacity to maintain balance, to strive towards a condition of homeostasis, is a characteristic of such living bodies. The living body is thus recognised as not just a container of so many organs, but one in which the organs within body systems and the systems in turn are organised or ordered in highly sophisticated ways to serve the common purpose of living.

We now find that the words mechanical and organic were no longer synonyms (meaning the same thing) but in fact antonyms (meaning opposite ideas). Entities that were termed organic were by definition capable of growing, changing, working as complex interacting and self-correcting systems. They were anything but mechanical, unchanging and automatic in their workings. As biological meanings took hold, the term organic tended to be reserved for things that possessed properties of life. Because living 'organisms' are made up of chemical compounds that by definition include the element carbon, biological chemistry was defined as carbon chemistry or organic chemistry (concerned with living things that occurred naturally rather than artificial manmade things). This association with things natural is found today in our reference to organic foodstuffs that are said to be grown naturally and not modified in any way by artificial substances. In the twenty-first century these distinctions become even more blurred when we find that living organisms can in fact be constructed artificially in the laboratory, and when foodstuffs such as grains can be genetically modified. Williams (1983) provides a particularly useful exploration of the etymology of the term organic and its associated terms (including 'organisation').

Of particular interest in the origins of the word 'organisation', is its application to social groups. This first emerged in the work of two of the founding fathers of modern sociology: Ferdinand Tonnies (in Germany) and Emile Durkheim (in France). Both authors carried forward their main work more than a century ago, although English language versions of their work have been produced more recently. Tonnies ([1887] 1955) suggested two forms of social life. One of these he termed *gemeinschaft* (community); the other he termed *gesellschaft* (association). He suggested that modern society was characterised by a movement away from community and towards association. In *gemeinschaft,* relationships are direct, intimate, enduring and often all-embracing (extending into family, work and recreational activities). In such 'communities'

people tend to live, be educated, work, marry, have families, care for the old and sick and be cared for when their time comes, and die and be buried all within the community. Ties of kinship and neighbourhood are strong and supportive. Such communities are distinct from all others and are to varying degrees self-sufficient. In *gesellschaft,* there tends to be a lack of such intimate and enduring relationships. People *are*, of course, interconnected in various circumstances, but the connection is one of 'association' rather than close and intimate relationships. This association tends to be of a contractual nature. Thus, our milk is delivered by a delivery person who is contracted by us to do so; he may not be well known to us, and more often than not lives in a different locale. So too with the plumber and the ambulance driver. It is characteristic of such social structure that there is an interdependence between different communities and between individuals who do not live in the same communities.

Durkhein ([1895] 1974) similarly proposed two forms of social life. He spoke of *mechanical solidarity* and *organic solidarity*. In mechanical solidarity, small, locality-based groups exist as self-contained communities that are essentially similar in a number of ways to Tonnies' ([1887] 1955) description of gemeinschaft. Because such 'communities' are geographically self-contained and usually, to a large extent, self-sufficient, Durkheim used the analogy of a mechanism of interconnected parts, but with the whole being an entity separate from other similar communities. In organic solidarity, there is an interconnection of people across localities. Again, this is similar to Tonnies' ([1887] 1955) conception of gesellschaft. Here people often live, work and play in different locations. Taken to its extreme it may be the case that as people spend little time within the locality they live, they may not even be acquainted with each other, as in modern housing complexes where people sometimes do not even know their next-door neighbour. Durkheim used the analogy of a living being, wherein the organs are interconnected and support each other in particular ways. Within such a social structure, while we may not be acquainted with other people outside our own family or primary group, we are dependent on many others for our survival. Doctors and nurses will treat us in hospital when we are ill, a water corporation will deliver our water supplies, an educational system will educate our young. This *division of labour* is characteristic of this form of organic solidarity.

Within those social structures that Tonnies defined as gesellschaft and Durkheim defined as organic solidarity, whose old style close face-to-face communities are less common, there tends to be social bodies established to meet various social needs, from managing our stocks and shares to burying our dead. Such formal structures, established within modern 'organic' societies to meet specific needs or provide specific services, are organisations. Drawing upon the above statements, we might suggest the following as being characteristic of the modern organisation:

- A social group makes up the membership of an organisation: individuals become members of such an entity by virtue of some specific function they will have within the organisation.
- The organisation performs some specific function/s within the wider society, and this 'division of labour' extends across broad areas of society (so that we have 'organisations' dedicated to particular social functions, such as schooling, or health provision, or money management).
- The organisation is therefore ordered or designed specifically to undertake the functions in an effective way.
- Because of the dependence of members of the wider social group upon the services or functions of the organisation, an organic relationship exists between the organisation and the wider society.
- The organisation is governed by certain rules and principles that pertain directly to its functions, and all members of the organisation share a commitment to these rules and principles.

- Members usually do not live within the organisation, but participate as members only when the particular goals are being pursued.
- In modern, complex societies, people may be in membership of more than one organisation. They may be employed and *work* within one organisation, they may participate in a religious organisation that serves a spiritual function, they may also be involved in recreational organisations such as golfing organisations, and at the same time be active in a voluntary organisation such as Age Concern. It is therefore a feature of modern societies that they become more and more 'organised' and that people increasingly hold multiple organisational membership.

It will be readily appreciated that a vital aspect of the organisation is the way in which it has sets of principles, rules of conduct, ordered ways of working that sustain it in achieving its specific purpose. In the context referred to earlier, this is a 'framework' that sustains the organisation in attaining its goals and the members of the organisation work co-operatively within this framework.

Study Activity 28.2

Consider your own home neighbourhood (the place where you live).

- Determine whether this neighbourhood conforms with organic or mechanical solidarity.
- Reflect upon how living in each of these ways may impact upon health and well-being.

Questionable assumptions

It may be assumed from the characteristics of the modern organisation outlined above, that all elements of the organisation work to a common purpose. In reality, however, this tends only to be true to a certain extent. It is often the case that the goals of an organisation, and the rules and principles under which it works, are only shared by a few of the most powerful and senior members of the organisation. People, who are themselves complex and self-interested, do not always fit so conveniently into the 'organic' features of the organisation. It turns out that even this organic model of organisations is too mechanical to explain the complexities of human nature! A significant example of this is the cult television series *The Office* which has achieved a mass following in the first years of this new millennium. This is a caricature of how not only are the goals of the organisation rejected by the office workers, but they are most often held in disdain and actively undermined. This position is made worse in no small way by the empty, ineffective and insincere machinations of the senior manager. The success of the series owes much to the way in which people recognise it as a cringingly accurate reflection of real life in modern organisations.

In some instances, the membership of an organisation consists of groups that have their own goals that may not always be in line with those of the organisation. In *The Office* discussed above, the office staff, to a large extent, reflect a homogenous group that are broadly similar in their degree of acceptance and rejection of the organisational position. But in other more complex organisations there are often powerful pressure groups that themselves have considerable power. Modern health care organisations are a particularly good example of such circumstances. The members of such organisations consist of numerous occupational groups. Among these are the health care professions (mainly medicine, nursing and those professions allied to medicine that are now termed health professions in the UK), themselves highly organised and with their own principles, rules and goals. In some instances these groups may work against each other, as 'turf wars' are fought out. Indeed, they may on occasion work to their own agenda and against the aspirations of the organisation as a whole, when it is felt that those organisational aspirations work against the interests of the profession and/or its clients.

It may also be assumed that in more

controlled and efficient organisations there is a greater likelihood that all the members will show commitment to the organisation's objectives, and that human activity will in general be geared towards these goals. This is often the premise within 'closed' or 'total' organisations. The common examples of these are those social entities that have been termed 'total institutions'. Here, the institution is completely closed off from the wider society and the members, to a large extent, not only work but also live within the institution. Examples of these are prisons, monasteries of closed religious orders, and the large mental institutions of the past. Goffman (1968) carried out extensive participant observation in such an institution and found that below the official life of the organisation a highly active under-life persisted, with its own rules and principles and working to its own ends. Even in the most controlled situations, it would seem that it is a part of human nature to at times go against the rules, to seek alternative interests and ways of living. In George Orwell's (1949) famous futuristic novel *Nineteen Eighty-four*, despite the highly ordered lifestyle rules that even prohibited heterosexual relationships, the main protagonist rebels against the oppressive regime and enters into such a relationship, with disastrous consequences.

The '1984' phenomenon demonstrated another feature of organisations that in fact speaks against the premise that such entities are organic in their capacity for growth and development. Because the rules and principles of the organisation tend to sustain the interests and goals of the most powerful members, there is in fact a vested interest in avoiding change, in maintaining a *status quo*. This manifests itself in a resistance to change that often causes the organisation to stagnate and in extreme cases even leads to its downfall. Of particular interest here is the current concern with modernising health services. This is, of course, a complex area, and the motives behind programmes of modernisation may include political agendas aimed at achieving the aspirations of one group over others under the apparently legitimate claim that the organisation *must* 'modernise'. This is an issue we discussed in some depth in Chapter 19 and later in Chapter 44. Notwithstanding such motivations, there is a demand that an organisation whose very *raison d'etre* is the health, well-being, safety and survival of those it serves must be a modern and efficient undertaking. This becomes highly problematic when powerful interests within the organisation (whether these are influential senior members or professional groups) resist the modernisation process.

The latter assertion assumes that such modernisation processes are universally desirable. It must be recognised, as referred to above and as detailed in Chapter 19, that the idea of modernisation is sometimes a flag under which other political motives sail. Of significance here is the economic model of health care provision that in recent years has increasingly incorporated formulae for rationing health care. This raises the issue of the ethical or moral principles upon which an organisation rests. It is certainly the case that in recent times organisations have recognised the importance of having a declared ethical position, and the areas of business ethics and health care ethics are rapidly growing areas of organisational activity (*see* Chapter 13). It is nevertheless the case that, in general, organisations operate on principles of utility, geared towards the achievement of organisational objectives. As such, they seldom devote significant time and resources to the moral dimensions of their activities. The result of this can be the possibility that those interests within membership of organisations that resist initiatives can be labelled as simply resisting modernisation when in fact they are presenting legitimated concerns that the powers that be are choosing to ignore. With such considerations in mind, we might add the following two items to the seven characteristics of organisations listed in the previous section:

- Organisations are composed of members and interest groups which may have their own goals or interests. In addition, because organisations exist within wider social systems, they

are often subject to outside influences. Organisations are thus by definition complex political entities.

- Because organisations *are* entities with specific functions, their activities impact upon their own membership and the wider society. There is thus always a moral dimension to the activity of an organisation that is often not fully attended to in terms of ethical choices.

Study Activity 28.3

In this and the preceding section we have identified nine characteristics of organisations. Using your library, identify key texts defining or describing organisations.

- As you work, note the key characteristics that emerge from the literature.
- Compare the results of your work with the characteristics identified in this chapter, and construct your own statement on the characteristics of an organisation. You may find it helpful to compare with fellow students who have also undertaken the activity, or seek a critical opinion from your personal tutor.

TOWARDS ORGANISATIONAL FRAMEWORKS

Coping with complexity within health care organisations

One of the difficulties of establishing frameworks for care centres upon the issue of complexity. It will be clearly seen from the previous section that while at first the phenomenon of the 'organisation' in modern society is a fairly straightforward concept, in reality it is a much more complex state of affairs. An organisation may have a clear organisational purpose, and be structured to achieve that purpose. But in reality, there are many variables at play. We have already noted that organisations are highly political social systems, and as such the interests of individuals or groups within *and* outside an organisation may conflict with the formal goals of the organisation. However, other factors not guided by political motives may also impact upon an organisation. Later, in Module 10, we will consider the impact of global influences on a particular nation or society, on communities within it, and even on individuals. Organisations are no less sensitive to such influences. A prime example of this was the terrorist attack on the New York World Trade Center in September of 2001. This alone had a massive impact upon world economies and indeed led to the collapse of many organisations. In a world that in late modernity has moved from a relatively stable state to one that is characterised by volatility and constant major change, it becomes more and more difficult to maintain organisational stability. In the new millennium successful organisations are characterised by their orientation to change and their ability to recognise rapidly changing patterns and respond rapidly to these.

Health care organisations are particularly vulnerable in such circumstances. The rapid advances in health technology, the equally rapidly changing patterns of health care needs, and the increasing demands of society, make such organisations particularly vulnerable to rapid change. It is not just the speed of change that is at issue here. It is the aforementioned complexity, the sheer difficulty of being able to predict what will come next in the modern world, which makes it more difficult for organisations to manage and survive (Giddens, 1991). It has become increasingly common to see situations that are complex, unstable and difficult to predict as moving towards chaos characterised by disorder and confusion. But it is important to recognise that the modern world of rapid change is *characterised* by disorder that often appears confusing. Waldrop (1992) refers to the way in which coping within complex and unstable situations demands a responsiveness that can be described as managing or surviving at the edge of chaos:

> Since the systems that are capable of the most complex, sophisticated responses will always have the edge in a competitive world . . . then frozen systems can always do better by

> loosening up a bit, and turbulent systems can always do better by getting themselves a little more organised. So if a system isn't on the edge of chaos already, you'd expect learning and evolution to push it in that direction. And if it is on the edge of chaos, then you'd expect learning and evolution to pull it back if it ever starts to drift away. In other words, you'd expect learning and evolution to make the edge of chaos stable, the natural place for complex, adaptive systems to be.
>
> (Waldrop, 1992, p. 295)

Against such a background, the way we use frameworks that will guide health care services is what becomes important. We must, of course, develop frameworks that do work. But we must also recognise that, such is the speed of change and the volatility of the health care environment, what works today may not work tomorrow. In such circumstances, the successful organisation is one that can transform itself into a *learning* organisation. That is, one that is constantly reviewing changes and developments in the environment and constantly looking to what adaptations the organisation must make in responding to such changes. This may even involve, as intimated by Waldrop (1992), the capacity to unfreeze (disengage from set structures and procedures that restrict organisational development) and then to take entirely new directions. In effect, the most important framework of all is that which we might describe as a learning framework. This involves not only the promotion of a learning orientation of the members of the organisation (in this case including the health care managers and professions), but also what literally amounts to a transformation: an *organisation* that is *itself* a learning organisation (Argyris and Schön, 1996).

Patient/client-centred frameworks

One such transformation may be that which involves a shift in perspective from addressing problems or issues from the point of view of the health care providers to that which centres upon the point of view (and needs) of the patient, client, or 'user' of our health services. This, in effect, involves a movement from a situation where, for example, health care professional groups, such as nursing, concentrate on what are essentially *nursing* problems, to a situation within which all the care providers, together, concentrate on patient or client problems. On the premise that no one perspective can accommodate such a broad orientation, or the depth of expertise needed across all the problems that arise, all must work together. This is the basis for that framework that is typically described as multidisciplinary team working. This is not a new concept, and the idea of health care teams has been around for many years. However, the notion of a team in which the members are co-equal partners, and one which might involve members from outside the health care system (such as social workers, teachers, police officers, housing officials) and also the patient/client, is often a more difficult goal to achieve.

More often than not, the situation is one in which a 'team' has closed membership and a designated manager or leader. In such circumstances, the likelihood is that the team may be more successful in some circumstances than others. In an alternative and more responsive framework for team working:

- The team may have a core membership, but would vary in membership according to the health care problem being addressed.
- The active involvement of the patient (or where this is not possible his/her representative or guardian) would be an essential aspect, allowing for the individual to participate in decisions concerning their own care.
- There would be a true commitment to equal partnership in which all would have co-equal rights to participate in the decisions.
- By definition, the team would be open, non-hierarchical and inclusive, rather than closed, hierarchical and exclusive.
- While there may be administrative responsibility vested in individual/s, the leadership or key worker role would be determined by the

particular health care issue rather than organisational edict.
- The decisions taken, and care implemented, would draw on the resources and expertise of the team as a whole.

Study Activity 28.4

The idea of a team approach to care is not new to nursing, and team nursing has been contrasted with task-orientated nursing over many years. One particular development in nursing equated broadly with the notion of a key worker, and indeed precedes such thinking. This is the concept of *primary nursing*.

- Using your library sources, construct a brief (two page/500-word) description of the primary nursing concept. A useful starting point may be the seminal text by Manthey (1992), who is in fact credited with inventing primary nursing.
- Consider how the concept 'primary nurse' related to the concept of 'named nurse' introduced in the UK health services.
- Compare and contrast the idea of the 'primary nurse' in nursing with that of the 'key worker' in multidisciplinary team working.
- Reflect upon how the nursing concept of primary nursing may function within organisations that have adopted multidisciplinary team working.

System-wide health care frameworks

The latter example illustrates a situation in which the strategy is essentially unfreezing in order to develop a new, more responsive framework based upon concepts of team working. Another transformation pertains to the need to balance such advances with a degree of organisational order, which Waldrop (1992) also advocated. A primary example of this within the UK health services is the development of what are known as National Service Frameworks (*see also* Chapter 19). Particularly within the English National Health Service, there are now such national frameworks for care groups or services (such as coronary care, mental health, care of older people). These frameworks provide guidelines or a blueprint for service provision established upon best standards of care. These in turn have been established through comprehensive research and development and health technology assessment procedures (Department of Health, 1998).

Fundamental to such organisation-wide frameworks is the fact that they are orientated towards the management of care at different levels. The ways by which such management is defined varies widely and there are many systems of health care management presented in the literature. However, it is possible to make a broad distinction in terms of level. Although there is nothing like a universal agreement on such definitions, it is useful to recognise systems that are based upon *care management* and systems that are based upon *case management*. In general, the idea of 'care management' refers to system-wide or organisation-wide initiatives for managing health care. It characteristically involves establishing a programme of care or caring services for a particular client group (e.g. care of older people, mental health, etc.). In this context, establishing a National Service Framework for such a group, as referred to above, would be one such example. The idea of 'case management' is established at the level of direct care provision, and relates to managing the care of a particular client or patient. The orientation here is that rather than different professionals providing their specific input in varying degrees of isolation, a 'case manager' develops planned care for the individual, and in so doing involves others as appropriate (Aliotta, 2001). The idea of a case manager is similar to that of 'key worker' referred to earlier, and it tends to be the mode of operation within modern team working approaches (as discussed earlier). To a large extent the 'primary nurse' is a nursing operationalisation of this concept. It may, however, be argued that the use of the term 'case' carries the risk of objectification of the patient or client, and similarly 'management' may convey a mechanical and recipe-like approach to care. If you have completed Study Activity 28.4 you will

have established that in 'primary nursing' there is a commitment to personalising care that may avoid such depersonalisation of the patient *and* the nurse.

It is again important to recognise that there is little consensus about the meaning of the above terms and how they are operationalised in practice. For example, even the latter distinction between care management and case management does not have universal agreement. Indeed, as Payne (2000) points out, in the UK public services there is a tendency to use the terms interchangeably, or to use the term 'care management' as the British term for 'case management' (a concept widely adopted in North America and in British social work). However, a more recent variant, and one that to an extent cuts across both these terms, is the term *managed care* (Cochrane, 2001). Managed care has been established largely against a backcloth of the discourse on best practice versus best value discussed in the introduction to this chapter. Essentially, in its various applications it involves planned programmes that specify what will be provided, the range of interventions (diagnostic tests, treatments, etc.) that will be provided, and sometimes also procedures to be followed in providing the services. Care provision is, therefore, determined by guidelines which in some circumstances may be precise. These can range across:

- broad *guidelines*, that state the general range of provision and provide some guidance on delivery
- *care pathways,* that state the activities that will take place at each stage in the course of care of a particular type of patient or client
- *protocols,* that are highly specific requirements in respect of interventions – stating what diagnostic tests can be used, identifying medicines that may be prescribed and in what dosages, etc.

It is often the case that managed care incorporates elements of all of these. There are clear advantages in such an approach, as care is standardised, usually on the basis of best evidence. However, concern is often expressed that such approaches work against clinical freedom and fail to take account of the specific circumstances. This is particularly the case in very controlled situations wherein any variation from the care pathway or protocol must be authorised in advance; indeed, in some circumstances expensive interventions allowed within protocols require prior approval in any case.

While the National Health Service National Service Frameworks referred to earlier tend to operate at the level of broad guidelines, they are nevertheless largely within a managed care philosophy. Furthermore, the use of care pathways and protocols is increasingly common within the UK health services. The introduction of organisational frameworks – national frameworks, managed care, care pathways and protocols, multidisciplinary team working, etc. – means that nursing can no longer conceive of itself as operating in a caring vacuum. Increasingly, how we organise our approaches to care must take account of wider organisational frameworks and constraints. In addition, as key health care personnel, nurses are increasingly involved in the formulation of frameworks at the organisational level. Such developments should be viewed as a challenge rather than a threat to nursing. Where care is increasingly standardised within frameworks at the organisational level, nurses must ensure that this incorporates and values the personal caring that is central to the nursing purpose.

Study Activity 28.5

Those who support managed care argue that this is justified so that best practices and best value can be incorporated in care. Those who are critical of the approach are concerned that health care is becoming increasingly economics driven, and that managers and economists are curtailing the clinical freedom necessary to promote effective health care.

- Using your library resources, carry out a brief review of the literature on managed care. Write a brief statement (about two A4 pages/500–600 words) presenting the potential strengths and

weaknesses of the approach. You may find it helpful to discuss this with a colleague or personal tutor/mentor.

SUMMARY

In this chapter we have considered the issue of frameworks that may guide service provision at organisational levels. In doing so, we have considered the nature of the social phenomenon called the 'organisation'. We have noted that at one level organisations are orderly social groupings established to achieve certain ends. However, not only do such organisations turn out to be more complex in reality, but increasingly they must survive and function effectively within a complex and rapidly changing social world.

A key premise put forward in the chapter is that in such circumstances health care organisations must be change-receptive and capable of themselves learning, growing, and adapting to complex, changing health environments. This was approached at two levels: the level of the caring interface, and the need for more effective team working; and, the society or nation-wide level, and the need to maintain a degree of order and assurance of quality and standards in volatile situations. In this latter context, frameworks for managing care at organisation-wide levels were considered, with particular reference to the concept of managed care. Consideration was given to the strengths and weaknesses of such frameworks and the extent to which they may impact upon clinical practice and nursing practice.

In the opening quotation to this chapter (Friedman, 1999), we noted that managed care, the example of an organisational framework for care that is probably the most extensive, is a strange experience for people. Indeed, all organisational frameworks impose some constraints and lead to reactions extending from perplexity through to the most hostile rejection. In such circumstances, we as nurses may beg questions as to the relevance of our own frameworks within these wider organisational contexts. The argument here is not that specific frameworks for guiding nursing practice (as discussed earlier in the module) are ineffective or that they should be discarded. On the contrary, it is recognised that these frameworks are essential guides to best nursing practices. Rather than detracting from high-quality care, such *nursing* frameworks enhance the nursing contribution within wider organisational frameworks.

REFERENCES

Aliotta, S.L. (2001) Case management of 'at-risk' older people. In: Cochrane, D. (ed.) *Managed Care and Modernization*, Open University Press, Buckingham

Argyris, C. and Schön, D. (1996) *Organizational Learning II: Theory, method, and practice*, Addison Wesley, Reading, MA

Cochrane, D. (2001) *Managed Care and Modernization*, Open University Press, Buckingham

Department of Health (1998) *A First Class Service: Quality in the new NHS*, Department of Health, London

Durkheim, E. ([1895] 1974) *The Social Division of Labor in Society*, The Free Press, New York

Friedman, E. (1999) Managed care: devils, angels, and the truth in between, *Health Progress* 80(3), 22–6

Giddens, A. (1991) *Modernity and Self-identity: Self and society in the late modern age*, Polity Press, Cambridge

Goffman, E. (1968) *Asylums*, Penguin, London

Jary, D. and Jary, J. (1995) *Collins Dictionary of Sociology* (2nd edn), Harper Collins, Glasgow

Manthey, M. (1992) *The Practice of Primary Nursing*, King's Fund Centre, London

Orwell, G. (1949) *Nineteen Eighty-four*, Martin Secker and Warburg, London

Payne, M. (2000) *Teamwork in Multiprofessional Care*, Palgrave, Basingstoke

Poole, L. (2000) Health care: New Labour's NHS. In: Clarke, J., Gewirtz, S. and McLaughlin, E. (eds) *New Managerialism, New Welfare?* Sage, London

Tonnies, F. ([1887] 1955) *Community and Association*, Routledge and Kegan Paul, London

Waldrop, M. (1992) *Complexity: The emerging science at the edge of order and chaos*, Penguin, Harmondsworth

Williams, R. (1983) *Keywords: A vocabulary of culture and society* (rev. edn), Flamingo-Fontana, London.

MODULE 6: FRAMEWORKS FOR PRACTICE

REFLECTIONS

This module marked a transition in the book, reflected in a movement from theoretical or knowledge concerns to modules that will primarily address practice issues. In this, the first of these modules, there was also recognition of a more subtle transition, that might indeed represent a paradigm shift in the relationship between knowledge and practice. In the past, it was common to utilise constructions known as *nursing models* as frameworks for guiding practice. These were in effect specific forms of *conceptual* models, as described within Chapter 14 of this book. However, you may recall that there we considered the use of conceptual or theoretical frameworks in principle rather than specific *nursing* models or theories. This reflects a growing conviction that, in a rapidly changing health care world, the use of static models that purport to inform the nursing project is limited. Indeed, in some American nursing schools, such 'models' are no longer taught.

This module took a similar stance by considering frameworks that may have more relevance in modern health care contexts. Across five chapters you were introduced to three of the major orientations:

- Frameworks that largely derive from a rational or logicopositivist perspective, significantly represented by problem-solving and competency-based approaches.
- Frameworks that largely derive from a more experiential orientation, significantly represented by the reflective practice movement and tacit and intuitive approaches to clinical reasoning.
- Frameworks that are established on an organisational level and largely derive from a quality agenda emphasising organisational or even national standards and practice protocols.

It is easy to see these major threads as being incompatible by virtue of being derived from different value systems. Indeed, there is some evidence to sustain this in the ways in which advocates of the perspectives establish lines of opposition. However, you may find it useful to reflect on the possibility that all three perspectives are essential and indeed complementary. Indeed, such complemetarity is proposed in the final chapter of the module.

Module 7: Therapeutic modes

Introduction

As a nurse, you bring to each nursing act a complex array of qualities that might be described in terms of self and role. This means that within your professional role you bring personal qualities, which mark you as someone whose natural tendency is that of reaching out to others in need. You also possess a certain body of knowledge and skills that you have learned and developed to levels of competence and beyond. It is vitally important to recognise this in nursing, where the work is carried out in the context of a close and intimate relationship between the nurse and the patient.

Up-to-date knowledge and a high degree of technical skill are essential and in many instances they are indeed life-saving. However, were these to be brought to bear through a distanced and rigid role, the nurse would be little more than an automaton. The coming together of role and self, or technique and relation, is the primary focus of this module.

29 THE THERAPEUTIC RELATIONSHIP

Carol Kirby

> *Humanisation is a reciprocal thing. We cannot know ourselves or declare ourselves human unless we share in the humanity of another.*
>
> (Brian Keenan, 1992)

> *The face of the neighbor signifies for me an unexceptionable responsibility, preceding my free consent, every pact, every contract.*
>
> (Emmanuel Levinas, 1991)

LEARNING OUTCOMES
After studying this chapter, you will be able to:

- Define the terms 'therapeutic' and 'relationship'
- Understand the integral elements of a therapeutic relationship
- Recognise the importance of 'openness' to the therapeutic relationship
- Discuss the role of the nurse in such a relationship
- Describe the nature of the personal relationship between nurse and patient
- Begin to apply therapeutic relating within your practice.

INTRODUCTION

Therapeutic relationship has its origin in a sincere respect for the absolute dignity of human life, for its personal meaning, significance and continual possibility. Beginning in human obligation and responsibility, in being-for-the-sake-of-another, it is realised through skilled compassionate caring. Within reciprocal human relations we come to know ourselves, our humanity. The meaning we find in life is discovered, not in individual freedom and power, but in ethical living relation *with* another, in 'unexceptionable responsibility' *to* the other. We co-exist in life and through the connection of relation we live in and understand the world; we live our humanity as one – human and all part of one another.

RELATIONSHIP AS THERAPY

The significant aspect of therapeutic relation is intensity of thought, feeling, reason and compassionate caring. The word 'therapy' derives from the Greek word *therapeia*, which means 'care'; the word *therapeutikos* refers to the person who provides that care for another. Therapy in recent times has been associated with a concept of treating or healing. The latter concept may suggest treatment that is medical in focus, or refer to a holistic understanding of a healing process that extends beyond a specific medical paradigm.

The word 'relationship' derives from the Latin word *relatus*, denoting 'connection'. In a human context, the connection is between persons, signifying perhaps genetic, legal or cultural relation, or distinctive group relation, based for example on ethnicity, profession or occupation. In such relation, there may not be of necessity any interpersonal participation between those who are connected. The nursing relation is one of therapeutic connection; it is both deeply personal and interpersonal. It is an emotional, cognitive and spiritual interconnection. In defining 'relationship', Janet Surrey (1991) speaks of an experience of emotional and cognitive intersubjectivity; of the ongoing, intrinsic inner awareness and responsiveness to the continuous existence of the other, or others, and of the expectation of mutuality in this regard. The therapeutic nursing relationship connects people in a purposeful dynamic of care. It is a relationship characterised by two defining conditions:

1 It is a professional relationship, an encounter of the 'one-caring' with the person 'cared-for'.
2 It is a relationship that protects patients from the inherent danger of vulnerability, keeps them safe during illness, and strengthens and generates healing.

The term therapy may designate a specific treatment orientation or practice aligned to a medical curative, rather than carative, orientation. In this sense, therapy signifies treatment. It may be used as a postfix or linked to other terms to indicate specific treatment, such as radiotherapy, chemotherapy, occupational therapy, art therapy, physiotherapy, or psychotherapy. In some instances (for example, in psychiatry) the postfix is used in classifying treatment modalities:

● Somatatherapy – physical methods of treatment
● Chemotherapy – chemical, or pharmaceutical methods of treatment (in general medicine the term is often reserved for chemical interventions in cancer treatment)
● Psychotherapy – methods that essentially use interpersonal communication or 'talk' as a treatment modality.

In all medical practice and the nursing interventions associated with it, the issue of relationship and consequential therapeutic potential is highly important. There exists a constant that extends across approaches demonstrating the importance that patients (clients) attach to the way in which they are related to by those who have helped them. Carl Rogers (1958) reported the way clients felt, irrespective of the approach to their treatment:

... the attitudinal elements in the relationship accounted for the changes which had taken place in themselves: the trust they had felt in the therapist; being understood by the therapist; the feeling of independence they had in making choices and decisions.

(Rogers, 1958)

More recently, Wheway (1999) has also emphasised the importance of dialogue and sharing as an important influence within successful therapeutic relationship.

Study Activity 29.1

● Reflect upon the elements distinguished by Carl Rogers (1958) – trust, being understood, and a sense of independence or empowerment – identifying the views of patients (clients). Observe the way in which nurses and doctors within your clinical placement areas relate to patients (clients), and reflect on your observations.
● Ascertain clear, observable instances where nurses and doctors made visible attempts to gain trust, to understand properly how the patient felt, to involve the patient in decision-making. Consider the extent to which these endeavours were present or absent. Reflect upon the reasons as to why they may have been absent.

EVIDENCE SUPPORTING THERAPEUTIC PRACTICE

The principle at the heart of this chapter is the fact that relationship in the sense of interpersonal relating is in itself therapeutic, having a helping or healing intention and influence. The studies by Rogers (1958, 1960, 1967) and Wheway (1999) provide important supporting evidence. Such research may be perceived as simply presenting the views or opinions of patients (clients). In a health service increasingly requiring an evidence-based approach to health care, there is a demand for strong outcome evidence to support investment in what are often determined to be expensive treatment approaches. To date, most research into the efficacy of therapeutic relation-ships has been conducted in respect of the specific application of such relationships in psychotherapy.

The research has shown that, while there is evidence to suggest that therapists and the general public value therapy (Rogers, 1967; Hollon, 1996; VandenBos, 1996; Mace, 1999), large-scale analyses of accumulated research evidence have not demonstrated a clear and significant positive outcome from such interven-tion (Eysenck, 1994; Linfors *et al.*, 1995; Tan, 1996).

Research into the effectiveness of trained and experienced psychotherapists when compared to untrained helpers has not demonstrated signifi-cant therapeutic advantage provided by the expert interventions (Burlingame and Barlow, 1996; Diamond, 1997).

While research has yet to demonstrate the supremacy of specific therapeutic intervention, there is evidence affirming that the quality of the therapeutic relationship or alliance has a signifi-cant and consistent positive impact upon outcome (Hays, 1995; Martin *et al.*, 2000; Ackerman and Hilsenroth, 2001; Kieffer, 2001).

While there is a dearth of evidence in this area, and much of it is conflicting, the following summary of research findings justifies to some degree the following affirming statements:

- Lack of expertise is not a justification for avoiding the use of therapeutic relating and even inexperienced practitioners can engage in relationship as an effective therapeutic medium.

- Therapeutic relating can and should be an integral part of the nurse's approach, as it is the essence of the relationship and its healing, supporting and empowering potential that is the constant therapeutic influence, rather than any particular 'technique' or specific inter-vention.

- It is possible, on the latter basis, to identify important elements of the relationship (or, as some therapists define it, the 'alliance'), which can and should be developed.

Study Activity 29.2

Undertake a search of the nursing literature on the essence and efficacy of therapeutic relationship as it is applied in nursing. Compare your findings with those reported above.

THE THERAPEUTIC RELATIONSHIP IN NURSING

Therapeutic relation sources and inspires hope. It has as its goal the opening to human potential and transformative possibility and the realisation of possibility within a caring dialogue. Through a collaborative and participatory healing process, which recognises the wholeness of human being and the distinctiveness and interdependence of each person, hope is brought forth and inten-tional therapeutic outcome is realised.

Nurses enter the therapeutic relationship with authentic and compassionate regard for the deeply personal and individual life of the person (the patient), honouring the uniqueness and inherent healing capacity of their life. They hear the person's story, their belief about what is happening to them. They listen with care to what is being said, grasp the meaning, and attempt to understand and to respond. It is acknowledged that the person is the expert on their own life, on how they experience what they are going through. With each other, they discover possibility, imagine the future and generate meaning. Nurses, in healing presence, are often helping people whose lives are in shreds, who are at the edge or even over the edge of endurance. In being there, they attempt to restore joy and equilibrium; they create a healing space, and provide the protection and peace of mind that set in motion the process through which life heals, in which the person grows strong and faces life renewed.

Milton Mayeroff's testimony (1990) of the meaning and importance of caring relation has a clear application to the therapeutic encounter. In his view, to care for another person in the most significant sense is to help them grow and actual-ise self. According to Mayeroff, through caring for certain others, and serving them through caring, one lives the meaning of one's life. We are at home in the world, not through dominating, or explaining or appreciating, but through caring and being cared for. The caring ingredients specified by Mayeroff (1990) provide a unity of elements essential to therapeutic relation:

- *Knowing* – 'to care for someone, I must know many things ... who the other is, what his powers and limitations are, what his needs are and what is conducive to his growth; I must know how to respond to his needs, and what my own powers and limitations are'.
- *Alternating rhythms* (the rhythm of moving back and forth between a narrower and wider framework) – 'I cannot care by sheer habit; I must be able to learn from my past. I see what my actions amount to, whether I have helped or not and, in the light of the results, maintain or modify my behaviour so that I can better help the other'.
- *Patience* (giving time and thereby enabling the other to find self in its own time) – 'patience is not waiting passively for something to happen, but is a kind of participation with the other in which we give fully of ourselves ... by patiently listening to the distraught man, by being present for him, we give him space to think and feel'.
- *Honesty* (being honest with oneself) – 'in caring I am honest in trying to see truly'. We are genuine in caring for the other when we 'ring true'.
- *Trust* – trusting the other to grow: realising that one is trusted has its own way of activating the person cared for to justify such trust and to trust oneself to grow.
- *Humility* – '[the one] who cares is genuinely humble in being ready and willing to learn more about the other and himself, and what caring involves ... through caring I come to a truer appreciation of my limitations as well as my powers; my limitations are neither resented nor glorified and I take pride in the successful use of my powers'.

- *Hope* – '[is] an expression of a present alive with possibilities, rallies energies and activates our powers; it is not a passive waiting for something to happen from the outside ... it is not simply hope for the other, it is hope for the realisation of the other *through* caring'.
- *Courage* (in going into the unknown) – 'courage is not blind; it is informed by insight from past experiences, and it is open and sensitive to the present ... the greater the sense of going into the unknown, the more courage is called for in caring.' (Mayeroff, 1990, pp. 19–34)

The elements are not in their enactment separate, rather they are integral to the wholeness of relation. There cannot be truth without humility, and hope will not be realised without courage: thus as relation unfolds, we are called to respond with consciousness and spirit in the caring moment. The essence of man, which is special to him, can be known only in living relation. Martin Buber (1947) asks us to:

> ... *consider man with man, and you see human life, dynamic, twofold, the giver and the receiver, he who does and he who endures, the attacking force and the defending force, the nature which investigates and the nature which supplies information, the request begged and granted – and always both together, completing one another in mutual contribution, together showing forth man.*

Study Activity 29.3

Martin Buber, a Jewish scholar and a most influential figure in the twentieth century, speaks of 'man' as synonymous with being human. Ignoring the gender bias in what was the accepted language of his time, consider the following questions:

- Do women relate differently to men?
- Are women more compassionate, with a greater capacity to empathise?

- Do women and men relate differently to those of their own gender and to those of the opposite gender?
- If gender differences exist, what is the implication for *therapeutic* relation?
- Reflect critically upon these questions and record your response.

You are required, as part of the educational process, to think critically, and to base your practice on the best available evidence. In this sense, your answers will not be considered scientific evidence. However, the patients you relate to in the future will all have their own views on these issues. In each nursing encounter, it is your views and those of the particular patient that are significant to the unfolding relationship.

Life is lived in relation, in living human relationship. A therapeutic environment has to be created, cultivated and nurtured if therapeutic potential is to be realised, and healing generated and sustained. McMahon and Pearson (1998) affirm that therapeutic nursing requires nurses creatively to assist patients in their quest for health and for healing. Løgstrup (1997) declares that we constitute one another's world and destiny and in so doing he provides a critical and essential caution:

> A person never has something to do with another person without also having some degree of control over him or her. It may be a very small matter, involving only a passing mood, a dampening or quickening of spirit, a deepening or removal of some dislike. But it may also be a matter of tremendous scope, such as can determine if the life of the other flourishes or not.

It is vital for nurses to recognise the extent to which what they say and do impacts upon the peace of mind, the joyfulness, or otherwise, of those for whom they purport to care. Our way of being with the patient can either inspire or dispirit them, can either create and sustain environments generating healing, or induce demorali-

sation. Through sincere belief that what happens to the patient really matters to us, we pay special attention to them; we listen to and learn with them, ensure that what they feel is understood. The importance of dialogue, of the patient being heard and understood, to successful therapeutic relationship has been emphasised by Carl Rogers (1958) and Wheway (1999), and is in accord with Sidney Jourard's belief that:

> ... one of the events which we believe inspires faith and hope in a patient is the conviction that someone cares about him. If this proves true, it implies that the quality of the nurse–patient relationship is a factor in the patient's recovery. Direct contact with a patient somehow increases his sense of being
> a worthwhile individual person, and this experience inspirits him – it does something to the body which helps it to throw off illness.
>
> (Jourard, 1971)

THE SPIRIT OF THERAPEUTIC RELATION

The therapeutic relationship begins in the discovery of the need that we have for each other. It is in the knowledge that each person – patient and nurse – matters; in an ability to invest someone with hope and to evoke a healing faith from within the person; in the commitment of the nurse to become fully engaged in a process of responding with responsibility; and in an understanding that it is the quality and integrity of the personal encounter that is of the utmost significance to the realisation of therapeutic intent. It requests involvement with a person, family or community in an evolving, unfolding movement that aims for personal growth and *becoming*.

Nurses must stake nothing less than their wholeness, their realness into the relationship. They must enter with fullness of attitude, knowledge and skill. Their central responsibility is to understand the person and to communicate understanding. The nurse is a vital link in human healing, and in the healing power generated within the compassionate experiencing of relationship.

The focus of the relationship is upon actualisation of dignity and autonomy, and the realisation of the potentials and possibilities of the patient. It requires the moral integrity, wisdom, responsibility, conscientious action and complex competencies of the nurse. It centres upon the whole person – mind-body-spirit. It is a relationship of invitation, an unconditional acceptance and confirmation of the person.

The therapeutic relationship has begun in the nursing encounter, person-with-person. It is witnessed in a nursing moment, when a son leaves his mother, who has been admitted to the psycho-geriatric ward, and glances over his shoulder. He is too broken and sore to take a fuller look. He begs you through his pain, 'Please nurse, please do everything that you can for her, for me – she's my mother.' You do not speak. Words do not carry a big enough message, and relieve no pain. You reach out and grasp his hand in your free hand, still holding his mother's hand. In silence you have told him that you have heard his cry for understanding, that you do understand his pain, his experience of guilt, even though it is essential for him to leave his mother with you. You have told him that you will do everything that you can do for his mother, and for him. The essential spirit of nursing is evident – the genesis of possibility and the movement to hope is unfolding; it can and will be realised.

OPENING THE HEART AND THE MIND

Every person's foremost task in life is to find the meaning in life and to actualise unique possibilities and potential. Nurses who have found such personal meaning communicate it in their nursing life. They are centred as a person and as a nurse, and are whole. Their personal and professional life are one, connected and interconnected. They are central to the realisation of therapeutic relationship, and fundamental to the humane realisation of the possibility and potential of the patient.

As nurses they have found a personal nursing faith – a reasoned rational faith – born out of intuitiveness, nursing knowledge and experience, and a critical analysis of these. This gives them confidence in their thoughts and feelings. Their caring action is moral action and they accept responsibility for it. In their journey to understanding they have reflected upon community life, and upon the wisdom that life has communicated to them. They have interpreted the messages and translated them into personal understanding. They have shared their story and their experience with others. They understand and are understood. They believe in themselves and in the other person. They have continually reached out to the other, and were there when needed. They are inspirited and hopeful. They have become a certain kind of person – a nurse confident to use self therapeutically.

According to Barbara Carper:

> ... the nurse in the therapeutic use of self rejects approaching the patient client as an object and strives instead to actualise an authentic personal relationship between two persons. The individual is considered as an integrated, open system incorporating movement towards growth and fulfilment of human potential. An authentic personal relationship requires the acceptance of others in their freedom to create themselves and the recognition that each person is not a fixed entity, but constantly engaged in the process of becoming.
>
> (Carper, 1978, p. 9)

Martin Buber (1953) describes an authentic personal relationship between two people, which is in essence a creation of freedom for personal growth, which upholds the dignity of the human being through unconditional positive regard and confirmation of personhood, as an 'I-Thou' relation. Buber distinguishes between man's two primary approaches to existence through 'I-Thou' and 'I-It' relationship. The difference in essence between these relationships is not, as is often thought, inherent in the nature of the object to which one relates; it is in the relationship itself. Friedman (1972) explains:

> I-Thou is a relationship of openness, directness, mutuality and presence … I-It, in contrast, is the typical subject–object relationship in which one knows and uses other persons or things without allowing them to exist for oneself in their uniqueness … I-Thou and I-It stand in fruitful and necessary alternation with each other. Man cannot will to preserve in the I-Thou relationship. He can only desire again and again to bring the indirectness of the world of It into the directness of the meeting with the Thou and thereby give the world of It meaning. So long as this alternation continues, man's existence is authentic. When the It swells up and blocks the return to the Thou, then man's existence becomes unhealthy, his personal and social life inauthentic.
>
> (Friedman, 1972, pp. xiv–xv)

Dialogue in therapeutic relation requires the nurse's willingness to respond with their 'whole being' to the unique experience, never 'apart from' but, rather, through engaged mutual contact, trust and faith. Carl Rogers (1990) spent his entire professional life in 'dialogue' – devoted to enhancing human communication through striving for and promoting the characteristics of helping relationships. He believed that the presence of certain attitudes in the therapist, when communicated to and perceived by the person, affect successful therapeutic relation. Rogers believed in the worth and dignity of the individual and of the therapist's capacity to provide a relationship of safety and freedom in accord with his respect for the person. He proposed three conditions central to therapeutic movement:

1 The therapist's congruence or genuineness
2 Unconditional positive regard, complete acceptance
3 A sensitively accurate empathetic understanding.

In conversation with Martin Buber on what he perceived to be the essential and effective moments in a therapeutic relationship, Rogers (1990) stated:

> … I feel, too, that when I am most effective, then somehow I am relatively whole in that relationship, or the word that has meaning to me is transparent. To be sure there may be many aspects of my life that aren't brought into the relationship, but what is brought into the relationship is transparent. There is nothing hidden. Then I think, too, that in such a relationship I feel a real willingness for this other person to be what he is. I call that acceptance. I don't know that that's a very good word for it, but my meaning there is that I'm willing for him to possess the feelings he possesses, to hold the attitudes he holds, to be the person he is. And then another aspect of it which is important to me is that I think in those moments I am able to sense with a good deal of clarity the way his experience seems to him, really viewing it from within him, and yet without losing my own personhood or separateness in that. Then, if in addition to those things on my part, my client or the person with whom I'm working is able to sense something of those attitudes in me, then it seems to me that there is a real, experiential meeting of persons, in which each of us is changed. I think sometimes the client is changed more than I am, but I think both of us are changed in that kind of an experience.
>
> (Rogers, 1990, p. 48)

Study Activity 29.4

- Comment on the relative importance of each of the three conditions Carl Rogers deemed central to therapeutic movement. Begin by reflecting upon and recording what each – genuineness, unconditional positive regard, and empathy – means to you.

- Consider some person (a patient or someone in your personal life) whom you found to be unpleasant or difficult, and whom you found difficulty in relating with. Reflect upon the challenge of how you would fulfill these three conditions in your relationship with such a person. Record your thoughts in this regard.
- Consult Felicity Stockwell's influential and important nursing study *The Unpopular Patient* (1971). Consider the study's main findings and relate them to your earlier reflections.

The wish to help others, and to do so with informed, compassionate, skilled care, is at the heart of the relationship of nursing, a relationship of such deep intimacy and trust that the person feels secure to expose *real* self – needs, fears, brokenness and suffering, joy and happiness. It is a relationship of suffering and hope, of anxiety and joy, but essentially of deep personal connection and experience of patient, family and community with nurse, with *nursing*. In the opinion of Tillich (1964), 'men usually live in the common experiences of daily life, covering over with talk and action their real inner personal experience'. Many patients who have spoken of their experience in hospitals have spoken of their need to 'cover over' their real personal experience. Indeed, one person's experience of a psychiatric hospital led her to say that for her 'the trick was to keep breathing' (Galloway, 1991).

Through the words of Phaedrus, Robert Pirsig (1993) testifies as follows:

> *When you're in agreement with the sane they're a great comfort and protection, but when you disagree with them it's another matter. Then they're dangerous. Then they'll do anything. The sinister thing that struck the most fear in him was what they'd do in the name of kindness. ... He saw that the sane always know they are good because their culture tells them so. Anyone who tells them otherwise is sick, paranoid and needs further treatment. To avoid that accusation*

> *Phaedrus had had to be very careful of what he said when he was in the hospital. He told the sane what they wanted to hear and kept his real thoughts to himself.*
>
> (Pirsig, 1993, pp. 372–3)

Nursing must unfold in such a way that people do not feel the need to 'cover over'. Rather, they need to experience a relationship and a therapeutic space in which experiencing is shared, confirmed and understood. Pirsig (1993) asserts that 'the most moral activity of all is the creation of space for life to move forward'. Such space, within which patients are empowered to decide about their own life, is central to their finding meaning in the experience of life. This is particularly significant for those patients who feel vulnerable, and for whom the meaning of their life, indeed often their very existence and survival, is in question. It is essential for the nurse to experience each person as a unique person, a particular person in a particular time with particular experiences which must be listened to, heard and responded to. The experiences that people have, and the meaning that they have given to their experience, are sacred and precious to them. It is their particular experience that must be understood. Nurses must create and sustain a therapeutic environment in which they can tell their story, and, in order to be of any help to them, must hear it, feel it and understand it.

Helping is a powerful process. Unskilled and unprincipled helpers can do a great deal of harm. (Carkhuff and Anthony, 1979; Egan, 1986). Helping is never neutral action and must never be taken for granted. It is a moral act connecting rational thought and feeling with reflective consciousness, principle and compassionate care. Genuine responsibility exists only where there is real responding and genuine dialogue where 'each of the participants really has in mind the other or others in their present and particular being and turns to them with the intention of establishing a living mutual relation' (Buber, 1953). The patient must be engaged and participate knowingly in the collaborative helping process, feel into the unfolding possibility and become empowered without the burden of judgement or of having to be any way other than their own way.

The heartbeat of therapy is a process of learning and becoming a person, together with others. It is learning that never ends:

> What I say and do in therapy is aimed at promoting understanding: a 'conversation', a meeting between two experiencing subjects (I and Thou) here and now, in such a way that the learning can be effective in other relationships ... the important therapeutic factor is not so much what is said but rather how it is said. In an unrepeatable moment, I hope to respond to my unique client by sharing in an ongoing act of creation, expressing and shaping immediate experience in the making and remaking of a verbal and non-verbal language of feeling. It is not only a matter of 'knowing about' someone but also, and mainly, of sharing a language of 'knowing'. Personal knowing has a 'logic' but it is not discursive, not set out in straight lines; it is an artistic all-at-once presentation of 'forms of feeling'.
>
> (Hobson, 1989, p. xiii)

Hildegard Peplau (1987), reflecting on what the future holds for psychiatric nurses, drew on a profound experience of nursing:

> Knowledge coupled with skill is required in order to foster favourable changes in patients. This means that an observing nurse will be aware of concepts that may explain the difficulties which patients show during a nurse–patient interaction. It is knowledge of the nature of presenting phenomenon – what it is, how it works, what purposes and functions it serves for the patient – which determines the particular skill to be used. Such knowledge of clinical phenomena, by a nurse, is to understand what has been noticed and use that understanding to choose the psychiatric nursing skill that would be most appropriate. This is skill application that requires considerable intellectual competence.
>
> (Peplau, 1987, p. 24)

Peplau brings attention to the importance and significance of knowledge and skill. A knowledge of the social and behavioural sciences is necessary to inform understanding, both of the human mind and of the ways in which people influence and relate to each other. Similarly, we need knowledge of the biological and medical sciences, so that we can interpret and respond to any pain and physical discomfort experienced by the patient. We also require skill, or the capacity to respond with confidence and competence. This is essential to the interpersonal skills of relation – the perceptual skills of observing and listening with attention, the skills of questioning and responding, and the skills of interpreting and responding to important non-verbal modes of communication.

This knowledge and skill can be diminished and made ineffective, perhaps even resulting in a negative effect, if they are not integrated within harmonious ethical caring practice. Peplau (1987) speaks in effect of an opening of mind. In responding with care we are concerned also with an opening of the heart. Knowledge and skill can be applied within mechanistic and impersonal restrictions behind the façade of a clinical role, or presented within connected person-with-person relationship. The alternative is nursing's *only* way, which is to engage with wholeness in inspiriting and enduring relation, and to create a relation that can move the mountains of human despair.

DEEPENING HUMAN-WITH-HUMAN RELATION

The therapeutic relationship begins with being a person in deep human and intimate connection with another. Within human-with-human relation, the patient, family or community experiences a sense of unity, completeness and dignity. The elements of such a therapeutic nursing relationship include:

- *authenticity of being* – realising potentials, renewing being
- *conscience* – consciousness of, engagement in moral activity, awareness of creation
- *commitment* – advocate with the other, 'with' when the other has no choice but to be there
- *presence* – being with, confirmation of the other person, constancy and immediacy of relationship
- *compassion* – the interdependence, feeling for and with, and concern of care
- *empathy* – involvement with, acceptance of, understanding of the way of the other person
- *empowerment* – liberation, freedom to realise potential, mutual understanding and confirmation.

These elements are inextricably interwoven. They are connected in the human act of caring at the heart of therapeutic relationship. They resonate with those referred to by Mayeroff (1990). They are proposed as the cornerstone of the nurse-patient relationship (Kirby and Slevin, 1992).

Authenticity of being

Authenticity of being begins in the knowledge that one's life is one's own life, that it cannot be lived by another person. We are the 'uncontested author', ultimately responsible for our life and for the living of it with freedom and responsibility, and constantly becoming self. It is the 'I' of the nurse in tune with self and with others, not hiding behind a mask, role, code or ritual. It means relating to others with the whole of oneself, the nurse with the patient – giving and receiving – in the alive nursing moment. The nurse in touch with self, relating to self, a 'source' for self, can become a 'source' for the patient – therapeutically-using-self. Connecting with self in this way enables one to be *for* another, but never in an over-involved way. They are their source of authentic being.

Conscience

Conscience is the call *of* and *to* care. It is primary to being and a source of being. It is a reaction of self-for-self, self thinking and judging moral issues and taking informed compassionate decisions. Conscience is not something that exists outside of us. Rather, it is with us in everyday down-to-earth actions; it *is* us. It is our sincerity, authenticity and it is obvious when we are who we say we are, and live as we say we do, as nurses caring – therapeutically relating.

The word 'con-science' refers to inner knowing, and extends beyond this to a knowing of who we are and what we stand for. It is the moral ground that we share, which holds us to doing what we know to be the right thing to do. It involves accepting responsibility for self and others.

To the Freudian psychoanalyst the conscience is the superego, the morals and standards of a culture that has become internalised through socialisation, and holds one to account. To the Jungian therapist the conscience is deeply embedded in the human spirit, and, rather than being consequential to the internalisation of external standards, it is a fundamental part of being human, and a constant call. J.E. Roberts (1990) believes that a caring consciousness should be inherent in the way that nurses practise nursing, and in doing what they do. In acting in this way, they provide care by virtue of a caring conscience. Sister M. Simone Roach, speaking of the human act of caring, believes conscience to be integral to personhood; a state of moral awareness and compass directing behaviour according to the fitness of things; a responding to something that matters, to a value as important in itself (1992, and personal correspondence 2001).

When a person exercises conscience they are not involved in some abstract cognitive endeavour. Rather, they are looking to their inner self and seeking direction from inner conviction. They are deepening human-with-human contact. Conscience, the invitation to responsible action, is at the core of the caring-healing dynamic of the nursing relationship.

Commitment

Commitment is the dynamic of caring conscience; it is the decision to act in accord with conscience. It is neither a mindless conception of duty nor obedience to another power or other minds. Commitment requires 'the willingness to enter with the patient that predicament which he cannot face alone as an expression of moral responsibility; the quality of the moral commitment is a measure of the nurse's excellence' (Levine, 1977). It is in essence advocacy with another – 'with', when the other often has no choice but to be there. Commitment as a specific act of caring has been spoken of by Roach (1992) as

> *... a complex affective response characterised by a convergence between one's desires and one's obligations, and by a deliberate choice to act in accordance, with them ... Commitment is a quality of investment of self in a task, a person, a choice of career, a quality which becomes so internalised as a value that what I am obligated to do is not regarded as a burden. Rather it is a call which draws me to a conscious, willing and positive course of action.*

The committed are united in conviction. They do not kill time, but live it in full accord.

Presence

The nurse being present to and in contact with the other person is at the heart of therapeutic nursing relation. Something of immense importance, it is both simple and complex. It is through contact with the real presence of the nurse that the patient can achieve what is for all a most important need – to be understood and to feel understood.

Not being present does not mean being absent. There can be an absence-of-presence in a relationship, when two people are together and interacting, and there is a presence, but not one that understands or attempts to understand. This can results in a sense of emptiness and, depending upon the person's vulnerability, a feeling of hurt.

There is joy in being a real presence with the patient. A real presence is an immediacy,

openness, awareness, freedom of expression, spontaneity and aliveness. The person who is present adds something just by being there, gives of themselves, welcomes your presence and is real to you. You feel real in their company, know that there is no 'proper' way but many ways, and that your way is as important as their way. You know that it is OK to be yourself. You feel understood. They have cared more about you in the moment of relating than about themselves. In so doing, they have told you without words how much you matter. Importantly, to be present as a nurse is not just to be there with fullness of feeling, but also with reason, knowledge and skill. Nursing presence is one person connecting with another in the therapeutic moment.

Compassion

Compassion is central to therapeutic relation. It is 'a way of living born out of an awareness of one's relationship to all living creatures; engendering a response of participation in the experience of another; a sensitivity to the pain and brokenness of the other, a quality of presence which allows one to share with and make room for the other' (Roach, 1992). Compassion speaks to the heart of the therapeutic encounter, and to the openness to love and life, in all of its joys, diversity and suffering. In essence, compassion involves not only concern and deep feeling for the suffering of another, but going to the other, not only to share in their suffering but also to ease their burden through sharing and skilled intervention.

Empathy

Empathy is an involved way of being, thinking and feeling, which enables one to see to the heart of the other. It is an engagement through which the patient is understood and feels understood. Empathy is understanding gained with the patient from their perspective, leading to an understanding of *their* way. Such understanding can only happen when we listen with understanding and when we care. Solomon (1991) explains:

If I want to know what you're thinking right now, all I have to do is care more about what you're thinking than what I'm thinking ... As soon as I care more what you're thinking than what I'm thinking I will give up my thoughts and I will absorb yours, and I will understand you.

Empathy involves going from oneself, from one's own thoughts and feelings and thinking and feeling, into the inner life of another in order to understand them more fully. It is an attempt to stand 'inside skin', to 'touch' the feelings of the other. It is intuitive in that it is dependent upon one's capacity to feel emotion or a situation and to convey that understanding to the other person. In empathic understanding we 'walk with the patient', creating space to generate healing. This is not simply a cognitive understanding; it is an understanding of wholeness and a capacity to feel for the pain of the other. In this context, Heidegger (1971) reflected:

How could cheerfulness steam through us if we wanted to shun sadness? Pain gives of its healing power where we least expect it.

Empowerment

Empowerment is care realised. It is the liberation of people so that they have the freedom to realise their potential with dignity in a personally responsible way. Through engagement in nursing dialogue each person gains awareness of self and of each other. In talking with the patient in a spontaneous way, things spoken of can be reflected upon rationally, verifying together what was meant, felt and experienced. In so doing, a deeper understanding can be attained. The patient is realising possibility, *becoming*. Liberation is expressed through self-care:

The concept of self care implies that the individual explore his possibilities, choose his actions, create his values. The individual is continually in-process: making himself,

seeking his own being. The provision of ready-made answers or absolutes only impoverishes Man, detracts from his authenticity. The recognition that Man is always in-process, always becoming, has implications for viewing the client who seems hopelessly fixed, immobilised in their situation. If the client is not categorised as an object but viewed as a being who resists definition, who is fluid and ever-reaching, his potential for achievement of wellbeing seems likely to be realised.

(Gulino, 1982, pp. 352–7)

The patient liberated to achieve their personal well-being and *more-being* is in enactment, which is an 'alive' process of empowerment.

Study Activity 29.5

- Consider the elements presented as the cornerstone of therapeutic nursing relation. Make personal records and brief summary statements to describe each element.
- Reflect upon your statements, then consider a personal relationship you have experienced (with a patient or with someone in your personal life) and establish whether each or any of the elements are present or absent.
- Use your personal record as a basis for discussion with nursing colleagues on the relevance of 'authenticity' of being and 'presence' to the therapeutic relationship.

CONCLUSION

The therapeutic relationship is a process of responding with responsibility, which begins with examining, understanding, affirming self and individual life; it requires commitment to the growth of personal possibilities and potentials, so that one can help others fulfill their life in an enriched, extended and personally chosen way. It is a responsibility commanding faith in oneself and in nursing life – a rational faith realised within informed, compassionate and skilled caring relation. It requires rational, critical reflection and an openness to renewal.

The nurse is a professional, a person in the world of nursing with specific purpose and conviction, present in living relation, and creating and sustaining nursing in such a way that it evokes healing, inspires hope, and helps people find meaning in their living and their dying. The therapeutic relationship is a fundamental mode of human relatedness, of self with other, with family or community. It is a relationship in which the duration of involvement is of less significance than the integrity and quality of the experiencing. It is a collaborative action with others, a relation of intense personal and professional being, a commitment to others, and a dignity of living and dying. It is in essence a manifestation of human love. In conclusion, it is worth considering Willard Gaylin's (1976) influential thought and wisdom on human caring:

> If we bend our nature too far, if we allow . . . technology, like the horns of the elk, to lead to an evolution too far from our basic needs and pursuits, we will be destroyed. We must, above all, respect the forces that bind us to others with love and concern, for that ensures the survival of a social matrix on whose existence we as a species depend for life. Caring and loving we are, and caring and loving we must be – caring and loving we will be as long as we so perceive ourselves. In other ways we are free to change, modify, adapt, and move. We are changing the rules of existence. We should change the rules of existence. We have a right to do so, and in certain cases, even a need to do so. Our nature will evolve in yet unanticipated ways, and that is as it should be. But to caring we should cling.
>
> (Gaylin, 1976, p. 180)

More than 30 years after Willard Gaylin's study, his anticipation of great technological advancement has been realised. Within modern health care services technological interventions have advanced beyond what may have been imaginable 30 years ago. To the patient surrounded by and attached to monitors, pumps and tubes, the potential alienation and depersonalisation of technology can be their reality. As the person listens to the beat and echo of technology resonate in silent space, the nursing voice speaks in the name of humanity. The human heart opens and responds in a caring-healing presence in a sacred space.

REFERENCES

Ackerman, S. and Hilsenroth, M. (2001) A review of therapist characteristics and techniques negatively impacting the therapeutic alliance. *Psychotherapy* **38**(2), 171–85

Buber, M. (1953) *I and Thou* (transl. Smith, R.G.), T & T Clark, Edinburgh

Burlingame, G.M. and Barlow, S.H. (1996) Outcome and process differences between professional and non-professional therapists in time-limited group psychotherapy. *International Journal of Group Psychotherapy* **46**(4), 455–78

Carkhuff, R.R. and Anthony, W.A. (1979) *The Skills of Helping: An introduction to counseling*, Human Resource Development Press, Amherst, Mass

Carper, B.A. (1978) Fundamental patterns of knowing in nursing, *Advanced Nursing Science*, **1**(1), 13–23

Diamond, J.A. (1997) The relationship between professional training, therapist skillfulness, and patient response to treatment. *Dissertation Abstracts International, Section B: The Sciences and Engineering*, **58** (4-B)

Egan, C. (1986) *The Skilled Helper: A systematic approach to effective helping*, Brooks/Cole, Pacific Grove, CA

Eysenck, H.J. (1994). The outcome problem in psychotherapy: what have we learned? *Behaviour Research and Therapy* **32**(5), 477–95

Friedman, M. (1972) In: Buber, M. (1972) *Between Man and Man* (transl. Smith, R.G.) Macmillan, New York

Gaylin, W. (1976) *Caring*, Alfred A. Knopf, New York

Galloway, I. (1991) *The Trick is to Keep Breathing*, Minerva, London

Gulino, C.K. (1982) Entering the mysterious dimension of the other: an existential approach to nursing care. *Nursing Outlook*, June 1982, 352–7

Hays, V.L. (1995) The effects of therapeutic alliance and social support on therapy outcome and mental health of women, *Dissertation Abstracts International, Section B: The Sciences and Engineering*, 55 (8-B)

Heidegger, M. (1971) *Poetry, Language, Thought* (transl. Hofstadter, A.), Harper and Row, New York

Hobson, R.E. (1989) *Forms of Feeling, the Heart of Psychotherapy*, Tavistock Routledge, London

Hollon, S. (1996) The efficacy and effectiveness of psychotherapy relative to medications. *American Psychologist* 51(10), 1025–30

Jourard, S.M. (1971) *The Transparent Self* (rev. edn), van Nostrand Reinhold, New York

Keenan, B (1992) *An Evil Cradling*, Hutchinson, London

Kieffer, K.M. (2001) The importance of therapeutic alliance precepts based on the theoretical orientation of licensed clinical and counseling psychologists. *Dissertation Abstracts International, Section B: The Sciences and Engineering*, 61 (7-B)

Kirby, C. and Slevin, O. (1992) A new curriculum for care. In: Slevin, O. and Buckenham, M. (1992) *Project 2000: The teachers speak*, Campion Press, Edinburgh

Levinas, E. (1991) *Otherwise Than Being, or Beyond Essence*, Kluwer Academic Publications, London

Levine, M. (1977) Nursing ethics and the ethical nurse. *American Journal of Nursing*, May 1977, 845–9

Linfors, O., Hannula, J., Aalberg, V. *et al.* (1995) Assessment of the effectiveness of psychotherapy. *Psychiatria Fennica* 26, 150–64

Logstrup, K.J. (1997) *The Ethical Demand*, University of Notre Dame Press, Paris

Mace, C. (1999) *Heart and Soul: The therapeutic face of philosophy*, Routledge, London

Martin, D.J., Garske, J.P. and Davis, M.K. (2000) Relation of the therapeutic alliance with outcome and other variables: a meta-analytic review. *Journal of Consulting and Clinical Psychology* 68(3), 438–50

Mayeroff, M. ([1971] 1990) *On Caring*, HarperColllins, New York

McMahon, R. and Pearson, A. (1998) *Nursing as Therapy*, Stanley Thornes, Cheltenham

Peplau, H. (1987) Tomorrow's world. *Nursing Times*, 7 June 1987

Pirsig, R.M. (1993) *Lila, an Inquiry into Morals*, Black Swan, London

Roach, Sister M. Simone (1992) *The Human Act of Caring*, Canadian Hospital Association, Ottawa

Roberts, J.E. (1990) Uncovering hidden caring. *Nursing Outlook* 38(2), 67–9

Rogers, C. (1958) The characteristics of a helping relationship. *Personnel and Guidance Journal* 37, 6–16

Rogers, C. (1967) *On Becoming A Person: A therapist's view of psychotherapy*, Constable, London

Rogers, C. (1990) *Dialogues*, Constable, London

Solomon, P. (1991) Paul Solomon speaks on spiritual roots and the journey to wholeness. *Human Potential Magazine* 16(3), 28–32

Stockwell, F. (1971) *The Unpopular Patient*, Royal College of Nursing, London

Surrey, J. (1991) The self in relation: a theory of women's development. In: Jordan, J.V., Kaplan, A., Miller, L. *et al.* (eds) *Women's Growth in Connection: Writings from the Stone Center*, Guildford Press, New York

Tan, S-Y. (1996) Process and outcome in psychotherapy: summary of consistent research findings for effective clinical practice. *Journal of Psychology and Christianity* 14(3), 263–8

Tillich, P. (1964) *Theology of Culture*, Oxford University Press, New York

VandenBos, G.R. (1996) Outcome assessment of psychotherapy. *American Psychologist* 51(10), 1005–6

Wheway, J. (1999) The dialogical heart of intersubjectivity. In: Mace, C. (ed.) *Heart and Soul: The therapeutic face of philosophy*, Routledge, London

30 THERAPEUTIC INTERVENTION IN NURSING

Oliver Slevin

> My interest in psychotherapy has brought about in me an interest in every kind of helping relationship. By this term I mean a relationship in which at least one of the parties has the intent of promoting the growth, development, maturity, improved functioning, improved coping with life of the other. The other, in this sense, may be one individual or a group.
>
> (Rogers, 1958)

LEARNING OUTCOMES

After studying this chapter you will be able to:

- Define the term 'therapy'
- Describe common means of classifying therapy
- Explain how psychological processes and relationships are engaged in that particular form known as psychotherapy
- Discuss appropriate therapeutic responses in the context of specialist, eclectic, and integrated interventions
- Explain the theoretical underpinnings and methods of common therapeutic approaches
- Identify empirical evidence for the efficacy of established therapeutic interventions
- Utilise such interventions appropriately in nursing practice situations.

INTRODUCTION

The Greek root of the word therapy is 'to take care of' or 'to tend to'. In the context of modern-day health care, this is interpreted as 'curing' or 'healing'. This latter word appears to get closer to the real meaning of therapy, as healing is a term which infers more extensive and holistic processes. It has connotations which go beyond a narrow notion of treatment or curing the body to a healing of the body *and* soul (or mind), aiming for a presence of well-being in the whole person.

In the broadest sense, therapy or healing extends across a wide range of interventions. An understanding of this range can be gained through a consideration of methods by which therapies are classified, and this is addressed below. It is important to note at this point that the range of meanings extends from the broadest (where therapy is simply a synonym for medical treatment of any type) to the narrowest (where therapy is intended to mean a specific approach). However, we can also recognise a continuum extending from a limited *treatment* perspective to a more holistic *healing* perspective, as intimated above. It is this latter sense of the term that is particularly relevant to nursing, and it is this that we attend to in this chapter. More specifically, we are addressing the healing (or making whole in a health context) that is achieved through the way we relate to those in our care. In this sense, we are concerned with that form of 'therapy' that is an integral part of what Rogers (1958) refers to as a helping relationship in the above opening quotation. The premise here is clear. It claims that the way in which we relate to our patients or clients is in itself capable of bringing about healing, or comfort, or improvement in the individual's condition or state of health and well-being.

IS THIS A MATTER FOR NURSES?

We hear these claims. Nurses are not therapists in their own right; their role is to support those who are qualified and licensed to provide therapy or treatment. Ordinary nurses should not be doing psychotherapy; this is a highly specialised area of treatment requiring trained personnel (who are usually not nurses). Ordinary nurses should not be dabbling in counselling; this is a specialist activity which should only be undertaken by trained counsellors. Nurses should not attempt to utilise behavioural techniques; these should only be undertaken by qualified behavioural therapists. Utilising art and drama as therapeutic interventions are the domain of the occupational therapist and no concern of the nurse. Family-centred therapeutic interventions belong to the realms of psychiatric medicine, clinical psychology and social work, and are not within the competence of nurses.

These latter statements are inaccurate and misleading. They are also highly dangerous to the profession of nursing and highly threatening to those who are nursed. They are dangerous and threatening on two counts. First, every person receiving care (and thus by definition needing help) has psychological and social as well as physical needs. The response to these needs is through helping relationships that are by definition – if they are successful – therapeutic; they are in fact *psycho-therapeutic* (or, in the case of social needs, socio-therapeutic). It would be quite wrong to suggest that nurses should not respond to the psychological and social needs of their patients, that they should not be psychotherapeutic in their interventions. This would relegate nursing to a concern only for providing physical care, and result in some of the most important needs of patients not being met. Second, there is a danger in not recognising the range of expertise possible in such helping relationships. Visualise for a moment, the nurse who sits quietly and holds the hand of a tearful and distressed patient. Who could deny the therapeutic, indeed the *psychotherapeutic*, value of this intervention? Yet it has all the appearance (although in this case, appearances may be deceiving) of being a simple thing. This does nevertheless illustrate that there are different *levels* of intervention.

There is in fact a continuum, at one end of which it is possible to provide psychological or emotional support without advanced levels of training and expertise in complex therapeutic techniques.

But what of the more advanced in-depth therapeutic interventions, involving deeply subjective relationships or complex psychological mechanisms? Common sense suggests that a nurse who does not have training and experience in such advanced practice techniques should not be indulging in them. Indeed, the American Psychiatric Nurses Association (2001) takes the view that in the mental health nursing field only advanced practitioners, specialist nurse practitioners or psychiatric nurse practitioners should undertake psychotherapy (these designated roles, which have broad equivalents in the UK and other European and Australasian countries, generally refer to roles beyond initial registration or licentiate level). But a lack of competence in such techniques is not the exclusive domain of nurses. Most doctors, occupational therapists and social workers also do not possess such competency. In nursing, as indeed for these other professional groups, there are limits to the helping interventions that can be used without further training. However, every nurse must have the capacity to respond appropriately to the psychological and social distress or needs of her patients. This is as true for the adult/general, learning disabilities or children's nurse as it is for the mental health nurse.

EMBRACING THE CONCEPT

In the course of the remainder of the chapter, words like counselling, psychotherapy, behaviour therapy, helping relationship, and therapeutic relationship will enter our debate. No apology is made for this. These terms, and involvement in the activities they signify, are an integral and essential aspect of the nurse's role. Nurses cannot abdicate their responsibility to provide psychological, social and even spiritual help and support to their patients through the vehicle of relationship and interpersonal interaction. Note carefully the words in this latter sentence: to provide psychological help and support ... through the vehicle of relationship and interpersonal interaction.

This is in fact quite a good definition of psychotherapy and fits in well with Rogers' (1958) statement in the opening quotation to this chapter. In essence, nurses must not only be concerned with physical care; they must also be psychotherapeutic in their interventions.

It is almost reflective of a mass phobia that in nursing we shy away from such jargon when other professional groups embrace it and in some cases lay claim to it as their own exclusive professional domain. It is, of course, right to be critical of jargon which is obscure and which is confusing to both our patients or clients and ourselves. However, this is no excuse for rejecting perfectly clear technical terminology that clarifies and defines rather than obscures. And it is indefensible if nurses not only shy away from the terminology, but also from the practices and interventions this terminology designates, to the disadvantage of their own patients or clients. In this regard, O'Toole and Welt (1994) have stated:

> The use of the term psychotherapy in nursing is a recent development. When Peplau first wrote about psychiatric nursing, she termed interventions with individual patients nurse–patient relationships. Later it was called one-to-one relationship, then counselling, and finally psychotherapy. Later definitions of the work emphasised the difference between specialists and generalists in the field; that is, specialists were able to conduct psychotherapy, generalists counselled and conducted nurse–patient relationships. Resistance of other mental health professionals, as well as other psychiatric nurses, to nurse psychotherapists contributed to the use of euphemisms for psychotherapy because other terms were less threatening and more acceptable.
>
> (O'Toole and Welt, 1994, pp. 360–1)

These comments are not a prelude to a crash course in psychotherapy and counselling. It would indeed not be possible in a single chapter to do more than scrape the surface of these broad areas. This is not a specialist book on psychotherapies, nor indeed is it a specialist book on mental health nursing. What is provided here is a presentation in respect of common and useful interventions which can be carried forward on the basis of the therapeutic relationship addressed in Chapter 29. The chapter should, therefore, be read in conjunction with the latter chapter, and should also be revisited when reading Chapter 39, which overviews mental health nursing. It should also be noted that in the next chapter, complementary therapies are considered. Such therapies extend across a range that includes the use of massage, reflexology, natural herbal remedies and other approaches. These are seen as different to, sometimes alternatives to, but more frequently complementary to, mainstream medical or health care approaches. You should recognise the links between these various orientations. In particular, three broad points are worth keeping in mind:

1 In both mainstream medicine *and* complementary therapies, a therapeutic relationship is an essential underpinning that facilitates and indeed enhances the efficacy of these other approaches. We shall justify this claim presently.
2 The need for nursing support extends from skilled physical care through effective interpersonal relationships (and the deliberate harnessing of these as therapeutic tools), to the use of a much wider range of 'complementary' interventions than is often envisaged as included in the nursing role.
3 In effect, the nurse draws on a wide repertoire of knowledge and skills in her/his work, and what determines nursing activity becomes the health care needs of the patient or client, rather than any limiting prescription of roles.

Study Activity 30.1 _____

Before we proceed to consider in greater detail the meanings attributed to the term 'therapy', reflect briefly on your own understanding of this term. Note down your ideas about the meaning or meanings you attribute to it. Keep your notes for further consideration in Study Activity 30.3.

CLASSIFICATIONS

Classification according to methods

In further exploring what we mean by 'therapy' and that particular orientation where the medium of helping is interpersonal relating, clarity can be aided by considering the matter of classifications. Here therapy can be subdivided into broad areas of intervention in accordance with the methods or types of intervention involved. In a comprehensive review of therapies in mental health, the National Health Service Executive (1996) in England simply referred to psychological methods (broadly speaking, psychotherapy) and physical methods (including the use of drugs or medicines). However, there may be five or more subdivisions in this classification (according to how they are subdivided).

Somatotherapy

This relates to physical interventions that aim at healing the physical body and/or the mind. In this broad sense of the term, surgery is somatotherapy; so too is the administration of medicines, sometimes referred to as chemotherapy (although this term is now commonly reserved for the drug treatment of cancer, where the drugs are predominantly cytotoxic drugs designed to kill cancer cells). To avoid the latter confusion, some suggest the use of the term pharmacotherapy (to specifically refer to the use of drugs or medications). Within the mental health field, the term psychopharmacology is also used, while others see drugs or medicines that treat the mind or mental functioning as psychotropic therapies. In psychiatry, somatotherapy refers to physical treatments that aim to treat mental illness and alleviate mental distress. This encompasses such methods as medicines (e.g. tranquillisers or antidepressant drugs – referred to above as 'psychotropic' medicines), electric shock treatment (electroconvulsive therapy) and psychosurgery (surgery which invades the brain structures to modify thinking, feelings and/or behaviour).

Psychotherapy

This relates to using psychological processes as therapy. It involves verbal or non-verbal interventions by a therapist that will influence healing, or improve or bring about well-being. The term psychotherapy has broad and narrow meanings.

In the broader sense, psychotherapy includes literally all non-physical treatments. This encompasses that type of therapy known as behaviour therapy (or the narrower approach of behaviour modification) which involves the use of learning theories as a treatment approach, and which tends to be objective, scientific and to depend little on relationships. The concern is modification of behaviour through learning. It also includes psychotherapeutic interventions that are based on therapeutic relationships, which are more subjective and humanistic and which are interpretive rather than scientific. The concern is understanding and coping with feelings, cognitions, and conflicts (conscious and unconscious) that emerge as anxiety or other mental 'symptoms'. The use of psychotherapy in this broader sense (i.e. encompassing both of these orientations) reflects an uneasy peace. In the past, orthodox behaviourists (e.g. Skinner, 1953) have rejected as being unscientific the interpretive approaches of humanistic therapists such as Victor Frankl (1969) and psychoanalytical therapists such as Sigmund Freud (1933). Conversely, some of these more humanistic therapists have rejected behaviourism as being simplistic and ineffective. They argue that humans are intelligent beings capable of cognitive and intentional processes that invalidate crude learning theory as an exclusive basis for treatment.

In the narrower sense, behaviour therapy is viewed as separate from psychotherapy, with the latter term being reserved for therapeutic interventions based on interpersonal relationships and interpersonal interaction. Some people attempt to clarify this distinction, by describing the latter as *verbal psychotherapy* or *talking therapies,* because of the use of interpersonal communication as the major therapeutic device. The Tavistock Clinic, a world-famous psychotherapy organisation, describes such approaches under the title *Talking Cure* (Taylor, 1999). Such therapies are, of course, not exclusively 'verbal'. They encompass verbal *interpersonal* or communication skills (such as listening, communicating verbally, responding, etc.) *and* non-verbal interpersonal or communication skills (such as observing cues from expression, gaze, tone of voice, touch, and non-language verbal cues such as sobbing, groaning, laughing, etc., as well as making use of these same modes of communication). But they also involve *intrapersonal* skills (such as insight, understanding, empathy, etc.), which are essential in interpreting what emerges and creatively harnessing these interpersonal processes to desired therapeutic outcomes.

Sociotherapy

Here the interventions are very similar to those of the behavioural and verbal psychotherapeutic approaches, in that they often employ learning theories and/or interpersonal relationships as the vehicles for bringing about healing or improvement. For this reason, the term sociotherapy is not so widely used and is often seen as a variant of psychotherapy, in the narrower sense of the term as described above (i.e. as one of the 'verbal' or 'talking' therapies). In essence, sociotherapeutic interventions are those that bring into play social or group influences as their major therapeutic device. There are three broad traditions here. One derives from social psychology and social learning theory and is variously described as *social milieu therapy* (the

word *milieu* meaning environment), or the *therapeutic community* approach (Jones, 1953, 1968). The basic idea is to bring the influence of the group into play. This is in an attempt to modify behaviour through such mechanisms as compliance with and internalisation of group norms and values, and modification of behaviour through the influence of social sanctions and social reinforcement. The second tradition derives from a bringing together of social role theory and psychodynamic principles and is described as *psychodrama* or *sociodrama* according to its ultimate goals (Moreno, 1952). The approach uses structured role-play techniques. These may be used to help resolve emotional conflict and problems by acting out situations in which fellow group members participate in acting the roles of significant others with whom the individual is in conflict. This is the emphasis in psychodrama. Alternatively, such role-play may be utilised as a vehicle for developing or learning social skills and competence, as in sociodrama. The third broad tradition also emphasises social learning. However, this is not exclusively limited to approaches that utilise social role theory as the medium for promoting learning or change. Other social learning approaches, such as training in communication and relational skills, may also be utilised. Some people prefer to describe social learning techniques such as this as *social skills training* (Trower *et al.*, 1978).

Complementary or alternative therapy

It may also be useful to recognise that complementary therapies (addressed in more detail in the next chapter) span a range of therapeutic interventions that are somatotherapeutic (such as reflexology, chiropractics and massage), pharmacotherapeutic (such as herbal remedies) and also involve psychotherapeutic influences (such as when used with aromatherapy or in relaxation therapy). In terms of *method*, the main differentiation would be that in these complementary approaches there tends to be a wider range of approaches. These extend well beyond what is narrowly encompassed in conventional medicine, and extent into the use of Eastern and New World philosophies and spiritual approaches to care.

Counselling

Even though we discuss counselling below (as a perspective), it may also merit inclusion in terms of method. In a sense, counselling goes a step further than complementary therapy in that it is largely non-medical in its orientation. Indeed, most counselling occurs outside of health care settings and some view the very term – counselling – as significant in that it identifies something that is different to 'therapy', which is viewed as a synonym for medical treatment. However, a real difficulty emerges here. In practice, methods included under psychotherapy and sociotherapy are very similar if not identical to those used in counselling (at least as it is understood by some). That is, methods of interpersonal communication and relationship building are used to help resolve difficulties in both cases. Thus, when reference is made to client-centred *psychotherapy*, the methods involved (which are discussed later), are virtually identical to those

employed in client-centred *counselling*. It may be argued that as the counselling perspective is not specifically concerned with treating problems of ill-health (as discussed below), and perhaps not even concerned with health in any context, the methods tend to be more generic and less technical than in psychotherapy. However, as counselling becomes more professional this differentiation is becoming less sustainable. Indeed, counselling is sometimes presented as extending across a range of activities. At one extreme is a particular understanding of counselling as 'guidance', as in highly structured roles involving information distribution and demanding little in terms of competencies beyond good communication skills. At the opposite extreme is a particular understanding of counselling as a form of therapy, demanding not only competence in communication and interpersonal skills, but the harnessing of these to complex helping relationships. As indicated in Fig. 30.1, this range extends from activity that might hardly justify the term counselling at all, to therapeutic activities that may go beyond the usual understandings of this term.

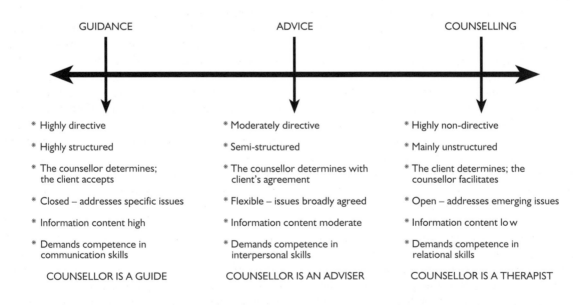

GUIDANCE	ADVICE	COUNSELLING
* Highly directive	* Moderately directive	* Highly non-directive
* Highly structured	* Semi-structured	* Mainly unstructured
* The counsellor determines; the client accepts	* The counsellor determines with client's agreement	* The client determines; the counsellor facilitates
* Closed – addresses specific issues	* Flexible – issues broadly agreed	* Open – addresses emerging issues
* Information content high	* Information content moderate	* Information content low
* Demands competence in communication skills	* Demands competence in interpersonal skills	* Demands competence in relational skills
COUNSELLOR IS A GUIDE	COUNSELLOR IS AN ADVISER	COUNSELLOR IS A THERAPIST

Figure 30.1 The range of counselling activities

Classification according to perspective

The classification of 'helping' interventions according to perspective calls into question the very term therapy itself. The helpers themselves and their particular professional or occupational value and belief systems largely determine the perspectives of such helping interventions. In some instances these do not always incorporate a notion of 'therapy', particularly where this word is taken as a synonym for treatment. In other instances, perspectives (and methods) overlap and at the boundaries 'turf wars' break out between the proponents. It is possible to identify at least three broad perspectives.

The medical perspective

Here the perspective is one that sees therapy as in essence synonymous with treatment. The result here is that only those therapies that fit into a medical model of disease, diagnosis, treatment and cure are recognised as therapy. Other types of intervention are seen as invalid and often their practitioners castigated as heretics (in the medical sense) or at best eccentric quacks. Into the broad fold of acceptable therapies comes not only the broad range of biological or physical medicine (including psychiatry), but also some psychotherapeutic techniques. By the mid-twentieth century, psychoanalysis had achieved medical respectability and acceptance. By the 1960s and 1970s, behaviour therapy was gaining acceptance. During the 1980s and 1990s, cognitive therapies gained membership of the club, and with the approach to the millennium and entry to the new twenty-first century, approaches that mixed approaches became more acceptable. Indeed, these more eclectic approaches – and that particular mixing of approaches that is known as cognitive-behavioural therapy – had become the most common form. A corollary of this acceptance is a territorial claim; the therapies which are accepted become medical treatments and can only be practised by doctors or the professions which supplement the practice of medicine or are allied to it (and thus supposedly under the ultimate control of doctors). These include clinical psychologists, nurses, physiotherapists, occupational therapists and sometimes social workers or teachers.

The medical adjunct perspective

Herein lies a range of therapies which either are not yet quite accepted by medicine or which are at the periphery of mainstream medical practice. They are often described as complementary, supplementary or alternative therapies, and (as suggested above) the term alternative medicine is sometimes used. In terms of method, these can range across the somatotherapeutic, psychotherapeutic and sociotherapeutic domains and range from those which are close to full acceptance as medical practice, such as acupuncture and homeopathic medicine, through reflexology, aromatherapy, therapeutic touch etc., to faith healing. Many of these have limited, although in some cases increasing, acceptance. However, they all tend to share a common perspective that is still a treatment – cure orientation. A number of these therapies are validated by a growing body of research evidence, and some will be considered in the next chapter.

The non-medical perspective

These approaches share a common outlook which is essentially non-medical in that they do not address disease and illness as such, but prefer to view the situation as one in which people are being assisted with personal problems of living. The medical model of disease, diagnosis, treatment and cure is not considered relevant, and indeed some of the proponents of these approaches are not merely non-medical but overtly anti-medicine in their outlook. They speak of coping and personal growth rather than treatment and cure, and those they help are clients not patients. The argument here is that labelling those who seek help as being ill is often both inaccurate and dysfunctional, more often than not requiring of 'patients' compliant behaviour and learned helplessness rather than the empowerment and autonomy needed to solve their own problems. It is also possible that for the patient or client, terms such as treatment and therapy may suggest mental imbalance and its associated stigma. Examples of such approaches include:

- the counselling movement, particularly that part of it influenced by the client-centred, person-centred or non-directive approach of Carl Rogers (1951, 1961, 1980, 1986)
- those adherents of the so-called anti-psychiatry movement (many of whom, such as Ronald Laing, were themselves qualified psychiatrists), who often employ existential approaches as an alternative to orthodox empirical psychiatry (*see*, e.g. Laing, 1960; Frankl, 1964, 1969)
- those also involved in the mental health field who view mental health problems as social skills deficits rather than illness and employ educational or social skills training approaches to what are seen as 'person' not 'illness' problems, particularly advanced in the UK by the psychologist Michael Argyle and his associates (Trower *et al.*, 1978).

MEANINGS

Range

It should become apparent that whichever classificatory system we utilise, the situation as it exists in reality tends to be more complex. This is clear when we realise that there is much inconsistency in what people mean when they use terms such as therapy, psychotherapy and counselling. Even a crude differentiation into those approaches that are medical and those that are non-medical does not suffice. At first glance, medical treatments such as surgery seem clearly to be exclusively somatotherapeutic. However, many forward-thinking and progressive surgeons recognise the value of complementary therapies such as relaxation or psychotherapies such as cognitive-behavioural approaches and incorporate these in their treatments. Similarly, many counsellors work with people who clearly suffer an illness or disability such as a phobia or autism.

How then does a consideration of the above two classificatory approaches help us in our understanding of therapy? First, it is clear that therapy can have a broad spectrum of meaning. If it is recognised as all forms of helping intervention that are related to the treatment of illnesses *and/or* helping people with problems or difficulties of daily living, therapy encompasses an almost infinite range of physical, psychological, social and even spiritual interventions. Second, if it extends beyond a concern with treatment and cure it is not necessarily confined to the practice of medicine, but raises the possibility that health, well-being and successful living can be attained by non-medical intervention. We are faced, in reality, with a range of activities, all of which to a greater or lesser extent span the medical or health care divide, as illustrated in Fig. 30.2.

What does seem to be clear is that therapy is in one sense of the word more than just treatment or curing. It has a more holistic and humanistic sense in which it is 'carative' and 'healing' in the mind/soul as well as body sense. This was most appropriately explicated by His Royal Highness, the Prince of Wales (1991) when in a keynote speech to the Royal College of Psychiatrists, he stated:

> *Caring for people who are ill, restoring them to health when it is possible, and comforting them always, even when it is not, are spiritual tasks. Training people for your profession and maintaining professional skills are not simply about understanding and administering the latest drugs but about therapy, in the original Greek sense of healing – physical, mental and spiritual. If you lose that foundation as a profession, I believe there is a danger you will ultimately lose your way.*
>
> (HRH The Prince of Wales, 1991)

For we nurses, who espouse a commitment to caring for patients and clients as people not cases, this is a valid and indeed highly important warning.

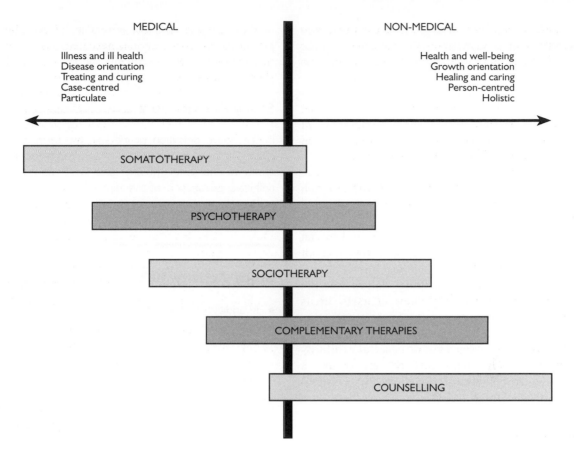

Figure 30.2 The therapeutic range

Definitions

It has been noted that for various reasons there is a reluctance to use the term therapy in regards to nursing. This is particularly the case when specific forms of therapy are contemplated. This has also been considered above, in regard to the reluctance to use the term *psychotherapy* in nursing and the various euphemisms which are used in its place. It is interesting to note this reluctance of nursing to embrace the therapeutic nomenclature, when, for example, in one highly influential publication Podvoll (1990), an American psychiatrist and therapist, described psychotherapy as 'nursing of the mind'. The pioneering psychiatric nurse Hildegard Peplau (1952) emphasised

the therapeutic dimension in her definition of nursing when she stated that:

> *Nursing is a significant, therapeutic, interpersonal process. It functions co-operatively with other human processes that make health possible for individuals in communities. Nursing is an educative instrument, a maturing force, that aims to promote forward movement of personality in the direction of creative, constructive, productive, personal and communal living.*
>
> (Peplau, 1952, p. 16)

However, Peplau's definition raises its own tautological problems. If nursing is a therapeutic interpersonal process, are all therapeutic interpersonal processes nursing? This is clearly not what Peplau is saying; nursing is *a* therapeutic process, and there are of course others. But this does beg a question as to how therapy can be defined. Taking into account the comments above, particularly those of Rogers (1958) in the opening quotation to this chapter, and those of the Prince of Wales and Peplau above, we can propose the following definitions.

- *Therapy* – the process of helping within which the clear intention is to promote the health and well-being of the whole person in his/her physical, psychological, spiritual and social contexts. This helping may take the form of physical, psychological or social interventions, or consist of the helping nature of the relationship between persons in itself. In its truest sense it incorporates curative and carative elements in a striving towards holistic healing, personal growth or peaceful death. By virtue of its helping nature, therapy involves a helper (the therapist), a client (a person in need), and the process (interaction) that takes place between them. It is thus a helping relation.
- *Nursing therapy* – involves all instances of therapy, as it is defined above, in which the helper is a nurse. As so defined, all nursing intervention is therapy and the nurse–patient (or nurse–client) relationship is by definition a therapeutic relationship.

The main concern in this chapter is those therapies wherein the intervention is in fact the therapist–client (or nurse–patient) interaction itself, i.e. the communications that occur within the therapeutic relationship. In the context of the definitions of therapy and nursing therapy presented above, the main (and sometimes exclusive) helping intervention is in fact 'relating'. Caroline Garland, a therapist at the Tavistock Clinic in London, describes it thus: 'It's the most intimate relationship you will ever have with another human being. You know your patients better than anybody else in their lives' (Garland, 1999; see also Taylor, 1999). It thus ties in closely and builds upon the discussion presented in the previous chapter. It is also, if the therapeutic function is accepted as an integral part of the nurse's role, specifically about nursing as psychotherapy and counselling.

Study Activity 30.2

In the above definition of therapy, the term 'holistic healing' is used. Carry out a library search for references to the term 'holism' and write up a clear, definitive explanation of this term. Relate your explanation to the notions of totality and simultaneity paradigms in nursing, as discussed in Chapter 9.

Study Activity 30.3

- In addition to the above definitions of therapy and nursing therapy, various other statements have been made about the nature of therapy. In addition to the library search in the previous Study Activity, seek out and note down six other definitions of the term 'therapy'. Compare these with the above definitions and also with your own initial views, as noted under Study Activity 30.1. Reflect on all of these, and attempt to improve on the above definition of therapy, drawing from your accumulated knowledge in undertaking these activities.

THERAPEUTIC ORIENTATIONS

Modes

The mode of responding to the patient's or client's need for help is an issue which requires attention. The response should be determined by the patient and the nature of their need for help. However, in many instances the mode of responding is determined by other factors. For example, in the UK National Health Service, the highly expensive psychoanalytical forms of intervention are seldom available to the poorer sections of society and can only be accessed through private practice by the very wealthy (*see*, for example, Pilgrim, 1990).

An important influence on the mode of responding is that of the professional attitudes and skills of the 'helpers' or therapists themselves. Thompson and Kahn (1988) describe this situation well in their account of inward-looking and outward-looking professions.

Inward-looking professions

The perspective here is that of a special and narrow approach to therapy. These therapists have developed a high degree of expertise in a particular approach and they only treat patients for whom that approach is suitable. For example, a psychoanalyst will usually agree to treat clients with particular forms of neuroses, but will refer a client with a phobia to a behavioural therapist. There are, of course, those inward-looking professionals who are so committed to their particular perspective that they do attempt to treat everyone via their particular therapeutic approach, irrespective of its suitability in some cases. However, this is not just inward-looking therapeutic practice, it is bad and unethical practice!

Outward-looking professions

Here it is not any particular therapeutic method which determines the therapeutic intervention, but the needs of the patient or client. The 'therapist' selects an appropriate intervention from within his/her existing repertoire and has an orientation towards looking outwards for alternative therapeutic strategies to include in this repertoire. While such therapists may develop competence in different therapeutic modalities, they tend to be *generalists* while inward-looking professionals are by definition *specialists*. The more generalised approach tends to take one of two forms: eclectic or integrated therapy.

Eclecticism and integration

By the latter third of the twentieth century there were in effect a number of divides in British psychotherapy and there existed a preoccupation with professional boundaries and rivalries, rather than with the issues of providing high-quality therapy. A resolution to this conflict was found in the notion of eclecticism. Today most therapists would – while they may have a particular orientation – advocate an eclectic approach, and indeed the majority of therapy is now of an eclectic nature.

The idea of eclectic therapy is more complex than it may seem. Such a bringing together or integration can occur at various levels and involve different degrees of integration (Garfield, 1995; Lazarus, 1996):

- *Eclectic diversity* – simply implies openness to the use of different methods as indicated by particular contexts. Here there is no attempt to integrate or combine methods in any way, but simply recognition that for different patients or clients, in different contexts, with different problems, different methods may be advocated.

- *Eclectic integration* – assumes that across all the theoretical underpinnings of the various therapies there may be common sound principles that can be integrated into one overriding 'meta-theory' with its associated integrated method of therapy. However, the orientations of different therapies often include very divergent and indeed opposing worldviews that make such eclecticism an unlikely achievement (Weinberger, 1995). For example, behavioural therapies adopt a view of the individual as a predictable being whose behaviour can be modified and shaped, and the therapist is a skilled behavioural technician. Conversely, client-centred/non-directional therapies adopt a view of the individual as a complex person capable of making personal choices, and the therapist is a sympathetic companion and facilitator. It is difficult to contemplate how common principles might emerge from such diverse positions to form a new encompassing theoretical and therapeutic perspective.

- *Technical eclecticism* – an endeavour to combine *methods* in therapy. The term technical is used to indicate that there is no attempt to achieve theoretical integration; indeed, theory is largely ignored. The concern is primarily with the efficacy or effectiveness of techniques or methods. That is, for a particular individual, assessment may indicate the value of different techniques and these are brought together in a mixed approach to therapeutic intervention. When therapists refer to eclectic therapy, it is usually a reference to this approach.

The idea of technical eclecticism has a longer tradition in the USA, and was advocated as far back as the 1970s and beyond by therapists such as Grinker (1970) and Thorne (1973). As such, eclectic therapy involves selecting what is useful for a particular client from all available methods. It is thus to all intents and purposes the approach adopted by outward-looking professionals. It has been suggested, particularly by the inward-looking professionals, that eclectic therapy is a hodgepodge of approaches adopted by amateurs who cannot possibly have clinical competence across an almost infinite range of highly complex activities. There is some merit in such criticism; there is in fact no specific therapeutic modality that is *eclectic therapy*, as it involves (in the case of technical eclecticism) selecting therapeutic methods from a menu of therapies to suit the individual case. Indeed, eclecticism is an orientation rather than a specific type of therapy. It is also true that the capacity to be highly competent across the full range of therapies, which literally extends into hundreds of different approaches, would be humanly impossible. Nevertheless, in recent years most therapists adopt some degree of eclecticism in their work (Norcross and Goldfried, 1992; Stricker and Gold, 1996; Woolfe and Palmer, 1999).

The nursing dilemmas

The dilemma of expertise

The above comments beg major questions in regard to how nurses as therapists can respond to their patients' or clients' need for help. The answer to such questions may be found in a fairly common sense approach. This would involve ordinary professional practitioners meeting the day-to-day needs of patients by utilising a range of therapeutic interventions at a level which is commensurate with their degree of skill or competence. Other practitioners may adopt specialist nurse therapist roles involving the provision of specific therapies at more advanced levels. The position thus advocated is as follows: all nurses should have an eclectic repertoire of therapeutic-relational skills that allows them to respond to the psychosocial needs of their patients.

Some patients (particularly in the mental health field) develop more serious psychosocial difficulties and perhaps even full-blown mental illnesses and in these situations more *specialised* therapeutic intervention becomes necessary. In this instance it is essential that trained psychotherapists undertake or supervise the interventions, and such therapists would include nurses with specialist training.

One useful source of guidance is a report on the provision of psychological treatments in the English National Health Service (National Health Service Executive, 1996). While this relates specifically to mental health services, it is useful in that it provides a straightforward framework for modes of therapy provision within the National Health Service:

- *Type A: psychological treatment as an integral component of mental health care* – this relates to therapeutic interventions as an integral part of an overall programme of care. Thus, while a patient or client may be receiving medication and perhaps other forms of physical therapy, a carer (e.g. nurse, doctor, social worker, or occupational therapist) may also provide psychological therapy, such as supportive, behavioural or cognitive therapy (see below for outlines). Indeed, in the course of care, a number of such interventions may occur at different times or even concurrently. It is assumed that such professionals will be able to utilise such skills within the context of the general management of the patient and as part of their general repertoire of helping skills.
- *Type B: eclectic psychological therapy and counselling* – a complete and discrete

treatment intervention, usually provided over a number of sessions by someone who is appropriately prepared to provide such therapy. However, such therapy is typically eclectic and may draw from different theoretical perspectives and use techniques drawn from different therapeutic modalities.

- *Type C: formal psychotherapies* – a discrete therapy within a particular therapeutic modality is provided by a qualified therapist. This includes the various specialist therapies, such as psychoanalysis and cognitive-behavioural therapy, and the therapist typically is employed or commissioned to work only within this therapeutic modality, for which he or she has specialised training.

Clearly, in respect of nursing, only mental health nurses who have undertaken advanced specialist training would be involved in type B and C therapies. However, in respect of type A therapies, all mental health nurses would be required to have the capacity to respond to patients' or clients' needs through such therapeutic intervention. Indeed, as patients or clients in other areas of care (including adult, children's and learning disabilities care) would similarly have social and psychological needs, such capacity is important in all branches of nursing. In line with such an approach, the non-specialist professional practitioner is (in responding as in type A above) also adopting what is essentially an eclectic position.

The dilemma of choice

Until the twentieth century, religion was the source of our succour and our salvation. By the twentieth century, medicine (and science) had become the new religion: science would construct a new and better world and medicine would cure our diseases, extend our lives and construct a happy and distress-free existence. But as we entered the new millennium, the failures of the new religion became apparent. Science indeed constructed a better world, but one fraught with risks and environmental threats. Medicine did not produce a disease-free

and distress-free utopia, and indeed constructed new medicine-made or *iatrogenic* disorders to complement those already available to us. In this world of disappointment, alienation and disempowerment constructed by the very tools of modernity that we hoped would save us, a new religion emerges – that of therapy. Now, rather than turning to the priest or the traditional physician (including the psychiatrist), we increasingly turn to the healer, the counsellor, the therapist.

The range of therapies mushrooms at an exponential rate, with a new modality that promises effective outcomes emerging almost daily. And the complexity of choice increases. We have counselling psychologists and psychological counsellors, psychoanalysis of multifarious colourings, and a whole range of cognitive, cognitive-behavioural, and cognitive-emotive therapies. With the notion of eclecticism we discussed earlier, all sorts of combinations become possible. And, even if we pin one 'method' down, it is almost impossible to find two therapists who totally agree on its theoretical underpinning and practice methods. Over 20 years ago an old standard (*The Psychotherapy Handbook*) listed over 250 different forms of psychotherapy, after excluding many that were less well known or duplicative of other entries (Herink, 1980). Since then further forms have appeared with increasing regularity. More recently, the Department of Health in England (Department of Health, 2001) identified 14 forms of psychotherapy commonly practised in the English National Health Service, including forms they termed eclectic and integrated (referred to earlier) which may incorporate a variety of approaches. They also recognised the wide usage of counselling and an additional 16 examples of psychotherapies that were practised in the National Health Service, although not as commonly as the other forms. Indeed, Mellor-Clarke (2000) reported that between 1990 and 1998 there was an increase from 31 to 51% of general practitioner practices in England offering a counselling service, with psychosocial problems being the second most common presenting problem in general practices. Given the massive and increasing volume of possible therapeutic interventions, the issue of choice becomes a real dilemma.

It is important to recognise that only a limited number of the more common and effective therapeutic approaches are included below. In addition, it should be recognised that the examples outlined below are largely individual therapy approaches where there is an individual therapist and a single patient or client. More systemic approaches, where clients are treated as groups, as in family therapy, therapeutic community or social milieu therapy, psychodrama, and other forms of 'group therapy', are not addressed. Such approaches are not unimportant. However, they are excluded not only because of space, but because they are less useful in demonstrating therapeutic techniques that nurses might use in their day-to-day work. Notwithstanding this latter assertion, it *is* important that the nurse is aware that the patient's context or background is important. Behind the highly anxious patient suffering from coronary artery disease may be an overly demanding wife and troublesome children. In such circumstances alleviating short-term anxiety through individual approaches may be less important in the longer term than one that treats a dysfunctional family group.

To this confusing array, we must also recognise that many therapies utilise modes of action that are not based exclusively on person-to-person verbal and non-verbal interaction, but emphasise other modes of human expression. Examples of such approaches include the use of drama (as in psychodrama, already mentioned above as a group technique), art, music, and dance. These latter two are particularly notable. The impact of music and dance as a therapeutic or healing influence has been recognised for centuries. For example, de Martino (1966) described the pizzica-tarantella, a form of dance to musical accompaniment traditional in parts of southern Italy. This finds its origins at the time of the Christian crusades, when it was believed that those bitten by tarantula spiders could only be saved by dancing to this rhythmical music for

extended periods. It is possible that this extreme activity had a physiological effect, helping to excrete the poisons. But irrespective of its 'magical' curative influences, it clearly also had a *psychotherapeutic* effect.

There is also some evidence indicating that there is therapeutic use of music and dance in nursing. Carol Picard (1994) described the influence of dance in healing and McCaffrey and Good (2000) have shown how music soothes, provides pleasure, and distracts from pain and discomfort. In this modern age, music and dance have attained very high levels of significance, particularly in the younger population. There is evidence that in an alienating and depersonalising modern world, this sustains a very high proportion of the younger population, and indeed may in some instances have reached levels of over-dependence: the modern-day equivalent of the pizzica-tarantella is alive and growing in the night clubs of Ibiza and in every city and village across the land. It might be argued that as we proceed with more traditional forms of therapy, the young have already chosen their alternative. It may seem that importing such a medium into health service therapy services is a little unrealistic. However, anyone who has observed the enlivening impact of an old-time waltz therapy session in a ward for older persons will need little convincing of the value of such interventions. We now proceed to consider a number of therapies, some of which are complex and 'intellectual'. However, it should not be forgotten that often the simple things – a song, the invitation to dance, the gentle touch – are also profoundly effective.

THERAPEUTIC INTERVENTIONS

The therapeutic relationship

In most of the 'therapies' outlined in this section (with the possible exception of some forms of behavioural therapy), the intervention is essentially relational. That is, the therapy is not only conducted within a relationship between the client/patient and therapist, but the interactions within this relationship are themselves intended to have a helping or healing influence. This highlights the fact that there are two aspects of any therapeutic intervention. First, there is an issue of relationship, or the nature of the association or bond between the two people involved (or in the case of group-orientated approaches referred to above, between the group members). Second, there is an issue of technique, or the nature of the technical skills being applied by the therapist.

This highlights an important consideration in the debate on therapeutic efficacy or effectiveness, and it is one of considerable controversy. The issue is essentially this. Is the main therapeutic influence the nature of the relationship or bond between the therapist and the patient/ client, or is it the technique that is used, or is it some combination of these two? The implications behind this question are considerable. If it were to transpire that the main impact is attributable to the relationship or bond, then the important thing would be to emphasise relationship building in therapeutic theory, practice and training, rather than emphasising a particular technique. The empirical evidence in respect of the impact of these two variables (relationship and technique) is important, and we address this below. However, as will be seen, irrespective of the weighting that is attributed to it, the relationship is of significant importance. It is therefore useful to link this consideration of the therapeutic relationship to the more in-depth examination provided by Carol Kirby in the previous chapter.

A fundamental aspect of such a relationship, as highlighted in the previous chapter, is its 'helping' nature. Irrespective of the attitude of the therapist (or nurse) to the client, and irrespective of the technique that is utilised, there is always an intention to *help* the other. However, beyond this more or less universal condition there is a wide range of views about what is the appropriate relationship or bond between the patient/client and the therapist. This matter of course has its parallel in nursing, where the appropriate relationship between the *nurse* and the patient has long been a subject of debate.

Essentially, the issue often comes down to two positions, and indeed points that may be taken on a continuum between them. At one end of the axis there is the view that the relationship should be intimate and subjective, akin to the relationship between close friends, partners or relatives. At the opposite end is the view that the relationship should be detached and objective, where the therapist is simply a professional delivering another treatment modality. The position taken on this matter tends to depend on two broad areas of consideration:

- the appropriateness of the professional relationship between the patient/client and the therapist/nurse, irrespective of the nature of the treatment or therapy
- the specific therapeutic method or technique involved. As will be seen in the subsequent outlines of therapeutic methods, some approaches depend on objectivity and detachment, while others depend on more subjective and intimate relationships. For example (as will be seen), in an orthodox traditional behavioural therapy approach, subjectivity and intimacy may even be considered to compromise the therapeutic interventions.

In general, therapists will tend to adopt therapeutic methods that are compatible with their attitudes on the correctness of a professional relationship, and at the same time they will be influenced by their commitment to a particular therapeutic approach. This situation is usefully illustrated by the position taken by various nursing theorists and 'therapists'. Hildegard Peplau (1952, 1962, 1988) is widely recognised as one of the pioneers of psychiatric or mental health nursing. Her interpersonal model of nursing (and therapy) is influenced by psychodynamic psychology and therapy (see below), particularly that approach developed by the psychiatrist Harry Stack Sullivan (1953). Peplau advocated a therapeutic relationship that she described as *professional closeness*. This essentially requires of the nurse/therapist that while there is an attempt to understand the patient, a degree of personal distancing should be maintained. Intimacy is discouraged and the nurse/therapist should never indulge in self-disclosure; it is (the argument runs) inappropriate to burden an already overburdened and distressed patient with the nurse's concerns (Peplau, 1965).

The psychiatric nurse/therapists Paterson and Zderad (1976, 1988) took an essentially opposing position. They advocated an existential theory and therapy (see below), in which intimacy is an essential prerequisite for an empathic and empowering relationship (Zderad, 1978). They drew extensively on the work of the existential thinker Martin Buber (1987) and especially his views on human relating. Buber differentiated between an *I-It* relation, in which the 'other' is viewed objectively and with a degree of detachment, and an *I-Thou* relation, in which the person goes out to the other as person-to-person. Here the participants do not think about or analyse the relationship in action, they are in the mode of *experiencing* the other, of being with and for them in that instant. The designation of the other as *Thou* is an expression of this profound intimacy. In that instant that we become conscious of the relation, that we actually *think* about it, we immediately move into the *I-It* mode. The other becomes in effect an *It,* an object of our attention. The difference here is significant, such that the current author has spoken of an I-It *countenancing* as opposed to an I-Thou *relating* (Slevin, 1999). It is important to note (as do Paterson and Zderad) that Buber was not presenting two opposing and alternative modes of being with others. He recognised that in different instances we must come out, to the *I-It* mode, to observe or countenance the other and attempt to reason and understand their position and how best *we* might relate to *them*, so that we can again in another instant the better enter the *I-Thou* relation of being with and for the other.

Study Activity 30.4

Reference is made above to the nursing approaches or models proposed by Peplau (1952, 1962, 1965) and by Paterson and Zderad (1976, 1988). These are among the most notable and influential models. They are also notable in being very different in their orientation.

- Using any of the standard texts detailing nursing models and theories, carry out detailed reviews of the two models. Contrast them by constructing two columns presenting the differences.
- Reflect upon the essential features and differences, and indicate what you feel are the strengths each may bring to a therapeutic nursing relationship.
- A more recent mental health model, known as the tidal model (Barker, 2000, 2001), also adopts a person-centred approach similar in some respects to the approach of Paterson and Zderad. It will be recalled from Chapter 14 that often so-called models of nursing are derived from other sources, and attention is drawn there to the need to be sceptical of mechanistic approaches to the framing of nursing care. Look up the tidal model and what it states about the nature of the therapeutic relationship between persons. Compare Barker's work with the person-centred approach of Carl Rogers (1986, which we discuss below) and the model proposed by Rosemarie Parse (1995), known as the 'science of human becoming'. Identify what, if anything, is innovative about the tidal model. A useful critique by Noak (2001) may be helpful in this respect.

As we shall see below, some therapeutic approaches are largely based upon the concept of intimate helping relationships, as explicated by Carol Kirby in the previous chapter. However, others are based on a more technical orientation, and the premise that 'relationship' is unimportant if not indeed dysfunctional. We must recognise this range of orientations, as illustrated in Fig. 30.3.

All this may, of course, leave the reader in something of a quandary. What sort of relationship *should* the nurse attempt to build and, on its foundations, which of the techniques that we discuss below should he or she adopt in nursing work? These questions can be answered to some

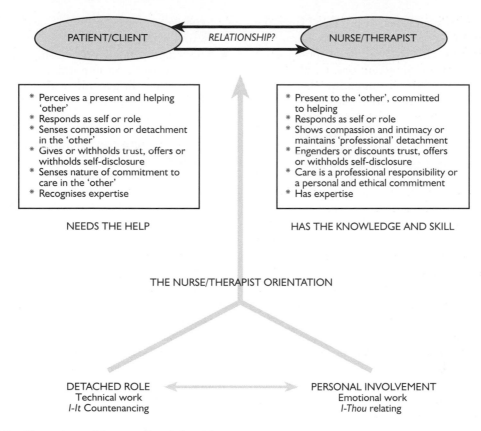

Figure 30.3 The nature of therapeutic relationships

extent by considering two factors: the evidence underpinning therapeutic work and the particular nature of nursing work.

Evidence

As we have progressed through the late twentieth century and into the new millennium, research into psychotherapy has increased significantly. Psychotherapy has become increasingly recognised as an important 'mainstream' treatment at the same time as an evidence base for all health care interventions progressed from an aspiration to an imperative. It is beyond the space available in the present chapter to review more than a small amount of this research. It is furthermore necessary to appraise such research with a particularly critical eye. Much of the research available is based on traditional scien-

tific research methods popular in medicine and experimental psychology, but not necessarily valued by therapists. This is partly because the most common form – the randomised controlled trial – may not be particularly suited to investigating a phenomenon that is by its nature complex and subject to contextual variations where eclectic methods are utilised. In essence, the controlled study of a particular therapy type that may never exist in such a controlled manner in the real world may be of limited practical value. The gap between *efficacy* claims under controlled and artificial circumstances may be far removed from *effectiveness* in real-world contexts. But even if the research evidence is accepted, there is controversy about what it tells us. In a controversial review, the distinguished psychologist Hans J. Eysenck (1995) claimed that the bulk of such research produced since the 1950s failed to demonstrate that psychotherapy showed greater effectiveness than spontaneous remission or placebo interventions. (A placebo is an intervention with no intended therapeutic effect. It is usually used to compare with, and highlight the effectiveness of, an intervention that is expected to be effective. For example, a chalk pill may be administered to a control group while the *real* medicine is given to an experimental group, to measure the difference between the medicine and what is in effect no treatment.) In yet another interesting study, Diamond (1997) found that the success rates for less experienced therapists with less training equalled and sometimes surpassed those of more well-qualified and experienced therapists.

The message here is clear. This is a particularly difficult area to research and it may be less well-suited to traditional research methods. This does not mean that we ignore all the available research. But it does mean that we must view it with a sceptical and critical eye. However, two publications have made important and momentous contributions in this area.

In the first of these, Roth and Fonagy (1996) conducted a very extensive review of psychotherapy research (indeed perhaps the most extensive study of its kind conducted before or since). In this they were able to demonstrate some significant patterns, of which the following are particularly important:

- There was a pattern demonstrating the effectiveness of therapeutic techniques such as interpersonal therapies, psychodynamic therapy approaches, behavioural, and cognitive-behavioural approaches across a range of conditions. Examples included the effectiveness of cognitive-behavioural approaches in depression and behaviour therapy techniques in phobias.
- Neither the training of the therapists nor the extent of their experience in general resulted in more successful outcomes than for less well-trained or experienced therapists, although some evidence suggested that

experience and training were important factors with more severely disturbed patients.
- The therapeutic relationship or alliance appeared to be an important factor in respect of outcomes in general, with more successful therapists being those who developed close personal relationships with their clients.

This latter pattern has been a notable finding in a number of other studies, some of which indicate that the relationship or alliance is *as important if not more important* than the technique used (e.g. Hays, 1996; Lindfors *et al.*, 1996; Tan, 1996).

In the second of these publications, the Department of Health (2001) presented guidance on clinical practice for therapy, drawing on the work of Roth and Fonagy (1996) and others. This publication also drew extensively on research findings, with the assistance of the British Psychological Society Centre for Outcomes Research and Effectiveness. As in the case of Roth and Fonagy's study, clear patterns emerged and were formulated into guidelines. Important findings were:

- evidence suggesting the efficacy of particular techniques for particular 'conditions'
- no strong evidence that the skill and the experience of the therapist are strong outcome indicators, other than the opinion of clinical experts that skill is significant in the treatment of more serious disorders
- support from some high-quality randomised controlled trials research for the therapeutic alliance (relationship between client and therapist) being a strong positive outcome influence
- indication that patients with more severe mental disorders benefit from longer term specialist therapy, while people facing difficulties in adjusting to life events (illness, disabilities, loss and bereavement) benefit from shorter term brief therapeutic support and counselling.

On the basis of the available research, we might reasonably make the following statements:

- Much of the distress that nurses meet in their day-to-day work can be addressed by shorter term therapeutic or counselling interventions. These activities can and should be incorporated into the normal repertoire of nursing activities (as in the type A psychological interventions described by the National Health Service Executive, 1996, and outlined earlier).
- The lack of advanced training is not a contra-indication to nurses' involvement in such work. Indeed, given the continuity of their contact with patients, they may be best placed to provide such support.
- The relationship that is established as the basis for such interventions is at least as important as the technique the nurse may utilise.

Nursing work

The latter of these three assertions of course brings us back to the issue of the nature of the relationship. Should the nurse maintain a professional distance in operating the technical approaches we describe below, or should he or she establish a more intimate helping relationship with patients or clients. The work of Hochschild (1983) is informative in this respect. In this seminal work, entitled *The Managed Heart*, Hochchild described the work of female airline flight attendants (air stewardesses) as being essentially emotional work. There was an expectation on the part of employers and travellers that attendants would maintain a pleasant and cordial countenance. This involved being pleasant to people even when they were unpleasant or difficult. In one sense, this was almost always an enforced and inauthentic pleasantness or façade – it was what they were paid to do. The dissonance between this enforced pleasantness and what the attendants really felt placed a high degree of emotional strain on them. Although her work did not include detailed study of nurses, Hochchild did draw comparisons. More recently, Bolton (2001) has described how nurses adopt various strategies to cope with the high emotional content of the work they do. These included strategies ranging from profes-

sional distancing to intimate relating (*see* Fig. 30.3), and included reactions ranging from cynicism to humour to indifference, sometimes presenting as hard and critical or soft and accepting.

What such studies do demonstrate is that nursing is unavoidably emotional in its context. Importantly, it involves a high degree of continuity of relationship with patients or clients who are in various states of emotional imbalance, ranging from mild unease to extreme emotional turmoil. While a degree of professional distancing, or at least objectivity, is essential, it cannot be denied that patients or clients expect their nurses to care and to show care. In this sense, the prospect of withholding emotional content is unrealistic. The nurse cannot choose as a permanent mode of relating either the close emotional involvement or the extreme professional detachment presented as a continuum in Fig. 30.3. For each patient, and at different times, there is a call for a particular mix or balancing of detachment and involvement, and indeed a movement between the two. In practice, the nurse will move in and out, between what (as discussed earlier) Buber (1987) described as the *I-It* and *I-Thou* relation. In doing so, the following rules of engagement would apply:

- The posture of standing back (as in the *I-It* countenancing) must not be a choice to be uninvolved, to reject the person or self of the other or withhold the person or self of the nurse. It has a purpose: to observe, assess, analyse; to determine what is to be done, what help can be proffered. In so far as it may be done in a mechanical way, with distancing and detachment its clear footing, it may in fact foil its purpose by creating unresponsiveness in the other.
- The posture of entering into engagement with the other (as in *I-Thou* relating) is not a choice to become involved in a relationship that is gratifying to the nurse/therapist or the patient/client in the context of erotic or filial love or attachment. It also has a purpose: to respond to the health needs of the other, in a

personal and caring way. As such, it must be recognised as a real and genuine concern for the other. The term *agapé* has been used to describe this form of love or caring for the other. It is a state of compassion that involves not only caring about and feeling with and for the other, but a commitment to helping that demands no reciprocal gratification (erotic, familial or otherwise).

By relating in this responsive and informed manner, the nurse establishes a personal alliance with the patient, within which the latter becomes aware of the nurse's acceptance and genuine concern. While this relationship may be therapeutic in itself, the techniques that are now outlined may enhance the effectiveness of the therapeutic relationship.

Supportive and existential therapy

Supportive therapy

Supportive therapy is essentially existential in its orientation, although this orientation has not always been recognised in this context. As its name suggests, the therapeutic intervention involves giving sympathetic support to a patient who feels distressed, or frightened, or alone as he or she faces the threat of mental or physical illness, trauma, or even death.

The approach is existential in that it follows phenomenological precepts. The patient is essentially alone in experiencing the threat which has come into their consciousness. The purpose of supportive therapy is to go out to the patient in their state of need, as one person to another, to convey to them that you, the nurse, care for them and that you are there for and with them. This involves three aspects (and it may be recalled that these were also identified in the previous chapter):

- *Congruence* – the capacity to convey to the patient that you have a genuine concern and regard for them as a person. You are going out to them as one person to another, not as a nurse in an impersonal and prescribed role,

who is relating to them in accordance with set rules of behaviour simply because that is what the job requires.

- *Unconditional positive regard* – conveying to the patient that you value and respect them as a person, irrespective of who and what they are. This is a non-judgemental way of being with the patient in which their importance to you as a person is clearly conveyed.
- *Empathy* – making a genuine attempt to understand how the patient is feeling *and* the capacity to convey this understanding to the patient.

Through these three processes the nurse is able to be present with and for the patient, to be in true relation with them. The *presence* emphasised in this approach would involve the capacity in the nurse to convey to the patient that she is really there, a presence to and for them. This can be conveyed by showing obvious non-verbal cues that they are being actively attended to. We attend in how we look, how we approach, the very posture we adopt. And also in the way we show that we are actively *listening* to what the patient says to us. It is important to recognise who we are interacting with in such circumstances. This person may have discovered a lump in her breast, or have been experiencing blackouts. She awaits a diagnosis and in this state she is acutely aware of her body, of the threats to it, of this strange environment and the (perhaps to her) strange people in it. In this heightened awareness the patient will discern perhaps more acutely than others, the extent to which we are attending with care and concern. The coming into presence with the other marks the commencement of *dialogue*. In the supportive therapy context, centred on conveying understanding and a sense of supportive 'being with and for' the patient, it may not even require *verbal* dialogue. The nurse may sit silently with the patient, holding their hand, acknowledging quietly their distress and sharing this with them. This may all sound simple and lacking in scientific sophistication and therapeutic technique, but it is often one of the most difficult things to do and its benefit to the patient in distress can be powerful.

Existential therapy

Existential therapy involves utilising similar approaches, but requires proceeding from providing support to facilitating the patient in bringing about change and growth. This is achieved through an in-depth addressing by the nurse-therapist and the patient-client of the meanings attached to the patient's reality *as it is experienced by them*, in the 'here-and-now'. This is essentially an interpretative approach that is described as *hermeneutic* (a term describing the reflective interpretation of phenomena). It differs from psychoanalytical interpretation discussed below, where the patient's experiences and thoughts are interpreted in terms of psychodynamic theory. Here the patient's experience is interpreted exclusively in terms of what it means to them. When these meanings are faced and explored, the nurse and the patient can then explore possibilities in regard to coming to terms with this reality and coping with it in the future.

Existential therapy is largely lacking in technique and structure. However, some existential therapists (*see*, for example, Yalom, 1980; May and Yalom, 1985) advocate an approach which addresses four 'worlds' – the *physical* world (including the physical environment and the patient's own body), the *social* world (including relations with others), the *psychological* world (the individual's identity and sense of self) and the *spiritual* world (which, as discussed in Chapter 23, is the largely unknown world, related to in terms of religious belief or the sense of meaning attached to existence). By exploring such worlds or dimensions, the patient may attain truthfulness to self, and clarity in regard to present and future existence. The goal is not so much to modify and change *behaviour*, but rather to assist the person to come to terms with *reality*, to achieve a capacity to not only face the future but to grow in terms of inner strength and confidence.

It is important to remember here that not everyone has the courage to face up to the frailty and temporary nature of their own existence. In fact, most people tend to shy away from this confrontation with the true self and the nature of its existence in the world, and instead hide behind the illusion of the routine, within safe and prescribed roles and norms of behaviour. To enter into such murky waters can be highly traumatic. It would be most unsafe, and indeed highly unethical, to impose upon a patient a confrontation with such issues when he or she has not got the courage and strength to face up to them. For example, a patient who has been told that he is terminally ill may be totally unable to face up to this reality. To impose on him a detailed discussion of this awareness and what it means to him could be disastrous. But the nurse who has true empathy with her patient will know when he is ready to discuss such issues. Until such time as this is totally clear, interventions must be limited to supportive therapy.

Psychodynamic therapy

Theory

Psychodynamic approaches to therapy are based on psychoanalytical theory. This assumes that our minds have conscious and unconscious elements. Sigmund Freud (1933), who invented this approach, suggested three aspects of mind. The *ego* is the conscious, everyday mental state of which we are fully aware – it is the known self, within which we are fully conscious of our thoughts and feelings. The *id* is the unconscious mind of which we are largely unaware. It is the deep recesses from which emerge our instincts for survival or destruction (Freud termed these the drives of *Eros* and *Thanatos,* after the gods of love and survival, and of death and destruction). The *super ego* is that part of the mind that is visualised as spanning our conscious (ego) and unconscious (id) states. In a sense it polices our mind, and is the moral conscience – suppressing or repressing unacceptable thoughts and feelings within our unconscious and judging how we consciously behave. However, unpleasant or threatening thoughts that are pushed into our unconscious are not gone, they are still there and can be a source of unease, anxiety or distress. Thus, in the Freudian theory, we can be experiencing extreme anxiety, or obsessional behaviour, or depression, without actually knowing why. This is because the cause is held from our consciousness: we experience the symptoms, but we do not know the source, and this in itself can be a source of profound distress.

Technique

In psychoanalysis, various techniques are utilised to uncover the unconscious conflicts that cause the conscious symptoms. Such techniques include searching for symbols in the patient's free associations – the accounts of his life or dreams. In some instances, hypnosis may be used to explore such depths of consciousness. As unconscious sources of distress are uncovered, the therapy usually proceeds by working through solutions. Here also a repertoire of techniques is used. A common approach is the use of *transference*. Here, where the unconscious conflict relates to difficulties or conflicts with another individual, the therapist takes the role of that person – in effect becomes that person – so that the sources of the conflict and possible solutions can be explored. A significant risk is that of *countertransference*. Here the *therapist* starts to experience emotional attachment to or involvement with the patient. This is why authors such as Peplau (1965) have advocated a degree of professional distancing. While most nurses will not be involved as psychoanalysts, it is important to be aware of the countertransference risk in day-to-day work: the child we nurse is not our own baby; and the adult we nurse must not become the object of our erotic desires.

Mental defence mechanisms

It will be clear that such therapy is highly complex. Analytical therapists undertake a training extending over many years, during which they are themselves required to undergo psychoanalysis. There are various approaches to psychodynamic therapy or psychoanalysis, and all tend to involve intensive therapy over extensive periods. Because of its complexity, and because nurses would not normally be involved in such work unless they also undertook the extensive training, we do not detail its possible applications in this chapter. However, there is one aspect of psychodynamic theory and therapy that is worthy of further attention, particularly as nurses will meet this in their day-to-day work in any health care setting. This is the phenomenon known as mental defence mechanisms (also termed ego defence mechanisms). Within psychodynamic theory, it is postulated that we develop various defensive mechanisms as a means of protecting the psyche (mind) from anxiety, shame, guilt, or similar distressing experiences. Some of the more common of these are presented below.

- *Repression* – any unpleasant thoughts or feelings that may be distressing if we are conscious of them, are unconsciously repressed or pushed out of our consciousness. Of course, such thoughts or feelings do not disappear. They continue to exist at the unconscious level of the psyche, or mind, where they may still be the source of tension and anxiety now or at a later time; and, when such anxiety or tension emerges, we cannot associate it with anything, because its cause is within the unconscious mind. As nurses, when a patient is confronted with distressing circumstances (e.g. bad news) but seems not to be exhibiting any adverse reactions, we should be aware that they might be repressing such material. The dilemma faced here is whether or not to attempt to halt or reverse this process. It is important to be aware that it *is* a defence mechanism, and at the time it may be the patient's only means of surviving. If the patient is not prepared to confront the adverse situation, it may cause great distress to attempt to force this issue and it may be best to defer the matter until later. In addition, as this is an unconscious process, the patient may deny that it is happening, and indeed become agitated or angry at suggestions to the contrary.

- *Regression* – in the face of some real threat the patient may regress (or go back to) earlier or child-like forms of behaviour. This may present as an adult who begins to cry, or thumb-sucks, or who indulges in childish tantrums, or whose speech takes on a child-like or whining quality. It is important that such behaviour is not treated with impatience or discounted as irresponsibility and immaturity. In one sense regression is all of these things. But the patient is not doing this in a contrived way. Such behaviour is a sign of real distress and the individual is not consciously aware of what is happening. Where the nurse observes behaviour that is indicative of regression, she should respond in a supportive way, utilising such approaches as those outlined under supportive therapy above.
- *Denial and suppression* – these defence mechanisms sometimes occur together, but may present separately. In denial, the patient determinedly refuses to face the true nature of issues they are confronted with. Thus, a patient who is informed that they have a progressive neurological illness may stead-fastly see it as a matter of little relevance, perhaps even telling their family and friends that the diagnostic procedures had after all shown up little, and the doctors were not really sure what had been wrong with them. They may even proceed beyond this to a state of suppression, forcing all conscious consid-eration of the problem from their life and getting on with other things. This is similar to repression, but here the person is making a conscious effort to 'forget about' the issue. Where these defence mechanisms occur, the nurse must again make a decision about how the patient will be approached, and this can only be informed within a close caring relationship with the patient. It may be the case, particularly in the initial stages, that the patient is not ready to face up to the problem. However, where the problem is likely to continue, as in the example cited here, at some stage – particularly as deterioration progresses – this must be confronted. Within a close interpersonal relationship, the nurse will come to know when the patient is ready for this, and at that stage the patient will respond by a willingness to confront the illness, and from here proceed with the nurse to consider ways of coping.
- *Aggression* – sometimes the patient may go beyond simple denial to demonstrating extremely aggressive and hostile behaviour to those around them. This may sometimes occur when an individual is presented with a sudden threat to health, such as a stroke or a diagnosis of terminal cancer. The reaction is typified by a 'Why me?' response in which the patient hits out at those around them and indeed themselves. This may present as verbal aggression or sometimes even violent behaviour. It is important that the nurse recognises this as a reaction arising from extreme fear, dread and distress. Such situa-tions can be most difficult to manage. A frequent reaction to aggression is to respond with hostility. Clearly, this will only increase the extent to which the patient feels threa-tened. However, at the same time, it is likely that while in this state any attempts to express understanding or sympathy may be equally provocative. It is important that the nurse maintains a neutral yet non-judgemental attitude, while ensuring that the patient does not harm himself or others. By simply demon-strating a care and concern for the individual, without being intrusively sympathetic, the individual comes to know that the nurse is there for them. This is important, as such aggressive reactions tend to be short-lived and followed by periods of extreme distress, at which stage support will be essential.
- *Rationalisation* – perhaps the most common of all defence mechanisms, similar in many respects to denial and suppression. However, in this rather more sophisticated (and thus more effective) mechanism, the patient develops arguments to justify a position they have taken. These can be quite sophisticated arguments that sometimes seem on the surface to be convincing. Of course, the patient is

aware at the unconscious level that the arguments are flawed. However, they are not lying or attempting to mislead others; they are in effect 'kidding' themselves, and rationalisation is a technical word for self-deception. For example, a person who is grossly overweight may claim that they are not overeating and that their metabolism is at fault. Or a nurse working in intensive care may argue that in this highly stressful situation she needs her cigarettes for their calming effect. Where such rationalisation may impact on health, at some stage it must be confronted by the patient, with the help and support of the nurse. However, here again, it is important to recognise that the patient had a need to rationalise, and until they are ready, any challenge to this may lead to extreme distress.

- *Intellectualisation* – like rationalisation this involves the use of cognitive processes and arguments to avoid emotional distress. For example, a young man may be informed that he has an inoperable brain tumour, after which modern forms of palliative treatment proceed. In the course of this he may exhibit an intense interest in the nature of his disorder and in the various techniques (some of them complex and sophisticated) that are being used in his therapy. It becomes clear that he is desperately immersing himself in all this science and technology to avoid the emotional confrontation with his death in a few short weeks. The problem is that those around him, also desperately avoiding any allusion to this distressing spectre in the background, seem to reinforce and support this unemotional way of being. However, eventually, as the situation worsens, the fact of approaching deterioration and eventual death must be confronted. Again, the nurse should not try to force the patient to face this before they are ready. As in all the defence mechanisms, this is a method the individual is using because they cannot, at that time, face the truth. But the time comes when the patient is ready, and here again within a close therapeutic relationship the nurse will be aware of

this. She must make it clear that she is present for the patient, and through gentle encouragement she can help them come face-to-face at last with their own destiny. Of course, when this happens, emotions will flood in, and those approaches described under supportive therapy above will become important.

- *Projection* – the reaction common in the scapegoating process, whereby we project our own weaknesses (contained within our own unconscious mind) unto others. In effect, we 'accuse' them of urges or tendencies that are contained deep in our own unconscious. Thus, the 45-year-old man who has been admitted with a severe myocardial infarction will later say it was his wife's fault; she insisted on serving up high-fat meals and fried foods. Of course, the fact that this is what *he* preferred to eat, perhaps *only* would eat, is not acknowledged. It is important to recognise that the patient is not deliberately lying to others here, or at least not only to others: he is primarily deceiving himself and he is making these claims sincerely. It is also important that from the early stages of his convalescence and rehabilitation, this patient must make major changes to his diet and lifestyle. There is little point in the nurse confronting the patient by *accusing* him of projection or even rationalisation (he is unlikely to understand, and more likely to respond with hostility and hurt). However, the nurse can confront the patient at the cognitive level, helping *him* to see that he is responsible for his lifestyle, that his previous lifestyle was unhealthy, and that there are ways of improving upon this.

- *Sublimation and compensation* – it is useful to consider these two mechanisms together, as they are similar, yet have subtle and important differences. In *sublimation*, unconscious impulses that are often unacceptable are channelled into conscious behaviour that is acceptable. The standard examples of the boxer who uses a sport to channel his aggressive urges, or the male nurse who channels homosexual urges into the nursing of male patients, are unfortunate. They do provide possible examples of the sublimatory process, but through their inappropriate and derisory use, devalue many boxers and male nurses! In *compensation*, a weakness in one area is 'made up for' or compensated by developing strength or excellence in another area. A common example here is the student who is weak (or thinks he is weak) at mathematics, developing a high degree of knowledge and ability in literary subjects. Within health care contexts, these processes can be recognised in many situations, and it is sometimes helpful to promote and support their development. For example, a psychiatric patient whose condition included strong aggressive urges may be helped to change his job from a highly frustrating environment to one where there is less frustration and more opportunities to redirect or sublimate psyche energy into intensive physical activity. Similarly, a person who was an active sports person and suffered a paraplegic injury may be encouraged to develop compensatory strengths in other areas, such as relating to people (perhaps becoming a Samaritans counsellor).

- *Dissociation* – this is a very extreme defence, whereby a very highly charged conflict or experience is completely detached or bracketed off from consciousness. This is often experienced consciously as amnesia, or lack of memory, for the emotional conflict or traumatic event – thus the term 'dissociative amnesia'. For example, the police may pick up a young woman wandering the streets – she does not know her name, or where she came from. Her belongings disclose her identity, but neither she nor her family know where she has been for two or three days and she is admitted to hospital. It later transpires that she had been the victim of a multiple rape by a gang. Clearly, in this situation very specialised medical and psychiatric help is necessary, and this is beyond the skills of the adult nurses who initially cared for her. However, it is important that where patients present with amnesia or confusion, the nurse is aware that a dissociative reaction may be occurring.

- *Conversion* – as in dissociation, the individual has been faced with some major conflict or a distressing situation. Indeed, dissociation and conversion are the two mechanisms that occur in what are known sometimes as *hysterical states* or *hysterical neurosis*. However, in conversion the escape route is by developing a physical rather than a mental response. The typical classical example is the student who awakes on the morning of an examination with a paralysis in her writing hand! But this is not malingering. In conversion there is a real paralysis of a limb, or blindness, or deafness, or difficulty in breathing. However, the 'realness' is not based in actual anatomical defects, but in functional deficiencies. For example, a wife whose husband is threatening to leave her may become paralysed in her lower limbs. But the distribution of paralysis may not follow anatomical pathways as in an organic paralysis. In this case, the wife may exhibit a paralysis that stops halfway up the thigh of each leg at a very precise level. She literally cannot move her limbs below this level and she has genuinely no feeling (that she can consciously respond to) below this level. However, this is, of course, an anatomical impossibility. Given the nerve distribution of the legs, such a paralysis just could not occur. But for most people, the unconscious mind that constructs this paralysis has no expert anatomical knowledge! Such *conversion* paralysis of the limbs is often called *glove and stocking* paralysis because it does not conform to anatomical possibilities, but follows instead the distribution of a glove or stocking. As in the case of dissociation, the treatment of conversion is a complex matter requiring expert intervention. However, it is important that the nurse recognises how such phenomena may occur and – where it is recognised – seek expert help. It is also important to recognise that not all physical changes brought about by mental processes are examples of conversion. In some instances, prolonged mental stress *can* produce actual organic changes to the body. In these instances, unlike in conversion, there is a real and definite physical illness, with actual pathological body changes. Such illnesses, which may include peptic ulceration, skin rashes and perhaps even (some would argue) some forms of cancer, are defined as *psychosomatic disorders*.

The examples of mental or ego defence mechanisms presented above are not necessarily a definitive set. A scrutiny of a standard dictionary of psychology or a comprehensive textbook of mental health nursing, such as that of Shives and Isaacs (2002) will identify others. Indeed, the listing of these may vary from authority to authority. The important point here is that while the registered nurse (or indeed any other health care professional) would not provide psycho-analytical therapy until after many years of training, all nurses will frequently meet up with patients who are using such mechanisms as means of dealing with their personal problems. The nurse must be able to recognise at least the most common of these mechanisms and be able to respond to them within the context of normal day-to-day nursing care.

Person-centred therapy

The terms client-centred counselling, client-centred therapy and non-directive counselling are also used. However, as the practitioners of the approach reject a narrow medical/disease-orientated application of the method, the term 'therapy' is sometimes avoided.

The method is largely derived from the work of its inventor, the American psychologist Carl Rogers (1951, 1961, 1986). Its theoretical orientation is that of humanistic psychology and in particular the individual's *self-concept*. The self-concept is different to the real or organismic self; it is essentially how the person sees himself. This can be influenced by significant others who may condemn or blame the individual and also by feelings of helplessness or worthlessness in the individual himself. The outcome may be that the self-concept is one characterised by a view of self which is different to that of the real self, which is always in fact (in the philosophy of Rogers), that of a truly worthwhile individual. Where there is a low self-esteem or a deficit of self-concept, person-centred therapy is of particular value.

The emphasis, as the title suggests, is on the person and their natural capacity to wish to come to terms with and solve their own problems. The approach requires that the therapist or counsellor does not instruct, guide or advise the client – thus the titles 'non-directive therapy or counselling'. The person may have extreme feelings of worthlessness and helplessness in terms of managing their own life and solving their own problems. This may seem insurmountable to them, perhaps even to the extent that their self-concept is so low that they are in a state of abject despair and contemplating self-destruction. But even in such instances the person-centred philosophy is one of faith in each human being's real worth and in their wishes and capacity to pursue a healthy and worthwhile existence. On this basis, the therapist or counsellor is a facilitator, acting as a catalyst for change in the client. The belief is that each person has within them the capacity to solve their own problems, to heal themselves. The therapist's role is not to guide and control the situation, but to enable the person to solve their own problems in their own way, to enable that person to find and release their own potential for self-healing or problem-solving.

The same basic tenets of congruence (conveyed genuineness), unconditional positive regard (acceptance) and empathy (conveyed understanding) described in supportive therapy above, are applied by the therapist here. Indeed, it was Carl Rogers who originally formulated these three elements as the fundamental basis of his person-centred approach. When the nurse-therapist goes out to the patient-client with these three attitudes, a relationship based on intimacy and mutuality develops. Essentially, what happens in such encounters is that the patient-client talks and the therapist listens. But the therapist is not a passive listener in the extreme sense. By conveying empathy through verbal and non-verbal acknowledgement, the therapist lets the client see that their ideas and feelings are not only understood but accepted as legitimate.

Furthermore, by putting back to the client their expressions, the therapist enables the client to achieve a truer understanding of their self-concept deficit and the reasons for this. The therapist does this by two techniques. One is literal *repetition*, in which the therapist repeats exactly what the client says. Under some circumstances this may seem a mechanistic and condescending device. However, if congruence and unconditional positive regard for the client have been demonstrated, this will be accepted as a genuine helping response. The other device is that of *reflection*. The essential thing in reflection is that the client's *meaning* is reflected back. Sometimes this may be a revelation to the client, as they have not yet confronted the actual meanings implicit in their own statements. For example, the client may say 'It is not really the sort of thing you can discuss with him'. In 'repeating' the therapist would repeat the exact words back to the client. But in reflecting, the therapist may say 'You have difficulty in discussing sexual matters with your father; this seems to worry you'. In reflection, not only is what the client is really saying explicated more fully, but its emotional content is made clear. In reflecting this more holistic statement back to the client, they have an opportunity to address it in full. They can accept it as a full explanation of what they have said (and this may be difficult, as the realisation of this truth may be a revelation to them of something they knew yet had not consciously acknowledged), or they may reject it and the subsequent discussion with further repeating and reflecting may clarify the real difficulty being encountered by the client.

The ongoing therapeutic encounter, characterised by a warm and accepting relationship, and subjected to increasing clarity through repeating and reflecting, enables the client to proceed towards not only recognising problems but also forming their own solutions to them. In this endeavour the therapist *never* leads or advises, but has complete faith in the client's capacity to arrive at the best solutions. Through the experience of being accepted and respected as a person of worth, who is listened to with genuineness and concern within the therapeutic situation, a sense of worth and a reduction of self-concept deficit is nurtured. Through arriving at their own solutions and the acceptance of the validity of these by the therapist, the client achieves a new sense of confidence and a reduction in felt or learned helplessness. It will be noted that such person-centred approaches are highly relevant to the nursing process of encouraging self-care.

Study Activity 30.5

Note the following statements made by the client in a person-centred counselling session. He is speaking about his work situation, which he is contemplating returning to after he recovers from his myocardial infarct and is discharged from hospital.

'Sometimes I just dread going back. The stress is so intense and everyone seems to be at each other's throats all the time'.

'I think about just leaving, not going back at all! In my old job I was much happier, but of course the money was considerably less'.

- In the first of these statements the client is conveying feelings about his job and in the second he is surmising on possible solutions (although he may not be fully aware of this). Write down a *reflective* statement, which the therapist (or nurse) may make in reply to each statement.

Behaviour therapy

Learning theory
Behaviour therapy aims at modifying behaviour through the application of learning theory in the treatment setting. There is a wide range of behavioural approaches, most of which require specific behavioural knowledge and skills on the

part of the therapist. Only two illustrations are presented here, based on two main strands of learning theory.

- *Classical conditioning* – also known as *Pavlovian conditioning* (after the Russian physiologist Ivan Pavlov). Classical conditioning is based on normal unlearned stimulus–response sets which are often in fact reflex actions. An unconditioned stimulus, such as the smell of food, will usually bring about an unconditioned or unlearned response of salivation. When a neutral stimulus (one which by itself would not normally produce a particular response) is paired or occurs contingently with the unconditioned stimulus on a number of occasions, this neutral stimulus will by itself produce the same response as the unconditioned stimulus. The person or animal thus learns to respond to this neutral stimulus – which is now called the conditioned stimulus – with the same response – which is now called the conditioned response.

For example, each time a dog is presented with food (an *unconditioned stimulus*) it responds by reflex salivation (an *unconditioned response*). However, each time the food is presented, a bell is sounded (a *neutral stimulus*, which by itself would not cause salivation). After this occurs a number of times it is found that if the bell is sounded without food being presented the dog will start to salivate. It has learned to associate the bell (now a *conditioned stimulus*) with food even if the food does not appear and it will start to salivate (this response now being termed a *conditioned response*). Much of our learning is based on classical conditioning. For example, a child may experience pain and discomfort on a number of visits to the dentist. On the occasions this has happened, the child is surrounded by people wearing white and using silver-coloured utensils. Following such exposure, any environment in which people wear white and use silver-coloured instruments, such as a butcher's shop or the hairdresser's salon, may distress the child.

- *Operant conditioning* – also known as *instrumental*, *operant* or *Skinnerian conditioning* (after the American psychologist B. F. Skinner). This is not based on reflex or automatic stimulus–response reactions, but on purposive or *operant* acts carried out by the animal or person – thus the term operant or instrumental conditioning. Here the reinforcer or cause of the behaviour is made contingent not on the stimulus (as in classical conditioning) but on the response. What happens here is that the person or animal, by virtue of a natural (inborn) activity drive, indulges in random activities all the time. If one of these random activities results in a rewarding or positive reinforcement and if this occurs on a number of occasions, the incidence of that behaviour will increase significantly.

For example, a rat in a cage may be indulging in a number of random activities. One of these is to pull a lever in the cage. If, on each occasion the lever is pulled, a food pellet is deposited in the cage, the rat will indulge in lever pulling as a frequent and purposive activity. As long as the positive reinforcement (food pellets on lever pulling) is provided, the learned response will endure. The rat will indulge in lever pulling more frequently than other random behaviour and will indulge in increased lever pulling each time it is hungry and needs food. This behaviour will continue even when food is only deposited on some occasions. It is only after a protracted period of always failing to obtain food on lever pulling that this learned response would become extinguished.

Operant conditioning can also occur as negative conditioning. Here, using the same example as above, negative reinforcers (i.e. those which are punishing rather than rewarding) can also modify behaviour. In the above example, the rat may be subjected to electric shocks passed through the floor of its cage each time it pulls the lever. After experiencing this a few times the rat will avoid pulling the lever and will even become intensely fearful if it is forced into the vicinity of the lever. As can be imagined, the use of negative reinforcers, particularly where these involve causing pain or discomfort, raises serious ethical questions.

- *Practical applications* – the nurse-therapist can utilise behavioural approaches in a wide range of everyday nursing activities. Because of its ascendancy as a therapy modality in the 1960s and 1970s, a number of specialist courses were introduced in the UK specifically to train nurses as specialist nurse-therapists utilising such approaches. There are a number of such courses still in existence, although they have developed as more eclectic programmes which do not limit their range of therapeutic interventions to those based on a narrow behavioural perspective.

The principles of learning theory are used in a wide range of situations. In addition, there is a large range of perspectives within the behaviour therapy field with the result that a large number of specific behaviour therapy techniques are described in the literature. Two broad approaches are described here.

Classical conditioning methods

- *Systematic desensitisation* – as has been noted earlier, individuals often develop irrational fears (phobias) by associating fear, discomfort or pain with a particular stimulus–response situation which does not normally evoke such extreme reactions. In an example above, a child associated the experiences of white uniforms and silver-coloured instruments in the dental surgery with pain and discomfort and generalised this fear into all situations of white uniforms and silver instruments. This child may while in hospital have an absolute dread of being taken to the treatment room to have his surgical dressings changed.

The aim in *systematic desensitisation* is to break this conditioned link and to associate the feared situations with pleasant rather than unpleasant stimuli. This is in fact a process of *counterconditioning*. The patient is gradually introduced to the feared situation and on each occasion the exposure is presented in the presence of pleasant rather than unpleasant experiences. In the example being illustrated here, the child may initially be taken to the closed door of the treatment room. He may be crying and upset. The nurse cuddles him and talks gently to him, and then takes him away. After doing this a few times she takes him to the open door of the treatment room, letting him see in, while all the time cuddling him and talking gently to him. This may also be repeated a few times. Gradually the nurse proceeds, in subsequent sessions, to move the child into the room, perhaps sitting in there for a period and reading him a story, then letting him explore the room, touching and exploring the instruments etc. She may then show him what the instruments are for, and how they are used, perhaps stroking his skin gently with a forceps and swab. If at any session the child becomes very distressed the nurse immediately takes him away from the treatment room and reassures him, so that he develops confidence in her and trusts her not to expose him to danger. After repeated sessions of *graded exposure,* the child will associate the treatment room with pleasure and not pain, and full counterconditioning will have occurred.

Systematic desensitisation therapy can be used in a wide range of situations. For example, it may prove successful with adults who fear going to the operating theatre, or with long-stay patients who have agoraphobia (fear of open spaces) and fear leaving the hospital. An example nurses sometimes meet in the community is that of the house-bound wife, which is another manifestation of agoraphobia.

- *Flooding* – the patient is exposed to the feared situation in its totality all at once. They are prevented from avoiding or escaping the situation. At first there is intense fear and panic, but as it is discovered that disaster has not struck, that pain or discomfort does not occur, the panic subsides. In the example above, the child may in fact be taken straight into the treatment room and held there. The nurse is gentle and talks quietly and reassuringly to the child, holding him to her and cuddling and stroking him. But she does not let him leave. Gradually the crying and screaming will subside and the nurse can walk the child around the treatment room, letting him see and explore its contents, as in the final stages in systematic desensitisation. Thus in a very short time, perhaps in just a few minutes, counterconditioning will have been achieved.

There are obviously ethical considerations in flooding, and some people would see the approach in the example given here as being tantamount to child abuse! In addition, there can be dangers in flooding. In a middle-aged patient, a heart attack might be induced; in the example above, an asthmatic attack may be induced in the child. This stresses the need for a full assessment of the patient before any nursing intervention, but particularly in those such as systematic desensitisation or flooding where anxiety and panic may be induced.

Operant conditioning: behaviour modification

As will be recalled, the principle here is that behaviour which is rewarded will be repeated more frequently, that which is punished will occur less frequently, and that which is neither rewarded nor punished will only occur randomly, if at all. Generally speaking, the use of aversive stimuli (punishment or negative reinforcement) is now seldom used for two reasons. First, there are ethical implications of 'punishing' people, particularly if they are patients or clients; and, second, the use of negative reinforcement has been found to be less effective, with a greater tendency for the person to revert to former behaviour when the negative reinforcer is removed.

The approach usually adopted is that of rewarding or positively reinforcing the required behaviour. Each time the behaviour occurs, a reward is given. The problem here is controlling the system of rewards. There are three useful techniques.

1   *Shaping* – the problem in behaviour modification is often waiting on the desired behaviour so that it can be rewarded. As behaviour is occurring randomly, this could take some time. What the therapist does is start off by rewarding behaviour that approximates to the desired behaviour. When this behaviour increases, only that which more closely approximates the desired behaviour is rewarded, and so on until the actually required behaviour occurs and then only it is rewarded. In other words, the required behaviour is shaped through reinforcing behaviour as it approximates the eventual required target behaviour.

2   *Extinction* – where any behaviour occurs and is not rewarded it will eventually become extinct or only occur randomly on rare occasions. The technique here is to be sure that when the behaviour to be reduced occurs, it is not positively reinforced in any way. As indicated above, research has indicated that the use of negative or punishing reinforcers is ineffective. However, the withholding of positive or rewarding reinforcers, as in extinction, is effective. Of course, the problem here is whether the withholding of some positive reinforcement, such as affection, may not in reality be a negative or punishing experience.

3   *Schedules of reinforcement* – it is obvious that if behaviour is positively reinforced every time it occurs and if this is carried on indefinitely, the therapy would be costly and time-consuming. Initially, it is of course important that each instance of the target behaviour is reinforced positively. However, subsequently schedules of reinforcement can be used. There are essentially four types of schedule. In the *fixed interval schedule*, reinforcement occurs at fixed time intervals, perhaps once every hour on the hour (i.e. the first time the required behaviour occurs after expiry of each hour). In the *variable interval schedule*, reinforcement occurs after varying time intervals, which can be randomly distributed. Thus, the subject may receive

reinforcements at 9 a.m., 9.20 a.m., 10.05 a.m., 11.30 a.m., 11.35 a.m., 13.40 p.m., and so on. However, to achieve the same or similar levels of behaviour modification, the average number of reinforcements over the period would have to be similar to the number of reinforcements in the fixed interval schedule. In the *fixed ratio schedule*, reinforcement occurs after each set number of instances of the target behaviour, perhaps on every 10th occurrence. In the *variable ratio schedule*, the average number of reinforcements would be the same as the number for the fixed ratio but the occurrence of reinforcements would be randomly distributed. The therapist would make sure that *on average* reinforcements would occur at the rate of one for each 10 occurrences of the behaviour, but they would be provided randomly. It has been found that with human subjects, such schedules are as effective over a period as continuous reinforcement, and that in fact reinforcement by such methods is more resistant to extinction. In the nursing situation, where constant and controlled observation of behaviour is not always possible, variable interval schedules are usually the most practicable approach.

Behaviour modification can have a wide application in nursing. For example, on an elderly care ward, one of the patients may demonstrate disruptive behaviour by incessantly shouting loudly. The nurses adopt the strategy of not responding to him at all when he shouts loudly at them, unless it is absolutely necessary in an emergency. This will promote *extinction*. When the patient lowers his voice to some extent, the nurses immediately go to him, attend to what he is saying and respond by smiling, touching him, responding immediately to his requests. They might even administer a material reward, such as a sweet or cup of tea. This is *shaping*. It should be found that when the patient wishes attention he will speak in a lower tone. As shaping proceeds, only lower and then lower still verbal behaviour from the patient is reinforced. At first,

on all occasions the patient speaks in a normal tone, without shouting, positive reinforcement is provided. When the desired effect has been achieved, the nurses can then adopt a *variable interval schedule*, not reinforcing each occurrence of the behaviour, but doing so at random times on 20 occasions each day.

A final point should be noted here. Humans are more complex than animals. It is therefore often difficult to identify positive reinforcers or rewards. For a child, this may be a little cuddle or a sweet. For a long-stay patient in an elderly care ward, this may be a fill of his pipe or a cup of tea. Most people will respond to social reinforcers such as personal attention – being smiled at, talked to, etc. The important thing is to identify what *is* rewarding for the individual, and this may vary from person to person. Here, once again, the importance of assessment is obvious, as the nurse must know what the patient will find rewarding before she can implement behaviour modification therapy. A means of circumventing this difficulty is the particular therapy known as *the token economy*. Here, in a special treatment unit, the rewards provided are in fact tokens in the form of plastic disks, stamps or some other means of identifying the accumulation of points. The patient or client can trade these points or tokens for real rewards that are gratifying to him or her. There is evidence that more sophisticated clients do not take well to token economy approaches, but it has been used extensively in the learning disabilities nursing field.

Study Activity 30.6

● Select a patient on your ward. If you are not on a ward placement, select a friend or acquaintance. When you are in their company and they say something to you, respond with smiling, nodding in agreement, making your attention to them very obvious. What you are doing here is applying positive reinforcement of the person's 'speaking' behaviour using social rewards. You should find that the individual responds to this reinforcement by talking more to you. Repeat this with several different patients or acquaintances, and you will find the pattern repeating itself. You are in fact applying a behaviour modification technique.

- Now try adopting a different strategy. When your acquaintances say something to you do not smile, nod in agreement or overtly show full attention. The pattern should now be different, and the duration and frequency of their verbal statements to you will decrease. You are again applying a behaviour modification technique, this time using the principle of extinction. But a word of caution here. It is important that you restrict your actions to withholding positive reinforcement. If you turn your back on your subject, or walk off while he is still speaking, this is in fact negative reinforcement. In such circumstances, adults are likely to take offence and instead of producing your target behaviour, the result may be distress or an aggressive reaction.

Cognitive therapy

This therapeutic approach is based on cognitive theory and its application in therapeutic interventions as developed in the work of Bandura (1977) and Beck (1976). The specific therapeutic method is mainly associated with the latter author, and Aaron Beck is widely recognised as the originator of this approach.

It is often found that more intelligent and sophisticated individuals do not respond well to behavioural techniques and indeed may find them demeaning and offensive. This draws attention to the fact that in human beings, intellect and thinking processes are in themselves important determinants of behaviour.

The premise in cognitive theory and in cognitive therapy is that every person is an active, thinking agent who interacts with his world. In the course of this interaction and his thinking about that which he perceives to be true about himself and the environment, the individual forms viewpoints or beliefs about these issues. He also has affect or feeling about these issues and his thoughts and feelings to a large extent interact with his behaviour or actions; each to an extent influences the other. On the basis of past cognitions and experiences, the individual develops outlooks or *cognitive schemata*, which are ways of thinking or habitual perspectives on himself and his world. For example, an individual may have developed a pessimistic outlook on how he can control his own destiny; he may feel this is controlled by others and he himself is incapable of exerting control. This is the *cognitive schema* of learned helplessness. In fact, in such situations, individuals often develop negative and devalued views about themselves which present as spontaneous thoughts of low self-esteem and lack of personal worth. In cognitive therapy, these are called *negative automatic thoughts*. The occurrence of negative schemata and negative automatic thinking can lead to emotional distress, anxiety, depression, etc.

The goal in cognitive therapy is to assist the patient or client to identify and analyse negative cognitions, to subject these to a process of reality testing and to challenge and then modify these faulty thinking processes. The very process of examining negative cognitions, for example by counting them and then describing each one in detail, has the effect of helping the client to distance himself from them and to examine them analytically and dispassionately. When the illogicality and lack of evidence to support negative schemata and automatic cognitions are exposed, the client's natural human tendency to think rationally will cause him to review his thinking. This is in fact tantamount to reviewing and modifying his understanding of himself and his social world. The rationale is that by removing the thinking distortions, emotional well-being will automatically follow. However, it must also be acknowledged that some of the client's cognitions are not the result of negative schemata or negative automatic thinking. For example, a person may really be in an environment in which he is undervalued and in which he lacks real control. In this context, the cognitive therapy incorporates a problem-solving aspect, in which client and therapist consider how such circumstances can be modified or avoided.

The technique employed by the therapist is largely determined by the therapeutic goal and techniques described above. The therapist adopts a collaborative relationship with the client, in which he encourages the client to identify cognitions or areas of thinking and belief which cause him concern. When such issues are identified the therapist uses a technique known as *Socratic questioning* (after the Greek philosopher, Socrates), which involves asking the client to describe and then explain and justify his negative, self-devaluing thoughts. As the client attempts to do this, he begins to see that his assumptions are illogical and do not stand up to detailed rational examination. From such challenging, the discourse proceeds to identify more realistic interpretations of self, self-worth and world. The client develops a new sense of worth and a new confidence, and his emotional distress becomes dispelled.

A useful nursing application here may be the situation of a young adult patient who has had a lower limb amputation. It may become obvious that he is depressed and has given up any real attempts to respond to physiotherapy and rehabilitation. In discussion, the nurse discovers that he feels he is a cripple, that he will never work again and that he is a burden to his wife and children. The nurse can ask the patient to identify these thoughts and to describe them to her. In her 'Socratic questioning' she can ask the patient to explain why he feels he will never work again: what evidence has he to justify this? Do they both not know other amputees who work, drive cars, even take part in sports? Does his wife think any less of him now? Do his children not love and need him as much as ever? This should lead to the patient reviewing his ideas towards more positive cognitions on the basis of the rational evidence he himself has disclosed in the course of being questioned. This is a more powerful influence for modifying thinking than someone else lecturing to the patient or, even worse, criticising his defeatism, thus increasing his low sense of worth.

In the course of therapy, real problems will of course arise, and discussion may have to involve problem-solving: Will he be able to drive his own car? Will he need a modified vehicle? How will this be paid for – will he be entitled to motability (disabled car driver) allowances? Here again, the nurse works as a collaborator, encouraging the patient to participate actively in the problem-solving. This not only helps to solve the problems, but also continues the process of re-establishing self-esteem.

It is often the case that therapists combine these cognitive techniques with behavioural techniques. Thus, in the course of therapy the nurse may utilise positive reinforcement, systematic desensitisation, etc., in combination with cognitive techniques. Such approaches, known as *cognitive-behavioural therapy,* have increased in popularity in recent years, as more eclectic rather than purist attitudes developed in the therapeutic community.

Study Activity 30.7

Carry out a literature review on the topic cognitive-behavioural therapy. Useful original references will be found under the authorship of Donald Meichenbaum (1977) and Michael Mahoney (1974), the main advocates of this approach. Briefly write up the approach. This write-up should include: a description of the theoretical underpinning; an explanation of the main techniques employed; and a suggested application in nursing practice.

SUMMARY

In this chapter, the use of the therapeutic relationship, as presented in Chapter 29, was elaborated upon. The chapter concentrated on those therapies that utilise as their main therapeutic device the therapist–client or nurse–patient relationship itself, and the interpersonal communication that occurs within the relationship. These interventions are those which are usually described as psychotherapy or, when a non-medical perspective is being adopted, counselling. The term psychotherapy was interpreted widely to incorporate behavioural techniques and those therapies in which cognitive processes and interpersonal dynamics are the main techniques involved, in so-called 'talking' or 'verbal' therapies.

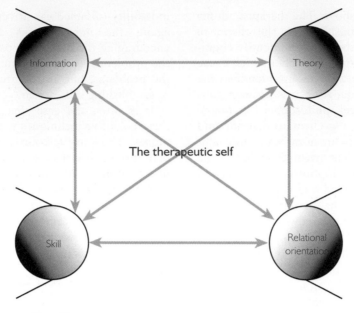

Figure 30.4   The therapeutic self

In seeking a depth of understanding of such therapies, attention was given to the nature of therapy, the different perspectives, and the interplay between what we termed the therapeutic relationship and specific therapeutic techniques. In considering these issues, we looked to the empirical evidence and theoretical perspectives that may inform how therapeutic interventions may operate effectively within therapeutic relationships. We also addressed a number of therapeutic methods or techniques that might usefully inform nursing practice. This centred our attention upon the practice of nursing and the responsibilities of the nurse in responding to the psychological, social and spiritual needs of patients and clients. In essence, the central concern of the chapter was the nurse as a therapeutic self, as one who must reach out to the other in need, as one whose *raison d'etre* is in fact a helping relationship with others. In drawing together the various strands discussed, the foundations of this therapeutic self can be seen as based upon interrelated elements of information, theory, skill and relational orientation, as illustrated in Fig. 30.4.

At the commencement of this chapter, we recognised that there are various shades of meaning to the term 'therapy'. In one of these, the term is taken to be synonymous with treatment or medicine in their widest contexts. In this latter sense, there are many involved in therapeutic work. For some of these, such as the pathologist working in a medical science laboratory, the orientation is exclusively objective, impersonal and scientific. The patient is far removed, seldom if ever seen. This work is no less valuable for this: it also serves humanity and the individual whose biopsy or blood specimen is being analysed. However, for others, and indeed for nurses more than all others, the situation is entirely different. The nurse cannot hide behind objective science, biological specimens, electronic readings and paper documentation. She (or he) is thrown into the presence of the patient. This presence, in its very existence, is a demand and it is ever-present in the lifelong working day of the nurse. It is a demand directly from the person that is the patient to the person that is the nurse. In this situation, questions about the relevance of therapy, in the sense of one helping the other, are in reality irrelevant. For each nurse, in each instance, with each patient, the very next thing the nurse does will have a therapeutic impact. There is no hiding place. In such circumstances we must embrace the concept of the nurse as a therapeutic self, and we must ensure the effectiveness of our interventions in easing the pain of those we care for. This chapter should, at the very least, act as a source of information and reflection on how we might respond to this challenge.

REFERENCES

American Psychiatric Nurses Association (2001) *Psychiatric–Mental Health Nursing Practice*, American Psychiatric Nurses Association, Arlington, VA

Bandura, A. (1977) *Social Learning Theory*, Prentice Hall, Englewood Cliffs, NJ

Barker, P. (2000) The tidal model of mental health: person centred caring within the chaos paradigm. *Mental Health Care* 4(2), 59–63

Barker, P. (2001) The tidal model: developing a person-centred approach to psychiatric and mental health nursing. *Perspectives in Psychiatric Care* 37(3), 79–87

Beck, A.T. (1976) *Cognitive Therapy and Emotional Disorders*, International Universities Press, New York

Bolton, S.C. (2001) Changing faces: nurses as emotional jugglers. *Sociology of Health and Illness* 23(1), 85–100

Buber, M. (1987) *I and Thou*, T&T Clark, Edinburgh (first published in German, 1923)

de Martino, E. (1966) *La Terre du Remords* [The Land of Self-affliction] (trans. Claude Poncet), Gallimard, Paris

Department of Health (2001) *Treatment Choice in Psychological Therapies and Counselling: Evidence based clinical practice guideline*, Department of Health, London

Diamond, J.A. (1997) The relationship between professional training, therapist skilfulness, and patient response to treatment, *Dissertation Abstracts International: The Sciences and Engineering* 58(4-B)

Eysenck, H.J. (1995) The outcome problem in psychotherapy: what have we learned? *Behaviour Research and Therapy* 32(5), 477–95

Frankl, V.E. (1964) *Man's Search for Meaning*, Hodder & Stoughton, London

Frankl, V.E. (1969) *The Will to Meaning: Foundations and applications of logotherapy*, New American Library, New York

Freud, S. (1933) *New Introductory Lectures on Psycho-analysis*, Norton, New York

Garfield, S.L. (1995) *Psychotherapy: An eclectic-integrative approach*, Wiley, New York

Garland, C. (1999) Talking cure. BBC television series – BBC 2: *Talking Cure,* November 1999

Grinker, R.R. (1970) The continuing search for meaning, *American Journal of Psychiatry* 127, 25–31

Hays, V.L. (1996) The effects of the therapeutic alliance and social support on therapy outcome and mental health of women. *Dissertation Abstracts International: The Sciences and Engineering* 55 (8-B)

Herink, R. (1980) *The Psychotherapy Handbook*, New Amerian Library, New York

His Royal Highness The Prince of Wales (1991) Lecture to the Royal College of Psychiatrists. *British Journal of Psychiatry* 159, 763–8

Hochschild, A. (1983) *The Managed Heart: Commercialisation of human feeling*, University of California Press, Berkeley, CA

Jones, M. (1953) *The Therapeutic Community*, Basic Books, New York

Jones, M. (1968) *Beyond the Therapeutic Community*, Yale University Press, New Haven, NY

Laing, R.D. (1960) *The Divided Self*, Penguin, Harmondsworth

Lazarus, A.A. (1996) The utility and futility of continuing treatment in psychotherapy. *Clinical Psychology: Science and Practice* 3, 59–68.

Lindfors, O., Hannula, J., Aalberg, V. *et al.* (1996) Assessment of the effectiveness of psychotherapy. *Psychiatria Fennica* 26, 150–64

McCaffrey, R.G. and Good, M. (2000) The lived experience of listening to music while recovering from surgery. *Journal of Holistic Nursing* 18(4), 378–90

Mahoney, M.J. (1974) *Cognition and Behavior Modification*, Ballinger, Cambridge, MA

May, R. and Yalom, I. (1985) Existential psychotherapy. In: Corsini, R.J. (ed.) *Current Psychotherapies*, Peacock, Ithaca

Meichenbaum, D. (1977) *Cognitive-behavior Modification*, Plenum, New York

Mellor-Clarke, J. (2000) Developing practice and evidence for counselling in primary care: the agenda. *British Journal of Guidance and Counselling* **28**(2), 253–66

Moreno, J.L. (1952) *Who Shall Survive?* Beacon House, New York

National Health Service Executive (1996) *NHS Psychotherapy Services in England: Review of strategic policy*, Department of Health, London

Noak, J. (2001) Do we need another model for mental health care? *Nursing Standard* **16**(8), 33–5

Norcross, J. and Goldfried, M. (1992) *Handbook of Psychotherapy Integration*, Basic Books, New York

O'Toole, A.W. and Welt, S.R. (1994) Editors' summary. In: O'Toole, A.W. and Welt, S.R. (eds) *Hildegard E Peplau, Selected Works*, Macmillan, Basingstoke

Parse, R.R. (1995) *Illuminations: The human becoming theory in practice and research*, National League for Nursing, New York

Paterson, J.G. and Zderad, L.T. (1976) *Humanistic Nursing*, John Wiley, New York

Paterson, J.G. and Zderad, L.T. (1988) *Humanistic Nursing*, National League for Nursing, New York (a re-issue of their 1976 text)

Peplau, H.E. (1952) *Interpersonal Relations in Nursing*, Putnam, New York

Peplau, H.E. (1962) Interpersonal techniques: the crux of psychiatric nursing. *American Journal of Nursing* **62**, 50–4

Peplau, H.E. (1965) Professional closeness, *Nursing Forum* **8**(4), 342–59

Peplau, H.E. (1988) *Interpersonal Relations in Nursing*, Macmillan, London (a re-issue of her 1952 text)

Picard, C. (1994) The healing power of dance. In: Gaut, D.A. (ed.) *Caring as Healing: Renewal through hope*, National League for Nursing, New York

Pilgrim, D. (1990) British psychotherapy in context. In: Dryden, W. (ed.) *Individual Therapy: A handbook*, Open University Press, Milton Keynes

Podvoll, G.M. (1990) *The Seduction of Madness*, Harper Collins, New York

Rogers, C. (1951) *Client Centered Therapy*, Houghton Mifflin, Boston, Mass

Rogers, C. (1958) The characteristics of a helping relationship. *Personnel and Guidance Journal* **37**, 6–16

Rogers, C. (1961) *On Becoming a Person*, Houghton Mifflin, Boston, Mass

Rogers, C. (1980) *A Way of Being*, Houghton Mifflin, Boston, Mass

Rogers, C. (1986) A client-centered/person-centered approach to therapy. In: Kutash, I. and Wolf, A. (eds) *Psychotherapist's Handbook*, Jossey Bass, San Francisco, CA

Roth, A. and Fonagy, P. (1996) *What Works for Whom? A critical review of psychotherapy research*, The Guilford Press, London

Shives, L.R. and Isaacs, A. (2002) *Basic Concepts of Psychiatric-Mental Health Nursing*, J.B. Lippincott, Philadelphia, IL

Skinner, B.F. (1953) *Science and Human Behaviour*, Macmillan, New York

Slevin, O. (1999) The nurse–patient relationship: caring in a health context. In: Long, A. (ed.) *Interaction for Practice in Community Nursing*, Macmillan, London

Stricker, G. and Gold, J.R. (1996) Psychotherapy integration: an assimilative, psychodynamic approach. *Clinical Psychology: Science and Practice* **3**, 47–58

Sullivan, H.S. (1953) *The Interpersonal Theory of Psychiatry*, Norton, New York

Tan, S-Y. (1996) Process and outcome in psychotherapy: summary of consistent research findings for effective clinical practice. *Journal of Psychology and Christianity* **14**(3), 263–8

Taylor, D. (1999) *Talking Cure*, Duckworth, London

Thompson, S. and Kahn, J. (1988) *The Group Process and Family Therapy*, Pergamon, Oxford

Thorne, F.C. (1973) Eclectic psychotherapy. In: Corsini, R.J. (ed.) *Current Psychotherapies*, Peacock, Ithaca

Trower, P., Bryant, B. and Argyle, M. (1978) *Social Skills and Mental Health*, Methuen, London

Weinberger, J. (1995) Common factors aren't so common: the common factors dilemma. *Clinical Psychology: Science and Practice* **2**, 45–69

Woolfe, R. and Palmer, S. (1999) *Integrative and Eclectic Counselling and Psychotherapy*, Sage, Thousand Oaks, CA

Yalom, I. (1980) *Existential Psychotherapy*, Basic Books, New York

Zderad, L.T. (1978) From here-and-now to theory: reflections on how. In: *Theory Development: What, why, how?* National League for Nursing, New York

31 Complementary therapies

Lynn Basford

LEARNING OUTCOMES

After studying this chapter you will be able to:

- Understand holistic nursing used within the context of complementary therapies
- Describe the philosophies and principles underpinning complementary therapies
- Describe the different techniques of chiropractic, osteopathy, massage, aromatherapy, therapeutic touch, shiatsu, reflexology, acupuncture, yoga, hypnosis and relaxation techniques
- Give examples demonstrating clinical application
- Describe the nurse's role and accountability when providing complementary therapy services to patients
- Understand the moves towards integration within the framework of the NHS
- Understand the need to practise, or be informed of, the evidence base of complementary therapies.

INTRODUCTION

Over the past twenty years there has been an increased demand for and use of complementary therapies (Endcott, cited in Wells and Tschudis, 1994; Vincent and Furnham, 1999, Department of Health, 2000; Richardson, *et al.*, 2001), to promote and enhance well-being, maintain health equilibrium or act as a healing catalyst. For example, Thomas and colleagues (2001) point out that in 1998 over 31 million visits were made to complementary therapists in the UK, who practised in the following domains: acupuncture, chiropractic, homoeopathy, hypno-therapy, medical herbalism, osteopathy, reflex-ology and aromatherapy.

The phenomenon has many explanations that are polar opposites. Views range from the belief that complementary therapies are increasingly popular because of patient dissatisfaction with traditional western medicine, or that the therapy has more efficacy in promoting health and healing than its traditional counterpart, to perceptions that there is a sympathetic need to engage in therapies that relate to the values and beliefs espoused by holistic care (physical, social, psychological and spiritual dimensions of care) (Kelner and Wellman, 1997).

It is suggested that in the UK one in three adults engage in acupuncture, osteopathy, chiro-practic, herbal medicine, hypnotherapy, homo-eopathy, reflexology and aromatherapy (Department of Health, 2000). This figure could be even higher if other, less familiar, therapies were added to the list; these might include relaxation therapy, art therapy, music therapy, spiritual healing, reiki, Indian head massage, nutrition therapy, Swedish massage, non-touch therapy, Ayurveda, traditional Chinese medicine, shiatsu and yoga.

The growth of interest is similar in the United States, where Eisenberg and colleagues (1998) found that 60 million people reported using one or more forms of 'unconventional medicine'. This figure they claimed exceeded the numbers of American people visiting a primary care practitioner. It is a staggering reve-lation that requires an explanation. Kelner and Wellman (1997) contend that it is because of a resurrection of thought and practice about health and illness that has been forgotten. In Switzerland, Rohrbach (1999) identified that some 40 per cent of the population used complementary therapies as part of their health care provision.

A high percentage of people within western communities are accessing some form of complementary therapy, therefore, and the opinion must be that complementary therapies contribute significantly to health care. If this is the case, these therapies should be respected for their actual and perceived value and effectiveness within a range of health conditions. Nonetheless, the choice to seek out complementary care remains firmly centred with the patients, who, for the most part, finance the service themselves.

From this position, complementary therapies are used instead of conventional medicine, or as an adjunct to medical models of health care that have been prescribed by the health care practitioner. There are concerns expressed with such an approach, in that complications may arise due to negative interactions between conventional and complementary models of health care. This situation could have legal and ethical implications as we move further into the clinical governance agenda. The health care professional and governing bodies are therefore seeking to change this dualistic pattern, and to offer a health service that integrates the best from conventional and unconventional modes of therapeutic interventions. Such developments are supported by patient advisory bodies, popular demand, professional groups, complementary therapists, and advocates of unconventional therapies such as the Prince of Wales. In 1993, at the International Nurses Conference, the Prince declared his support for further integration, suggesting that:

> ... the best of conventional clinical medicine combined with the best of complementary therapies and coordinated via enlightened, better-educated doctors and primary care professionals was the way forward
> (Wells and Tschudin, 1994, p. lx)

To offer a theory and practice of nursing that excludes a reference to these modes of therapeutic interventions would be unsatisfactory,

given the phenomenal increase in demand for complementary therapies. While it is unreasonable to expect that all nurses would become complementary therapists, it would be a rare situation for a modern-day nurse not to engage with patients who are either using complementary therapies, or who expect to have the choice of complementary therapies as part of their conventional treatment. In 1995, for example, 70 per cent of cancer centres in England and Wales offered complementary therapies as part of an integrated approach to health care (White, 1998). In addition, 22 per cent of women with breast cancer have consulted a complementary therapist as part of their overall treatment, or to relieve symptoms of chemotherapy and radiotherapy treatment. It is therefore necessary for nurses to have at least an understanding of complementary therapies if they are going to be able to prescribe the most effective treatments available from a diverse range, or to give appropriate and effective advice to patients. Gaining an understanding also means knowing the evidence that will address 'issues of effectiveness and harm' (Richardson, 2000, p. 99).

This chapter aims to give you an understanding of some key complementary therapies. Through wider reading and observations in practice, you should be able to debate the use of complementary therapies used in health care.

DEFINITIONS OF COMPLEMENTARY THERAPIES

The broad church that classifies therapeutic interventions that are unconventional, in the sense of opposing western medical views of health care, are colloquially known as 'complementary'. The Cochrane Collaboration defines 'complementary' or 'alternative' medicine, as follows:

> ... a broad domain of healing resources that encompasses all health systems, modalities, and practices and their accompanying theories and beliefs, other than those intrinsic to the politically dominant health systems of a particular society or culture in

a given historical period, complementary therapies includes all such practices and ideas self-defined by their users as preventing or treating illness or promoting health and well-being.

(Cited in DoH, 2000, p. 2)

Broadly speaking, the term 'complementary therapies' refers to a group of therapeutic interventions that are not conventionally taught or used in mainstream practice (*see* Table 31.1). In the 1970s and 80s they were collectively known as 'alternative medicine', but, as the system became increasingly used as an adjunct to conventional medicine, it was felt that 'complementary' best described these activities (Zollman and Vickers, 1999). Debatably, this is a simplistic position that does not give a comprehensive overview through which a universal understanding can be gained. It has been suggested that the term has been complicated over the intervening years by its use as an overarching umbrella to define a group of disciplines. Further to this, the move towards a common understanding and meaning has been undermined by the terminology being used interchangeably, which has added to the confusion.

Table 31.1 A selection of complementary therapies

Acupressure	Hypnosis
Acupuncture	Indian head massage
Alexander relaxation technique	Massage
Anthroposophic medicine	Meditation
Aromatherapy	Naturopathy
Autogenic training	Nutritional therapy
Ayurveda	Osteopathy
Chiropractic	Reflexology
Cranial osteopathy	Reiki
Healing therapies	Relaxation
(touch and non-touch)	Visualisation
Herbal medicine	Shiatsu
Homoeopathy	Yoga

THE CONCEPT OF HOLISM

Principally, the values and beliefs underpinning complementary therapies are rooted in holistic frameworks, which view man's health from a physical, psychological, sociological, environmental and spiritual framework that exists within universal energy fields (Rankin-Box, 1992). Holism is concerned with the unity of life and the fundamental principle of all systems. Illness occurs if there is an imbalance of the flow of energy within and external to the physical form. If the blockage is sustained, disease is manifested, which can be either an acute episode or of a chronic nature.

Many complementary therapies promote the belief that the body has the capacity to heal itself and the therapies are a catalyst to promote, restore or maintain health equilibrium. This is really not too far-fetched – certainly, the body is able to begin its own healing process when the flesh is cut or a bone is broken. In normal circumstances, people assume that the cut finger will heal itself, or that the bone will mend. However, when the damage is more complicated than a cut finger, as with cancer, or chronic illness, then therapeutic intervention is required to facilitate the body's own natural processes to restore health.

Using a framework of holism the complementary therapist will assess the patient and may prescribe a range of actions. These might include modification of lifestyle, nutritional correctness, exercise regimen, breathing and relaxation, as well as more specific treatment. Holistic assessment and execution of treatment are inherent values and principles of practice that the modern-day nurse should hold. From this position, their philosophy and principles of practice can be said to be more akin to those of the complementary therapist than of the physician who only treats the presenting health condition.

Complementary therapies and the concept of holism clearly have a symbiotic relationship with one another. As long ago as 2000 BC, the Chinese philosophers believed that, when a disease is treated, it is necessary first to treat the mind; there are no diseases, 'only people with disease' (Baumann, cited in Dossey *et al.* 1998). From the beginning of human existence, man has pursued the panacea of health and, ultimately, life itself. It has been a journey that has followed many paths and encountered many changes. Primitive men dug for medicinal plants, while the ancient Egyptians described the value of essential oils used in conjunction with massage, bathing, ingestion and inhalation. The Ayurvedic manuals of ancient India described botanical drugs, used in the context of a fascination with magic and mythology, while the ancient Chinese visualised man as a reflection of the universe, complete with the essential life-giving property of *qi*, or vital energy (McGilvery *et al.*, 1993).

The principles inherent within ancient and Eastern health care practices have evolved over time and remain in accordance with the various belief systems from which modern-day complementary therapies are derived. The knowledge base has been extended through practice and scientific enquiry and as such the therapies have become more attuned and sophisticated to reflect health needs within contemporary practice. For example, through trial and error, acupuncturists have identified the best spots to target in order to reduce pain levels during childbirth. Their knowledge and techniques have evolved over time to such an extent that there is now a high degree of success, which can be replicated.

THE NEED FOR A COMPLEMENTARY APPROACH

A scientific, technological and reductionistic model that has evolved over the last 200 years predominantly underpins conventional provision of health care in the developed world. Undeniably, the advances in immunology, genealogy and parasitology, the discoveries of antibiotic drugs, vitamins, insulin and growth hormones, and the improvements in surgical intervention made possible by antiseptics, anaesthesia and technological advancements, have all contributed to the enormous improvements in health care. Nonetheless, it is an approach that perceives the human body primarily as a physical entity and a highly complex machine that can be understood and, as appropriate, treated, modified and repaired. This approach denies exploration of the psychological, sociological and spiritual dimensions that contribute to the health state of the individual and the community. It relies heavily on advanced technological innovations, invasive therapies and toxic drugs, which, when administered, incur high costs and require highly qualified human resources. It is an approach that defies universal application (Rankin-Box, 1992; Wells and Tschudin, 1994).

The medical model also adopts a patriarchal and paternalistic approach to health care, which usually assumes that responsibility, and, therefore, power and control, rest firmly with the doctor. It is an approach that encourages the individual to relinquish all personal responsibility, cultural values and beliefs in the pursuance of health care. In short, the patient becomes the passive recipient of care, which is in opposition both to government directives and to moral codes.

Dissatisfaction with the above approach and political concerns related to the spiralling costs of health care have served to promote investigation into and use of alternative models. As a result, complementary approaches have found renewed favour with politicians, professionals and governing bodies. Nevertheless, some skeptics remain, who think that complementary therapies are 'hocus pocus', and demand evidence to prove that complementary therapies can deliver safe, effective care that is more economical than conventional treatments (Zollman and Vickers, 1999). Such challenges have provoked the need for practitioners working with complementary therapies to provide the evidence base through which they practice, and to identify a range of professional competence that can be regulated and monitored. While this could be seen as a biased demand, the same criteria and request is made of conventional practice that still lacks sufficient empirical evidence.

NURSING AND COMPLEMENTARY THERAPIES

Nursing in the twenty-first century is embracing a wide diversity of knowledge and skills in the implementation of its practice. The skills range from engagement in highly sophisticated technical interventions, via those more centred on the notion of caring, easing pain and suffering and promoting a dignified death, to those that promote health at the individual and community level. Whatever the branch of nursing, there are some fundamental principles that inform its practice. Essentially, these are based around assessing and caring for the patient and their significant others in a holistic manner, which is informed by the best available evidence.

Using holistic frameworks to guide practice has, according to Pearson and MacMahan (1991), enabled the development of a therapeutic relationship that is therapy in its own right. Nursing as therapy offers a different dimension to what has gone before in the modern period. If, as many of the complementary therapies assert, each person is an energy form that exists within the context of universal energy, then it could be conceived that nursing as a therapeutic intervention is able to transfer energy, or to act as a catalyst for the individual's own energy fields to begin the healing process. Chopra (1990) has referred to the latter concept as 'quantum healing', using the explanations of quantum physics and Ayurveda therapy. Following this line of thought, it is assumed that the transference of energy between the giver (nurse) and recipient of care is through quantum mechanisms. In this sense, Basford (2001) contends that nursing is a quantum therapy and can be seen as complementary in nature to conventional practice.

The concept of therapeutic relationships within holistic frameworks confirms the opinion that nursing and complementary therapies have a symbiotic relationship with each other in principles of practice. The dichotomy is presented through traditional education and practice based on the medical model. However, the new reforms in health care provision provide the opportunity for nurses to extend their field of practice as independent practitioners. Some will have the licence to prescribe from a limited formulary, whilst others will prescribe from practice protocols. This means there can be more freedom to become competent to practise using a range of therapeutic techniques as an integrated holistic approach in health care. Watson (1988) contends that, when a nurse enjoys independence with responsibility and accountability, there is an increased sense of achievement and job satisfaction, and, as a result, improvement in the quality of patient care. Partnership between the nurse and recipients of care is improved and patient empowerment is increased, which secures a degree of control and independence. Choosing conventional or unconventional health care interventions can be discussed with the patient in an informed way if the nurse has the knowledge and wisdom to direct the discussion away from the dominant conventional model.

EVIDENCE-BASED PRACTICE

Conventional medicine and nursing have grown accustomed to the notion that they must, at all times, provide care that is delivered to high standards based on the best evidence of practice. What is considered 'best evidence' is largely based around the body of knowledge that health care has, derived from the process of randomised control trials. The methods of scientific enquiry have limitations when exploring aspects of health care that do not fit with these methodological processes. In truth, there remains a large area of health care practice that is not based on scientific evidence and the same can be said for complementary therapies. Although the Cochrane Library currently cites 5000 reports and over 60 systematic reviews on complementary therapies (MacDonald *et al.*, 2000; Richardson, 2000), there is a recognition that much scientific enquiry is still to be undertaken before the profession has a complete body of knowledge based on the evidence of practice (Zollman and Vickers, 1999). In support of this, Vickers (2000) points out that, in the space of five years, the number of randomised control trials into the field of complementary therapy has almost doubled. However, some concerns have been expressed with regard to the reliability and validity of the research process. Much of this criticism rests with the methods used and the small number of participants engaged in the research.

So, should health care practitioners be using complementary therapies if they have not been proved to be effective?

Although it may seem as though the development of complementary therapies has been relatively short-lived, without a period of evolution through effective use in clinical practice, in fact, they have evolved over centuries, pre-dating the notion of randomised trials. There is also a supposition that conventional medicine operates from the proof of efficacy. Dalen (1998) contends otherwise, suggesting that patients were treated for cardiovascular disease with coronary artery bypass grafts from as early as 1964, well before the evidence of effectiveness was obtained, in 1974. In the interim years, use of the treatment was based on nothing more than the evidence of clinical practice. In addition, Dalen contends that the procedure of bedside pulmonary catheterisation was first performed in 1970 and continues to be practised without scientific evidence that it improves patient outcomes.

It might be logical to argue that any practice that is not found to have a scientific correlation with the efficacy of care should be considered unconventional. This proposition is unrealistic, given the complexities and changing nature of health care. Instead, as a prime consideration, any therapeutic intervention should have a sound knowledge base that is formulated either through repeated clinical practice and (with intuitive knowing) is seen to have a positive health outcome, or through evidence produced in randomised trials.

The Cochrane Library now includes numerous systematic reviews on complementary therapies. For example, there is evidence that St John's wort (*Hypericum perforatum*) can have a beneficial effect upon mild to moderate depression, and that Saw palmetto (*Serenoa*

repens) works on benign prostatic hyperplasia (Wilt *et al.*, 2000), while acupuncture is found to be effective for pain relief (Ernst and Pittler, 1998; Melchart *et al.*, 1999) and nausea (Vickers *et al.*, 1998). Governing bodies such as the Royal College of General Practitioners strongly recommend that patients with back pain, who do not have complications, should receive either chiropractic, osteopathy or physiotherapy within six weeks of diagnosis (Zollman and Vickers, 1999). In the United States the Institute of Health supports the use of hypnosis and relaxation therapies for the relief of pain related to cancer (Grossman *et al.*, 1999).

The support for such complementary therapies within these statements has served to encourage the release of funds to support empirically based research into the field. This much-welcomed activity will add to the credibility of complementary therapies, and ease their integration into conventional medicine.

Study Activity 31.1

Search for systematic reviews on the following websites:
www.cochranelibrary.com;
www.rccm.org. uk/cochrane.htm and
www.compmed.unmc.umaryland.edu/compmed/ cochrane/cochrane.htm

MONITORING AND MAINTAINING STANDARDS

Regulation and legal frameworks

With the exception of osteopaths and chiropractors, there is no mandate for complementary practitioners to join any official governing body before they engage in clinical practice. As a result, there is a lack of public confidence in the monitoring of practitioners and the maintaining of standards. The situation is further confused by the number of different organisations with which practitioners have either affiliation or accreditation. Vickers (2000) cites that there are between 150 and 300 organising bodies with differing standards and size of membership. There is currently a strong lobbying for unification, with a common standard framework, disciplinary procedures, professional liability, standard entry criteria, and professional codes of conduct.

By contrast, the General Osteopathic Council and General Chiropractic Council are legitimised, along with other professional bodies such as the General Medical Council, through Acts of parliament. This framework affords the right to statutory self-regulation. Disciplines such as acupuncture, herbal medicine and homoeopathy are currently working towards this status. It would be neither feasible nor desirable to regulate all complementary therapies through Acts of parliament, but it is essential to acknowledge the importance of public safety through voluntary self-regulation. This should provide a monitoring service to ensure that clinical competence and minimum standards are upheld.

Nurses and doctors are accountable and responsible to their respective governing bodies if they offer complementary therapy services. The usual legal requirement remains – that they be competent to practise, having obtained training, and have the knowledge, skill and experience. Further, their practice must be based on the best evidence available and meet any standards set by the profession.

Education and training

In the UK it is an offence for a person to practise as an osteopath or chiropractor without first undergoing the prescribed education and training determined by the governing bodies, the General Osteopathic Council and the General Chiropractic Council. On successful completion of the course they are eligible to register and then given licence to practise.

This is not the situation for other complementary therapies, and training can range from a weekend course to a full-blown academic programme. Competence to practise is therefore variable, depending on the course or training programme the practitioner has undertaken.

Increasingly, complementary therapy programmes are undertaken in academic institutions. For example, the University of Westminster offers acupuncture, the University of Middlesex offers herbal medicine, and the University of Derby and the University of Exeter offer combined complementary studies. Nursing and medical programmes are also increasingly offering modules on complementary therapies as part of their undergraduate pre-qualifying programmes.

PROVISION OF COMPLEMENTARY THERAPIES WITHIN THE NHS

Whatever the perceived or actual reason for the increase in use of complementary therapies, evidence shows that patients are engaging in such therapies both inside and outside the NHS. In 1989 a survey demonstrated that 74 per cent of the public surveyed voted positively for complementary therapies being available on the NHS (MOIRA poll, 1989, cited in Department of Health, 2000).

Today, there is increasing evidence within the NHS of further integration of complementary therapies with traditional medicine (Dalen, 1998). The Department of Health report (2000) on complementary medicine illustrates the use and range of complementary therapies within the context of primary care. This study found that, in the primary care setting, 40 per cent of general practices offered access to a range of complementary therapies. Some were administered by members of the primary care team (doctors, nurses, physiotherapists, among others), others by independently employed complementary therapists or via direct referrals to such services. This picture is supported by a more recent study by Zollman and Vickers (1999), who suggest that 20 per cent of primary health teams use some form of complementary therapy within everyday practice.

There are a number of advantages in using complementary therapies in primary care: there is a demonstrable financial benefit, plus the knowledge that the patient has had a comprehensive assessment that meets conventional methods and those that relate to complementary therapies. Nonetheless, there are some disadvantages: the primary care team member may be inadequately trained to prescribe or give complementary therapy, or may have to limit the time for consultation and assessment because of the allocated time slots that are a feature of general practice.

Regardless of the perceived advantages and disadvantages of the emergence of Primary Care Trusts (April 2001), the direction for increasing integrated models of care as part of mainstream service is set to continue, given the authority invested in the Primary Care Trust to commission care that is commensurate with need. However, the concepts underpinning any policy-making will have to follow set criteria, which consider the efficiency, effectiveness and economy of any service, while giving meaningful consideration to the competence of the therapists and standards used within the broader arena of clinical governance (Department of Health, 2000).

Specialist provider units

Within the UK there are five homoeopathic hospitals that accept referrals from primary care practitioners under the same parameters afforded secondary care services. These are services that are wholly funded by the NHS and remain free at the point of care. In the hospitals, practitioners who are trained in conventional and complementary modes offer other complementary services to the patient, adding to the richness of the service provision. The provision is audited in line with any other health service provision (Zollman and Vickers, 1999).

Secondary and intermediate care

While the picture in the secondary and intermediate care sectors is not as progressive as in the primary care setting, there is evidence to suggest that complementary therapies are in demand and are increasingly used in certain settings. For example, obstetric departments use relaxation techniques, yoga, acupuncture and hydrotherapy

and visualisation techniques; pain clinics use acupuncture, visualisation and relaxation techniques; rheumotology departments use manipulative therapy from osteopaths, chiropractors and physiotherapists; hospices use aromatherapy, reflexology, massage, hypnosis, relaxation and visualisation techniques, healing therapies, acupuncture and homoeopathy; clinical psychology departments use hypnosis, relaxation techniques, massage and neuro-linguistic psychology; and elderly care services engage in the use of aromatherapy, massage, acupuncture, relaxation training, music therapy, reflexology visualisation, pet therapy and healing therapy.

Clearly, a number of therapies can complement conventional medicine, but the range is seemingly limited to the use of certain therapies that have gained more credibility with the medical profession: acupuncture, aromatherapy, osteopathy, chiropractic, herbal medicine, hypnotherapy and homeopathy.

Study Activity 31.2 _____

- It is suggested that the common philosophy and value systems of complementary therapies are akin to those of modern nursing. Discuss this suggestion, giving your reasons.
- The history of complementary therapies goes back thousands of years. Identify the similarities in thinking about health and healing. What are the merits and demerits of such fundamental thoughts?
- You may believe that myths, magic and symbols have no place in modern health care. Is this correct?

Consider the following scenario: a middle-aged woman has been diagnosed with breast cancer. Her first action is to pray, her second is to fantasise that it isn't happening to her. She engages in wishful thinking and tries to imagine that it is a mistaken diagnosis, and that it was for her neighbour, whom she does not like. She then buys a charm to bring her good luck, and does not walk underneath ladders. She visits a clairvoyant to ascertain her future. Finally, she starts to visualise the cancer shrinking. On examination two weeks later, this is indeed found to be the case.

Could any of this woman's actions or the events that ensue be considered within the ancient historical concepts about human life?

- In your reflective diary consider other activities that could be viewed as beliefs in myths and magic that were embraced in the past. In considering and identifying these issues, consult the body of evidence and establish whether any of these activities could be evidence of positive coping mechanisms and can assist individuals in having positive health outcomes.

COMMON COMPLEMENTARY THERAPIES

The following are examples of some of the most common complementary therapies that are used within the context of health care. The list is not intended to be exhaustive and students are encouraged to read more widely on the subject and observe the effects of such practices in a clinical setting.

Touch

We often talk about the way we talk, and we frequently try to see the way we see, but for some reason we have rarely touched on the way we touch.

(Desmond Morris, 1971, cited in Autton, 1989)

Touch is described as the universal language, having no barriers, regardless of age, culture, race, or religion. It is a form of communication that has meaning for each individual, an expression of sharing feelings with others, and, as Autton (1989) suggests, it 'links us to our humanness'. It is a reciprocal experience that transcends personal space; as one person touches another, so they are touched in return (Mazis, 1971). Through the medium of touch, emotions can not only be released but also shared; it is a powerful way of communicating with one another (Young, 1965).

Montague (1971) upholds this view by suggesting that touch is the 'mother of senses' and that, next to the brain, the skin is the most

important organ system. He places a great deal of importance on the therapeutic value of touch, especially as a means of alleviating the effects of tension. The act of physical contact is seen as a means of restoring homeostasis in response to physical tension and general stress, with an overall soothing result.

Clearly, connecting with another person through touch can be a simple expression of caring and a powerful therapeutic experience. Its use is, however, subject to cultural and societal differences in attitudes and accepted practices. In some cultures it is an inherent feature of everyday activity, in others there is reluctance, while in more extreme situations, it is totally taboo. The English, for example, are generally non-tactile while the Italians and the French tend to extend greetings in a highly tactile manner. Autton (1989) contends that these differences relate to the past in the mystical and magical moments associated with ancient healing and religious ceremonies.

Notwithstanding the above, the use of touch has a universal application within the context of healing. It is used to comfort and communicate, and to activate the body's self-healing properties. Therapeutically, the art of touch is used in a variety of ways. Some include the use of contact, such as massage, others are non-contact, as in therapeutic touch, which involves the therapist working within the patient's own energy field. Nursing practice is particularly suited to touch as a form of therapy because of the nurse's direct relationship with the patient during the caring activity.

Study Activity 31.3

- List nursing activities that could incorporate touch therapies as a means of improving nursing care and promoting self-healing and a sense of well-being. After reading this chapter, return to your list and identify the most appropriate therapeutic medium, giving your reasons.
- Write up a case example where touch has been used in your experience in the health field. Talk to

patients and ask them whether they have experienced any benefits from touch therapy.

- Read the psychological literature on touch and its influence on bonding. Consider the cultural variants relating to the use of touch.

Massage

Historical perspective

Historical records indicate that ancient societies were aware of the therapeutic value of massage. Hippocrates once stated that 'the physician must be experienced in many things, but assuredly in rubbing, for rubbing can bind a joint that is too loose and loosen a joint that is too rigid' (cited in Autton, 1989). Massage techniques are an inherent feature of traditional Chinese and Indian medical care therapies that have evolved over time, while in Europe in the eighteenth century Dr Hendrik Ling developed an approach to massage that is now known as the Swedish massage system. Ling believed that massage applied in a particular manner could assist healing and improve the circulation and lymph systems of the body. However, massage has not always enjoyed a positive position in the promotion of health. A number of cultures throughout history have thought of massage as a form of 'quackery'.

The revival of 'touch therapy' in the modern period is credited to Metzeger, a Dutchman with an interest in the 'natural therapies'. In Britain in the nineteenth century, women massage therapists were employed to provide massage therapy under the prescribed instructions of physicians for a range of medical complaints. By 1895, the skill of rubbing had been learned by a few nurses, who were employed as 'medical rubbers'. Standards of practice were introduced under the banner of the 'Society of Trained Masseuses', which in 1920 became the 'Chartered Society of Massage and Medical Gymnastics', the forerunner of the 'Chartered Society of Physiotherapy' (Mason, 1992). Physiotherapists use the art of massage today as a method of analysis and treatment, and it is used in a much wider context in beauty and remedial therapy (Pratt and Mason, 1981).

Techniques

Common to the different techniques are a number of underlying principles and guidelines to which practitioners should adhere. Patients are assessed within a holistic framework. Health problems that are not compatible with massage therapy, such as varicose veins, heart conditions, hypertension and acute asthmatic conditions, should be clearly identified. The environment should be warm, quiet and softly lit, and any equipment close to hand to avoid disruption. The patient should be well supported and comfortable, in a position that is suitable for massage therapy.

Prior to the massage, the therapist should take a few moments to create a bond with the client, to enable the client to feel secure and at ease. The therapist should 'focus' or 'centre' on themselves in the role of providing massage as a mechanism for healing. From that point, touch should become the medium of communication, with verbal interruptions only when necessary.

A massage medium, either talcum powder or oil, should always be used. Hand movements should be firm and purposeful and in total contact throughout the whole process. When manoeuvres change direction it should feel like a seamless progression.

There are three basic techniques – stroking, kneading, striking – incorporating a range of variations.

Stroking (effleurage) is a smooth, sliding, rhythmical movement, which always follows the direction of venous drainage towards the heart (*see* Figure 31.1). Pressure can either be light or deep, depending on the need, but it is an excellent technique for increasing the venous and lymphatic drainage, improving circulation and the function of the muscle. It is a technique that enables the therapist to assess skin condition, level of tension or relaxation, and the presence of any lumps underneath the skin.

Kneading uses firm hand pressure, as it will move skin on muscle, muscle on muscle, or tissue on tissue. The hands are placed side by side in a flat position and then moved in a circular fashion, either together or opposite to one another (*see* Figure 31.2). It is a particularly useful technique for relieving tension.

For the technique of **striking**, the outside edges of the hands are used to make short, sharp, hacking movements. Striking is useful in loosening congested secretions from the lungs, as

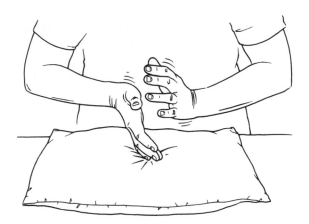

Figure 31.3 Practising hacking on a pillow

in cystic fibrosis. The hands are alternated in a quick repetitive manner (*see* Figure 31.3). Massage of a general nature (including thumbing) is usually completed using this method.

Massage in health care

Massage can have both physical and psychological benefits. In general terms, there is increased circulation and reflex activity in the central, peripheral and automatic nervous systems. More specifically, stroking aids venous return and the removal of waste products accumulated in the tissues; kneading and striking stimulate local circulation and mobilise soft tissues. The psychological benefits are connected with the reciprocity of touch and the relaxation process associated with massage.

Massage is useful for the promotion of health and well-being of individuals either as a separate therapy or as a complement to orthodox medicine. Clinically, massage can be used to reduce stress and promote the repair of tissue and muscle damage from traumatic injuries. It is claimed to promote relaxation and sleep and can relieve muscle cramp and aches. A randomised clinical trial conducted by Preyde (2000) on patients with sub-acute low back pain has shown that massage therapy can lead to improved function and less intense pain.

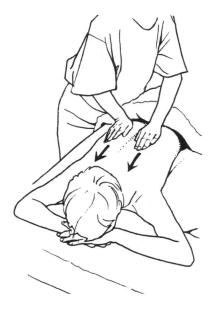

Figure 31.1 Effleurage to the back

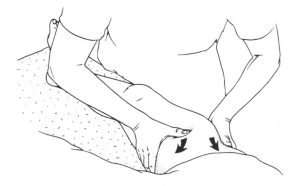

Figure 31.2 Double-handed kneading

Nurses are rediscovering the art of massage in a variety of specialties, from obstetrics to terminal care, as well as in the areas of mental health and learning disabilities. The therapy is useful because it can be incorporated into routine caring activities such as bed bathing and pressure area care, thus providing a more meaningful experience instead of seemingly perfunctory attention. Massage can be used as a technique on its own or combined with essential oils, offering a much wider therapeutic scope.

Study Activity 31.4

- With a colleague, find a suitable area and practise a range of massage techniques. Record your blood pressure before beginning and again at the end. At the end of the session, evaluate your own feelings and those of your partner.
- Consult with other people who have experienced massage in health care, document their experience and compare with your own and that of your partner.
- Examine the literature and identify the evidence of positive health outcomes when massage is used.

Aromatherapy

> *Look in the perfumes of flowers and of nature for peace of mind and joy of life.*
> (Wang Wei, eighth century AD, cited in Hildebrand, 1994)

Historical perspective

The value of natural plant oils in the promotion of health and well-being can be traced back to the beginnings of early civilisation. The Chinese recorded the medicinal properties of plants in about 4500 BC, while the ancient Egyptians exploited the physical and spiritual properties of aromatic oils, using them for medicinal purposes, food preservation, cosmetics and embalming. The Arabians used essential oils predominantly for the production of perfume, but the European countries barely made refer-

ence to them until the twelfth century, when the returning Crusaders extolled their virtues. Plant oils were subsequently used to ward off plague and illnesses and to disguise obnoxious smells.

By the seventeenth century, herbalists such as Culpeper made studies of the aphrodisiac and therapeutic qualities of oils. During the First World War, there was strong interest in their antiseptic and anti-inflammatory properties, and French surgeon Jean Valnet used essential oils to promote wound healing. In 1928, Rend Maurice Gattefosse first described the use of essential oils as a therapeutic aid in dermatology as 'aromatherapy'. Marguerite Maury went on to develop the technique of blending essential oils for use in therapeutic massage (McGilvery *et al.*, 1993).

Essential oils

Essential oils can be extracted from various parts of a plant through the process of distillation, expression, maceration, cold process or solvent extraction. The oils have a small molecular structure and are said to penetrate the skin, unlike vegetable oils, which can only lie on the surface. Through inhalation, essential oils can stimulate the olfactory stem, which transmits messages to the brain, releasing various neurochemicals that may be relaxant, stimulant, sedative or euphoria-inducing. Apart from their sensuous vapours, which are used in perfumes, the oils can also be ingested, added to baths, steam inhalations, combined with the technique of massage, and used in pot-pourri.

Aromatherapy in health care

The list of essential oils and their many uses is a long one, and it is impossible to give a comprehensive account here. Essential oils are generally used in health care to promote relaxation, reduce pain symptoms, treat muscular conditions, lower blood pressure, activate the immune activity, stimulate the digestive processes, release endorphins generating a feeling of well-being, and relieve colds and sore throats. They can act as an antiviral or antibacterial agent (Cosentino, 1999) and can reduce anxiety levels in intensive care units (Dunn *et al.*, 1995). They are also used in palliative care (Wilkinson, 1995) and in cardiac surgery environments (Stevenson, 1994).

Commonly used essential oils and their benefits
Basil is commonly used as a culinary herb, yet its essential oil is most beneficial when used as an anti-depressant or when combined with other oils such as thyme, which then acts as a powerful antiseptic. (Mode: inhalation and massage.)

Bay is a culinary herb with therapeutic properties that help relieve bronchitis, colds and influenza, and rheumatic aches and pains. (Mode: inhalation, baths and massage. Widely used in perfumes and exotic bath essences for its uplifting effects.)

Cedarwood is highly valued for its fragrance and its therapeutic qualities in dermatological practice, particularly in the treatment of acne, eczema and alopecia. It is also useful in relieving respiratory congestion due to bronchitis and catarrh. (Mode: inhalation and massage.)

Chamomile is a wild flower whose essential oil is renowned for its sedative properties and as an anti-inflammatory agent. (Mode: certain chamomile species are used for their herbal infusions such as tea, but the oil is used extensively for its anti-allergenic properties in cosmetic products for the body, bath and hair.)

Cinnamon is a spice that has a distinctive taste that is hot and peppery. Its oils are used as an anti-depressant, and for respiratory and digestive problems. It is also reputed to be an aphrodisiac. (Mode: inhalation and massage. Can also be used in pot-pourri.)

Comfrey is a wild plant, reputed to promote cell regeneration. It is therefore useful for the treatment of wounds and skin disorders. (Mode: massage, compresses and ingestion.)

Frankincense is the gum of a tree grown in Arabia, Africa, and China. Therapeutically its properties were recognised before the birth of Christ. It is said to aid concentration, preserve youthful skin, and act as a powerful expectorant. (Mode: inhalation, baths and massage.)

Lavender is a shrubby plant whose flower has a distinctive aroma. It is especially effective in harmonising the nervous and emotional systems. It is useful in alleviating migraines and can be used as an antiseptic and insect repellant. (Mode: inhalation, baths, massage.)

Lemon oil is obtained from the rind of the fruit and has a classic citrus aroma. It is a powerful antiseptic and astringent, and is widely used in skin problems. (Mode: inhalation, baths and massage.)

Rose oil is one of the most expensive essential oils. It is reputed to be a powerful aphrodisiac and mood enhancer. It is also used for circulatory problems and to relieve constipation. (Mode: baths, massage and pot-pourri.)

Ylang-Ylang is from a tropical tree native to Indonesia and the Philippines. It is generally used as a relaxant or for the treatment of high blood pressure. (Mode: baths and massage.)

Aromatherapy is a therapeutic medium, which allows personal choice both in the method of application and the essential oils used. When combined with massage, the time spent in the process of giving also enables the patient to share problems verbally, in the confidence that they will be heard sympathetically and without judgement. Through touch the therapist can share the experience of pain, developing a relationship that is empathetic to the patient's needs. In itself, aromatherapy is not a panacea, but it serves as a useful adjunct when combined with other therapies.

Study Activity 31.5 ─────────

- Visit a chemist or beauty shop where essential oils are sold. Smell the various perfumes and note those you like immediately and those you dislike. Read the literature available about them and identify their use, both as beauty aids and as therapeutic treatments.
- Collect information regarding the occasions when aromatherapy is used within nursing and health care practice. Visit the library and find relevant research papers on the efficacy of aromatherapy in health care.

- Identify any adverse indications (contraindications), when aromatherapy should not be used.

Therapeutic touch

Therapeutic touch is a concept that is growing in popularity. Alongside this, increasing numbers of people are visiting healers for therapy because they are dissatisfied with orthodox medicine (Wells and Tschudin, 1994).

Historical perspective

Therapeutic touch is a non-invasive therapy, which has its roots in China and India some 5000 years ago. Turton (1992) points out that both of these ancient cultures recognised the concept of 'vital energy' or 'life force' that could be channelled to enhance healing. In China this is known as *qi* and in India the term is *prana*. In ancient Greece, Hippocrates was renowned for his healing gift of 'touch', while the most famous healer known in the western hemisphere is Jesus Christ, and Christianity embraced the concept of healing through the 'laying on of hands'. Some who practised healing in this way were persecuted under witchcraft laws, but Turton (1992) points to one notable healer, Valentine Greatrake, who is recorded in historical documents of the seventeenth century as having cured many persons for a variety of ills through the laying on of hands.

In 1950, MacManaway was involved in two commissions on healing, one by the British Medical Association and the other by Bishops of Canterbury and York, the outcome of which concluded: 'any cure that is claimed to have resulted from healing is in fact due to wrong diagnosis, suggestion, remission, or spontaneous healing'. MacManaway (MacManaway and Turcan, 1983) points out that the concept of remission and spontaneous healing is only another way of accepting that something has happened for unexplainable reasons. By 1955, the National Federation of Spiritual Healers had been set up under the leadership of Harry Edwards, who was renowned for his gift of healing.

Dolores Krieger, Professor of Nursing in New York, showed interest in the concept of healing, and undertook a research programme using therapeutic touch as part of nursing practice (Krieger, 1981). She believed that an energy field that could be massaged and balanced by the hand surrounded all life. Her now-famous research study with persons suffering from myocardial infarction demonstrated that, after touch therapy, there was a rise in the patients' haemoglobin levels. The reasons for this rise have never been fully understood, but the results of the study were so significant that Krieger continued to instruct nurses in incorporating the technique into everyday practice.

Technique

Hippocrates recorded his perception of the healing process thus:

> *It is believed by experienced doctors that the heat which oozes out of the hand, on being applied to the sick, is highly salutary ... it has often appeared while I have been soothing my patients, as if there was a singular property in my hands to pull and draw away from the affected parts aches and diverse impurities, by laying my hand upon the place and by extending my fingers towards it.*
>
> (Cited in Harvey, 1983)

Contemporary descriptions of therapeutic touch imply a simple routine, but Krieger (1981) suggests that it should be much more complex. Wyatt (Wyatt and Dimmer, 1988) supports her argument, pointing out that:

> *therapeutic touch is performed on the human energy field, which is approximately three to five centimetres beyond the skin surface. It is an effort to balance this field and make it more uniform and smooth. This is achieved by the practitioner running her hands through the field in a head-to-toe direction.*
>
> (Wyatt and Dimmer, 1988)

There are six stages to the process, beginning with centering. In centering, the practitioner enters a relaxed state of mind and focuses on her breathing. Assessment of the patient's energy field, as identified by Wyatt, can then be made, with variations usually indicated as either hot or cold. These are noted mentally. Activation of the energy field will commence with brisk but smooth movement of the hands. Energy transference can now begin, with the practitioner visualising the energy, which is then drawn in through her head from the environment and directed to the depleted areas of the patient. The field is then balanced and smoothed to be as symmetrical as possible. Finally, the process is evaluated, to assess the amount of balance achieved.

Therapeutic touch and health care

Therapeutic touch is a non-invasive technique that is an excellent adjunct to traditional health care. Research has clearly demonstrated success in reducing anxiety, acute and chronic pain, and in reducing labour and delivery times in childbirth. Tinnerin (cited in Turton, 1992) provides the following example of the use of therapeutic touch in children's nursing:

> *Jamie had grossly inflamed intestines from Henoch-Schönlein's purpura. She found that following a couple of therapeutic touch sessions, Jamie had a virtually healed bowel. Clinically, Jamie presented a bewildering picture. The physicians were mystified and could not explain the negative findings, particularly when, three days earlier, his intestinal picture had been so glaringly poor. Tinnerin continued giving therapy and within two days Jamie's symptoms began to subside and eventually disappeared.*

Clearly, therapeutic touch can become an inherent feature of contemporary nursing practice. It is a therapy that considers patients as individuals with unique needs.

Study Activity 31.6

- Find information on therapeutic touch used in the UK and the USA. Discuss the advantages and disadvantages of this approach in contemporary health care.
- Find out if therapeutic touch is either used or recommended as a therapeutic medium in your clinical areas.
- If you have no skin sensitivity or contra-reasons why you should not experience aromatherapy, try massaging lavender oil into your skin at night after a stressful day. Write your own experience down in your reflective diary.

Shiatsu

Historical perspective

Shiatsu is a practice of Oriental origin that dates back over 5000 years. It is a form of healing that incorporates the use of touch of varying degrees of pressure to specific areas or points on the body. Shiatsu is a therapy more recently associated with Japan and officially licensed in 1957 by the Japanese Ministry of Health (Jarmey and Tschudin, cited in Wells and Tschudin, 1994). As with other complementary therapies, shiatsu encourages the activation of the body's self-healing properties. It relies on the ancient concepts of Do-In and Anma.

Do-In and Anma

Do-In is a form of self-application whereby the individual applies pressure to various meridian points through friction, percussion and stretching. It also involves the process of dynamic meditation, with breathing techniques being combined with physical activity. This practice is designed to promote a sense of mental as well as physical well-being.

Anma is an ancient technique used in the Orient as a form of daily healing and is practised to promote well-being, relieve tension, minor aches and pains, and prevent ill-health. Rankin-Box (1992) suggests that the practice of Anma is more akin to shiatsu and may be its precursor. It involves the use of pressure, kneading and stretching, and a general knowledge and understanding of the meridian system.

Yin and Yang

In Oriental healing, the notion of the human body's harmonious relationship is of paramount importance and is expressed through the concept of Yin and Yang. According to the concept, everything in the universe has opposing but complementary properties, and this is reflected in the Chinese symbol for Yin and Yang (*see* Figure 31.4).

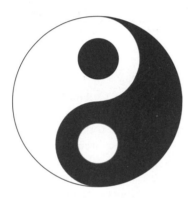

Figure 31.4   The Yin/Yang symbol

Yin is associated with cold, dark, rest and passivity, while Yang represents warmth, brightness, activity and movement. Jarmey and Tschudin (cited in Wells and Tschudin, 1994) illustrate the comparisons between Yin and Yang in Table 33.2.

If a person has too much Yin or Yang, they will succumb to ill-health. Restoring balance is therefore a necessary feature of shiatsu therapy.

Technique

In essence, shiatsu includes the use of the palms, thumbs, knees, forearms, elbows and feet. The Japanese Ministry of Health and Welfare describes shiatsu as follows:

> *Shiatsu therapy is a form of manipulation administered by the thumb, fingers and palms*

Table 31.2   The properties of Yin and Yang

Yin	Yang
Shade	Brightness
Female	Male
Moon	Sun
Rest	Activity
Material	Immaterial
Contraction	Expansion
Soft	Hard
Concerning the body	
Front	Back
Organ's substance	Energy supplying organ
Interior organs	Exterior tissue – skin
Blood and other body fluids	Ki
Moist	Dry
Slow	Rapid
Cold	Hot
Sinking	Rising
Clinical manifestations	
Chronic disease	Acute disease
Gradual onset	Rapid onset
Pale face	Red face
Not thirsty	Thirsty
Loose stools	Constipated
Cold	Heat
Sleepiness	Restlessness, insomnia

> *(plus elbows, knees and feet), without the use of any instrument, mechanical or otherwise, to apply pressure to the human skin, to correct internal malfunctioning, promote and and maintain health, and treat specific diseases.*
>
> (Jarmey and Tschudin, 1994)

Shiatsu is a process designed to restore the balance of the body's *ki* energy levels and, in so doing, release this energy from blocked channels, thereby relieving pain, correcting internal malfunctioning, and promoting a sense of well-being.

All functions and organs of the body are linked by meridian channels (*see* Figure 31.5). At certain strategic points, these channels are close to the surface of the body, enabling pressure to be exerted and *ki* energy to be released.

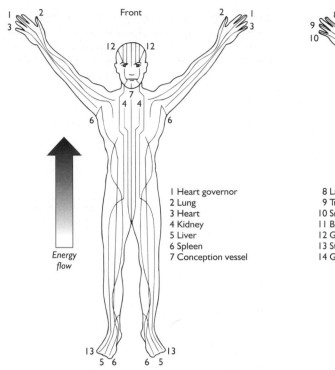
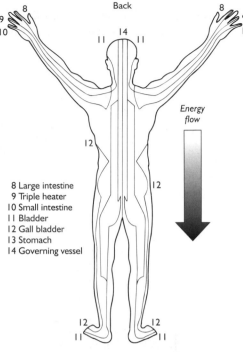

1 Heart governor
2 Lung
3 Heart
4 Kidney
5 Liver
6 Spleen
7 Conception vessel

8 Large intestine
9 Triple heater
10 Small intestine
11 Bladder
12 Gall bladder
13 Stomach
14 Governing vessel

Figure 31.5 The meridian system

In giving shiatsu therapy, the therapist must adhere to certain principles:

- Prior to the therapy a comprehensive assessment of the patient's health status must be undertaken.
- The therapist must be healthy, in order to enable an exchange of vital energy between the therapist and the recipient.
- The therapist should be relaxed and able to achieve a state of centredness.
- Pressure should always be applied at right-angles.
- The therapist must be competent to practice the art and technique of shiatsu.

Tonyfying

Tonyfying involves the application of stationary pressure at a specific point using thumb or fingertip for a maximum of two minutes. After this time, either a reaction will have been felt or the therapist will need to try a different position. Dispersing *ki* energy is released smoothly along the channel by applying pressure with the thumb or finger on the site, in a circular movement.

Calming

This is achieved by placing the palms over an area of high *ki* activity to induce a calming effect.

Shiatsu and health care

Shiatsu is a technique that has the potential to be used in the everyday practice of health care. It can be used to teach patients basic principles of self-healing as in Do-In, or practised by a therapist, who can activate the body to self-heal and promote a sense of balance or harmony. It is particularly beneficial in reducing the symptoms of stress-related illnesses such as back pain, in improving posture, stamina, digestion and libido, correcting menstrual disorders, easing childbirth, and relieving headaches.

As with most therapies, there are certain circumstances when the use of shiatsu is inadvisable. These include severe skin conditions, burns, high temperatures, bleeding, painful swellings, cancer, and degenerative diseases.

Study Activity 31.7

Visit a shiatsu therapist and explore the range of health problems for which shiatsu is used. If possible, ask to observe the technique being practised.

Acupuncture

Historical perspective

In acupuncture, a feature of Oriental health care that has evolved since the period between 8000 and 3000 BC, fine needles are inserted at strategic points in the body in order to achieve a therapeutic effect. There is evidence to suggest that primitive man used stone needles to puncture the skin, and these were later superseded by needles of bone and bamboo (Downey, 1992). Through the process of trial and error a comprehensive knowledge has developed, with the notion that pathways or channels possessing 'vital energy' circulate throughout the body. This concept was first recorded in the second century BC in a classic text known as the *Huang Di Nei Jing* (Wadlow, 1994, cited in Wells and Tschudin, 1994). The principles highlighted in this text remain the same today but some developments and refinements have occurred over the centuries.

The principles and philosophies of acupuncture are similarly expressed in other Oriental therapies such as shiatsu and reflexology, the main premise being that the body is endowed with *qi* energy that travels through channels in the body. This energy is harmoniously balanced through the position of Yin and Yang, so that when there is too much of either Yin or Yang the individual suffers from ill-health.

The meridian channels run close to the surface of the skin at strategic points and it is at these points that acupuncture needles can be inserted to unblock the channels and restore balance. Downey (1992) points out that there are twelve major meridians and eight minor ones. The major ones are identified either with Yin or Yang and have a corresponding organ (*see* Table 31.3):

Table 31.3 The organs associated with Yin and Yang

Yin	Yang
Lung	Colon
Spleen	Stomach
Heart	Small intestine
Heart governor	Triple heater
Kidney	Bladder
Liver	Gall bladder

Technique

As with all complementary therapies, the assessment process is detailed and exact. The first consultation may last for up to two hours, and will include a recording of past and present medical, dietary and social history, followed by a full examination, enabling the practitioner to make an accurate diagnosis. Prior to the beginning of treatment, the therapist will discuss any findings with the patient and then, with the patient's consent, commence treatment.

Acupuncture needles vary in size from 1.7 cm to 10 cm. They are very fine and solid. The most commonly used areas are the feet, lower leg, hands, and forearm. Treatment can last from a few seconds to an hour, depending on the nature of the problem. Insertion of the needles causes no pain but the patient may experience a tingling or numbing sensation.

Acupuncture and health care

In China today, acupuncture remains a central feature of health care (along with herbal medicine, massage, dietary therapy and therapeutic exercise, all of which represent Traditional Chinese Medicine). This approach to health care is not viewed as complementary to modern western medicine, but of equal contribution. Acupuncture is widely used in Asia to treat a myriad of conditions, and is often co-jointly used with other therapies including western medicine.

The World Health Organisation (WHO), recognising the growing interest in acupuncture worldwide, consulted with the Chinese Ministry of Health to share its experiences. As a result of the consultation, WHO (1979) went on to identify a range of diseases that could be usefully treated through acupuncture (Table 31.4).

In 1997, the US National Institute of Health conference on acupuncture concluded that research had provided a body of knowledge illustrating that the technique releases opiods and peptides in the central nervous system, and leads to changes in the peripheral and neuroendocrine function. From the growing body of evidence, it was identified that acupuncture can play a significant role when used either in an isolated way, or as an adjunct to conventional medicine. It was felt that acupuncture could be effectively used with addiction, stroke rehabilitation, headache, gynaecological problems, headaches, muscular problems, osteoarthritis, asthma, nausea and pain (Parker, 2000). A randomised control study on the use of acupuncture relating to stroke demonstrated that patients improved significantly better than the non-controlled group during a six-week treatment period, and had improved even further at the follow-up period of one year (Kjendahl *et al.*, 1997).

The 'Acupuncture trials' website lists more than 150 randomised clinical trials during the period 1995–8, which support the claim made at the 1997 acupuncture conference.

The growing body of evidence indicating the efficacy of acupuncture has led to an increase in the use of the technique throughout the western hemisphere. In the UK there are two schools of acupuncture: the traditionalists who base their work on Traditional Chinese Medicine and

Table 31.4 Disorders that can be treated by acupuncture

Upper respiratory tract Acute sinusitis Acute rhinitis Common cold Acute tonsilitis	Acute and chronic gastritis Gastric hyperacidity Chronic duodenal ulcer Acute bacillary dystentery Constipation Diarrhoea
Respiratory tract Acute bronchitis Bronchial asthma	**Neurological/muscular/skeletal disorders** Headache Migraine
Disorders of the eye Acute conjunctivitis Central retinitis Myopia (in children) Cataract	Trigeminal neuralgia Facial palsy Pareses following stroke Peripheral neuropathies Sequelae of poliomyelitis Menières disease
Disorders of the mouth Toothache Post-extraction pain Gingivitis Acute and chronic pharyngitis	Bladder dysfunction Enuresis Intercostal neuralgia Frozen shoulder Tennis elbow Sciatica
Gastrointestinal system Spasms of the oesophagus Hiccups	Low back pain Osteoarthritis

Reproduced with permission from the World Health Organisation (1979, cited in Wells and Tschudin, 1994)

those who practise the technique for the purpose of relieving pain, including doctors, dentists, nurses, midwives and physiotherapists. Increasingly, hospitals and health clinics operating within the NHS have established the use of acupuncture as a form of analgesia within daily practice.

Study Activity 31.8

- Observe an acupuncture therapist in action.
- Discuss the range of clinical use.
- Ask the patient to give an account of their experience.
- Explore the literature for evidence of positive health outcomes.

Reflexology

Reflex therapy relates to the notion that all organs, systems and structures of the body are 'reflected' on to the feet or hands. Therefore if pressure is exerted at a strategic point on either hands or feet, stimulus will occur in a corresponding organ or system (Figure 31.6). This stimulation of the organ or system activates the body's natural self-healing properties and the system's ability to maintain equilibrium (homeostasis).

The philosophical principles underpinning reflexology are based upon the ancient Oriental belief that energy pathways travel through the body connecting each part and terminating in either the hands or feet. Each part of the body is divided into ten zones, through which the energy travels in a longitudinal manner, and these zones are reflected in a specific area of the foot. In effect, the feet are a map of the body. If an organ or system is malfunctioning in any part of the zone, the energy flow is blocked, affecting all the other organs and systems that relate to that zone. By applying pressure in a specific way to

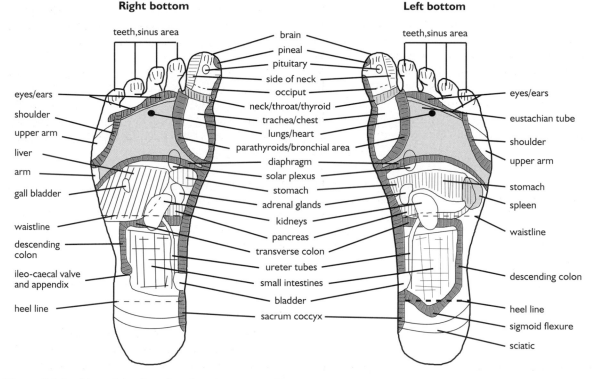

Figure 31.6 Map of the feet showing placement of organs

the zone's terminal reflexes (feet or hands), tension and congestion are released, allowing the energy to flow freely and restoring the body's harmonious, healthy relationship.

Historical perspective

Reflexology is a concept that has been understood and practised as a healing therapy for thousands of years. It appears in a wall painting in an Egyptian tomb dating back to 2300 BC. Early in the twentieth century doctors observed reflexology being used by the American Indians to relieve pain and promote a sense of well-being. A couple of decades later, Eunice Ingham Stopfel compiled charts locating the reflexes on the feet, which she used to develop a particular pressure technique. She was instrumental in drawing popular attention to the study of reflexology. The International Institute of Reflexology continues to research and develop the art and science of reflexology based on Stopfel's work.

Technique

Reflexology is a non-invasive therapy, which relies on the interconnectedness between two people, the receiver and provider. The therapist uses the art of touch in a caring and specific manner, recognising that the feet are particularly sensitive areas of the body. Prior to the commencement of treatment, the development of a rapport between the therapist and the patient is essential, and the environment should be conducive to relaxation. Ideally, the patient should be lying down, with the feet in alignment with the therapist's chest. Initial contact with the feet is important in setting the right tone. The therapist should hold both feet gently, to enable the patient to relax and to form a relationship. The following aspects of the feet are then examined:

- temperature
- skeletal structure
- tissue tonus
- the skin.

Reflex therapy involves the use of the thumb and fingers. The thumb, moving only the distal joint, moves in a caterpillar walk in a forward direction, usually beginning with the toes, followed by the sole, and then the ankle area. The movement is slow and rhythmic and the pressure is of an even nature. During the therapy, both hands always remain in contact with the feet, providing a sense of comfort and support.

Reflexology and health care

Reflexology promotes a sense of well-being and activates the self-healing properties of the body. It is of particular benefit in reducing stress and associated diseases. In addition, it can relieve depression, muscular spasm and pain, and restore hormonal imbalance in women suffering from dysmenorrhoea or menopausal symptoms. The use of reflexology in the control and relief of chronic and acute pain is growing in popularity. In midwifery, for example, reflexology is used during labour to relieve backache during the first stage, to sedate strong labour pains or to stimulate contractions during the second stage, and, if necessary, to stimulate the delivery of the placenta. Therapy can continue in the puerperium period as a relaxant, to relieve perineal discomfort, and to stimulate the flow of breast milk.

Reflexology can be given safely in conjunction with orthodox treatments. While it is not a panacea for all ills, it can activate each cell in the body to work in conjunction with one another, in order to promote total health and balance (Goodwin, 1992).

Study Activity 31.9 ────────────

- With a colleague, practise massaging each other's feet and evaluate the experience.
- Using Figure 31.6 opposite, identify the points in the foot that correspond to particular organs.

Hypnosis

Hypnosis is described as the inducing of an altered state of consciousness whereby the subject is not asleep but in a trance. Trances can be associated with daydreaming.

Historical perspective

Throughout history humans have indulged in the practice of hypnosis. Shamans and witch doctors commonly used it, while in ancient India, yoga transcripts described different levels of meditation, corresponding to different states of consciousness. The use of hypnosis in contemporary health care is said to have begun with Franz Mesmer in 1773. Because Mesmer relied on theatrical effect he was not taken seriously by his peers and was ultimately discredited. From this point, the recognition and value of hypnosis in health care has been a contentious issue (Tamin, 1992, cited in Rankin-Box, 1992).

In the nineteenth century James Braid examined the practice, and first referred to it as hypnosis. Freud, on the other hand, found no advantage with the therapy and his rejection was seen as a major setback in the development of its use. During the First World War, Ernst Simmel revisited the concept in an attempt to treat patients suffering from war neurosis. His work interested psychologists in the USA, including Erickson and Spiegel, who further developed techniques for use in health care practice. As a result, their work is said to have influenced and provided a foundation for contemporary practice.

Technique

A variety of techniques are employed to induce a hypnotic state, but most will aim to achieve the following:

- induce trance
- deepen the trance
- strengthen the ego
- allow post-hypnotic suggestion
- end the trance state.

A trance can be induced by asking a patient to fix on a point until the eyes feel heavy. When the eyes are closed, the patient is said to have begun entry into trance. Deeper trance states are achieved through the process of relaxation and visualisation of peaceful scenes such as walking on a beach or visiting a rose garden. The more vivid the sounds, smells and sensations become, the deeper the trance state. Ego strengthening can begin when the patient has reached a deep trance. This stage involves positive suggestions being offered to the subconscious mind. For example, the therapist may suggest that the patient is more relaxed and feeling in control of life, imparting a feeling of self-confidence and self-assurance. Post-hypnotic suggestions can reinforce the learning that has occurred in the trance by promoting a continued feeling of self-worth, but they will only work if the patient accepts them. Finally, the therapist concludes the therapy by gradually encouraging the patient to return to consciousness and a feeling of refreshment (Tamin, 1992, cited in Rankin-Box, 1992).

Hypnosis in health care

As with most complementary therapies, hypnosis can be used in a wide range of applications. It is increasingly used within the context of mental health, palliative care, midwifery practice, dentistry and minor surgery. A number of health problems can be treated through hypnosis:

- physical problems – such as intractable pain, hormonal dysfunction and migraine;
- psychological problems – such as behavioural problems, anxiety states and phobias;
- health problems associated with children – such as enuresis, tics and stammers.

Hypnosis can be used effectively as a means of complementary health care. Used in a therapeutic sense, it has a wide application and is free from side-effects. However, it is most effective in conjunction with orthodox medicine.

Study Activity 31.10 _____

- Sitting quietly, relax, take a few deep breaths, and allow your mind to wander to a recent pleasant experience. Note the detail and clarity with which you can recall the scene.
- List the range of clinical applications of hypnosis.

- Seek out relevant research papers.
- Debate the moral and legal implications of using hypnosis in health care.

Yoga

Historical perspective

Yoga is a philosophy, an art and a science, which has been a tradition in India for over two millennia. The word 'yoga' originated from the ancient Sanskrit *yuj*, meaning 'to join' or 'yoke'. On an individual level this refers to the notion that health is achieved when a person is united physically, psychologically and spiritually. In a much broader context, the philosophy of yoga perceives human life as a feature of universal law and requires the joining of each individual with the universal spirit to achieve self-realisation and the ultimate truth (McGilvery *et al.*, 1993).

Yoga philosophy has many different routes, or pathways, through which a practitioner can attempt to achieve universal harmony and enlightenment. However, they all feature a common ideological principle that seeks to attain the betterment of the individual and of humanity itself.

Archaeological records indicate that yoga was practised in India between 2500 and 1500 BC. In 220 BC, a scribe known as Patanjali wrote his treatise on yoga called *Yoga Aphorisms*, which is still considered an authoritative work today. Patanjali describes yoga as having eight limbs, all of which have equal importance and together make up the whole. McGilvery *et al.* (1993) describe them as follows:

- Five universal commandments (*yama*) aimed at creating a better world: not harming anyone or anything; truthfulness; not stealing; leading a godly; chaste life; and not grasping
- Five personal disciplines (*niyama*): cleanliness; contentedness; self-discipline; self-study and study of the Scriptures; and dedication to God
- Practice of postures (*asana*): devoted and conscientious practice of the various types of posture
- Practice of breath control (*pranayama*): practising breathing techniques with care and discrimination
- Detachment from worldly activities (*pratyahara*): developing a non-attached attitude of body and mind
- Concentration (*dharana*): being able to hold on to a subject mentally
- Meditation (*dhyana*): developing a quiet, meditative state
- Trance or a state of bliss (*samadhi*): reaching a state of absorption in a subject or in the Divine.

Technique

In the West the yoga techniques commonly practised are associated with different postures (*asana*) and breath control (*pranayama*).

Asana is a word taken from the Sanskrit language meaning 'to sit' or hold a posture or pose without discomfort to prepare the mind for meditation. Collectively, asanas are designed to stimulate and relax all the body's organs, systems, and structures, but each asana works on a specific area of the body. There are around 80 to 100 commonly known asanas. When practised regularly the therapeutic benefits are renowned. They work by stimulating the organs and systems of the body to increase their efficiency and effectiveness as a connected whole. This process facilitates an inner calm and a discipline of the mind in preparation for meditation (Bhole, 1974).

For the yoga practitioner, breath is a vehicle for vital force or energy. *Pranayama* is the control of that vital force, which permeates all elements of universal life. *Ayama* means control and *prana* is life force or vital energy. The effects of prana are believed to be therapeutic, and the more pranic energy received the less likely it is that the body will become ill.

Pranayama techniques require a prolonged exhalation and holding of the breath. There are several results of concentrating on breathing in this manner:

- It has a tranquillising effect and is particularly useful in anxiety states.
- Breathing is slowed, reducing the heart rate.
- Retention of the breath increases cellular breathing.
- It disciplines the mind between the subconscious and conscious psyche (Van Lysbeth, 1979).

Yoga and health care

Yoga is principally a way of life that promotes a holistic view of health within a universal context. Once they have been learned, individuals can adapt many of the techniques to suit their individual circumstances. It is used in health care to reduce the effects of modern-day stress and restore a sense of well-being. The practice of pranayama can create a sense of peace, reduce stress levels, slow the heart rate, and reduce blood pressure, while the practice of asanas can be used specifically to correct certain problems or to prevent ill health. Furthermore, yoga has been shown to be a powerful therapeutic tool for self-fulfilment and self-development, which, in a much broader context, can benefit humanity. Yoga has no age limit, nor is it focused only on the able-bodied. For example, individuals suffering from multiple sclerosis or arthritis can adapt certain asanas, which will prolong, or in some instances, increase the mobility of the joints and limbs (Widdowson, 1982).

Study Activity 31.11 ───────

- Describe the philosophies underpinning yoga.
- What are the therapeutic advantages of using yoga techniques?
- Practise the technique of pranayama daily and after two weeks evaluate your experience.
- Continue by combining pranayama with postural yoga poses for two weeks and evaluate your experience. (Postural yoga poses can be found in a range of self-help books. Choose one in your library and follow the instructions carefully.)

The manipulative therapies: osteopathy and chiropractic

Historical perspectives

Osteopathy and chiropractic share the same historical beginnings, both emerging from the folk tradition of 'bone setting'. In the late nineteenth century, US citizen Daniel Palmer developed a systemised approach that became known as chiropractic, while Andrew Taylor Still's similar system became known as osteopathy. The similarity is such that a number of textbooks refer to the systems collectively as 'the manipulative therapies'.

Techniques

Chiropractors and osteopaths use techniques that work on the soft tissue to increase a joint's range of movement or to relieve muscular spasm. The best-known technique is the 'high-velocity thrust', a short, sharp motion usually applied to the spinal region, and designed to release structures with a restricted range of movement. It is rather peculiar in that the thrusting action often produces a sound of a joint 'cracking', and this can be disturbing if the patient is unprepared. There are different methods associated with the 'high-velocity thrust' technique. Chiropractors more often use hand pressure on the vertebrae, whereas osteopaths favour the use of limbs to make a levered thrust.

Other models are commonly shared by the two professions, including the following:

- Soft-tissue techniques that use 'muscle energy techniques', technically known as 'proprioceptive neuromuscular facilitation', which is said to make use of post-isometric relaxation to increase the range of restricted movement
- Functional techniques, used to reduce pain – for example, in the hip joint – by applying a gentle, sustained pull to the limb (the leg, in the case of the hip joint), in conjunction with slow rotational movement. This technique requires an understanding of the neuromuscular behaviour and advanced palpatory skills

- cranial osteopathy, used by osteopaths, who place their hands on the cranium and sacrum and gently handle the bones of the skull. Skilled osteopaths can palpate the pulsation of the cerebrospinal fluid and, through correction to any disturbances detected, can restore balance to the neuromuscular system.

Chiropractic and osteopathy in health care

Both interventions are said to be complete systems of health care, based on the belief that any misalignment of the spine could have a relationship with most health conditions. However, most chiropractic or osteopath interventions are provided for musculoskeletal conditions. Lower back pain is a notable complaint and therapy (manipulative treatment) is highly recommended by the Royal College of General Practitioners, to be given within six weeks of pain symptoms. Reducing lower back pain symptoms through the application of manipulative techniques has been identified by Koes *et al.* (1992) and Meade *et al.* (1995), while Balon *et al.* (1998) have identified a positive health outcome in cases of childhood asthma. There are also said to have been health benefits in cases of sports injuries, neck injuries, repetitive strain disorder, arthritis, infantile colic and behavioural problems (treated with cranial osteopathy).

Study Activity 31 12 ————————

- Manipulative techniques such as osteopathy and chiropractic have reached integration with conventional medicine. Why do you think this is so?
- Reflecting on your patients who have had health conditions that relate to the muscular skeletal system or the neuromuscular system, describe the treatment given. Were any of the patients referred for manipulative therapy, or were they just given analgesia and advised to rest? Identify the rationale for the decisions made by the health care team.
- If conventional medicine was the only therapeutic intervention given, did the patient's symptoms improve?

- Explore the literature and seek out the recommended treatment for low, uncomplicated back pain.
- Try to find out how many working hours are lost in one year by employees who have low back pain.

SUMMARY

Western health care is beginning to embrace the concept of holism and technological intervention as a means of achieving a comprehensive integrated health care service. Individuals should consider in partnership with health care workers a range of therapies that may assist in the self-healing process. Nurses will play a significant role in this partnership, and should therefore have comprehensive knowledge and competence in a wide range of health care therapies.

Traditionally, nursing practice has reflected a medical model that relies heavily on technological intervention in the context of specialism. However, a human being is more than merely the sum of his parts, and health care provision needs to reflect this. A range of therapies are increasingly used as a complement to conventional medicine. Their roots are based within the concept of holism and within Oriental philosophies, which consider the physical, psychological, and spiritual factors of the body working harmoniously together.

Complementary therapies should not be seen as a panacea for all ills, or as a last resort when traditional therapies have failed. Nurses should not use these therapies because they are fashionable, but should consider them as a useful adjunct, or alternative, to conventional health care to facilitate the healing process. Kushi (1981) suggests that complementary therapies offer simplicity within a natural framework of explanation. Contemporary scientific knowledge, combined with intuitive knowledge that has evolved over time, has resulted in a wide-ranging repertoire that can contribute to the enrichment of health.

Nurse education has embraced the concept of total nursing care, in which the nurse is required to assess and respond to patients on every level, within a holistic, cultural and universal framework. This concept justifies complementary therapies and promotes a partnership arrangement in the delivery of health care. According to Vaughan (1988), a single step begins the journey of a thousand miles and in order to begin the process of healing, patients need to begin to heal themselves and their connections and relationships with their world. Achieving awareness of unifying consciousness empowers patients to engage with self-healing.

Complementary therapies are wide-ranging and can be used by all practitioners involved in health care. However, standards of practice vary, with educational programmes lasting from a weekend to several intensive years. Defining standards through legal regulation will ensure the safety of recipients and the accountability of individual practitioners.

REFERENCES

Autton, N. (1989) *Touch: An exploration*, Darton, Longman and Todd, London

Balon, J., Aker, P.D., Crowther, E.R. *et al.* (1998) A comparison of active and stimulated chiropractic manipulation as adjunctive treatment for childhood asthma. *New English Journal of Medicine* 339, 1013–20

Basford, L. (2001) Quantum healing: a nursing therapy (*www.shef.ac.uk/uni/projects/stti/*)

Bhole, M.V. (1974) *Therapeutic Importance of Yoga Practices*, University Yoga Publications, Connington, Cambridge

Chopra, D. (1990) *Quantum Healing: Exploring the frontiers of mind/body medicine*, Bantam Books, New York

Cosentino, B. (1999) Chiropractic: a new respect for an ancient treatment (*www.healthgate.com*)

Dalen, J.E. (1998) 'Conventional' and 'unconventional' medicine: can they be integrated? *Journal of Archives of Internal Medicine* [editorial] 158 (20)

Department of Health (2000) *Complementary Medicine*, DoH, London

Dossey *et al.* (1988) *Holistic Nursing: A handbook for practice*, Aspen Publishers, Gaithersberg, MD

Downey, S. (1992) Acupuncture. In: Rankin-Box, D.F. (ed.) (1992) *Complementary Health Therapies: A guide for nurses and the caring professions*, Chapman and Hall, London

Dunn, C., Sleep, J. and Collett, D. (1995) Sensing an improvement: an experimental study to evaluate the use of aromatherapy, massage and periods of rest in intensive care units. *Journal of Advanced Nursing* 1, 34–40

Eisenberg, D., Davies, R., Ettner, S. *et al.* (1998) Trends in alternative medicine use in the national survey, *Journal of American Medical Association* 11, 1569–75

Ernst, E. and Pittler, M.H. (1998) The effectiveness of acupuncture in treating acute dental pain: a systematic review, *British Journal of Dentistry* 184, 443–7

Goodwin, H. (1992) Reflex zone therapy. In: Rankin-Box, D.F. (ed.) (1992) *Complementary Health Therapies: A guide for nurses and the caring professions*, Chapman and Hall, London

Grossman, S.A., Benedetti, C., Payne, R. *et al.* (1999) NCCN practice guidelines for cancer pain. *Oncology* 13, 33–44

Harvey, D. (1983) *The Power to Heal: An investigation of healing and the healing experience*, The Aquarian Press, London

Hildebrande, S. (1994) Massage with essential oils: a quality of life, *Journal of Clinical Nursing* 1(3), 114–15

Kelner, M. and Wellman, B. (1997) Health care and consumer choice: medical and alternative therapies. *Social Science Medicine* 45, 203–12

Kjendahl, A., Sallstrom, S., Osten, P.E. *et al.* (1997) A one-year follow-up study on the effects of acupuncture in treatment of stroke patients in the subacute stage: a randomised controlled study, *Clinical Rehabilitation* 11(3), 192–200

Koes, B.W., Bouter, L.M., van Mameren, H. *et al.* (1992) Randomised clinical trial of manipulative therapy and physiotherapy for persistent back and neck complaints: results of one-year follow-up. *British Medical Journal* 304, 601-60

Krieger, D. (1981) *The Renaissance Nurse*, J.B. Lippincott, Philadelphia

Kushi, M. (1981) The Michio Kushi Institute of Great Britain, London. Cited in Rankin-Box, D.F. (ed.) (1992) *Complementary Health Therapies: A guide for nurses and the caring professions*, Chapman and Hall, London

MacDonald, R., Muirow, C. and Lau, J. (2000) Serenoa repens for benign prostatic hyperplasia. In: Cochrane Collaboration, Issue 2. Cochrane Library, Update Software, 2000, Oxford

MacManaway, B. and Turcan, J. (1983) *Healing*, Thorsons, Wellingborough

McGilvery, C., Reed, J. and Mehta, M. (1993) *The Encyclopedia of Aromatherapy, Massage and Yoga*, Acropolis Books, London

Mason, A. (1992) Massage. In: Rankin-Box, D.F. (ed.) (1992) *Complementary Health Therapies: A guide for nurses and the caring professions*, Chapman and Hall, London

Mazis, G.A. (1971) Touch and vision: re-thinking with Merleau-Ponty and Sartre on the carers. *Psychology Today* 23, 321–8

Meade, T., Dyer, W., Browne, W. *et al.* (1995) Randomised comparison of chiropractic and hospital outpatient management for low back pain: results from extended follow-up, *British Medical Journal* 11, 349–51

Melchart, D., Linde, K., Fischer, P. *et al.* (1999) Acupuncture for recurrent headaches: a systematic review of randomised controlled trials, *Cephalagia* 19, 779–86

Montague, A. (1971) *The Human Significance of the Skin*, Columbia University Press, New York

Parker, G.B., Tupling, H. and Pryor, D.S. (1978) A controlled trial of cervical manipulation of migraine. *Australian and New Zealand Journal of Medicine* 8(6), 589–93

Pearson, A. and MacMahan, R. (1991) *Nursing as Therapy*, Chapman and Hall, London

Pratt, J.W. and Mason, A. (1981) *The Caring Touch*, Heyden, London

Preyde, M. (2000) Effectiveness of massage therapy for sub-acute low back pain: a randomised controlled trial. *Canadian Medical Association Journal* 162(13), 1815–20

Rankin-Box, D.F. (ed.) (1992) *Complementary Health Therapies: A guide for nurses and the caring professions*, Chapman and Hall, London

Richardson. J., Jones, C. and Pilkington, K. (2001) Complementary therapies: what is the evidence for their use? *Journal of the Professional Nurse* 17(2), 96–9

Rohrbach, M.V. (1999) Complementary and conventional medicine: prejudices against and demands placed on natural care and conventional doctors, *Schweiz Med Wochenschr* 129(42), 1535–44. (*www.healthgate.com*)

Stevenson, C. (1994) The psychophysiosociological effects of aromatherapy massage following cardiac surgery. *Complementary Therapies in Medicine* 2(1), 27–35

Thomas, K.J., Nichol, J.P. and Coleman, P. (2001) Use and expenditure on complementary medicine in England: a population-based survey. *Journal of Complementary Therapies in Medicine* 9, 2–11

Turton, P. (1992) Healing: therapeutic touch. In: Rankin-Box, D.F. (ed.) (1992) *Complementary Health Therapies: A guide for nurses and the caring professions*, Chapman and Hall, London

Young, M.G. (1965) The human touch: who needs it? In: Stewart, J. (1965) *Bridges not Walls*, Addison-Wesley, Menlo Park, CA

Van Lysbeth, A. (1979) *Pranayama*, Unwin Paperbacks, London

Vaughan, F. (1988) Human survival and consciousness evolution. In: Grof, S. (ed.) Suny Press, Albany, New York

Vickers, A. (2000) Recent advances in complementary medicine. *British Medical Journal* 321, 683–6

Vickers, A., Ohlsson, A., Lacy, J.B. and Horsley, A. (1998) A massage therapy for premature and/or low birth-weight infants to improve weight gain and/or to decrease hospital length of stay. In: *Cochrane Collaboration*, Issue 3, The Cochrane Library, Oxford

Vincent, C. and Furnham, A. (1999) Complementary medicine: the state of evidence, *Journal of the Royal Society of Medicine* 92, 170–7

Watson, J. (1988) *The Philosophy and Science of Caring*, Associated University Press, CO

Wells, R. and Tschudin, V. (1994) *Wells Supportive Therapies in Health Care*, Baillière Tindall, London

White, P. (1998) Complementary medicine treatment of cancer: a survey of provision. *Journal of Complementary Therapies in Medicine* 6, 10–13

WHO (1979) cited in Wells, R. and Tschudin, V. (1994) *Wells Supportive Therapies in Health Care*, Baillière Tindall, London

Widdowson, R. (1982) *Yoga Made Easy*, Hamlyn Press, London

Wilkinson, S. (1995) Aromatherapy and massage in

palliative care. *International Journal of Palliative Nursing* **1**, 21–30

Wilt, T., Ishani, A., Stark, G. *et al.* (2000) Serenoa repens for benign prostatic hyperplasia. In: *Cochrane Collaboration*, Issue 2, Cochrane Library, Update Software 2000, Oxford

Wyatt, G. and Dimner, S. (1988) The balance of touch. *Nursing Times* **84**(21), 40–2

Zollman, C. and Vickers, A. (1999) ABC of complementary medicine: complementary medicine in conventional practice. *British Medical Journal* **319**, 901–4

Module 7: Therapeutic modes

Reflections

At the end of the previous module, we noted that the module marked a transition from earlier modules, which primarily (although not exclusively) addressed knowledge or theory concerns, to modules that primarily addressed practice issues. That module appropriately accommodated this point of transition in the book by addressing frameworks that might guide practice. Nurses are, of course, skilled practitioners and as such must bring high levels of competence to bear within highly complex health care systems. However, nursing is always in the context of relation, within which the nurse who is caring is thrust into helping relationships that in themselves have the power to exert positive influences. It is claimed (and hard evidence was presented within this module to sustain such claims) that these relationships can have healing influences. That is, they can be in and of themselves therapeutic. There is a clear logic in moving from frameworks, through relationships to the activities taking place within such relationships.

This module explored and presented arguments to sustain the premise that such relationships are therapeutic. The first chapter examined the nature of the therapeutic relationship. The second chapter explored the ways in which such relationships can themselves exert therapeutic influences. The third chapter extended the theme of healing by addressing the various complementary or alternative approaches that may be used as vehicles for realising this healing potential.

The claim that within our relationships with patients (using interpersonal processes alone, or complementary therapy aids), we have the capacity to heal, is a matter of some controversy. This may be in part a result of the suspicion many hold for healing terminology, with its links to some extreme fundamentalist religious movements and the various scandals associated with some of these. It may also of course be a reaction on the part of those who in the past held a monopoly on health care delivery and maintained this on a traditional scientific or biomedical science footing. You may find it helpful to reflect on the arguments for and against the idea that relationships can in themselves be therapeutic. In doing this, it might be helpful to consider:

- the ways in which some relationships have a negative influence on the partners, and sometimes even can be highly destructive;
- the argument that if evidence sustains such potentially negative influences, then the converse must logically apply.

MODULE 8: THE DELIVERY OF NURSING CARE

INTRODUCTION

Module 8 is concerned with aspects of the delivery of nursing care, commencing with an exploration of public health and the paradigms that underpin this concept. Indeed, public health is 'everyone's business', and should be a central theme that underpins the delivery of all nursing care. As part of promoting the health and well-being of individuals, nursing has a duty to provide a safe environment when care is delivered. We devote one chapter to this issue, recognising the duty of care and professional responsibilities of the nurse. In addition, we recognise the importance of giving assistance with daily activities of living when the patient can no longer undertake these all-important tasks themselves. In this module we recognise the nurse's role and include a chapter that relates to the concept of providing daily care to those vulnerable and sick individuals.

Next, the module raises the issues of managing and relieving pain and coping with death and bereavement. Both concepts are caring activities in which nurses have a pivotal role to play, and while they are significant nursing duties, in the past they have been severely under-addressed. There are many reasons for this, but in essence the main ones have been founded on the lack of knowledge and understanding of nurses themselves and the limited amount of available evidence to undertake their practice.

Finally, the module explores the dimension of caring in the community. This is a modern phenomenon that encourages health care professionals to care for their patients in a community framework as opposed to an institutional hospital setting. In your career, you will see an explosion of community developments, care pathways that require different organisational structures and the necessity of health and social care professionals working and learning together. Upon reading this chapter and applying the theories in practice to develop a comprehensive skill base, you will add to your repertoire of knowledge and understanding.

32 PUBLIC HEALTH: THE PROMOTION AND PROTECTION OF HEALTH

Ann Long

LEARNING OUTCOMES

After studying this chapter you will be able to:

- Define the term 'public health' in terms of its health concerns and public orientation
- Recognise that public health concerns extend beyond the immediate health concerns of the individual to the wider health concerns of communities, society as a whole, and even beyond national to international concerns
- Identify the factors that influence the health of the public
- Describe strategies designed to protect and improve the health of the public
- Outline the contribution of nursing to such strategies, particularly in respect of health promotion, health education and prevention
- Recognise an increasing global dimension in public health, and the implications of this for nursing.

INTRODUCTION

This chapter begins with presenting arguments on the definition and nature of health. It continues with examining the characteristics inherent in the global definition of public health and safety, including public health policies and future directions. The chapter proceeds with exploring the dimensions of health promotion and health education within the totality of public health and safety. A fervent argument on the topic of health empowerment is also presented.

HEALTH

There are many definitions of health. Indeed, scholars are now debating if it is a good idea to continue to strive to find a definition that suits everyone's taste and can be all encompassing (Fleming, 1999). The etymology of the word health suggests that it is related to words that mean 'wholeness', 'prosperity', and 'holiness'. Therefore, health, wholeness and sanctity are noted as being synonymous in the Germanic languages. Knowing this leads to a greater conundrum, as definitions of wholeness and sanctity are esoteric and nebulous. Ultimately, the concept of health is indefinite and cannot be categorised in the language of representational abstractions. Indeed, definitions of health that have not been rigorously analysed are little more than propositions that advocate well-meaning ideologies. Similar to beauty, which is in the 'eye of the beholder', health is a personal matter. Therefore, individuals define it according to their beliefs, values and satisfaction. Yet, it is one of our most valuable assets as it is a 'resource for everyday life: not the objective of living' (World Health Organisation, 1984, p. 23).

Examination of this definition means that health is a positive concept and without it we are not really living in the truest sense of the experience. It also means that in order to be and remain healthy, we need the physical capability as well as personal and social resources. Deeper examination of this concept of health reveals that the relationship between health and illness is not a bipolar one. Both health and illness are inextricably linked within the wider continuum of health. At one end of the continuum health is manifested in illness:

people who are disabled or have a chronic illness can be healthy by adopting health-enhancing behaviours and appropriate coping strategies that promote healthy living and improve the quality of their lives. At the other end of the health continuum, people who are healthy can be the carriers of the seeds of illness, which can be deprived of their potential threat by preventative action, healthy living and healthy lifestyles. Those who smoke or overindulge in any of the health-defying behaviours are examples of this group of people.

Health is also ascribed miscellaneous meanings according to the agenda of the particular groups who are describing it in society. Nurses might perceive health as the anticipated result of caring for patients. Politicians might regard it as a largely economic endeavour that should reap net gains from a defined financial investment and, in the long run, might save future government monies and encourage votes. To midwives, health might involve finding ways to marry the rights of women to choose their own types of care and delivery to the midwives' duties to provide safe and effective deliveries for mothers and infants. At times these interests converge (Fleming, 1999). The health of individuals, families, communities and the planet Earth is threatened from many sources. Therefore, it would seem appropriate to include all of these realities when defining our notion of health. Remember that over-reliance on textbooks for absolute definitions of abstract concepts sometimes leads to rigidity of thought and failure to tackle problems in a comprehensive and global way. This could result in nurses missing and therefore not addressing all the intrinsic and extrinsic factors that impact on an individual's health. Ultimately, health is a vital, alive and dynamic process that is forever changing and unique to each human being.

Study Activity 32.1

- Work with your peer group and create your own definition of health. Ensure that it covers cultural, socio/environmental, physical, psychological and spiritual dimensions of health.
- List five factors that impact on the health of the planet.
- What might you do to improve your health? List five factors that are blocking you from being healthy today.

PUBLIC HEALTH: A HISTORICAL OVERVIEW

During the nineteenth century, the natural environment was viewed as the potential source of ill-health. Dangers to health arose from the transmission of infections from one person to others they were in contact with. For example, tuberculosis existed within the body as a specific identifiable infection that was clinically treated by physicians. Health was a state that was either gained or lost by the disappearance of the infection. Little emphasis was placed on discovering and responding to the psychosocial spaces mapped out within close relationships, families, groups, communities and nations. Limited contemplation was given to finding ways of promoting the overall health of humankind and discovering what circumstances and events happen within and between people that impact on their health and well-being. For example, sexually transmitted diseases were manifested clinically in bodily responses and these were treated chemically in the hope of eradicating them. However, they also existed and spread through the medium of close physical relationships, the dynamics of which were analysed rarely except in art and literature. Preventive medicine eventually advanced and was no longer restricted to environmental questions such as sanitation, but became concerned with the minutia of social life and the ramifications of social behaviours. It became important to assess patients' contacts, family networks, and to provide home visits whereby health professionals could survey and constantly monitor the whole community in the hope of eradicating infections.

In the new public health agenda, inequalities,

inequities and poverty have been identified as being related to health (Benzeval *et al.*, 1995). The widening gap of inequality has moved the UK down the life expectancy ratings from 12th to 17th of the 24 member states, as indicated by the Organization for Economic Co-operative Development (Melling and Sutton, 1997). It is essential, therefore, to collect sound epidemiological data in order to design public health strategies that target and alleviate social needs.

PUBLIC HEALTH AND SAFETY

Within the UK, public health has been defined by the influential Acheson Committee (Department of Health and Social Security, 1988) as:

> *... the science and art of preventing disease, prolonging life and promoting health through organised efforts of society.*
> (Department of Health and Social Security, 1988)

Public health has been distinguished from health care interventions for individuals (whether they are in good health or ill-health) by its focus on community-wide or society-wide concerns. In this sense, public health is essentially about the prevention of ill-health at the societal level, and it is thus viewed as a health protection function. However, Downie *et al.* (1997) draw attention to the health promotion element in the Acheson Committee definition. Such health promotion also incorporates a specific targeted aspect that involves educational approaches, commonly referred to as health education. The bringing together of these protective, preventative, promotional and educational approaches under the public health banner draws attention to its proactive as well as reactive connotations, and identifies its level of operational activity as being at the level of the *public* (i.e. the community or society as a whole). It is often easy to link public health with terms such as primary care and community care. It is certainly the case that primary care is to a large extent preventative, while services provided for individuals and

communities within non-institutional settings share the term 'community' as an indicator of the target group. However, public health extends across non-institutional (community) and institutional (hospital, clinic, etc.) settings, across all age groups, and across the full range of environmental threats to physical and mental well-being. In addition, it takes in a wider range of health interventions, ranging from housing, water supply and sewage disposal (sometimes referred to as the environmental health element, and sometimes viewed as a separate area of functioning), through specific health interventions such as immunisation programmes, to health promotion approaches that include educational and public information activities.

Health protection is achieved through policy development at various levels from legislation to voluntary agreements and codes. The goal of public health and safety is to add to human comfort by preventing ill-health, promoting a return to good health and treating conditions for healthy living. Its aim is to generate organised community effort to address public concerns about health by applying scientific and technological change. Three interrelated pathways have been identified within the concept of public health (Cowley, 1999):

1 The traditional medical health as a product or outcome pathway – this aims to ensure that all dimensions of health are identified and problems treated, usually with medication.
2 A potential health as a beginning pathway – this aims to enable people to reach their optimum potential so that they can fulfil their opportunities in life, with identification and removal of obstacles that block health and well-being status.
3 Health as a process pathway – this places a holistic emphasis on the health and well-being of individuals, families and communities within their cultural/socio-economic environments, and the situations in which people live.

Synthesis of the concepts embraced in these pathways shows that public health is viewed as a 'population approach' as it aims to promote every individual's health. This contrasts with the approach that targets high-risk groups, which concentrates on those people who are supposedly at greatest risk of ill-health. The new public health agenda, therefore, is underpinned with the conviction that the health of every member of society is inextricably linked with the health of all other members. This means that the health of the whole society is dependent on the health of the poorest.

In addition, Antonovsky (1987) argues that attention should be focused on discovering how health is created and maintained rather than examining continuously illness and disease. This concept or model of 'health creation' encompasses three key elements: manageability, comprehensibility and meaningfulness. Manageability relates to the extent to which people feel they have the resources to respond to the conditions that arise in their daily lives. Comprehensibility relates to the degree to which people make sense of their social world when situations or events happen in their lives that impact on their health and well-being. Meaningfulness relates to the individual's ability to participate in the processes that might affect their future. In this model, people are the producers of health through healthy living and adopting health-protective behaviours.

Study Activity 32.2

- If nurses were to focus on the 'creation of health' model rather than the 'illness and disease model', how might interventions be changed?
- Would it be possible to use one model or are both models equally meaningful to nurses and patients?
- Give five reasons for your answer.

KEY DIMENSIONS IN PUBLIC HEALTH

There are four key interdependent dimensions included in the philosophical underpinnings related to public health and safety. They are: strategic directions for public health and safety;

health promotion; health education; and health empowerment.

Strategic directions for public health and safety

The *Health 21 – The health for all policy framework for the WHO European region* document (World Health Organisation, 1998) outlines the public health agenda until the year 2005. It highlights two goals, which are to promote and protect people's health throughout their lives and to reduce the incidence of the main diseases and injuries and alleviate the suffering they cause. The document identifies three key values: health as a fundamental human right; equality in health and solidarity in action between and within all countries and their populace; and participation and accountability of individuals, groups, institutions and communities for continued health enhancement.

The document provides detailed guidance for countries on how to formulate national health policies, focusing on the targets listed in Table 32.1. The targets add strategic direction for promoting public health and safety. Furthermore, the direction highlighted has a life of its own, which should be flexible enough to change proactively with emerging needs and aspirations.

In addition, health impact assessments and area regeneration will be encouraged to improve the socio-economic and environmental context for enhanced health chances.

In this new holistic agenda for public health, patients and their families/carers are part of the health-promoting network. They are no longer the passive recipients of care, but active participants within biographical and psychosocial spaces rather than within strictly anatomical boundaries. For the public health agenda to be effective, it is better to capture the voluntary element in human behaviour as individuals face more and more problems of coping and adjustment. The public health agenda can best be captured when people come to believe that they play an important part in creating and maintaining healthy relationships, healthy communication patterns and contented, healthy lives.

Table 32.1 Targets for health policies in European countries

- Closing the health gap between countries
- Closing the health gap within countries
- Creating supportive family policies that facilitate a healthy start in life
- Designing policies to reduce child abuse, accidents, drug abuse and unwanted pregnancies to promote the health of young people
- Creating health policies to improve health, self-esteem and independence in ageing
- Improving mental health
- Reducing communicable and non-communicable diseases
- Reducing injury from violence and accidents
- Promoting healthy and safe physical environments
- Promoting healthier living by designing fiscal, agricultural and retail policies that increase the availability of and access to fruits and vegetables
- Reducing harm from alcohol, drugs and tobacco
- Focusing on a 'settings approach' to health action, which means that homes and environments should be designed in a manner conducive to sustainable health
- Accepting a multi-sector responsibility for health
- Agreeing on an integrated health sector with much stronger emphasis on primary care
- Managing for quality of care using the European health for all indicators to focus on outcomes and compare the effectiveness of different inputs
- Providing equitable and sustainable funding
- Developing human resources such as educational programmes for providers and managers based on the principles of the health for all policy
- Advancing research and knowledge by providing health programmes based on scientific evidence
- Mobilising partners for health by engaging with the media/ television and the Internet

(From World Heath Organisation, 1998)

The ethos of health provision will also change as medical strategies shift from the pronouncements of experts towards concepts of 'informed choice', 'non-directive counselling' and the need for evidence-based, 'non-judgemental' health information that does not impinge on human rights or civil liberties as new empowering models of public health emerge (Kemm and Close, 1995; Simnet *et al.*, 1999; Scriven and Orme, 2001).

Two important reports have been issued recently that promote the public health agenda. They highlight the importance of integrating public health priorities within the primary care frameworks. Key recommendations include the need for health professionals to work together using a comprehensive, integrated approach to achieve the public health targets outlined in Table 32.1 (Department of Health, 1998; Taylor *et al.*, 1998). In the publication by Taylor *et al.* (1998), practical solutions were provided to help transpose the concept of public health into action at both national and local levels. It recommended strongly that organisations, communities and interest groups should work together to:

- tackle social and environmental issues
- focus on collaborative local strategies to achieve public health
- accept joint ownership for decision-making
- be collectively accountable at local and national levels, for identifying and evaluating health improvement
- develop outcome measures that are appropriate to measuring action on public health.

In 1999, the Government published a strategy to improve the health of everyone and particularly the health of people who are less secure financially (Department of Health, 1999a). This document focuses again on the axiom of working together and adds that some of the factors that harm people's health are beyond the control of any single individual. It provides examples such as housing, air pollution, unemployment, poor wages, crime and disorder. In addition, it advances guidance on designing and implementing measures for environmental protection. Equally important, it sets targets aimed at saving lives and preventing up to 300 000 untimely deaths by the year 2010:

- *Cancer* – to reduce the death rate in people under 75 years of age by at least one-fifth
- *Coronary heart disease and stroke* – to reduce the death rate in people under 75 years of age by at least two-fifths
- *Accidents* – to reduce the death rate by at least one-fifth and serious injury by at least one-tenth

- *Mental illness* – to reduce the death rate from suicide and undetermined injury by at least one-fifth (Department of Health, 1999b).

To achieve these targets, £21 billion was to be donated to the public health agenda with a focus on smoking as the single largest preventable cause of poor health. The Department of Health (1999a) report recommends that high standards must be set if these targets are to be achieved. They added the following recommendations for transposing the concepts to practice:

- establishing a new Health Development Agency described as a statutory body with the remit of raising the standards and quality of public health provision
- increasing education and training for health, with a new skill audit and workforce development plan and specific measures for all the disciplines of nursing and midwifery
- reviewing and critiquing public health information and establishing public health observatories in each National Health Service region, setting up disease registers and promoting research
- establishing a new public health fund.

Clearly the Government is committed to working towards improving the health and well-being of the total population by promoting healthy lifestyles, healthy environments and healthy working, as well as workable alliances between statutory, voluntary, community groups and all other interested parties and individuals. Influencing and transforming the new public health system is a dream of enlightenment that can become a reality for nursing. This is supported by the following citation:

> *Nurses have key and increasingly important roles to play in society's efforts to tackle the public health challenges of our time, as well as ensuring the provision of high quality, accessible, equitable, efficient and sensitive health services, which ensure continuity of care and address people's rights and changing needs.*
>
> (World Health Organisation, 2000)

This document continues with urging all relevant authorities in the World Health Organisation's European Region to step up their action to strengthen the nursing and midwifery contribution by: 'Ensuring a nursing and midwifery contribution to decision-making at all levels of policy development and implementation'.

This holistic concept of public health requires nurses to become competent in promoting and protecting people's health and safety throughout their lives, with the aim of contributing to 'health for all' (World Health Organisation, 1998). It recognises that the involvement of nurses in promoting health depends, to some extent, on how they are employed in the service (Gott and O'Brien, 1990). Thus, nurses in clinical areas will participate in health promotion at more face-to-face and group levels of provision, while those in management will have greater involvement with strategic and planning issues.

Health promotion

The nature and process of health promotion was formally recognised in the Ottawa Charter by the World Health Organisation (1986). Five key areas of health promotion were identified in the Charter:

- building healthy public policy
- creating supportive environments
- strengthening community action
- developing personal skills
- re-orientating health services.

Health promotion was defined as 'The process of enabling individuals to increase control over and improve their health' (World Health Organisation, 1986). The proposition relating to increasing control implies that individuals should be empowered through a range of health-promoting measures, which have policy, education and service provision implications. Moreover, most health-related activities assume that effective communication contributes to the process of moving health status beyond simple adherence to therapy (Ogden, 2000). This assumption is reflected in commonly used concepts such as 'process', 'enabling', 'facilitating', 'empowering' and 'control' as essential elements of health promotion (World Health Organisation, 1998).

Thus, health promotion has moved beyond the simple process of advice giving which sought to change health attitudes and behaviours. Indeed, Becker (1976) argued that people might be heavy smokers and also be aware of the consequences of their smoking but continue to value their smoking more than the projected life years they are sacrificing. It is very probable that most people have heard the health debates before they come into contact with nurses. Therefore, hearing them once again is unlikely to change their minds or influence their behaviours (Long, 2001). If nurses really want to promote health they must find out the reasons why people continue to engage in health-defying behaviours that they already know are damaging their health.

Study Activity 32.3

Work with your peer group and discuss:

- What do the terms 'enabling', 'facilitating', 'empowering', 'promoting' and 'control over one's health' mean to you?
- What do the terms 'informed choice', 'non-directive counselling' and 'non-judgemental health information' mean to you?
- What key communication skills do nurses require to participate in health promotion?
- Why do people continue to engage in health-defying behaviours such as smoking when they are aware of the risks associated with their behaviours?

Models and explanations of health promotion

Tannahill (1985) argued that health promotion consisted of the three overlapping dimensions of health education, prevention and health protec-

tion. During the next decade, a number of models and explanations of health promotion were advanced in UK literature (French, 1990; Ewles and Simnet, 1999; Tones and Tilford, 2001). Within these models it is acknowledged that health promotion focuses on individuals and incorporates lifestyle issues and structural (fiscal/ecological) elements. The French (1990) model of health promotion includes the four interlinked areas of disease management, disease prevention, health education and the politics of health. By including the dimension of disease management, French (1990) claimed that the cure or amelioration of disease raises, and therefore promotes, health status and consequently has a role to play in health promotion. Also included within the concept of disease management is the notion of relapse prevention, for example, the prevention of relapse in drug or alcohol abuse. Ewles and Simnet (1999), however, recognised the difficulty in embracing disease management within health promotion. On the one hand there are illness and disability services, and on the other 'positive health activities which are about personal, social and environmental changes to prevent ill-health and develop healthier conditions and ways of life' (pp. 22–3).

Hence, health education was also identified as a dimension within the broad umbrella term of health promotion (French, 1990). Including the dimension of health education was later supported by Ewles and Simnet (1999) and Downie et al. (1997).

In tandem with the development of these models and explanations, various strategic health promotion approaches have been developed. It is argued that traditional approaches to health promotion have proved ineffective in areas of social deprivation. Tones and Tilford (2001) claim that they are ineffective because they focus first on individuals and second on facilitating health gains through the mediums of education and behaviour change. Evidence shows that they have been unsuccessful in lowering the risk of illness from, for example, heart disease. By concentrating health promotion strategies on risk factors such as smoking, diet and exercise, wider issues were not addressed.

In addition, it is essential to note that these approaches contributed to the notion of 'victim blaming', which could be described as quasi-moral attempts to blame illnesses on certain lifestyles. Consequently, individuals are made to feel that they, personally, are the authors of their own ill-health. Linked to this have been several other developments that focused on different approaches to health promotion.

The 'settings' approach to health promotion was one such development that has been encouraged by the World Health Organisation (Scriven and Orme, 2001). The setting is viewed as any environment in which people spend significant parts of their lives, such as workplaces, schools, hospitals, prisons, cities and communities. The settings approach aims to enhance health status through the development of health-promoting environments, where health is facilitated by interdisciplinary and intersectoral approaches. A number of key settings have been developed, for example, promoting healthy cities (World Health Organisation, 1988), the health-promoting school (World Health Organisation, 1993) and the health-promoting hospital (World Health Organisation, 1994).

Community development approaches came into vogue in the 1980s. They were conceived from the belief that people, individually and collectively, have the person power to recreate and transform their own lives as well as the lives of others. These approaches embraced human principles such as hope, expectations, aspirations coupled with human action. For more detailed reading see Smithies and Webster (1998). The overall aim of community development is to address issues related to inequalities in health. The objectives are to:

- enable communities to gain ownership and some control over their environment
- set priorities and make decisions on improving health status
- plan, implement and evaluate strategies in order to achieve health gains in communities.

The health action zones approach is a recent policy initiative aimed at stimulating innovation and tackling health inequalities. It is recognised that health inequalities exist by income, occupation, gender, education, ethnicity, residency, age, weight and geographical locality. Studies demonstrate that many entrenched inequalities are actually widening (Acheson, 1998). Of notable concern are the health inequalities that are endured by groups who are marginalised by mainstream service provision and/or those experiencing social exclusion. The cornerstone of health action zone success is community participation, where all those contributing to the health and well-being of the population implement locally agreed strategies for improving the quality of health (Department of Health, 1998b).

Public health approaches advocate more innovative initiatives to delivering health promotion (Department of Health, 1999a). This report stresses that the fundamental role for the National Health Service is health improvement for the whole population – high health standards for all and not just for the financially better off. It advances the role that communities should play in public health and safety, with plans for people, communities and the Government to work together in partnership to improve the health status of the population.

Study Activity 32.4

Poor health springs from wider issues in the community.

- List six social/environmental factors that impact on people's health and well-being.
- If you had money and power, which of these factors would you attempt to redress first, and why?
- How might nurses contribute to the debate on influencing policies affecting health?

Health education

Health education is defined as: 'Any planned measure which aims to enhance health status/

awareness through increasing empowerment of targeted individuals/groups by the facilitation of learning' (Fleming, 1999, p. 64). Health education includes a number of activities that go well beyond the traditional notions of providing health information and takes place at primary, secondary and tertiary levels.

Primary health education focuses on providing scientific information on the risk factors associated with diseases such as smoking, diet, exercise, high blood pressure and related behavioural changes. It also involves providing knowledge on the services available and the development of life skills such as assertiveness, conflict resolution, negotiation, and lobbying.

Secondary health education is designed to provide health information on screen testing such as breast, cervical and testicular screening, as well as screening for sight and hearing loss. It is also related to the provision of monitoring techniques by environmental health departments and health and safety agencies to ensure the quality of air and water and hygiene standards in areas where food is prepared. The National Rivers Authority and various other regulatory bodies perform similar duties at a societal level through monitoring-related health and social issues.

Tertiary health education is related to the provision of health information for people who are living with established illnesses/disabilities. Tertiary health education aims to provide scientific information on the nature of the illness/disability, with expected outcomes and the nature of remedial/rehabilitation/relapse prevention measures.

Agenda setting is a further dimension of health education that is just outside the scope of the approaches described above. French (1990, p. 9) describes this as 'putting health on the agenda of policy makers'. It is also about helping people to develop their own health agendas. Tones and Tilford (2001) advanced this definition to include a process where governments evaluate and audit the public's acceptance of proposed health-related legislation. This leads us to the next key dimension in public health, health empowerment.

Health empowerment

Empowerment has been defined as 'a process of helping people assert control over the factors that affect their lives' (Sines, 1995, p. 31). However, this definition assumes that there is a very refined set of factors that affect people's lives. Therefore, if we do not control them, then there is something wrong with us. Nursing takes place within the context of power differentials and social inequalities and within the whims of political determination and economic change. Clearly, nursing does not take place in a vacuum; power dynamics are involved at all levels of life. For example, within the hierarchical nature of nursing itself, among nurses and other professionals, between nurses and patients/clients and also in the labelling process and the reconstruction of labels. Patients/clients/communities can also become the targets of inter-professional rivalry and conflict, which, in turn, renders them powerless and passive recipients of health information. In addition, power can be conveyed through the use of language such as medical jargon that professionals sometimes use to 'blind' others with. They use knowledge, skills and attitudes relating to scientific evidence that is not easily understood by the vast majority of people. An individual's sense of personal control over one's life is conditional on society's approval. Health empowerment is conditional on Government providing equality of opportunity to all members of the population in areas such as housing, education, employment, income, safety, civil liberties and health care. In the absence of such equality, health empowerment is merely a counterfeit exercise.

Study Activity 32.5 _____

It has been argued that empowerment means helping people gain control of factors that affect their lives. Discuss the following questions with your peer group:

- How do people control judgemental and discriminatory views and practices that are held in the wider community and beyond?

- How could nurses help to construct a culture of understanding, tolerance, acceptance and respect?
- How do we validate people who we 'socially construct' as different?
- How do we demonstrate that we are listening to their voices?
- How could we help make visible the invisible?

It seems evident that empowerment is difficult to define and even more puzzling to extrapolate to some areas of practice. However, the above readings mean that empowerment can also be seen as a political process whereby political power and its accompanying resources are transferred from service providers to service users. This quantum step means that service users would become stakeholders in the control of policy and not allow a charitable, professionally led agenda of what constitutes empowerment take over. In addition, it means that professionals should listen to people about their definitions of empowerment. Ultimately, this means sharing power with people who never had a legitimate access to power. Can you envisage a day when there will be user-led services? This type of initiative would seem to follow on from the current public health and safety agenda. It would require a shift in thinking from the dominating professional paradigms, which view health care as a discipline, to the axiom of health care as a gift and a generosity of spirit towards others. This type of ethos respects that each individual reacts to different situations and life-threatening conditions in their own unique way. It enables them to identify and own their personal thoughts and feelings, together with their culture, religion, sexual orientation and spirituality. It also respects and values their right to make decisions that affect their lives as well as their right not to make decisions. Therefore, in nursing, empowerment is very closely linked to anti-oppressive practice. Furthermore, it is associated with the practice of liberating people and promoting the social change that walks hand in hand with public health and safety. Finally, in the politics of nursing practice associated with public health and safety, who are the 'experts'?

Study Activity 32.6

Work with your peer group and discuss the following ethical issues:

- Are there times in people's lives when they cannot make decisions about their health and well-being?
- When might people have their right to make decisions denied for the 'common good'?
- List and discuss five other potential ethical dilemmas related to the promotion of public health and safety.

SUMMARY

This chapter examined notions of health, public health and safety and public policy in addition to health promotion and health education. It emphasised the need for a holistic approach to public health and safety that sought to promote the optimum health and full potential of the total population. The chapter continued with arguing for the need to work together to build healthy alliances with all other statutory, voluntary and community groups so that the services provided will eventually become people led, with professionals providing health knowledge and evidence from rigorous research to aid decision-making processes. Such an approach, supported by sound health legislation and financial support, would go some distance to improving the health of all members of the population. The provision of health-promoting opportunities targeted at individuals, families and communities provides nurses with exciting challenges as they continue to search for new and creative ways to promote, improve and maintain the health status of the population and of the planet (Craig, 2000; Mason and Clarke, 2001; Cowley, 2002).

REFERENCES

Acheson, D. (1998) *Independent Inquiry into Inequalities in Health*, HMSO, London

Antonovsky, A. (1987) *Unravelling the Mystery of Health: How people manage stress and stay well*, Jossey-Bass, San Francisco, CA

Becker, M.H. (1976) Sociobehavioral determinants of compliance. In: Sackett, D.L. and Haynes, R.B. (eds) *Compliance with Therapeutic Regimens*, Johns Hopkins University Press, Baltimore, Mass

Benzeval M., Judge, K. and Whitehead, M. (1995) *Tackling Inequalities in Health: An agenda for action*, King's Fund, London

Cowley, S. (1999) Purpose, process and power in public health nursing. *Nursing Review* 17(1/2), 30–4

Cowley, S. (ed.) (2002) *Public Health in Policy and Practice: A sourcebook for health visitors and community nurses*, Bailliere Tindall, London

Craig, P. (ed.) (2000) *Nursing for Public Health: Population-based care*, Churchill Livingstone, London

Department of Health (1998) *Shared Contributions, Shared Benefits. The report of the working group on public health and primary care*, Department of Health, London

Department of Health (1999a) *Saving Lives: our healthier nation*, The Stationery Office, London

Department of Health (1999b) *A National Service Framework for Mental Health. Modern standards and service models*, Department of Health, London

Department of Health and Social Security (1988) *Public Health in England. Report of the committee of inquiry into the future development of the public health function (Acheson Committee – Chairman Sir Donald Acheson)*, HMSO, London

Downie, R.S., Tannahill, C. and Tannahill, A. (1997) *Health Promotion Models and Values* (2nd edn), Oxford University Press, Oxford

Ewles, L. and Simnet, I. (1999) *Promoting Health: A practical guide* (4th edn), Scutari Press, London

Fleming, P. (1999) Health promotion. In: Long, A. (ed.) *Advanced Interaction for Community Nursing*, Macmillan, London

French, J. (1990) Boundaries and horizons: the role of health education within health promotion. *Health Education Journal* 49(1), 7–10

Gott, M. and O'Brien, M. (1990) The role of the nurse in health promotion. *Health Promotion International* 5(2), 137–43

Kemm, J. and Close, A. (1995) *Health Promotion Theory and Practice*, Macmillan Press, Basingstoke

Long, A. (2001) The labyrinth of health as perceived by two groups of community nurses. *Journal of Psychiatric and Mental Health Nursing* 7, 233–40

Mason, C. and Clarke, J. (2001) *A Nursing Vision of Public Health: All Ireland statement on public health and nursing*, DHSSPS, Belfast; DOH&C, Dublin

Melling, J. and Sutton, S. (1997) The information revolution, health reform and doctor manager relations. *Public Policy and Administration* 14, 1–13

Ogden, J. (2000) You're depressed? No I'm not. GPs' and patients' models of depression, *British Journal of General Practice* 49, 123–4

Scriven, A. and Orme, J. (eds) (2001) *Health Promotion: Professional perspectives* (2nd edn), Palgrave/Macmillan Press/Open University, Basingstoke

Simnet, I., Perkins, E. and Wright, L. (1999) *Evidence-based Health Promotion*, John Wiley, Chichester

Sines, D.T. (1995) *Community Health Care Nursing*, Blackwell Science, Oxford

Smithies, J. and Webster, G. (1998) *Community Involvement in Health: From passive recipients to active participants*, Ashgate Publishing, Aldershot

Tannahill, A. (1985) What is health promotion? *Health Education Journal* 44(4), 167–8

Taylor, P., Peckham, S. and Turton, P. (1998) *A Public Health Model of Primary Care – From concept to reality*, Public Health Alliance, London

Tones, K. and Tilford, S. (2001) *Health Education – Effectiveness, efficiency and equity* (3rd edn), Nelson Thornes, Cheltenham

World Health Organisation (1984) *Health Promotion: A discussion document on the concepts and principles*, WHO Regional Office for Europe, Copenhagen

World Health Organisation (1986) *Ottawa Charter on Health Promotion. An international conference on health promotion*, WHO Regional Office for Europe, Copenhagen

World Health Organisation (1988) *Healthy Cities, Papers 1, 2 and 3*, WHO Regional Office for Europe, Copenhagen

World Health Organisation (1993) *The Health Promoting School*, WHO Regional Office for Europe, Copenhagen

World Health Organisation (1994) *Health Promoting Hospitals – Aims and concepts, strategies and possibilities for participation in the network*, WHO Regional Office for Europe, Copenhagen

World Health Organisation (1998) *Health 21 – The health for all policy framework for the WHO European region*, WHO Regional Office for Europe, Copenhagen

World Health Organisation (2000) *Munich Declaration. Nurses and midwives: A force for health*, WHO Regional Office for Europe, Copenhagen

33 MAINTAINING A SAFE ENVIRONMENT

Clare Bale

LEARNING OUTCOMES

After studying this chapter you will be able to:

- Identify the areas of the biological sciences that are relevant to the control of infection
- Identify the main types of infection and their impact on health in the clinical setting
- Describe the various types of infection, in particular hospital-acquired infection and its implications in terms of human and financial resources
- Identify factors that contribute to patients' susceptibility to infections
- List and describe risk factors associated with certain body systems and clinical practices
- Identify the components of an effective infection control programme
- Explain the nurses' responsibility in infection control and the roles of the wider multidisciplinary team
- Discuss the ways in which the control of infection relates to the arena of professionalism and social policy.

INTRODUCTION

As we have already seen in earlier chapters, nursing activities incorporate the promotion of a broad concept of health, one that embraces wider definitions of well-being, as opposed to merely the absence of disease. The delivery of nursing care is informed by theoretical 'models' of care and the process of 'maintaining a safe environment' is one of the crucial elements within many of these frameworks.

The nurse has an obligation, both professional and social, to maintain safety. The genealogy of professional duty can be traced right back from the influence of the Hippocratic Oath, through Florence Nightingale's original edict that 'hospitals should do the sick no harm' (1863) and currently resides within the Nursing and Midwifery Councils *Code of Professional Conduct* (2002), in which nurses are guided to safeguard and promote the interests and well-being of patients and clients, through the identification of risk and action to minimise its effect. Socially, the framework to maintain safety resides within Government policy, legislation and National Health Service regulation, in particular the recently formed National Patient Safety Agency which acts as an independent body to encourage the National Health Service to learn from previous mistakes and prevent further erosion of patient safety.

Given that the nurse is arguably the most predominant 'formal' giver of care in Western society, she or he has the immediate capacity to facilitate the promotion (or reduction) of patients' health and well-being. Inextricably linked to this action is the duty to maintain a safe environment. However, evidence suggests that hospitals and health care are not always safe (Plowman, 1997). In fact, the formation of the National Patient Safety Agency devolved directly from statistics which illustrated that adverse events occur in around 10% of admissions a year. From this statement it may be inferred that there must be 'good' and 'bad' nurses – nurses who maintain safety and those who reduce it. Indeed, there are many moralistic or emotive ways in which one may view the professional activities of the nurse. For example, from the patients' point of view, the 'good' nurse may be one who is gentle, always smiling and who takes time to answer any concerns and worries. The importance of these altruistic elements is widely recognised by members of society (not only at a professional level but particularly by those who have experienced the need for them). In light of this, the role of the nurse as advocate for patients is of paramount importance when considering the issue of safety.

The aim of this chapter, however, is not to validate value judgements around the notion of good or bad care, but to examine the knowledge base and skills required for the nurse to promote safety.

There are many aspects to the maintenance of a safe environment of which you as a student nurse must be aware (*see* Table 33.1 for a summary of these). The concept of maintaining a safe environment incorporates many elements integral to the delivery of 'patient' care, both physical and psychological. For example, physical activities such as moving and handling, wound care and intravenous therapy, as well as the less tangible activities of consent, advocacy, confidentiality and equal opportunities. All of the above have the potential to impact upon the physical or emotional well-being of the patient. In addition, the modern discourse of work-related health and safety means it also involves the occupational maintenance of safety for nursing staff and other health care employees. Therefore, issues such as stress management, adherence to policy and procedure and record keeping are now part of

Table 33.1 Elements influencing the safety of the environment

Building and planning
Control of Substances Hazardous to Health (COSHH)
  regulations
First aid (including CPR)
Fire prevention
Ionising radiation
Infection control
Moving and handling
Nutrition and food hygiene
Pollution control
Stress at work
Violence and aggression
Work-related injury

the safety agenda and crucial to the protection of both patients and staff alike. The maintenance of a safe environment cannot be discussed without awareness of such issues. However, for the duration of this chapter, you are invited to concentrate upon the vehicle of infection control in the acute setting, and upon the importance of the nurse's professional role in controlling and reducing risk to well-being. It will examine the routes and mechanisms through which the maintenance of a safe environment and infection control may be promoted, as every aspect of patient care has infection control implications. There is no longer room for complacency with regards to compliance (Ward, 1994), as infection control is an important issue permeating through theory and to the activity of nursing itself.

Study Activity 33.1

Using Table 33.1 as a guideline, liaise with environmental health and your local infection control team to source the formal legislation that governs each element of safety provision. Through open discussion with your clinical mentors and colleagues, consider and reflect upon where these various pieces of legislation interface with nursing care and management.

INFECTION AND THE BIOLOGICAL SCIENCES

Infection is defined as 'the entry and multiplication of an infectious agent, such as a micro-organism, in the tissue of a host, resulting in disease' (Williams *et al.*, 1960). Apart from the serious disease-causing microbes, healthy people and most micro-organisms coexist in harmony most of the time. Any disruption, however, of the equilibrium between the two enables the micro-organism to penetrate the body's defence mechanisms and cause infection. There are many factors which contribute to the acquisition of infection in an individual, such as age, nutritional status and medical intervention; these will be discussed later in the chapter. Before examining these factors, let us first consider the various types of infection that exist.

In order to be conversant in the theory of, and apply an effective approach to, infection control care, the nurse must be aware of the four areas of biological science which relate to the subject (Horton, 1995). These can be defined in the following way:

- Anatomy and physiology (how the body works)
- Basic microbiology (characteristics of micro-organisms and their effect on the body)
- Applied microbiology (how micro-organisms behave in the clinical setting)
- Pharmacology (the response of the body to the introduction of drugs).

INFECTIONS CAN BE EITHER 'ENDOGENOUS' OR 'EXOGENOUS'

When the micro-organisms responsible for infection are 'resident', that is they belong to the patient's own microbiota or flora, the infection which results is classed as *endogenous*. There are a number of micro-organisms which exist naturally on or within the human body. These are classed as 'natural flora' and in the healthy individual exist without the individual being aware of their presence. Skin flora or 'resident' micro-organisms may be transferred from one body part to another, for example, from the nose, to the hand and then onto a vulnerable site such as a wound. Resident organisms rarely cause significant problems in healthy hosts, but will exploit vulnerabilities in the weakened host. If the delicate balance between the natural flora and the body's defence mechanisms is disrupted, for example when the immune system is compromised through illness, then symptoms of infection may occur.

The body has an effective shield in place to protect itself – the skin. The skin is the largest organ in the body and normally presents an effective barrier to the penetration of the underlying structures by harmful micro-organisms. This shield is of further use because skin flora

produce substances known to have anti-microbial properties, and these prevent or retard colonisation by other *exogenous* micro-organisms (i.e. organisms from an external source).

Because microbial cells are much too small to be seen with the naked eye, different types of micro-organism can be differentiated using stains and microscopic investigation. Gram's reaction is used to highlight and contrast various cell structures and therefore types of micro-organism. Gram-positive bacteria have a thick protective cellular wall, whereas Gram-negative bacteria have a thin inner cell wall and an outer membrane.

Many varieties of both Gram-positive and Gram-negative micro-organisms exist on the skin and can be found at any site on the body, including the perineum. Up to half the population is thought to carry *Staphylococcus aureus* in their anterior nares (Williams *et al.*, 1960). Some harmful micro-organisms known as '*clinically significant*' are frequently encountered in clinical practice.

When the microbiological source is external, the resulting infection is classed as *exogenous*, and there are a number of micro-organisms which can cause disease or infection should they be transferred to a susceptible human host. The micro-organisms responsible for exogenous infection are '*transient*' in that they may be passed from one patient to another through a variety of mediums, including the nurse. The human body is familiar, and able to cope with, its own resident organisms. If though, the host is compromised by illness, as is likely within secondary or acute settings, cross-infection or hospital-acquired infection is likely to be the result. Table 33.2 (overleaf) lists some of the main micro-organisms and the possible infections they are associated with.

Study Activity 33.2 —————

- By reading basic textbooks on microbiology, source the following information to underpin your knowledge and skills related to infection control:

Table 33.2   Some of the most common infections

Staphylococcus aureus (Gram-positive)	Bacteraemia, sepsis, septic shock toxic shock syndrome, skin and soft tissue infections, impetigo, burns, folliculitis, furuncles and carbuncles, cellulitis, bite wound infections, lymphadenopathy, lymphadenitis, lymphangitis, infective endocarditis, osteomyelitis, infectious arthritis, diskitis, myositis suppurative, bursitis, neonatal mastitis.
Escherichia coli (Gram-negative)	Acute enteritis, prostatitis, epididymitis, urinary tract infections, renal abscess, neonatal mastitis.
Pseudomonas aeruginosa (Gram-negative)	Urinary tract infections, renal abscess.

- – The classification of micro-organisms
- – The characteristics of micro-organisms
- – Micro-organisms of clinical significance
- – The pharmacology of antibiotic therapy.
- • List three Gram-positive and three Gram-negative micro-organisms, identify their normal habitat, the type of infection they may cause and the current options for treatment.

ANTIBIOTIC RESISTANCE

The accidental discovery of penicillin in 1928 by Alexander Fleming signified a massive breakthrough in the treatment of disease, which prior to the prevalent use of antibiotic therapy resulted in highly significant levels of mortality (Porter, 1997). In the twentieth century, however, began the emergence of highly infectious viral diseases, resurgent diseases and mutating bacteria, causing a crisis within the realms of health care provision and public health. Antibiotics, once considered heroic against infection, are now loosing their effectiveness, and antibiotic resistance is fast becoming a national and a global problem. The often indiscriminate and widespread use of antibiotic therapy, both in animals and humans (Garrod, 1972), together with microbiological practice in the conjugation of bacteria's genetic material, are thought to have exacerbated the rapid spread of resistance (Mendoza, 1985).

Antibiotic resistance can be found in all micro-organisms, bacteria, fungi, viruses, parasites and prions. Bacteria, however, in particular

Gram-negative bacteria (normally inhabiting the gut but causing urinary tract infections, lower respiratory and wound infections) and methicillin-resistant *Staphylococcus aureus* (MRSA; Fig. 33.1) (Mimms *et al.*, 1993), because of their involvement in high levels of *nosocomial* (hospital-acquired) infections, are of paramount concern for the nurse and the promotion of effective infection control.

Staphylococcus aureus, as we have already seen, is part of the natural flora usually found on the skin and mucosa. The resistant form emerged in 1961, only a short time after methicillin was first used, and increased to an estimated 20–40% of all *Staphylococcus* infections (Ayliffe, 1986).

MRSA infections are likely to occur in the nose and skin lesions, as well as indwelling devices such as catheters. The impact of anti-

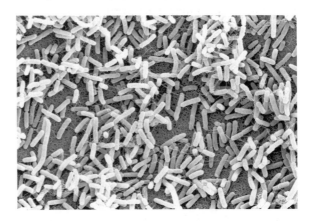

Figure 33.1   Methicillin-resistant *Staphylococcus aureus* (MRSA)

biotic resistance to the individual and state include higher mortality rates, longer hospital stays, increased severity of disease, and more debilitating disease (Twomey, 2000) which collectively raise financial costs and drain resources. Twomey also argues that the contemporary trend towards the minimum stay in hospital, e.g. out-patient surgery and treatment, may contribute to bacterial resistance if health care professionals do not maintain rigid standards in infection control techniques when caring for surgical patients in this new dynamic setting.

HOSPITAL-ACQUIRED INFECTION

Hospital-acquired infections are also known as *nosocomial* infections and are classified as infections acquired in the hospital by a patient who was admitted for other reasons. In contrast, an infection which is present on admission, or becomes evident within 48 hours of admission, is called *community acquired*. Hospital-acquired infection occurs 48 hours after the incubation period, or follows an invasive or manipulative procedure. Examples of common hospital-acquired infections are surgical wound infections, infections of the urinary tract, lower respiratory tract (especially pneumonia), and blood (bacteraemia or septicaemia); the last two are the main causes of infection related to morbidity. Other infections include infections of the skin, eyes, mouth, and intravenous infusion site. The incidence of in-patients who have a nosocomial infection in the UK is currently estimated to be 10% (Plowman, 1997), in other words, a patient admitted to hospital has a one in 10 chance of contracting an infection during their stay in hospital. Nosocomial infections also carry a significant risk of morbidity and death (Selwyn, 1991). Plowman (1997) claims that 6000 deaths per year are caused by hospital-acquired infections.

Emmerson *et al.* (1996) identified the main types of hospital-acquired infection (*see* Fig. 33.2).

The 'real' cost of nosocomial infection to the state is difficult to define. Ayliffe *et al.* (1990)

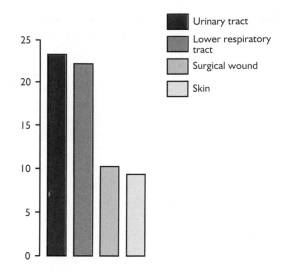

Figure 33.2 The main nosocomial infections (Emmerson *et al.*, 1996)

consider the costs to relate to three main areas:

- Cost to the patient and family through loss of physical function, suffering, anxiety and loss of earnings
- Cost to the hospital through the increased use of drugs, especially antibiotics and dressings, increased medical and nursing time, and prolonged bed occupancy (it is estimated that an infected patient stays an average of four days more than normal in the hospital)
- Cost to the state through tax loss, benefit payments (the employer bearing the cost of sick pay), the extra costs to the National Health Service and community health requirements.

Recent studies suggest that the annual economic burden is considered to be around £930.6 million for in-patient costs, not to mention the subsequent financial implications for general practitioners and community care (Plowman, 1997). In light of these figures, it is easy to understand the huge economic burden that nosocomial infection places upon National Health Service resources. Plowman suggests that a 10% reduction in hospital-acquired infection would result in the release of monetary resources amounting to £93.1 million and free approximately 364 000 bed-days for use by other patients.

In a study conducted by Glynn *et al.* (1997), the use of invasive devices was identified as the most significant risk factor associated with hospital-acquired infection, increasing infection rates from 1 in every 100 to 7.2. The nurse's first-line involvement in the management of invasive devices such as urinary catheters and intravascular cannulae, means that she/he can implement effective infection control practices to reduce such risk.

PATIENT SUSCEPTIBILITY

Having identified some of the micro-organisms causing infection and the various classifications of infection, let us now go on to consider factors which contribute to an individual's likelihood or risk of acquiring infection.

In order for an infection to occur, there are five predisposing factors that must be present:

1 Micro-organisms likely to cause infection
2 A reservoir where the infectious agent can survive and multiply
3 Portals of exit or a path by which the infectious agent can leave the reservoir
4 A mechanism for the transfer of the infectious agent from the reservoir to the susceptible host
5 A portal of entry or path by which the agent enters the host.

These five factors constitute a process which is known as the chain of infection (*see* Fig. 33.3). Given that the vast majority of hospital patients are admitted with an existing condition which

has probably impacted upon their general state of health, natural equilibrium and ability to fight disease, together with the increased prevalence of micro-organisms in the hospital setting, the risk of acquiring infection in secondary care is high.

There are several factors which predispose patients to the risk of developing infection (Ayliffe, 1986; Donowitz, 1987):

- Age extremities (such as babies and the elderly)
- Congenital abnormalities (giving structural/ functional difficulties)
- Family history of particular infections
- Previous attacks of serious infection (the patient's medical records may indicate a particular susceptibility)
- Prolonged or intense exposure to a source of infection
- Malnutrition or obesity
- Poor personal hygiene, incontinence or general debility
- Immune suppression by either therapy or disease
- Recent antibiotic therapy
- Vascular or urinary catheterisation, surgical drains
- Poor skin integrity via trauma, surgery or chronic disease
- Haematoma or bruising
- Poor respiratory function
- Metabolic disorders (e.g. diabetes mellitus, cystic fibrosis, generalised arteriosclerosis)
- Implanted prosthetic materials, foreign bodies in a wound
- Malignant disease.

In infectious diseases, the final outcome can depend as much, if not more, on the susceptibility of the host as upon factors relating to

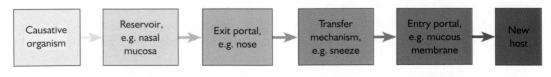

Figure 33.3   The chain of infection

micro-organisms. Many, possibly unknown or not immediately obvious, elements in the patient's constitution can predispose them to infections. The nursing assessment of a patient upon admission and during ongoing evaluation and planning of care provides a valuable opportunity for the nurse to identify any such factors and integrate appropriate strategies into the planning of patient care.

Study Activity 33.3

Using an appropriate anatomy and physiology textbook or electronic learning aid, identify the body systems that contribute to the fight against infection and the ways in which these mechanisms may be compromised.

RISK FACTORS ASSOCIATED WITH CERTAIN BODY SYSTEMS AND CLINICAL PRACTICES

The genitourinary system

As has already been identified, the genitourinary tract is the most common site of nosocomial infection; they account for 23% of hospital-acquired infections in the Plowman (1997) survey. In the UK and the USA it is estimated that 86% of urinary tract infections are associated with instrumentation, usually catheterisation (Johnson, 1986). The most common micro-organism responsible for urinary tract infections is said to be *Escherichia coli*, an organism commonly found in the large intestine (*see* Fig. 33.4) (Williams *et al.*, 1960).

These infections have a clinical significance for patient morbidity; they can become a reservoir for multiple drug-resistant organisms requiring highly toxic and expensive antibiotic therapies. A number of factors have been identified as contributing to urinary tract infections (Stamm and Turk, 1981; Clifford, 1982; Crow *et al.*, 1986):

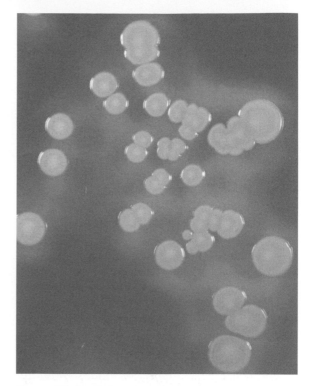

Figure 33.4   *Escherichia coli*

- The indiscriminate use of catheters: 500 000 patients are thought to be catheterised per annum
- A lack of expertise and aseptic technique during catheterisation, resulting in trauma to the meatus or the urethra, which leads to contamination of the drainage system
- A lack of maintenance of the integrity of the drainage system
- The duration of catheterisation: the risk of infection doubles after the first week
- The number of catheter and drainage bag changes.

The high incidence of hospital-acquired urinary tract infections informs the nursing care given and Roe (1992) recommends the use of soap, water and clean wash cloths, particularly for patients with long-term catheters, while the Department of Health Drug Tariff (1992) recommends changing drainage bags only every

5–7 days, as it is suggested that more frequent changing does not reduce the risk of infection. It is also important for the nurse to encourage the patient to perform as many self-caring activities as is reasonable, for the more the patient is responsible for his or her care, the less likely they are to be exposed to the chain of infection.

The respiratory system

Respiratory infections, in particular those of the lower tract, e.g. pneumonia, carry a high mortality rate and account for 22% of hospital-acquired infections in Plowman's (1997) survey. Lifestyle factors, some of which are host related (such as smoking and industrial disease), interfere with a patient's respiratory function. Other pathophysiology is the result of hospital procedures and treatments, such as reduced mobility following surgery. Even nasogastric tubes have been associated with hospital-acquired pneumonia. Adherence to the principles of *asepsis* and utilising the principles governing *decontamination* (cleaning), *disinfection* and *sterilisation* when dealing with equipment and wounds, such as tracheostomy incisions, are paramount in the reduction or avoidance of this type of infection.

The gastrointestinal system

There have been many well-publicised incidents of food poisoning, including the 2002 Scottish outbreak in which 12 hospitals and a school were hit by a virus which originally closed an infirmary in Glasgow and forced the cancellation of 240 admissions. These have resulted in not only the scape-goating of eminent politicians such as Edwina Curry in the case of the risk of salmonella in egg yolks, but also in increased awareness among health providers about the possible hazards of gastrointestinal infections. Such incidents illustrated the far-ranging and catastrophic economic and bio/psycho/social effects that the transmission of infection may cause.

Since losing Crown immunity, food safety within the National Health Service is now regulated by the Food Safety Act, and all hospitals follow stringent protocols regarding the preparation, storage and consumption of food in the health care setting. While nurses are no longer responsible for the preparation of food, they may be involved in storing patients' own food that has been brought in by visitors. It is important, therefore, that you as a student nurse identify and adhere to the policies set out by the organisation regarding the storage and handling of food. Guidelines to food handling can be found in a document published by the Hospital Caterer's Association (1998). Major gastrointestinal infections include gastroenteritis and enteroviral infections such as rotavirus and other small, round structured viruses. All patients can be susceptible to these infections, although the elderly, children, infants and pregnant women are considered to be most at risk (Jarvis *et al.*, 1984).

The vascular system

Glynn *et al.* (1997) identified the relationship between invasive procedures and the increased risk of hospital-acquired infections. Intravenous therapy particularly involves a high risk of introducing micro-organisms, initially at the time of insertion and subsequently through contamination of the device in the management of the system. Intravenous device-related infections are known to originate from the patient's own flora or from micro-organisms transmitted from the hands of the person inserting the device. These devices also provide a direct pathway for micro-organisms between a person's external environment and the bloodstream (Maki, 1982). The term *bacteraemia* means that micro-organisms have entered the patient's blood and can be life-threatening.

The insertion of intravascular devices was traditionally carried out by medical staff. However, with the changing scope of practice, this procedure is now commonly performed by nurses. It is therefore essential that nurses are aware that the majority of intravenous site infections can be attributed to micro-organisms such as *Staphylococcus epidermidis* which are found on human skin. The importance of hand washing and cleaning the insertion site cannot be over-emphasised, as well as the promotion of asepsis principles. Other activities to reduce the risk of intravenous site infection are as follows:

- Non-touch techniques should be employed when changing infusion bags.
- Equipment should be checked for any damage or contamination during manufacture or transport.
- Cannula sites should be regularly observed and the changing regime specified in the hospital protocol should be adhered to.
- Any indication of infection, such as localised inflammation and/or swelling, should instigate removal of the cannula and further investigation (Maki, 1982; Goodison, 1990).

Surgical wounds

In the Plowman (1997) study, surgical wound infections were one of the four largest categories of hospital-acquired infection, and as such this category of infection requires specific analysis and consideration. Wound infections cause the healing process to be delayed, thereby prolonging hospitalisation and placing demands on nursing and medical resources. They also cause considerable psychological and physical distress to the patient through high levels of discomfort and pain, indignity, and dependency. A reduction in the incidence of surgical wound infections is highly desirable, as is the prompt and appropriate treatment of existing or new infections.

There are three main routes by which a wound may become infected:

1 self-contamination from surrounding skin or the gastrointestinal tract
2 airborne contamination from dust or water droplets
3 contact contamination from clothing, equipment or contact with carers' hands.

As the major carer responsible for the everyday management of wounds, the nurse must be aware of the signs and symptoms of early infection. Such signs include localised swelling, redness, heat and pain, accompanied usually by pyrexia. The severity of these symptoms will usually increase as infection progresses, and frequently strong odour and increased amounts of exudate and pus will be present. Rapid identification of infection by observing for these signs, and obtaining microbiological cultures (Cutting and Harding, 1994) mean that subsequent treatment can be implemented to minimise the negative effects of wound infection and reduce the risk of cross-infection to other patients.

Kingsley (2001) suggests the use of a systematic infection continuum and algorithm tool as means to improve practice and care in the realm of wound infection. He argues that nurses need to be confident in their ability to diagnose and treat infected wounds and this can be aided by the use of clear (theoretical) frameworks. He states that, nurses who have a good knowledge of the principles of infection control on tissue viability will be more assertive when negotiating the initiation of medically prescribed therapy for patients. Kingsley, therefore, is recommending that with a sound knowledge base constructed from best evidence, the nurse is in a position to act as patient advocate in the management of infection.

Skin

Meers et al. (1981) showed that 13.5% of patients with hospital-acquired infection suffered from skin infections. Dispersal of micro-organisms from these patients, as well as that of the normal skin flora, has implications for nursing practices such as the timeliness and methods of bed making and wound dressing. Bacteria often accumulate in large numbers in hospital bedding, and bed making has been shown to result in the dissemination of micro-organisms into the air. The shaking of bedclothes is therefore undesirable. Air counts of *Staphylococcus aureus* of more than 50 particles per cubic foot have been found during bed making. Because organisms settle on the floor, bedclothes should not touch the floor during bed making.

A patient can become colonised with the hospital flora within days of admission. The skin, including the hands, and mucous membranes of older and more debilitated people are likely to become colonised with Gram-negative organisms (Johanson, 1969; Chin and Davis, 1978). The colonised patient can become infected or the organisms can be transmitted to other susceptible patients. Infections through the skin may also result due to the fact that the patient has already received a traumatic injury before admission or that the integrity of the skin is compromised through diagnostic or therapeutic procedures such as surgical incisions, aspirations, biopsies, injections, cannulations and debridement.

Study Activity 33.4

Drawing on the most common nosocomial infections identified in Fig. 33.2 – urinary tract, lower respiratory tract, surgical wound and skin – describe possible chains of infection that may exist for these infections to have developed.

Infection control policy

In the quest for optimum service provision, it may be useful to see infection control as a continual, ongoing process, which incorporates many elements, non-clinical and clinical (*see* Fig. 33.5).

In order for the spread of hospital-acquired infection to be minimised or reduced, it is essential that the factors detailed in Fig. 33.5 are incorporated into nursing practice within every hospital and every department.

Infection control, however, is not a solo activity and the nurse is well placed to harness the skills and expertise of the multidisciplinary team to compliment his/her professional skills in implementing an effective approach to infection control. There are a number of strategies that

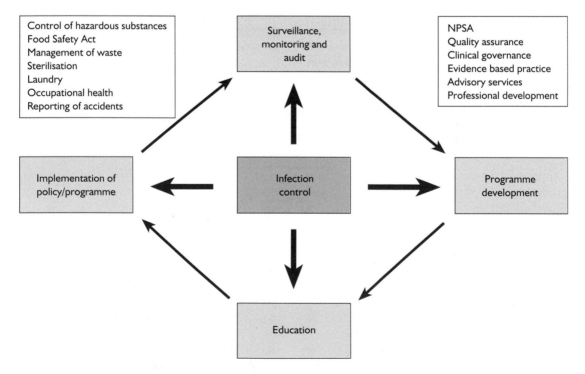

Figure 33.5   The infection control process

nurses may carry out to improve practice through a multidisciplinary approach, such as recruiting the help and advice of infection control staff, health and safety officers and microbiologists, consulting with and utilising the risk management team and analysing statistics and complaints to examine practice issues relating to infection control. Through critical analysis of research, and personal and organisational reflection relating to infection control, the nurse can play a pivotal role in the dissemination and advancement of good practice.

Study Activity 33.5 ———————

- Make a list of all the health care team, clinical and non-clinical, and their responsibilities in relation to the maintenance of a safe environment.
- Are there any ways in which nurses could develop stronger links with these workers to strengthen the maintenance of an infection control policy?

The nurse's responsibility

As stated at the beginning of this chapter, the nurse has an obligation to maintain a safe environment, and to do no harm to the patient. This obligation has taken on new meaning and pertinence with the rise of 'evidence-based practice', in which the clinician uses the best evidence available, in consultation with the patient, to decide upon the option which suits the patient best. When considering the safety of the environment, the nurse must now use consultation and available evidence to inform and develop practice; making it relevant and appropriate for the situation, the patient and the event. This view is reinforced and cemented not only by the United Kingdom Central Council Code of Conduct, clause 3 (UKCC, 1996) which states that 'as a registered nurse, midwife or health visitor, you are personally accountable for your practice and, in the exercise of your professional accountability, must maintain and improve your professional knowledge and competence', but also by the Government White Paper: *The New*

NHS: Modern, dependable (Department of Health, 1997), *The NHS Plan* (Department of Health, 2000), the National Institute of Clinical Excellence, the Centre for Health Improvement, and the National Patient Safety Agency which initially developed and now regulates statutory obligation to ensure that high-quality and clinical care and quality standards are met by trusts.

Finding evidence to support the maintenance of a safe environment can be problematic. There can often be a shortage of published information, and the quality of any research must always be critiqued. The organisation's infection control policy will have written guidelines on most activities that are undertaken in clinical areas, and when you first enter a clinical area you must make yourself aware of these.

McCulloch (1998) identified seven principles for infection control, which are a useful framework to support infection control policies and which you may find useful when analysing core elements of any infection control regime:

1 Safe hands
2 Safe equipment
3 Safe environment
4 Safe practice
5 Safe disposal
6 Safe linen
7 Safe clothing.

Safe hands

Physical contact with patients is one element of the nurse's work activity which remains constant and unchanging in its intensity. Touch and handling have long been associated with the notion of caring and/or healing throughout history, for example in the 'laying on of hands' or in Monica Dickens' autobiography *One Pair of Hands* (1958). The appropriate use of touch has the ability to enhance the therapeutic relationship that exists between patient and nurse. As well as being necessary to perform physical tasks, touch can communicate empathy and support. However, contact between patient and nurse can also have negative consequences as micro-organisms can be passed on from patient to nurse or nurse to patient, creating opportunity for the spread of infection (Reybrouk, 1983). This process is known as *cross-infection*.

Hand washing is one of the key methods of reducing or preventing infection (Richie *et al.*, 1993). However, it has been identified that some health care workers do not wash their hands as often as they should (Emmerson *et al.*, 1996). This failure to comply with one of the main principles of infection control may be attributed to various reasons, such as inadequate training, lack of resources, chapped hands and insufficient support (Heenan, 1992). As a method of overcoming this fact, a patient education model is valuable in increasing hand washing compliance. In their study, patients were educated to partake in an activity by which they asked carers whether they had washed their hands before making physical contact. The results of the study showed that empowering patients to 'take charge' was indeed effective, so much so that soap consumption rose by 34% during the trial period.

Hand washing, using the proper technique and for the required length of time, will remove the transient micro-organisms which pose a threat to staff and patients alike (Taylor, 1978). Taylor's studies into hand washing illustrated that 89% of staff failed to completely clean the whole of the hand during hand washing, the most frequently missed surfaces being the back of the thumbs, the nail beds and in between each finger. Figure 33.6 shows the correct method for washing hands.

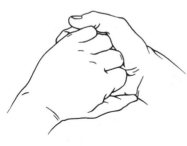

1 Palm to palm.

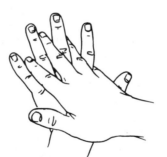

2 Right palm over left dorsum, left palm over right dorsum.

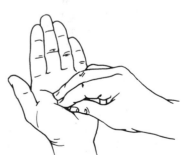

3 Palm to palm, fingers interlaced.

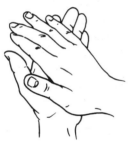

4 Backs of fingers to opposing palms with fingers interlocked.

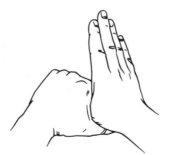

5 Rotational rubbing of right thumb clasped in left palm and vice versa.

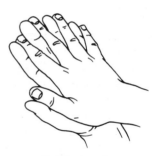

6 Rotational rubbing backwards and forwards with clasped fingers of right hand in left palm, and vice versa.

Figure 33.6   Hand washing technique (adapted from Ayliffe *et al.*, 1990)

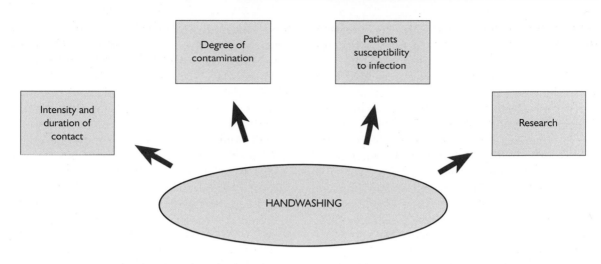

Figure 33.7 Factors to consider before hand washing

There are several factors which need to be taken into consideration when hand washing (*see* Fig. 33.7).

It is important that effective hand washing is supported by practices which are equally as useful in the prevention of cross-infection, such as the avoidance of wearing jewellery and nail polish and adequate rinsing and drying of the hands with disposable towels. Use of the appropriate washing agent is also a factor for the nurse to consider. There are generally three types of cleansing agent: regular soap, antibacterial scrubs and hand sanitisers. Transient bacteria can almost totally be removed by soap and water alone, whereas the removal of resident skin flora requires the use of an antibacterial alcoholic agent (Lowbury *et al.*, 1974). There are three main types of hand washing (Lowbury, 1991), social, clinical and surgical, and one must utilise the correct method for the task to be performed. The time required to wash hands should be 1–15 seconds for socially clean hands, 15–30 seconds when undertaking dressings or wound care and 2–5 minutes prior to surgery. The nurse needs to be aware of the effects on the skin of inappropriate hand washing and the need to care for the hands. Up to 85% of nurses experience some type of work-related skin problem, and one in four develop

significant skin damage (Larson *et al.*, 1997). Soaps and detergents strip the skin on the hands of its protective fat, moisture and acid content, interrupting the pH balance and leaving the skin prone to inflammation and bacterial invasion. It may take up to 30 minutes for the skin to return to its natural balance after hand washing. Therefore, washing not less frequently but more appropriately is one of the key areas to reducing nosocomial infection.

The Center for Disease Control (1986) suggests that hands should be washed:

- After prolonged and intense contact with any patient
- After removal of gloves
- Before and after entering or leaving source isolation rooms
- Before and after patient contact
- Before handling food
- Before all clean procedures
- Before aseptic procedures
- Before any invasive procedure
- Before contact with any immunosuppressed patient.

Safe equipment
There are three main methods of decontamination within the health care setting. These are

cleaning, disinfecting and sterilisation. Cleaning involves the removal of up to 80% of micro-organisms through the use of a detergent and water, and is a visible, socially acceptable level of cleanliness. The process of disinfection can be carried out by various methods such as heat and chemicals. It relates to the removal of harmful micro-organisms (but not bacteria). Sterilisation means the total removal or destruction of harmful micro-organisms, including bacterial spores (Xavier, 1999), through steam pressure (autoclave), dry heat (hot air oven) or gas exposure. Some argue, however, that complete sterility is unattainable (Kelsey, 1972).

The method used is dependent upon the activity being carried out and the degree of risk. The legal documents relating to decontamination are the Health and Safety at Work Act (1974), the Public Health (Infectious Diseases) Regulations (1988), the Management of Health and Safety at Work Regulations (1992) and the Control of Substances Hazardous to Health (COSHH) regulations (1994).

Asepsis is the prevention of microbial contamination of living tissue/fluid or sterile materials by excluding micro-organisms. Aseptic techniques are used by nurses to prevent contamination of the patient or equipment, for example when carrying out a wound dressing or invasive procedure. They should be used in any activity which bypasses the body's natural defences such as the skin or mucous membranes (Mallet and Bailey, 1996). This can be achieved by the use of gloves or forceps, taking care to ensure that gloves are intact and that forceps do not damage tissue. Either way, a no-touch technique should be employed, and protocols for utilising this approach can be found on all wards.

With regards to the safety of specific equipment, the Medical Devices Directive 93/42/EEC (Medical Devices Agency, 1995) regulates the re-use of medical equipment and all equipment is designated as either for single or multiple use. The central sterile supplies department normally provides sterile supplies of dressing packs and instruments. However, there are real risks of cross-infection associated with the re-use of other equipment, for example through the communal use of creams and wound tapes (Oldman, 1987) together with inappropriate or inadequate cleaning of equipment between patients (Castille, 1999) such as nebuliser equipment, washbowls (Bowell, 1993) and commodes. Recent studies have shown that despite guidelines to the contrary, many hospitals are still using surgical equipment which should be disposed of, and that only a third of respondents said their hospital's infection control policy reflected day-to-day activity (Institute of Sterile Services Management, 2001). These figures highlight the need for an evaluation of practice, as well as the difficulties of enforcing policy.

Study Activity 33.6

- Discuss what you understand by the 'principles of asepsis'.
- List three patient care activities where these principles should be utilised.
- List three patient care activities where these methods are not necessary, and any alternative approaches that may be used instead.

Safe environment

The caring environment is the nurse's professional domain, and although there are organisational and professional responsibilities and regulations set in place, it is the nurse who bears a high proportion of the responsibility for maintaining safety. Ayliffe *et al.* (1992) identified the environment as a source of infection. Tracing the modern genealogy of nursing, there are activities which historically have always been the concern of nurses, such as taking care to prevent falls, dealing with spillages of potentially hazardous substances or body fluids and serving food. As already discussed, these are now governed by Government legislation such as the COSHH regulations, the Food Safety Act as well as local infection control policy and protocols. In fact, many of these activities are now becoming the domain of other health care workers and not specific to the nurse. Moving through time, other areas relating to safety and hospital-acquired infections are now becoming increasingly well known, and are commonly addressed in literature and textbooks, for example the need to protect mattresses which, when damaged by phenols and alcohols, harbour micro-organisms (Department of Health, 1991). The contemporary era, however, has taken the subject of safety into another dimension, and includes the need to deal with physical abuse, the problem of contaminated computer keyboards (Bures *et al.*, 2000), the need for electronic security tags in the hospital environment, the disposal of body parts and dealing with stress. The nurse must be aware of the policies pertaining to all elements of safety, psychological and physical, within the work environment in order to promote personal safety and well-being, and that of patients, visitors and colleagues.

Study Activity 33.7

- By locating and reading infection protocols pertaining to dealing with hazardous waste from your work area, describe how, as a nurse, you would deal with the following events, and your rationale for doing so:
- A spillage of blood
- Bed linen soiled with faeces
- Spilled contents of a catheter drainage bag.

Study Activity 33.8

- Based upon your understanding of evidence-based practice and ritualised behaviour, try and identify three patient care activities throughout nursing history that may have been carried out in a manner which under current practices did not promote the reduction of infection.
- In what ways has practice changed from these instances, and what lack of skills or knowledge has been addressed?

Safe disposal

The reasons why the waste generated in hospitals and the health care environment is classified, divided into different categories and regulated, are those of safety and economics. The correct disposal of waste at the point of generation is thought to be able to reduce costs by £10 million per annum and organisations failing to comply with the Environmental Protection Act (1990) are open to costly prosecution.

Some non-clinical household waste such as flowers, paper towels and newspapers can be sent to a local landfill or be recycled in the normal manner. Other clinical waste is potentially dangerous, risking infection, and must be dealt with in a safe manner. It may be contaminated with blood, faecal matter, human tissue, etc. This waste must be contained, usually within a yellow bag, and incinerated on site.

The disposal of 'sharps' is of particular concern, because of the risk of needlestick injury and the transmission of blood-borne diseases such as HIV and hepatitis B. Sharps bins are provided in every health care setting, and it is the personal responsibility of the nurse to ensure that they are used and disposed of in the correct manner. Immediately after use, sharps must be placed into the sharps disposal box, which when full must be carefully sealed and sent for incineration (Health and Safety Commission, 1982). Under no circumstances must needles be re-sheathed, as this practice greatly increases the risk of injury, and accounts for 15–41% of all needlestick injuries (McCormick amd Maki, 1981). One way of avoiding the likelihood of injury is to attach the sharps bin directly to the trolleys or to place them at the bedside (Hart, 1990). Interestingly, on 28 November 2001, the Department of Health changed its policy on disclosure, based upon research carried out by the Expert Advisory Group on Aids/UK Advisory Panel. Health care workers infected with blood-borne viruses are no longer required to disclose if they are suffering from HIV. Not a single case of transmission from health care worker to patient has ever been detected in the UK. If correct preventative measures are taken to reduce risk then neither patient nor carer should be at risk from the other.

Study Activity 33.9

- Write down a list of all the things that you dispose of during your everyday practice as a nurse. These may include clinical and non-clinical waste.
- Consider how many people come into contact with this waste prior to and after you.
- In what ways might this waste be hazardous to other professionals and members of the public?
- What policies and procedures are put in place to reduce these risks, and are they adhered to?

Safe linen and clothing

Linen and clothing, like all other pieces of equipment in the health care setting, are a likely source for the transmission of micro-organisms if not treated with care. The Government regulates the treatment of hospital linen through environmental legislation (primarily the Environmental Protection Act 1990) and, as with waste disposal and food handling, organisations who fail to comply with the law are open to prosecution. The laundering of hospital linen is carried out by the laundry department, where infected linen is processed at a higher temperature than non-infected linen. For this reason, and also to protect laundry staff from the risk of exposure to pathogenic organisms, the nurse has the responsibility of ensuring that linen is identified using the standardised system of colour-coded or algeanate bags. Barrie (1994) suggests several methods for providing safe linen, five of which are particularly relevant to nurse–patient care:

1 Change bedding carefully do not shake sheets to reduce airborne organisms.
2 Bag linen at the bed side into a washable or disposable container.
3 Place linen that is contaminated with potentially infected substances (blood, diarrhoea, exudates) into a dissolvable liner and secure tightly.

4 Wear gloves and aprons for handling contaminated linen.
5 Use the National Colour Coding System.

The transfer of micro-organisms from patient to nurse via the nurse's uniform and plastic aprons has been investigated (Lidwell *et al.*, 1974; Babb *et al.*, 1983; Wong *et al.*, 1991), and it has been advocated that the colonisation of uniforms is reduced by the wearing of protective aprons. However, this opinion has been recently disputed by Callaghan (1998) who found that the wearing of aprons was not associated with significantly less bacterial contamination on uniforms, and that the plastic aprons themselves were heavily contaminated. Uniforms were found to be heavily contaminated with micro-organisms throughout the shift, and although hospital laundering systems render uniforms sterile at the end of the washing cycle, home laundering could offer no such reassurance. This study has implications for the use of protective clothing and equipment and also for the laundering of uniforms. White plastic aprons should be used during direct patient contact including bed making, cleaning and toileting. They should be discarded after a single use with an individual patient. Blue plastic aprons should be worn when handling food and then discarded.

Nurses' uniforms should be laundered using specialised hospital facilities whenever possible, or if laundered at home, organisational guidelines for this activity should be adhered to.

Other items of protective clothing include eye protection, face masks, foot protection and fluid repellant gowns. However, the use of any protective equipment is only one of the principles of good infection control and must be used in conjunction with other techniques such as hand washing.

SUMMARY

The risk of acquiring infection within the hospital setting is a costly reality, and nurses must be aware of their responsibilities with regards to patient care, professional relationships and self-protection. This awareness will enable them to perform a high standard of care and adhere to the strict code of conduct by which they are regulated. Maintenance of a safe environment in respect of infection control and all other aspects of health and safety can only be promoted if the nurse is equipped with a sound theoretical knowledge base on which to base actions. As a student nurse, throughout professional development and ongoing education, you must ensure a knowledge progression from a basic understanding of policy and underlying principles of risk and acquisition of infection, to that of skilled practitioner, able to apply and evaluate scientific knowledge in practice. There are many support networks available within the health care and academic setting to support the nurse along this journey. By harnessing the skills and utilising the skills of the multidisciplinary team, and by reflecting upon your own learning needs and achievements, you can make a real difference to the safety of the clinical environment.

Study Activity 33.10 ━━━━━━━

A male diabetic patient, aged 72 years, has been admitted to your ward following an above right knee surgical amputation under general anaesthetic. He has returned to the ward with an intravenous infusion and wound drain. He is doubly incontinent, and has a long-term indwelling urinary catheter *in situ*.

- From your nursing assessment, what do you consider to be the risk factors of your patient developing an infection?
- What types of infection is he at risk from, and what are the organisms responsible?

REFERENCES

Ayliffe, G.A.J. (1986) Guidelines for the control of epidemic methicillin resistant *Staphylococcus aureus. Journal of Infection* 7, 193–201

Ayliffe, G.A.J., Collins, B.J. and Taylor, L.J. (1990) *Hospital Acquired Infection: Principles and practice*, Wright, Bristol

Ayliffe, G.A.J., Fraise, A., Geddes, A.M. *et al.* (1992) *Control of Hospital Infection: A practical handbook* (3rd edn), Chapman & Hall, London

Babb, J.R., Davies, J.G. and Ayliffe, G.A. (1983) Contamination of protective clothing and nurses' uniforms in an isolation ward. *Journal of Hospital Infection* 4, 149–57

Barrie, D. (1994) How hospital and linen services are provided, *Journal of Hospital Infection* 27, 219–35

Bowell, B. (1993) Preventing infection and its spread. *Surgical Nurse* 6(2), 5–12

Bures, S., Fishbain, J.T. and Uyehara, C.F. (2000) Computer keyboards and faucet handles as reservoirs of nosocomial pathogens in the intensive care unit. *American Journal of Infection Control* 28(6), 465–71

Callaghan, I. (1998) Bacterial contamination of nurses' uniforms: a study. *Nursing Standard* 13(1), 37–42

Castille, K. (1999) Infection control: to reuse or not to reuse – that is the question. *Nursing Standard* 13(34), 48–52

Center for Disease Control (1986) Guidelines for hand washing and hospital environment control. *Infection Control* 7(4), 231–5

Chin, P. and Davis, D.G. (1978) Hand flora. *Journal of Hygiene* 77, 93–6

Clifford, C.M. (1982) Urinary tract infection: a brief selective review. *International Journal of Nursing Studies* 19, 213–22

Crow, R.A. *et al.* (1986) *A Study of Patients with an Indwelling Catheter and Related Nursing Practice*, Nursing Practice Unit, University of Surrey

Cutting, K. and Harding, K. (1994) Criteria for identifying wound infection. *Journal of Wound Care* 3(4), 198–201

Department of Health (1991) *Hospital Mattress Assemblies: Care and cleaning*, SAB (91) p. 65, Department of Health, London

Department of Health (1992) *Drug Tariff*, HMSO, London

Department of Health (1997) *The New NHS: Modern, dependable*, The Stationery Office, London

Department of Health (2000) *The NHS Plan*, HMSO, London

Department of Health (2001) *The Kennedy Report*, HMSO, London

Dickens, M. (1958) *One Pair of Hands*, Michael Joseph, London

Donowitz, G.R. (1987) The immunosuppressed patient. In: Farber, B.F. (ed.) *Infection Control in Intensive Care.*

Emmerson, A.M., Enstone, J.E. and Griffin, M. (1996) The Second National Prevalence Survey of infection in hospitals. *Journal of Hospital Infection* 32(3), 175–90

Garrod, L.P. (1972) Causes of failure in antibiotic treatment, *British Medical Journal* 4, 473–6

Glynn, A. *et al.* (1997) *Hospital Acquired Infection: Surveillance policies and practice,* Public Health Laboratory Service, London

Goodison, S.M. (1990) Keeping the flora out. *Professional Nurse* **August**, 572

Hart, S. (1990) Clinical hepatitis B: guidelines for infection control, *Nursing Standard* 4(45), 24–7

Health and Safety Commission (1982) *The Safe Disposal of Clinical Waste*, London, HMSO

Heenan, A. (1992) Handwashing practices, *Nursing Times* 88(34), 70

Horton, R. (1995) Infection control in nurse education and practice, M.Phil thesis, University of Bradford

Hospital Caterers Association (1998) *Good Practice Guide: Food service standards at ward level*, Hospital Caterers Association, Sittingbourne

Institute of Sterile Services Management (2001) *The Decontamination of Surgical Instruments*, UKCC press release 14 November 2001

Jarvis, W.R., White, J.W. and Munn, V.P. (1984) Nosocomial infection surveillance. *Morbidity and Mortality Weekly* 33, 955

Johanson, W.G. (1969) Changing pharyngeal bacteria of hospital patients. *New England Journal of Medicine* 28, 1137–40

Johnson, A. (1986) Urinary tract infection. *Nursing* 3, 102–5

Kelsey, J.C. (1972) The myth of surgical sterility. *Lancet* 2, 130–1

Kingsley, A. (2001) A proactive approach to wound infectionl *Nursing Standard* 15(30), 50–8

Larson, E., Friedman, C., Cohran, J. *et al.* (1997) Prevalence and correlates of skin damage on the hands of nurses. *Heart Lung* 26(5), 404–12

Lidwell, O.M., Towers, A.G., Ballard, J. *et al.* (1974) Transfer of microorganisms between nurses and patients in a clean air environment. *Journal of Applied Bacteriology* 37, 649–56

Lowbury, E.J. (1991) Special problems in hospital antisepsis. In: Russell, A.D. (ed.) *Principles and Practice of Disinfection, Sterilisation. Blackwell Science, Oxford*

Lowbury, E.J. *et al.* (1974) Disinfection of hands: removal of transient organisms. *British Medical Journal* 2, 230–3

Maki, D. (1982) A semi-quantitative culture method for identifying intravenous catheter related infections. *New England Journal of Medicine* 296, 1305–6

Mallet, J. and Bailey, C. (eds) (1996) *The Royal Marsden NHS Trust Manual of Clinical Procedures*, Blackwell Science, Oxford

McCormick, R.D. amd Maki, D.G. (1981) Epidemiology of needle-stick injuries in hospital personnel. *American Journal of Medicine* 70, 928–32

McCulloch, J. (1998) Infection control: principles for practice, *Nursing Standard* 13(1), 49–56

Medical Devices Agency (1995) *The Reuse of Medical Devices Supplied for Single Use Only, Medical Device Bulletin MDA DB 9501*

Meers, P., Ayliffe, G.A.J., Emmerson, A. *et al.* (1981) Report on the national survey of infection in hospitals. *Journal of Hospital Infection* 2(Suppl), 1–51

Mendoza, M.C. (1985) Evidence for the dispersion and evolution of plasmids from *Serratia marcescens* in hospital. *Journal of Hospital Infection* 6, 147–53

Mimms, C.A. *et al.* (1993) *Medical Microbiology*, Mosby, London

Nightingale, F. (1863) *Notes on Hospitals*, Longman, London

Nursing and Midwifery Council (2002) *Code of Professional Conduct*, Nursing and Midwifery Council, London

Oldman, P. (1987) An unkind cut. *Nursing Times* 83(48), 71–4

Plowman, R. (1997) *Hospital Acquired Infection*, Office of Health Economics, London

Porter, R. (1997) *The Greatest Benefit To Mankind – A medical history of humanity from antiquity to the present*, Harper Collins, London

Reybrouk, G. (1983) The role of hands in the spread of nosocomial infection. *Journal of Hospital Infection* 90(30), 63–4

Roe, B.H. (1992) Use of indwelling catheters. In: Roe, B.H. (ed.) *Clinical Nursing Practice: The promotion and management of continence*, Prentice Hall, Hemel Hempstead

Selwyn, S. (1991) Hospital infection: the first 2500 years, *Journal of Hospital Infection* 18(Suppl. A)

Stamm, W.E. and Turk, M. (1981) Nosocomial infection of the urinary tract. *American Journal of Medicine* 70, 651–4

Taylor, L.J. (1978) An evaluation of handwashing techniques. *Nursing Times* 74, 108–10

Twomey, C. (2000) Antibiotic resistance – an alarming health care issue, *AORN Journal* **72**(1), 63–80

United Kingdom Central Council for Nursing, Midwifery and Health Visiting (1992) *Code of Conduct*, UKCC, London

United Kingdom Central Council for Nursing, Midwifery and Health Visiting (1996) *Guidelines for Professional Practice*, UKCC, London

Ward, K.A. (1994) A community perspective. In:

Worsley, M.A. *et al.* (eds) *Infection Control*, Daniels Publishing, Cambridge

Williams, R.E.O., Blowers, R., Garrod, L.P. *et al.* (1960) *Hospital Infection: Causes and prevention*, Loyde-Luke, London

Wong, D., Nye, K. and Hollis, P. (1991) Microbial flora on doctors' white coats. *British Medical Journal* **303**, 1602–4

Xavier, G. (1999) Asepsis. *Nursing Standard* **13**(36), 49–53

34

HELPING WITH THE ACTIVITIES OF LIVING

Marlene Sinclair

LEARNING OUTCOMES

After studying this chapter you will be able to:

- Make definitive statements concerning self-care, self-care requisites and health deviation self-care deficits
- Outline the activities of living associated with self-care
- Present a case for nursing as an activity concerned with providing help, in line with the statements of Virginia Henderson and Dorothea Orem
- Have a deeper understanding of self and others when giving and receiving care
- Recognise the importance of providing help on the basis of the best available evidence
- Apply knowledge to the practice of nursing in line with common self-care requisites
- Utilise holistic and reflective approaches to care delivery
- Utilise Internet research skills to support nursing practice.

INTRODUCTION

This chapter is about nursing in practice. It is designed to develop nursing knowledge, skill, and attitudes in a personal and professional manner. We can conceive of nursing as an activity concerned with caring in a health context. In effect, the nurse helps the patient in those aspects of living where it becomes apparent that he or she cannot cope on their own. Perhaps the most well-known definition of nursing comes from Virginia Henderson (1966):

The unique function of the nurse is to assist the individual, sick or well, in performance of those activities contributing to health or its recovery (or to peaceful death) that he would perform unaided if he had the necessary strength, will or knowledge and to do this in such a way as to help him gain independence as rapidly as possible.

Henderson's definition is still the most widely quoted because it provides a succinct statement that reaches to the very heart of what nursing is about. The three essential elements of her definition cover the full range of what nursing involves:

1 It *frames* nursing as assisting or helping in relation to activities that relate *specifically* to contributing to health or its recovery or, importantly, to peaceful death.
2 It sets specific *parameters* by stating that this help is only provided in circumstances where the one cared for cannot perform the health-maintaining or health-recovering activities unaided.
3 It emphasizes an *approach* that such help as is needed is provided so that it includes developing capacity for self-help to as great an extent as possible.

Study Activity 34.1

Log on to the following websites for further information about Virginia Henderson:
   – International Nursing library
   – Tribute to Virginia Henderson 1897–1996.
Note: In some instances in this chapter addresses are given for websites. Where this is not so, the website can be reached using a fast search engine, such as Google or BBCi.

Clearly, where individuals are acutely ill they may be unable to contribute significantly to their own care. This may be the case particularly where the health interventions are highly complex and involve the use of complicated technology. However, apart from situations where the individual is unconscious, there is almost always some way in which the individual can participate. Nowadays, it is common practice to involve patients in their own care even from the early stages of an acute illness such as stroke or heart attack. This is linked to a philosophy of commencing rehabilitation from the very beginning of such an interlude and recognises the healing influences that underlie the prevention of learned helplessness and the promotion of independence. The American nurse Dorothea Orem spoke of such helping in terms of the concept of self-care. Orem (1985; 1995) presented a number of self-care requisites, as follows:

- Universal self-care needs
- Self-care needs as a result of health care disturbances
- Development-related self-care needs.

She extended these by referring to health deviation self-care requisites, which relate specifically to needs that emerge when health and well-being are under threat, i.e. when a person is disabled, injured or generally unwell. At a basic level this may involve the person treating their health problem by going to a pharmacist and purchasing medication over the counter for flu-like illnesses. On another level the person with chest pain will seek medical help.

Study Activity 34.2

- Log on to the following website for further information about Dorothy Orem's theory of self care:
  - International Orem Society for Nursing Science and Scholarship.
- From this, make brief notes outlining Orem's model of nursing.

This chapter does not attempt to produce a manual of procedural skills for the practice of nursing, but rather will focus on principles of practice. In a rapidly changing health care world new evidence and new technologies are constantly modifying day-to-day practice. Furthermore, many aspects of practice involve the potential risk of harm. For example, faulty lifting and moving techniques can lead to injury of patients and staff. Nowadays, health care agencies tend to provide staff specifically to train practitioners in such procedures, and there are usually specific protocols, established by policy at local level, which must be followed. Students should use these for guidance on such matters, rather than standard textbooks. For the most part, this chapter concentrates on the general principles of assisting patients in their day-to-day need for care.

These practical activities should not be considered as merely the learning of psychomotor skills, although these are important. In high-quality care, the nurse is bringing together best knowledge and practice, and integrating them into the art and science of *doing*, an integration that is sometimes referred to as 'praxis'. This involves not simply mindlessly doing but the process of reflection before, during and after these acts of doing. Indeed, as experience is developed, there is also a tacit dimension to such doing, where the nurse knows intuitively what is to be done. This highlights an important principle. While the information presented in the chapter provides knowledge relating to practice, it is only *in* that practice that the knowledge becomes fully realised and integrated. It is therefore important that the student supplements the chapter with practice learning; a reflexive movement between the text and practice and back from that practice to the text is vital for the optimal level of practice learning to be achieved.

Study Activity 34.3

We have spoken of helping in nursing in terms of Orem's self-care framework. We might alternatively view these as activities of living, the approach taken by Roper, Logan and Tierney (1980; 1996).

- Using your library and textbook sources, conduct a brief review of Roper *et al.*'s description of activities of living. Write this up as a 400-word (one A4 page) account.
- Compare the approach of these authors with that of Orem. Reflect on the similarities and differences and consider which framework you feel might be most useful.

THE PRINCIPLES OF GOOD PRACTICE

Thinking and doing

The modern nurse practitioner must be a thinking person who possesses analytical skills. For her to be deemed a competent practitioner, however, she must also base nursing practice on sound research and evidence wherever possible. The current preparation of nurses for practice should include a combination of education and training.

The nurse must be able to care for the patient as an individual from a holistic point of view, and be sensitive to all his physical, psychosocial, and spiritual needs:

> *In holistic theory, all living organisms are seen as interacting, unified wholes that are more than the mere sum of their parts. Viewed in this light, any disturbance in one part is a disturbance in the whole system.*
>
> (Ham Ying, 1993)

Nurses must be doers as well as thinkers; they must do the caring and learn from a range of real-life caring situations. The nurse practises her profession in the process of doing. The nurse that values the personal, individualised and human character of her profession gives holistic rather than disease-centred care. Therefore, in theory, the emphasis in nursing should be on caring for the individual, with the person (not the disease) as the focus of care. The nurse's role is to care for the patient, using the nursing process to aid him or her to attain his personal best in health and illness.

As yet, there is no unifying theory for the complex business of nursing, as 'it demands a variety of theories with which to view its reality and structure' (Castledine, 1994). Castledine refers to paradigms offering new solutions to unsolved problems. He states that conceptual models can also be seen as paradigms. 'So as each new model emerges – Peplau, Rogers, Orem and Roy – there are shifts and changes in acceptance and dominance by such models' (Castledine, 1994). He emphasises the fact that 'we may never find an all-embracing model and to search for such a goal is inappropriate given the complex nature of nursing'.

Therefore, as a practitioner one must not be afraid to utilise a variety of models or to use an eclectic approach, taking parts of models and combining them to develop a conceptual framework that suits a particular patient or group of patients in a particular care setting. However, Castledine (1994) does propose 14 statements about the properties of nursing that contribute to our understanding of its nature, as follows:

1 Nursing is culturally and economically determined.
2 In a complex society, nursing is divided up into various specialist roles.
3 As nursing becomes acceptable in a society, so it develops and seeks a knowledge base, which eventually becomes more exclusive and concerned with professionalisation.
4 The root meaning of the word 'nurse' is to nourish, and a simple definition of nursing is closely related to nurturing.
5 Nursing has to do with meeting the problems and concerns related to bodily human functioning.
6 Nursing is also concerned with mental and emotional health, and spiritual problems and concerns.
7 One of the major goals of nursing is to help a person with his physical, emotion, and mental health concerns, thus enabling him to adapt and cope with change.
8 Nursing is about being available and sensitive

to those who are having difficulties or problems in caring for themselves.

9 Nursing is an interactive process emphasising an interpersonal relationship and a shared experience in health-related matters.

10 Nursing has high moral and ethical standards, of which accountability, autonomy, advocacy, collaboration, and a duty to care are key elements.

11 Nursing aims to protect the public and respect the laws of the land.

12 There is a nursing role in educating for health, i.e. aiding health promotion and disease prevention.

13 Nursing is concerned with social policies and political decisions that may affect the health of those who are being cared for.

14 Nursing uses an eclectic approach to its understanding of its aims in society and its development as a service to people.

Study Activity 34.4

Nursing is a service that:

- helps people as individuals, families and communities to achieve and maintain good health
- supports, assists, and cares for people during illness or when their health is threatened
- enhances people's ability to cope with the effects of illness and disability
- ensures (as far as possible) that death is dignified and free from pain.

Nursing achieves these goals by applying knowledge and skills gained through education and training, updated and tested by research. It is this combination – along with the desire to care for others – that provides the basis of nursing.

- Why did you enter the profession of nursing?
- How will you translate what you think and feel now into practice?

Knowledge for practice

Problem-solving processes

By far the most common presentation of an approach to solving nursing problems is that described as the 'nursing process' method (*see* Chapter 24). In general, this is a process involving four stages:

1 assessment
2 planning
3 delivery of care (implementation), and
4 evaluation (of effectiveness of care).

More recently, this has been divided into five stages, whereby assessment provides information for a second stage – making nursing diagnoses or identifying nursing problems – followed by a third stage of constructing a plan of care, a fourth stage of implementing the planned care, and a fifth stage of evaluating that care. In general, the second stage is referred to as *nursing diagnoses* in the USA and *nursing problem identification* in the UK, but both approaches are commonly found in the UK. This additional stage emphasises the fact that the nursing process viewed in traditional problem-solving terms can be a staged and sequential process. However, it is important that the process of solving nursing problems is not so rigidly linked to a problem-solving formula that it works against flexible and reflective practice.

The nursing process has been used to teach nursing for almost 20 years, but has recently come under scrutiny. Benner and Tanner (1987) and Benner, Tanner and Chesla (1996) found that experienced nurses developed their own intuitive problem-solving approaches to care and did not separate problem-solving into the distinct steps of assessing, planning, implementing and evaluating. In their study of nurses' problem-solving abilities, Hurst *et al.* (1991) found that many nurses used different approaches, depending on the type of patient and the situation. Therefore, to suggest that a general model of four or five stages of problem-solving would invariably work was inappropriate for the experienced nurse. Field (1987) identified the need for an initial framework to guide the novice but not to be used by the expert practitioner. Fonteyn and Cooper (1994), writing about the usefulness of the written nursing process, suggested that 'the focus should be on nursing action in practice, not on written theory of practice'.

In Australia, nursing teachers are also using the problem-based learning (PBL) approach. The problem is introduced before any preparation or study has occurred and in as real a manner as possible. Students are encouraged to think on the spot, as they would when dealing with real clinical problems. According to Creedy *et al.* (1992), 'PBL approaches encourage students to be active creators rather than passive receptors of knowledge.' Similar approaches in Canada emphasise the importance of situating problem-based learning within the practice situation (Morales-Mann and Kaitell, 2001)

Study Activity 34.5 _____

You are a student on a ward for the first time, along with a staff nurse. One of the patients in a bed nearby shouts out that he needs to go to the toilet. The possible immediate responses to this situation could be:

a) Ignore the request; you are not a real nurse yet.
b) Pretend you are busy and let the auxiliary or staff nurse deal with the patient.
c) Call one of the others and tell them that the patient needs to go to the toilet.
d) Tell the patient to get up and go to the toilet, giving verbal directions to the nearest toilet.
e) Just go and get the bedpan or the commode.
f) Talk to the patient and give him what he/she wants, i.e. a bedpan or commode or assistance.
g) Assess the whole patient. Utilise all available knowledge of his/her mental, physical, or psychological status. Ensure safety. Consider whether the patient's request matches his current dependency level and your own competence, then negotiate action with the patient.

● Which one of these options would you choose? Briefly write down the reasons behind your choice.

Study Activity 34.6 _____

When you have completed your education you may automatically choose item g) and go even further as

your ability to solve problems becomes more sophisticated. You will be more aware of the patient's rights, your professional responsibilities, the ward philosophy of caring, standards of care, and the involvement of the multidisciplinary team in rehabilitation care. In short, you will have developed your own beliefs and values in caring for individual patients. You may observe that an experienced nurse seems to have adopted action e) in the list under Study Activity 34.5. When you ask why they took this course of action, the answer may be something like, 'I don't know – it just was the right thing to do at the time.'

The implication here is that the nurse seems to have acted intuitively. In one sense this term means something like a sixth sense, some almost mystical power. But in another, it means that the person is so experienced, so aware of previous instances of a situation, so 'tuned in' to the particular patient, that she is not ignoring a problem-solving approach, but in fact short-circuiting what would otherwise be a ponderous and disjointed process.

● Using your library and the internet, research the term 'intuition' and write a brief 400-word (one-page) statement on the meaning of the term.
● Review the work of the nursing scholar Patricia Benner and her ideas on intuitive practice or clinical wisdom (e.g. Benner, 1984; Benner *et al.*, 1999). Reflect upon how Benner's approach and a nursing process approach may be complementary in arriving at a decision about delivery of care. List your main points and discuss these with your fellow students and/or teacher.

Whatever approach is taken to identify and resolve nursing problems, or determine nursing actions, any solution must be considered in a critical manner. *Critical thinking* is vitally important in nursing. It demands a questioning attitude, not accepting concepts as automatically given but seeking to establish their validity rationally (Duchscher Boychuk, 1999). This develops with experience, and through such approaches as concept clarification, concept analysis and theory evaluation (*see* Module 3). Facione and Facione (1996) describe a *critical spirit*, a cautious, reflective and questioning attitude to problems and their resolution or responses.

Nursing frameworks

It is important that our delivery of care, whichever nursing process we use, is situated within a wider context and informed by knowledge from a range of areas. It is vitally important that we use the best available knowledge to inform our practice, and this is frequently derived from research. We refer to this as an evidence-based practice approach. However, if the reader reflects further on the latter Study Activity, it will be clear that there are other ways of 'knowing' that may inform our practice: intuitive knowing is an intensely personal process embedded in reflection and often derived from the wisdom emerging from extensive experience. Such knowledge is also important, particularly where 'evidence' or sound research is not available to guide our practice.

Even when we are dealing with meeting a patient's needs for the basic activities of living (breathing, eating, personal hygiene, etc.), it is important that we use effective theoretical or knowledge frameworks to guide our practice. These can be divided into broad theoretical frameworks, which give general direction to our practice, and specific theoretical frameworks, which guide that practice in more concrete ways.

In Module 3, we found that diverse forms of knowledge can inform nursing, and it is essential to have a well-structured and developing body of knowledge that is pertinent to the activity of nursing. Carper (1978) and Fawcett (1995; 2000) provide two such broad frameworks.

Study Activity 34.7 ———————

An older, confused patient in your ward repeatedly attempts to get out of bed and because she is frail and unsteady on her feet there is a real danger that she may fall and injure herself. At the same time, you know that any form of physical restraint may be distressing to her and could be viewed as unacceptable.

- Review Carper's patterns of knowing (1978), as presented in Chapter 9. Carper identified four such patterns: empirical, ethical, personal and aesthetic. (Module 3 devotes one chapter to each of these patterns.) Identify how each of Carper's patterns might inform how you would care for this patient.

Study Activity 34.8 ———————

A young man on your ward is confined to bed and requires a bed bath. You are already aware that he is shy and a little introverted. When you explain what is about to happen he becomes visibly embarrassed.

- Review Fawcett's metaparadigm of nursing (1995; 2000), as introduced in Chapter 9. The metaparadigm is a statement of the fundamental concerns of a discipline. Fawcett proposed four such elements: person, health, environment, and nursing.
- Each must be taken into consideration in each nursing situation. For example, questions may be raised about this person or 'patient' and his social background or environment. Use Fawcett's metaparadigm to identify and list considerations that might inform how you approach this nursing activity with this particular patient.

Frameworks such as those proposed by Carper and Fawcett provide general direction to our nursing activities. But it is also argued that there is a need for more specific frameworks to guide how we proceed to carry out nursing work. In Chapter 14 we considered how theoretical frameworks described as nursing models may inform this process. One of the difficulties with such models in the past was a tendency to adopt one model, such as that of Orem (1995) or Roper *et al.* (1996) and expect this to guide all nursing work for all patients in all situations. Together with a lack of strong empirical evidence to establish the efficacy of such models, this led to a decrease in their popularity. However, there is now a much more creative and flexible approach to the use of such models, as suggested by Aggleton and Chalmers (2000), and nurses are more innovative in adopting different models and adapting them to fit in with their particular nursing challenges.

From knowing to doing

We have considered the application of knowledge (or theory) to our practice and the use of processes and frameworks that may guide that practice. However, to view nursing as exclusively the application of knowledge to the nursing situation puts it at risk of becoming mechanical and impersonal. When we speak of nursing *care* we assume a concern on the part of the one caring for the person being cared for. This involves not only a commitment to help that arises out of concern and compassion for the other, but also a recognition of the other as a person with whom we share a caring relation (*see* Chapter 2). As Kitson (1985) stated:

> *A consciousness of caring would seem to grow from within the person and also from without. We cannot care without having been cared for, nor can we care without first having sensed what matters to us.*
>
> (Kitson, 1985)

Where Kitson refers to a consciousness of caring growing in part from without, a significant element of this 'without' is the person being cared for. In a true caring orientation we must recognise the primacy of this person and, in our own appreciation of what it is to be cared for, recognise why it is important to establish what they would need or wish. The recognition of the primacy of this person incorporates a recognition of their need to return to full personhood (to as great an extent as possible), or to approach a peaceful and pain-free death. This orientation is fundamental to an acceptance of the principle of self-care and moves away from the view of the patient as a passive recipient of care to a person with rights, who must be empowered with the responsibility for their own care wherever possible. The nurse's role involves promoting autonomy and defending the patient's right to this is part of the concept of advocacy, equally central to the nurse's role.

Study Activity 34.9

- Log on to the Nursing and Midwifery Council (NMC) website and read the document *Requirements for Pre-registration Nursing Programmes* (Nursing and Midwifery Council, 2001). Note the content at paragraph 20, as follows:

> *Provision of care*
> *Orientation must be towards practice, which is responsive to the needs of various client groups across different care settings. This will be reflected in the capacity to assess needs, diagnose and plan, implement and evaluate care in such circumstances. Care practice must not only reflect collaborative working with other members of the care team but must also empower patients and clients, and their carers, actively to participate in the planning, delivery and evaluation of care. These principles must be reflected in all programmes of preparation leading to entry to the register.*

- Discuss ways in which Orem's theory about self-care (1995) applies to this statement.
- Explain how the notions of autonomy and advocacy can be important in empowering the individual as a self-carer.

STANDARDS OF CARE

So far we have explored a variety of ideas about nursing and you have written lots of notes for reflection. You should reread these notes on a regular basis. They will demonstrate a development in your personal knowledge, skill, and attitude. Your awareness of the intimacy of nursing and your hunger to develop competences in nursing practice will gradually increase. This will contribute towards establishing a high quality of care.

Much of a nurse's work involves helping patients with personal functions. Using everyday nursing skills to help with such activities may seem mundane, but again, it is vital to the quality of care. The term 'everyday nursing skills' is in itself problematic. In the first edition of this book this chapter was entitled 'Basic daily care'. In a recent publication entitled *The Essence of Care* (Department of Health, 2001), reference is made to:

> *. . . the fundamental and essential aspects of care . . . what might be described as the softer aspects of care, which are nevertheless crucial to the quality of care patients experience.*
>
> (Department of Health, 2001, p. 8)

In the foreword to this publication, Sarah Mullally, the Chief Nursing Officer at the English Department of Health refers to:

> *. . . those core and essential aspects of care that quite rightly matter so much to patients and their carers, yet which rarely attract the attention they should during the quality improvement process.*
>
> (Mullally, 2001, p. 2)

While none of these terms may adequately describe the aspects of care being referred to, there is a general recognition that they concern assisting individuals with activities of living or with basic human needs in such areas as biological functions (breathing, elimination, etc.), nutrition, hygiene, alleviation of pain and discomfort, and alleviation of psychological distress. There is increasing recognition that these apparently routine or taken-for-granted aspects of care are powerful determinants of quality of care and indeed powerful influences upon health and well-being. They also demand high levels of skill, sensitivity and thoughtfulness. Assisting a teenage boy with a bedpan is no less complex a skill than the erection of an intravenous infusion.

Another problematic area is that of establishing standards and guidelines for delivering such care. No attempt is made here to present the full range of such care in terms of specific guidance or detailed procedures. Such guidance would quickly become out of date. Establishing standards and then producing guidelines for practice is an undertaking that demands a high

level of resources and expertise, which is not always available to health care providers at a local level (McClarey and Duff, 1997). There is therefore an increasing movement towards establishing benchmarks for such guidance at national level. The idea implicit in such approaches is that these benchmarks (standards against which care can be compared or assessed) are developed on the basis of best evidence and identification of exemplars of good practice by expert groups. The most influential of these has been the initiative of the Department of Health (2001), which has now been incorporated into the agenda of the NHS Modernisation Agency and also informs monitoring standards of the Commission for Health Improvement (Cham-bers and Jolly, 2002). *The Essence of Care* (Department of Health, 2001) presents a benchmarking toolkit covering eight areas of care as follows:

1 Principles of self-care
2 Food and nutrition
3 Personal and oral hygiene
4 Continence and bladder and bowel care
5 Pressure ulcers
6 Record keeping
7 Safety of patients with mental health needs in acute mental health and general hospital settings
8 Privacy and dignity.

It is important to note three points about this list:

1 Emphasis is given to the importance of self-care.
2 The list should not be taken as comprehensive; within this general area of basic or fundamental care there are a number of other important aspects of care. For example, the toolkit is to be extended in the near future to include communication with patients and communication with carers.
3 Reference to communication draws attention to the importance of teamwork. The Department of Health guidelines and toolkit (2001) are being developed not just as a

nursing initiative, but as one that involves all the members of the health care team.

Study Activity 34.10 ─────────────

This is a lengthy activity that will take up 1–2 hours of study time. Obtain access to the Department of Health document *The Essence of Care* (2001). If this is not available in your clinical area, an Adobe PDF file copy can be downloaded from the Department of Health internet website (it is a hefty document of almost 200 pages so you may wish to read and use it on-screen).

- Read the sections covering each of the eight benchmark topics in the publication, making notes as you go along.
- Establish whether the clinical areas you are working in or have access to use the benchmarking tools or whether they use a different set of national guidelines.
- Compare the benchmarks in this document to the clinical guidelines in the clinical area you are considering, evaluating how comprehensive these are and how they compare with the benchmark equivalents in citing underpinning evidence for best practice.
- Where there are no direct or closely comparable guidelines or standards, reflect upon how the benchmarks might improve care delivery in that setting.

How do such guidance or benchmarks inform practice at the nurse–patient interface? While such benchmarks can give broad guidance, each individual patient is different and each set of circumstances within which a particular aspect of care is being delivered is to some extent unique. This was recognised in initial work on such guidelines by the United Kingdom Central Council for Nursing, Midwifery and Health Visiting (1996), and subsequently incorporated in the new Nursing and Midwifery Council's *Code of Professional Conduct* (2002). A fairly straightforward formula could be proposed for the use of such guidelines. This would state that:

- National standards as reflected in benchmarks established upon best evidence and practice provide an overall source of guidance to those managing services at local levels.
- Those responsible for services at local level must also establish guidance for best practice within their area of accountability (trust, hospital, clinic, community setting). Under requirements for effective clinical governance, which places accountability for clinical standards upon chief executives and health service managers (Department of Health, 1998), there is a responsibility to ensure that such guidance is in place. It should draw upon the national benchmarks but be adapted to the local health care setting, as appropriate.
- Practitioners involved in direct care should base their care on the guidance provided within their health care setting. Where this is not available, it is important that national guidelines or benchmarks or, in their absence, other sources of evidence, are consulted. In any case, the practitioner must recognise that guidance derived from such sources must be adapted to suit the particular patient in the particular circumstances.
- Individual practitioners must recognise their responsibility to ensure that their own practice is based upon the best available evidence and other sources of valid and reliable information on best practice. The availability of guidance at local or national level does not remove the responsibility to critically appraise such information and evaluate its relevance and safety to the care they are delivering.

Finally, in adapting such practices, the views, and indeed rights, of the patient are of the greatest importance. Couchman and Dawson (1990) draw attention to the patient's rights:

- not to be harmed
- to be given informed consent
- to be given privacy
- to self-respect and dignity
- to refuse care or treatment
- not to be denied services.

In order to deliver effective and efficient care to patients in today's nursing climate, it is important that patients recognise that their rights have been taken into consideration (Department of Health, 1991). The rights of individual patients along with the Nursing and Midwifery Council's *Code of Professional Conduct* (2002) constitute a sound basis for the delivery of health care.

THE DELIVERY OF CARE

Common aspects of care

It will now be clear that the approach advocated is that of looking for carefully developed up-to-date guidelines, rather than looking to textbooks that may rapidly pass out of date. The following examples give guidelines for care in broad terms so that the student can begin to establish a basis for the delivery of such care. However, these are presented as illustrative examples only and up-to-date guidelines should be consulted for current evidence-based approaches to the interventions being addressed. Furthermore, the initial assessment of a patient is extremely important because essential details can be collected that will help the nurse to act in the patient's best interest. A move from independence to dependence by the patient can occur as a result of acute illness during surgery or in the progressive deterioration of a chronic condition such as multiple sclerosis, AIDS or cancer. In some care situations the patient may become unconscious and unable to speak. It is on the basis of careful assessment as a source for establishing nursing problems or diagnoses that effective, planned practice interventions can be determined.

The four fundamental aspects of care related to activities of living are:

- the need for bodily cleanliness
- the need to eat and drink
- the need to eliminate body waste
- the need for relief from pain and discomfort.

INDIVIDUALISED PERSONAL HYGIENE

Individuals have different attitudes towards washing their bodies. Cultural and social differences exist and patients must have their right to consent to treatment respected. The nurse should conduct a full assessment of the patient's current health status, which should include the level of independence plus any special needs, such as cultural washing practices. In addition, the nurse must act as a member of a caring team and be sure that the choices she offers to the patient are reasonable, safe, effective, and therapeutic.

It is particularly important in maintaining personal hygiene to promote a viable and healthy skin. The skin is one of the body's first defences against injury and infection and without it the body would not survive for more than a few minutes. The skin is a complex organ, consisting of different structures, tissues and glands, many of which have exceptional protective properties. (You may wish to review your human biology of the skin and its structure here.) If skin is allowed to become dirty and infected, or if damaged areas are not treated or areas of risk (known as pressure areas) exposed to excessive or prolonged pressure, the skin may break down. In assisting with personal hygiene, attention should be paid to the tissue viability of the skin.

Study Activity 34.11 ———————

Skin breakdown due to excessive pressure on its surface is a particular risk when there is prolonged bed rest, in neurological malfunction or paralysis, during prolonged anaesthesia, where there is body emaciation, or poor states of nutrition or hydration. Such breakdowns are commonly referred to as pressure ulcers, pressure sores, decubitus ulcers or 'bedsores'.

- Do a literature review on this topic. Useful starting points are:
  - Waterlow (1988)
  - Braden (1989)

– NHS Centre for Reviews and Dissemination (1995)
– Wellard and Lo (2000)
– Morison (2001).

• Write a brief description of a pressure ulcer.

• The Waterlow and Braden references relate to two of the most widely used assessment scales in the area of pressure ulcer prevention and care. Look these up and compare them.

• Using your library sources and local clinical guidelines for pressure ulcer care, list:

– the five most important preventative measures
– the five most effective treatment interventions
– the five most useful devices for relieving pressure at vulnerable areas of the body surface.

Handwashing

One of the most fundamental aspects of professional nursing practice is infection control and hand hygiene is the single most important principle of safe infection control. In all the interventions that follow it is important to remember that in moving from person to person the nurse's hands are a potential source of spread of infection. It is therefore vitally important that hands are washed and thoroughly dried using clean disposable towelling before and after any practice procedure and at other times before and after handling equipment, medicines, antiseptics and therapeutic substances.

Study Activity 34.12

• Obtain the following article on hand hygiene and read it carefully:

Gould D (2000) Hand hygiene research: past achievements and future challenges. *British Journal of Infection Control* 1(1), 17–22.

Hygiene preferences: personal cleansing and dressing

Consideration of the following details can improve the quality of care experienced by the patient and are incorporated into many nursing assessments:

• patients' preference for soap, emollients and skin cream
• the use of deodorants, antiperspirants, and powder
• the use of depilatory cream, shaving stick, foam, or waxing
• the use of special hair treatment, and shampoo preference
• the use of tampons or sanitary towels
• the use of make-up, skin cleanser, and toner
• nightwear or daywear
• nail care (including feet as well as hands)
• normal bathing routine (shower or wash down).

Guidelines for bathing

• Assess the mental and physical condition of the patient.
• Remember that the patient has rights – to consent to treatment, to individuality, to safety, and to information.
• Remember that patients have choices.
• The role of the nurse involves education of the patient, and every opportunity to provide health information must be taken.
• Patients should be given information about the purpose of bathing, e.g. to cleanse the skin, to reduce the risk of infection, to improve general well-being, or as a skin treatment.
• Preparation of the patient and the environment reduces wasted time and promotes efficiency.
• The patient's preferences about water depth, temperature, use of cleansing lotions, etc. should be taken into account where possible. However, in all instances the temperature of the water must be accurately measured by a bath thermometer.

- Assistance with bathing is provided when the patient is unable to care for himself. Where this involves lifting and moving the patient the nurse must ensure that she has adequate assistance and that those involved are adequately trained in the use of lifting and moving apparatus.
- The nurse must prioritise her actions on the ward so that she has time to devote to such assistance.
- In no circumstances should frail or confused patients or those at risk be left alone during the bathing routine.

Spiller (1992) reminds us that 'despite the current emphasis on individualised, patient-centred care, examples of nursing practice based on ritual and routine are still common'. Greaves (1985) demonstrated that patients were often dirtier after being washed, as a result of *Pseudomonas* growing on wet washcloths and washing basins. However, Nightingale (1859) believed that leaving a patient unwashed was as injurious to the natural process of health as if the patient were given poison.

Study Activity 34.13 _____

In the past, patients have been scalded by being immersed in bath water that was of too high a temperature. In modern health care facilities within the NHS it is usual for hot water supplies to bathrooms to have thermostatic controls. However, this is not always the case and patients also have varying tolerance to the temperature of water. Water that is too hot can injure, but water that is of too low a temperature can also have harmful effects.

- Check the guidance in your clinical area on the temperature of bath water.
- Review the literature on bathing, with particular attention to bathing scalds, temperature of bath water, and means of ascertaining temperature.
- Write out the main safety points you have uncovered and discuss these with your mentor, clinical supervisor or ward manager.

Showering

The popularity of the shower is increasing and, with the use of shower chairs and restraining equipment, many patients opt to shower. Another reason for this is the reduced risk of hospital-acquired infection. The nurse must ensure that the patient is capable of going to the shower and must provide assistance if required. It is essential that all hospital showers have fully operational heat regulators. Adequate nurse call systems must also be in place.

Again, preparation of the patient and the environment can save valuable time. If the patient requires the use of restraining equipment to protect them from falling or damaging their limbs, they must never be left alone in the shower. The nurse must always remember to attend to all the patient's hygiene needs.

The traditional bed bath

The skill of performing a safe, effective and therapeutic bed bath is necessary for all nurses (*see* Table 34.1). This intimate task makes demands on the nurse's knowledge, skill, and attitude. The central focus of nursing is caring and performing for the individual those things that he or she cannot do. However, the nurse must be careful to avoid routinised bathing rituals, as highlighted by Spiller (1992).

The bed bath is usually given to patients when self-care is limited or impossible, e.g. to those who are unconscious, febrile, postoperative, or in a plaster cast. Again, the assessment of the patient's strengths and weaknesses, as well as the inclusion of hygiene preferences, is essential. It is also essential for the nurse to ensure that the patient who has just had surgery has been given adequate analgesia prior to carrying out the procedure. The nurse needs to be certain that she understands the safety needs of the patient with regard to joint mobility, body alignment, and any special instructions. Patients who are in the intensive care unit also require a full explanation of the procedure prior to commencement, and a warning should be given that their breathing may be compromised when they are turned on their side to have their back washed. A great deal of thought and care is required to complete a bed bath that leaves a patient feeling refreshed and comfortable. The competent nurse would choose a unique way of caring for each individual patient.

Study Activity 34.14

Review the article by Casey (2002) The physiology of the skin. *Nursing Standard* **16**(34), 47–51. Use the key words 'anatomy and physiology' and 'skin and skin disorders' to search out further articles on this subject on the internet.

Table 34.1 Preparation for a traditional bed bath

Checklist for preparation of the environment
- Ensure that the room temperature is adequate.
- Provide adequate privacy.
- Position items of furniture to provide adequate space (care is very often provided in the patient's own home).
- Check bathing equipment and ensure that the water is at a suitable temperature (35–40°C).
- Ensure that there is a separate bag for dirty linen and waste material.
- Obtain the patient's wash cloths, cleansing agents, etc.
- Check that the patient has clean clothes to put on afterwards.

Preparation of the patient
- Obtain consent from the patient.
- Provide a full explanation of the proposed procedure.
- Give an approximate length of time for completion.
- Ensure that there is adequate privacy.
- Keep the patient as comfortable as possible.
- Observe patient requests.
- Identify areas that the patient will wash himself.
- Provide assistance where necessary.
- Allow plenty of time for the patient to use the toilet.
- Provide analgesia if necessary.
- Check that the patient is not expecting visitors and that the doctor's round is not due.
- Try to provide individualised care within the confines of the environment.

Study Activity 34.15

- Read the article by Spiller (1992), For whose sake – patient or nurse? Ritual practices in patient washing. *Professional Nurse*, **7**(7), 431–4.

- Read about methicillin-resistant *Staphylococcus aureus* (MRSA) by Makoni (2002) in MRSA: risk assessment and flexible management. *Nursing Standard* **16**(28), 39–41. Discuss the implications for practice with peers, lecturers and mentors.

Table 34.2 gives the protocol and rationale for bed bathing.

When the bed bath is over the patient should be left feeling revitalised, clean, warm and comfortable. An alternative to the traditional bed bath is the towel bath (refer to Wright, 1990). Finally make sure you have used the bed bath as an opportunity to check for tissue viability (*see* Study Activity 34.11).

Study Activity 34.16

Write notes on the following situations.

- An 18-year-old male is paralysed from the neck down, due to a fracture at the level of C7, and requires a bed bath. How would you involve him in his care?
- A 42-year-old female with a severe learning disability is first day post-op. after undergoing an appendectomy. She requires her personal hygiene to be attended to. How would you obtain consent to provide care for this patient?
- A 62-year-old senile, bedridden gentleman is being nursed at home, with care being provided by the care co-ordinator. He is often aggressive and refuses to be washed by the visiting nurse. How do you think you could cope with this problem?

Female perineal care

Table 34.3 gives the protocol and rationale for female perineal care.

If patients are menstruating, remember to place a clean sanitary towel in position and secure with sticky adhesive, or attach to sanitary belt. All blood-stained materials need to be placed in the appropriate disposal bag to reduce risk of blood-borne disease.

Table 34.2 Bed bathing

Protocol	Rationale
1 Remove top blankets and sheets. Fold individually from top to bottom and in half again. Place at the foot of the bed on extension rail or over a chair.	1 Keeps linen dry for replacement and saves time and energy when remaking the bed. Ensure that linen does not lie on the floor, to prevent infection, and dispose of soiled or dirty linen in the appropriate bags.
2 Place a large, clean, dry towel or bath blanket over the patient's chest and ask him/her to hold it in place. Pull the top sheet from under the blanket and fold it in two.	2 Provides warmth and privacy for the patient.
3 Position the patient as close to your edge of the bed as possible, remembering to adhere to guidelines for handling and moving patients.	3 Prevents unnecessary stretching and damage to your back.
4 Remove the patient's clothing, maintaining his/her privacy and dignity.	4 Keeping the towel in place prevents overexposure and embarrassment for the patient.
5 Place the patient on his/her back and provide at least one pillow.	5 Patients feel more comfortable with at least one pillow, and some patients may request elevation of the bed if they have breathing difficulties.
6 Pay particular attention to the safe positioning of IV lines, drains, and catheters.	6 To prevent dislodgement of items, and to maintain a safe environment for the patient.
7 Converse freely with the patient – talk about hobbies, radio, TV, etc.	7 Relieves patient anxiety, and helps to reduce embarrassment. If the patient is unconscious it is essential to continue to stimulate him.
8 Use the patient's preferred cleansing agent.	8 Many people suffer from dry skin after using soap, especially the elderly (Carnevali and Patrick, 1993), and many women use a cleansing lotion or cream (Gooch, 1987).
9 Place a face towel under the patient's head and carefully wash their face, ears, and neck. It is best not to use soap. The eyes should be given special care, using a solution of normal saline for patients who are unconscious or those who have eye infections.	9 Protects the bed; soap is an irritant.
10 Remove the towel and place it under the arm furthest away. Commence washing with soap or patient preference, beginning under the arm and working down towards the hand. Repeat for the other arm.	10 Protects the bed. Prevents the arm nearest to you from becoming wet.
11 The hands can be placed in the basin of water to wash them.	11 Stimulates sensation in unconscious patients. Provides extra cleanliness, particularly if a nail brush is needed to clean under nails.
12 The patient's body is washed from the neck to the abdomen and the body towel is kept in position between the wash, rinse, and dry periods.	12 Provides privacy and warmth, and prevents overexposure and embarrassment.
13 Place the towel under the leg furthest away from you, as close to the groin as possible and repeat the washing procedure. Repeat for the other leg.	13 Prevents the leg nearest to you from becoming wet as you reach across to do the other.

(cont.)

Table 34.2 Bed bathing (*cont.*)

Protocol	Rationale
14 Feet may be immersed in the wash basin.	14 Extra cleansing of feet may be necessary. Provides stimulation.
15 Change water, change wash cloth, check temperature, and leave the patient to wash the genital area if capable. Wash the genital area if the patient is unable. Wash from the umbilicus down.	15 The perineal area is considered to be infection-bearing, and clean, discardable cloths are required to reduce the risk of infection. The patient must be allowed the maximum amount of privacy.
16 Cleanse from front to back in the female.	16 The anal area contains numerous bacteria. These bacteria can travel into the female urethra or the vagina, where they can cause infection.
17 Cleanse the penis tip without soap, gently pulling back the foreskin, if present, and cleansing carefully. Wash, rinse and dry.	17 The top of the penis is sensitive and easily damaged. Debris tends to collect here and needs to be removed. The foreskin of the penis must be pulled back into place once cleaned.
18 Discard water and cloths.	18 Reduces the risk of infection.
19 Turn the patient on to his/her side, and place the towel lengthways on the bed, against the back.	19 Protects the bed.
20 Ensure that the bath blanket is still in place.	20 Provides privacy and warmth, and reduces overexposure.

Table 34.3 Protocol and rationale for female perineal care

Protocol	Rationale
1 Explain the procedure to the patient.	1 Treats the patient with respect. Encourages independence.
2 Take fresh, warm water (35–40°C) and a clean wash cloth and some soap.	2 A warm solution provides comfort to the patient.
3 Place a towel underneath the patient. Bend the patient's knees and open the legs gently.	3 Protects the bed.
4 Wearing gloves, begin to wash the urethra or pubic area, remembering to wash towards the anal area.	4 Gloves protect the nurse from harmful bacteria. Reduces risk of anal contamination of urethra or vagina.
5 If there is a catheter in situ, open the labia gently, expose the meatus and cleanse thoroughly, removing any encrustations. Wash from the meatus outwards, down the catheter tube. Wash, rinse and dry.	5 Catheters are notorious sources of infection and require scrupulous cleansing.

Study Activity 34.17 _____

Write notes on the following:

- What type of patient do you think is likely to require female perineal care?
- Do you think that male students should carry out female perineal care?
- Would it be less embarrassing to carry out care of the perineal area if the patient was unconscious, mentally confused, or suffering from a learning disability?

Oral health care

The aim of good oral hygiene is to maintain the condition of the mouth in a state of health and cleanliness. Table 34.4 gives the protocol and rationale for cleansing the mouth area.

Mouth care or oral hygiene demands special skills of observation and a sound theoretical knowledge from the nurse. Nurses have been accused of giving little attention to the importance of this everyday practice, but this is not necessarily true. Nurses are recognising the need for more research into practice, hence the many research reports that focus on this area; for example Trenter-Roth and Creeson (1986), Miller and Rubenstein (1987), Shepherd *et al.* (1987), Walsh and Ford (1989), Hatton-Smith (1994) and Kay and Locker (1997).

Study Activity 34.18 _____

The objective of this Study Activity is to increase your awareness of the importance of carrying out mouth care with the appropriate knowledge, skills, and attitude.

- Review the following articles on mouth care and make notes for your practice:

 Peate, I. (1993) Nurse-administered oral hygiene in the hospitalized patient. *British Journal of Nursing* **2**(9), 459–62.
 Hatton-Smith, C.K. (1994) A last bastion of ritualised practice? A review of nurses' knowledge of oral healthcare. *Professional Nurse* **9**(5), 305–8.
 Kay, W., Locker, D. (1997) *Effectiveness of Oral Health Promotion: A review*. Health Promotion Effectiveness Reviews, No. 7, Health Education Authority, London.

Care of prostheses

Many patients today wear a prosthesis of some kind. This may be something as simple as a pair of spectacles or as complicated as a facio-maxillary appliance. There are many different forms of prostheses, and it is important to make sure they are cared for properly. Information is best obtained from manufacturers or the prostheses unit within your health care trust or hospital. However, the nurse should also consult the patient about care and preferences.

Table 34.4 Protocol and rationale for mouth care

Protocol	Rationale
1 Inspect the lips, teeth, tongue, palate and surrounding tissue.	1 Identifies any broken or damaged teeth, or any infections, so that treatment can commence and the risk of disease is halted.
2 Remove any dentures or plates, and cleanse thoroughly with a solution of the patient's usual preference. Rinse the teeth.	2 Thorough cleansing reduces the risk of mouth infection, ulceration, gingivitis or thrush (Shepherd *et al.*, 1987).
3 Rinse the mouth with mouth wash. Replace teeth.	3 Chlorhexidine is extremely useful. It has a pH of 7 and is a popular choice.
4 Provide the patient with a dish to spit into, clean water, toothbrush, and toothpaste. Assist with brushing and rinsing if needed.	4 Use a non-abrasive toothpaste.

Study Activity 34.19

Find out how many different types of prosthesis are generally available today. Obtain data about the numbers of people in your area who have false limbs. Try to find out whether there is a central register that contains this type of data on a national level.

Eye care

Most patients will not require the nurse to provide special assistance with this activity. Patients who may require assistance are those who are too young (e.g. babies), those too ill to do it for themselves, those who suffer neurological disease, unconscious patients, paraplegics or those who need to be taught specific eye care following surgical procedures, such as corneal grafts and laser therapy. Table 34.5 gives the protocol and rationale for eye care.

Nasal care

Those requiring assistance with, or education about nasal care are babies or small children, patients who are unconscious, or who have had oral surgery or oesophageal surgery and need to have a naso-gastric tube in situ for a long time. Table 34.6 gives the protocol and rationale for nasal care.

Table 34.5   Protocol and rationale for eye care

Protocol	Rationale
Equipment: sterile or non-sterile cotton balls; sterile or non-sterile container; gloves; normal saline; towel.	
1 Explain the procedure to the patient.	1 Treats the patient with respect. Encourages independence.
2 Wash your hands. Decide on the need to use sterile materials or clean materials. Put on appropriate gloves.	2 Reduces infection. Use sterile material when the patient has a high risk of obtaining an infection, e.g. if he or she has had eye surgery. Otherwise, wear clean, disposable gloves.
3 Place a towel or a basin to the side of the patient's face. He/she may sit up or lie on the side that requires cleansing.	3 Protects the patient's clothing and bed linen. If one eye is infected, it is important to protect the other eye from receiving the overflow, thus also becoming infected.
4 *Option 1*: Using sterile gloves, dip sterile cotton balls into a sterile solution of warm, normal saline. Squeeze off excess water.	4 *Option 1*: Sterile materials are expensive and are not necessary with every patient.
Option 2: Using clean gloves, dip clean cotton balls into clean, warm tap water and squeeze off excess water.	*Option 2*: Read Clulow, M. (1994) A closer look at disposable gloves. *Professional Nurse* **9**(5), 324–9.
5 Cleanse the eye, starting from the inside near the nose, and moving near the temple to the outside in one gentle movement. Discard the cotton ball. Repeat until debris and encrustations are removed.	5 Cleansing the eye from the inner to outer aspect prevents the solution from entering the lacrimal duct.
6 Repeat the procedure for the other eye. Encourage the patient to practice the procedure.	6 Many patients still require scrupulous attention to eye hygiene after discharge from hospital, so you must ensure that the patient is capable of self-care.

Table 34.6 Protocol and rationale for nasal care

Protocol	Rationale
Equipment: a small bowl of warm water (35–40°C); gauze; gloves; cotton buds; suction apparatus.	
1 Explain the procedure to the patient.	1 Treats the patient with respect. Encourages independence. Make it into a playful experience for small children.
2 Wash hands and wear gloves.	2 Reduces infection.
3 Take a small bowl of warm water (35–40°C) and moisten cotton buds. Gently insert them into the nostrils and remove any hard, dry secretions.	3 It is essential to be gentle as the mucous membranes of children are easily damaged.
4 Cleanse the naso-gastric tubing with moistened gauze, cleaning from the nostril out along the tubing, and dry. Gentle suction may be necessary when patients who have copious secretions are unable to clear their own noses.	4 Naso-gastric tubes often become encrusted with secretions that dry, harden and can pierce the skin, causing bleeding, pain, discomfort and infection. Children do not usually learn to blow their nose until they are 5 years old.
5 Apply moisture cream around the nostrils.	5 Keeps skin moist and intact.

A cultural perspective

In today's multicultural society, nurses need to aware of cultural differences, so that individual care can be provided. The three main cultural groups will be discussed briefly in relation to hygiene practices.

Moslem

Moslem patients like to wash in running water, so a shower or wash down with running water needs to be provided. They also like to wash their genital area after using the toilet, and need a wash basin or a bidet for this. The left hand is used for this practice and the right hand for eating. The mouth, hands and feet are washed five times a day, prior to praying, for which a jug and basin are needed. The female body is usually covered from head to toe, so long operation gowns must be provided, or individuals should be allowed to wear their own clean clothes. Men wear caftans or pyjamas.

Study Activity 34.20 _____

- If a Moslem was going to the operating theatre, why would it be valuable to know which hand was used for what?

- How do Moslem ladies cope with keeping their body covered when they are having a baby?

_____

Hindu

Showering under running water is important, so adequate facilities should be available. Hindus require to wash their genitals after using the toilet, so a jug and bowl at the bedside are needed. The nurse may have to perform the cleansing if they are incapable. Women must cover their legs, breasts and upper arms and may require their own clean clothing during operations. Some wash before they pray, but unlike Moslems, they do not have set times for prayer. They may need help with washing.

Sikh

Sikhs have similar practices to Hindus and Moslems. They too prefer to shower, and to wash after using the toilet. Long hair, beards and turbans are worn by the men, while women wear their hair in a bun, kept in place by a 'Kangha'. The hair is never cut and the head is the most sacred part of the body. Devout Sikhs never completely take their underpants off, and these 'kacchas' are pushed down, left over one ankle and recovered when the clean ones are on the other leg. They also wash before they pray, usually once or twice a day.

Study Activity 34.21

Read Narayanasamy, A. (1993) Nurses' awareness and educational preparation in meeting their patients' spiritual needs. *Nurse Education Today* **13**, 196–201. Use the questionnaire to test your own knowledge about spiritual care.

A summary of personal hygiene

Attendance to patients' basic hygiene is a core nursing skill that demands the following:

- superb practical skills
- sound theory and knowledge
- awareness of relevant research
- an individual approach
- attention to small detail
- a cultural awareness
- a kind, gentle, compassionate nature.

Study Activity 34.22

Read the following quotation attributed to the nursing pioneer, Virginia Henderson (1966):

The nurse is temporarily the consciousness of the unconscious, the love of life of the suicidal, the leg of the amputee, the eyes of the newly blind, a means of locomotion for the new-born, knowledge and confidence for the young mother, a voice for those too weak to speak.

- Write a short essay of 500–700 words on how you think you will develop the necessary knowledge, skills and attitudes to become the consciousness of the patient.

NUTRITIONAL ASPECTS OF CARE

Dietary intake

Eating and drinking are essential to living. Most of us eat our three meals a day with little concern. When we are ill, however, we may require a modified diet, or even naso-gastric feeding if we lose our independence due to ill health. Therefore nurses must be able to understand basic nutritional requirements in order to provide an adequate dietary intake for the patients under their care (Lask, 1986; Scanlan *et al.*, 1994; Barasi, 1997).

Study activity 34.23

- Find out as much information as you can about the nursing care of a patient receiving total parenteral nutrition.
- Describe how you would tackle the problem of obesity with a 60-year-old man who has high blood pressure and a previous history of myocardial infarction and lives on his own in a council flat.

Vitamins and minerals

A balanced diet must include protein (to build up body tissue), carbohydrate or sugar (for rapidly accessibly energy) and fat (as an additional source of energy, a source of stored energy in the body and for utilisation of fat-soluble vitamins). In addition to vitamins (vital amines or organic substances needed in small amounts to govern body activities and metabolism) we need minerals – chemical substances that become electrolytes when dissolved within the body. They are important for the maintenance of healthy body tissue and fluid balance as well as nerve conduction and blood clotting. When working on the wards you will see patients having blood taken to check their electrolytes. Those who are not eating or are unable to eat a balanced diet due to illness will have these tests. Doctors prescribe intravenous solutions that contain potassium and sodium to solve the problem.

A balanced diet must also include sufficient fluid intake, as water or other beverages: the human body can service up to several weeks without food, but a much shorter period (a few days, according to climatic conditions) without water. Fibre, in foods such as whole grain cereals, fruit, and some vegetables, provides the bulk that helps digestion and cleanses the gastrointestinal tract. Fibre may also assist in preventing diseases of this tract, such as cancer or diverticulitis.

Study Activity 34.24

Consult the recommended text on nutrition and dietetics for your course of study, or if no specific text is recommended, find one in your library that has been published within the past 5 years. Write brief outlines of normal dietary requirements under headings for the main nutritional categories – proteins, carbohydrates, fats, vitamins, minerals, fluid intake and fibre. The concept of a 'normal diet' depends on the individual, the activities they undertake, and factors such as need to replenish damaged tissues after injury or surgery. This should lead to the concept of a 'balanced diet', which relates to the specific demand placed on the individual in terms of growth, replenishment, homeostasis and energy outputs.

Assisting with dietary intake

Patients will normally prefer to feed themselves, and where possible this aspect of self-care must be promoted. However, in some instances the nurse must assist the patient. How the patient is fed depends very much on his condition and dietary requirements; in some instances more specialised techniques such as naso-gastric or trans-abdominal tube feeding may be required.

Study Activity 34.25

• Read through Table 34.7, and see if you can find any evidence from the literature that would back it up:

Table 34.7 Principles for dietary provision

- Assess the patient's normal diet and his record.
- Pay special attention to children and the elderly.
- Assist individuals to select a nutritious diet from the menu when in hospital.
- Check that the patient gets the correct meal ordered.
- Check that the patient consumes the food provided.
- Observe the patient at meal times.
- Ensure that meals are hot and attractively presented.
- If relatives bring in food from home, don't forget to cancel the ward meal.
- Remember to check the nutritional value of food brought in and offer advice if necessary.
- Promote a healthy diet by providing information on recommended low fat, high fibre, low salt, and low sugar diets.
- Contact the dietician if patients are unable to eat a normal diet, so that soft or puréed food can be provided. The dietician will also provide a weight reduction or a weight increase diet.
- Patients on naso-gastric or gastric feeding will require a visit from the dietician to recommend the appropriate liquid diet.
- Encourage patients to be independent and to feed themselves.
- Provide extra time for those who have a disability or those in the rehabilitation phase.
- The occupational therapist may be called to provide adapted cutlery and plates for a patient with motor problems.
- Record the food and dietary intake of individuals who are dependent on you to provide their dietary intake.
- Encourage patients to eat together at a table if they can do so.

(Adapted from Francis, 1985; Dickerson, 1986; Patients' Association, 1993 and Barasi, 1997)

The following are important considerations:

• Ask the patient for his preferences and ascertain whether he has any dislikes in terms of the food being served. Do this before the meal is served; most modern health care facilities have a menu choice, which is offered to patients in advance.

- Present the food as attractively as possible. While it may be necessary to 'spoon feed' or use feeding cups, where possible use normal dining utensils: soup spoons, knives and forks, dessert spoons, glasses, cups and saucers. Take time to arrange the meal on the tray – small touches such as a flower in a small vase can have significant psychological benefits.
- Where relatives are participating in care, encourage them to feed the patient or help with this activity. However, where patients are seriously ill or at special risk, always ensure that there is adequate support and supervision.
- Ask the patient whether they like condiments, sugar in tea or coffee and ensure that their tastes are being catered for (unless contra-indicated, as in a low-salt diet).
- Do not rush the event – 'shovelling' food into the patient is unethical, distressing and may even be dangerous.
- Make sure the patient is supported in a comfortable, upright position, and sit in a relaxed posture at the same level, with the meal on a bed table so that the patient can see it.
- Place a serviette loosely around the patient's neck.
- Always include a glass of water with a meal (irrespective of other beverages being served) and offer sips frequently, particularly if the patient is having difficulty swallowing, and at the end of a meal.
- If possible, assist the patient to feed himself by supporting and directing his arms and helping him raise the food and drink to his mouth.
- Ensure that only small amounts of food or fluid are fed at a time, and place food at the top of the tongue to stimulate the swallowing reflex.
- It is important that food and drinks are served at the correct temperature. Cold food or beverages such as tea or coffee could distress the patient, and if they are too hot there is a risk of injury, particularly where the patient has neurological complications.
- Constantly pat lips and chin dry with a serviette if the patient cannot do this unaided.

Remember that the patient may be uncomfortable or distressed if food or fluids are allowed to dribble.
- Observe carefully throughout for difficulties in swallowing. If there are signs of obstruction (choking noises, signs of distress, changes in complexion or level of consciousness) immediate emergency action to clear the airways is needed. Always ensure that when patients are seriously ill or at special risk (as with stroke patients), suction apparatus and oxygen are readily available. In such an emergency you should always call for assistance immediately.
- Treat the event as a social occasion, an opportunity to speak with the patient. Remember that dining is an important social event, enjoyable in most cultures – an opportunity to meet and share with others (Wykes, 1997).
- On completion, ensure that the dining table or tray is cleared away and that the patient is left clean and comfortable.

Cultural considerations

Eating is essential to human life. The individual's cultural background affects the type of food eaten. Many people adapt to the Western lifestyle, others do not, so always assess – never assume. Some food differences between cultures are given below.

Moslem

Moslems fast during Ramadan, eating when the sun goes down. Pork and all pork products are forbidden. Meat can be eaten if the blood has been drained according to halal ritual. Moslems usually eat vegetarian food when hospitalised.

Hindu

Some fast at regular periods and eat a restricted diet. No beef is eaten, and some do not eat eggs.

Chinese

There are no notable periods of fasting. Rice is eaten at most meals. Special teas and herbal remedies are common and sometimes taken for their healing properties (see Chapter 31).

ELIMINATION

Using the toilet is a private matter for everyone. We base some perceptions about our current health status on our observation of the waste products left in the toilet and it is a function we like to perform alone. It is hardly surprising that most people suffer acute embarrassment if they require assistance with any aspect of toileting, especially when incontinence is a problem. Patients may need assistance in going to the toilet or in the use of the bedpan, urinal or commode. Safe lifting and moving skills are required. Privacy is also a requirement and where bedbound patients are using a bedpan or commode, the area must be carefully screened. Odour is often embarrassing to the patient and it is important to ensure good ventilation and to use safe air freshners. Assistance in cleansing after using the toilet or after a bout of incontinence requires particularly sensitive intervention on the part of the nurse. This activity must be accomplished gently but efficiently, and the patient must always be left dry and comfortable.

Study Activity 34.26 ————————

- How do you think you would cope with not being in control of your bladder or bowel?
- Do you think it would be easier to be elderly and incontinent or young and incontinent?
- Is incontinence a national problem?
- Can people with learning disabilities control their bowel and bladder?

The characteristics of normal urine and urination in healthy adults

Output of urine ranges from 1500 ml to 2000 ml per day, depending on the amount of fluid consumed. Adults normally urinate 3–6 times a day (except when they have a urinary infection or are stressed), passing 300–600 ml on each occasion. Oliguria is the term used to describe the passing (micturition) of a small amount of urine, a total daily output of less than 500 ml. This can be due to retention of urine, kidney or heart disease, excessive vomiting, diarrhoea or perspiration. Polyuria is the term used to describe the micturition of too much urine – this is often a sign of diabetes or pituitary malfunction.

The colour of urine varies from pale lemon to golden amber. When it is more concentrated, it is darker in colour and stronger in smell. Dark brown, frothy urine usually indicates the presence of bilirubin. Red or pink colouration usually indicates blood in the urine caused by menstruation or infection, or by eating beetroot. Mahogany-coloured urine is usually caused by urobilinogen, the incomplete breakdown of red blood corpuscles.

The most common method of testing urine is by using reagent strips, which provide instant information on the characteristics of the urine (*see* Table 34.8).

Table 34.8 Characteristics of urine, as shown by reagent strips

Content	Result
Protein	Should read negative. If present, it suggests a urine infection or impaired kidney filtration, and further tests are required.
Glucose	Should read negative. If present, it suggests a recent high sugar intake or diabetes, and further tests are required.
Ketones	Should read negative. If present, they indicate that the person has not eaten for some time, and that their body fat is being broken down to provide energy.
pH balance	Should be acidic, as this discourages bacterial growth (average pH of 6).
Specific gravity	Should be approximately 1.000 to 1.030.

As well as using reagent strips, the nurse can use her sense of smell when testing urine. A sweet smell usually indicates sugar, the pungent smell of acetone is often associated with ketones and a fishy smell is often present when urine is infected. In the case of abnormal urine, many tests can be carried out in the laboratory, and the nurse needs to be able to obtain a mid-stream specimen of urine. This should be collected in a sterile container in the middle of the urination process, after the genitals have been cleansed. The person should stop urinating in mid-flow, place a sterile container to catch the flow and then recommence urination. Only a small amount (enough to give 20 cc of urine) needs to be collected. The container should be removed without touching the inside, and given to the nurse to bottle and label before it is sent to the laboratory.

Study Activity 34.27

This exercise requires a disposable container.

● Using the minimal guidelines to obtain a mid-stream specimen of urine, take one from yourself, pretending that the container is sterile. Think about the information provided and ask yourself whether it is sufficient. Evaluate your skill in performing the task. Use your eyes and nose to identify character-istics present in the urine. Imagine how patients would deal with this request, and write a short report on the event.

Table 34.9 gives the protocol and rationale for promoting urinary continence.

The characteristics of faeces

Faeces are subject to the same observational criteria as urine. The volume should be between 200 and 300 gm daily. This amount may be increased if food is insufficiently digested, as in the case of reabsorption problems caused by intestinal disorders, diarrhoea and pancreatitis. A decreased volume occurs when fluid and fibre intake is low, causing constipation. Frequency should be one or two motions per day, but for some people it will be every 2–3 days. Diarrhoea or loose stools can be due to infection, stress or bowel disorders such as Crohn's disease. Table 34.10 gives the characteristics of normal faeces.

Study Activity 34.28

● Write approximately 500 words on the observa-tional skills required by the nurse when assessing problems associated with elimination in the following patients:

  – an 18-year-old Down's syndrome patient admitted with constipation
  – a 30-year-old female who has had a colectomy for Crohn's disease
  – an elderly, confused patient admitted with a possible bowel obstruction.

Remember that incontinence can be extremely embarrassing for the client, so the nurse must practise good communication skills, and be gentle and consid-erate.

Study Activity 34.29

● Read the following research articles and discuss the implications for your nursing practice.

  – Cox et al. (1989) Infection of catheterised patients: bacterial colonisation of encrusted Foley catheters shown by scanning electron micro-scopy. *Urological Research* **17**(6), 349–52.
  – Thornburn, P. et al. (1992) Undercover trials. *Nursing Times* **88**(13), 72–8.
  – Simpson, L. (2002) Collectable guide on inter-mittent self-catheterisation. *Nursing Standard* **16**(29) [collectable guide insert].

Table 34.9 Promoting urinary continence

Protocol	Rationale
1 Seek the patient's consent.	1 It is essential to obtain the patient's cooperation from the beginning. Ensure privacy and confidentiality.
2 Identify the incontinence pattern.	2 There are numerous causes, ranging from retention of urine to neurological spasms. A detailed history helps to clarify the problem. Stress incontinence is a common side-effect of childbirth and can be decreased with pelvic floor exercises. People with neurological disorders such as motor neurone disease or multiple sclerosis often suffer from neurogenic bladders, which can be treated with antispasmodic drugs.
3 Examine the lower abdomen.	3 Ensure that the bladder is not full and that the incontinence is not caused by overflow of urine from a distended bladder.
4 Commence observation and recording of incontinence (fluid balance chart).	4 It is important to have accurate assessment details to identify patterns of behaviour.
5 Inform the patient of the reasons for the measures being taken.	5 Patients have the right to information and should have some control over nursing assessment, observation and recording of data.
6 Encourage the patient to comply with a 2–3 hourly toilet regime.	6 Bladder retraining can alleviate the problem.
7 Provide privacy.	7 Using the toilet is a private business. Patients may request help when going to the bathroom.
8 Encourage the patient to perform simple pelvic floor exercises.	8 Pelvic muscle tone can be improved with exercise (Wells, 1990; Roe, 1991).
9 Ensure that the patient remains clean, dry and comfortable.	9 Skin integrity can be damaged by the ammonia in urine and can lead to infection.
10 Provide incontinence pads or waterproof underwear.	10 Helps the patient to relax and reduces anxiety. Some products can reduce skin damage.
11 Offer males a disposable padded urinal or an external catheter or tubing.	11 The padding may be soft cotton, which will protect the penis from chaffing. Helps to retain dignity and comfort.
12 Refer the patient to a urologist.	12 The reason for prolonged incontinence must be identified so that long-term care can be planned.
13 Perform catheterisation.	13 This is an emergency procedure to relieve urine retention or control incontinence if there is serious skin breakdown. Intermittent catheterisation can be performed by the patient or caregiver to promote continence.

Table 34.10 The characteristics of normal faeces

Characteristic	Description
Colour	Normally brown. Light-coloured, fatty stools are usually associated with a lack of bilirubin. Black faeces may be due to taking iron in the diet or to intestinal bleeding. The latter is known as melaena and has a distinct, pungent smell. When suspected, three samples of faeces should be sent to the laboratory for analysis of occult blood. Red faeces can be as a result of eating beetroot. Fresh blood streaks on the outer surface of the stool indicate anal bleeding, often due to haemorrhoids. Green, loose faeces indicates infection and samples must be sent to the laboratory.
Smell	Normally smell of rotten food. Certain foodstuffs (garlic, onions, cabbage and leeks) can make the smell very unpleasant. Foul smells are associated with infection and blood.
pH balance	Faeces are normally neutral.
Abnormal content	Blood, mucus, pus and worms are abnormal and require further investigation.
Shape	Usually semi-solid sausage shape. Long, tapered stools can be indicative of fissures or tumours. Porridge-like, fatty stools indicate malabsorption of fats.

- Search the following websites about incontinence and discuss the quality of the evidence and the benefits of patient information on-line:
  - Association for Continence Advice
  - Continence Promotion Committee of the International Continence Society
  - Digestive Disorders Foundation
  - Disabled Living Centres Council
  - ERIC (Enuresis Resource and Information Centre)
  - The Ileostomy and Internal Pouch Group
  - National Association for Colitis and Crohn's Disease (NACC)
  - Promocon (continence product information sheets and display)
  - Spinal Injuries Association
  - Multiple Sclerosis Society.

If the patient suffers from constipation, the nurse must begin care by assessing the normal pattern of bowel movement and taking details about the daily dietary consumption of fibre and fluid. Most constipation problems can be alleviated by dietary intervention and a few lifestyle adjustments, such as more exercise and fresh air. Laxatives, suppositories or enemas are given to relieve the acute problem, but are definitely not recommended on a long-term basis. A full investigation and medical examination are required to rule out the possibility of bowel tumours or diverticulitis. Table 34.11 gives the protocol and rationale for promoting bowel continence.

Vomiting

Vomiting is not normal. It is a frightening experience for the patient and usually occurs involuntarily, although it can be induced by those who suffer from eating disorders such as anorexia or bulimia. Whatever the cause, the nurse needs to comfort the patient by placing her hands on the forehead and the occiput to support and protect the head. Vomiting can be vigorous and forceful, and the presence of a nurse with a calm, confident approach can ease the fear in this situation and a gentle, quiet and reassuring voice can have a positive psychological effect. The nurse must always be aware of her own non-verbal signals, as patients can be very sensitive.

Study Activity 34.30

- Write short notes on the nursing care of:
  - the patient who is vomiting postoperatively

Table 34.11   Promoting bowel continence

Protocol	Rationale
1 Seek the patient's consent.	1 It is essential to obtain the patient's full cooperation and to ensure privacy and confidentiality.
2 Identify the incontinence pattern.	2 Some people use laxatives on a regular basis.
3 Observe the faecal material.	3 Patients with neurological problems can lose sphincter control. Gross constipation can lead to leakage of faecal material. Infection can cause diarrhoea.
4 Record stools on a chart. Measure diarrhoea and fluid.	4 Patients can become very ill if they have continuous diarrhoea. Parenteral nutrition may be necessary to relieve symptoms and restore fluid and electrolyte balance (Bladen, 1986; Dewar, 1986). Special dietary attention is also necessary.
5 Seek the patient's participation in a toilet regime. Provide dietary advice.	5 Identify pattern and take the patient to the toilet to encourage defecation. Gentle massage of the lower abdomen can stimulate a motion. After dietary assessment, provide information on nutrition, high-fibre bulk foods and a high fluid intake (Andrews, 1993; Mead, 1994). A semi-solid movement is easier to manage than a loose, watery one.
6 Promote skin integrity.	6 Provide incontinence pads. Use a barrier cream around the anus to prevent excoriation. Wash and dry the whole genital area after an episode of incontinence.

– the patient vomiting as a result of raised intra cranial pressure
– the patient admitted for care because of bulimia and anorexia nervosa.

Sputum

Sputum is often described by new students as the most difficult aspect of elimination for them to face. The sound of someone getting ready to spit, and the colour and the stickiness of it take some time to get used to. However, a patient may need assistance with expectoration of sputum, especially following surgery. Before chemical expectorants are used, it is preferable to provide warm drinks, support the patient's chest and shoulders if needed, and provide encouragement. Gone are the days when it was the role of the most junior nurses to collect and empty sputum cartons. But perhaps the practice

had a hidden value in that the junior nurses learned very quickly that the variety of contents in the container was important. Expectorating sputum is the respiratory system's mechanism for eliminating unwanted organisms. The body will not dehydrate as a result of copious expectoration of sputum but it does indicate that there is something wrong. The nurse's observation skills should be used to aid diagnosis and provide treatment. Table 34.12 gives the characteristics of sputum.

PAIN RELIEF

Under most conditions pain is a protective mechanism and an aid or indicator for medical diagnosis. Following surgery, however, when the cause is obvious and usually temporary, its prevention and alleviation is the sole purpose of a nursing intervention. If pain is left untreated, it interferes with all activities of living, particularly

657

Table 34.12 Characteristics of sputum

Characteristic	Description
Amount	Small amounts of white or yellow occur in the sputum of many individuals on a daily basis. Catarrh is a very common problem, but copious amounts indicate a more severe condition, such as cystic fibrosis or a chest infection.
Colour	Blood-stained sputum must be investigated, to identify whether the bleeding has occurred from the respiratory tract, lungs or as a direct result of trauma to the upper respiratory tract by the coughing action. Cancer of the lung is associated with fresh, blood-stained sputum. Green sputum indicates a lung infection. Brown sputum can be caused by an old bleed in the respiratory tract.

sleeping, and tends to reduce the patient's morale and motivation to participate in his care. A number of studies have commented on the under-use of analgesia for patients with pain following surgery (Cohen, 1980; Donovan *et al.*, 1987; Seers, 1988). In a published report, the Royal College of Surgeons and Anaesthetists (1991) observed that up to 75 per cent of patients complained of continuous moderate to severe postoperative pain. The report suggested that analgesia tended to be withheld by medical and nursing staff until patients displayed obvious or observable signs of pain. The reasons for this practice seem to be threefold.

1 It is difficult to assess precisely the nature and extent of the patient's pain.
2 The staff may have an exaggerated concern about potential iatrogenic problems, such as addiction or respiratory depression through the use of opiate-based analgesics (Weiss *et al.*, 1983).
3 Patients can be reluctant to ask for analgesia for a range of personal reasons (Teske *et al.*, 1983; Walker and Campbell, 1988).

Kitson *et al.* (1993) identifies two means by which the existence of pain may be effectively measured: the differing perception of pain between the nurse and the patient, and the effect of medical and nursing interventions. Kitson goes on to describe a range of useful tools. For example, the patient is asked to respond to Likert questionnaires, which use sets of descriptive words such as no pain, mild or very severe pain. Alternatively, a visual analogue scale is used (sometimes called a pain-ometer), which comprises a perpendicular line containing no leading words or numerals between the end points, asking the patient to mark the line with a cross at a point which best reflects his present level of pain.

Study Activity 34.31

For a recent update on the best evidence for the use of analgesia visit the Bandolier site at *http://www.jr2.ox.ac.uk/bandolier/* and conduct a search on best analgesia for postoperative pain. The following excerpt demonstrates the type of data to be found: *www.jr2.ox.ac.uk/bandolier/booth/painpag/wisdom*

Abstract: Postoperative analgesia
High-risk patients undergo simple operations as well as complicated ones. Optimal analgesia for simple procedures can be deduced from systematic reviews. For simple drug treatments we know that oral NSAIDs are the most effective, and that injected opioids need to be given at higher doses to beat the oral NSAIDs. For patients who cannot take NSAIDs combinations of paracetamol and opioid are the second best choice. For high-risk surgery spinals and epidurals, using combinations of local anaesthetic and opioid may enable radical change in hospital stay and morbidity from the procedure. Against this must be set any risk from the spinal or epidural itself.

HJ McQuay, DM, Clinical Reader in Pain Relief

Self-administered or patient-controlled analgesia

The nurse's responsibility for controlling the patient's postoperative pain should focus on enabling patient-centred decision-making. This may take the form of providing the patient with options of one or more forms of pain-relief, for example a combination of traditional pharmacology with complementary therapies (massage, aromatherapy, and reflexology). Patients are increasingly encouraged to self-administer and evaluate the effectiveness of prescribed analgesia. Dallison (1991) describes the benefits of patient-controlled analgesia in terms of increased patient morale and empowerment, but also outlines the difficulties if it is practised without a philosophy that values patient participation, or if the patient is not totally committed to the practice. However, Dallison (1991) asserts that problems of compliance by patients need not necessarily materialise if the patient is well prepared and supported throughout the practice, and informed consent to participate is obtained.

In view of the risk that the patient may self-administer an excessive dose of medication, it is not always necessary for him to receive strong narcotics such as morphine or papaveretum for postoperative pain relief (Closs, 1990). Given the non-therapeutic sedating effects of these drugs, the Royal College of Surgeons and Anaesthetists (1991) recommends the use of milder analgesia (non-steroid anti-inflammatory medication such as indomethacin) for both minor surgery and day surgery cases. Alternatively, the patient can be offered a patient-controlled analgesia system (PCA), which delivers analgesia via an intravenous infusion when the patient presses a hand-held button attached to a computer-controlled pump (Trounce and Gould, 2000). The pump has an automatic lock-out time, which prevents the patient from self-administering an excessive level of the drug, without compromising his control over the administration. Thomas and Rose (1993) argue that PCA is an optimum method for adminis-

tering analgesia, in that it ensures a correlation between the degree of pain reported and the amount of analgesia administered. Although comparative studies undertaken between PCA and standard intra-muscular injections do not reveal any significant difference in postoperative complications (Kleiman et al., 1987; Bollish et al., 1988), there is some evidence to suggest that patients may require less postoperative analgesia (Lange et al., 1988), and that the period of hospitalisation can be reduced (Clarke et al., 1989; Thomas, 1991). Additionally, PCA is popular among patients (including young children), relatives, and nursing staff because it is relatively simple to operate, it encourages patient participation, it resolves the perennial reluctance of patients to ask the nurse for analgesia, and it eliminates the previous labour-intensive nursing task of administering an intramuscular injection containing a controlled drug.

> *Patient-controlled analgesia with opioid produces modest improvement in pain relief compared to the same opioid given conventionally. Patients preferred it, and there were no more or fewer adverse events reported.*
>
> (Walder et al., 2001)

Study Activity 34.32

- Log on to the internet and read the following Bandolier update on patient-controlled analgesia (PCA):
  - *www.jr2.ox.ac.uk/bandolier/booth/painpag/ Acutrev/Other/PCAup.html*
- Also visit the following page:
  - *www.jr2.ox.ac.uk/bandolier/booth/painpag/ Acutrev/Other/PCAup.html*

SUMMARY

With the growing use of the internet the general public are routinely logging on to retrieve information about all aspects of self-care. Therefore, it is essential for all nurses to become familiar with the internet and develop skills in reviewing health information from public sites. You will quickly learn that the majority of sites available for public access are maintained by national or international charities. These can be extremely valuable resources for many people and help lines, chat rooms and e-mail are becoming common forms of electronic social support.

This chapter has described how nursing care can help to maintain the basic or fundamental daily care activities of hospitalised patients and clients. Emphasis has deliberately been placed on personal nursing care, such as toileting, bathing, and feeding, which in conventional hospital nursing has tended to be the province of untrained or junior staff. However, this is a highly important area of nursing care that impacts directly on quality. That is why the Department of Health, in its document *The Essence of Care* (2001) now places such emphasis on establishing benchmarks for this type of care.

In modern health care systems the emphasis on high technology intervention, rapid turnaround and shorter periods of stay in hospital often appears to leave little time for the more personal aspects of care. Yet modern medicine is greatly limited in terms of the health care experience if the patient is lying in an uncomfortable or painful state, wet and cold with incontinence, or suffering from thirst or hunger and becoming increasingly frail and dehydrated. Within such systems, patients feel alienated and uncared for, treated as cases or problems rather than as individuals who deserve dignity and respect. While full attention is given to diagnostic procedures and therapeutic interventions, the important aspects of comforting the sick and assisting with those personal needs they can no longer meet themselves is also of importance. This chapter provides the basis from which the student can progress towards developing competence in these vitally important nursing activities, and a concern for individuals that ensures they will be carried out with compassion and sensitivity.

REFERENCES

Aggleton, P. and Chalmers, H. (2000) *Nursing Models and Nursing Practice* (2nd edition), Macmillan, London

Andrews, C. (1993) Mixed meals (ileostomy diet). *Nursing Times* 89(43), 50–8

Barasi, M.E. (1997) *Human Nutrition: A health perspective*, Edward Arnold, London

Benner, P. (1984) *From Novice to Expert*, Addison Welsey, Menlo Park, CA

Benner, P. and Tanner, C. (1987) Clinical judgement: how expert nurses use intuition. *American Journal of Nursing* 87, 23–31

Benner, P., Tanner, C. and Chesla, C. (1996) *Expertise in Nursing Practice*, Springer, New York

Benner, P., Hooper-Kyriakidis, P. and Stannard, D. (1999) *Clinical Wisdom and Intervention in Critical Care*, W.B. Saunders, Philadelphia, IL

Bladen, L. (1986) Eternal feeding. *Nursing: The add-on journal* 3(1), 281–5

Bollish, S.J., Collins, C.L., Kirking, D.M. *et al.* (1988) Efficacy of patient-controlled versus conventional analgesia for postoperative pain. *Clinical Pharmacology* 4, 48–52

Braden, B.J. (1989) Clinical utility of the Braden scale for predicting pressure sore risk. *Decubitus* 2(3), 44–51

Carnevali, D. and Patrick, M. (1993) *Nursing Management for the Elderly* (3rd edition), Lippencott, Williams and Wilkins, Philadelphia, IL

Carper, B.A. (1978) Fundamental patterns of knowing in nursing. *Advances in Nursing Science* 1(1), 13–23

Casey, G. (2002) The physiology of the skin. *Nursing Standard* 16(34), 47–51

Castledine, G. (1994) Nursing can never have a unified theory. *British Journal of Nursing* 3(4), 180–1

Chambers, N. and Jolly, A. (2002) Essence of care: making a difference. *Nursing Standard* 17(1), 40–4

Clarke, E., Hodsman, N. and Kenny, G. (1989) Improved postoperative recovery with patient-controlled analgesia. *Nursing Times* 85(9), 54–5

Closs, S.J. (1990) An exploratory analysis of nurses' provision of postoperative analgesic drugs. *Journal of Advanced Nursing* 15, 42–9

Clulow, M. (1994) A closer look at disposable gloves. *Professional Nurse* 9(5), 324–9

Cohen, F.L. (1980) Post-surgical pain relief: patients' status and nurses' medication choices. *Pain* 9, 265–74

Couchman, R. and Dawson, S. (1990) *Nursing and Healthcare Research*, Scutari Press, London

Cox, A.J., Hukins, D.W. and Sutton, T.M. (1989) Infection of catheterised patients: bacterial colonisation of encrusted Foley catheters shown by scanning electron microscopy. *Urological Research* 17(6), 349–52

Creedy, D., Horsfall, J. and Hand, B. (1992) Problem-based learning in nurse education: an Australian view. *Journal of Advanced Nursing* 17, 727–34

Dallison, A. (1991) Self-administration of oral pain relief. *Nursing* 4(35), 30–1

Department of Health (1991) *The Patients' Charter*, HMSO, London

Department of Health (1998) *A First Class Service: Quality in the new NHS*, Leeds NHS Executive, Leeds

Department of Health (2001) *The Essence of Care*, DoH, London

Dewar, B. (1986) Total parenteral nutrition at home. *Nursing Times* 82(28), 35–8

Dickerson, J. (1986) Hospital-induced malnutrition: a cause for concern. *Professional Nurse* 1(11), 293–6

Donovan, M., Dillon, P. and Maguire L. (1987) Incidence and characteristics of pain in a sample of medical–surgical in-patients. *Pain* 30(1), 69–78

Duchscher Boychuk, J.E. (1999) Catching the wave: understanding the concept of critical thinking. *Journal of Advanced Nursing* 29(3), 577–83

Facione, N.C. and Facione, P.A. (1996) Externalising the critical thinking in knowledge development and clinical judgement. *Nursing Outlook* 44, 129–36

Fawcett, J. (1995) *Conceptual Models and Contemporary Nursing Knowledge* (3rd edition), F.A. Davis, Philadelphia, PA

Fawcett, J. (2000) *Analysis and Evaluation of Contemporary Nursing Knowledge: Nursing models and theories*, F.A. Davis, Philadelphia, PA

Field, P.A. (1987) The impact of nursing theory on the clinical decision-making process. *Journal of Advanced Nursing* 12, 563–71

Fonteyn, M.E. and Cooper, I.F. (1994) The written nursing process: is it still useful to nursing education? *Journal of Advanced Nursing* 19, 315–19

Francis, D. (1985) Food, fats and facts for nutrition in children. *Nursing: The add-on journal* 2(39), 1149–52

Gooch, J. (1987) Skin hygiene. *Professional Nurse* 3, 77–8

Gould, D. (2000) Hand hygiene research: past achievements and future challenges. *British Journal of Infection Control* 1(1), 17–22

Greaves, A. (1985) We'll just freshen you up dear. *Nursing Times* 81(10) [Supplement], 3–6

Ham Ying, S. (1993) An analysis of the concept of holism within the context of nursing. *British Journal of Nursing* 2(5), 771–5

Hatton-Smith, C.K. (1994) A last bastion of ritualized practice? A review of nurses' knowledge of oral healthcare. *Professional Nurse* 9(5), 304, 306–8

Henderson, V. (1966) *The Nature of Nursing: A definition and its implications for practice, research and education*, Macmillan, New York

Hurst, K., Dean, A. and Trickey, S. (1991) The recognition and non-recognition of problem-solving stages in nursing practice. *Journal of Advanced Nursing* 16, 1444–55

Kay, W. and Locker, D. (1997) *Effectiveness of Oral Health Promotion: A review*, Health Promotion Effectiveness Reviews, No. 7, Health Education Authority, London

Kitson, A. (1985) On the concept of nursing care. In: Fairburn, G. and Fairburn, S. (eds) *Ethical Issues in Nursing*, Avebury, Aldershot

Kitson, A., Harvey, G., Hyndman, S. *et al.* (1993) A comparison of expert and practitioner-derived criteria for postoperative pain management. *Journal of Advanced Nursing* 18(2), 218–32

Kleiman, R.L., Lipman, A.G., Hare, B.D. *et al.* (1987) PCA versus intramuscular injections for severe post-operative pain. *American Journal of Nursing* 87(11), 1491–2

Lask, S. (1986) The nurse's role in nutritional education. *Nursing: The add-on journal* 3(8), 296–300

Makoni, T. (2002) MRSA: risk assessment and flexible management. *Nursing Standard* 16(28), 39–41

McClarey, M. and Duff, L. (1997) Making sense of clinical guidelines. *Nursing Standard* 12(1), 34–6

Mead, J.O. (1994) An emphasis on practical management. *Professional Nurse* 9(6), 405–6

Miller, R. and Rubenstein, L. (1987) Oral health care for hospitalised patients. *Journal of Nursing Education* 26(9), 362–6

Morales-Mann, E.T. and Kaitell, C.A. (2001) Problem-based learning in a new Canadian curriculum. *Journal of Advanced Nursing* 33(1), 13–19

Morison, M.J. (2001) *The Prevention and Treatment of Pressure Ulcers*, Mosby, St Louis, IL

Mullally, S. (2001) Foreword. In: Department of Health (2001) *The Essence of Care*, DoH, London

Narayanasamy, A. (1993) Nurses' awareness and educational preparation in meeting their patients' spiritual needs. *Nurse Education Today* 13, 196–201

NHS Centre for Reviews and Dissemination (1995) *The Prevention and Treatment of Pressure Sores*, Effective Health Care Bulletin, University of York, York

Nightingale, F. (1859) *Notes on Nursing: What it is and what it is not* (reprinted 1970), Duckworth, London

Nursing and Midwifery Council (2001) *Requirements for Pre-registration Nursing Programmes*, NMC, London

Nursing and Midwifery Council (2002) *Code of Professional Conduct*, NMC, London

Orem, D. (1985) *Nursing: Concepts of Practice* (3rd edition), McGraw-Hill, New York

Orem, D. (1995) *Nursing: Concepts of Practice* (5th edition), Mosby, St Louis, IL

Patients' Association (1993) *Caring for Patients in Hospitals*, Patients' Association, London

Roe, B.H. (1991) Benefits of bladder re-education. *Nursing* 4(39), 11–13

Roper, N., Logan, W. and Tierney, A. (1980) *The Elements of Nursing*, Churchill Livingstone, Edinburgh

Roper, N., Logan, W. and Tierney, A. (1996) *The Elements of Nursing*, Churchill Livingstone, Edinburgh

Royal College of Surgeons and Anaesthetists (1991) *Report on the Working Party on Pain After Surgery. Commission on the Provision of Social Services*, Royal College of Surgeons and Anaesthetists, London

Scanlan, F., Dunne, J. and Toyne, K. (1994) No more cause for neglect: introducing a nutritional assessment tool and action plan. *Professional Nurse*, 9(6), 382, 384–5

Seers, K. (1988) Factors affecting pain assessment. *Professional Nurse* 3(6), 201–6

Shepherd, G., Page, C. and Sammon, P. (1987) The mouse trap. *Nursing Times* 83(9), 24–9

Simpson, L. (2002) Collectable guide on intermittent self-catheterisation. *Nursing Standard* 16(29) [collectable guide insert].

Spiller, J. (1992) For whose sake – patient or nurse? Ritual practices in patient washing. *Professional Nurse* 7(7), 431–4

Teske, K., Daut, R.L. and Cleland, C.S. (1983) Relationships between nurses' observations and patients' self-reports of pain. *Pain* 16, 289–96. Cited in: Closs, S.J. (1990) An exploratory analysis of nurses' provision of postoperative analgesic drugs. *Journal of Advanced Nursing* 15, 42–9

Thomas, V.J. (1991) Personality characteristics of patients and the effectiveness of patient-controlled anaesthesia. Unpublished PhD thesis, Goldsmith's College, Univeristy of London. Cited in: Thomas, V.J. and Rose, F.D. (1993) Patient-controlled analgesia: a new method for old. *Journal of Advanced Nursing* 18(11), 1719–26

Thomas, V.J. and Rose, F.D. (1993) Patient-controlled analgesia: a new method for old. *Journal of Advanced Nursing* 18(11), 1719–26

Thornburn, P., Cottenden, A. and Lodger, D. (1992) Undecover trials. *Nursing Times* 88(13), 72–8

Trenter-Roth, P. and Creeson, N.S. (1986) Nurse administered oral hygiene: is there a scientific basis? *Journal of Advanced Nursing* 11(3), 323–31

Trounce, J. and Gould, G. (2000) *Clinical Pharmacology for Nurses* (16th edition), Churchill Livingstone, Edinburgh

United Kingdom Central Council for Nursing, Midwifery and Health Visiting (1996) *Guidelines for Professional Practice*, UKCC, London

Walder, B., Schafer, M., Henzi, I. *et al.* (2001) Efficacy and safety of patient-controlled opioid analgesia for acute postoperative pain. *Acta Anaesthesiologica Scandinavica* 45, 795–804

Walker, J. and Campbell, S. (1988) Pain assessment and the nursing process. *Senior Nurse* 8(5), 28–31

Walsh, M. and Ford, P. (1989) Rituals in nursing. *Nursing Times* 85(41), 26–35

Waterlow, J. (1988) The Waterlow card for the prevention and management of pressure sores: towards a pocket policy. *CARE – Science and Practice* 6, 8–12

Wellard, S. and Lo, S.K. (2000) Comparing Norton, Braden and Waterlow risk assessment scales for pressure ulcers in spinal cord injuries. *Contemporary Nurse* 9(2), 155

Wells, M. (1990) Stress incontinence and pelvic floor exercises. *Professional Nurse*, 6(3), 151, 154–6

Wright, L. (1990) Bathing by towel. *Nursing Times* 86(4), 36–9

Wykes, R. (1997) The nutritional and nursing benefits of social mealtimes. *Nursing Times* 93(4), 32–4

35

COPING WITH DEATH AND BEREAVEMENT

Jo Cooper

LEARNING OUTCOMES

After studying this chapter you will be able to:

- Recognise and monitor the physical manifestations of decline and death
- Understand the psychological processes of death, including the emotional reaction of the individual and the defence mechanisms commonly encountered
- Discuss the reactions of formal/professional carers, informal carers and relatives to the dying process
- Adopt a holistic approach to the dying process, which integrates physical, psychological, social and spiritual dimensions and takes account of the interactions between them, as manifest in the processes of death and bereavement
- Address ethical considerations in death and bereavement, drawing upon appropriate frameworks for moral decision-making
- Reflect upon and identify key attributes of the caring relationship between the nurse and the dying patient and their relatives/loved ones
- Describe effective nursing interventions in helping the individual towards as peaceful and pain-free a death as possible
- Identify and describe effective strategies for supporting relatives/loved ones during the dying process and the period of bereavement
- Present a convincing argument for team approaches to palliative and terminal care that draw on the experience and expertise of all members of the health care team and also involve and empower the patient and his/her relatives or loved ones.

INTRODUCTION

The process of physical deterioration varies and depends largely on the nature of the disease and the circumstances of care and treatment (Copp, 1999). Changes can be subtle and minimal or deterioration can be more obvious. Most people experience some or all of the following symptoms:

- Pain
- Incontinence
- Nausea and vomiting
- Breathlessness
- Noisy breathing
- Inability to swallow
- Feelings of weakness and malaise (Lichter and Hunt, 1990: Lindley-Davis, 1991; Back, 1992).

Excepting situations of sudden death, such as that due to accident or violence, death generally occurs progressively because of failure of the normal physiological functioning of cardiovascular and respiratory systems. Hinton (1984) pointed out that diseases such as cancers, vascular disorders and strokes either interrupt or damage blood supply, leading to eventual death when the damage is extensive. Acute infections may kill either by damaging body structures directly or through the spread of toxic products that damage vital centres such as the brain stem. Some malignancies secrete hormone-like substances that have direct effects on nutrition, immunity and other vital metabolic functions in the body (Nuland, 1994). Nonetheless, towards the end of life a number of vital processes often decline simultaneously. The view that the flow of vital fluids is crucial to life and that stopping the movement of liquids and gases at a cellular and organism level constitutes death has long served as a distinguishing feature for advocates of the traditional concept of death (Copp, 1999).

The psychological processes of death appear to be linked with the perception of death and dying and the emotions that may be evoked (Copp, 1999) and the nature of death and dying is paradoxically linked to individuals' fear of them, giving rise to anxiety and dread. It is uncommon to find that a life-threatening condition, such as a diagnosis of an incurable disease, may precipitate a psychological crisis by arousing anxiety (Copp, 1999). When anxiety is evoked in a death or dying situation, defences are activated simultaneously in an attempt to control that anxiety, and this intricate interplay of anxiety and defences is important as a function for survival. Some of the defence mechanisms observed include denial, repression, projection, reaction formation, regression and rationalisation (Qvarnstrom, 1978). Of these, denial appears to be the most frequently used, suggesting the inherent anxiety that consistently recurs when someone has to confront mortality. Denial is a useful coping strategy. It allows people to buy time and to process some of the more difficult information they are receiving. It allows them to gain a sense of control and normality. Many people oscillate between denial, or partial denial and acceptance of the situation. Health care professionals view denial negatively (Rainey, 1988; Russell, 1993; Smith, 1993). Copp (1999) suggests that this was further compounded by Kübler-Ross's labelling of denial as an individual's initial response to terminal illness (1969). Denial came to be perceived as negative – the least mature response to a terminal illness. In contrast to this view, acceptance of dying had positive implications.

Some commentators (Weisman and Hackett 1967; Weisman, 1974; Rainey, 1988; Smith 1993) make the valid point that denial operates not just to avoid something that feels threatening but also to preserve existing relationships.

Study Activity 35.1

The preceding paragraphs made reference to defence mechanisms, which are also sometimes referred to as mental defence mechanisms. Particular attention was paid to the defence mechanism of denial, but reference was also made to repression, projection, reaction formation, regression, and rationalisation. Carry out the following activities:

- Go to your library or psychology textbook/s, seek out and write down brief definitions of these terms. As you do this, reflect on the meaning of each term. If any are still difficult, search the literature further and refine your defining statements for these terms.

- When you feel reasonably confident that you understand each term, reflect upon any examples of individuals using the mechanisms, from either your nursing or personal experience. You may find it particularly helpful to extend this by reflecting upon any instances where you may have used one or other of these defence mechanisms yourself.

- The latter specific form of self-reflection is sometimes referred to as (or associated with) another mental mechanism known as introspection. Now look up this term as well, and consider its usefulness in your work of nursing dying patients.

Retain your notes on this exercise. They will be referred to again at Study Activity 35.2.

NURSING CARE

The main goals in nursing are:

- promoting and restoring health
- preventing illness and caring for the sick (Watson, 1985).

Care delivery can take many forms, ranging from being alongside someone, to listening, performing and advocating. Thus the concept of caring has been highlighted as central to nursing (Watson, 1985; Benner and Wrubel, 1989). Caring is seen as relational and rooted within nurse–patient interactions, giving rise to a relationship where people are engaged in giving and receiving help. There has been much written on the nature of the nurse–patient relationship and much has centred on the therapeutic nature of the relationship in nursing (McMahon and Pearson, 1998). Morse (1991) describes the dynamic nature of the nurse–patient relationship. She identifies relationships as being clinical, therapeutic, connected or over-involved, and they are dependent on the levels of contact between the nurse and the patient.

In a study by Samarel (1991), which looked at the involvement of nurses with dying patients, it is clear that nurses find it difficult to care and at the same time to remain emotionally uninvolved with patients. Indeed, in a seminal piece of research, Menzies (1961) demonstrated how nurses often use what she termed 'social defence mechanisms' to avoid the anxiety and trauma associated with close personal contact and identification with the patient. She showed that nurses often use such devices as ritual, a preference for task-centred as opposed to patient-centred approaches, and rigid adherence to highly structured professional roles, in order to maintain personal distance. Mander (1994), who also refers to Menzies' work, reports how the midwives in her study of perinatal bereavement found it difficult to remain untouched by the stress and grief. Indeed, the midwives expressed concerns about the extent this impacted upon their capacity to care for the bereaved parents. While the death of a newborn baby or child is likely to be a particularly distressing situation, any dying or bereavement process is highly emotive.

Emotional involvement has traditionally been identified as an unavoidable aspect of caring for the dying, particularly by those working in hospices. However, emotional involvement underpins much of the caring behaviour identified by Davis and Oberle (1990), showing that building an open and trusting relationship was valued highly by patients. In their study, Davis and Oberle (1990) highlighted that the essence of emotional involvement lies in the giving of self. Caring for the dying involves being alongside the individual, and being exposed to individ-

dual vulnerabilities that are specific to dying people, which are not met in normal circumstances. They suggest the following features of working with the dying:

- *Valuing* – respecting others and the patient as individuals
- *Connecting* – establishing and continuing a good relationship with the family
- *Empowering* – facilitating strengths within the family by encouraging and defusing
- *Doing for* – enabling the patient by controlling pain and resolving problems
- *Finding meaning* – helping to focus on living and acknowledging death
- *Preserving own integrity* – valuing oneself as a nurse and being aware of one's own needs and attachments.

Although Davis and Oberle imply that these features define the role of the specialist nurse, they are just as likely to be experienced in general nursing work and so do not appear to be exclusive to those who work with the dying (Copp, 1999).

In a study by James (1986), it was suggested that nurses used several strategies to manage their feelings when caring for the dying. The more mature staff had thought about their own deaths, and most nurses used their own life experiences in empathising with patients' feelings. Smith (1993) highlighted that some student nurses felt cheated when patients they had been caring for died when they were off duty. This feeling was intensified when ward staff failed to let the students know of the deaths. Smith related the feeling of being cheated out of the opportunity to conclude the care that the student had begun. Some nurses see performing last offices for the person who has died as part of completing care. The act of closure of any relationship is important (Copp, 1999).

Nursing care involves not only the care of the patient, but also that of the family. Ensuring that their needs are met and that their views and feelings are taken into account is pivotal in ensuring a holistic approach to care-giving. When a patient's condition deteriorates, families may still want to be involved in care provision. They often feel guilty in spending time on themselves. An important feature of the relationship between nurses, patients and their families is that eventually the involvement with the patient and family members ends when the patient dies. Davis and Oberle (1990) call this 'breaking the connection'. This may be perceived as an important aspect of emotional involvement, particularly in the way nurses contain grief and transitions in the course of their professional work.

Study Activity 35.2

Consider again Isobel Menzies' ideas on 'social defence mechanisms' (Menzies, 1961). You may wish to reread the preceding section referring to her work, or indeed obtain a copy of her paper. Although this was written many years ago, it is a famous and seminal piece of research, still commonly cited today.

- Observe nurses on your ward/placement area, and consider whether they use the sort of social defence mechanisms referred to by Menzies. Watch out for the following pointers:
  - Do you find that some of the nurses you observe feel more comfortable with routine, task-centred approaches?
  - To what extent are the nursing activities you observe based upon ritual?
  - Do any of the nurses you observe seem to prefer sticking to rigid and prescribed roles, and are there any who seem to be willing to go beyond this to a more personal approach? If this is the case, how do these nurses differ?
- Make brief notes of your observations. You should try to do this at the time of the observations or as soon as possible after each one. Reflect on your findings. It might be useful to go back to your notes for Study Activity 35.1 at this point. Consider now if you feel that nurses (as opposed to patients or clients) should use mental or social defence mechanisms, and how this may be particularly problematic in the case of death and bereavement. You may also find it helpful to discuss these issues with your fellow students and mentor.

Buckman (1993) outlined a three-stage model of the process of dying:

1 Initial stage
2 Chronic stage
3 Final stage.

He suggests that when confronted with impending death people react in a way consistent with their character and with the way they have coped with difficulties in the past. During nursing assessment, which is always an ongoing dynamic process, a useful question to ask the individual is 'How have you coped with crises in the past?' This provides both you and them with some insight into past difficulties, their coping behaviour and how they might view their present difficulty. Buckman suggests that it is more useful to perceive a patient's emotions as sources of insight into their personality, rather than as indicators of the stage they are passing through. He describes the initial stage as a mixture of reactions characteristic of the individual, which may include any or all of the following:

1 Initial stage:
  - fear
  - anxiety
  - shock
  - disbelief
  - anger
  - denial
  - guilt
  - humour
  - hope
  - despair
  - bargaining.
2 *Chronic stage (being ill):*
  - resolution of those elements of the initial response that are resolvable
  - diminution of intensity of all emotions.
3 Final stage (acceptance):
  - defined by the patient's acceptance of death; not an essential stage, provided that the patient is not distressed, is communicating normally and making decisions normally.

Eleven emotions are listed in the initial stage and Buckman states that a person can be considered to have entered the chronic stage when elements of the initial emotions have resolved, with or without assistance. The chronic stage may or may not occur, depending on whether the person resolves their emotions. If this does not happen, the chronic stage does not exist for the person and Buckman advises the professional dealing with such a patient to seek help for them. In the third and final stage, the patient appears to experience less emotional intensity and this is defined by acceptance of the impending death, although acceptance is not perceived to be an absolute necessity.

RELATIONAL ASPECTS

Kessler (1997), suggests that caring for the dying person is not so much about talking, as about listening. A person has the right to hope, but hope often changes – a hope of a cure; a hope not to have pain; a hope of not loosing control; a hope not to die alone. We rob the dying of the right to hope when we insist that they face reality. Hope improves the quality of life.

Our own discomfort of death can make it difficult to talk with a dying person about what is happening. Often family and friends talk about everything except the fact that someone is dying. Most of us are afraid that what we say will be either too threatening or too trivial. It is best to be honest and say, 'I don't know what to say to you'. Often this opens up communication and that person will give some guidance for future dialogue. There are no rules and we take our lead from the person themselves. Every situation has to be assessed individually. Sometimes, we get it wrong. Listening is the key – often friends and families feel panic-stricken, thinking they must 'do something' and end up rushing around but achieving very little. Often, there is nothing to 'do'. They just need to 'be'; to sit quietly, to listen and not to abandon that person but to just 'stay with it', however uncomfortable and painful it will feel, is the best response of all. Do not be afraid of silence. Holding the hand of a person or just being close by will communicate all that needs to be said

(Kessler, 1997). Touch is a very powerful tool that tells a person how much we care.

Sometimes, answering a person's questions honestly can upset them, or their family. Some people wish afterwards that they had not asked. When we feel that the person really wants to talk about their dying, then we do not have the right to deny them of the opportunity, though the family may wish to protect the individual from reality. It undervalues their feelings and emotions if we are not prepared to be open and authentic in our communication with the dying person.

It is important that both the person who is dying and their family are helped by facilitation to say what they feel needs to be said. This is about getting to know your patient and the family. It is important to take the time to build a relationship of trust and openness and to use your intuitive knowledge to find a way of helping and supporting them. Kessler (1997) suggests there are people who do not want to talk about death or dying. Talking about it means facing the fact that they are going to die. Sometimes people are afraid that talking about it will make it happen. However, it can be an empowering experience to openly be able to discuss the 'how' and the 'where' of dying and to not only participate actively in making these decisions but to know that choices have been heard and respected. As a person's disease advances and cure is no longer the goal, the disease-modifying therapies diminish in importance and care that was initially curative in its goal changes to care that is palliative (Copp, 1999). The goal of palliative care is to achieve the best quality of life for patients and their families by providing relief from pain and other distressing symptoms and offering a support system that integrates physical, psychological, social and spiritual aspects of care (World Health Organization, 1990).

Study Activity 35.3

In the discussion above you will have noted the emphasis on such activities as listening, sitting with, being with, attending 'in silence', touching and holding.

These allude to some of the most intimate nursing activities. Yet, though these can be powerful means of supporting, and indeed powerful healing influences, they are also areas with which many nurses have difficulty. Indeed, nurses may often use the defence mechanisms referred to in Study Activities 35.1 and 35.2 to avoid what they find to be painful or embarrassing encounters with their patients.

- Reflect on these aspects of relating to your patients. In doing so, you might consider the following:

  - factors that may distract you when you are listening to your patient, and how you might cope with these
  - differences between doing things *to* the patient, doing things *for* the patient and doing things *with* the patient
  - knowing when to say or do something and knowing when it is just important to be there as a silent but receptive presence
  - cultural characteristics or personal attitudes that may influence how nurses and patients feel about touching and holding.

ETHICAL CONSIDERATIONS

At the end of life, relief of suffering is of the utmost importance, as preserving life becomes impossible. Four cardinal principles apply (Gillon 1994):

- *Patient autonomy* – respect for the patient as a person
- *Beneficence* – to do good
- *Non-maleficence* – to do no harm
- *Justice* – fair use of available resources.

The four principles need to be applied against a background of:

- respect for life
- acceptance of the inevitability of death.

When a person is close to death, the use of invasive interventions, such as intravenous infusions, antibiotic therapy and cardiopulmonary resuscitation is inappropriate.

It is difficult to describe the 'usual' death. Each death is different and unique. It does not follow an exact series of events. Many people ask 'How will it be at the end?' Few people have a peaceful death, or die in their sleep. Many people seem to have a struggle near the time of death and this can be very painful and distressing for the family and carers, both professional and informal. It is normal for the systems of the body to become less efficient, and although it is difficult to diagnose the onset of dying as a physical process, it may be helpful to say it begins when medical treatment cannot halt the course of a disease.

As death approaches, the person may become more tired and spend more time in bed, where they are more physically comfortable, and they may slip into a semiconscious or unconscious state. This is normal. Although the person is often unable to respond, it is believed that hearing is still acute. Relatives often want to see the person eating normal-sized meals, feeling that everything will be all right if food is eaten. For the person approaching death, food does not provide any interest and often only small sips of water can be tolerated. Mouth care becomes important, to maintain oral hygiene and rehydration of the oral mucosa. Breathing patterns change. There is no set order of events. For many, there seems to be such a strong will to live that it is not easy to die and it often takes longer than predicted. The aim is always to provide comfort, both emotional and physical.

Maintaining a person's dignity within the medical culture can be difficult. People are often stripped of their dignity when they agree to coming into hospital. Small but important ways in which we can help to see that they are treated with dignity include:

- Knocking at the door before entering
- Making sure we introduce ourselves properly
- Always using a person's proper name, or asking how they would like to be addressed

- Making sure that we really listen to what they are saying
- Making the 'little things' count.

It is not so much 'what' we do but 'how' we do it. It is how we use our own body language and the tone of our voice that convey messages more loudly than words. Macleod (1994) asserts that the 'little' things within the partnership count, because they make a difference to the patient. They are imbued with knowledge and skill and are described as 'intentional' actions. Benner (1984) describes these as the hallmark of nursing 'expertise'. Everyday occurrences, such as adjusting a pillow, admiring a family photograph, and making sure the family are taking care of themselves, hold a position of equal value to our empirical knowledge and skills when we are caring for a person approaching death. Ersser (1998) asserts that patients value the presentation of the nurse and that ones attitudes and demeanour matter more than the 'way' one performs tasks. By being attentive to a person's thoughts, feelings and needs, we demonstrate that we are paying them respect and saying, 'I am with you, I am available to help' (Egan, 1982).

Kessler (1997) suggests that death is one of the most isolating experiences in life. One dies alone. Without realising it, we can easily add to their isolation. We no longer include them in conversations and no longer listen to them. We can exclude them physically and emotionally. We fail to tell them what is going on in our everyday lives. Some individuals will want to talk about their death; most will ask how it might happen and what it will be like. Family members, often try to discourage frankness and openness, fearing that it will upset the person who is dying. They often feel that they do not want the person to 'give up the fight for life', or may try to say that 'everything will be fine'. It is sometimes difficult for them to face reality. Colluding with the frightened, dying patient that they will get better and 'everything will be all right' is not necessarily helpful. It is easy for the family and the community professional to collude with the patient when they are unsure about what to say or do. However, colluding may serve to undervalue their feelings, and block any useful communication, thus making 'letting go' difficult (Cooper, 2000). Sometimes the patient needs to be 'given permission' to die by the family. People often wish to hold on to what they know and love. It can be a struggle for both parties to let go, but it is sometimes sufficient for the family to tell the patient that it is all right for them to die (Callahan and Kelly, 1992).

The success of any intervention with the dying person and their family lies in the effective use of communication skills; in recognising one's own role and personal limitations (Macleod Clark et al., 1991). This is paramount in helping these people to explore, discover and clarify the meaning of their own life and to enable a greater sense of well-being. Enabling the patient and the family to discuss emotive issues does not just happen; it requires skills of facilitation and an ability to bring about the situation in a positive direction, thus enhancing disclosure.

Benner (1984) makes the point that individuals who exercise their own independence and need for strong personal control may not recognise that they are being helped. To some patients this might seem like nothing more than having a chat. The person may be unaware that the situation is continually being assessed and evaluated and that the skills of negotiation, active listening and decision-making are being carried out. The principle of the Calman-Hine report (1995) on cancer services relating to good communication and psychological support are essential for patients and their families. Attention to a connected reciprocal personal relationship that will ultimately benefit the patient, family and the health care professional is pivotal if we are aiming for excellence in care delivery.

Dying may give rise to many repressed emotions: sadness, numbness, guilt and jealousy of those who are well (Rinpoche, 1998). It is often helpful to the family for them to understand that being open and honest with the patient can open up channels of communication and this may be facilitated by an appropriate professional (Cooper, 2000). The patient is nearly always in a position to help and guide the family and the professional, if asked. It is sometimes, very difficult, especially for the inexperienced practitioner, to explore a person's feelings and thoughts. We are often afraid that we may say the wrong thing. Listen to yourself; your intuitive knowledge: if it feels right, then generally it is right. What is often not right is to say nothing, to avoid painful issues. Then nothing useful is achieved.

When you sit with a person who is facing death, you can see and feel their emotional pain. This is distressing for the health care professional and provokes feelings of helplessness and fear. There is a temptation to run away whenever we feel we cannot make the situation 'better'. Try to sit with your uncomfortable feelings; acknowledge them to yourself instead of ignoring them, and take them to clinical supervision. It may be that the only thing you can give to this person is 'yourself'. Sit with it, feel it and reflect on it. This is one of the most helpful interactions when you are dealing with another person's grief. People will value you for your humanness and for being yourself, just as much as they will for your clinical expertise and knowledge. As Carper (1978) suggests, the care provided should result from the sensitive blending of knowledge from both humanistic and natural science. To develop the 'artistic' and 'ethical' components of nursing demands the engagement of the nurse's self, as expressed through body movement, tone of voice, eye contact, facial expression and touch (Benner and Wrubel, 1989).

Study Activity 35.4 ⸻

In the passage above, there is a reference to Carper's work on patterns of knowing (1978). In her work she discusses empirical, ethical, personal and aesthetic ways of knowing.

Carper's patterns of knowing have also been discussed in Module 3. Indeed, that whole module was largely structured around her four ways of knowing.

- Revisit this module and refresh your memory on Carper's proposals for the four ways of knowing.
- When you have done this, consider how you might use Carper's patterns as a framework for caring for the dying patient. In doing this, you should make notes under four columns, briefly indicating the main ways in which each 'way of knowing' might inform your practice.

MANAGING SYMPTOMS

Patients with a life-threatening condition will often present with multiple symptoms. Table 35.1 highlights those most frequently encountered, together with their prevalence in a hospice population.

Table 35.1 Prevalence of symptoms most frequently encountered in patients with life-threatening illness

Symptom	Percentage of patients
Pain	82%
Nausea and vomiting	59%
Dyspnoea	51%
Constipation	51%
Weakness	64%
Anorexia	64%
Depression	40%
Confusion	20%

(From Donnelly and Walsh, 1995)

All symptoms are controllable, even if they cannot be eliminated. However, the reality is that some symptoms are difficult to control and treatment should be planned using holistic and eclectic approaches, again paying attention to detail. Continuous nursing assessment and evaluation is the key to effective symptom management, remembering that needs may change very quickly, demanding rapid response. It is not the intention of this chapter to look at symptomatology, but we must recognise that the person approaching death may experience one, several or all of the above symptoms and it is the remit of the multi-disciplinary team to ensure that all symptoms are identified and given appropriate care and treatment. Some of the physiological processes that occur when death is close will now be discussed to enable the practitioner to appreciate their significance and normality.

Breathing

This continues to be normal until very close to the end (Kessler, 1997). If it does change – and mostly towards the end of life, it does – this can be frightening to those observing. If the person has respiratory disease or lung cancer, they may have lived with changes in breathing pattern for several months or years. The breathing may become laboured, with short breaths, which takes a great deal of effort from the patient and can be very distressing for the family. The person often feels that they are going to suffocate and it is a very frightening experience. The most important thing is not to leave the person alone and to reassure them that they will always have enough breath for their needs and will not suffocate. Anxiolytic drugs are often used in this situation to reduce panic and anxiety. Noisy, distressed breathing often accompanies approaching death, often referred to as 'terminal rattle'. This is due to secretions that collect in the pharynx. Actions to take include the following:

- Ensure that the patient is not distressed.
- Try to reposition the patient to relieve the breathing.
- Explain the problem to the relatives – they are often more distressed than the patient.
- Consider giving a subcutaneous injection of hyoscine hydrobromide, butylbromide or glycopyrronium. This can be given as an immediate dose or via syringe driver.
- Gentle suction can be helpful if the patient is deeply unconscious.

Sleeping

This usually increases in the days and hours preceding death, when the body systems are closing down. This is normal and it is helpful to

confirm the normality of this to the relatives. During the final hours, the person may become semiconscious or unconscious. It is important to behave as if they can still hear you, gently speaking to them and including them in conversations.

Nutrition

As a person approaches death, his interest in hydration and nutrition often becomes minimal. It is not helpful to insist that the person take food and fluids: their disinterest should be seen as part of the process of letting go (Twycross, 1997). It is important that oral hygiene is maintained, with rehydration of the oral mucosa and lips.

Incontinence

There may be loss of bladder and bowel control. This may cause some physical discomfort, as well as compromised dignity and privacy. Caring for and maintaining the dignity of a person who may be distressed or in pain requires skill, patience and time. The goal of care is comfort. Soft pads can be placed underneath the patient to maintain tissue viability and integrity. An indwelling urinary catheter may be appropriate, following a continence assessment.

Cyanosis

This is due to a lack of oxygen in the blood, together with increased carbon dioxide, and can result in a bluish discoloration of the skin and mucous membranes. At this point, the functioning of the circulatory system is impaired, which is a normal part of the process of dying.

Hypoxia

The inefficient use of oxygen can cause behavioural changes. These include poor judgement, decreased alertness, headaches, confusion, and drowsiness (Kessler, 1997). Hypoxia can also lead to convulsions, unresponsiveness and cyanosis. Nursing intervention includes maintaining the individual's safety, and administering appropriate, medications to reduce physical symptoms, such as headaches and confusion.

Restlessness

This is often part of the transitional process. A person may be unaware that they are trying to get in or out of bed without a purpose; plucking at the sheets; rambling in their speech; confused as to their environment; unable to relax or find a comfortable position. The mainstay of treatment is usually a benzodiazepine such as Midazolam, which will sedate them, or Haloperidol to help clear the confused mind. Management of terminal restlessness focuses on both pharmacological and psychological intervention to minimise the distress of the patient and relatives (Cooper, 2000).

Body temperature

A high temperature is normal as the individual approaches death. This is sometimes accompanied by perspiration. Nursing intervention includes comfort measures and gentle repositioning. As the circulatory system shuts down, the extremities become colder than usual. As circulation is compromised, the heart can no longer pump blood throughout the body, and it is pulled to the lowest part of the body by gravity (Kessler, 1997).

Skin changes

Unexplained bruising may appear at various points in the body. This is due to failure of platelet mechanisms. Tissue viability and the prevention of pressure damage will have been negotiated earlier in the illness trajectory and are helpful in maximising comfort.

Vision and hearing

These senses decrease and the individual may notice that their vision is blurred or appears to be fading. It is widely believed that hearing is the last sense to go, which is why it is important to behave as if people can hear right up until the end of their life.

The moment of death

When life has left the body there will be no heartbeat, pulse or breathing. There will be no response when spoken to or touched. The eyelids may still be open and these can be gently closed. The jaw will be relaxed and open and the skin will have lost any colour. It is important to take time and allow the relatives to do the same. Preparation of the body should be unhurried and calm, allowing the family to remain with the person for as long as possible. There is often such a rush during the week following a death and so many things to attend to, but the moment around and following a death should remain as private, personal, dignified and compassionate as when the person was living. Events at this time will stay with the family for the remainder of their lives and the focus of care should ensure that their needs are identified and met.

TRANSCULTURAL ISSUES

Koffman (2001) suggests that within many cultures, family members, friends and leaders within the community are an important component of caring for a dying person. An individual's extended family may wish to visit at regular and frequent intervals and perhaps stay for long periods. Therefore, accommodation of a large number of visitors may be anticipated. Close relatives may wish to be present at the time of death and their cultural norms should be explored and respected as far as possible.

There is literature available elsewhere that can provide clarity and a framework for understanding ethnic minority groups (Cooper, 1993; Field et al., 1997). Within all nursing care the emphasis should be on the individual. This ensures greater compassion and cultural understanding of the diverse requirements of minority groups.

CLINICAL SUPERVISION

Using the process of regular clinical supervision and reflection enables clinical practice to remain within clinical boundaries. The importance of self-care and supervision should not be underestimated in helping to prevent burn out and stress. Nursing people with life-threatening illness carries a high emotional cost and supervision can offer a means of protection (Butterworth and Faugier, 1992); being close and helpful without feeling personal distress requires self-awareness and respecting one's own feelings (Larson, 1992). Support from colleagues and work in collaboration with the multi-disciplinary team is paramount to both the patient and the health care professional in maintaining well-being.

MULTI-DISCIPLINARY TEAMWORK

Team working and maintaining good working relationships is vital in order to provide the best possible eclectic care. This focuses on the needs of the patient and the family. The needs of the patient can be overwhelming and regular nursing assessment and evaluation will help to identify multi-factorial problems. It is often helpful to ask the patient 'What is the worst thing for you at the moment?' This helps to prioritise problems and prevents the health care professional from forming their own agenda. The nurse will then work in partnership with the patient and with the multi-disciplinary team, which brings its own rewards. It must be possible to discuss care strategies within the team without any individual feeling threatened, and the sharing of ideas and feelings leads to an optimum level of care for the patient and family (Booth, 2000).

Listening to the patient and working with them and the family provides enrichment and personal growth in one's own life experiences. Learning is not a one-way process – the patient and family can teach us, the carer, so much of what we need to know and understand.

BEREAVEMENT

Personal crisis

Bereavement is the greatest personal crisis many people ever have to face, and grief has been described as a transition process (Parkes, 1986).

By grieving, the person is able to adjust to the loss and the meaning of that loss in his life.

Even when death is expected, there may be a sense of shock, disbelief and denial. These feelings are likely to last longer with an unexpected death. During the acute distress that usually follows, bereaved people often experience physical and emotional reactions to grief. These may be due to anxiety or may mimic the symptoms of the deceased (Sheldon, 1998).

Common emotional reactions to grief are given in Table 35.2:

Table 35.2   Common reactions to grief

Emotional	Physical
• Sadness	• Feeling lost
• Helplessness	• Weakness and fatigue
• Yearning	• Sleep disturbances
• Confusion	• Loss of appetite
• Hopelessness	• Sighing
• Guilt	• Tension
• Anger	• Self-neglect
• Bitterness	• Increased blood pressure
• Relief	• Poor resistance to illness.
• Peacefulness	

Some people may question their faith or for some their faith may become even more important and play a major part in the healing process. Bereavement can present an opportunity for life changes and reflection on experiences. For most people adjustment to the situation and a slow return to normality are usual. Often family events, anniversaries and celebrations may cause painful memories and feelings, and as Sheldon (1998) notes, 'in this sense grief never really ends'.

There is often a search for meaning and understanding about the death. This is even more marked in a person who is young. Often sudden and unexpected death is associated with long-lasting levels of distress, especially if it is associated with violence, suicide, or substance misuse (Sheldon, 1998). When a person has been ill over a long period of time, death is often expected, especially by health care professionals.

However, this does not automatically mean that the family expects the death; often they are unaware that the person is close to death. Some families will deny death until it actually happens and then the shock can be tremendous. It is important to remember that the death of someone with terminal illness can still be unexpected (Twycross, 1997).

Vulnerable groups

There are certain groups within our society that are more vulnerable than others. These include:

- *Children* – who are often protected by adults from difficult and painful events, in order to shield them from emotional pain (Sheldon, 1998). It is easy for a child to feel excluded from the situation and they will have little idea about what is going on around them. Children are very insightful; they see and they feel. However, children cannot always express these feelings, and are consequently often left in isolation. Children begin to understand some aspects of death and bereavement as early as 2 or 3 years old; by the age of 5, over half will have some degree of understanding. By involving the child in the reality of the death, there is the opportunity for the child to tell the person how much they care about them (Faulkner, 1995). The child needs to be given the opportunity to ask their own questions and to be given simple, truthful answers in a sensitive way, helping them to gain understanding of a situation that should be viewed as normal. A question that often arises is, 'Should the child attend the funeral service?' The short answer to this is yes because they should be given the opportunity to say their own goodbye and this forms part of the grieving process. Parents often find taking a child to the funeral difficult. They often may not want to display their own grief in front of the child and may feel inhibited in doing so. These feelings can often be fully explored with the parent and the parent helped to make a decision that feels right for them and their family. Teenagers often find it difficult to express their emotions, especially to their parents. Friends of their own age may act as supporters and provide them with the help needed.

- *Confused elderly people and people with learning difficulties* – their needs may be ignored, because they are unable to express their feelings verbally (Sheldon, 1998). They will benefit from continuing support and simple clear explanations, often at regular intervals. They should be given the opportunity to attend the funeral service and their wishes asked for and respected. In a study by Hollins and Esterhuizen (1997), fifty people with learning difficulties who were being cared for in the community and who had recently lost a parent were compared with 50 others who had not been bereaved. Those who had been bereaved were unlikely to have been warned of the coming death of their parent and to have been taken to visit the grave, and only half were known to have attended the funeral. They had much higher scores on measures of anxiety, depression, hyperactivity, stereotyped movements and other indicators of distress. Despite this, most of the professional and family carers were unaware of their distress and did not attribute their symptoms to bereavement.

Some losses will pass unrecognised. This results in a lack of support to those who suffer those losses. This is termed disenfranchised grief (Doka, 1989). Hidden losses may arise when a relationship has been a secret, when the ending of the relationship cannot be acknowledged, or when the loss is associated with feelings of embarrassment or inadequacy (Parkes, 1998). For example, in the case of a homosexual relationship, the partner may be unable to express grief openly for fear of being castigated. This can cause particular difficulties where the person has died from HIV infection or other sexually transmitted diseases. People may isolate themselves, withdrawing from their usual social circle and refusing any offer of support from health care professionals. Parkes (1998) makes an interesting point that mothers who have babies are under considerable social pressure to rejoice rather than grieve. Pregnancy may be unplanned and unwanted and even if planned, the mother may need to grieve for the many losses that can result from it.

Health care professionals often ignore their own need to grieve. Basic training teaches us to cope with whatever is thrown at us and not to show or to give way to displays of emotion. Acknowledging our own grief and allowing ourselves to be vulnerable enables our own emotional growth to occur. We are then in a stronger position to offer optimal support and concern for those within our care, and for those with whom we work.

Models of grief

The process of grief has been described in different models.

Phases of grief (Parkes, 1986)

Initially, bereaved people can often feel as if they are detached from reality. The reality of the death has not yet penetrated their awareness; they may appear outwardly to have accepted the loss. Shock, sadness and numbness gradually give way to intense feeling and searching behaviour is common, for example:

- Seeing the dead person in or out of the home situation
- Dreaming about the deceased
- Going back to places they had visited together and hoping to see them.

Despair sets in when the person realises that the deceased will not return. Emotional and physical reactions to grief can then occur. Depression and emotional liability may last for over a year following the bereavement. Life transitions are eventually progressed and the bereaved enters the phase of resolution. At this point, the bereaved person is able to remember the deceased without feelings of overwhelming despair and is ready to re-invest in the world.

Tasks of mourning (Worden, 1991)

Worden (1991) describes the process of grief as a series of tasks, which have to be worked through by the bereaved, to enable them to move forward. These tasks include:

- Accepting the reality of the loss
- Experiencing the pain of grief
- Adjustment to an environment in which the dead person is missing
- Withdrawing emotional energy and re-investing in other relationships and activities.

It is possible to facilitate the process of grieving by helping the bereaved person to work through the tasks of mourning. Many hospices have bereavement services that include one-to-one counselling from a bereavement worker and group support, facilitated by appropriately trained professionals. This type of group provides a safe environment whereby people can openly talk about their feelings and experiences with others in similar situations and have their feelings acknowledged and understood, in a way that is not judgmental.

Dual process (Stroebe, 1994)

This model acknowledges that most bereaved people oscillate between acknowledging the grief and avoiding it. Avoidance includes actively aiming to keep fully occupied, either socially or by a rapid return to work. Memories are blocked out because they provoke painful feelings that the person is unable to deal with. This is described as loss-oriented and restoration-oriented behaviour. Loss-oriented behaviour focuses on the loss and the emotional reaction to it. In restoration-oriented behaviour, there is some degree of suppression, distraction and 'taking time off' from grief (Twycross, 1997). This enables people to proceed with normality as much as they can. Most people oscillate between the two styles of coping. On one day, the person may be appearing to cope well and to have adjusted to their recent loss. On another, their grief may completely engulf them.

Study Activity 35.5 _____

Consider a bereaved person you have encountered in your work as a nurse or in your personal life. Reflect upon their reaction to the loss, and which one of the above models (or indeed which mix of them) would have most adequately provided a framework for intervention.

Outcomes

There are several aspects associated with a good or poor outcome. These can be identified at the time of bereavement and can be used to focus resources in order to prevent long-lasting or complicated grief (Parkes, 1990):

How the person died

- Was it was timely or untimely?
- Was it expected or unexpected?
- Was it unduly disturbing for the relatives?

Deaths that are untimely, unexpected or unduly disturbing are likely to cause more severe and more prolonged grief (Twycross, 1997).

Relationship between the deceased and the bereaved

How ambivalent was the relationship. All relationships have a degree of ambivalence. However, in cases where there has been an insecure attachment to the deceased, or a relationship where one person had been overly dependent and the other dominant, there are likely to be problems in readjustment (Penson, 2000).

Support

- Can the bereaved share their feelings with family and friends?
- Do they have the support from health care professionals?
- Do they 'feel' supported?

Anticipatory grieving

Bereavement starts at the time the relative knows that the patient is not going to recover (Penson, 2002). Periods of denial are normal and often necessary during a terminal illness, but an excessive use of denial may make it harder for the bereaved person to start sharing with others after the death (Twycross, 1997). The bereaved person may feel angry: this not only prevents normal grief from taking place, it also serves to isolate the person from other family members and friends who do not want to be the target of this anger.

Previous losses

It is useful to have some information about how the person has coped with previous losses or crises in their life and whether or not this loss will determine any unresolved grief.

The most positive factor in favour of a good outcome is a supportive family or close friend who is able and willing to allow the bereaved to 'be themselves', to talk about the loss, or not to talk about it, and to accept and respect the bereaved person's wishes.

Helping the bereaved provides a challenge to all of our skills. It challenges us personally and we need to be prepared to feel the pain of another person's distress. How can we help the bereaved person through a smooth transition of adjustment?

Bereavement visiting

The objective of the bereavement visit (Faulkner 1995) is to assess whether:

- grieving has commenced
- grieving is within normal limits
- there is any sign that adaptation has commenced.

Identifying people potentially at risk and referring them to the appropriate agency for support may make the adjustment less traumatic, giving them information about how they might feel and reassuring them that grief is a normal process, shared by everyone at some time or another. Giving them a list of support agencies, such as Cruise, or a contact telephone number may help them to feel less isolated in their grief.

Negotiate the time of the bereavement visit, so that the person knows you are coming, rather than just arriving on the doorstep. It is very easy for the visit to become social, over a cup of tea and a chat. It is important to remind the person why you are there and to stay focused as to the reason of the visit. There is only a thin line between friendship and a therapeutic relationship (Penson, 2000). There is a danger of being unable to let go as we, as health professionals, become attached to certain families. This would not be conducive to forming a therapeutic relationship.

How does the bereaved person relate to the deceased? Do they talk about them in the past or the present? Is the room as it was before the deceased died with nothing being moved or altered? If the person is blocking, it is important to explore relevant factors and to see how they feel in the 'here and now' (Faulkner, 1995). Are there any children in the family and how are they getting along; do they need more help? What plans do they have, if any, for the future? Do they feel like going out and meeting people or have they withdrawn into their own environment?

At the time of the assessment, it is important to look for a change in the level of feelings over the last few weeks. You might ask the person to compare how they feel now to how they felt at the time of the death, to elicit emotional changes that are slowly taking place. If there are feelings of anger or guilt, these can be gently explored and the person helped to understand these normal reactions to grief.

Your assessment will reveal whether the pattern of grief is normal or abnormal. Has the individual been able to talk openly about the deceased? What have they done about the clothing and possessions? Is the bereaved person able to think or speak about the future?

If the pattern of grief is abnormal, the feelings will be just as intense, or more so than they were initially (Faulkner, 1995). They may not be able to talk about the deceased at all and the future may be hanging over them like a black cloud. Does the person seem clinically depressed?

Faulker (1995) offers the following advice:

- If you feel satisfied that grief is within normal limits, then there is no need for further action, but leave your phone number anyway.
- If you have identified the need for further support then negotiate another bereavement visit.
- If your assessment reveals the absence of grief, or is outside normal parameters, then refer to other agencies.

Boundaries for visiting should be negotiated and set early on. This lets the person know that your visits will have a natural conclusion. To keep visiting will encourage dependence, which will be difficult to break, making closure of the relationship for both parties a painful, rather than a positive experience.

Study Activity 35.6

In the above section, we discussed situations in which there may be a need to refer the bereaved person to another agency or source of support. Earlier in the chapter, we also referred to the importance of teamwork. Where professional helpers and others involved with the patient or client work in teams, such decision-making is made significantly more effective. This is particularly the case where a nurse accepts responsibility for managing the care of the patient or client (dying patient or bereaved person), as is reflected in approaches such as primary nursing.

- Do a search in your library and on the Internet for these two concepts: *team working* (you might use such search terms as 'team working', 'team nursing', 'teamwork', 'team management', 'inter-professional collaboration', 'multi-disciplinary working'), and *primary nursing* (you might use such search terms as 'primary nursing', 'named nurse', 'patient-centred care', 'holistic nursing'). Make brief notes on these, refining your notes through further searching and reading until you are satisfied you have a fundamental understanding of the two concepts.

- Now do a critique of how each of these two approaches may work in the care of the dying patient and his/her relatives, and the subsequent care of the bereaved person. You may find it useful to undertake this using the SWOT framework, which includes:

  Strengths – ways in which the approach may be useful/effective

  Weaknesses – ways in which the approach may hinder the effectiveness of care

  Opportunities – the extent to which this particular area of care provides occasion for the utilisation of the approach

  Threats – the factors within the environment of care that may limit or make the approach less effective.

- Consider how these two approaches may be complementary or, alternatively, incompatible. You might find it helpful to seek the views of experienced nurses in this area of care.

- Finally, reflect on how team-orientated approaches may support staff in caring for terminally ill patients.

Implications for practice

The implication for nursing practise is to recognise that responses to loss are always complex and both socially and culturally shaped according to the mode of death and the relationship of attachment to the deceased (Costello and Kendrick, 2000). We are all unique in the way we handle grief. There is no single intervention that will benefit everyone (Sheldon, 1998) Thorough assessment and evaluation, framed in a sensitive and thoughtful way, using the skills of listening and empathy, will help us to recognise what action will be of help to each individual. We must respect the fact that not every bereaved person will want or need support from health care professionals. There are people who find the strength to cope within themselves or within their own family group and their wishes should always be respected. It is only when we truly listen and understand that we can offer the help and support that is really needed.

SUMMARY

This chapter has discussed the observable responses the nurse can make when working alongside people who are dying and their family, and the appropriate nursing interventions aimed at improving quality of life.

The skills and knowledge we have gained from this chapter can also be applied when caring for any individual experiencing loss following illness that has influenced his or her life. Patients and family experience similar emotional responses regardless of the nature of the illness. Here, the insight gained into the concerns of those facing bereavement will help the nurse to identify those issues important to the individual and family that require specialist interventions.

Penson (2000) reminds nurses of their facilitative and explorative role. The art and skill of professional practice is about supporting the individual and family when life's experiences are difficult. The challenge and reward for the nurse is the ability to have a meaningful impact when caring for the person who is dying, who may be experiencing distressing symptoms and facing multiple losses.

To achieve this we need not only to listen, but to hear what is said and (just as important) what is not said. The skill is to turn this knowledge into a meaningful and constructive intervention that aids the individual and family at the time it is most needed by them. To do so, we must communicate, appreciate, understand and act upon the issues that impact on the person and family coping with death and bereavement.

REFERENCES

Back, I.N. (1992) Terminal restlessness in patients with advanced malignant disease. *Palliative Medicine* 6(4), 293–8

Benner, P. (1984) *From Novice to Expert: Excellence and power in clinical practice*, Addison-Wesley, Menlo Park, CA

Benner, P. and Wrubel, J. (1989) *The Primacy of Caring*, Addison-Wesley, Menlo Park, CA

Booth, R. (2000) Spirituality: sharing the journey. In: Cooper, J. (ed.) *Stepping into Palliative Care: A handbook for community professionals*, Radcliffe Medical Press, Oxford

Buckman, R. (1993) Communication in palliative care: a practical guide. In: Doyle, D., Hanks, G.W.C., MacDonald, N. (eds) *Oxford Textbook of Palliative Medicine*, Oxford Medical Publications, Oxford

Butterworth, T. and Faugier, J. (1992) *Clinical Supervision and Mentorship*, Chapman and Hall, London

Callahan, C. and Kelly, P. (1992) *Final Gift*, Poseidon Press, New York

Calman-Hine (1995) *A Policy Framework for Commissioning Cancer Service*, Department of Health, London

Carper, B.A. (1978) Fundamental ways of knowing in nursing. *Advances in Nursing Science* 12(2), 1–8

Cooper, D.B. (1993) Transcultural issues and approaches. In: Wright, H., Giddy, M. (eds) *Mental Health Nursing*, Chapman and Hall, London

Cooper, J. (2000) Terminal restlessness. In: Cooper, J. (ed.) *Stepping into Palliative Care: A handbook for community professionals*, Radcliffe Medical Press, Oxford

Copp, G. (1999) *Facing Impending Death Experiences of Patients and Their Nurses*, Nursing Times Books, London

Costello, J. and Kendrick, K. (2000) Grief and older people: the making or breaking of emotional bonds following partner loss in later life, *Journal of Advanced Nursing* 32(6), 1374–82

Davis, B. and Oberle, K. (1990) Dimensions of the supportive role of the nurse in palliative care. *Oncology Nursing Forum* 17(1), 87–94

Doka, K. (1989) *Disenfranchised Grief*, Lexington Books, Lexington, MA

Donnelly, S. and Walsh, D. (1995) The symptoms of advanced cancer. *Seminars in Oncology* 22, 67–72

Egan, G. (1982) *The Skilled Helper*, Brooks/Cole, CA

Ersser, S.J. (1998) The presentation of the nurse: a neglected dimension of therapeutic nurse–patient interaction? In: McMahon, R. and Pearson A, (eds) *Nursing as Therapy* (2nd edn), Stanley Thornes, Cheltenham

Faulkner, A. (1995) *Working with Bereaved People*, Churchill Livingstone, New York

Field, D., Hockey, J. and Small, N. (1997) (eds) *Death, Gender and Ethnicity*, Routledge, London

Gillon, R. (1994) Medical ethics: four principles plus attention to scope. *British Medical Journal* 309, 84–188

Hinton, J. (1984) *Dying*, Penguin, Harmondsworth

Hollins, S. and Esterhuizen, H. (1997) Bereavement and grief in adults with learning disabilities. *British Journal of Psychiatry* 170, 497–501

James, N. (1986) Care and work in nursing the dying: a participant study in a continuing care unit. Unpublished PhD thesis, University of Aberdeen, Aberdeen

Kessler, D. (1997) *The Rights of the Dying*, Ebury Press, London

Koffman, J. (2001) Rituals surrounding death in the black Caribbean community. *Palliative Care Today* X, 1–7

Kübler-Ross, E. (1969) *On Death and Dying*, Macmillan, New York

Larson, D.G. (1992) The challenge of caring in oncology nursing. *Oncology Nursing Forum* 19(6), 851–61

Lichter, I. and Hunt, E. (1990) The last 48 hours of life. *Journal of Palliative Care* 6(4), 7–15

Lindley-Davis, B. (1991) Process of dying – defining characteristics. *Cancer Nursing* 14(6), 328–33

Macleod Clark, J., Hopper, L. and Jesson, A. (1991) Progression to counselling. *Nursing Times* 87(8), 41–3

Macleod, M. (1994) It's the little things that count: the hidden complexity of everyday clinical nursing practice. *Journal of Clinical Nursing* 3, 361–8

Mander, R. (1994) *Loss and Bereavement in Childbearing*, Blackwell Scientific, Oxford

McMahon, R. and Pearson A. (1998) *Nursing as Therapy* (2nd edn), Stanley Thornes, Cheltenham

Menzies, I. (1961) *The Functioning of Social Systems as a Defence Against Anxiety*, Tavistock, London

Morse, J. (1991) Negotiating commitment and involvement in the nurse–patient relationship, *Journal of Advanced Nursing* 16, 455–68

Nuland, S. (1994) *How We Die: Reflections on life's final chapter*, A.A. Knopf, New York

Parkes, C.M. (1986) *Bereavement: Studies of grief in adult life* (2nd edition), Pelican, London

Parkes, C.M. (1990) Risk factors in bereavement: implications for the prevention and treatment of pathologic grief. *Psychiatric Annuals* 20, 308–13

Parkes, C.M. (1998) Coping with loss: facing loss. *British Medical Journal* 346(5), 1521–4

Penson, J. (2000) Bereavement. In: Cooper, J. (ed.) *Stepping into Palliative Care: A handbook for community professionals*, Radcliffe Medical Press, Oxford

Penson, J. (2002) A hope is not a promise: fostering hope within palliative care. *International Journal of Palliative Nursing* 6(2), 94–8

Qvarnstrom, V. (1978) *Patients' Reactions to Impending Death*, Institute of International Education and Department of Medicine, Stockholm

Rainey, L. (1988) The experience of dying. In: Wass, H., Bernardo, F. and Neimeyer, R. (eds) *Dying: Facing the facts* (2nd edn), Hemisphere, Washington DC

Rinpoche, S. (1998) *The Tibetan Book of Living and Dying*, Ryder, London

Russell, G.C. (1993) The role of denial in clinical practice. *Journal of Advanced Nursing* 18(6), 938–40

Samarel, N. (1991) *Caring for Life and Death*, Hemisphere, London

Sheldon, F. (1998) ABC of palliative care bereavement. *British Medical Journal* 31(6), 456–8

Smith, D.C. (1993) The terminally ill patient's right to be in denial. *Omega* 27(2), 115–21

Stroebe, M. (1994) Helping the bereaved to come to terms with loss: what does bereavement research have to offer? *Proceedings of the First St George's Conference, 'Bereavement and Counselling'*, St George's Hospital Conference Unit, London

Twycross, R. (1997) *Introducing Palliative Care* (2nd edition), Radcliffe Medical Press, Oxford

Watson, J. (1985) *Nursing: The philosophy and science of caring*, Little, Brown, Boston, MA

Weisman, A.D. (1974) *The Realisation of Death: A guide for psychological autopsy*, Jason Aronson, New York

Weisman, A. and Hackett, T. (1967) Denial as a social act. In: Levin, S. and Kahana, R. (eds) *Psychodynamic Studies on Aging: Creativity, reminiscing and dying*, International Universities Press, New York

Worden, J.W. (1991) *Grief Counselling and Grief Therapy* (2nd edn), Tavistock, London

World Health Organisation (1990) *Cancer Pain Relief and Palliative Care: Report of a WHO expert committee*, Technical Report Series, World Health Organisation, Geneva

36

CARING IN THE COMMUNITY: A NURSING PERSPECTIVE

Ann Long

LEARNING OUTCOMES

After studying this chapter you will be able to:

- Outline the development of policy for care in the community
- Relate these developments to health care goals of quality, effectiveness and efficiency
- Identify the specific health orientation of community nurses
- Describe the five principles underpinning community nursing
- Identify specialisms within community nursing in the UK
- Outline the generic activities of community nursing roles within collaborative and partnership working.

INTRODUCTION

The NHS and Community Care Act (Department of Health, 1990) and its attendant White Papers outlined the strategic framework for the provision of all health and social care services in the UK. It emphasised the importance of caring for people in the community. This, in turn, led to reduced dependency on secondary health care provision in favour of developing a range of flexible options based on local needs as well as patients' rights and choices. Following this, *The New NHS, Modern, Dependable* (Department of Health, 1997) document identified the need to implement robust indicators of National Health Service performance. In addition, it recommended that 'organisational barriers should be broken down and stronger links forged with Local Authorities' hence placing the needs of patients at the centre of the care process. The publication of this paper supported the view that care in the community can empower people who are disadvantaged, marginalised or socially excluded by providing more flexible and responsive services that are planned, designed, evaluated and controlled in partnership with service users (Ovretveit, 1998).

In 1998, the Government called for providers to ensure the 'existence of clear, national standards, supported by consistent, evidence-based guidance to raise quality in the NHS': *A First Class Service: Quality in the new NHS* (Department of Health, 1998). The paper again highlighted the principle that the total care process should be shared with patients and their families/carers and that positive partnerships should be developed between statutory agencies, voluntary services, the independent sector and representatives of the communities in which patients live. Thus, the reconstruction of the patient's identity to one that views them as active participants in their own health care is one of the dominating features of New Labour's health care plan.

However, the reality of community care has not always matched this ideal. Ovretveit (1993) claimed that the history of community care is one of competition for finance between acute hospital care and primary health care. The New Labour Government is determined to remove the competitive image of care provision that has been depicted by previous governments by promoting their ethos of 'an open economy' in care provision. However, an accusation that is often levied at community care is that while it is successful at meeting the needs of a patient with a single need it often fails to meet the needs of patients with multiple or complex needs (Ovretveit, 1998).

THE INTRODUCTION OF PRIMARY CARE GROUPS AND TRUSTS

The Health Act (1999) built on the Health Act (1996) which issued a mandate for the creation of new primary care groups and trusts (and their associated primary care teams). The 1999 Act made provision for community health care trusts and general practitioner fundholding practices to apply for primary care group/trust status to replace the concept of general practitioner fund-holding. Such emergent trusts will account to local health authorities and will be monitored by the National Health Service Executive through its associated regional offices. The key responsibilities of these new primary care groups/trusts are to evaluate and effectively provide health care to locally defined populations and to ensure that they do so in accordance with service users' wishes and aspirations.

To enable the primary care groups/trusts to carry out their role effectively means that each primary care group/trust searches for and compiles health and social information to act as a baseline for advising on the actual and potential health and social needs of local populations. Primary care groups/trusts must also demonstrate trans-sector and trans-professional co-operation and collaboration. In this new health agenda the care of people who are ill is no longer dominated by the solitary figure of the general practitioner. Rather there is a large network of health and social care professionals working collaboratively for an integrated and comprehensive health care system. Community nurses are part of this network. So, too, are patients, their families and informal carers. The successful realisation of this philosophical and pragmatic agenda has implications for the education and training of a multidisciplinary workforce that can provide 'the necessary capacity, skills and diversity' to work, in partnership with representatives of local communities (Department of Health, 1999). The overall goal is to meet the holistic needs of patients, families/carers and the wider community if the ultimate strategy for improving the health and social well-being of the population is to be achieved (Department of Health, 1999).

QUALITY, EFFECTIVENESS AND EFFICIENCY

The Government's investment in quality and standards will influence significantly the health care environment in which primary care teams will work. In particular the emphasis on clinical governance and clinical effectiveness demands the design and implementation of new models of role and functional accountability for all members of primary care teams. The National Institute for Clinical Excellence is expected to provide a strong lead on clinical and cost-effectiveness by developing and disseminating guidelines and by auditing methodologies to prevent duplication and fragmentation of care provision. At all levels of care, effectiveness and quality are stressed as much as efficiency in this proposed framework for assessing performance. The Institute will serve to develop new evidence-based service frameworks that will embody the best practice in any given service. It also aims to secure nationally uniformed standards of care. Consequently, each member of the primary care team is responsible for the way care is delivered. In addition, clinicians and managers are accountable for the quality of patient care. It is vitally important that the Institute recognises the ongoing work that community nurses have already undertaken in promoting clinical effectiveness and that all of the profession's work is reflected adequately and developed further. Moreover, it is crucial that greater efforts are made to ensure that all information is distributed promptly to practitioners.

The need to develop outcome measures is paramount as these proposals roll out. Health improvements, including equitable access to services, which embrace individual differences and the needs of minority groups, including children, are central. Within this remit the need to improve convenient access to information on all aspects of health, healing and recovery is essential. Relevant information must be designed and made readily available to the public. The overall aims of the Institute are to audit meticulously and research rigorously the effective provision of health and social care, efficiency, outcomes, and patient/carer expectations and satisfactions.

Examination of the above documents demonstrates that the focus of care has been placed justly within communities. The expectation is that resources will be deployed to meet identified health and social care needs through the provision of integrated public health initiatives: *Making it Happen* (Department of Health, 1995), and *A Public Health Model of Primary Care* (Public Health Alliance, 1998). In addition, a range of professionals including doctors, community nurses, social workers, clinical psychologists, educational psychologists, paramedics and others will provide holistic, therapeutic care. This shift of emphasis is the result of enlightened thinking and changing political ideologies relating to the concepts of illness and the provision of health care. Primary care teams will continue to provide the first point of contact for patients and their families/carers and the acute sector will support and complement their work.

Overall, a range of initiatives surrounding public health, a reduced reliance on the in-patient sector and the development of community care have resulted in an acceleration of primary care activities. Consequently, the provision of nursing care in the community is reliant on the acquisition and development of competence in different specialist areas of expertise.

Study Activity 36.1 _____

- Review the definitive statements on public health in Chapter 32.
- Identify perceived differences and similarities between the concepts 'public health' and 'primary care'.
- Identify how the term 'community care' relates to the concepts 'public health' and 'primary care'.

- Write three brief statements on public health, primary care, and community care. Your statements should each be about 200 words and should demonstrate the main emphasis in each concept.

COMMUNITY NURSING

Community nurses are in the privileged position of being 'professional guests' who are invited into the sanctity and privacy of other people's homes. Therefore, the provision of community nursing care begins with reflecting on what it means to have that honour and privilege bestowed upon them. The provision of high-quality therapeutic activities requires community nurses to use responsive, proactive skills such as health surveillance, risk analysis, social action, therapeutic communication skills, as well as a range of specialised therapeutic interventions designed to meet the expectations, aspirations and needs of service users (United Kingdom Central Council, 1994). Specialist areas of community nursing have been identified by the United Kingdom Central Council (1994) as:

- public health nursing (health visiting)
- district nursing
- occupational health nursing
- community learning disability nursing
- community children's nursing
- school nursing
- community mental health nursing
- general practice nursing.

Study Activity 36.2 _____

In this chapter we do not go into detailed consideration of the eight community nursing specialties within the UK. However, to orientate yourself to these roles, carry out a brief library search for information on each. Write up the results of your searches as eight brief statements of approximately 50 words, each outlining one of the eight roles. Each statement should:

- briefly define the role in terms of its client group or area of practice;
- outline the specific defining characteristics of the role that differentiate it from the other roles.

Society, the nursing profession and people who are ill (as well as their carers) need to be aware of the drive by community nurses to provide health and nursing care to patients, families and communities which is evidence based and founded on a code of professional conduct. The primary objectives of community nurses are to:

- respect, value and facilitate the inherent healing resources that reside (sometimes dormant) within individuals, families, groups and nations
- advocate proactively on behalf of people who are ill and their carers and promote self-advocacy
- promote health and prevent ill-health
- provide systematic, high-quality, therapeutic care to people who are ill and their carers.

THE PRINCIPLES OF COMMUNITY NURSING

Five principles underpin the professional practice of community nursing. Community nurses use these principles to explain, guide and predict their practice. They are operationalised continuously and simultaneously and it is their dynamic combination in practice that depicts the distinctive nature of community nursing. The principles are based on the belief that health is *a human right* and a *resource for life* and not the objective of living (World Health Organisation, 1998). In their uniqueness, community nurses provide systematic care for the diversity, breadth and depth of health and social care needs. The Department of Health and Social Services Northern Ireland (1995) defined the five principles of Community Health Nursing as:

- the search for recognised and unrecognised health needs
- the prevention of disharmony in health

- the facilitation of health-enhancing activities
- the provision of therapeutic approaches to health care
- the influence of policies affecting health.

The search for recognised and unrecognised needs

The search for and identification of recognised and unrecognised health needs is the foundation on which all care provided is built. This principle highlights a needs-based approach to the provision of services. It is the first step towards entering into partnerships with patients, families/carers and communities, as people are usually best placed to identify their own needs. At a micro-level, all community nurses compile and update annually health and social profiles of their caseloads and of certain marginalised groups, such as the travelling community, non-nationals or those families currently enduring or recovering from domestic violence. At a media-level, community nurses, in partnership with other professional groups, begin with compiling health and social profiles of the general practitioner practice populations for which they are responsible. At a macro-level they work in partnership with clients, carers and representatives of community groups and voluntary organisations to compile health and social profiles detailing the health and social needs of the community or ward they serve.

After compilation, these profiles act as an information source for prioritising, planning, implementing and evaluating care. They also provide information where the data gathered in one caseload, practice population or community are compared with others in different communities throughout the UK. Indeed, the data collected are also compared with those found in other countries thus fulfilling the World Health Organisation target, which suggests reducing the health gap within the UK and also between the UK and other countries (World Health Organisation, 1998).

Health and social well-being cannot be divorced from the socio-economic and cultural context in which it is experienced (Long, 1997).

It is difficult, if not impossible, for people who are ill or disabled to heal and recover and retain their dignity in a climate where poverty and unemployment are paramount. It is even more perplexing when there is gross inequality and social exclusion and where those who belong to minority groups are undervalued and deprived of equitable opportunities and equal civil liberties for personal, social, educational and futuristic self-growth and development (Long, 1997). Health and social profiles are essentially contextualising profiles as they bring health information into the social context. They provide community nurses with an overview of the socio-economic distribution of wealth and an awareness of how people's experiences of poverty and deprivation shape the quality of their lives and affect their health. Community nurses, therefore, have a role in promoting the human rights of all individuals (Human Rights Act, 1998).

In addition, public policy impacts disproportionately on people who are already disadvantaged by their illness or disability. Therefore, equity features strongly in the compilation of health and social profiles. Consistent with the adoption of an equity-focused approach to the compilation of profiles is the use of participatory models that fully involve people who are living with their illness or disability at every stage of the process of care delivery and evaluation. The final compilation of profiles is open to public scrutiny.

Profiles help to shift the emphasis from the simple recording of the activities and skills of individual practitioners to the preparation of evidence for evaluating service provision and subsequent health outcomes. Hence, they can be used as performance measurement tools as required by the Government. The Office for Public Management (2000, p. 40) stated that community nursing must be 'measured not by the activity it undertakes but by the difference it makes'.

It is important to emphasise that the compilation of health and social profiles is not strictly a science, although they draw on a wide range of demographic, economic, psychosocial, epidemio-logical and environmental data as well as hereditary and health care evidence, which are known to impact on health. Profiles, therefore, can never be 100% accurate. However, they are a creative and collaborative form of enquiry, which are uniquely placed in terms of time, space and local conditions, and the rigour with which the data are gathered can be evaluated.

Overall, health and social profiles that are carried out on an annual basis provide evidence on the centrality of human concern for people with health and social needs and their carers and they also demonstrate respect for individuals, families and communities. They confirm that the providers of health services genuinely listen to people who are ill or disabled and their families/carers with the aim of proactively responding. In response to using the principle *the search for recognised and unrecognised health needs* as a guide to practice, profiles are used as reliable resources to:

- confirm that the views and perceptions of patients, their advocates and their families/carers are paramount
- provide a systematic needs-based approach to practice
- help with the critical assessment and allocation of resources
- act as a basis for planning, developing and evaluating proactive and responsive community services
- enable community nurses to target and prioritise their services effectively
- improve, change and expand services to meet individuals' and families'/carers' needs, preferences and aspirations
- identify measurable health outcomes.

The prevention of disharmony in health

The Caplan (1961) model of primary, secondary and tertiary prevention is used as a practical guide to explain this principle. During the twentieth century, the role and function of community nurses in the UK expanded both in scope and scale, including their key role in health promotion and prevention. Health promotion has been defined as 'the process of enabling individuals to increase control over and improve their health' (World Health Organisation, 1984, p. 16). The use of the term control implies that community nurses adopt facilitatory approaches that empower individuals to maintain and sustain healthy lifestyles within health-promoting environments. This model of health promotion is, therefore, individual/group/community led. Examples of health promotion activities facilitated by community nurses and designed to enrich the quality of the lives of individuals and groups are:

- pre-conceptual health care
- the promotion of self-efficacy
- the promotion of healthy bonding
- the promotion and maintenance of healthy relationships
- the promotion of positive parenting
- the promotion of healthy communication patterns
- the promotion of self-worth, self-valuing and self-nurturing
- the promotion of a healthy lifestyle
- human sexuality and education for love
- death, dying and letting-go as natural experiences of living.

Health-promoting environments

Examples of health promotion activities that advance the concept of health-promoting environments and community development have been highlighted by the Ottawa Charter (World Health Organisation, 1986) as:

- building healthy public policy
- creating supportive environments
- strengthening community action
- creating health action zones
- promoting health in schools, colleges and workplaces
- developing personal skills
- re-orientating the health services to community care.

Community nurses are educated and trained in the following skills:

- practising in an anti-discriminatory manner
- lobbying for the provision of new services or changes to existing services
- forming self-help and residents groups
- negotiating for changes in the environment and communities at local and national levels
- advocating on behalf of marginalised groups and their carers
- challenging oppression, inequality and deprivation
- promoting human rights
- focusing on social and environmental justice
- collaborating and co-operating with other professional, voluntary and private agencies
- identifying potential positive and negative indicators to health
- assessing the risk indicators posed by providing care in the community
- designing care pathways that prepare patients for a smooth transition from hospital care to care in the community.

These skills enable community nurses to facilitate the process of developing health-promoting environments and community developments.

Secondary prevention

Secondary prevention activities involve screen testing for indicators of illness or disability with the aim of providing the best possible interventions as early as possible. While the process of screening for illness is still in its infancy, nonetheless, such screening provides useful indicators on the overall health status of individuals and groups. For example, reliable and valid instruments are used by community nurses to screen test for:

- hearing and vision
- phenylketonuria
- thyroid deficiency
- anaemia
- cholesterol
- breast, prostate and testicular cancer
- HIV and Aids
- cystic fibrosis
- post-natal depression
- anxiety and stress management

- risk factors for self-destructive and self-mutilating behaviours
- the early identification and remediation of alcohol and drug abuse
- depression
- Alzheimer's disease
- referral for dental, nutritional, blood pressure, cardiovascular disease, and other physical health needs.

It is impossible to consider using all screen testing measurements that are currently in vogue. However, service providers are encouraged to prioritise or rank those they consider to be clinically appropriate and match the demographically and epidemiological findings of the area serviced.

Tertiary prevention

Tertiary prevention involves planning health care in a way that the services provided are designed to prevent further deterioration in severe and enduring health problems. To practice this role effectively, community nurses are skilled in monitoring health outcomes, evaluating the therapeutic care they provide and assessing patient and carer satisfaction with the care provided. The principle *the prevention of disharmony in health* also embraces the notion that community nurses are competent and confident to assess, monitor and evaluate the uses, benefits and side-effects of prescribed medications. In addition, community nurses have a firm knowledge of the interactions that might occur when two or more medications are prescribed.

The facilitation of health-enhancing activities

There are many definitions of health (Fleming, 1999). Scholars are now debating if it is a good idea to continue to strive to find a definition that suits everyone's taste and which can be all-encompassing (Kemm and Close, 1995). The etymology of the word health suggests that it is related to words that mean 'wholeness', 'prosperity' and 'holiness'. Therefore, health, wholeness and sanctity are denoted as being synonymous in the Germanic languages. Examination of this proposition shows that health is one of our most valuable assets and without it we are not living in the truest sense of the experience. Community nurses translate the third principle to practice, for example, by designing health and self-awareness programmes that improve the quality of people's lives and enable them to reach their full potential as recommended by the Department of Health (1998). Such programmes are implemented to facilitate people to:

- accept themselves and others as unique individuals
- embrace and integrate their physical, sexual, cultural and religious identities and respect that others differ
- appreciate the beauty and wonder of nature and how human beings are connected with it;
- improve relationships
- become aware of their inner strengths and resources as well as their emotional pain and distress
- realise their creative potential
- appreciate the need for self-reflection, intimacy, solitude and inner peace
- value the need for leisure time activities
- develop coping strategies for dealing with maturational and life crises
- increase their understanding of life's meaning and purpose.

Study Activity 36.3

Consider the above statements about how health is defined and experienced. Review earlier statements about definitions of health in Chapter 32.

- With all these statements in mind, carry out library and Internet searches for meanings of the term 'health'.
- On the basis of these various sources and your reflections upon them, write a brief referenced article (of approximately one A4 page/400 words) that reviews the concept of health and how it has

varied across place and time. Retain this article for future reference and refinement.

The provision of therapeutic approaches to health care

The role of community nurses has undergone significant change as community health care services have continued to expand and develop. Community nurses provide care for a wide variety of patients and their carers in the community. It is clear, therefore, that as generic community nurses they are specialist practitioners who 'nurse' individuals, families, groups and communities. Community nurses, therefore, are provided with a solid generic educational foundation in the biopsychosocial-political and spiritual dimensions that impact on the population's health and well-being. In order to practice at this depth and breadth, community nurses are educated and trained in a wide range of contemporary therapeutic approaches to care. This type of education and training provides them with the essential 'tools' (skills) to practice an eclectic and integrated approach to nursing care that is quality driven and tailor made to match each individual's and family's unique needs and aspirations.

The use of presence and the therapeutic relationship

Most nurses enter the nursing profession with a strong belief in the ideology of caring for other people. Community nurses espouse the caring ethos as the axiom of their practice. For the purpose of practising the fourth principle, a person-valuing paradigm is recommended as the theoretical model upon which community nursing care is built. The person-valuing paradigm has its foundations in, and was developed from, a synthesis of philosophies on human existence. For example, the theory of human becoming (Parse, 1995), the human science perspective of a unitary human being (Rogers, 1980), notions on existential phenomenology (Sartre, 1969; Merleau-Ponty, 1974; Heidegger,

1987), philosophies on dialogicalism (Marcel, 1949; Buber, 1958). Put simply but deeply, these writers believed in the sacredness of all life and the absolute worth of every individual. The person-valuing paradigm provides guidance on the importance of the therapeutic use of self and the therapeutic relationship in community nursing. The characteristics, knowledge and skills that community nurses bring with them to the therapeutic relationship can be the greatest catalyst of all in moving the healing process forward for those in need (Long, 2001).

The re-emergence of 'therapeutic caring relationships' has been well synthesised and debated in nursing circles by reputable academics such as Watson (1988), Kitson (1993), Parse (1995) and Barker (1998). This interest provides an indication of the profession's view of the centrality of 'human presence' as the fundamental foundation of nursing care (Slevin, 1999a). The use of presence as a therapeutic guide to the development, maintenance and closure of therapeutic relationships involves nurses embracing humanistic values, which, according to Kitson (1993), subsequently change nursing practice to one that embraces an ethical caring position. Community nurses are fully committed to the humanistic mode of practising nursing and, therefore, embrace the person-valuing model of care. Using this model means that relating with people is an ethical virtue and, hence, the practice of community nursing takes on a moral rightness (Slevin, 1999b). The use of this term may be justified in terms of respect for others, dignity and human rights.

When engaging in a therapeutic relationship, community nurses demonstrate that they are open to listening authentically to the patients' sharing of experiences. Patients are aware of the community nurses' authenticity by observing descriptions of their lived experiences being validated in the caring eyes of non-judgemental nurses. This means that community nurses have the ability to convey accurate empathy with patients' descriptions of their lived experiences and their personal life stories of pain and distress. Chronic ill-health is inextricably embroiled within each person's search to find the meaning of life and the purpose of living.

Community nurses begin nursing care by creating a therapeutic ambience and providing a high degree of emotional nourishment. They accept patients, families/carers as they are and not as how they would like them to be. They convey genuine compassion for and empathy with patients, families/carers in terms of their healing and recovery (or dying and death). As catalysts for healing and change, community nurses have the ability to begin the journey from within the patients' frame of reference and subsequently rely on patients for the direction, pace and movement of the healing process (Rogers, 1997).

Assessment

Regardless of which type of therapeutic intervention is used, all care begins with making an initial assessment of the patient's and family's biopsychosocial, spiritual and cultural needs as well as their health service needs. Assessment can be carried out in a structured way. For example, they might decide to use an appropriate nursing model such as Peplau (1958), Roper *et al.* (1996), Robinson (1997), and Barker (1998), to assess needs.

Assessment tools, however, do not pick up everything that is going on in an interview. How patients say something is often more important than what they say or what they cannot say at an initial interview. People show their distress nonverbally by the way they sit, for example, or by crying, joking, day dreaming, having sudden lapses of memory, sighing, or by becoming fatigued while speaking about a particular topic. Community nurses are aware of these aspects through their skills of observation and listening. Overall, no one form of assessment provides a complete picture but used in conjunction with the community nurses' clinical expertise and judgement it is possible to gain sufficient information to process, integrate and interpret patients' needs. Once needs have been assessed the next step in the process is to provide the therapeutic care appropriate to the needs identified using best practice methods.

Risk assessment

Clearly the health outcomes to be achieved by providing community care, including the increased social inclusion of people who are chronically ill or disabled and their carers, far outreach the deficits. The implementation of the care programme approach involving the concept of the 'named' key worker, requires community nurses to offer more formal specifications of their risk assessment methods, including the criteria used to underpin their clinical judgements. This is especially true in the area of child protection. *Working Together Under the Children Act 1989* is a guide to arrangements for interagency co-operation for the protection of children from abuse and harm (Department of Health, 1991). The document does not attempt to give guidelines on the practice of individual professions in the recognition of child abuse or subsequent care. However, the aspect of child protection should be at the forefront of every community nurse's mind. Therefore, an overall strategy for risk assessment and risk management is one of the key functions of all community nurses.

Risk management falls into three distinct categories: before, during and after an incident or event. Prevention is the key as neither practitioners nor patients, families/carers wish to be on the giving or receiving end of serious harm. The content of the care plan also helps to prevent risk. Risk assessment is carried out through the conduit of assessment and re-assessment of holistic needs, together with an open policy on information sharing and exploration of the thoughts and feelings of patients, families/carers together with openness to mutual learning. Risk management is either an implicit or explicit goal for all interventions. The most appropriate activity to minimise risk is initiating and maintaining a safe and therapeutic relationship within a framework which provides services that respond proactively to patients', families'/carers' needs in an equitable manner, for example, assertive outreach (Allen, 1998; Morgan, 1999) and positive parenting (Irving and Long, 2001).

Paradoxically, risk taking is also an important part of risk assessment and management. Positive risk taking means supporting patients, families/carers to make and take decisions about their lives, explore and test out their choices and learn from the experience of 'failure' when the decision they take does not work out. This is, after all, what living is about. This suggests that community nurses also take positive risks and, therefore, is another reason why they require sound systems that support them in their professional and personal development, including structured clinical supervision (Cutcliffe and Butterworth, 2001).

Individuals, families/carers and world-wide approaches to therapeutic care

Community nurses are specialist nurses who work in the community setting. Therefore, they are educated and trained in the skills and knowledge required to practise an eclectic and integrated approach to care, which is drawn from a wide range of therapeutic interventions. The primary aim of this generic training is promoting health, healing and recovering at individual, family/carer, community and global levels.

The therapeutic care of individuals

Each of the eight specialist disciplines of community nursing is educated and trained in a range of therapeutic interventions appropriate to their specialist areas. Many of the interventions overlap. For example, the promotion of the health of schoolchildren will not differ radically from the promotion of the health of children who are being cared for by community children's nurses or health visitors. Furthermore, the care of women will not differ significantly when it is provided by occupational health nurses or general practice nurses. However, each discipline of specialist community nursing is equipped with specific therapeutic interventions to match the unique needs of their patient/client group. For example:

- Health visitors provide behavioural management programmes for children with behavioural problems.
- Community learning disability nurses provide therapeutic interventions for individuals presenting with challenging behaviours.
- Occupational health nurses provide therapeutic interventions which deal with stress management techniques in the workplace.
- Community mental health nurses provide a range of psychotherapeutic and psychosocial interventions to individuals with mental health problems.
- District nurses provide therapeutic care for individuals who are terminally ill.
- Community children's nurses provide therapeutic care for children with cystic fibrosis.
- General practice nurses provide therapeutic care for individuals with chronic heart disease.
- School nurses provide therapeutic care for children with asthma.

The therapeutic care of families

As families and carers provide most of the essential psychosocial care for patients/clients, working with and caring for families are essential components of the community nurses' role. The potential to engage with families and carers in a meaningful way contributes significantly to the healing process or to peaceful dying and death. One of the most important roles of community nurses is to provide effective therapeutic care without usurping the family's role in the caring process. Community nurses have a responsibility to provide accurate information to families at each stage of the healing process. They also have a teaching responsibility, for example, teaching carers how to provide effective and safe mouth care. In addition, they use their counselling skills to listen to and reflect upon the families'/carers' needs, fears, anxieties and aspirations.

A knowledge and understanding of family communication patterns and family dynamics and the integration of theory with practice adds to the community nurse's repertoire of skills, which they draw on and use to add to their integrated and eclectic approach to care.

The therapeutic care of communities

Community nurses promote health and prevent illness at community level. This is synonymous with their role in public health and public protection. The aim of public health is to create environments that promote healthy living and are conducive to human comfort. In such health-nurturing communities, people who are ill are facilitated to reach their optimum potential and are accepted and valued as equal citizens within the community they live and also within society. In addition, community nurses use their advocacy role to safeguard, protect and defend the rights of their patients/clients and to assist, enable and empower them to ensure that their needs are met. People who are ill and their families/carers have the right to liberty, equity of services, acknowledgement of their illness, and access to self-help groups. They also have the right to refuse an assessment or treatment, and families/carers have the right to refuse to care (British Medical Association, 1992). Advocacy, therefore, and the promotion of self-advocacy are essential components of community nursing to ensure that people's strengths and aspirations and not only their diagnoses are recognised.

At a wider level, community nurses use their advocacy skills to address public concerns about health. This means that community nurses work with other agencies in order to provide a holistic focus, which includes not only caring for individuals and families/carers but the entire socio-economic environment and situation in which people live, including their housing and leisure time activities. In order to carry out their public health role effectively, community nurses use the following values to underpin their practice:

- an anti-discriminatory code of practice
- equity and social inclusion
- participation, collaboration, community development and community empowerment
- social and environmental justice and health as a human right.

Community empowerment emphasises community participation and ensures that the voice of residents is heeded in the decision-making process. True participation means that the Government would recommend a multi-agency responsibility for health.

Sarason and Duck (2001) have edited a valuable resource book on clinical and community psychology and point out that the multifaceted role in relationships in conjunction with social support perceptions can enhance understanding of the process of social support and the potency of its effects. They present research findings on the effects of social support on health and well-being and on tried and tested interventions from the personal relationships realm that have been applied to a wide range of clinical and community issues within the context of communal coping.

The therapeutic care of the globe

Health and social inclusion have been highlighted as key priorities for care at the global network of the World Health Organisation collaborating centres for nursing and midwifery (World Health Organisation, 1999). Six priority areas were emphasised to advance and strengthen trans-national co-operation, invigorate new activities and redefine priorities in health care. This European initiative provides a forum for listening to the voice of the 'real experts' in mental health (i.e. people with mental health problems), their carers and health care staff. It also supports the World Health Organisation (1998) document, which outlines targets for health policy in European countries. It is recognised that all countries have a role in shaping and influencing the service delivery of the future. Priorities are:

- enhancement of the value and visibility of health for all
- development of health indicators
- promotion of the health of children and young people
- mobilising partners for health (engaging with the media/Internet)

- promotion of health in old age
- promotion of health during working life and influencing employment policy
- reduction of harm from alcohol, drugs and tobacco
- closing the health gap between countries.

Study Activity 36.4 ⎯⎯⎯⎯⎯⎯

In the past it was not considered important that community nurses working in the field (or indeed nurses in general) should concern themselves with global issues. However, now we are expected to recognise global impact on our practice, and to respond to such influences. One facet of this is sometimes described as 'the death of distance', a concept that includes how individuals and materials (organic and inorganic) can easily traverse national and continental divides, sometimes at supersonic speed.

- Reflect upon the consequences of this for community nursing, and in so doing identify at least five instances of global influences impacting upon the health of communities.

Responding effectively to policies affecting health

Health is political. It cannot be divorced from the decisions made by local county and urban councils or from policies created and legislated at Government level. Using the principle of *the influence of policies affecting mental health* as a guide to practice means that community nurses are political – although specifically non-aligned, and concerned only with advancing the twin causes of freedom and justice. They must have the courage to take on parties or institutions, irrespective of size or power, and confront key issues affecting health in the public arena. The community nurses' *raison d'être* is to represent people who are ill or socially excluded (for whatever reason) and their families/carers. This model of community nurses is brave and articulate. He or she cares. They have the ability to

see and to comprehend the wider picture of health and health care provision. All too often service users and their families/carers have been the subject of research, providing intimate details of their lives to be used by others. Rarely have their expertise and experience been used to influence service development and treatment response. In this respect, voluntary groups and pressure groups add an important dimension to the debate. With the current emphasis on co-operation and collaboration and with the plurality of statutory, voluntary and private sectors, this stimulates a need for quality assurance and clinical governance, which hopefully will increase the choices available to individuals. Moreover, to ensure those services are proactive and acceptable to users, their needs and aspirations should also be sought and cognisance taken of them.

Community nurses and other health professionals could set about designing strategies to meet some of the Government's challenges, which aim to:

- tackle the causes of inequality
- ensure fast and easy access to a range of therapeutic interventions
- inform patients fully at all stages of their illness and the recovery process
- involve patients in their own care by working in partnership with them and planning their care with them
- advance and enhance the clinical performance and the productivity of all staff employed by the National Health Service
- promote flexibility of education and training and also promote reflexive and reflective working practices
- remove fudged professional boundaries to ensure that the right skills are organised in the right way, to deliver equitable, quality-driven, patient-centred services
- create and utilise local networks with the aim of influencing the political agenda and promoting positive images of people who are ill, disabled or socially excluded, including the services that are provided.

A voice for women

There is a need to critique and recast assumptions about women's health in ways that elevate their experiences. Women frequently find their views being undervalued and discounted. Community nurses provide a voice for women who are disadvantaged, ill or disabled. They can be instrumental in highlighting the real concerns of women's issues. Moreover, community nurses are taught to identify gender differences relating to ill-health and disability, and where necessary, ensure that services are designed that are appropriate to meet women's needs. It is essential to hear and value women's perceptions of where their concerns, problems and pains are coming from. Therefore, further research needs to be carried out in this area. Community nurses play a significant role in representing women who are ill, disabled or socially excluded and work ardently at influencing policies affecting their health and well-being.

Study Activity 36.5 _____

It has recently been suggested that, as women's health is at last being recognised as a special area requiring attention, the matter of men's health is in danger of being overlooked. Indeed, recently interest in 'men's health' has also come to the fore.

- Carry out a brief library and Internet search under the terms 'women's health' and 'men's health'.
- Identify at least three specific aspects of women's health and three specific aspects of men's health, which in each case is not a major issue for the opposite gender.

A forum for children and young people

The promotion of children's and young people's health and well-being is fundamental to enable them to reach their full potential. Adults are response-*able* for the health and social well-being of future generations. This means that we are collectively responsible for creating healthy families, environments, schools and play areas, as well as a healthy globe. The needs of children world-wide cannot be overlooked because they live in a different country. As one humanity living on Earth at this moment in history, the children of the world are equal in their need for health and social care. Therefore, all children should be prized and cherished. The ultimate aim of such a world-wide project would be to facilitate children to reach their full potential.

The effectiveness with which children's needs are assessed is the key to the effectiveness of subsequent interventions, the provision of services and ultimately the health, growth and development of our children. The duty to protect children from the emotional challenge and pain of starvation, illness and stress demands sensitivity, knowledge, understanding and a multidisciplinary approach to care. Determining who is in need and what those needs are and providing services to safeguard and care for these children requires urgent attention. All adults must strive to ensure that children are conceived, born and grow up in environments consistent with safe and effective care (Department of Health, 1994).

A platform for older people

Images of old age that evolved within the political and socio-medical arena have been forceful. Older people have become both a 'problem' and a 'burden' to society after they are economically inactive following retirement. Many degrading and offending labels have been levelled at the older populace, including 'geriatrics', 'the elderly', 'the elderly mentally infirm', 'psychogeriatrics' and the new term of 'elder abuse'.

Despite pleas from senior citizens not to have these labels attached to them, professionals and others continue to use them, resulting in the marginalisation of older people. Community nurses have a role in promoting the self-esteem of older people. They could begin this process with flicking the tail of the coin that depicts negative images and negative affirmations of older people on to its head, which should portray positive images and positive affirmations. This simple gesture could help to raise society's awareness of older people's wisdom and experience through respecting and acknowledging the creative, inherent resources in human beings at all stages of their life span, especially when their self-esteem with the outside world becomes threatened. Community nurses are aware that varied support networks do make it easier for older people to live comfortably and safely within the community. In addition, improved awareness of the subtleties of older people's and families'/carers' relationships, as well as the tensions that exist in such relationships, would help the professionals' assessment of needs and, hence, their provision of care. Further research is required into promoting the quality of life for older people and their families/carers. In the meantime, more effort should be made by community nurses to promote positive representations of older people rather than continuing to ostracise them through the ramifications of the labelling process.

Summary

Contemporary, effective, caring, quality-driven community nursing services are organised in a way that helps to accomplish the vision expressed about 'health for all' that has been expressed throughout this chapter. Community nurses engage in and strive to enhance the full spectrum of nursing care throughout the life span. This generic way of working enables the creative potential of professional practice to be fulfilled. The key features addressed in this chapter emphasise the following:

- the fundamental principle that the perceptions and opinions of patients/clients, their families/carers and their advocates are paramount
- the empowerment of patients/clients, families/carers, communities and people with health problems and disabilities world-wide
- the education and training of community nurses to work as specialist practitioners
- the primacy of health promotion and prevention at individual, family/carer, community, European and global levels

- the interface between acute care and community care and between other agencies and voluntary services
- the expertise of community nurses and their unique and dynamic combination of therapeutic skills and therapeutic approaches to care
- the provision of proactive and responsive services designed to meet the assessed needs of patients, families/carers and communities
- the axiom of working in a collaborative, co-operative and flexible way.

Finally, partnership between Government, local councils, the voluntary, statutory and private services and community groups, both at national and local levels, is vital to ensure the delivery of the best possible services. Ultimately, the overall aim is to improve the health and well-being of the population.

References

Allen, D. (1998) *Mental Health and Nursing*, Sage, London

Barker, P.J. (1998) *Assessment in Psychiatric and Mental Health Nursing: In search of the whole person*, Stanley Thornes, Cheltenham

British Medical Association (1992) *Targets on Community Care: Targets for service provision*, British Medical Association, London

Buber, M. (1958) *I and Thou*, T&T Clark, Edinburgh

Caplan, G. (1961) *An Approach to Community Health*, Tavistock, London

Cutcliffe, J. and Butterworth, T. (2001) *Clinical Supervision: Principles, processes and practice*, Routledge, London

Department of Health (1990) *NHS and Community Care Act*, HMSO, London

Department of Health (1991) *Working Together Under the Children Act 1989*, HMSO, London

Department of Health (1994) *Working in Partnership: A collaborative approach to care*, HMSO, London

Department of Health (1995) *Making it Happen*, The Stationery Office, London

Department of Health (1997) *The New NHS, Modern, Dependable*, HMSO, London

Department of Health (1998) *A First Class Service: Quality in the new NHS*, Leeds NHS Executive, Leeds

Department of Health (1999) *Making a Difference: Strengthening the nursing, midwifery and health visiting contribution to health and healthcare*, HMSO, London

Department of Health and Social Services Northern Ireland (1995) *Action Plan for Community Nurses, Midwives and Health Visitors*, Department of Health and Social Services, Belfast

Fleming, P. (1999) Health promotion for individuals, families and communities. In: Long, A. (ed.) *Advanced Interaction for Community Nurses*, Macmillan, London

Heidegger, M. (1987) *On Being and Acting: From principles to anarchy* (trans. R. Shurmann), Indiana University Press, Bloomington, IL

Irving, P. and Long A. (2001) Critical incident stress debriefing following traumatic life experiences. *Journal of Psychiatric and Mental Health Nursing* 8(4), 307–14

Kemm and Close (1995) *Health Promotion: Theory and practice*, Macmillian, London

Kitson, A. (1993) Formalising concepts related to nurisng and caring. In Kitson, A. (ed.) *Nursing: Art and science*, Chapman and Hall, London

Long, A. (1997) Avoiding abuse amongst vulnerable groups in the community: people with a mental illness. In: Mason, C. (ed.) *Achieving Quality in Community Health Care Nursing*, Macmillan, London

Long, A. (2001) Mental health nursing. In: Sines, D., Appleby, F. and Raymond, E. (eds) *Community Healthcare Nursing*, Blackwell Science, Oxford

Marcel, G. (1949) (trans. Farer, K.) *Being and Having*, Dacre Press, London

Merleau-Ponty, M. (1974) *Phenomenology of Perception*, Humanities Press, New York

Morgan, S. (1999) *Assessing and Managing Risk*, Pavilion, London

Office for Public Management (2000) *Leading the Future*, T.G. Scott, London

Ovretveit, J. (1993) *Coordinating Community Care: Multidisciplinary teams and care management*, Open University Press, Buckingham

Ovretveit, J. (1998) *Evaluating Health Interventions*, Open University Press, Buckingham

Parse, R.R. (1995) Human becoming: Parse's theory of nursing. *Nursing Science Quarterly* 5(35), 35–45

Peplau, H. (1958) *Interpersonal Relations in Nursing*, Putman, New York

Public Health Alliance (1998) *A Public Health Model of Primary Care*, Department of Health, London

Robinson, K. (1997) *Family Needs Assessment*, Routledge, London

Rogers, C.R. (1997) *Client Centred Therapy*, Constable, London

Rogers, M. (1980) Nursing: a science of unitary man. In: Reihl, A. and Ray, C. (eds) *Conceptual Models for Nursing Practice*, Appleton-Century, Crofts, New York

Roper, N., Logan, W. and Tierney, A. (1996) *The Elements of Nursing* (4th edn), Churchill Livingstone, Edinburgh

Sarason, S. and Duck, S. (2001) *Community and Clinical Psychology*, Routledge, London

Sartre, J.P. (1969) *Being and Nothingness*, Routledge, London

Slevin, E. (1999a) Use of presence in community health care nursing. In: Long, A. (ed.) *Interaction for Practice in Community Nursing*, Macmillan, Basingstoke

Slevin, O. (1999b) The nurse–patient relationship: caring in a health context. In: Long, A. (ed.) *Interaction for Practice in Community Nursing*, Macmillan, Basingstoke

United Kingdom Central Council (1994) *The Future of Professional Practice – The council's standards for the education and training following registration*, United Kingdom Central Council, London

Watson, J. (1988) *Nursing: Human science and human care*, Appleton-Century-Crofts, New York

World Health Organisation (1984) *Summary Report of the Working Group on Concepts and Principles of Health Promotion*, World Health Organisation, Copenhagen

World Health Organisation (1986) *Health for All. Declaration of WHO Conference on Primary Health Care, Alma Ata*, World Health Organisation, Geneva

World Health Organisation (1998) *Health 21: The Health for All policy framework for the WHO European region*, World Health Organisation, Copenhagen

Module 8: The delivery of nursing care

Reflections

The concept of public health draws out the social conscience and collective responsibility in improving the health and well-being of individuals, communities and nations. This module has focused on these domains, offering insights into the central role nurses have within these frameworks of care. Having a public health perspective addresses social inequalities in health, social exclusion and isolation. As the famous writer John Donne has poetically established, 'no man is an island'. With the technological revolution and people's increased mobility, the public health agenda is firmly with us and as a new nurse it is imperative that you have a full and clear understanding of the nurse's role and responsibilities to prevent disease and promote health.

The notion of health inequality is a complex phenomenon that defies a common understanding. However, this has not prevented governments from addressing the issues of social deprivation, lifestyle and living conditions in their attempt to improve the health of individuals and populations. While studying this module you will have explored the wider issues of public health and the political directives of governments and global health communities. Before advancing your studies, it may be useful to reflect on the UK's public health agenda, your local agenda and the public health agenda of the World Health Organisation.

This module also focused on death and dying and pain management. We are privileged as a profession to witness and be engaged with those in our care from birth to death. Continuing our health paradigms, we acknowledge that birth is a healthy (normal) activity and by the same token death should also be viewed in this sense. The concept of ensuring everyone is entitled to a healthy death should be the norm. It should be pain free with a sense of peace and dignity. Consider this concept and when you go about your nursing business, strive to ensure this happens.

We have mentioned that health care in the UK is increasingly undertaken in the community setting. You will therefore be increasingly exposed to working in a range of settings that are not institutions. From your reading, can you list health care that was once delivered in hospital settings alone, and which is now undertaken in general practitioners' surgeries, or in the patient's own home?

When you have the opportunity to apply the knowledge gained from this module you will have advanced your competence to care for people who are most vulnerable and dependent. Do not underestimate the privilege it is to give someone the care they need without taking away their dignity.

MODULE 9: NURSING PERSPECTIVES

INTRODUCTION

This module is concerned with perspectives on nursing and largely follows the branch paradigms of the pre-registration nursing programmes, i.e. adult nursing, mental health nursing, children's nursing and learning disability nursing. We have included here a section on gerontological nursing because of its increasing importance in the care we give to an ageing population and the necessity for you to understand how older people have different health needs than those of younger cohorts.

After reading this module you will be conversant with the philosophical intents and core nursing practices in each of these nursing domains. In addition, you will have gained a useful insight into fields of nursing that you have not chosen to study, but during your career you may come across individuals that are outside of your sphere of practice and will at least have an understanding of their care needs.

37 Adult nursing

Marlene Sinclair

LEARNING OUTCOMES

After studying this chapter you will be able to:

- Understand the basic principles of the provision of nursing care for adults
- Differentiate between adult nursing and the other branches of nursing in the UK
- Recognise the difference between adult nursing as a main branch of nursing, and more advanced and specialist roles, such as that of a midwife
- Describe the nature of services available for adult patients
- Discuss the role and function of the nurse caring for adult patients
- Search the Internet for up-to-date information and best evidence relevant to aspects of adult nursing.

INTRODUCTION

This chapter presents a brief outline of the adult branch of nursing, which is concerned primarily with the care of adults in terms of physical health and well-being. However, although there is a branch of nursing concerned with mental health, this does not mean that adult nursing excludes a concern for mental health and well-being in adults. Indeed, it would be impossible to isolate a concern with physical health from concerns about the psychological, social, and spiritual health and well-being of individuals and communities. Modern nursing tends to adopt a more holistic approach, considering the health care needs of the whole person. Furthermore, there is usually a direct link between physical and mental health, wherein each influences the

other; not only can poor physical health affect our mental state, but emotional distress and anxiety can also affect our physical health. Indeed, some physical disorders are recognised as having a significant psychological cause or aetiology, and are thus termed psychosomatic disorders.

This aside, adult nursing is nursing that takes place in health care settings concerned primarily with physical health and well-being of individuals within the adult age ranges. Such care occurs within hospitals and institutions and in community settings. The purpose of the current chapter is to position adult nursing within the general range of nursing provision and to identify the main orientations within the adult nursing perspective.

It is not intended that the chapter will provide a detailed presentation of all the activities that come within the adult nursing role. There are textbooks that attend specifically to this purpose. However, in a rapidly changing health care world, it is no longer possible to detail specific nursing approaches and procedures that could be identified as best practice for any significant period of time. The constant emergence of new evidence and the commitment to evidence-based practice (EBP), discussed in Module 4 of this book, bear witness to the fact that procedures, techniques, and recognised therapeutic interventions are constantly changing. It is increasingly important that nurses base their specific interventions on best practice, established through EBP, and contained within procedure manuals and practice protocols agreed within the local health care setting.

All aspects of basic nursing care are continually changing, with new research information arriving on a daily basis via the Internet. Therefore, this chapter focuses on providing key

Internet references to enable students to seek essential and relevant information.

Adult nursing is practised across both institutional settings (hospitals and nursing homes, etc.) and community settings (primary care trusts and health centres, etc.). The delivery of care in community settings has been considered in Chapter 36 so will not be discussed here.

Adult nursing covers all age ranges apart from children. A particular grouping within this range is that of older people, and because this particular age range presents major challenges for health care provision, Chapter 41 is devoted to this topic, and, again, will not be discussed in detail here. However, it should be noted that the care of older people – where attention is primarily focused on physical health and well-being – formally comes within the responsibility of adult nurses. Similarly, where attention is primarily toward the mental health of older people, this comes under the mental health branch of nursing.

BACKGROUND TO ADULT NURSING

The subdivision of nursing into branches is peculiar to the UK and one or two other countries (such as the Republic of Ireland). In most other countries, the level of Registered or Licensed nurse is not subdivided in this way. For example, in North America, all nurses are general nurses at the point of initial qualification; that is, they are prepared to address the full range of health needs (physical, mental, social) across all age ranges. It is perhaps more accurate to describe such nursing as generic rather than general, particularly as in the past the term 'general nurse' in the UK related to nurses who were concerned (as are adult nurses) with physical care. In those other countries where the level of registered practitioner is generic, specialization occurs following registration, and is by definition at a higher level than the baseline generic registration level. Thus mental health, paediatric, learning disabilities nursing, etc. are by definition specialist in those countries, while in the UK they are simply

another 'branch' or 'division' of nursing at the registered/non-specialist nursing level.

It is useful to briefly consider the historical background. You may have come across terms such as State Registered Nurse (SRN), Registered General Nurse (RGN) and, for more recently qualified nurses, Registered Nurse (RN). Prior to the 1980s, nursing in the UK was regulated by councils in the four UK countries, the largest and best known being the General Nursing Council (GNC) for England and Wales. Under these regulatory bodies there were two levels of licensed nurse: registered and enrolled (the latter being a more practical level, requiring shorter training). Midwives were regulated by separate regulatory bodies (except in Northern Ireland). For registered nurses, the divisions were as follows:

- State Registered Nurse (SRN) – concerned primarily with general or physical care across all age ranges
- Registered Sick Children's Nurse (RSCN) – concerned with the care of children, particularly sick children
- Registered Mental Nurse (RMN) – concerned with the care of the mentally ill, across all age ranges (including children)
- Registered Nurse (for the) Mentally Handicapped (RNMH) – concerned with the care of people then termed mentally handicapped, or persons requiring special care
- Registered Fever Nurse (RFN) – concerned with the care of people suffering from communicable diseases.

The division of Registered Fever Nurse gradually lapsed as modern health care overcame the major threats from communicable diseases such as tuberculosis, poliomyelitis and typhoid. Other forms of practitioner were the Health Visitor (a registered practitioner with further training in public health and child care) and District Nurse (a registered practitioner with further training in home nursing). In both these instances, these were not actually divisions of a nursing register, but came largely within the area of post-registration qualifications. By this time other post-registration specialties were also emerging in such areas as intensive care and coronary care, most notably under a Joint Board of Clinical Nursing Studies established within the English National Health Service.

Following the Nurses, Midwives and Health Visitors Act (1979) all the nursing, midwifery and health visiting regulatory bodies were drawn into a more unified framework of a United Kingdom Central Council for Nursing, Midwifery and Health Visiting (UKCC) and four National Boards for Nursing, Midwifery and Health Visiting (one in each of the four UK countries). At this time a new Register of Nurses, Midwives and Health Visitors had the following *nursing* divisions:

- Registered General Nurse (RGN) – concerned primarily with physical care, but limited specifically to adults
- Registered Children's Nurse (RCN) – concerned with the physical and mental health of children (no longer specifically designated as a sick children nursing role)
- Registered Mental Nurse (RMN) – concerned with the mental health of adults and children
- Registered Nurse (for the) Mentally Handicapped (RNMH) – concerned with the care of people then termed mentally handicapped, or persons requiring special care.

But by this time (the 1980s) the term 'mental handicap' (and earlier terms such as 'mental deficiency' and 'mental subnormality') were being discarded in favour of a less stigmatising label: 'learning disability'. The UKCC also eventually adopted the term 'learning disability nursing'.

In the latter half of the 1980s, the UKCC reviewed nurse education in a major study known as *Project 2000* (UKCC, 2001). The aim of *Project 2000* was to ensure that best knowledge and practice were integrated in education and practice that would be centred upon the individual or community receiving care. Very similar nursing branches were identified in a new single Register of Nurses, Midwives and Health Visitors, as follows:

- Registered Nurse (adult nursing)
- Registered Nurse (children's nursing)
- Registered Nurse (mental health nursing)
- Registered Nurse (learning disabilities nursing).

The UKCC did permit nurses already on the register to use their previous designations. As a result, an adult nurse may currently be using the designation SRN, RGN, or RN. While *Project 2000* retained the divisions in modified form, it did introduce a new training whereby all nursing students undertook an 18-month Common Foundation Programme, followed by an 18-month Branch Programme in one or other of the four divisions. This established a generic or common caring base across all four branches or divisions. This common base addressed not only physical but also psychological, social and spiritual aspects of care. It also provided a foundation in terms of orientation towards the needs of adults, people with mental health issues, children and people with learning disabilities, as well as in the areas of community care, maternity care and the care of older people.

By now you may have noted two subtle peculiarities of the British system:

1 While adult and children's nursing are determined by age ranges, mental and learning disabilities nursing are determined by a particular service for clients or patients across all age ranges.
2 While it is recognised that each individual must be approached as having physical, psychological, social and spiritual needs, adult and children's nursing are concerned primarily with physical care (although children's nurses are in fact also trained to deal with emotional care and the mental health of children and their families).

At the turn of the millennium, a further major review of regulation took place, resulting in the establishment of a new Nursing and Midwifery Council for the whole of the UK, which came into being in April 2002. Around the point of changeover, a further review of nursing practice and education had taken place. This retained the latter four divisions, but for training reduced the Foundation Programme element to one year, with a consequent increase of the Branch Programmes to two years. This was based on evidence that more time was required to adequately prepare nurses for a specific branch. It also had the consequence of significantly reducing the 'common' or 'generic' element of nurse education.

A significant concern, and a debate that will undoubtedly continue, is whether like most other countries, we should have a generic nursing in the UK, a broad-based general training, with specialisation in such areas as mental health, learning disabilities or paediatrics (children's health) taking place after registration. This is the model followed in medicine, where the number of specialties has indeed increased in recent years. It is also the common model in most other professions, such as engineering and law. However, to date we continue to have four branches in nursing, and our concern in this chapter is with that branch or subdivision of nursing known as adult nursing.

It should also be noted that although the regulatory bodies adhered to four different branches or divisions of nursing at basic registered practitioner level, the need for specialisation in some areas of practice following registration continued to be recognised within a Post-Registration Education and Practice (PREP) system. Under this system nurses and midwives could be trained as Specialist Nurse Practitioners or Specialist Community Nurse Practitioners, and have such qualifications recorded (as opposed to registered) on the single professional register. Indeed, in England by the end of the 1990s, a clinical structure was established on a four-tier basis, as follows:

- Health Care Assistants (non-registered nursing assistant personnel)
- Registered Practitioners
- Senior Registered Practitioners (which included ward managers and recorded specialist practitioners)

- Nurse Consultants (largely involved in practice development, research and leadership roles).

Study Activity 37.1

- On the basis of your current knowledge of nursing, reflect upon the issue of nursing being subdivided as opposed to being a generic profession at the entry level.
- Compare how nursing is structured differently to other health professions, such as medicine, which are generic at the entry level.
- Identify arguments for and against specialisation at entry level, as opposed to at a more advanced post-registration level.
- Visit the UK Centre for Interprofessional Education at *http://www.caipe.org.uk/* and consider the benefits of multi-professional education for doctors, nurses, midwives and other professions allied to health. Discuss them with lecturers, mentors and peers.
- Read the Cochrane review on interprofessional education:

  Zwarenstein, M., Reeves, S., Barr, H. *et al.* (2002) *Interprofessional Education: Effects on professional practice and health care outcomes* (Cochrane Review), The Cochrane Library, Issue 1, Update Software, Oxford.

THE ROLE OF THE ADULT NURSE

As noted above, the primary orientation of adult nursing is that of physical health and well-being. But, as stated above, this does not mean that the adult nurse ignores the psychological, social and spiritual needs of patients and clients. Threats to physical health bring with them varying degrees of mental, social and spiritual distress, and a holistic orientation to nursing requires attention to all these facets of personal care. Furthermore, distress in these areas may not only have a detrimental effect on physical health, but in some circumstances may actually cause physical ill health (which we termed above as psychosomatic disorders).

The role of the adult nurse extends across a number of dimensions, among which the most important are:

- The full range of health and well-being, from good health to poor health and extending into actual physical illness
- The full range of adulthood, extending from adolescence through young adulthood and middle age to the later stages of life
- The provision of care that extends from health promotion and health education through to the care of individuals with actual physical illness or disability
- The provision of care across a range of settings, from acute hospitals and other institutional settings, through to the care of individuals in their homes.

CARE IN THE GENERAL HOSPITAL SETTING

In modern health care facilities there is an increasing tendency towards specialisation. Several decades ago hospital treatment and care was largely administered under the supervision of a medical consultant – either a general surgeon (in the case of surgical intervention) or a general physician (in the case of medical or non-surgical intervention). Beyond this there were a few specialties, such as cardiac or neurological surgery, or medical specialties such as geriatrics or dermatology. With advances in medical science and technology it became increasingly clear that consultants could only maintain expertise in very specific areas, and as a consequence specialisation increased so that today general surgery or medicine is less common, particularly in highly advanced health care systems.

These same advances have also created significant changes in the patterns of health care provision. For example, there has been a significant increase in day treatment and much more rapid turnaround times. Thirty years ago a routine surgical intervention involved as much as 3–4 weeks of in-patient care. Today a patient may arrive in the morning, be treated in a day surgery unit, and return home the same day. In some instances, as more flexible approaches to primary care are developed, patients may now even be treated at home under hospital-at-home schemes. In the future, much minor surgery will be conducted at the general practitioner's surgery and many nurses are being trained to undertake minor surgery, such as the removal of warts and the removal of objects from nasal or ear passages.

Specialist roles for nurses are developing rapidly. Practice nurses are experts at dealing with wound care and procedural issues in the treatment room, while nurse practitioners are experts in health assessment and care and take on their own patient/client caseload.

However, there are still common patterns to the treatment of adults in general (physical care) settings. Such approaches are outlined below. There are specialist texts for in-depth treatment of such topics as surgical or medical nursing, and the intention here is to present a general view of what adult nursing involves.

SURGICAL NURSING

Approaches

Surgical treatment usually involves some form of surgical intervention, where the treatment involves an invasion of or entry into the body for purposes of some manipulative procedure designed to occasion repair and healing and/or alleviate suffering. In common parlance, this is referred to as an 'operation', which is most frequently carried out under a general anaesthetic (the administration of substances that induce unconsciousness, remove sensitivity to pain, and control body processes to make the surgical intervention safer and more effective). Nowadays, such intervention may take place using laser technology or microsurgery using fibre optics so that incisions are minimal or absent. Surgical nursing involves the care of patients undergoing such treatments. This is commonly divided into pre-operative care, care in the intra-operative period, and post-operative care.

Nursing assessment and pre-operative care

The pre-operative assessment of patients involves the identification of possible post-operative physiological and psychological risk factors, as well as the collection of data that would be useful for the care of the patient post-operatively. In some settings this information is collated by the 'anaesthetic nurse', who is specially trained to provide care for individuals preparing for surgery. Although much of the data collected at this stage is routine and usually collated in standardised form, the nurse must consider the information obtained as unique to the patient. The pre-operative assessment can be classified into the following three sections:

1 The assessment of surgical risk
2 Baseline observations
3 Pre-operative information and educational needs.

Assessment of surgical risk

The age of the client
Both the very young and very old (for differing reasons in terms of their physiological response to surgery), are considered to be more at risk than adults. The old may have circulatory system impairments, such as cardiac disorders or reduced metabolic rates. The very young are considered at risk because of their limited fluid reserves and the fact that their circulatory and renal systems have not yet fully developed.

Nutritional status
The nurse must consider the patient's pre-operative nutritional status. Patients who are malnourished have particular difficulties with surgery, as they are more likely to suffer post-operative complications. For example, protein deficiencies affect the healing process; vitamin C is important for the laying down of collagen fibres and capillary strengthening; low carbohydrate intake will result in shortages in glucose reserves; dehydration can predispose the patient to shock. Generally, if the patient is nutritionally com-promised, core body temperature becomes lowered, which can have an affect on wound healing (Poulton, 1991). Additionally, other studies (Powell-Tuck, 1983; Gorse et al., 1989) have found a correlation between poor nutrition, wound infections, and delayed healing. Given the extent of these potential problems, Millar (1991) suggests that all patients who are about to have surgery require a comprehensive pre-operative nutritional assessment. This should include the patient's present and perceived normal weight, his normal dietary intake and food habits (likes, dislikes, and preferred times for eating) and any recent changes in appetite. This information should be combined with a physical examination and laboratory data obtained through blood and urine samples.

Stress
The combined effect of illness, hospitalisation, and pending surgical intervention can increase stress and anxiety and produce a physiological or psychological imbalance affecting an individual's homeostasis (Boore, 1978). Therefore, the pre-operative assessment of a patient is an appropriate opportunity for detecting the presence of stress and identifying its cause and nature. Wilson-Barnett and Fordham (1983) found that providing patients with adequate information about their treatment and dealing effectively with any other fears significantly reduced pre-operative stress, which in turn, reduced post-operative discomfort and promoted recovery. Thompson (1990) contends that in the immediate pre-operative period the patient feels particularly vulnerable, yet tends to be given minimal nursing care, often by the least skilled nurses. Interestingly, various other studies reveal no significant correlation between stress and the nature or type of surgery that the patient is about to undergo. Hayward (1975) found that all patients benefit from pre-operative information. Janis (1958) noted that anxiety and stress are just as prevalent whether patients are having major or minor surgery. During the pre-operative period, the nurse should pay particular attention to non-verbal cues that may suggest

discontent (body posture, facial expression, and eye contact), and utilise effective communication skills (for example questioning, listening, paraphrasing and observation) to encourage the patient to express fears about aspects of his care in hospital. It is not sufficient for the nurse simply to recognise the presence of stress. In order to enable the patient to deal with it, she must draw on additional specific stress-reducing skills, such as the use of touch, music therapy, massage, aromatherapy, or relaxation exercises (Caunt, 1992).

Medications

Because some medications adversely react with anaesthetic agents, the nurse should ascertain which medications the patient has previously taken, prescribed or otherwise. This information should be recorded and made available to the doctor and anaesthetist.

Baseline observations

Baseline observations on the patient (temperature, pulse, blood pressure and respirations) are taken and recorded. The skin is observed for colour and unusual marks, in order to provide the nurse with comparable data post-operatively. The nurse should routinely screen the patient's urine for the presence of abnormal constituents to discount such things as diabetes or the presence of a urinary tract infection. The doctor will carry out a full physiological and neurological examination and organise a range of investigations (including blood tests, electrocardiographs, and chest X-rays) to ensure that the patient is fit for anaesthesia and surgery.

Pre-operative visits

For patients who are about to have elective surgery, a pre-operative visit by a specialist nurse is an increasingly common occurrence. Preoperative visits can take many forms. Theatre staff may visit the patient in the ward; the patient may visit the ward before admission to meet nursing staff; or a specialist nurse could visit the patient at home in advance of admission to hospital.

A visit by the theatre nurse before surgery is useful for three reasons. First, it allows the development of a meaningful relationship between the patient and the nurse, as well as simply providing a familiar face. Second, it is an opportunity to give the patient specific information about his care in the immediate recovery period. Third, during this visit the theatre nurse can form an early assessment of the patient's own interpretation of feelings regarding his imminent surgery, and allay any fears or worries the patient may have. Furthermore, Lewis (1994) argues that because the amount of time patients spend in hospital has been substantially reduced both pre- and post-operatively, the theatre experience has become a proportionately more significant part of the patient's stay in hospital. Day-surgery care provides the most tangible example of this, in that patients are often not formally admitted to a ward at all. Preoperative assessment by theatre staff is therefore particularly important for the early detection of either post-operative changes or complications.

For patients who are about to have major surgery, pre-admission visits to the hospital are considered invaluable by both the patient and staff for facilitating post-operative self-care and adaptation. In some hospitals women who are to have a hysterectomy are sometimes invited to meet their primary nurse 2 weeks prior to their surgery. This allows the woman to become oriented to the hospital ward prior to admission. She can meet other patients having similar surgery, possibly at around the same time, and also be given information about the kind of care given immediately before, during and after surgery. For patients who may require stoma surgery, home visits by a stoma nurse have proved invaluable. Black (1994) contends that home visits allow these patients to be more relaxed and to retain control during interview sessions. They are more open and ask questions of a more intimate nature as a result.

Pre-operative fasting

Given that general anaesthesia depresses gastrointestinal functioning, there is a danger that the patient may aspirate and inhale gastric contents during administration. As this can have fatal consequences, patients are usually asked to fast 6–8 hours before surgery. The patient and his relatives are informed of this need and a sign to this effect is usually placed at the head of the patient's bed. During the fasting period the patient can be offered mouth rinses to moisten and relieve discomfort of the oral cavity. While pre-operative fasting is universally accepted, the nurse must also ensure that the patient's fasting time is not excessively prolonged. According to Hung (1992a, b) the dangers of prolonged fasting can range from mild discomfort, irritability, and dehydration to more serious post-operative complications, such as shock.

Study Activity 37.2

Read through the recommendations for pre-operative fasting on the Internet at www.anesthe sia.psu.edu/intranet/guidelines/npo

Preparation of the skin

Pre-operative skin preparation contributes significantly to the establishment of an area of asepsis (i.e. one free of infection) around the site of surgery. It also reduces the risk of post-operative infections of the wound. Hair is removed because micro-organisms readily cling to it, thus providing an obvious environment for infection. Aside from reducing the risk of infection, shaving the area also helps to create a clear field of vision for the surgeon. Hair may be removed using a wet or a dry razor, electric clippers, or a depilatory cream. Close shaving with the use of a razor requires careful attention because it can cause soft tissue abrasion, also creating a potential source of infection (Cruse and Foord, 1980; Tunevall, 1988). Alternatively, Kovach (1990) makes the comment that using electric clippers is inconvenient because they must be completely disassembled and sterilised before being used on another patient. Depilatory creams can cause allergic reactions in

some patients. Irrespective of how the nurse opts to remove hair in preparing the patient for surgery, it is important that she displays a degree of sensitivity, particularly for patients undergoing neuro-surgery, where all the hair is removed from the scalp.

There is a general consensus about the value of total body washes pre-operatively, in terms of reducing skin flora, although showers are considered to be more effective than baths. Patients need to be reminded to wash their hair thoroughly, to pay particular attention to cleaning the more hidden areas of the body (under the breasts and nails, and the umbilicus), to remove all make-up, and afterwards to dry themselves with a freshly laundered towel (McKenzie, 1988; Kalideen, 1990).

Consent to treatment

Study Activity 37.3

- Before proceeding into this section, write a brief note of your own understanding of 'consent'. Explore the sources below, and then revisit your initial statement to see how you might amend this.
- Visit the United Kingdom Parliament site and familiarise yourself with the recent Patient Consent Form Bill that went through parliament in January 2002 at www2.york.ac.uk/inst/crd/ehcb.htm
- Read the Health Technology Assessment on informed decision making at www.hta.nhs-web.nhs.uk/execsumm/SUMM301.HTM
- Read the article in the British Medical Journal about consent for intimate examinations on the BMJ website at www.bmj.comColdicottetal.326(7380): 97
- What should you do when a patient refuses consent to medical treatment? Read the data on www.offsol.demon.co.uk/tlr98803.htm

All hospitals require adult patients who are fully alert (or next of kin in certain circumstances) to sign consent forms for surgery, which are countersigned by a doctor. The purpose of a signed consent form is twofold. The patient is protected from having surgery to which he has not agreed, and the doctor and the hospital are protected against claims that unauthorised surgery has been performed. Much has been written about the value of providing patients and their families with information about an operation and its contribution to promoting recovery. However, it is very rarely considered as an integral part of the process of attaining consent for surgery. While the consent forms may provide tangible evidence that a patient and his family understand the nature and expected result of surgery, in practice it is usually necessary for further explanations to be given to ensure the patient's full understanding. Therefore, obtaining the patient's consent for surgery should be perceived by the nurse as more than simply a mechanism for protecting against litigation. Castledine (1988) points out that providing effective pre-operative teaching to patients and their families facilitates involvement in all aspects of care, including the patient's ability to consent to surgery.

Brewster (1992) uses her experiences in a busy genito-urinary unit to describe how careful planning between the primary nurse, the anaesthetist and the doctor, acting for the surgeon, can prepare the patient for surgery, and at the same time make the exercise of giving consent more meaningful and valuable to the patient. First, Brewster describes how, through informal teaching sessions and a specially designed pre-operative booklet, the nurse can ensure that the patient has an understanding of the specific post-operative aspects of prostate surgery (trans-urethral resection), such as catheter care and through drainage, eating and drinking regimen, and potential sexual difficulties (for example, retrograde ejaculation). Next, Brewster describes how, by carrying out a similar exercise, the anaesthetist ensures that the patient also understands the anaesthetic. Finally, the doctor provides appropriate information about the nature of the surgery before co-signing the consent form with the patient. Brewster argues that by this strategy the patient is provided with a clear and comprehensive out-line of the operation and is given the opportunity to ask pertinent questions during any stage of the process, before eventually consenting to surgery.

Depending on the nature of the surgery, special precautions and limitations of movement will need to be adhered to (for example following a total hip replacement), which requires pre-operative understanding and agreement.

Care immediately before surgery

The care given before surgery should be smoothly planned and organised in such a way that the nurse and patient are working in partnership as far as possible. The patient should be assisted to feel in control of the situation at all times, and privacy and confidentiality will be maintained.

Before administering the pre-medication to the patient, the nurse should ensure that the following actions have been taken:

- The bed should be freshly made and the patient asked to empty his bladder and put on a theatre gown, to minimise the risk of infection or urinary incontinence.
- All prostheses, including dentures, should be removed for the patient's safety.
- The patient should be fitted with anti-embolitic stockings. Circulatory problems could be exacerbated through surgery or the patient could go on to develop a deep venous thrombosis. The stocking's elasticated material compresses the veins of the leg, facilitating venous return and preventing stasis, or the pooling of blood.
- Thorough oral hygiene should be offered or carried out to prevent the risk of the patient aspirating food particles, and to make him more comfortable.
- Jewellery and valuables should be removed for safe-keeping to prevent them from being misplaced during surgery.
- The prescribed pre-medication should be administered to promote rest and reduce anxiety.

Study Activity 37.4 ⎯⎯⎯⎯⎯⎯⎯

- Using a role-play situation, practice carrying out a pre-operative assessment, and collating some of the information discussed in this chapter, with one of your student colleagues.
- During your assignment to a surgical area, set a clinical objective with your mentor that you will both observe and practice preparing a patient for surgery.
- Read the following research article:

  Jester, R. and Williams, S. (1999) Pre-operative fasting: putting research into practice, *Nursing Standard* 13(39), 33–5.
- Discuss the implications for putting research into practice with your clinical mentor.
- Log on to the Royal College of Nursing website for the *Nursing Standard* journal on line (*www.nursing-standard.co.uk*) and search for articles on surgical nursing, pre-op care, wound management and post-operative pain management.

Intra-operative and critical care nursing

When a patient goes for surgery he becomes the responsibility of the anaesthetic room and theatre nurse. Thereafter, depending on the nature of the surgery, he may be temporarily transferred to either a recovery room or an intensive care unit for close monitoring. Throughout this period patients are extremely vulnerable. Thus, the nurse must act for the patient in terms of providing total protection and care. The role of the theatre nurse has been a source of considerable debate. If a reductionist interpretation of nursing is taken (i.e. that theatre nursing is principally about assisting the surgeon and ensuring that he is handed the appropriate instrument at the proper time), then it would be hard to justify differentiating between the role of nurses and other staff, such as operating department assistants (ODAs). Conversely, if theatre nursing is interpreted as a continuation of the total package of care, mutually agreed with the primary care nurse from the outset of the patient's stay in hospital,

then the presence of a theatre nurse would not only be justifiable but essential. Within this framework, the theatre nurse is perceived as a clinical specialist, with a focused nursing expertise, who is acting in the position of locum primary nurse (Evans, 1991; Tudor, 1992).

Evans (1991) describes some of the professional functions proper to theatre nursing as follows:

- *Planning* – nursing care is underpinned by the process of nursing, through a comprehensive assessment via pre-operative visits, providing care by competent and confident practitioners, and using professional judgement to evaluate the effect of nursing interventions.
- *Communication* – ensuring accurate communication creates continuity of care between theatre and ward staff.
- *Multi-disciplinary team* – apart from her discrete professional tasks, the nurse has a responsibility to work alongside other health care professionals in a co-operative way, in order to provide a smooth theatre service (Henderson, 1979).
- Quality assurance – through monitoring care, the theatre nurse sets standards, and ensures that the nursing care provided contributes to the overall quality of service for the patient.

The theatre nurse ensures that the following information is documented and communicated to the receiving nurse:

- The site of incision and operation procedure
- Evidence of verified post-operative counts (wound swabs)
- Diathermy pad site and condition of the skin
- Disposal of specimens (biopsies)
- The number and position of any implants, catheters or drains
- Any specific instruction from the surgeon (such as care of the wound site).

Study Activity 37.5 ⎯⎯⎯⎯⎯⎯⎯

- During your surgical placement, arrange with your clinical teacher to follow a patient pre-operatively through his period in theatre and the recovery room.

- Discuss with your colleagues and a teacher the special role of the theatre nurse.
- Visit the following websites, search for information relevant to your current level of study and bookmark for future reference:

  - British Association of Critical Care Nurses at *www.baccn.org.uk/*
  - European Federation of Critical Care Nurses at *www.efccna.org/*
  - American Association of Critical Care Nurses at *www.aacn.org/*

Post-operative nursing care

Wound closure

Following surgery the surgeon will close the patient's wound in order to restore normal anatomy. This step is achieved using sutures made of either natural or synthetic materials, which are either absorptive or non-absorptive (non-absorptive ones have to be manually removed). As an alternative, the surgeon may choose to use stainless steel clips, staples, or skin closure strips along with sutures. Because stitches leave a tract that can become a focus for infection or a source of skin irritation, close observation of the wound site is necessary. Irrespective of which material is used, removal usually takes place 7–10 days post-operatively if the wound is healing sufficiently (Nightingale, 1990).

Wound assessment

The first phase of wound care involves an assessment of the wound, which enables the nurse to establish with the patient realistic and measurable goals for wound healing specifically, and post-operative care generally. If the wound is assessed and documented accurately, subjective and intuitive evaluation is not necessary. Sutton (1989) identifies some observable and measurable factors that can act as indicators for asses-

sing wound healing: blood supply to the wound site, the presence of infection, the local environment (particularly if the wound is around the perineal area, where healing is difficult and the risk of infection is increased), nutritional status of the patient, and psychological aspects such as motivation to comply with treatment in order to recover fully. In taking a more holistic interpretation of wound assessment, Dealey (1991) considers it important to monitor the wider physiological and psychological effects, including the effect on the patient of reduced mobility, elimination, personal cleansing, and dressing caused by the presence of a wound, as well as the psycho-sexual effects of coming to terms with disfigurement.

Wound care

A wound is a loss of continuity of skin or mucous membrane due to either accidental injury or surgery. Wound healing involves the replacement of destroyed tissue with a similar type of living tissue. Healing can be either by partial or complete regeneration or repair. Regeneration implies a total restitution of the original structure of tissue. Healing by repair involves the formation of a new permanent structure of scar tissue. Although there is evidence of wound care dating back to Ancient Egypt, the Greeks, and throughout the Renaissance Period, it is only in relatively modern times (from the nineteenth century) that recognisable practices have appeared. Much of this progress can be attributed to early microbiologists such as Joseph Lister, Louis Pasteur, Ignaz Semmelweiss, and Joseph Gamgee.

Wound dressing and drainage

A wound dressing is a covering applied to a wound to protect it from further harm while, at the same time, aiding the healing process. There is an endless range of options from which a nurse may choose when selecting an appropriate dressing for a wound.

Quite often during surgery the surgeon will insert a drain into the wound site. This encourages the discharge of pus from an abscess or removes normal body fluid that has made its way into the wrong body compartment, such as blood due to bleeding, or urine appearing in the peritoneum following trauma to the bladder (Nightingale, 1990). There are two types of wound drainage: open drains and closed drains. The drain is placed into the wound just before closure, and is then attached to a sealed vacuo-container, which attracts the drainage from the wound site. It is the responsibility of the nurse to monitor the drain, ensuring that drainage is not impeded, observing and documenting the amount of drained fluid, examining the insertion site to ensure that it is properly secured, and providing specific care to the patient to explain her actions.

As the biology of wound healing processes unfolds we have a proliferation of different therapies and strategies aimed at improving patient care. The latest of these is vacuum therapy (total negative pressure TNP). For the latest information visit their website at *www.vacuumtherapy.co.uk/protocols.htm*

Study Activity 37.6

Search the following key Internet resources for the most up-to-date information on wound care:

— Electronic journal on worldwide wound management at *www.worldwidewounds.com/*
— The Wound Management Forum at *www.smtl.co.uk/cgi-bin/HyperNews/get.cgi/wounds.html* For useful reference information on wound dressings visit *www.dressings.org/Dressings/calaband.html*
— European Tissue Repair Society at *www.etrs.org/*
— Wound Management Practice Resource Centre at *www.smtl.co.uk/WMPRC/index.html*
— Oxford International Wound Healing Foundation at *www.oxfordinternationalwoundfoundation.org/*.

General post-operative care

Collect the patient from the theatre
The patient should be collected from the theatre by an experienced nurse, who should ensure that airway maintenance equipment is available, and that information is collected from theatre staff. This nurse's task is to effect a safe transference from theatre to ward, and to re-establish a good rapport with the patient post-operatively (Allin, 1991).

Prevent obstruction of the patient's airway
To maintain a clear airway and minimise the patient's discomfort, place him initially in the recovery position and observe that normal respirations are maintained. When his cough reflex has returned, offer small amounts of fluid if the nature of the surgery allows.

Vomiting
If vomiting occurs, maintain the patient in the recovery position. An anti-emetic may be prescribed and administered to maintain the patient's safety, alleviate his distress and prevent further vomiting.

Haemorrhage
The nurse should monitor the patient's pulse, blood pressure, amount of wound drainage and oozing of exudate from the suture line, in order to detect early signs of post-operative bleeding.

Prevention of secondary complications

Chest infection
To encourage self-care in minimising the development of specific post-operative complications, support the patient's deep breathing exercises, and encourage him to expectorate excess sputum.

Difficulty in passing urine
To permit the early detection of either urinary retention or a reduced renal output because of the non-therapeutic effects of anaesthetic (O'Reilly, 1991), monitor the frequency and amount of urine passed by the patient.

Mobility
To encourage self-care and prevent the formation of either pressure sores or deep venous

thrombosis, encourage limb physiotherapy (putting the limbs through all their normal movements), and relieve pressure areas by assisting the patient to change position every 2 hours.

Personal hygiene
To maintain the patient's personal dignity assist him with personal hygiene until self-care has been achieved.

Postoperative pain

Pain is defined as 'an unpleasant sensory and emotional experience associated with actual or potential tissue damage'. It is a complex process, influenced by both physiological and psychological factors. In the past, management of post-operative pain has sometimes been shown to be inadequate. It is important that such pain is managed effectively as, in addition to the physical and psychological distress, it can affect organ systems in the following ways:

- *Respiratory* – reduced cough, atelectasis, sputum retention and hypoxaemia
- *Cardiovascular* – increased myocardial oxygen consumption and ischaemia
- *Gastrointestinal* – decreased gastric emptying, reduced gut motility and constipation
- *Genitourinary* – urinary retention
- *Neuroendocrine* – hyperglycaemia, protein catabolism and sodium retention
- *Musculoskeletal* – reduced mobility, pressure sores and increased risk of deep venous thrombosis
- *Psychological* – anxiety and fatigue.

When assessing pain, bear the following points in mind:

- Pain is a subjective experience. Observer assessment of patient behaviour is unreliable.
- Pain should be assessed and recorded by visual analogue scales, a verbal numerical reporting scale or a categorical rating scale.

Non-pharmacological methods of pain relief include:

- Preoperative explanation and education
- Relaxation therapy
- Hypnosis
- Cold or heat
- Splinting of wounds, etc.
- Transcutaneous electrical nerve stimulation (TENS).

Pharmacological methods of pain relief include simple, stronger or specialised analgesia. A simple analgesia is paracetamol, a weak anti-inflammatory agent that can be administered orally or rectally, and is best taken on a regular rather than 'as required' basis. Opiates are stronger analgesias, of which the most commonly used drugs are diamorphine, morphine and pethidine (in descending order of strength). Specialised analgesias include the administration of medicines directly into nervous tissue or muscles, or the use of epidural anaesthesia (Rigg *et al.*, 2002).

Study Activity 37.7

- During a surgical clinical placement observe the strategies used by clinical staff to evaluate the effectiveness of the prescribed regime for wound care.
- List any five products that are currently used in wound dressing.
- List any five observations that the nurse should make when caring for a patient with a Redi-vac drain in-situ.
- Discuss with your colleagues/link tutor and mentor the value of using patient-controlled analgesia in a surgical ward.
- Conduct an Internet search for on-line references related to nursing and post-operataive pain management, and make notes for yourself on useful resources for you and for your clients. A useful starting points is *www.surgical-tutor.org.uk/default-home.htm? core/preop2*

MEDICAL NURSING

Approaches

There tends to be a slight confusion over the term 'medical'. In one sense it describes the overall discipline of medicine, but in another it relates to the diagnosis and treatment of disease, injuries or disabilities by methods other than surgery. This second definition (all medicine other than surgery) is, of course, very broad, including disciplines such as psychiatry. However, where the work of the doctor known as a physician is considered, this usually involves diagnosis and treatment that is primarily concerned with physical disease, injuries or disabilities. It is this area that is usually alluded to when the terms 'medicine' and 'medical' are used to differentiate a treatment modality from surgery.

In recent years medicine has become more specialised. It is now uncommon to find a consultant physician working at a generic level. As for surgery, general medicine has given much ground to the burgeoning advances of specialisms. This is not necessarily a bad thing. As with surgery, as medical science and technology have advanced at ever-increasing rates, it would be difficult for the single physician to maintain high levels of knowledge and skill across broad areas. The area of cancer care is a good example, where the levels of sophistication of chemotherapeutic and radiotherapeutic treatment and pain relief demand highly specialised skills.

As with surgery, the patterns of treatment in medicine have shifted radically in recent years. Here also, there are increasing usages of approaches such as day treatment and outpatient care, and treatment at home. While in medicine, as for surgery, the average lengths of in-patient stays in hospital have reduced, the pattern is less dramatic. When patients are admitted for medical (as opposed to surgical) treatment the range of diagnostic activities tends to be greater, and the treatment interventions (utilising drugs and other therapeutic substances) tend to require longer periods in many instances.

However, it is important that the student gains some insights into the general approaches adopted in medicine (as opposed to surgery). The following sections are not intended to provide a detailed account of medical nursing, but rather to assist you in understanding the role of the nurse in this area of work within adult nursing.

Rehabilitation and adaptation

Nursing in medical units requires the nurse to provide care for patients with a range of diseases and conditions. These diseases include infectious diseases, acute conditions that respond quickly and positively to treatment, as well as degenerative conditions that often result in the patient becoming chronically debilitated. While rehabilitation and facilitating individual adaptation is a philosophical foundation for all aspects of nursing practice, it tends to have special relevance to medical nursing, as it enables patients with chronic and debilitating conditions to attain a level of well-being, while at the same time accepting a constant level of physical limitation. Rehabilitation involves optimising the patient's existing abilities and utilising them creatively along with available aids, thus minimising the amount of nursing or informal care support. From this premise, specialised nursing interventions such as the prevention of pressure sores or bowel and bladder care have an added dimension, as promoting the return of control over these functions provides the patient with a perception that well-being or adaptation has been maximised. Footner (1992) suggests that primary nursing provides an ideal framework for organising rehabilitation effectively. In allotting a named primary nurse to be responsible and accountable for the planning and delivery of care, a more therapeutic relationship is created, patients' needs are interpreted more accurately, the supportive role of rehabilitative nursing in terms of counselling becomes more meaningful, and communication with other members of the multi-disciplinary team is made easier.

Effective rehabilitation also depends on the ability of the nurse to think critically, creatively, and flexibly. Miller (1992) describes critical thinking as the ability to process information by using intuitive, logical, and analytical problem-solving strategies and recognising that rigid adherence to old practices tends to stifle creativity. Benner (1984) identifies the ability to think laterally as marking the difference between the competent and the expert practitioner. According to Benner, the expert nurse is able to confront and handle situation-specific nursing problems by utilising critical thinking skills. Rehabilitation programmes can focus first on ascertaining the individual's perceptions of his disability, using an appropriate assessment framework. Then prescribed nursing interventions and objectives can be agreed within a partnership relationship (Christensen, 1993), and the full involvement of the patient's family can be encouraged. This is particularly important given the family's invaluable knowledge of the patient, and it can enable the nurse to obtain an accurate assessment from which appropriate interventions can be prescribed. Furthermore, early involvement in providing care will assist the family in the longer term to assume the position of principle caregiver for the patient.

Study Activity 37.8

Visit the following website and create your own database of information:
Rehabilitation Nursing Forum: *www.rehabnursing.org.uk/*

Patients with chronic or long-term debilitating diseases

Chronic illness refers to any altered health state that cannot be immediately alleviated by either surgery or a short course of medical treatment. Three features of chronic illness have been identified:

1 The symptoms interfere with normal activities and routines.
2 The effectiveness of medical treatment is limited.

3 Medical treatment, although intended to relieve symptoms and improve the patient's well-being, invariably disrupts the patient's usual lifestyle.

In terms of the residual effect on patients, Lubkin (1986) describes chronic illness as an irreversible accumulation of impairments involving the patient's capacity for self-care, adaptation and prevention of further disability. Physical incapacity also creates additional psychological stress for patients. For example, Strain (1979) outlines a number of commonly occurring features, including lowered self-esteem (given that the patient may feel that the integrity of his body has been compromised), fear of loss of interdependent contact insofar as his affective needs are changed by illness, or guilt if the patient interprets the development of his disease as some kind of divine retribution. Miller (1992) contends that the principle underlying the problem, in terms of nursing patients with chronic illness, is the loss of control. While adaptation to the effects of incapacity will be the long-term principle focus of prescribed nursing interventions, Feldman (1974) points out that in the initial stage it is more pertinent to enable the patient to come to terms with the reality of his disability, and to discard any false hopes that he will, some day, be cured or awake from a dream. This step requires the nurse to use specific interventions, which foster a spirit of positive adjustment. Education enables the patient to be aware of the purpose of his treatment, in terms of the prognosis and expected therapeutic and non-therapeutic side-effects. Teaching the necessary skills for the patient to be in personal control of his disability helps to motivate him towards achieving full compliance with treatment programmes, which will maximise potential progress (Thorne, 1993).

Recent studies confirm that giving comfort and reassurance are essential nursing skills, particularly during this early phase of disability, so that the patient feels secure and at ease. In an age of high technology care, patients can unwittingly be reduced to no more than disease processes. It has been argued that comforting by the nurse is particularly important. It should not be interpreted as a passive or purposeless exercise inherited from a by-gone age of nursing, but as a dynamic process designed to engender within the patient a positive perception of his chronic debility (Teasdale, 1989; Cameron, 1993).

Table 37.1 gives a list of some of the most common chronic diseases.

Table 37.1 Examples of chronic diseases

Endocrine disorders
Diabetes mellitus
Hypo- and hyper-thyroidism
Circulatory disorders
Coronary heart disease
Peripheral vascular disease
Renal and genito-urinary disorders
Renal failure
Incontinence
Impotence
Respiratory disorders
Chronic obstructive airways disease
Locomotor and Neurological disorders
Spinal injury
Rheumatoid arthritis
Multiple sclerosis
Gastro-intestinal disorders
Ulcerative colitis
Stoma

The Chronic Disease Prevention (CDP) databases were developed to provide access to information on chronic disease prevention and health promotion to health professionals responsible for supporting, planning, developing, implementing, and evaluating chronic disease prevention and risk reduction efforts. The databases provide bibliographic citations and abstracts of various types of materials, including journal articles, monographs, book chapters, reports, curricular materials, fact sheets, and proceedings. Full text is provided for selected publications. The databases also contain descriptions of chronic disease prevention and health promotion programmes. You can visit the website at *www.cdc.gov/cdp/he.htm*

Members of the multi-disciplinary team involved in rehabilitation include the following:

- Physiotherapist
- Occupational therapist
- Medical social worker
- Dietician
- Speech therapist
- Disability resettlement officer
- Medical staff.

Study Activity 37.9

- With your colleagues, select any one chronic disease or condition and identify 10 aspects of normal lifestyle that may potentially be affected.
- Briefly describe the measures that could be implemented in order to help a patient with a long-term and possibly debilitating condition to come to terms with changes in lifestyle.

Patients with infectious diseases

An infection is an invasion and proliferation of pathogenic micro-organisms within the body. An infectious disease occurs when an invading micro-organism results in a detectable alteration of normal tissue function. Micro-organisms vary in their virulence (their ability to produce disease).

The course of an infection has three stages:

1 *The incubation period* – the time between the organism's entry to the host (the patient) and the onset of symptoms.
2 *The prodromal period* – the time from the onset of non-specific signs and symptoms (including fatigue, elevated temperature and irritability) to the specific symptoms of the infection.
3 *The illness period* – the point at which local specific signs and symptoms combine with a generalised feeling of being unwell (systemic effects). The patient will often complain of headaches and severe fatigue, and may suffer additional psychological and social problems,

which the nurse must address when prescribing and providing care.

HIV infection and Aids

HIV was first isolated in 1983 and belongs to the group of viruses known as retro-viruses. All viruses are relatively small life forms, composed of a core (nucleic acid) surrounded by protein and fat. The nucleic acid is the virus's essential pre-requisite for life, as well as containing its capacity for reproduction, although this will occur only within another cell. Retro-viruses are so-called because of their unusual ability to change their nucleic core backwards, so that they fully integrate into the nucleic acid of the host human cell. Depending on their type, all viruses are attracted to and ultimately destroy different human cells. In the case of HIV, the virus is believed to be attracted to both the brain and the helper cells (T4 lymphocytes) of the immune system. Because helper cells contribute to defending the body against infection and cancers, HIV's affinity for this group of human cells may predispose patients to the more characteristic problems of Aids.

Transmission

Although HIV has been isolated in a wide range of body fluids, it has been indicated that transmission of the virus is restricted to blood, semen, vaginal secretions, donor organs and breast milk. The possible spread of the virus from one individual to another would therefore be confined to direct contact via three principle modes: unprotected penetrative sexual intercourse (either heterosexual or between homosexual men); the transfusion of infected blood or blood products (including that of HIV drug abusers through the use of infected needles); during childbirth or, post-natally, through breast feeding.

Diagnosis

The diagnosis of Aids or HIV disease is often made when a patient infected with HIV displays a combination of certain constitutional changes related to the fact that the patient's immune system has been compromised. The patient may complain of persistent swelling of the lymph glands, marked weight loss, thrush, night sweats or specific opportunistic infections or tumours. Opportunistic infections include pneumonia, toxoplasmosis, or herpes, while Kaposi's sarcoma is the most frequent form of tumour formation. Kaposi's sarcoma is a malignant and aggressive form of cancer that, when associated with Aids, can be widely disseminated throughout the body, including the skin, lymphatic, pulmonary, and central nervous systems, as well as the gastro-intestinal tract.

Treatment

As yet there is no definitive cure for either HIV infection or HIV disease. Although patients are currently given the compound drug AZT (zidovudine), which supposedly acts by slowing down the virus's ability to replicate, recent reports suggest that it has limited effect. There is no vaccine available that has the ability either to encourage natural immunity through the production of antibodies, or prevent the virus from attaching itself to human cells. Thus the treatment at the moment, and for the foreseeable future, focuses on preventing the spread of the disease, treating the presenting signs and symptoms, and caring for the person with the disease.

Study Activity 37.10

Log on to the British HIV Association website for evidence-based guidelines on the treatment of patients with HIV at *www.aidsmap.com/about/bhiva/guidelines.pdf*

Nursing the patient with Aids or HIV disease

When a patient tests positively for the presence of HIV it means that he will remain infected and be a source of infection for the rest of his life and that there is a possibility that he may develop Aids. Therefore nursing the patient with this disease must include precautions to prevent further transmission of the virus (for example, the use of gloves and adhering to local policy when carrying out venepuncture, cleaning spillages, disposing of waste, using any sharp instruments and reporting needle stick injuries, minimising the potential risk that the patient may develop other HIV-related problems).

Meeting the patient's physical, social and psychological needs

UKCC guidelines, citing evidence from a number of Public Health Laboratory Service Publications, confirmed that the risk of practitioners contracting HIV from patients was very remote if universal precautions are diligently followed. Nevertheless, because of inaccurate and irresponsible media coverage, there has been a tendency for the general public to adopt a victim-blaming attitude to patients with HIV infection. The Nursing and Midwifery Council Guidelines (NMC, 2001) go on to remind practitioners of the importance of confidentiality and non-discriminatory care when caring for patients with HIV or Aids. Nurses are not immune to negative prejudices, but they need to accept that showing them can compromise effective care. In 2001 the NMC stated that:

> *From now on the risk of HIV transmission to patients will be assessed on a case-by-case basis. Patients will no longer be automatically informed and whether patients are notified will depend on the level of risk. The change of policy was announced by the Department of Health in a press release issued on 28 November. The decision was made in the light of the fact that, in spite of extensive research, not a single case of transmission of HIV from an infected health care worker to a patient has ever been detected in the UK. The new DoH policy is based on advice from two agencies: the Expert Advisory Group on AIDS and the UK Advisory Panel on Health Care Workers Infected with Blood Borne Viruses*
>
> (NMC, 2001, *www.ukcc.org.uk/cms/content/home/ search.asp*)

Previously, all patients in the UK had been notified regardless of their level of risk. Mandatory testing for HIV status is an ongoing debate fuelled by a recent incident in Wolverhampton when 10 South African nurses were discovered to be HIV positive. The NMC view is that the key point about HIV is that 'employees with the virus should be honest with their employer about the issue. Having the virus should not, by itself, bar someone from practice'.

Study Activity 37.11

- Briefly describe the policy in your area in relation to minimising the risk of contracting HIV and procedures in the event of a needlestick injury.
- Discuss with your colleagues and a nurse teacher how you would react if you found out that a patient you were nursing was found to be HIV positive.
- Discuss whether nurses should be allowed to continue practising if they are HIV positive.
- Visit the following Internet sites and discuss the implications of HIV/Aids for your practice:
  - The National HIV Nurses Association (UK) *www.nhivna.org.uk/articles.htm*
  - BMJ Collected Resources *www.bmj.com/collections*
  - British HIV Association *www.aidsmap.com/about/ bhiva/bhivagd.asp*

CHILDBIRTH AND MATERNITY SERVICES

The provision of childbirth services provides a focus for the debate as to whether some physical phenomena should be considered healthy or unhealthy. The discussion centres on the points where expert medical advice supersedes the mother's subjective experience or interpretation, where uniform universal provision fails to accommodate diversity and individual choice, and the circumstances when the mother can be permitted to retain total control over her pregnancy. These questions are frequently asked in relation to practices associated with childbirth, including home deliveries, pain relief during labour, the presence of the family at the birth of the baby, and dealing with stillbirth or neonatal death.

The development of midwifery services

Charting the changes in the provision of childbirth services shows the increasing involvement of the medical profession, bringing with it a specifically disease-oriented approach to health. In medieval times, although the church tended to control specific areas such as conception and reproduction, it took little interest in the actual maternal process of bearing and giving birth to children. This was generally perceived to be the domain of women and was left to female kinsfolk or the earlier form of midwife, the handy woman (Shorter, 1983). During the nineteenth century it was still left to the midwife to deal with most deliveries, although the medical profession had begun to become involved in the form of higher status male practitioners – 'accouchers' – who were permitted to use forceps in the delivery of babies, although midwives were prohibited from using these instruments (Donnison, 1977). By the middle of the twentieth century childbirth services had become integrated into the value system of medicine.

The trend towards medical care was a form of self-fulfilling prophecy because the increased involvement of the medical profession in childbirth services created a public perception that childbirth was a pathological condition, rather than a naturally occurring event, and therefore automatically required medical management. The majority of births had taken place in the home, helped by the midwife, but after medically controlled hospitals had become more freely available and accessible, providing high standards of hygiene, surgical procedures and modern anaesthesia, the trend changed to an almost total situation of hospital care. By the 1960s, hospital and medically controlled childbirth had acquired the status of agreed public policy, principally because of its apparent association with safer childbirth and a decreased neonatal mortality rate. For example, the Peel Report recommended that by the 1990s all maternity care should be provided through hospitalisation (Peel Report, 1970, cited in Tew, 1990).

It is argued that doctors have quite different ways from women of looking at both pregnancy and antenatal consultations, and also have differing expectations and interpretations of events during pregnancy. To demonstrate these differences they provide a number of examples.

Women see themselves as experts in what is uniquely happening to their bodies during pregnancy, and this expertise is often not adequately recognised.

Women wish to control what happens to them during pregnancy, but doctors sometimes act as if all decisions are theirs. For mothers, the outcome of a satisfactory pregnancy is assessed not just by the criteria of a live baby and mother, but by a satisfactory personal experience.

Oakley (1993) asserts that hospital-based medical care and the growing use of technological equipment, albeit necessary, further contributes to dehumanising the mother and decreasing the importance of her role during childbirth. In support of this view, Jones (1993) argues that hospital-centred maternity services have served to dismiss intuitive caring, subjective knowledge or experience as old wives' tales, which have been replaced by rational, expert knowledge. Jones also suggests that giving birth at home, if the mother so desires, contributes to feeling safe and more content because she is in a familiar environment, usually her own bed, surrounded by friends and family. In terms of midwifery practice the trend towards medical care seemed to reduce the midwives' relative autonomy which, according to Jones (1993), resulted in their becoming not only regulated by medicine, but directed by it, particularly in the delivery suite. More recently, however, there has been an increasing realisation among health service providers that childbirth services need to be more accommodating of the holistic requirements of women, and that midwifery resources need to be more fully utilised.

Changing childbirth

The Nuffield Institute (Ball *et al.*, 1992) published a discussion document containing a revised framework for midwifery practice in 1992. Among its main proposals was a recommendation that clients of midwifery services (mothers) should be offered the opportunity for almost total care from one primary provider, who may be a midwife, a general practitioner or an obstetrician. Total care would include the provision of appropriate care during pregnancy, labour and delivery, as well as the puerperal period (immediately following delivery). If necessary, the client would be referred to an obstetrician but, even in this event, the primary provider would continue to be available to offer the client support and guidance. In order to help midwives assume the role of primary provider, the Nuffield Report (Bell *et al.*, 1992) recommended that midwifery services needed to be more flexible in their staffing systems. Midwives should be able to provide clients with appropriate care whether at home, in community, ante- or postnatal clinics, delivery suites, operating theatres or maternity hospital wards. The document argued that the benefits of such a move would be a better retention level of midwifery staff, a more effective use of midwifery knowledge and resources, and, most importantly, an increase in satisfaction for the client.

The government expert group on maternity care published a report entitled *Changing Childbirth* (Department of Health, 1994), which led to a dramatic change in the power base for maternal care, with a shift from the professionals to childbearing women. As a result, women have been given the three Cs: Choice, Control and Continuity of carer. The term 'woman-centred care' depicts post-modern women making informed choices about every aspect of their maternity care, taking control over their labour and birth and deciding on their lead professional themselves (i.e., midwife, GP or consultant obstetrician).

The beginning of pregnancy

The female genital tract is divided into a number of internal and external reproductive organs (*see* Figure 37.1a and b). Internal organs are contained in the small pelvis and external organs are collectively referred to as the vulva. The vagina is a passage running upwards and back-

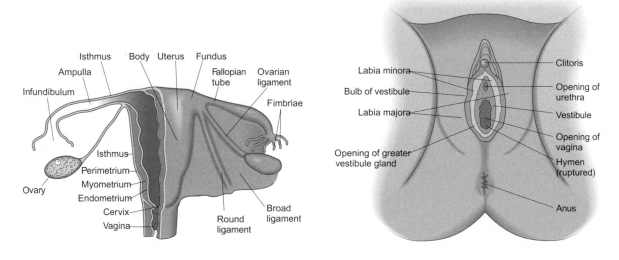

Figure 37.1 The female reproductive organs a) internal organs; b) external organs

wards, leading from the vulva to the uterus. Its walls consist of connective tissue, weak muscle, and a lining of stratified epithelium formed into folds (rugae). The uterus (womb) is a hollow, muscular, pear-shaped organ situated in the true pelvis between the bladder and the rectum. The function of the uterus is to receive a fertilised ovum, to provide nourishment for the foetus during pregnancy, and to expel the foetus by contracting its muscular wall at the end of pregnancy. Through a process of oogenesis, ova are produced and eventually released by the ovaries during ovulation, after which they are transported to the uterus via the Fallopian tube (uterine tube). Conception occurs when the ovum is fertilised by the male spermatozoa, and is the key process in the creation of new life.

Human beings require 46 chromosomes, arranged into 22 pairs of autosomes and one pair of sex chromosomes. Chromosomes carrying essential genetic information come from both parents. The developing ovum initially has 44 chromosomes but, in preparation for combining with a spermatozoon, it reduces this number to 23 chromosomes. During fertilisation two unique half-sets of genetic material from the ovum and the spermatozoon combine into a new and unique full set. The sex of the baby is determined by the father at conception, as the sperm cell contributes one of its two sex chromosomes, X for female or Y for male, to the X chromosomes already present in the ovum.

Signs of pregnancy

The term 'pregnancy' is used when the fertilised ova (blastocyst) establishes itself against the wall of the uterus in a process called nidation. The gestation period for the development of a human foetus is around 266 days. The expected date of delivery is usually calculated from the first day of the last menstrual period. Signs of pregnancy are classified into two groups: during the period of presumptive or probable signs, the mother may suspect that she is pregnant, because of a number of physiological changes. These include the cessation of menstruation, due to the release of human chorionic gonadotrophin (HCG) and

the fact that during nidation the corpus luteum remains intact and ovulation temporarily ceases. Breast changes begin to occur, and superficial veins become more obvious, pigmentation appears around the areola tissue and colostrum is produced, a chloasma or the pregnancy mask appears, and the mother may complain of morning sickness and frequency of micturition. For a confirmation of pregnancy, the presence of chorionic gonadatrophin hormone (CGH) in the urine of a woman is the earliest positive indicator. The Gravindex slide test involves mixing one drop of urine with one drop of prepuerin on a slide, and if agglutination does not occur CGH is said to be present. From this point the positive signs of pregnancy become more obvious: the mother feels foetal movements, the nurse or midwife can detect a foetal pulse and ultrasound scan can demonstrate graphically the existence of a foetus.

Study Activity 37.12 ───────────

- Briefly describe the anatomy of the female reproductive system.
- List the early indicators of pregnancy.

─────────────────────────────

Antenatal care

Antenatal care is the care provided in the interest of both the mother and the baby throughout the nine months of pregnancy. At the beginning of the century antenatal care was virtually non-existent. A mother-to-be made a booking with either a doctor (if she could afford one) or a midwife (if she couldn't) to assist her only at the point of beginning labour. Early antenatal services were introduced to identify the relatively small percentage of women who could be considered at risk, in order to provide the necessary attention. In contrast, today all mothers are encouraged to make an early appointment to attend antenatal clinics. Women can go directly to a midwife for midwife-led care, they can attend their GP and midwife for shared care or their GP, midwife and hospital for hospital-shared care. Women with high-risk pregnancies complicated by underlying pathology such as diabetes, cardiac problems, epilepsy, or complications associated with the pregnancy itself such as twins, hypertension, or threatened miscarriage, must attend a consultant-led unit for care.

The aims of antenatal care are:

● To maintain the full health of the mother
● To effect a safe and emotionally satisfying pregnancy and the delivery of a healthy baby
● To identify any deviation from the normal and provide appropriate care
● To prepare the mother for a normal labour and successful feeding and caring for the baby
● To provide parents with information in order to reduce their knowledge deficits.

In the UK, the National Perinatal Epidemiology Unit maintained that there was no evidence to support the claim that hospital was the safest place in which to give birth. They also recommended that the closure of small obstetric units on the grounds of safety be stopped. Zander and Chamberlain (1999) acknowledged that 75% of care given to pregnant women came from midwives and that the midwifery model of care could become the dominant model for the future. They perceived consultant input to be changing and moving more towards that of other consultants working in the NHS – supervising medical staff and becoming a referral point of contact for all women who require specialist input. These major changes in the delivery of maternity care have been in effect for many years. A major influence on practice was the Department of Health report *Changing Childbirth* (1994), in which there was a shift in emphasis from the medical model of care to the woman-centred model. *Changing Childbirth* stated:

> *The woman must be the focus of maternity care. She should be able to feel she is in*

> *control of what is happening to her and be able to make decisions about her care based on her needs, having discussed matters fully with the professionals involved.*
>
> (Department of Health, 1994)

Providers of antenatal services have been accused of over-medicalising what should be for most people a healthy and normal physiological state. The report of the World Health Organisation – *Care in Normal Birth – A practical guide* (1999) – states that the current medical approach to childbirth has the potential to:

● turn a normal physiological event into a medical procedure
● interfere with the freedom of women to experience the birth of their children in their own way and in the place of their own choice
● lead to unnecessary interventions because of the need for economies of scale.

Although antenatal care is unquestionably invaluable to both the mother and the foetus, the nature of its organisation and provision has been criticised.

The World Health Organisation (1999) report states that childbirth is a physiological process and the use of routine interventions should be questioned, as they can cause more harm than good.

Study Activity 37.13

● Visit the website for the World Health Organisation at *www.who.int/health_topics/pregnancy/* and search for information on normal birth and technological birth. Discuss your findings with your midwifery mentor and visiting lecturer/link teacher.

The midwifery model and the medical model

Midwifery is concerned with normal childbirth and obstetrics is concerned with pathological or abnormal birth. For the majority of women, giving birth is something natural. A woman's body is designed to cope with physiological birth, including the release of endorphins for pain relief in labour. Ideally, the two approaches to care ought to complement each other, the midwife providing care to normal women and doctors providing care to those who need their expert training in that which is abnormal.

The midwifery model of care is now being accepted by doctors as being the best choice for 'low-risk' women (Zander and Chamberlain, 1999) and in many primary care settings midwives have the main responsibility in caring for normal women in birth. The establishment of birthing centres in the 1980s in the USA and in the 1990s in the UK has led to increasing satisfaction for some women, role expansion for some midwives and in many cases changes in the delivery of medical care for some doctors (Walker, 2001).

Midwives and midwife-led care

Midwives who practise in birthing centres or midwife-led units are less reluctant to interfere with nature and tend to use less technology and more personal skills (Walker, 2001). An independent evaluation of Edgware Birthing Centre provides solid evidence of the benefits of the service to women and to the NHS, including a significantly lower episiotomy rate of 1.6% (7 in 400 births) and a higher breastfeeding rate of 85% of women who gave birth in the centre. With the nearest acute centre 5 miles away, the intrapartum transfer rate was 12% (589 births) and 19% were transferred antenatally for obstetric/medical problems. Of these, 19% were transferred for induction of labour.

The website Birth Choice *www.birthchoice uk.com* provides information on 418 units providing maternity care in the UK. Of these, 60 units provide stand-alone midwifery care (these units are managed by midwives). The website provides essential information for any woman wanting to choose a place of birth and the database contains contact details for each unit, as well as birth statistics.

The first antenatal visit

The first antenatal visit is, in many ways, the cornerstone for effective antenatal care, given that it is probably the earliest tangible indicator that the woman is going to have a baby. During this visit, it is important for the woman to be made to feel special by the midwife, and allowed to express her feelings about being pregnant in a non-judgemental environment. It is also an opportunity for the midwife to obtain a full obstetric and medical history, including personal data, her full name, age, marital status and next of kin, her menstrual history, the date when menstruation stopped, details of her personal menstrual cycle and the method of contraception that she has used, her obstetric history, the number and dates of previous pregnancies and any difficulties with them. Details should also be obtained of weight, gender and method of feeding her babies, her medical history, the details of all childhood diseases that the mother had, as well as all medical and surgical problems. A physiological assessment to assist in either the early detection of any abnormal physiological change or to anticipate possible future difficulties should be carried out. This includes recording the woman's weight, height, shoe size, temperature, pulse, and blood pressure, observing her general physical condition such as her oral cavity (including her teeth), hair, skin, and any physical deformities (spinal curvature, limb shortening or limps), and carrying out an abdominal examination. A blood sample should be taken for grouping, rhesus antibodies and haemoglobin count, as well as a hepatitis, VDRL and HIV screening (after having obtained the woman's consent). Urine will be tested for the presence of protein, sugar, or acetone, and if any of these are present the woman will be asked to provide an MSSU for further investigation. In most maternity units all of this data is stored electronically and a working copy is kept in the woman's notes. Women are encouraged to carry their own case notes wherever possible.

Study Activity 37.14 ————————

- Discuss with your colleagues the reasons why the first antenatal visit is so important for both partners and the midwife.
- During your maternity care placement, arrange with your clinical mentor to observe a first antenatal visit.
- Recently, antenatal care has been extended to include the preconception period. Couples who are planning to become parents are referred to midwifery teams and offered a range of specific information, such as health education (smoking, use of alcohol and diet) and genetic advice, as well as physical examinations to detect potential difficulties. Discuss with your colleagues and your link teacher the value of this strategy.

Labour

At the end of pregnancy the foetus, placenta, and membranes are expelled from the uterus by the onset of labour or childbirth. Labour is divided into three stages.

First stage of labour

During this stage regular contractions of the uterus occur (the uterus begins to slowly reduce in surface size); these contractions become stronger and more painful, the cervix becomes dilated and there may be a vaginal loss, or show. This is a mucoid plug that has previously sealed the cervix throughout the pregnancy.

It is essential to check a woman's birthing plan when she comes into labour as the woman may have made special requests such as her partner cutting the cord, not wanting the cord to be clamped immediately after birth or wanting to take the placenta home. These requests should be taken very seriously and every attempt is made to accommodate the woman's wishes.

An abdominal examination is undertaken to ascertain the lie, presentation and position of the foetus and a vaginal examination assesses the cervical dilatation and position of the presenting part.

The method and frequency of the auscultation of the fetal heart depend on the state of the woman and whether or not she is having a technological birth. A technological birth is one in which the woman is induced, has an IV infusion of syntocinon, continuous electronic fetal monitoring and in most cases requires epidural analgesia. In normal physiological birth a woman can labour using water, massage, relaxation, aromatherapy, inhalation and intramuscular pain relief. The fetal heart is monitored half-hourly using a pinards stethescope or a sonicaid machine.

Contractions will be observed for length, strength and frequency. Baseline observations are important and should be undertaken regularly. They record the temperature, pulse, respirations and blood pressure of the mother.

Women are encouraged to make use of toilet facilities and urinary output will be measured and tested for the presence of proteins or ketones. Women are also encouraged to use water to provide pain relief and relaxation. In some units women give birth in specially designed birthing pools.

Second stage of labour

When the cervix is fully dilated, the foetus is passed into the extended vagina by the expulsive contractions of the uterus. As the foetus descends, its head pushes against the perineum and finally pushes through the vulva, followed by the shoulders and the rest of the body. During this stage the external genitalia of the mother should be cleansed with an aseptic solution. The midwife should put on a sterilised gown or apron. When the baby is born, its eyes, face and head are dried quickly, as babies lose heat rapidly. This is one reason why the birthing room is kept warm at the time of birth. Usually, the cord is clamped quickly after birth. This is carried out using two pairs of artery forceps to clamp the cord and then it is cut with sterile scissors. The Apgar score is taken at 1 minute and at 5 minutes. This assessment includes body tone, colour, respiratory rate, heart rate and reflexes. Provided the baby is well, it is given to its mother as quickly as possible. Skin-to-skin contact is encouraged and if the mother wishes to breastfeed she is supported by the midwife and the baby is helped to the breast.

Third stage of labour

During this stage the placenta and membranes are expelled from the uterus. In the majority of cases active management of this stage is the norm, with the woman consenting to receive an injection of syntometrine with the birth of the shoulders. When the baby is born, the uterus quickly reduces in size, with a simultaneous reduction in the amount of available attachment area for the placenta, causing it to separate from the uterine wall. Indications that the placenta has separated include a small amount of bleeding, an observable lengthening of the cord and the fact that the uterus rises as a hard round ball. The placenta is then removed by the midwife, who examines it carefully before depositing it in a yellow hazard bag for incineration.

Postnatal care

A woman may stay in hospital for anything from 6 to 24 hours or more after birth, depending on her well-being and that of her baby. Women who have a forceps, vacuum or caesarean birth will usually stay for 3–6 days.

Generally speaking, the postnatal period lasts for 6–8 weeks. During this time the reproductive organs return to their pre-pregnancy state, and the other physiological changes caused by pregnancy disappear. In the immediate postnatal period, the midwife ensures that any suture sites are cared for, and do not become either inflamed or infected, and that the mother is allowed to rest. The midwife also encourages the mother to bond with her new baby, and helps her overcome any difficulties with breastfeeding or bottle feeding.

Study Activity 37.15 _____

Discuss with colleagues your preferred birth choices related to place of birth, birth attendant, pain relief,

position in labour, infant feeding, and search for evidence on each of these. Make notes and discuss your findings with colleagues, lecturers and midwives.

The safety of childbirth

The significant reduction in the mortality rate of mothers and babies during pregnancy and childbirth is indisputably linked with the contribution made by health legislation and administrative changes, such as higher professional standards, improved education and training for doctors and midwives, and better arrangements for the care of pregnant women in terms of hospital provision and specialist services (DHSS, 1976). On the other hand, Chalmers et al. (1980) note that in situations where babies still continue to die or suffer postnatal problems, the blame falls on women. Mothers may be accused of wilfully putting their babies at risk by smoking, bottle feeding, or choosing the wrong diet during pregnancy, not attending antenatal clinics, or by insisting against professional advice on a home confinement.

Lewis (1980) and Chalmers et al. (1980) question whether maternity policies are the principal contributors to the decline in infant and maternal mortality. In the first instance, Lewis affirms that prior to the provision of services middle-class women faced equal problems in childbirth. Therefore, alternative causative factors, such as poor nutrition and poverty, were conveniently avoided by both professional and political bodies. Second, Chalmers et al. suggest that the reasons why many women choose to ignore health education advice may not be different from those in the population as a whole. As Townsend and Davidson (1982) argue, an unhealthy lifestyle is often predetermined by low self-esteem caused by social and economic conditions, over which individuals have little control.

Study Activity 37.16 _____

Discuss with your colleagues and lecturer the statement in the Black Report (Townsend and

Davidson, 1982) that the amount of attention given to health education information is determined by the client's social and economic circumstances.

Obstetric care and the diversity of modern society

In sociological terms, the traditional image of childbirth occurring within a conventional family surrounded by an extended family framework no longer exists in many areas. The nature of what constitutes a family unit has been redefined. While there is no single causative factor, the proportionate increase in the incidence of contributory factors has played a significant part. These include the accessibility and rate of divorce, the number of single parents, the number of families reconstructed because of the remarriage of either partner or both, and situations where the guardians of children may be in a homosexual relationship. Alongside this, midwives should be aware that the resident population of most cities includes women from a range of ethnic, racial, and cultural backgrounds. Their particular religious beliefs and customs must be understood and respected. Although contraception has been relatively freely available for almost 20 years and abortion is legally accessible for women, it cannot be assumed that all pregnancies, even when completed, are planned or wanted.

Study Activity 37.17

- Briefly describe society's changing interpretations of what constitutes a family.
- Reflect on your own beliefs as to what a family should be, and discuss with your colleagues how negative attitudes can affect the nurse's ability to provide objective care.

Future maternity services

The professional response to the future of midwifery services in the UK is clearly articulated in the Royal College of Midwives document *Vision 2000* (Royal College of Midwives, 2000) where there is a description of a future service that is 'high quality, cost-effective, evidence-based and a service that is responsive to individual needs and preferences whilst promoting and sustaining public health'.

Study Activity 37.18

- In 2002, the RCM launched its Virtual Birth Institute, designed to promote normal birth. Log on to the RCM website and familiarise yourself with this new initiative designed to promote normal and natural birth for women in the twenty-first century.
- Visit the following websites and build your knowledge base prior to going on your maternity placement:

    – For access to position papers on homebirth, normal birth, waterbirth, etc. and general information on midwifery, visit the Royal College of Midwives website at *www.rcm.org.uk/*
    – For problems with breastfeeding, see the National Childbirth Trust website at *www.wisdom-net.co.uk/breast.html*
    – For information on all aspects of childbirth, see the *Dr Foster Good Birth Guide 2002* at *www.home.drfoster.co.uk/birth/drfosterbookshop.htm*
    – Visit the part of the The National Electronic Library for Health (NELH) for access to data on all aspects of midwifery at *www.midirs.org/nelh/nelh.nsf/welcome?openform*
    – For information on consumer participation in health visit the Australian website at *www.participateinhealth.org.au/index.asp*
    – For a deeper understanding of the current debate on normal versus technological childbirth read the on-line article by Goer (2002) The assault on normal birth. *Midwifery Today* **63**: *www.midwiferytoday.com/articles/disinformation.asp*
    – Visit the English Department of Health website for national data on infant feeding practices at *www.doh.gov.uk/public/infantfeedingreport.htm*
    – If you wish to read about current breastfeeding initiative 'Babyfriendly status' visit the UNICEF website at *www.babyfriendly.org.uk/*

— For important information on the management of teenage pregnancies visit the website for the Teenage Pregnancy Unit at *www.teenagepregnancyunit.gov.uk/*

SUMMARY

This chapter has presented the principles of adult nursing, including the role of the nurse in surgical and medical environments of care. Surgical nursing, such as pre- and post-operative care, and problems specific to medical nursing have been discussed, with illustrative examples. Childbirth and maternity care focuses on aspects of pregnancy (prenatal care, labour and postnatal care), with attention given to current changes in the provision of maternity care.

With the growing body of knowledge currently available on-line, references to websites are provided wherever possible. The reason for this is twofold: you need to gain confidence in using the Internet and developing key skills in searching databases for best evidence in relation to all aspects of your nursing practice; also, research evidence is arriving on our desks and machines every day, resulting in frequent changes to practice. Therefore, this chapter provides the basic principles and where possible, references to specifics.

It is not our intention that in completing this chapter and its study activities you will have attained an in-depth knowledge of adult nursing, but rather that you will have a broad overview of this branch of nursing and the role of the nurse within it. Within the current education for nurses in the UK, a one-year Foundation Programme is followed by a two-year Branch Programme in a particular division of nursing (in the case of this chapter, adult nursing). Such is the nature of modern health services that the following circumstances apply:

- The speed of change and the rapid advance in health technology make it impossible for a textbook in nursing, medicine, or for other health professions to be fully up-to-date.

Indeed, it is more likely to be the case that significant changes would occur even in the period during which the text is being written!

- Increasing specialisation requires that nurses continue to learn and update themselves on an ongoing basis, and indeed that they receive additional formal training to function in key posts within such specialties.

It is hoped that in this changing and increasingly specialised arena, this chapter will provide you with an overview of adult nursing and the skills to continue updating, even beyond the point of registration.

REFERENCES

Allin, K. (1991) Postoperative handover. *Surgical Nurse* **4**(3), 23–7

Ball, J., Flint, C., Garvey, M. *et al.* (1992) *Who's Left Holding the Baby? An organisational framework for making the most of midwifery services*, University of Leeds, The Nuffield Institute, Leeds

Benner, P. (1984) *From Novice to Expert*, Sage, Menlo Park, CA

Black, P. (1994) Management of patients undergoing stoma surgery. *British Journal of Nursing* **3**(5), 211–16

Boore, J. (1978) *Prescription for Recovery*, Royal College of Nursing, London

Brewster, J. (1992) Operations explained. *Nursing Times* **88**(39), 50–2

Cameron, B.L. (1993). The nature of comfort to hospitalised medical surgical patients. *Journal of Advanced Nursing* **18**, 424–30

Castledine, G. (1988) Preoperative information. *Surgical Nurse*, October, 11–13

Caunt, H. (1992) Preoperative nursing interventions to relieve stress. *British Journal of Nursing* **1**(4), 171–4

Chalmers, I., Oakley, A. and Macfarlane, A. (1980) Perinatal health services: an immodest proposal. *British Medical Journal*, **280**, 842–5

Christensen, J. (1993) *Nursing Partnership: A model for practice*, Churchill Livingstone, London

Coldicott, Y., Pope, C. and Roberts, (2003) The ethics of intimate examinations: teaching tomorrow's doctors. *British Medical Journal* **326**, 97–100

Cruse, P.J. and Foord, R.N. (1980) The epidemiology of wound infection. *Surgical Clinics of North America* **60**(1), 27–40

Dealey, C. (1991) Assessing wounded patients. *Nursing* **4**(25), 27–8

Department of Health (1994) *Changing Childbirth*, HMSO, London

DHSS (1976) *Priorities for Health and Personal Social Services: A Consultative Document*, HMSO, London

Donnison, J. (1977) *Midwives and Medical Men*, Heinemann, London

Evans, E. (1991) Nurses in the operating theatre. *Surgical Nurse* **4**(2), 10–14

Feldman, H.R. (1974) Chronic disabling illness: a holistic view. *Journal of Chronic Disease* **27**, 287–91

Footner, A. (1992) *Orthopaedic Nursing*, Baillière Tindall, London

Goer, (2002) The assault on normal birth. *Midwifery Today* **63**, **10–14**

Gorse, G., Messner, R. and Stephens, N. (1989) Association of malnutrition with nosocomial infection, *Infection Control and Hospital Epidemiology* **10**(5), 194–203

Hayward, J. (1975) *Information: A prescription against pain*, Royal College of Nursing, London

Henderson, V. (1979) Preserving the essence of nursing in a technological age. *Nursing Times* **75**(20), 12

Hung, P. (1992a) Pre-operative fasting. *Nursing Times* **88**(48), 57–60

Hung, P. (1992b) Preoperative fasting of patients undergoing elective surgery. *British Journal of Nursing*, **1**(6), 86–287

Janis, I.L. (1958) *Psychological Stress*, Wiley, New York

Jones, L. (1993) *Health as a Contested Concept*, The Open University Press, Milton Keynes

Kalideen, D. (1990) Preparing skin for surgery. *Nursing* **4**(15), 28–9

Kovach, D. (1990) Nip it in the bud. *Today's OR Nurse* **12**(9), 23–6. Cited in: Freshwater, D. (1992) Preoperative preparation of skin: a review of the literature. *Surgical Nurse* **5**(5), 6–10

Lewis, J. (1980) *The Politics of Motherhood*, Croom Helm, London

Lewis, M. (1994) Communication in theatres. *Surgical Nurse* **7**(1), 27–9

Lubkin (1986) *Chronic Illness: Impact and interventions*, Jones and Bartlett, Boston, Mass

McKenzie, I. (1988) Pre-operative skin preparation and surgical outcome. *Journal of Hospital Infection* **11**, 27–32

Millar, B. (1991) Nutritional assessment. *Surgical Nurse* **4**(5), 21–5

Miller, J. F. (1992) *Coping with Chronic Illness* (2nd edition), F.A. Davis, Philadelphia, IL

Nightingale, K. (1990) Wound closure. *Nursing Times* **86**(14), 35–7

NMC (1994) *Acquired Immune Deficiency Syndrome and Human Immuno-deficiency Virus Infection (AIDS and HIV Infection): The Council's position statement*, Annexe 1 to Registrar's Letter 4/1994, NMC, London

O'Reilly, P.H. (1991) Postoperative urinary retention in men. *British Medical Journal*, **302**, 864

Oakley, A. (1993) The limits of the professional imagination. In: Beattie, A., Gott, M., Jones, L. *et al.* (1993) *Health and Wellbeing*, The Open University Press, Milton Keynes

Poulton, L. (1991) Preoperative bowel preparation. *Surgical Nurse* **4**(2), 12–14

Powell-Tuck, J. (1983) Parenteral Nutrition, Paper presented at the annual symposium of the Infection Control Nurses Association. Cited in Kingley, A. (1992) Assessment allows action on risk factors. *Surgical Nurse* **7**(10), 644–8

Royal College of Midwives (2000) *Vision 2000*, RCM, London

Rigg, J.R.A., Jamrozik, K., Myles, P.S. *et al.* (2002) Epidural anaesthesia and analgesia and outcome of major surgery: a randomised trial. *Lancet* **359**, 1276–82

Shorter, E. (1983) *The History of Women's Bodies*, Allen Lane, London

Strain, J. (1979) Psychological reactions to chronic medical illness. *Psychiatric Quarterly* **51**, 173–83

Sutton, J. (1989) Accurate wound assessment. *Nursing Times* **85**(38), 68–71

Teasdale, K. (1989) The concept of reassurance in nursing. *Journal of Advanced Nursing* **14**, 444–50

Tew, M. (1990) *Safer Childbirth? A critical history of maternity care*, Chapman and Hall, London

Thompson, R. (1990) Preoperative visiting. *British Journal of Theatre Nursing* **27**(4), 8–9

Thorne, S.E. (1993) *Negotiating Health Care: The social context of chronic illness*, Sage, London

Townsend, P. and Davidson, N. (1982) *Inequalities and Health: The Black Report*, Penguin, London

Tudor, M. (1992) The endangered species. *Nursing* **5**(7), 24–7

Tunevall, G. (1988) Procedures and experiences with preoperative skin preparation in Sweden. *Journal of Hospital Infection* 11, 11–14

UKCC (2001) *Project 2000*, UKCC, London

Walker, J. (2001) Edgware Birth Centre: what is the significance of this model? *Midirs Midwifery Digest* 11(1), 8–12

World Health Organisation (1999) *Care in Normal Birth – A practical guide*, WHO, Geneva

Wilson-Barnett, J. and Fordham, M. (1983) *Recovery from Illness*, Wiley, Chichester

Zander, L. and Chamberlain G (1999) ABC of labour care. *British Medical Journal* 318, 721–3

Zwarenstein, M., Reeves, S., Bar, H. *et al.* (2002) *Interprofessional Education: Effects on professional practice and health care outcomes* (Cochrane Review), The Cochrane Library, Issue 1, Update Software, Oxford

FURTHER READING

American Society of Anesthesiologists Task Force on Preoperative Fasting: Practice (1999) Guidelines for preoperative fasting and the use of pharmacologic agents to reduce the risk of pulmonary aspiration: application to healthy patients undergoing elective procedures. *Anesthesiology* 90, 896–905

Audit Commission (1986) *Making a Reality of Community Care*, HMSO, London

Audit Commission (1991) *Community Care: Managing the cascade of change*, HMSO, London

Audit Commission (1992a) *Homeward Bound: A new course to community health*, HMSO, London

Audit Commission (1992b) *The Community Revolution: Personal social services and community care*, HMSO, London

Audit Commission (1992c) *Lying in Wait: The use of medical beds in hospital*, HMSO, London

Benson, S. (1994) Sniff and doze therapy. *Journal of Dementia Care* 2(1), 12–14

Bollish, S.J., Collins, C.L., Kirking, D.M. *et al.* (1988) Efficacy of patient-controlled verses conventional analgesia for postoperative pain. *Clinical Pharmacology* 4, 48–52

Bowers, L. (1992) Ethnomethodology 2: A study of the CPN in the patient's home. *International Journal of Nursing Studies* 29(1), 69–79

Brook, P., Degun, G. and Mather, M. (1975) Reality orientation: a therapy for psycho-geriatric patients: a controlled study. *British Journal of Psychology*, 127, 42–5

Castledine, G. (1982) Sorry, I haven't got time. *Nursing Mirror* 155(13), 17–20

Challis, D. and Davies, B. (1986) *Matching Resources to Needs in Community Care*, Gower, London

Cheah, Y.L. and Moon, G.M. (1993) Specialism in nursing: the case of nursing care for elderly people. *Journal of Advanced Nursing* 18, 1610–16

Clarke, E., Hodsman, N. and Kenny, G. (1989) Improved postoperative recovery with patient-controlled analgesia. *Nursing Times* 85(9), 54–5

Closs, S.J. (1990) An exploratory analysis of nurses' provision of postoperative analgesic drugs. *Journal of Advanced Nursing* 15, 42–9

Cohen, F.L. (1980) Post-surgical pain relief: patients' status and nurses' medication choices. *Pain* 9, 265–74

Cumberlege, J. (1986) *Neighbourhood Nursing: A focus for care*, Report of the Community Nursing Review, HMSO, London

Dallison, A. (1991) Self-administration of oral pain relief. *Nursing* 4(35), 30–1

Davies, B. (1986) American lessons for British policy and research on the long-term care of the elderly. *The Quarterly Journal of Social Affairs*, 2(3), 321–55

Department of Health (1989) *Working for Patients*, Cmnd 555, HMSO

Department of Health (1989) *Caring for People: Community care in the next decade and beyond*, Cmnd 849, HMSO, London

Department of Health (1991) *Nursing in the Community*, HMSO, London

Department of Health (1991) *The Patient's Charter*, HMSO, London

DHSS (1976) *Provision and Health: Everybody's business*, HMSO, London

DHSS (1977) *The Way Forward – Priorities in the Health and Social Services*, HMSO, London

DHSS (1990) *The National Health Service and Community Care Act*, HMSO, London

DHSS (1992) *Maternity Services*, Health Committee (2nd report), HMSO, London

Dietch, J.T., Hewett, L.J. and Jones, S. (1988) Adverse effects of reality orientation. *Journal of the American Geriatrics Society* 37, 974–6

Donovan, M., Dillon, P. and Maguire, L. (1987) Incidence and characteristics of pain in a sample of medical-surgical in-patients. *Pain* 30(1), 69–78

Edwards, N. (1987) *Nursing in the Community: A team approach for Wales. Report of Community Nursing in Wales*, Welsh Office, Cardiff

Garrett, G. (1991) *Health Needs of the Elderly* (2nd edition), MacMillan, London

Goate, A., Chartier-Harlin, M.C. and Mullan, M. (1991) Segregation of a missense mutation in the amyloid precursor protein gene with familial Alzheimer's disease. *Nature* 349, 704–6

Griffith, Sir R. (1988) *Community Care: Agenda for action*, HMSO, London

Hancock, A. (1994) How effective is antenatal education? *Modern Midwife* 4(5), 3–15

Harding ,W.G. (1981) *Report of a Joint Working Group on the Primary Health Care Team*, HMSO, London

Harvard Davis (1971) *The Organisation of Group Practice: A report of a sub-committee of the Standing Medical Advisory Committee*, DHSS and Welsh Office, HMSO, London

Henderson, A.S. (1988) The risk factors for Alzheimer's disease: a review and a hypothesis. *Acta Psychiatrica Scandinavia* 78, 257–75

Hughes, E. (1990) *Enhancing the Quality of Community Nursing*, Kings Fund, London

Kargar, I. (1993) A cause for concern. *Nursing Times* 88(44), 46–8

Kitson, A. (1990) The dialectics of dementia, with particular reference to Alzheimer's disease. *Ageing and Society* 10, 177–96

Kitson, A., Harvey, G., Hyndman, S. *et al.* (1993) A comparison of expert and practitioner derived criteria for postoperative pain management. *Journal of Advanced Nursing* 18(2), 218–32

Kitwood, T. (1993) Discover the person, not the disease. *Journal of Dementia Care* 1(1), 16–17

Kleiman, R.L., Lipman, A.G., Hare, B.D. *et al.* (1987) PCA versus intramuscular injections for severe post-operative pain. *American Journal of Nursing* 87(11), 1491–2

Krebs, D. (1983) Nursing in Primary Health Care. *International Nursing Review* 30(5), 141–5

Lange, M.P., Dahn, M.S. and Jacobs, L.A. (1988) Patient-controlled analgesia versus intermittent analgesia dosing. *Heart Lung* 17, 495–8

Leininger, M. (1984) *Care: The essence of nursing and health*, Slack, NJ

Loyd, C. (1987) Postoperative nausea and vomiting. *Senior Nurse* 7(4), 25–6

Mackie, I. (1992) A milieu approach to dementia day care. *Nursing Standard* 6(5), 32–5

Maxwell, R. (1989) Strong Medicine for the NHS. *The Observer*, London, 5 February

Morton, I. and Bleathman, C. (1988) RO: does it really matter whether it's Tuesday or Friday? *Nursing Times* 84(6), 25–7

NMC (2001): www.ukcc.org.wk/cms/contemt/home/search.asp

Norman, A. (1980) *Rights and Risks*, Centre for Policy on Ageing, London

Oakley, A. (1980) *Women Confined*, Martin Robertson, Oxford

OPCS (1991) *Base National Populations Projections*, Series 2, 17, HMSO, London

Orem, D. (1985) *Nursing: Concepts of practice*, McGraw Hill, New York

Pearson, A. (1988) *Primary Nursing: Nursing in the Burford and Oxford Development Units*, Chapman and Hall, London

Royal College of Nursing (1990) *Standards of Care for District Nursing*, District Nursing Forum, Royal College of Nursing, London

Royal College of Nursing (1992a) *A Powerhouse for Change*, Draft Document, RCN, London

Royal College of Nursing (1992b) *Focus on Restraint* (2nd edition), Scutari, London

Royal College of Surgeons and Anaesthetists (1991) *Report of the Working Party on Pain After Surgery*, Commission on the Provision of Social Services, Royal College of Surgeons, London

Rubin, V. (1994) How validation is misunderstood. *Journal of Dementia Care* 2(2), 14–16

Seers, K. (1988) Factors affecting pain assessment. *Professional Nurse* 3(6), 201–6

Shaw, H. (1983) What aspects of the nursing process are applicable in theatre nursing, and how can they be implemented? *NAT News*, May, 11–13

Skeet, M. (1985) *Some International Concepts of Old Age*, Baillière Tindall, London

Smith, J. (1994) Reading around risk and restraint. *The Journal of Dementia Care* 2(1), 18–19

Teske, K., Daut, R.L. and Cleland, C.S. (1983) Relationships between nurses' observations and patients' self-reports of pain. *Pain* 16, 289–96

Thomas, V.J. (1991) Personality characteristics of patients and the effectiveness of patient-controlled anaesthesia. Unpublished Ph.D. thesis, Goldsmith's College, University of London. Cited in Thomas, V.J. and Rose, F.D. (1993). Patient-controlled analgesia: a new method for old. *Journal of Advanced Nursing* 18(11), 1719–26

Thomas, V.J. and Rose, F.D. (1993) Patient-controlled analgesia: a new method for old. *Journal of Advanced Nursing* 18(11), 1719–26

Titmuss, R.M. (1968) *A Commitment to Welfare*, Allen and Unwin, London

Tobianski, R. (1993) Understanding dementia. *Journal of Dementia Care* 1(1), 26–8

Trounce, J. (1992) *Clinical Pharmacology for Nurses* (13th edition), Churchill Livingstone, Edinburgh

Ungerson, C. (1981) *Women, Work and the 'Caring Capacity of the Community': A report of a research review*, Report to the SSRC, Mimeo, University of Kent, Canterbury

Wagner, G. (1988) *A Positive Choice*, NISW, HMSO, London

Walker, J. and Campbell, S. (1988) Pain assessment and the nursing process. *Senior Nurse* 8(5), 28–31

Weiss, O.F., Sriwatanakul, K. and Alloza, J.L. (1983) Attitudes of patients, housestaff and nurses towards post-operative analgesic care. *Anaesthesia and Analgesia* 62, 70–4

Wells, T. (1980) *Problems in Geriatric Nursing Care*, Churchill Livingstone, Edinburgh

World Health Organisation (1946) *World Health Organisation Constitution*, WHO, Geneva

World Health Organisation (1978) *Alma-Ata, Primary Health Care*, Health For All Series, No.1. WHO, Geneva

Wilson, M. (1973) Caring for an aged population. The problem of society. *Nursing Times* 69(14), 486–91

Woods, B. (1994) Reading around reality orientation. *Journal of Dementia Care* 2(2), 24–5

Zerwekh, J. (1991) A family caregiving model for public health nursing. *Nursing Outlook* 39(5), 213–17

CHILDREN'S NURSING

Denise Burgin

LEARNING OUTCOMES

After studying this chapter you will be able to:

- Identify the historical milestones that led to the hospitalisation of children, and children's nursing
- Discuss the role of the children's nurse
- Describe the disadvantages of hospitalisation for children and the special needs of the adolescent or young person in hospital
- Discuss the development of community children's nursing
- Identify the optimum organisational culture for the development of reflective practice.

INTRODUCTION

This chapter provides an overview of children's nursing from the opening of the first children's hospitals to the present day. It provides an insight into how children's nursing has developed, and highlights the fact that children are different from adults and have special health care needs. Information is included about the reduction in child mortality rates and the increasing morbidity related to the improved survival rates of children suffering from chronic illness. The shift to primary care is noted, with details of the development of community children's nursing services. The complexities of the role of the community children's nurse is discussed, with a consideration of the difficulties associated with the nurse's presence in the family home. The difficulties associated with the interpretation and implementation of the concept of family-centred care, over 25 years after its inception, requires special consideration and debate. Specific groups

of children have been discussed separately, either because they present differing problems or because their needs are often overlooked: these are hospitalised adolescents, children with mental health needs, children in ethnic minorities and those requiring protection. Finally, the development of children's rights and their increasing visibility within society and within contemporary child health care is discussed.

THE HOSPITALISATION OF CHILDREN

The concept of childhood is socially constructed and as we know it, essentially a creation of the twentieth century. In the middle ages, children were totally immersed in the adult world from about the age of 7 years and were not given any special status (Aries, 1962). Fortunately, moral reformists in the late seventeenth century recognised that children were not ready to participate in adult life at this age, and recommended education and special treatment. This ultimately resulted in an extension of childhood for the upper and middle classes. For the lower classes, however, this extension was short. With the increased demand for workers brought about by the Industrial Revolution, children were seen as cheap labour, working appallingly long hours in poor conditions. New legislation in 1833 prevented the employment of those under 9 years (Armitage, 1998), until the 1920s; nonetheless, many still faced the harsh realities of full-time labour at the age of 12 or 13 years (Aries, 1962; Humphries *et al.*, 1988).

Study Activity 38.1 _____

- Try to define the words 'child' and 'childhood'.
- Visualise a child or young person that you know aged 12 years. Reflect upon their daily lives, the

pattern of their day, and the things they consider to be important.

- Imagine that same child or young person working full time in a local factory.

It appears that the hospitalisation of children only began in England with the opening of children's hospitals in the mid-1800s. The first was the Hospital for Sick Children, Great Ormond Street (GOS), which opened in 1852 and was followed by others in Liverpool, Norwich and Manchester in 1853. In Scotland, children's hospitals were opened in Edinburgh, Glasgow and Aberdeen in the 1860s, followed by a further six new hospitals in London around the same time. Similar hospitals were founded in Wales and Northern Ireland. Prior to this time only outpatient treatment was available (Miles, 1986a). In London this service was provided from three dispensaries founded by Dr George Armstrong (1719–1789). Armstrong was very opposed to the hospitalisation of children, stating that 'to take a child away from its parents or nurse would break its heart immediately'. However, Dr Charles West, founder of Great Ormond Street Hospital, felt that the current outpatient provision was insufficient and that the benefits of inpatient treatment, the psychological trauma of separation, and the physical dangers associated with hospitalisation were a real situation and a learning experience for children.

The opening of children's hospitals established a need for the special training of sick children's nurses. The call for such training was recorded in the nursing record by the Lady Superintendent of GOS in 1888. To love little children and to want to take care of them were considered to be the right motives for entry into children's nursing at this time. Increased demand for beds in the children's hospital in the early twentieth century necessitated extensions to the buildings. Fortunately recruitment did not appear to be a problem at this stage, as nursing was becoming a respectable occupation, children's nursing eminently so. At the opening of the National Register for Nurses in 1919, it was recognised that special provision was needed to meet the requirements of sick children, and a special part of the Register was created especially for sick children's nurses (Miles, 1986b). The question of the future of specialised children's nurses has arisen at various times over recent years, particularly regarding the discussions relating to professional mobility within the European Community. Fortunately, the specialist requirements of children are recognised within Diploma programmes, and reassurance has been offered that there are no plans to end child branch pre-registration education (Mullally, 2001).

THE EFFECTS OF HOSPITALISATION

Almost a century after Dr Armstrong expressed his concern about the emotional effects of hospitalisation on children, the Curtis Committee (Ministry of Health, 1946) claimed that two of the most destructive elements for deprived children were separation and an unfamiliar environment. However, it was some time before it was realised that the Curtis Committee report also applied to children in hospital. This situation not only caused separation from family, and an unfamiliar environment, but the added stress of painful, distressing experiences.

The increasing concern about the effects of parental separation and hospitalisation was highlighted by Bowlby, whose influential book, *Child Care and the Growth of Love* (1965), was to have a profound effect on the way children were cared for in our hospitals. Bowlby emphasised the importance of the continuing mother–infant relationship to the mental health of the child in later years. Bowlby stressed that long-term psychological damage could occur in children due to separation from the family in a strange environment. Evidence of the observed stages of separation anxiety was presented, bearing witness to the potential psychological damage, which could occur through any kind of institutionalisation. Further support for Bowlby's findings came in 1952, with James

Robertson's film *A Two-Year-Old Goes to Hospital* (1953), which gave a heart-rending account of the experiences of a little girl admitted to hospital for the repair of an umbilical hernia. Pressure for change was mounting.

Amidst growing concern, the government convened a committee, chaired by Sir Harry Platt, to examine the hospital care of children. The report of this committee, *The Welfare of Children in Hospital* (Ministry of Health, 1959), and its many recommendations, formed the basis for radical change. The report was aimed at reducing the emotional distress of children during hospitalisation. Criticism was made of hospital rituals and disciplines, and a recommendation was for home-care or day-care facilities where possible. It was also recommended that the care of children should be in bright, cheerful children's wards with toys, a playroom, and possibly a nursery nurse allocated to help occupy younger children. Major issues raised were the need for unrestricted visiting, preventing separation of mother and child whenever possible, and the appointment of a Registered Sick Children's Nurse to be in charge of every ward.

Progress towards these changes was steady but slow, with a great deal of pressure from concerned professionals and pressure groups such as the National Association for the Welfare of Children in Hospital (NAWCH), now Action for Sick Children. The charter produced by this group incorporated the Platt recommendations and was adopted as a basis for quality children's care in many areas. Various reports since Platt (Committee on Child Health Services, 1976; NAWCH, BPA and RCN, 1987; Department of Health, 1991a; House of Commons Select Committee, 1997) have recognised progress but still express concern at the lack of facilities and services in many areas. A common element in all of these publications is the recognition that children have special health care requirements. Unfortunately, none of these reports attempted to define the specific role a children's nurse would perform.

THE ROLE OF THE CHILDREN'S NURSE

Very little change occurred in the role of children's nurses from the beginnings of hospitalisation until the reforms brought about as a consequence of the Platt report in the 1960s. For very many years the role of nursing staff was purely concerned with saving lives and trying to prevent the spread of infection. Death was a common occurrence in children's wards, and hospital stays were lengthy even for quite minor procedures. In addition, visitors were seen as an interruption to the hospital routine and were severely restricted. The effect this had on the children was quite profound and often detrimental to the child's recovery. The culture that prevailed was paternalistic and bureaucratic, with many rules and regulations, which nurses dutifully obeyed.

Gradually the focus of health care for children moved away from just saving lives to helping each child, whatever their condition or disability, to achieve their maximum potential. Implementation of the Platt report caused major changes in how children's nurses went about their duties, as have shorter hospital stays, increased day-care provision, and recent advances in technology, chemotherapy, and transplantation.

Many children's nurses experienced a sense of loss, as they gave up many of the most satisfying aspects of their role to enable parents – rightfully – to care for their own child. The nurse is now required to be educator, counsellor, and advocate, as well as expert communicator and highly skilled technician. The knowledge necessary to undertake this unique role is obviously extensive. The child branch diploma programmes therefore allow for this essential broad education. Further, with the increasing recognition that a child's health is an important indicator of health in later life, an awareness of the impact of poverty and social exclusion on health (Department of Health, 1999; Scottish Executive, 1999) and the worsening effects of health inequalities (Department of Health, 1998), a considerable amount of the pre-registration curriculum is dedicated to understanding child health and the children's nurse's role in health promotion.

The context of children's nursing practice is both complex and challenging, with a demand for high-quality care, based on evidence rather than ritual or custom. Nurses at every level of the organisation are increasingly accountable and involved in decision-making through the mechanisms of clinical audit and shared governance. The concept of reflection has emerged over recent years as a means of facilitating the nurses' effectiveness within these situations, as well as contributing to the effectiveness of clinical supervision and practice development. Reflective practice offers an excellent framework through which care can be critically examined (Dearmun *et al.*, 1996). Unfortunately, its adoption is problematic and influenced greatly by the organisational culture that pervades. Clarke and colleagues (1996) identified that organisational cultures, which stress collaboration as a way of working, are likely to encourage reflective practice. In addition to a commitment to working together with others, these organisations exhibit features such as respect for and promotion of autonomy and a commitment to continuous improvement. However, organisational cultures that are judgemental are likely to inhibit reflective practice. The nature of reflective practice is in essence concerned with acting with certainty on a basis of uncertainty. An over-emphasis on judging performance will discourage reflection and encourage rule-based, non-reflective practice. Equally, developmental cultures that recognise the problematic nature of professional competence and the difficulty of learning to perform competently are more likely to encourage reflective practice than non-developmental cultures.

CHILDREN ARE DIFFERENT

Children are vulnerable because of the complex development that occurs at each stage of childhood and adolescence. Their limited experience affects their understanding and perceptions of the world. Children are also more physiologically vulnerable than adults. The onset of illness for them is often sudden, and deterioration can be rapid. Contributory factors are immature respiratory and cardiovascular systems, which have fewer reserves than those of the adult, together with a faster metabolic rate, which requires a higher cardiac output, greater gaseous exchange and a higher fluid and calorie intake per kilogram body weight than adults (Hazinski, 1992).

Vulnerability to water imbalance in infants is due to the amount and distribution of body water. An infant's body is composed of 70–75% water, compared to 57–60% in an adult. In children, most of this fluid is in the extra-cellular fluid compartment and is therefore more accessible. Relatively moderate fluid losses may therefore seriously reduce the blood volume, resulting in shock, acidosis and death. Infants also have a larger surface area in relation to body weight, which allows more fluid as well as heat to be lost through evaporation from the skin, and creates intolerance to extremes of temperature.

CHILD HEALTH

Comprehensive information relating to the overall incidence of illness in children is not available. However, the state of a nation's health is usually reflected by mortality and morbidity statistics; these figures show that mortality at all ages is falling. The infant mortality rate – a particularly important indicator – is at an all-time low (Office for National Statistics, 2001). In contrast, morbidity has increased over recent decades. The prevalence of chronic illness in childhood more than doubled between 1972 and 1991. Contributory factors include the improved chances of survival for very low birth-weight babies (under 1500 g), and for those suffering from chronic childhood illnesses such as cystic fibrosis and asthma. Overall data about the prevalence of disability in children is difficult to obtain. This is partly due to debates about what constitutes disability in childhood. In 1993, 3% of children under 15 years (360 000) were classified as being disabled. The definition of disability used was taken from the World Health Organisation, who stated that disability was, 'a restriction or lack of ability to perform normal activities which has resulted from impairment of a structure or function of the body or mind'. The most prevalent types of disability relate to behavioural problems, continence, locomotion, and intellectual functioning. Some children have multiple disabilities.

Many families describe positive feelings of joy and satisfaction related to caring for their sick or disabled child (Beresford, 1994; Dobson *et al.*, 2001); however, the impact of caring can have a profoundly negative effect on all aspects of family life, especially the development of siblings. An additional burden for these families is reduced income. There is increased expenditure associated with the needs of a child with chronic illness or disability. It has been identified (Dobson *et al.*, 2001) that parents of disabled children spent on average twice as much on comparable items, i.e. children's possessions, medical items and toiletries, than other families. More items were also required to amuse, occupy and stimulate their children. Unfortunately, many of these items were reported as being more expensive than those used by non-disabled children. A key factor, which contributes to this low income relates to fact that the demands of caring for a disabled child make it difficult for both parents to work. A lack of practical and emotional support further compounded the financial worries of these families.

COMMUNITY CARE

In 1955 the World Health Organisation (WHO) stated that the best place for sick children to be cared for was at home. For a number of years children's community care received a very low priority. The first community paediatric schemes were established in 1948 in Rotherham, and in the 1950s in Paddington and Birmingham. The schemes were primarily concerned with providing an alternative to hospital care for the acutely ill child. In Rotherham the scheme was instituted in an attempt to reduce the high infant mortality rate, thought to be due to the effects of cross-infection in hospital. After 3 years the infant mortality rate had halved, although it is not clear whether there were other public health measures undertaken at this time, which contributed to this outstanding success. Following these early schemes, there was very little development for the next 20 years. Five schemes existed in Britain in 1970 and seven in 1980. By 1991, however, there were 46 general schemes and 30 specialist schemes (Lessing and Tatman, 1991); this had increased to 130 in 1994 (Royal College of Nursing, 1995).

This large increase in the number of community children's nursing services resulted from many factors, including the shift to primary care within the health service reforms following the NHS and Community Care Act (1990), the potential to reduce costs by shortening the length of stay in hospital, and the demands for ongoing specialist care and support in the home arising from the increased survival of children with chronic or life-threatening illness and disability. However, service provision is still 'patchy', with only 50% of health authorities purchasing them and only 10% of children in the country having access to a 24-hour service (Department of Health, 1997), and they appear to have developed in a 'piecemeal' fashion. Primarily the services are based either within the acute sector, i.e. hospital paediatric unit, or in the community, i.e. health centres (Winter and Teare, 1997).

Paediatric Community Nurses (PCNs) provide home care for children suffering from a wide variety of conditions, many of which are highly dependant and require complex equipment. Education of the child and family is an essential part of the role, since this enables them to undertake more advanced tasks such as intravenous drug and tracheotomy care, thereby preventing repeated hospital admissions for the child. Nurses also act in liaison with the hospital, general practitioners, and other special-ist services. To date the service has received very little evaluation and the costing information available is conflicting, although it is generally felt that the service is cost-effective. It could be argued that the advantages of home care should not be measured purely in financial terms and that there are other advantages, including the prevention of admission to hospital and the continuity of family life, which are of equal importance.

The demand for more children's community nursing is on-going, but the service is not without problems and certain factors appear to be crucial to its effectiveness. These include the need for practitioners to be fully integrated into a community children's nursing service, with managerial support and flexible exper-ienced nursing staff committed to promoting the family's ability to manage all aspects of care, which can be very complex. Furthermore, while it is recognised that the community children's nurse plays a vital role in supporting families in their own home, the very presence of the nurse is disruptive to family processes, especially when nurses remain in the family home (Coffman, 1997). The need for the nurse to find a balance between being with the family in a supportive way and being separate (not being viewed as one of the family, which is intrusive and threatening to the family unit) is very important (Patterson *et al.*, 1994).

Study Activity 38.2

- Quickly jot down what the word 'home' means to you.
- Make a list of the people that you welcome into your home.
- Are there parts of your home that you consider to be more private than others?
- How would you feel if you had to have strangers in your home 24 hours a day, 7 days a week?
- How would you feel if those strangers had access to the most private parts of your home?

HOSPITAL CARE

Despite the increasing amount of community support, over 1.5 million children under 15 years are admitted to hospital each year (Office of National Statistics, 2001), Various statistics related to the causes of admission demon-strate that respiratory illnesses were the most common cause of admission for children under 4 years old, while between the ages of 5 and 14 years injuries exceeded respiratory problems.

Most paediatric wards have made efforts to provide a relaxed, friendly environment. Contemporary practice is based on the concept of individualised, family-centred care, the ultimate aim being a partnership between the nurse and family that should form the basis of quality paediatric care. This is the idea under-lying the implementation of the American concept 'care-by-parent' in British hospitals. The underlying idea is that parents bear total responsibility for their child's hospital care, providing that the child's condition is not critical and that the parents are willing to accept the arrangement. The schemes were reported to succeed and the results were satis-factory, but the programmes were not main-tained because of lack of commitment on the part of the nursing staff. It has been suggested for many years (Darbyshire, 1995) that nurses often appear to pay lip service to the notion of partnership based on equality and mutual respect and that parents are not included in decision-making. Some parents believe that they are there merely to substitute for lack of staff (Audit Commission, 1993).

It is argued (Darbyshire, 1995) that both the concept of family-centred care and its implemen-tation are infinitely more problematic than the literature suggests; also that paediatric nursing has over-simplified the complexity of the rela-tionships and encounters between children, parents and nurses within a children's hospital. In describing the struggle of nurse educational-ists to move the concept of family-centred care into the twenty-first century, Coleman *et al.*

identifies that one of the key barriers to practice is the lack of empowerment of nurses themselves, who are therefore unable to facilitate a reciprocal social process in which children and their families are helped to take control over their stay in hospital.

A further consideration in promoting the concept of family-centred care is to ensure that the notion of family is not oversimplified to present an idealised image. Notions of male breadwinner, female housewife and two children currently represent only a small population of families. The number of dependent children living in lone parent households doubled between 1971 and 1991 from 1.0 million to 2.2 million, respectively (Botting, 1995). It is argued that the notion of family is highly controversial (Gittins, 1995) and full of ambiguities and contradictions. Children's nurses must therefore be able to differentiate between the ideology and the actual ways in which individuals interact and live together.

A primary nursing system, which requires total responsibility and accountability to be taken by one named nurse for each patient cared for, is only partially in place. This is probably because of the traditional problems associated with a consistent provision of nurses, but the situation could also derive from a lack of trained staff with the essential expertise and ability. In many areas where primary nursing is being implemented, an adapted method is in operation, in which a core team of nurses share responsibility for the care of a group of children. There are some who believe that the concept of primary nursing was the template for the introduction of the 'named nurse' (Department of Health, 1991b) and clearly influenced by the incentive for increased quality and accountability. However, Steven (1999) argued that problems can arise when ideas from one concept (i.e. primary nursing) are transferred to that of another – 'the named nurse'.

Nursing process documentation is evident in all clinical areas, but there is a lack of evidence-based information to support its impact on patient care. There is also very little paediatric nursing theory from which conceptual models of care can be developed. As a consequence, adult models are being used for paediatric care. While conceding that the use of adult conceptual models provides a logical framework in the absence of more appropriate ones, these models cannot truly represent or enhance contemporary children's nursing practice.

One area consistently surrounded by uncertainty is the assessment and control of children's pain. Many hospitals now employ specialist teams to assess and manage children's pain and to advise other professionals on effective pain control methods. Some of the misconceptions related to children and pain, including those maintaining that the inadequate myelination of nerve cells in the infant means that they cannot feel pain, or that narcotics are more dangerous for children or more likely to lead to addiction, are beginning to be dispelled. A commitment to improving the quality and standards of care under the umbrella of clinical governance was a major theme of the Government's proposals to 'modernise' the National Health Service (Department of Health, 1997). Towards this end the Royal College of Nursing produced 'clinical practice guidelines for the recognition and assessment of acute pain in children' (Royal College of Nursing, 1999).

Ethical dilemmas are part of everyday paediatric nursing practice, and an awareness of these issues is essential for today's practitioner. Increased levels of knowledge, coupled with increasing technology have increased the complexity of the decision-making process. More than ever, children's nurses must be aware of the influence they have on the decisions made by children and their families, who require information about care, presented in a way that allows them to fully participate in the decision-making process. It is recognised that the ethical issues involved in consent are complex and difficult and an understanding of moral theory, ethical frameworks and the way they can be applied in practice are essential to contemporary children's nursing practice.

Certain groups of children require specific discussion, either because of the particular problems they present, or because their needs have been overlooked, particularly hospitalised adolescents, children with mental health needs, and those from ethnic minorities.

HOSPITALISED ADOLESCENTS/YOUNG PEOPLE

The special needs of adolescents in hospital are receiving a higher profile at the present time, but there is still a great deal to be done. Adolescence signifies a period of rapid physical growth and development, more so than at any other time since early infancy. This period marks the transition from childhood to adulthood. The age of consent of adolescence varies according to the individual child, but may be as early as 10, and it can extend into the twenties, although 18 is usually thought to be the beginning of young adulthood. According to Erikson (1963) the key issues related to this stage concern resolving the confusion between identity and role. The overwhelming question that becomes central to the adolescent at this time is 'Who am I?' The tremendous physical, mental, and social changes experienced by the adolescent cause an identity crisis. Its resolution involves the development of sexual identity, including a mature role concept and some understanding of personal sexuality, the development of an occupational identity related to the conceptualisation of themselves as adults, and the development of an ideological identity touching on beliefs, attitudes, and ideas (Bee and Mitchell, 1994).

Anything that interferes with this development, such as illness and hospitalisation, with their potential loss of independence and control, can seriously interfere with the individual's development, causing inner conflict, anger, withdrawal and impairment of long-term development. Careful assessment, coupled with an ability to make relationships on their level, the maintenance of privacy and the prevention of boredom are essential for nursing. In this situation the adolescent is extremely vulnerable – a fact that is often obscured behind a façade of overconfidence (Shelley, 1993).

The Platt report, referred to above, was the first to identify that adolescents have needs different from those of adults and children. This idea was further supported by Court (Committee on Child Health Services, 1976) who acknowledged that children's needs and problems were sufficiently different to warrant consideration as a distinct group for health care provision. However, the small numbers of adolescent patients made specialist care units impractical at that time. As the numbers of adolescents accessing health care services increases, as a result of the improved survival of those with chronic childhood illnesses, a ward or area specifically for adolescents is now justifiable.

A small number of adolescent units have been established in recent years, but for the majority the only choice is between adult or children's wards. The adolescent may feel equally misplaced in both areas. Research undertaken by Burr (1993) demonstrated that adolescents were best cared for in children's wards by children's nurses, as these nurses were more interested in them and had more insight into their needs. It would seem that in the absence of a special unit, separate areas and facilities within children's wards are acceptable. Guidance for the setting of hospital care standards for adolescents (NAWCH, BPA and RCN, 1991) affirms that adolescents will recover faster if they are in an environment specifically designed for them, particularly when their emotional, educational and social requirements are understood.

CHILDREN WITH MENTAL HEALTH NEEDS

Given the complex nature of adolescents' development, it is not surprising that they form a large percentage of the children with mental health needs. Although there are disagreements about the rates of child and adolescent mental health problems, most agree that the rates of recorded problems are rising (Scottish Executive, 2001). An Office of National Statistics survey (Office for National Statistics, 2000) reported the incidence of mental health problems in childhood and adolescence as 1 in 10, with boys from low income families most at risk. The overall level tends to be higher in adolescence because some disorders persist and others arise in this older age group (Health Advisory Service, 1995). Between the age of 5 and the onset of puberty, mental health problems are largely conduct disorders or emotional disorders specific to childhood (Woodroffe *et al.*, 1993). Major psychiatric disorders begin to occur from puberty onwards, the most common conditions being depressive disorders, which affect between 2 and 5% of adolescents. Suicide is rare before the age of 12 years. The rate in 15–19-year-olds is six per 100 000 for men and 1–2 per 100 000 for women each year. The suicide rate for 15–19-year-olds is about three per 100 000, and the rate for attempted suicide about 400 per 100 000 (Health Advisory Service, 1995).

A greater risk of mental health problems occurs in the following situations:

- Families suffering socio-economic disadvantage
- Families where there is discord and divorce
- Situations where the parents themselves suffer from psychiatric disorder, particularly maternal depression
- Abused children – research indicates that about 35% of all physically abused children show psychiatric disorders
- Physical illness – children suffering from physical illness, especially chronic illnesses such as cystic fibrosis, diabetes and childhood leukaemia; rates are particularly high in children with learning disability
- Children who have multiple disabilities
- Young offenders – a diagnosis of primary mental health disorder can be made in one-third of young men aged between 16 and 18 years who have been sentenced by a court (Health Advisory Service, 1995).

The importance of these factors to children's nurses is that the acute paediatric services are often the first point of contact into the health care system for these young people. Knowledgeable and sensitive handling of these situations

within the acute sector is essential if the existing problems are not to be confounded by inappropriate management. The select committee inquiry into health services for children (House of Commons Select Committee, 1996) repeatedly emphasised the importance of integrating services and criticised the current lack of integration. Nowhere is this integration more important than between the child and adolescent mental health team and the acute paediatric services (*see* Table 38.1).

Table 38.1 Factors affecting the mental health of children

- Family disadvantage
- Family discord or separation
- A parent having a mental illness
- Poor parenting skills
- Chronic physical illness in the child
- Chromosomal or other genetic abnormalities in the child
- Brain damage in the child
- Physical, sexual or emotional abuse
- Experiences of sudden or extreme trauma
- Learning difficulties or language or communication problems
- Bereavement

CHILDREN IN ETHNIC MINORITIES

An estimated 8% or 1.3 million children under 16 years of age in the UK may be considered to be in ethnic minority groups. At present relatively little is known about the differences in child health thought to be caused by ethnic factors. Information suggests that morbidity and mortality is higher in ethnic minority children than in others (Botting, 1995). Further, a study to determine the problems encountered by black and other ethnic minority families when they are admitted to hospital (Action for Sick Children, 1990) demonstrated that the main issues of concern related to the following factors:

- Information giving
- Food
- Facilities for parents
- Facilities for religious observance

- Staff attitudes
- Availability of interpreters
- Awareness of the need for multicultural play
- Ignorance of naming systems
- Care of children with blood disorders.

From these findings guidelines were produced to advise on improving all aspects of care. There is a lack of available evidence to identify whether these guidelines have had any impact on care provision to these families. Anecdotal evidence from children's nurses suggests that to date there has been very little change.

The National Health Service (Scottish Executive, 2001) has stipulated its beliefs of the right of everyone to be treated in an appropriate manner, which includes being treated in a way that is sensitive to their cultural, ethnic and religious background. Furthermore, a study sponsored by the Joseph Rowntree Foundation, describes ethnic minority families with a disabled child as 'living on the edge'. It was identified that families from these groups experience greater disadvantage and difficulties when caring for a severely disabled child than their white counterparts.

CHILDREN REQUIRING CHILD PROTECTION

Great controversy surrounds the subject of child abuse. There seems to be no agreement about what it is, why it happens and what we should do about it. However, there is agreement that abuse causes severe physical and psychological problems for children. The abuse of children is not confined to one social group but it is more common in families subjected to environmental stresses and strains associated with socio-economic deprivation. The term 'child abuse' is a relatively new term within British culture and it was not until the early 1970s that formal procedures were implemented for the management of children suspected of being abused. For the first time, child abuse was recognised as a societal problem and not a private family matter, as had been believed for centuries previously. This recognition did not include sexual abuse,

and it was not until the late 1980s that the existence of widespread child sexual abuse was confirmed. Since this time studies of sexual abuse in the UK have emphasised an apparently persistent increase in the number of detected and reported cases (Monck *et al.*, 1996). The number of children on at-risk registers is reported to be 30 000, but it is impossible to estimate the true incidence of abuse as increased awareness could account for the increased reports.

The law relating to safeguarding and protecting children changed dramatically with the introduction of The Children Act (1989), The Children (Scotland) Act (1995) and The Children (Northern Ireland) Order (1995). Within this legislation a radical shift occurred in relation to the role of parents with regard to their children, and the law. No longer were children seen as the 'belongings' of their parents. Parental rights became parental responsibility. From a nursing perspective protecting children requires that every nurse, wherever they practice, has a clear understanding of their duties and responsibilities (Department of Health, 1992). For everyone concerned it has become increasingly recognised that the best position to view child protection from is in the context of children's rights.

CHILDREN'S RIGHTS

In the 1980s it was increasingly recognised that childhood had become a period of dependency and powerlessness and that children were an oppressed group (Frost and Stein, 1989). Formulating and adopting rights for children has been seen by many advocates as a way of addressing this oppression and powerlessness, both nationally and internationally. The British Government ratified the UN Convention on the Rights of the Child in 1991. In committing themselves to these goals, the participating governments have agreed to be guided by the principle that children's essential needs should be given a high priority in the allocation of resources at national, international and family levels.

Although the convention is not part of UK domestic law, any legislation brought before parliament must be compatible with the treaty. Child health nurses can use the principles of the convention to raise concerns and to advocate on behalf of children (Royal College of Nursing, 1998) The three central tenets of the agreement are that all the rights in the convention apply to all children regardless of racial origin, sex, religion, language, disability, opinion, or family background, that all decisions made on behalf of children must be in their best interests, and that children have the right to participate in decisions affecting them. Alderson (1995) argues that whenever adults define children's best interests, these can be very different from the way children experience their own best interests. Transmitting this language of children's rights into everyday child health practice is a challenge to every child's nurse. Apart from confusion between perceived interests and rights, there can be conflict between different rights. Does the terminally ill child have a right to heroic treatment or a right to die (Alderson, 1995)?

Issues around the child's right to consent to treatment occupy much of the discussions surrounding the implementation of children's rights into health care practice. Consent is not just about major decisions; it is about smaller choices, such as going to theatre on a trolley or

which hand is preferred for blood to be taken from (Brook, 2000). According to Atherton (1994), the question nurses must ask themselves is how often they seek the consent of the child before carrying out interventions, whether it be administering medication, bathing or taking a temperature (Royal College of Nursing, 1998).

The Royal College of Nursing's philosophy of care for paediatric nursing is shown in Table 38.2.

SUMMARY

This chapter has charted the shift in society's attitude to children and childhood from the early recognition of childhood as a distinct entity, the oppression and exploitation of the nineteenth and early twentieth centuries to the adoption and promotion of children's rights into the early twenty-first century. The relationship between the state of a child's health to their future health as an adult and hence to the health of the nation is now well established. The importance of equality and the inclusion of all sections of society is a key factor within this. The role of the children's nurse in promoting health, identifying ill-health and its contributory factors is essential. Children are distinctly different from adults. They are vulnerable because of their immature physiological systems and develop-

Table 38.2   The RCN philosophy of care for paediatric nursing

The needs of the child as an individual	Partnership with the family
In working towards the provision of appropriate facilities for sick children, nurses should: • Recognise each child as a unique, developing individual, whose best interests must be paramount • Listen to children, attempt to understand their perspectives, opinions and feelings and acknowledge their right to privacy • Consider the physical, psychological, social, cultural and spiritual needs of children and their families • Respect the right of children, according to their age and understanding, to appropriate information and informed participation in decisions about their care.	Nurses should: • Recognise that good health care is shared with families – who should be closely involved in their child's care at all times unless, exceptionally, this is not in the best interests of the child • Promote the active participation of children and their families in care and by providing teaching and support, assisting them to be partners in care • Promote the right of children to have a parent accompany them during hospitalisation and treatment.

(From Royal College of Nursing, 1995)

mental stage; consequently, they have different health care needs, requiring the employment of specially qualified nurses.

The practice of children's nursing is complex and challenging but it is also stimulating and immensely satisfying. The lack of theory or practice-based research is currently a serious impediment to its development. There has been some improvement in recent years, with the increase in nurses entering academic departments; however, many still appear to view with suspicion the development of a research base from which to inform practice. Reflective practice offers an ideal mechanism to develop practice-based theory, but its implementation depends on an organisational culture that is non-judgemental and fosters respect for autonomy.

The future is uncertain. What is clear is that the demand for quality and excellence is unlikely to reduce. Public accountability for the services provided is a key factor in contemporary health care practice. Issues relating to children are particularly emotive and receive a lot of media attention. Political awareness is essential for children's nurses, so that they can represent children's interests and influence policy making. The demand for strong leadership within children's nursing has never been greater and it is essential that individuals with leadership potential are identified and developed as early as possible.

REFERENCES

Action for Sick Children (1990) *A Study To Determine the Problems Encountered by Black and Other Ethnic Minority Families When Their Children Enter Hospital*, Action for Sick Children, London

Alderson, P. (1995) What right to health care? *Health Matters* **20**, 18–19

Aries, P. (1962) *Centuries of Childhood*, Cape, London

Armitage, G. (1998) Analysing childhood: a nursing perspective. *Journal of Child Health Care* **2**(2), 66–71

Atherton, T.M. (1994) The rights of the child in health care. In: Lindsay, B. (ed.) *The Child and Family: Contemporary nursing issues in child health and care*, Baillère Tindall, pp. 3–21

Audit Commission (1993) *Children First: A study of hospital services*, HMSO, London

Beresford, B. (1994) *Positively Parenting*, Social Policy Research Unit, University of York, York

Botting, B. (1995) *The Health of Our Children*, decennial supplement, OPCS survey, London

Bee, H.L. and Mitchell, S.K. (1994) *The Developing Person*, Harper and Row, London

Bowlby, J. (1965) *Child Care and the Growth of Love*, Pelican, London

Brook, G. (2000) Children's competency to consent. *Paediatric Nursing* **12**(5), 31–5

Burr, S. (1993) Adolescents and the ward environment. *Paediatric Nursing* **5**(1)

Clarke, B., James, C. and Kelly, J. (1996) Reflective practice: reviewing the issues and refocusing the debate. *International Journal of Nursing Studies* **33**(2) 171–80

Coffman, S. (1997) Home-care nurses as strangers in the family. *Western Journal of Nursing Research* **19**(1), 82–96

Committee on Child Health Services (1976) *Fit for the Future* (The Court Report), HMSO, London

Darbyshire, P. (1995) Family-centred care within contemporary British paediatric nursing. *British Journal of Nursing* **4**(1)

Dearmun, A., Atkins, S. and Murphy, K. (1996) Reflective practice. *Paediatric Nursing* **8**(2), 29–33

Department of Health (1991a) *The Welfare of Children: Young people in hospital*, HMSO, London

Department of Health (1991b) *The Patient's Charter*, HMSO, London

Department of Health (1992) *Child protection. The Children Act (1989): Guidance for senior nurses, health visitors and midwives*, HMSO, London

Department of Health (1997) *The New NHS: Modern, dependable*, The Stationery Office, London

Department of Health (1998) *Independent Inquiry into Inequalities in Health Report* (The Acheson Report), Department of Health, London

Department of Health (1999) *Saving Lives: Our healthier nation*, The Stationery Office, London

Dobson, B., Middleton, S. and Beardsworth, A. (2001) *The Impact of Childhood Disability on Family Life*, Joseph Rowntree Foundation, London

Erikson, E.H. (1963) *Identity and the Life Cycle*, International Universities Press, New York

Frost and Stein (1989) *The Politics of Child Welfare*, Harvester Wheatsheaf, London

Gittins (1995) *The Family in Question*, Macmillan, London

Hazinski, M.F. (1992) *Nursing Care of the Critically Ill Child* (2nd edition), Mosby, St Louis, IL

Health Advisory Service (1995) *The NHS Health Advisory Service: Together we stand. The commissioning, role and management of child and adolescent mental health services*, HMSO, London

House of Commons Select Committee (1996) *Fourth Report, Session 1996–97: Child and Adolescent Mental Health Services*, The Stationery Office, London

Humphries, S., Mack, J. and Perks, R. (1988) *A Century of Childhood*, Sedgwick and Jackson, London

Lessing and Tatman (1991) Paediatric home care in the 1990s. *Archives of Disease in Childhood*, 66, 994–6

Miles, I. (1986a) The emergence of sick children's nursing (Part 1). *Nurse Education Today* 6, 82–7

Miles, I. (1986b) The emergence of sick children's nursing (Part 2). *Nurse Education Today* 6, 133–8

Ministry of Health (1946) *Report of the Care of Children Committee* (The Curtis Report), HMSO, London

Ministry of Health (1959) *The Welfare of Children in Hospital* (The Platt Report), HMSO, London

Monck, E., Bentovim A., Goodall G. *et al.* (1996) *Child Sexual Abuse: A descriptive and treatment study*, Department of Health, London

Mullally, S. (2001) Report of Royal College of Nursing Conference, Manchester. *Paediatric Nursing* 13(7)

NAWCH, BPA and RCN (1991) *Caring for Children in the Health Service*, HMSO, London

Office for National Statistics (2001) *The Mental Health of Children and Adolescents*, Office of National Statistics, London

Patterson, J.M. Jernell, J., Leonard, B.J. *et al.* (1994) Caring for medically fragile children at home: the parent–professional relationship. *Journal of Pediatric Nursing* 9(2), 98–106

Royal College of Nursing (1995) *RCN Philosophy of Care for Paediatric Nursing*, Royal College of Nursing, London

Royal College of Nursing (1998) *The Socio-Political Context of Care*, Royal College of Nursing, London

Royal College of Nursing (1999) *Clinical Practice Guidelines For the Recognition and Assessment of Acute Pain in Children*, Royal College of Nursing, London

Robertson, J. (1953) *A Two-Year-Old Goes to Hospital*, Child Development Research Unit, Tavistock

Scottish Executive (1999) *Towards a Healthier Scotland*, The Stationery Office, Edinburgh

Scottish Executive (2001) *Fair for All: NHS Scotland and people from ethnic minorities*, The Stationery Office, Edinburgh

Shelley, H. (1993) Adolescent needs in hospital. *Paediatric Nursing* 5(1)

Steven, S. (1999) Named nursing: in whose best interest? *Journal of Advanced Nursing* 29(2), 341–7

Winter, A. and Teare, J. (1997) Construction and application of paediatric community nursing services. *Journal of Child Health Care* 1

Woodroffe, C. Glickman, M., Baker, M. *et al.* (1993) *Children, Teenagers and Health – The key data*, Office of Population Censuses and Surveys, 1990, Office of Population Censuses and Surveys, London

World Health Organisation (1955) *WHO Bulletin 12*, WHO, Geneva

FURTHER READING

Children in Scotland (1999) *Review of the Mental Health (Scotland) Act 1984*, Report for The Milan Committee of a consultation seminar, Children in Scotland, Edinburgh

Department of Health (1989) *The Children Act: A new framework for the care and upbringing of children*, HMSO, London

Department of Health (DoH) (1991) *Health and Personal Social Services Statistics for England (HPSSS)*, *Common Services Agency (CSA)*, Hospital Statistics for Scotland, Scottish Crime and Health Department, Edinburgh

Henderson, J., Goldacre, M. and Griffith, M. (1990) Time spent in hospital by children: trends in the Oxford record linkage study area. *Health Trends* 22(4), 166–9

Kurtz (1992) *With Health in Mind*, Action for Sick Children, London

Slater, M. (1990) *Health For All Our Children: Achieving appropriate health care for black and ethnic minority children*, Action for Sick Children, London

Smith, M. and Robus, N. (1989) *The Financial Circumstances of Families with Disabled Children Living in Private Households*, OPCS Surveys of Disability in Great Britain, Report 5, HMSO, London

Woodroffe, C. and Kurtz, Z. (1989) *Working for Children?* National Childrens Bureau Publications, London

Whiting, M. (1988) *Community Paediatric Nursing in England*, Royal College of Nursing, London

UNICEF (1990) *First Call for Children: Convention on the rights of the child*, UNICEF, Geneva

39 MENTAL HEALTH NURSING

Ann Long

LEARNING OUTCOMES

After studying this chapter you will be able to:

- Define and describe the characteristics of mental health and mental ill-health as the field of concern in mental health nursing
- Identify factors that impact upon mental health
- Describe the common manifestations of mental ill-health that the mental health nurse may encounter
- Identify skills that are important within the role of the mental health nurse
- Explore the therapeutic relationship that is fundamental to the role of the mental health nurse.

INTRODUCTION

The nature of mental health and illness has been discussed and theorised about for centuries across disciplines and cultures. Human beings struggle to create order out of chaos and a fear of the unknown or the irrational leads people to construct their personal stories about the experiences that happen in their lives. When people explore their stories with others (such as a nurse), it helps them to make sense of their world, as experiences occur in seconds, minutes or years and each of these time scales, when added together, constitutes each human being's lifetime. The sharing of experiences with others is one of the most significant ways to explore, construct and express meaning and it helps people to realise they are not alone (Mishler, 1986). Moreover, the meanings inherent in the sharing are conveyed through the use of

language which is 'our means of ordering, classifying and manipulating the world' (Spender, 1995, p. 3).

Various influences impact on our mental health, for example, personality (Bruner, 1987), attitudes/beliefs/culture (Hinton and Levkoff, 1999), gender (Bushfield, 1996; Crowe, 1996), cognition (Sparkes, 1994), mood (White and Epston, 1990; Polkinghorne, 1996) and social context and relationships (Sarason and Duck, 2001). The quest to find personal meaning in a social world is inevitably influenced by cultural and political forces (Saris, 1995). The dynamic interplay of these factors impacts on mental health and well-being and is covertly or overtly displayed in the coping strategies that individuals adopt to help them make sense of their unique experiences in their world.

Study Activity 39.1

Write brief statements on how you consider the following factors might impact on mental health and well-being:

- gender
- ethnicity
- culture
- class
- politics
- education
- language.

People with mental health problems experience phenomena which are disconcerting to them and/or their environments and they often struggle to make sense of their experiences of altered mental states in order to gain psychological equilibrium (Kleinman, 1988; Smale, 2000). Examination of this proposition means that the term psychological equilibrium is concomitant with the concept of mental health. However, a search of the literature shows a deficit of definitions of mental health. Long and Chambers (1993) made a brave attempt to define it as:

> *A process of equilibrium both within and between the inner and outer self, the social environment and the natural world in which people live. Self-awareness, self-acceptance and the ability to adapt and cope with changing life circumstances are manifestations of mental health. In addition, there is a personal recognition and acceptance of inner strengths and resources and a desire to aim for continuous personal potential and development throughout life.*
>
> (Chambers, 1993, p. 7)

These authors speak of mental health as a 'process of [psychological] equilibrium' and emphasise the dynamic interplay between the internal and the external world. Literature reveals that a variety of terms have been used to denote mental health problems, including mental illness, mental distress, psychic pain, madness, insanity and mental pain. They indicate the diversity and complexity of interpretations of this phenomenon among those who are experiencing mental health problems and those hoping to help them. No one term is privileged over another because all are equally meaningful (or meaningless) depending on the individual's perceptions and experiences. These complexities lead us to your second Study Activity.

Study Activity 39.2 ———

Continuum

Mental health ⟵⟶ Mental illness

- Write brief statements and discuss with your peer group what the following terms really mean to you. Consider what these terms might mean to people who are enduring mental ill-health, their families and their carers:

- insanity;
- mania;
- schizophrenia;
- depression;
- anxiety neurosis.

- After carrying out a library search of these terms and discovering how other authors have described them, place each of these terms where you think they fit on the mental health, mental ill-health continuum above.
- Give reasons for your decisions, which should always be open to change over time.

> *The realm of meaning is not static: it is enlarged by the new experiences it is continuously configuring as well as by its own refiguring process which is carried out through reflection and recollection.*
>
> (Polkinghorne, 1988, p. 15)

When exploring perceptions of mental illness, it is important to recognise that members of the anti-psychiatry movement argued that *mental illness* is not an illness *but a problem with living* (Szasz, 1961) causing a disequilibrium between the inner and the outer world in which people live. Achieving equilibrium or a balance between the inner and the outer world is more difficult for some than others. We may, in fact, be living in a society that positively gives rise to mental health disequilibrium. There is growing recognition of the relationship between behaviour and environment, collectively as well as individually. Society places emphasis on the power of wealth, the importance of material possessions and the relevance of educational qualifications. However, it is hard for some people to sustain and maintain mental health in a climate where poverty and unemployment are paramount, where there is gross inequality and social injustice. In addition, people who are marginalised, undervalued, deprived of equitable opportunities and equal civil liberties for personal, social, educational, and futuristic self-growth and development have difficulty achieving mental health or reaching their potential.

All this, coupled with the pressures of advertising, with its indoctrination about norms of happiness, weight, friendship and sexual satisfaction and the subsequent feelings of inadequacy and failure among those who have not accomplished, and possibly will never achieve those social and advertiser norms. It is both humane and realistic to offer high-quality nursing care to people who exhibit these mental health indicators. This leads to Study Activity 3.

Study Activity 39.3 _____

Continuum

Mental health ←——————→ Mental illness

- How might the following factors impact on mental health? Where might you place them on the continuum? Give reasons for your decisions.

    - Unemployment
    - Domestic violence
    - Child abuse
    - Homelessness
    - Addiction
    - Broken relationship
    - Loss of a loved one
    - Diagnosis of a terminal illness
    - Sexual abuse
    - Attempted suicide/suicide.

- These are only some of the painful experiences that happen in people's lives and affect their mental health, either in the short term or the long term. What other experiences would you add to the list?
- Work with your peer group and consider how some of these experiences might affect different people.
- Where might you place yourself on the mental health, mental ill-health continuum today?
- Discuss your findings with your peer group or during a seminar facilitated by your lecturer.

How we feel today, right now, is not static, we are constantly changing. This means that our mental health is not static, it is moving and changing continually. Ultimately, the concept of mental health is difficult to define. Perhaps it is best explored and examined by the person in need of help. However, interestingly, a search of the literature shows a scarcity of service users' interpretations of their experiences of mental health problems.

EMOTIONAL PAIN AS A HUMAN CONDITION

For the purpose of this chapter the phenomenon of mental ill-health is considered a euphemism for *emotional pain* that is endured intrinsically by human beings. Core, painful feelings that people experience within the gestalt of emotional pain are examined to support this argument. It is further argued that the two people involved in the nurse–person relationship are co-equal in their humanness and both are absorbed in the culture of emotional pain, albeit on different sides of the healing relationship.

Figure 39.1 illustrates this equality, and also that the nurse has worked at resolving her emotional pain during self-awareness programmes, the channel with the nurse is open and receptive to listening to the person's life history of pain and distress, and that she has the core human qualities to provide feedback and hope for the person. Throughout this, the nurse needs clinical supervision to maintain mental health and well-being.

Study Activity 39.4 _____

It has been argued that mental health and mental ill-health are part and parcel of the human condition and inextricably linked with the meaning of life and the purpose of living. Discuss the following philosophical arguments with your peer group and/or in seminars facilitated by your lecturer.

What does it mean to be human?
What does it feel like to be a man/woman?
What is the meaning of life?
What is the meaning of suffering?
What does the term 'emotional pain' mean to you?

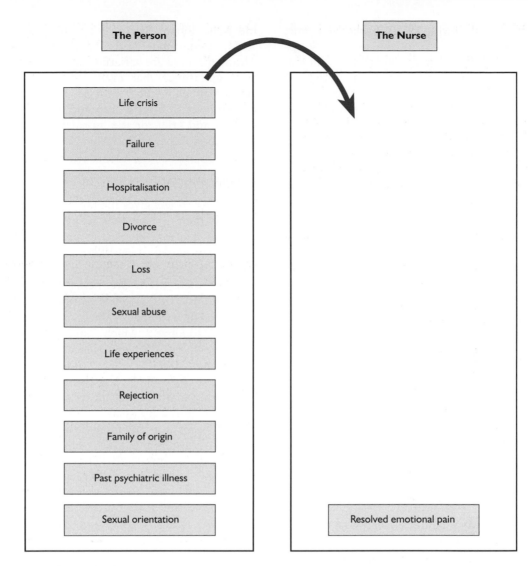

Figure 39.1 Containers of emotional pain

Enduring emotional pain is the most profound experience in human existence. It is difficult to touch, impossible to convey and so indescribably painful it cannot be shared in words. An intense feeling of coldness affects the total being leaving it lifeless, frozen and numb (Long, 1997a, 1998). Trying to explain the human phenomenon of emotional pain through the channels of speech and language serves only to dilute and dissolve its meaning to the people involved.

Emotional pain has a life of its own that has to be embraced sequentially, felt, experienced and lived through (Long, 1997a, 1998).

Emotional pain is especially confusing and troublesome when no eye can see it, no ear can hear it and no mind can conceive the internal trauma and unhealed wounds (Heidegger, 1962). Given time people try to come to terms with and make sense of the experience and some finally accept the reality of life's endless blows (Long,

1999; Long and Slevin, 1999). In the meantime, the world insists on revolving and life keeps moving forward ... for everyone else. Unfortunately, for people who are in the throes of emotional pain, the carnival of life has come to a halt and everything in it is shaken and jarred (Long, 1997b). During emotionally painful times, people stop living, they merely exist. It is as if the torment in their lives has the power to trap them in an emotional time warp (Long, 1998). Consequently until they have dealt with the pain they are unable to move forward in their lives (Long, 1998).

People who are enduring emotional pain have little energy to speak let alone weep. This lack of energy to cry out, which at least allows the pain to be acknowledged, also happens internally within the deeper self (Miller, 1983a, b; Long, 1997a). When people are weighed down with so much hurt, tears are normally impossible to shed, even within the secrecy and silence of their own hearts (Miller, 1983a, b). Individuals become locked into their lonely, isolated world of desolation (Long and Reid, 1996). It is impossible to be sure about anything as nothing is real. Indeed, sometimes the emotional pain is so intense that individuals are unable to discriminate between night-time and daytime, the sun and the moon, other people's voices in their heads or, their own internalised voices. Yet, within their consciousness people who are enduring emotional pain are aware that they are incomplete and that they must continue their search to find meaning (Long, 1998, 1999). Their main concern, therefore, is not being but becoming as 'becoming is superior to being' (Klee, 1969 cited in Powell, 1977).

EMOTIONAL PAIN AS LOSS OF 'NORMALITY'

Emotional pain is an inevitable feature in human life (Jung, 1958). Embedded within the rawness of emotional pain are feelings such as mistrust, shame, guilt, anger, remorse, sadness and grief (Long, 1997a, 1998). In addition to these painful emotions, some individuals may feel a sense of powerlessness and a strong belief that

life is no longer worth living (Reid and Long, 1993; Long and Reid, 1996; Long, 1998). Although, there are variations about the meaning and significance that each individual gives to emotional pain, both nurses and clients, as human beings, suffer a deep and intense sense of sadness and grief for the 'normality' of the way things used to be.

EMBRACING SADNESS AND GRIEF

The power to feel gives human beings the energy to know their spontaneous reality. Emotions are the tools that may be used to permit individuals to be fully aware of the 'here and now' and to know through their comfort or discomfort whether their needs are being fulfilled (Jung, 1958; Long, 1999). An E-motion is energy in motion. For example, sadness is the energy in saying 'goodbye' which allows people to complete one of life's experiences before moving on (Long, 1995, 1998). Indeed, life is a prolonged farewell. It is a continuous series of completing maturational life crises and progressing through the life span, as for example, when infants *become* toddlers and neophyte nurses become registered nurses. Similar transitions occur across Erikson's (1978) psychosocial stages of development. Individuals need to negotiate the first stage, *trust versus mistrust*, before they can move on to the second stage, *autonomy versus shame*, and the third stage, *initiative versus guilt*, and so on. Erikson (1978) claimed that those individuals who do not negotiate these stages successfully are unable to proceed emotionally to the next stage of development. When nurses have secured a knowledge of which stages of development clients have not successfully negotiated, they are in a prominent position to facilitate them to successfully work through these stages in the 'here and now' encounter (Long, 1999).

All human beings have to negotiate many of life's adversities. Human trials and tribulations that some of their clients have had to negotiate, such as the death of a loved one or becoming terminally ill, are examples of misfortunes that cause people to grieve for the 'normality' of the way things used to be. Grief and sadness, therefore, afford people the energy to complete the past and move on. Levine (1987, p. 142) has defined grief as 'the tearing open of the heart, leaving the heart vulnerable and exposed. And the deep lesson of compassion, for which we were born becomes evident'. Being allowed to grieve, therefore, grants people the fundamental energy required to move on in their lives, self-actualise and develop (Long, 1999). Wherefore, grief is a lot more than crying. It is a healing feeling (Long, 1995).

Remnants of mistrust, shame, guilt, anger and resentment as well as other painful emotions are skilfully repressed in 'internal containers' that all human beings use to store their emotional pain (Klein, 1969; Long, 1998) (*see* Fig. 39.1). During life crises in particular and transitional phases in general, these painful emotions appear in people's minds and hearts like phantoms haunting them and tormenting them (Klein, 1969). They are manifested in a range of unusual behaviours that people use especially during the 'letting go' stage of human relationships (Long and Slevin, 1999). Any of life's painful experiences, despite their torment and pain, cannot be relived, but if faced with courage need not be lived again and again.

Study Activity 39.5

- Write brief statements on what the world looks like viewed through the eyes of someone who is contiguously:

  - sad
  - depressed
  - angry
  - resentful
  - jealous
  - frustrated
  - lonely
  - guilty.

- Discuss your interpretations with your peer group or in a self-awareness seminar.

SELF-AWARENESS PROGRAMMES

Nurses might begin their education and training by exploring and synthesising the human condition and by discovering what it means to be human and what it must feel like to be labelled, for example, a schizophrenic. Explorations could take place in self-awareness programmes specifically designed to facilitate nurses to develop and grow personally and professionally (*see* Fig. 39.2 for examples of constructs to be explored).

Phenomena such as the meaning of life with all its pain and beauty, loving and being loved, relationships, rejection, abandonment and loss should be included in explorations. Following such programmes, nurses will then be in a better position to care for other human beings. The person-valuing paradigm forwarded by Long (2001) was designed to create a new way of thinking about nursing and a new way of perceiving people in need of care. Implicit within the paradigm is the notion that human beings have their own unique pathways in life. Nurses, as co-equals, must first learn to become self-aware and subsequently embrace the character ethic, aimed to equip them with the essential 'core human' care qualities and human principles required to work in the therapeutic relationship (*see* Fig. 39.3).

This type of preparation should enable nurses to work therapeutically with people who are in need of care. Another key reason for promoting self-awareness programmes is to give nurses safe opportunities to examine, explore and 'empty' the remnants of their unresolved pain that is stored within their 'emotional containers' (Long, 1998) (*see* Fig. 39.1). This form of exploration facilitates nurses to *become* mentally healthy enough to 'contain' other people's painful emotions and thoughts within the nurse–person relationship.

Figure 39.4 illustrates the multivariate pathway to nursing as a profession. Phase 1 of this pathway illustrates a selection of fundamental socialisation constructs and issues from within the family of origin to which neophyte nurses may have been exposed on their life

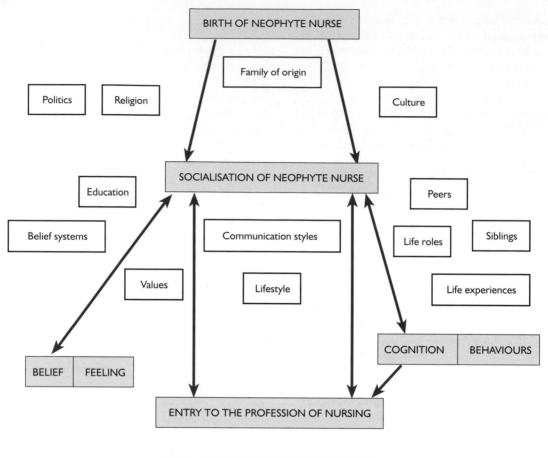

SELF-AWARENESS PROGRAMMES

Figure 39.2   The metamorphosis of neophyte nurses to the profession

journey to the nursing profession. It is suggested that neophyte nurses should be given opportunities to explore these constructs within self-awareness programmes (*see* Fig. 39.2). Phase 2 highlights a range of human principles and 'core, human' care qualities that Long considers being inherent within her philosophy of a 'character ethic' for mental health nurses. She suggests that these healing qualities should be examined within self-awareness programmes before neophyte nurses become accredited for working in the nurse–person relationship (*see* Fig. 39.2). Phase 3 examines the complex interaction

dynamics that are involved in initiating, maintaining and closing therapeutic relationships and links the key concepts with the need for nurses to attend lifelong personal clinical supervision.

Study Activity 39.6

• Look at Figs 39.2 and 39.3 and examine the core human care qualities and the human principles depicted. Most of these have been explored elsewhere in this book. The figures depict some essential qualities and skills that form the nucleus of

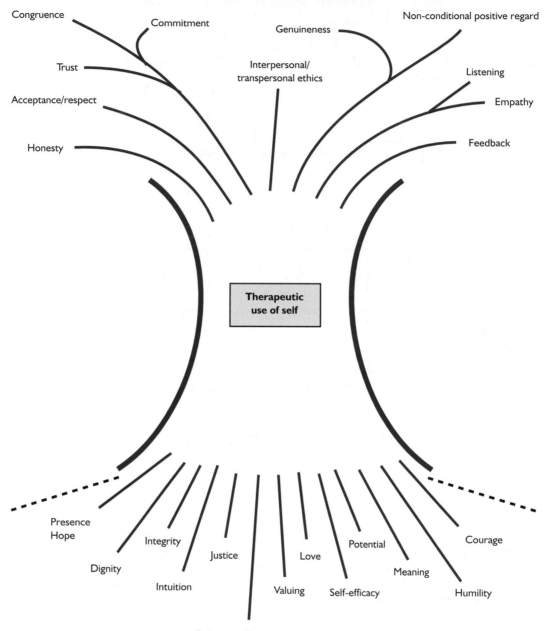

Congruence

Commitment

Genuineness

Non-conditional positive regard

Trust

Interpersonal/
transpersonal ethics

Listening

Acceptance/respect

Empathy

Honesty

Feedback

**Therapeutic
use of self**

Presence
Hope

Integrity

Justice

Love

Potential

Courage

Dignity

Meaning

Intuition

Valuing

Self-efficacy

Humility

Being moral/compassionate

HUMAN PRINCIPLES

Figure 39.3 Promoting a character ethic for mental health nurses

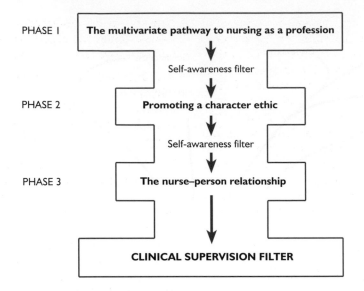

Figure 39.4   The multivariate pathway to nursing as a profession

the therapeutic use of self and they are collectively versatile.

- Reflect on Fig. 39.1 and identify how you might resolve some of the remnants of unresolved pain from your own 'container'.
- Explore these figures with a member/members of your peer group or within a self-awareness seminar.

THE THERAPEUTIC NURSE–PERSON RELATIONSHIP

Nursing care as an aesthetic activity involves guiding people from the actual reality of where they are in terms of suffering towards achieving their potential in terms of healing. Nurses help people to cope with and work through the emotional pain that resides within the realms of human distress and also with the profundity and aftermath of life crises. While nurses are not the sole navigators of caring they do hold a central position in the caring field.

With the aid of a non-judgemental co-traveller such as a mental health nurse, the work involved in exploring and resolving emotional pain can become a journey of rediscovery. Feelings,

thoughts and resulting reflections that give meaning to and make sense of the experiences require uncovering, naming, embracing and recognising before they are integrated into a new and liberated sense of self. At the end of this painful journey, people are greeted into the welcoming arms of self-acceptance, the disturbing passage closed but not forgotten as 'people do not solve problems they outgrow them' (Jung, 1958). The outcome of this work brings positive mental health and well-being. Long (1998) claimed that there are various stages in the healing process and that nurses can work with people enabling them to negotiate their own unique healing stages while on their journeys of recovery. The paper by Long (1998) should be read in conjunction with this chapter, which continues with advancing three therapeutic communication constructs as being intrinsic within the nurse–person relationship. They are therapeutic connecting, climbing healing steps towards recovery and the dance of recovery.

Therapeutic connecting: emotional touching
All relationships begin with one human being making a connection with another. The theore-

tical underpinnings of therapeutic connecting have their origins in the study of the bonding process that takes place in the mother–child relationship (Bee, 1998). Therapeutic connecting is one of the key interaction constructs in effective human-with-human relationships and Buber (1970) referred to this emotional bond as 'in-touchness'. Within the nurse–patient relationship each person has known and experienced a range of painful human emotions as well as a variety of positive ones that can be globally encapsulated within the gestalt of *loving and being loved*. The two people involved in the relationship are also endowed with a number of internal resources and strengths coupled with many talents and skills. However, it is expected that the nurse is the person who is congruent and the patient incongruent as he/she is enduring a vulnerable life crisis and is, therefore, in need of care. Consequently, when nurses work in a proactive way within the ethos of the person-valuing paradigm, they should bring the world of nursing to clients rather than expecting clients to leave their known world and enter the professional's demise. After all, the nurse and the client are also co-equal because both are coming afresh to a new relationship in their lives – the nurse–person encounter. Making an emotional connection with another is a happening for the two persons involved. Therefore, it is a valued life experience. Penn (1982, p. 13) submits that therapeutic connecting is 'a co-evolving for both people involved in the healing relationship'. Connecting is a deep and honest meeting and sharing of souls that may also occur in the group situation where feelings are honestly explored and identification and empathy occurs. Therapeutic connecting within nursing means that nurses must have the ability to *be there with the other* and *be there for the other* in the existential 'here and now' encounter – as the other is the sole focus of their contemplation (Sternberg, 1995; Long, 1998). As the result of therapeutic connecting, patients will then be able to share their emotional pain with nurses, thus allowing them to 'let go' of some of the repressed pain within their emotional containers (*see* Fig. 39.1).

Nurses may be described as emotional stepping stones, guides sometimes, emotional midwives at best, who are there to help people:

- understand and give meaning to some of their emotional pain
- alleviate some of their suffering
- enable them to work on strengthening the self.

Three fundamental dimensions are essential for successful rendition of therapeutic connecting as a compassionate communication activity in nursing. They are commitment, trust and feedback.

Commitment is a state of mind (Argyle, 1997). The main aim is for nurses to make a decision to stay with the relationship (Long, 1995, 1998). It provides a sense of stability and security for the other person as it is the bedrock on which trust is born. Commitment also means that 'all loose ends' must be dealt with before the other is referred to another professional, albeit temporarily. Preparation for letting go is a standard feature in commitment. Before ending any relationship, nurses must understand that this should never be done abruptly or without sensitivity, regardless of the way the ending has come about (Long, 1998). Commitment is an essential element in caring and when it is missing the other person may be left feeling abandoned. Past experience from working in psychiatric hospitals shows that many of the long-stay patients were treated in an 'I-It' manner (Buber, 1970) like *objects* when they were passed from one professional to another without regard to the additional emotional pain this may have caused. This may be explained pictorially by looking again at Fig. 39.1, where instead of facilitating people to 'empty' their emotional containers, some professionals further add to the pain. It is essential, therefore, for nurses to think wisely when committing themselves to the therapeutic relationship because if they cannot commit themselves totally to work with the person during the healing process they may end up causing people extra hurt and pain (Long, 1998).

Trust involves one individual relying on another to contain and validate the other's thoughts, feelings, behaviours as well as their recollections of life experiences (Klein, 1969; Long, 1995, 1999; Kapur, 1999). The meaning of 'containment' as conceived by Klein (1969) has been symbolically depicted in Fig. 39.1. An essential element in trust is the ability to convey to others that they are special, that they matter and the sharing of their life stories will be treated as sacrosanct. Other communication constructs involved in the phenomenon of trust include reliability, consistency, genuineness and dynamism (openness and frankness) (Long, 1997c). Trust also includes an element of risk-taking, in that other people open themselves up to facing uncertainty, vulnerability and loss should their trust be betrayed or violated (Long, 1995; Long and Slevin, 1999; Baxter, 1999; Slevin, 1999).

Feedback and reflection of thoughts and feelings are important communication elements in initiating, maintaining and closing a therapeutic relationship (Hargie *et al.*, 1994). When nurses skilfully utilise these communication activities they provide clarification, interpretation and a summary of how they non-punitively evaluate the other's feelings, thoughts and behaviours during the 'here and now' encounter (Klein, 1969; Long, 1999; Kapur, 1999). Feedback is an essential ingredient for *being in tune with*, or making an emotional connection with whatever is going on in the other's internal world at that moment (Long, 1997b).

In its entirety, therefore, therapeutic connecting is an essential component required in the nurse–person relationship which primarily enables nurses to gain entrance into the other person's emotional world. The aim of entering the person's world has been fluently portrayed by Thorne (1994, p. 112) who claimed that the fundamental essence of care is to:

> *Gain entrance into the world of the client through emotional commitment in which they [nurses] are willing to involve themselves as people and reveal themselves ... the primary*

> *goal is to see, feel and experience the world as the client sees, feels and experiences it.*
>
> (Thomas, 1994, p. 112)

It is clear that nursing is costly and demanding in terms of making emotional connections and offering oneself up to the care of others. There are two fundamental reasons for this. First, there are the inward pains that nurses bring with them to the job and second, there are emotional scar tissues that are intrinsically part of our human inheritance. Ultimately, caring nurse are those who have made a decision to care. In addition, nurses need to be facilitated to look within and explore their own emotional containers before they can provide effective human care, otherwise they may not have achieved the required state of congruence. This can be facilitated in self-awareness programmes. Consequently, Long and Chambers (1993) claimed that nurse lectures are responsible for creating and maintaining a therapeutic ambience within self-awareness programmes which might enable students to deal with some of the unresolved emotional pain within their own 'containers' before they attempt to enter the client's world. If students are not granted this opportunity in self-awareness programmes:

> *Certain conflicting material is excluded from consciousness because it is too painful. However, because it is emotionally charged, it remains active in the personality, and overt behavioral symptoms result from it. Full awareness, including allowing oneself to experience the emotions consciously, results in the alleviation of the symptoms.*
>
> (Freud, 1974, p. 71)

When nurses become congruent and discover how to enter the other person's world effectively, they are capable of exploring experiences of emotional pain 'with wide open eyes, with knowledge, facts, theories held at bay, looking at the experience with astonishment ... Becoming absorbed in the phenomenon' (Oiler, 1992, p. 180). Thereafter, when nurses have been accepted into the person's world they must 'let that which shows itself be seen from itself in the very best way in which it shows itself from itself' (Heidegger, 1962, p. 58).

Climbing healing steps towards recovery

The second construct to be explored is the proposition that nurses co-travel with people on their journeys towards healing and recovery (Long, 1999). Human beings grow only as much as their horizons allow. Metaphorically speaking, this strenuous journey towards mental health and recovery is analogous to having to climb a symbolic, emotional and spiritual ladder or mountain (Long, 1998). Vygotsky's (1962) work on the acquisition of knowledge is used here as a theoretical guide to support and advance this argument. Vygotsky (1962) argued that individuals move from their *actual potential state* in terms of knowledge and thinking to their *full potential*. He described teachers as guides who create an environment conducive to learning in which students grow towards their potential. Vygotsky (1962) used the analogy of intellectual 'scaffolding' that teachers erect to enable individuals to incrementally climb to reach their full potential. He further argued that each individual is unique. Therefore, each 'scaffold' must be different to match the person's exclusive needs (Reid and Long, 1993).

This concept of 'scaffolding' has been transposed to mental health nursing where it symbolically illustrates the healing steps that people negotiate on their journey from *actual* emotional pain towards their emotional and spiritual *potential*. It makes sense that following their own explorations during self-awareness programmes, nurses should have the ability to erect an 'emotional scaffold' containing unique healing steps for each of their clients to symbolically climb. This is a highly complex process but it is well worth the effort, as it is the phase at which the healing process begins to evolve (Long and Reid, 1996). Before erecting emotional scaffolding it is important for nurses to have an informed knowledge of various social interaction sequences that may be recognised in clients'

behaviours and that require nurses to respond in therapeutic ways and at the appropriate times (Hargie *et al.*, 1994). For example, sensitive nurses will know intuitively which healing step of the 'emotional scaffold' they should stand on when their clients are climbing. There will be times when nurses should stand on the same healing step as clients, directly beside them and become *a second self*. This movement may be required when people are unconscious, dying or have just attempted suicide (Long and Reid, 1996). At other times, nurses will know to stand on the healing step just ahead of clients, quietly motivating them, while anticipating and proactively attending to their needs. While on this healing step, people will often ask for guidance in a symbolic way by putting their hand out towards nurses. Interestingly, if nurses are too many steps ahead of people in terms of recovery, knowledge and perfect mental health, they may be too far forward for the person to make an emotional connection with them.

Compassionate nurses will know when to stand on the healing step directly behind clients, gently 'nudging' them towards independence, recovery, and potential. Of equal importance, there are times when people need to stand still and rest for a while as they embrace their emotional pain. Compassionate nurses will know to '*be there*' for them and '*be there*' with them on the same healing step of the 'emotional scaffold' while entering into quiet moments of communion or togetherness with them. Examples of this type of emotional connecting can be observed at funerals, where emotional support is that provided to those grieving – mainly by the presence of others – and is that which usually takes place in an ambience of silence. When nurses demonstrate this type of awareness it conveys to people that they have embraced human principles and qualities that empower them to accompany individuals up the healing steps of the emotional 'scaffold' of life – hence facilitating them towards their full potential (Long, 1998).

Reid and Long (1993) and Long and Reid (1996) in their research regarding nurses' attitudes to the nursing care of suicidal persons, found that nurses had great difficulty standing on the 'same step of the scaffold' as people who wished to take their own lives. The authors claimed that this group of nurses' inability to utilise therapeutic communication skills and accurate empathy might have become blocked as the result of their own belief and value systems about life and death issues as well as their personal interpretations regarding the fundamental meaning and purpose of life.

An interesting proposal forwarded by Long and Reid (1996) related to the theoretical speculation where people refer to having '*lost the will to live*', either owing to personal changes or because of unbearable life situations. Long and Reid (1996) advanced Assagoli's (1978) theoretical work on the development of the 'will' and suggested that nurses should be taught how to become confident enough to allow people to borrow their 'will to live' during those initial and critical days following suicide attempts. At times such as these, nurses should be standing on the step just behind people on the emotional 'scaffold' while gently motivating them to continue with their lives. Albert Camus (1983) had this to say:

> *Do not walk before me I may not follow*
> *Do not walk behind me I may not lead*
> *But, [nurses] walk beside me and be my*
> *friend.*
>
> (Canus, 1983, p. 53)

The proposition that nurses should build healing steps that form 'emotional scaffolding' intersects with Maslow's (1987) study of human nature. This work led Maslow to many conclusions, including the fundamental notion that human beings have an innate tendency to move towards higher levels of health, creativity and self-fulfilment. Both self-actualisation and health are synonymous and they have been defined by Maslow (1987) as:

> *The coming to pass of the fullest humanness,*
> *or as the being of the person, it is as if self-*

> *actualizing creativity (health) were almost*
> *synonymous with, or a sine qua non aspect*
> *of, or a defining characteristic of essential*
> *humanness.*
>
> (Maslow, 1987, p. 167)

It is difficult to become fully human when people are enduring emotional pain, especially when their depths are not available to them (Long, 1997a, b, c, 1998). Mental health nurses can co-travel with people on this journey by encouraging them to rediscover their natural path towards self-actualising and self-fulfilment. To facilitate healing, therefore, 'there is nothing that has to be done – there is only someone to be' (Small, 1987, p. 113).

The dance of recovery

As well as erecting emotional 'scaffolding' to enable people to climb towards their potential, nurses should be prepared to 'emotionally connect' with them in a 'healing' dance, a type of emotional interactional synchrony (Bee, 1998). This construct refers to a form of behaviour that is a characteristic of human communication. Whenever two people of the same culture group talk with each other a detailed analysis of their movements shows that they engage in a kind of dance with each other (Long, 1999). People are generally unaware that they engage in this complex dance routine, but it goes on nonetheless. It is fair to say that within the nurse–person relationship, both people involved belong to the same culture of emotional pain. However, in the dance of recovery, clients should be encouraged to take the lead.

At times, clients may guide the healing dance backwards, in other words they may regress (Freud, 1974). Caring nurses should not be afraid to risk entering into the essential spiralling movements of the various steps, taking cognisance of the emotional tempo and tapping into the emotional rhythm, while listening – with accurate empathy – to the music behind clients' thoughts, feelings and behaviours. It is also important for nurses to listen for other, perhaps hidden, agendas (unconscious defence mechanisms). Examples of these defence mechanisms are:

- stagefright, that is resistance (Waltzlawick, 1994)
- falling backwards, that is regression (Freud, 1974)
- blaming the world, other people or the nurse for their inability to move on, that is projection (Freud, 1974)
- laughing about the sadness of the music, that is repression (Freud, 1974).

Furthermore, nurses must also realise that people may mistrust them with certain aspects of their lives. The naive observer may label this complex construct as 'paranoia'. However, within the ethos of the person-valuing paradigm, mistrust might indicate that some people are not aware that nurses have the essential 'core, human' care qualities that enable them to enter into and sustain therapeutic dialogue, especially if quality time is not available and only social chit-chat is engaged in.

At a deeper and more profound level, nurses may also face the paradox of being guided backwards into the Sathya – the truth – which rests within the recesses of unknown and unseen territories of the mind (i.e. the unconscious) (Freud, 1974). Sathya, or truth, is what human beings search for and this notion has been depicted in a charismatic way by Browning (1812–1889) in *Paraclesus*, part 1:

> *Truth is within ourselves: it takes no rise*
> *from outward things, whatever you believe.*
> *There is an inmost centre in us all,*
> *Where truth abides in fullness; and around,*
> *Wall upon wall, the gross flesh hems us in,*
> *This perfect, clear perception – which is truth.*
>
> (Browning, 1812–89)

Nurses should not be afraid to journey with people into and through their pain, as knowledge and insight into the truth within sets them free – to *become* themselves (Long, 1999; Long

and Slevin, 1999). As painful and torturous as the emotional pain may be, it can show the way to the truth. Individuals will not, cannot, give up their search until they know and understand what it all means (Long, 1997a, b, c). Emotional pain is the doorway to 'self' and the truth about 'self' becomes the light at the end of the journey (Long, 1997b). Ultimately, making an emotional connection with another (the nurse) and climbing the healing steps of the emotional 'scaffold' and participating in 'the dance of recovery' is a revelation, a sacred, spiritual pilgrimage, it is supremely, the process of *'becoming a person'* (Roger, 1990).

It is crucially important that nurses take cognisance of three more premises. First, they should never flee from emotional pain, nor deny its existence. Nurses may take solace from Levine (1987) who claimed:

> *I cannot assuage your pain with any word,*
> *nor should I. Not that she … or I would*
> *inflict such pain by choice, but there it is.*
> *And it must burn its purifying way to*
> *completion … For something in you dies*
> *when you bear the unbearable. And it is only*
> *in the dark night of the soul, that you are*
> *prepared to see as God sees and love as God*
> *loves.*
>
> (Levine, 1987, p. 144)

Second, it is important that both the nurse and the client realise that healing does not mean discovering utopia, although it does represent a greater sense of mental health and well-being, based on spiritual insights and the emergence of an even more human-like identity (Long, 1997b, 1998). Paradoxically, to be spiritual means to be fully human and the converse is also true, with all its pain and beauty, sickness and health, living and dying (Long, 1997b). Nonetheless, as the result of working through the healing process with mental health nurses, people can begin to see themselves against the backdrop of a bigger picture – the wholeness of the human family (Long, 1997b).

Third, emotional pain should never be viewed with a keyhole mentality or as a series of still-shots, because the specific contents of painful experiences differ greatly from person to person.

SUMMARY

Nurses who have worked effectively in self-awareness programmes are in an ideal position to help people to listen to and explore their life stories of emotional pain and distress. 'One cannot choose wisely in life unless he dares to listen to himself, his own self, at each moment in life' (Maslow, 1987, p. xxxlll).

Nurses, as clinicians and clients, as people with emotional pain, hold the pivotal position – within the therapeutic encounter. 'For me the rainbow interprets this … the glory shining between two people which can exist only between them. Each human relationship should be … a glorious rainbow' (Lawrence, 1936). It must be stressed, however, that nurses need to be adequately prepared for this unique role. It is essential for nurses to work towards entering the client's world without expecting them to enter the world of professionals. Some people attend doctors in order to be prescribed a cure when, in reality, they bring their own cure with them in terms of the powerful healing resources that reside within every individual.

REFERENCES

Argyle, M. (1997) *The Psychology of Happiness*, Methuen, London

Assagoli, R. (1978) *Psychosynthesis*, Viking, New York

Baxter, R. (1999) Secrets and lies. In: Long, A. (ed.) *Interaction for Practice in Community Nursing*, Macmillan, London

Bee, H. (1998) *The Developing Child*, Harper Row, New York

Browning, R. (1812–1889) *Paraclesus*. In: Hawes, D. (ed.) *Poems Compared*, Bell and Hyman, London

Bruner, J. (1987) Life as narrative, *Social Research* 54, 11–32

Buber, M. (1970) *I and Thou*, T&T Clark, Edinburgh

Bushfield, J. (1996) *Men, Women and Madness: Understanding gender and mental disorder*, Macmillan, London

Camus, A. (1983) *The Outsider*, Penguin Classic, Harmondsworth

Crowe, M. (1996) Cutting up: signifying the unspeakable. *Australia New Zealand Journal of Mental Health Nursing* 5(3), 103–11

Erikson, E. (1978) *Dimensions of a Man*, Norton, New York

Freud, S. (1974) *The Standard Edition of the Complete Psychological Work of Sigmund Freud*, Vols 1–24, Hogarth, London

Hargie, O., Saunders, C. and Dickson, D. (1994) *Social Skills and Interpersonal Communication*, Routledge, London

Heidegger, M. (1962) *On Being and Acting: From principles to anarchy* (trans. R. Shurrnann), Indiana University Press, Bloomington

Hinton, W.L. and Levkoff, S. (1999) Constructing Alzheimers' narratives of lost identities, confusion and loneliness in old age. *Culture, Medicine and Psychiatry* 23(4), 453–75

Jung, C.G. (1958) *Modern Man in Search of Soul*, Constable, London

Kapur, R. (1999) Unconscious communication. In: Long, A. (ed.) *Interaction for Practice in Community Nursing*, Macmillan, London

Klein, M. (1969) *The Writings of Melanie Klein*, Vol. 3, Hogarth, London

Kleinman, A. (1988) *The Illness Narratives: Suffering, healing and the human condition*, Basic Books, New York

Lawrence, D.H. (1936) *Lady Chatterly's Lover*, Penguin, Harmondsworth

Levine, M. (1987) *Who Dies?* Anchor Books, New York

Long, A. (1995) Community mental health nursing. In: Sines, D. (ed.) *Community Health Care Nursing*, Blackwell Science, Oxford

Long, A. (1997a) Loss: the journey to recovery. *Journal of the British Association of Counselling* 6(1), 13–4

Long, A. (1997b) Nursing: a spiritual perspective. *International Journal of Nursing Ethics* 4(6), 496–510

Long, A. (1997c) Avoiding abuse amongst vulnerable groups in the community: people with a mental illness. In: Mason, C. (ed.) *Achieving Quality in Community Health Care Nursing*, Macmillan, London

Long, A. (1998) The healing process, the road to recovery and positive mental health. *Journal of Psychiatric and Mental Health Nursing* 7(4), 1–9

Long, A. (1999) *Interaction for Practice in Community Nursing*, Macmillan, London

Long, A. (2001) Mental health nursing. In: Sines, D., Appleby, F. and Raymond, E. (eds) *Community Healthcare Nursing*, Blackwell Science, Oxford

Long, A. and Chambers, M. (1993) Mental health in action. *Senior Nurse* 13(5), 7–9

Long, A. and Reid, W. (1996) An exploration of nurses' attitudes to the nursing care of the suicidal patient. *Journal of Psychiatric and Mental Health Nursing* 3(1), 29–37

Long, A. and Slevin, E. (1999) Living with dementia: caring for an older person and her family. *International Journal of Nursing Ethics* 6(1), 23–36

Maslow, A. (1987) *Personality and Motivation*, Harper and Row, New York

Miller, A. (1983a) *The Drama of the Gifted Child*, Basic Books, New York

Miller, A. (1983b) *For Your Own Good*, Farrar, Straus and Giroux, New York

Mishler, E.G. (1986) *Research Interviewing: Context and narrative*, Harvard University Press, Cambridge, MA

Oilier, J. (1992) *No Boundary*, Shambhala, Boulder, CO

Penn, P. (1982) Circular questioning. *Family Process* 21, 267–80

Polkinghorne, D. (1996) Transformative narratives: from victimic to agentic life plots. *American Journal of Occupational Therapy* 50(4), 299–305

Powell, J. (1977) *Why am I Afraid to Love?* Fontana Collins, Glasgow

Reid, W. and Long, A. (1993) Therapeutic approaches to the nursing care of the suicidal patient. *Journal of Advanced Nursing* 18, 1369–76

Roger, C.R. (1990) *Client Centred Therapy*, Constable, London

Sarason, S. and Duck, S. (2001) *Community and Clinical Psychology*, Routledge, London

Saris, A.J. (1995) Telling stories: life histories, illness narratives and institutional landscapes. *Culture, Medicine and Psychiatry* 19, 39–72

Slevin, O. (1999) The nurse–patient relationship. In: Long, A. (ed.) *Advanced Interaction in Community Nursing*, Macmillan, London

Smale, R. (2000) Peering through the darkness: the subjective experience of clinical depression. *Journal of Psychiatric and Mental Health Nursing* 7, 227–83

Small, J. (1987) *Transformers*, Devors, California

Sparkes, A. (1994) Life histories and the issue of voice: reflections on an emerging relationship. *International Journal of Qualitative Studies in Education* 7, 165–83

Spender, D. (1995) *Man Made Language*, Routledge and Kegan Paul, London

Sternberg, R.J. (1995) *In Search of the Human Mind*, Harcourt Brace, Texas, IL

Szasz, T. (1961) *The Myth of Mental Illness*, Harper, New York

Thorne, S. (1994) Person-centred counselling. In: Dryden, W. and Feltman, C. (eds) *Individual Therapy*, Open University Press, Milton Keynes

Vygotsky, L. (1962) *Thoughts and Language*, MIT Press, Cambridge, Mass

Waltzlawick, W. (1994) *Change: The principle of problem formation and problem resolution*, Norton, New York

White, M. and Epston, D. (1990) *Narrative Means to Therapeutic Ends*, Norton, New York

40 LEARNING DISABILITY NURSING

Eamonn Slevin

LEARNING OUTCOMES

After studying this chapter you will be able to:

- Understand what learning disability is
- Become familiar with what learning disability nurses do
- Discuss the central philosophical and theoretical aspects that underpin learning disability nursing
- Be aware of trends and policy that influence the care of people with learning disabilities.

Various Study Activities are presented throughout the chapter. These are designed to allow you to reflect on your understanding of what you read in the chapter. You will be able to undertake these 'thinking' activities as an individual, or alternatively some activities are designed for group work, or for directing what you do in practice.

INTRODUCTION

In this chapter, learning disability nursing is considered. The aim of the chapter is not to attempt to provide a comprehensive account of all that learning disability nurses do. But rather to provide a conceptual discourse of the philosophical and theoretical assumptions that underpin the role and functions of this group of professional carers. In order to enhance understanding, historical factors are considered and current and future policy are overviewed. The focus of learning disability nursing care, i.e. clients who have a learning disability and their family/carers,

is central to all that this group of nurses does. When the term 'client' is used in this chapter, it will most often relate to the client and their family or carer.

WHAT IS LEARNING DISABILITY?

Definitions

It is common, and perhaps of value to professionals, to be able to attach definitions to the client groups they care for. Definitions are also needed to allow for legislation and policy developments. The term *learning disability* in its widest context means that a person has a disability in learning that originates during the developmental stages of their life. The actual cause, if known, might be attributed to an occurrence at the pre-natal, peri-natal or post-natal stages of their development. The cause/s may be due to a chromosomal disorder, genetic, or environmental factors, or a combination of a number of complex and interrelated causes. The focus of this chapter is not to provide a detailed account of these causes; you can consult a text such as Watson (2000) for a detailed discussion on the causes of learning disability.

The overall outcome for the person is that they have a significant learning disability in relation to the following aspects of their life:

- Intelligence is below normal, identified by measurement of their intelligence quotient (IQ).
- They have problems of a significant nature with social skills and development.
- they have a need for support or guidance in some or a number of aspects of their life (*see* Table 40.1).

Table 40.1   ICD-10 classification of learning disability

ICD-10 classification	Approximate IQ range	Mental age in adult	Functional level and likely dependency
Mild	50–69	9 to <12 years	Likely to result in some learning difficulties in school. Many adults will be able to work and maintain good social relationships and contribute to society.
Moderate	35–49	6 to <9 years	Likely to result in marked developmental delays in childhood, but most can learn to develop some degree of independence in self-care and acquire adequate communication and academic skills. Adults will need varying degrees of support to live and work in the community.
Severe	20–34	3 to <6 years	Likely to result in continuous need of support.
Profound	<20	<3 years	Results in severe limitation in self-care, continence, communication and mobility.

Modified from Cooper (1994)

These three aspects might lead to the person having difficulties in a number of areas in their life, such as communication, motor skills, thinking and reasoning, sensory problems, forming relationships or attending to their personal care needs.

Most estimates of the number of people with learning disabilities indicate that 3 people per 1000 will have a learning disability. The prevalence of learning disability has been reported as 3.5 per 1000 of the population in Great Britain. This rate was found to fluctuate according to age as follows: 1.7 per 1000 for 4 year olds and younger, 6.3 per 1000 among 16–19 year olds, with a reduction to 2.8 per 1000 among people over 75 years old (Kavanagh and Opit, 1999).

Study Activity 40.1 ─────────

You will notice that the above aspects and the difficulties they might cause for a person with learning disabilities focus a great deal on the person him/herself.

● Do you think these difficulties might influence other members of society (who do not have a learning disability) in how they think about, feel or act towards someone who has learning disabilities? Discuss this question with a group of your colleagues.

Classification of learning disability

Learning disability can be further defined in terms of various classification systems, e.g. people may be described as having a 'learning disability', or with having a 'severe learning disability' (a two-group classification). There is a four-group International Classification of Diseases (ICD-10) system utilised widely and supported by the World Health Organisation. This system of classifying a person who has a learning disability is presented in Table 40.1.

It will be noticed that the ICD-10 classification is in fact an international diagnosis that places learning disability in a 'disease' category. This system is used widely for research purposes, to identify a person's condition in medical record systems and to facilitate possible identification of needs and treatments that a person may require. There is, however, a philosophical shift in the care of people with learning disabilities away from an over-focus on 'disability' towards a focus on 'ability' and promoting health (this will be discussed in a later section of this chapter).

Study Activity 40.2 _____

First meet with a small group of your colleagues. Arrange that each of you individually reflect on the two statements below, and following a period of thought on these two statements make two lists; one that lists the advantages of a classification system such as the ICD-10, and one that lists the disadvantages. Then meet as a group again, combine your lists, and compare the advantages and disadvantages. Finally, discuss your findings with your lecturer or clinical preceptor.

1 Classification systems are not useful as they place people within pigeonholes from which they may never escape.
2 Classification systems are useful as they can be used to identify nursing dependency levels of clients.

HISTORICAL ASPECTS RELATED TO LEARNING DISABILITY NURSING

In order to understand what learning disability nurses do, it is necessary to have a degree of awareness of historical aspects that have influenced this branch of nursing. Meleis (1997) suggests that nursing in general has undergone many ups and downs on the road to professional recognition. Learning disability nursing as a distinct branch of nursing has perhaps felt more turbulence over the years than the other branches. Emerging from psychiatry, where the care of people with learning disabilities initially rested, learning disability nursing developed. In 1919 the first learning disability nursing certificate was awarded (at that time called a Certificate for Nursing in Mental Deficiency). By the early 1950s, just over 5000 certificates in learning disability nursing had been awarded in Great Britain and Ireland (Mitchell, 1998). There are currently over 26 000 learning disability nurses

registered with the Nursing and Midwifery Council (NMC) within the UK as a whole.

As an emerging profession, learning disability nursing may be considered as a relative fledgling within the general family of nursing. In addition, it has been the focus of debate and uncertainty in terms of its continued existence as a distinct branch of nursing for many years. Mitchell (2000) provides a citation from the Chairman of the General Nursing Council, which stated 'mental deficiency nurses had no claim to be called sick nurses at all'. Some reports have recommended the abolition of learning disability nursing, with social care workers subsuming the care role of people with learning disabilities (Briggs, 1972; Jay, 1979). Every decade or so these issues have been raised.

However, when the UKCC (1986) established its new preparation for practice, *Project 2000*, learning disability nursing was integrated as an essential branch of nursing. The Cullen Report (Cullen, 1991), established by the four UK Chief Nursing Officers to consider the future of this branch of the profession, came out in general support of learning disability nursing and stated 'mental handicap nursing has much to offer as a role model' (Cullen, 1991, p. 10).

Parrish and Sines (1997, p. 1122) comment on how learning disability nurses seem to be 'the only group that is constantly being challenged to justify its existence...'. There are various reasons why learning disability nursing might have faced difficulties in the past, many of which are still present today. Some of these might be that the clients these nurses care for are not 'sick' or 'ill', their needs are quite often grounded in social circumstances and the total family is often the focus of care. Mitchell (2000) presents an interesting and thought-provoking analysis of one reason why learning disability nursing might have met with resistance throughout its history. In his article, 'Parallel stigma?', Mitchell (2000) forwards the suggestion that learning disability nurses may possibly be stigmatised due to their work with learning disabled people. In addition, he asserts that because of an apparent difficulty to adhere to the traditional 'treat and cure' role, learning disability nurses have found themselves marginalised within the general family of nursing.

Study Activity 40.3 _____

Consider the ideas expressed by Mitchell (2000) that learning disability nurses could be marginalised because they care for a group of people who are marginalised. The notion of one group of people facing stigma due to their alliance with another group who are stigmatised has been suggested before, e.g. by Goffman (1963).

- Spend some time on your own asking yourself the questions:

  1 Is Mitchell's assertion of 'stigma by association' a valid view?
  2 Can you think of any other groups of people who might be stigmatised because of their association with a particular group of people?
  3 Why might groups of people, communities or societies might stigmatise individuals or groups who are in some way different to them?

PAST, CURRENT AND FUTURE POLICY

McConkey (1998) suggests that people with learning disabilities have been segregated from others in society for at least 200 years. They, and their families, have been stigmatised and people were placed in institutions, usually for life, because of their disability. A range of policy legislative acts on education, and health and social service treatment policies since the 1880s and into the 1900s, led to slow but steady changes in the education and care of people with learning disabilities (Education Act, Department of Education, 1944, 1970) and (National Health Act, DHSS, 1949; Mental Health Act, Department of Health, 1983). These are only some of the reports. The influence of these for people with learning disabilities took many years to have impact. From the early education legislation of the 1800s that considered people with

learning disabilities to be uneducable, it took until the 1970 Education Act before opinion changed and the education of people with learning disabilities transferred from the health service to education authorities.

As with education provision, the various health and mental health legislations took many years to impact on the lives of people with learning disabilities. Early legislation dealt mainly with compulsory admission to hospital, guardianship, issues surrounding sexual conduct and terminology used to describe people with learning disabilities. For example, labels used to describe people with learning disabilities such as 'idiot' and 'imbecile' were replaced with 'feeble-minded', then 'subnormality' came into vogue (DHSS, 1959) followed by the term 'mental handicap' (DHSS, 1983). At the beginning of this new millennium, the term 'learning disability' is in vogue (Department of Health, 2001), but there is no reason to believe that in future years this term will also not take on a disparaging connotation.

What took place in the various social and policy evolutionary changes in the care of people with learning disabilities was separation of the care for this client group from that of psychiatry where it originally rested. Hospitals for people with learning disabilities developed separately from those for people with mental illness. This was seen as a positive step in service provision for people with learning disabilities. But as the years progressed, the negative effects of institutional living led to social and political pressure to move towards 'community care'. The greatest pressure for the transfer of care was not from governments and service employed policy makers, but from society, and in particular 'from parents and disabled people themselves' (McConkey, 1998, p. 72). It was recognised that people with learning disabilities had a right to live as others did in the general community. This social movement was also influenced by care philosophies in the USA and the Scandinavian countries (Nirji, 1969; Wolfensberger, 1983); these will be discussed in the next section. The net outcome was the acceptance by government of the need to promote community care for people with learning disabilities. Mulvey (1995), referring to the changes in the care of people with learning disabilities, comments on how the old Victorian hospital buildings are closing and a new era of community care is evolving.

Study Activity 40.4 ———————

It is stated above that there were negative effects of institutional living for people with learning disabilities. With a group of colleagues discuss what these negative effects might be.

———————————————————

The future care provision for people with learning disabilities is going to change a great deal. The report *Continuing the Commitment* (Department of Health, 1995), suggested that learning disability nurses should provide a health promotion focus, explicate their role to service users, empower clients and provide evidence-based interventions. The report, *Valuing People: A new strategy for learning disability for the 21st century* (Department of Health, 2001), forwards a number of principles and recommendations to guide future learning disability services (some of these will be expanded upon in the next section). *Valuing People* recognises the valuable input that the learning disability nurses can make. For example, in relation to health facilitation, the report states 'learning disability nurses will be well placed to fulfil this role' (Department of Health, 2001, p. 63).

PHILOSOPHICAL AND THEORETICAL ASSUMPTIONS

Due to the changing nature of current health care, there have been a number of changes in the philosophical and theoretical assumptions that underpin learning disability nursing. National policy and social change dictate that the locus of care of people with learning disabilities is transferring to the community. Learning disability nurses are adapting to meet the changing needs

of the people they care for (Parrish and Sines, 1997); the development of the community nurse for people with a learning disability is an example of a service response to the demands of community care.

The concept of 'clinical specialist', although recognised in the USA since the 1940s, is relatively new in the UK, only being recognised in the 1980s (Bousfield, 1997). It is characterised by reflective practice based in research, graduate education and a firm base in an applied specialist area (Bousfield, 1997). The community nurse for people with a learning disability is a recognised specialist in providing community care. Learning disability nurses may also become specialists in caring for people with learning disabilities who exhibit challenging behaviours, or who have a co-existing mental health problem. A clinical nurse specialist is equipped to 'intervene in more depth with more complex problems within a well defined speciality' (Dunn, 1997, p. 815). Learning disability nurses need to reflect on the care they provide and through use of reflection in practice articulate their unique role.

Kay (1995, p. 96) states 'the research base in our knowledge and understanding of learning disabilities comes from the professions of psychology, medicine and education'. This is indeed the case and much of the care of people with learning disabilities has been influenced strongly by philosophical assumptions that are grounded in the wider social sciences. A good example of this is the movement that has its routes in care philosophies in the USA and the Scandinavian countries (Nirji, 1969; Wolfensberger, 1983). These were known as 'normalisation', later changed to 'social role valorisation' by Wolfensberger as he felt there was a misunderstanding of the aims of normalisation. Following on from these, John O'Brien suggested the phrase 'ordinary life principles'. O'Brien forwarded what became known as 'five accomplishments' that services and professionals should strive to achieve in the care of people with learning disabilities. The five are choice, relationships, dignity and esteem, participation and integration, and competence (O'Brien and

Lyle, 1987). As indicated by O'Brien, these five aspects can be used by all professionals to measure the effectiveness of their interventions. The five principles provide a framework that learning disability nurses can use to guide their practice (*see* Fig. 40.1), and to evaluate the effectiveness of their interventions.

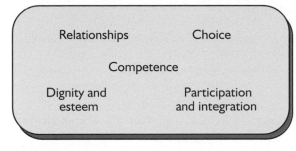

Relationships   Choice

Competence

Dignity and   Participation
esteem   and integration

Figure 40.1 The accomplishment framework (O'Brien and Lyle, 1987)

All the five elements in this framework are principles for empowered community living. Competence is placed in the centre, as a major role of the nurse is to use strategies and skills to enhance the competence of clients. This in turn empowers the client to make choices, form relationships and participate in their community with the ultimate outcome being affirmation of their dignity and self-esteem.

While it is appropriate that nursing should draw on an eclecticism of theory from other professions for its knowledge base, like all areas of nursing, learning disability nursing needs to develop its own discrete knowledge base. Many learning disability nurses still work in the hospital setting. Hospitals for people with learning disabilities will change dramatically over the coming years. They will no longer operate as 'long-stay institutions', many will close and those that remain will be much smaller in size and they will operate as specialist hospitals for short-term treatment and assessment. The division between these hospitals and community care will become blurred as a seamless service evolves. Learning disability nurses should not feel threatened by this, rather they should see it as an opportunity to develop their unique specialist skills. Clarke and

Cody (1994, p. 41) go as far as to suggest that 'Nursing theory-based practice is not feasible in institutions where medical orders overshadow all other disciplines'. To emphasise this point, Clarke and Cody (1994) compare the four meta-paradigm concepts that are the central concern of nursing – person, environment, health and nursing (Table 40.2).

Study Activity 40.5

With colleagues discuss the views of Clarke and Cody. If learning disability nursing is not overshadowed by medical orders, do you think clients will be advantaged, and if so how?

When care is transferred to a community setting, the four elements of the metaparadigm of nursing are directed by a changed contextual philosophy, as depicted in Table 40.2. The concept of 'client' takes on a broader meaning, in that family and even community, are considered as the client.

'Environment' is not seen in terms of a clinical or medical milieu. In the hospital setting the client adapts to the hospital environment, and this often leads to institutionalisation. In a community setting the opposite is the case in that the learning disability nurse needs to possess and apply the knowledge and skills required to adapt to the client's environment.

'Health' in the comparison between hospital and community also has a different focus, as can be seen in Table 40.2 (overleaf). Health does not focus on old definitions based on the medical model, i.e. 'absence of disease', but rather on the promotion of health and the social well-being of the client (in the broadest sense). The role of the learning disability nurse therefore moves to that of the promotion of quality of life from a holistic perspective.

'Nursing', as can be seen in Table 40.2, moves from dominance by medicine in a hospital setting to one of autonomous practice in the community setting. Elder (1996, p. 34) states 'Nurses can be instrumental in helping to reso-

Table 40.2 Comparison of metaparadigm concepts in hospital and home settings

Metaparadigm concept setting (home)	Hospital setting	Community setting (home)
Human being	Less than 1% of the population, separated from family and labelled with a disease entity	Over 95% of the population; person and family as client; group or community as client; personal and cultural identity easily seen
Environment	Standardised room, ward or specialised unit; a work setting for health care professionals, with access severely limited for most others (such as family and friends)	Natural sociocultural, and symbolic environment shared with family and community in dynamic interchange with human being. The client and environment cannot be separated and are not mutually exclusive
Health	Dichotomised with illness; considered its polar opposite and as such the goal of care; when health is objectively appraised as good the person is ejected (in the case of the learning disabled person this may be continued containment)	Includes illness as an aspect of life; goal of care most often viewed as the quality of life experienced by the person, family or community
Nursing	Activities largely delegated by physicians; centred on treatment of illness through medication, technology, predictable interventions	Largely autonomous practice; interventions tend to be mutually negotiated with clients, based on client values and require broad knowledge on the nurse's part; orientated towards quality of life

(From Clarke and Cody, 1994)

cialize families from a "treatment by professionals" model to a co-operative educational model'. This brings with it a major philosophical shift in responsibility and accountability. There is also a move towards shared planning with the client and family which involves the learning disability nurse who becomes more autonomous, sharing this new found autonomy with the client and family. Thus, the learning disability nurse is an empowered practitioner in the community and he/she in turn empowers the client and family.

The report, *Valuing People: A new strategy for learning disability for the 21st century* (Department of Health, 2001), forwards a number of principles and recommendations that are reminiscent of the care philosophies presented here. Some of these recommendations for people with learning disabilities are: enhancing choice, improving health, promoting partnerships, improving the quality of services, supporting carers, social inclusion, promoting equality and facilitating life transitions, i.e. child to adoles-

cent, to adult, to old age, in all aspects of life, social, recreational and occupational. To monitor and achieve this, 'person-centred planning' will be utilised for all people with learning disabilities and their families. This approach involves placing the client and family in a pivotal position and planning care not only *for* them but *with* them.

AN EXPLICATION OF THE ROLE OF LEARNING DISABILITY NURSING

The above discussion clearly indicates that learning disability nurses will need to have and continue to develop specialist skills. But there has undoubtedly been a past failure of the learning disability nursing profession to clearly explicate its role. There are reasons for this, for example the tacit and often intangible nature of what these nurses do for clients, which some refer to as invisible care (Parrish and Sines, 1997). The idea of 'invisible care' is not unique to learning disability nursing. Slevin and Buckenham (1992) suggest that it exists to an extent in all branches of nursing. The concept of the 'intuitive practitioner' also suggests an indiscernible element in nursing care provision (Benner, 1984; Benner and Tanner, 1987). Kitson (1987, p. 328) has referred to this as nursing's 'Achilles heel' and she suggests the need to demonstrate the therapeutic value of nursing interventions. Birchenall *et al.* (1993), commenting on learning disability nursing, suggest that failure to clearly define roles has 'misled many to consider that an untrained workforce ... would do the job as effectively'.

Study Activity 40.6 ──────────

With colleagues, organise a debate on the above citation by Birchenall et al. (1993).

───────────────

Some authors have responded admirably to the challenge of explicating the learning disability nurse's role. Baldwin and Birchenall (1993) present a framework for the role of learning disability nursing. They utilise Beck *et al.*'s (1988) holistic model of care that involves the overlapping elements of physical, emotional, intellectual, social and spiritual care. No single one of these elements takes precedence over the other as it is their interconnectedness within individuals which emphasises the 'holistic' nature of the model. Rather than remain at this abstract level of explicitness, which is what has frequently created difficulty in the identification of the role of the learning disability nurse, Baldwin and Birchenall (1993) build on this and develop a framework. The framework describes six roles of the learning disability nurse as: therapist, educator, manager, advocate, counsellor and clinician, which have been adapted from Peplau's (1952) role categories (Birchenall *et al.*, 1993). They then list the competencies of each of these roles within the nursing process framework. A commendable aspect of this model is that Baldwin and Birchenall (1993) do not 'pigeonhole' the clinician role of the nurse as

performing clinical procedures. This role is viewed by them as that which:

> *integrates theory and practice ... [by incorporating] a focus of care that covers all aspects of an individual's life i.e. the holistic health focus.*
>
> (Baldwin and Birchenall, 1993, p. 851)

The care of people with learning disabilities and their families is so complex that no one professional could provide all the care that they require. The learning disability nurse works as a central member of the multidisciplinary team with a range of other professionals and there is no doubt teamworking will continue to be a key skill requirement of this group of nurses. In the future, the term 'multidisciplinary' might well become redundant with regard to people with learning disabilities. A better term might be a 'co-operative team', i.e. one that involves people with learning disabilities and their carers/families as central players in all aspects of care.

While the issue of being an advocate is questionable for nurses, as they may frequently have to advocate for clients against the service that employs the nurse, Grace (2001) suggests that nurses are best positioned to take on a 'professional advocacy' role. Grace further suggests that this is at two levels, that of the individual client and at a micro-society level. Not forgetting the many difficulties learning disability nurses have faced that have been alluded to previously in this chapter, the learning disability nurse should also act as an advocate for the profession. Closely aligned to the skills needed to act as an advocate are those of leadership. Learning disability nurses now, and will in the future, need to have leadership skills.

Learning disability nurses will need knowledge and skills to use models of care that emphasise 'person-centred planning' for people with learning disabilities. It is beyond the scope of this chapter to detail the numerous approaches that fall within the general family of person-centred planning. Table 40.3 provides a listing of some approaches and you can consult the

Table 40.3 Approaches to person-centred planning

Approach	Underpinnings	Reference
Individual programme planning	Involves assessing, target setting and evaluation. Multi-disciplinary input is utilised. Not always regarded as person-centred planning	Crosby, 1976
Shared action planning	Small group planning, carer and client participation in plans of care, needs identified but wishes also considered. Relationships, vision planning and aims set.	Brechin and Swain, 1987
Essential life planning	Involves assessing aspects essential to life (positive and negative). Client involved in assessment, plan and implementation. Review meetings guide the process.	Smull and Burke-Harrison, 1992
Personal future plans	Used to plan for transitions from childhood to adulthood (mainly used in the USA).	Everson, 1996
Planning alternative tomorrows with hope	Used to plan and guide life changes, e.g. moving out of long-stay hospital.	Flavey et al., 1994

references to obtain further information on these.

Carper (1978) presented four patterns of knowing that offer a framework to encapsulate the role of nursing: empirics, aesthetics, ethics, and personal knowledge. These four patterns also frame what learning disability nurses do and the knowledge they need. These are discussed here as separate entities to facilitate their presentation, but in practice learning disability nurses will integrate all four patterns into their nursing actions.

Empirics

The learning disability nurse of today and the future will need to support their practice by evidence. Evidence-based practice in learning disability nursing requires specialist skills and knowledge. This knowledge is in two respects, one is the knowledge of how to find, critique and decide on the value of approaches to care (research knowledge), the second is the knowledge and skills to use the care approaches. Both of these endeavours require from the nurse a commitment to lifelong learning.

Some of the things learning disability nurses do are communicating, risk analysis, person-centred planning, and educating others. They will need to have knowledge and skills in various therapeutic interventions such as behavioural management, cognitive-behavioural therapy counselling, structured teaching approaches and family therapy. The learning disability nurse will also need advanced skills in ergonomic and environmental assessment to advise on residential living.

Aesthetics

Aesthetics may be considered the art of nursing and, thus, how skilled a nurse is at 'caring', and it relates to how he/she applies this skill. Johnson (1994) identifies five aspects that relate to the 'art' of nursing.

Grasping meaning

This has to do with a nurse's ability to observe and assess, and it has to do with feelings, imagination and understanding. Thus, it relates to self-awareness in the learning disability nurse and the ability of the nurse to see and understand the client holistically.

Connecting with clients

This involves the nurse being able to connect with the person with a learning disability at all

SUMMARY

Learning disability nursing has travelled a long distance since its inception, and it has faced many challenges. It is to the credit of this professional group that they have so often risen to these challenges and that they remain a unified strong branch of nursing. Also of credit to this group of nurses is their consistent wish to align themselves with the clients they care for and their carers/families.

There are going to be major changes in the care of people with learning disabilities in the future and there seems little doubt that learning disability nurses will play a key role in service provision. This group of nurses has offered a great deal in the past to the quality of life of the clients they care for and they will continue to do so in the future. In addition, learning disability nursing has much to offer to the general family of nursing.

REFERENCES

Baldwin, S. and Birchenall, M. (1993) The nurse's role in caring for people with learning disabilities, *British Journal of Nursing* **2**(17), 850–4

Beck, C.M., Rawlings, R.P. and Williams, S.R. (1988) *Mental Health Psychiatric Nursing* (2nd edn), C. V. Mosby, St Louis, IL

Benner, P. (1984) *From Novice to Expert: Excellence and power in clinical nursing*, Addison-Wesley, Menlo Park, CA

Benner, P. and Tanner, C. (1987) How expert nurses use intuition, *American Journal of Nursing* **8**(1), 23–31

Birchenall, P.D., Baldwin, S. and Birchenall, M. (1993) Preparing the advanced practitioner in learning disabilities nursing. *Nurse Education Today* **13**(4), 250–8

Bousfield, C. (1997) A phenomenological investigation into the role of the clinical nurse specialist. *Journal of Advanced Nursing* **25**(2), 245–56

Brechin, A. and Swain, J. (1987) *Changing Relationships: Shared action planning with people with a mental handicap*, Harper and Row, London

Briggs, A. (1972) *Report of the Committee of Nursing*, HMSO, London

Carper, B.A. (1978) Fundamental patterns of knowing in nursing, *Advances in Nursing Science* **1**(1), 13–23

Clarke, P.N. and Cody, W.K. (1994) Nursing theory-based practice in the home and community: the crux of professional nursing education. *Advances in Nursing Science* **17**(2), 41–53

Cooper, J.E. (1994) *Pocket Guide to ICD-10 Classification of Mental and Behavioural Disorders*, WHO, Geneva

Crosby, K.G. (1976) Essentials of active programming, *Mental Retardation* **14**(2), 3–9

Cullen, C. (1991) *Caring for People: Community care in the next decade and beyond – mental handicap nursing*, Department of Health, London

Department of Education (1944) *Education Act*, HMSO, London

Department of Education (1970) *Education Act (Handicapped Children)*, HMSO, London

Department of Health (1995) *Continuing the Commitment – The report of the learning disability nursing project*, HMSO, London

Department of Health (2001) *Valuing People: A new strategy for learning disability for the 21st century*, HMSO, London

DHSS (1949) *National Health Act*, HMSO, London

DHSS (1959) *Mental Health Act*, HMSO, London

DHSS (1983) *Mental Health Act*, HMSO, London

Dunn, L. (1997) A literature review of advanced clinical nursing practice in the United States of America. *Journal of Advanced Nursing* **25**(4), 815–9

Elder, J.H. (1996) Behavioural treatment of children with autism, mental retardation, and related disabilities: ethics and efficacy, *Journal of Child and Adolescent Psychiatric Nursing* **9**(3), 28–36

Everson, J. (1996) Using person-centred planning concepts to enhance school-to-adult life transition planning. *Journal of Vocational Rehabilitation* **6**(1), 7–13

Flavey, M., Forest, M., Pearpoint, J. *et al.* (1994) Building connections. In: Thousand, J., Villa, J. and Nevin, E. (eds) *Creativity and Collaborative Learning*, Paul H. Brookes, Baltimore, Mass

Goffman, E. (1963) *Stigma: Notes on the management of spoiled identity*, Penguin, Harmondsworth

Grace, P.J. (2001) Professional advocacy: widening the scope of accountability. *Nursing Philosophy* **2**, 151–62

Jay, P. (1979) *Mental Handicap Nursing and Care*, HMSO, London

Jenkins, R. (2000) Use of psychotropic medication in people with a learning disability. *British Journal of Nursing* 9(13), 844–50

Johnson, J. (1994) A dialectical examination of nursing art. *Advances in Nursing Science* 17(1), 1–14

Kavanagh, S.M. and Opit, L.J. (1999) The prevalence and balance of care for intellectual disability: secondary analysis of the OPCS disability surveys. *Journal of Applied Research in Intellectual Disabilities* 12, 127–48

Kay, B. (1995) Grasping the research nettle in learning disability nursing. *British Journal of Nursing* 4(2), 96–8

Slevin, O. and Buckenham, M. (eds) (1992) *A New Curriculum for Care. Project 2000: The teachers speak – innovations in the nursing curriculum*, Campion Press, Edinburgh, pp. 57–88.

Kitson, A.L. (1987) Raising the standards of clinical practice. *Journal of Advanced Nursing* 12(3), 321–9

McConkey, R. (1998) Community integration. In: Fraser, W., Sines, D. and Kerr, M. (eds) *Hallas' – The care of people with intellectual disabilities*, Butterworth-Heinemann, Oxford, pp. 69–89.

Meleis, A. (1997) *Theoretical Nursing Development and Progress* (2nd edn), J.B. Lippincott, Philadelphia, IL

Mitchell, D. (1998) The origins of learning disability nursing. *International History of Nursing Journal* 4(1), 10–16

Mitchell, D. (2000) Parallel stigma? Nurses and people with learning disabilities. *British Journal of Learning Disabilities* 28(2), 78–81

Mulvey, J. (1995) An overview of learning disabilities. In: Holt, G., Yan, K. and Bouras, N. (eds) *Mental Health in Learning Disabilities*, Pavilion, Brighton, pp. 3–9

Nirji, B. (1969) The normalization principle and its human management implications. In: Kugel, R.B. and Wolfensberger, W. (eds) *Changing Patterns of Residential Services for the Mentally Retarded*, Presidential Committee on Mental Retardation, Washington, DC

O'Brien, J. and Lyle, C. (1987) *Framework for Accomplishments*, Responsive Systems Service, Decatur, GA

Parrish, A. and Sines, D. (1997) Future directions for learning disabilities nursing. *British Journal of Nursing* 6(19), 1122–4

Peplau, H. (1952) *Interpersonal Relationships in Nursing*, G. P. Putnam, New York

Rogers, M.E. (1990) Martha Rogers' theoretical framework for nursing. In: Parker, E.M. (ed.) *Nursing Theories in Practice*, National League for Nursing, New York, pp. 5–11

Smull, M. and Burke-Harrison, S. (1992) *Supporting People with Severe Reputations in the Community*, National Association of State Directors of Developmental Disabilities, Virginia

United Kingdom Central Council (1986) *Project 2000: A new preparation for practice*, United Kingdom Central Council, London

Watson, D. (2000) Causes and manifestations. In: Gates, B. (ed.) *Learning Disabilities* (3rd edn), Churchill Livingstone, London, pp. 21–38

Wolfensberger, W. (1983) Social role valorization: a proposed new term for the principle of normalization. *Mental Retardation* 21(6), 234–9

41 GERONTOLOGICAL NURSING

Lynn Basford

LEARNING OUTCOMES

After studying this chapter you will be able to:

- Explain the concerns expressed with the perceived growth in the older population
- Identify the major causes of morbidity and mortality within the older population
- Understand the nature of positive and negative coping strategies with chronic illness
- Discuss the role of the nurse in promoting health for the older person
- Discuss the role of the nurse in chronic disease management
- Describe the standards identified in the *National Service Framework for Older People* (Department of Health, 2001)
- Promote and adopt an anti-discriminatory practice towards older people
- Reflect on practice when caring for the older person in any field of health and social care.

BACKGROUND

Gerontology is the study of age and the process of ageing, which embraces how and why some people age successfully while others succumb to increased morbidity and premature mortality. The term is generically used, regardless of the specific professional domain of individual scientists. In the field of health care the focus of study is directed upon the bio-psycho-social aspects of healthy ageing and the ways in which health interventions can restore or maintain health equilibrium.

While gerontology is the scientific term to categorise the study of ageing, it is useful to identify when a person has reached a chronological age that indicates they are now an older person. For official purposes it commences at retirement age, which varies between countries and between genders. For example, in the UK the current retirement age is 60 years for women and 65 years for men. However, upon reaching approximately three score years an individual is classified as being an older person. They belong to this category until the point of death – a period that can span four or five decades. Grouping and labelling older people under one umbrella simply does not reflect the physiological, psychological, social and spiritual differences that exist between the 'young old' and the 'oldest old'. It is a position which does not recognise that upon reaching retirement age many individuals are relatively healthy and active and will have different needs to those at the terminal point of their natural life. Conversely, the oldest old – octogenarians, noctogenarians and centenarians – are more likely to suffer from increased diminished functional capacity and some degree of disability (Hoffman *et al.*, 1996). At some point between these two parameters there will be a transitional phase where decline in health occurs and health and social care services are increasingly required.

Therefore this chapter focuses on identifying the reasons we should celebrate being an ageing society, while recognising the concerns and the challenges that present for the future. In recognising future trends, discussion centres on the need for Health and Social care reforms using the *National Health Service Ten-Year Plan* (Department of Health, 2000a) and the *National Service Framework for Older People* (Department of Health, 2001). Consideration will be given to some of the major incidences of chronic diseases that are prevalent in the older population, which contribute to increased morbidity and premature death. The ways in which older people cope with chronic illness will be discussed and the nurse's role will be analysed.

INTRODUCTION

In the twenty-first century it can be said that we have entered a post-modern period in which an unprecedented number of the world's population have reached the fabled 'three score years and ten'. The United Nations proclaims that within the next two decades the growth in adults reaching 60 years in developing countries is set to double the rate in the industrialised developed countries, while in developed countries themselves the number of individuals reaching 80 years and over will double (Alvarez, 1999). This is a pattern that is set to occur in England, in that it is predicted that between 1995 and 2025 the number of adults over the age of 80 will increase by one-half (Department of Health, 2001). In the USA the US Census (United States Bureau of the Census, 1996) identified that within 15 years there would be some 39 million people over the age of 65 years, a figure that is predicted to rise to 80 million by the year 2050. On a national and global scale these are staggering statistics that require a moment of celebration and yet, at the same time, they give rise for concern to governments, the World Health Organisation (WHO), health professionals, epidemiologists, economists, and the scientific community.

Celebrating an ageing society

The points for celebration are centred on the notion that we have at last witnessed the 'joyous' advent of an ageing society, with more and more people living a longer life, having escaped or survived a premature death. It is assumed that this 'ageing' phenomenon is largely due to scientific discoveries and technological innovations, therapeutic advancements and the increased moral and social conscience of governments (Maes *et al.*, 1996). Nonetheless, living a longer

life is not justifiable if all it means is living with increased disability and diminishing functional health. There is a vision associated with becoming old that is often portrayed by the public and professional bodies alike. Such perceptions are not entirely congruent with emerging research findings, which contend that functional health declines in old age are not absolutes and do not have inevitable associations with the process of ageing (Butler and Gleason, 1985). In this sense, living beyond 65 years should not be viewed negatively as, given the right environment and appropriate healthy lifestyle, older people can achieve 'healthy' ageing and remain free from disability until they reach the end of their natural lifespan.

An individual's genetic disposition is a predisposing factor in achieving a long, healthy life, but the individual's living conditions, lifestyle and social support are also important factors (Albert *et al.*, 1995; Seeman *et al.*, 1995; Basford, 2001). In recognising this, it is clear that the phenomena of ageing defy a simple explanation and as such require further investigation to establish the empirical features of longevity. It is a position that Ageing Research Institutions such as the National Institute of Ageing, USA, the Andrus Foundation for Ageing Research, USA, and the European Commission for Ageing Research have recognised.

Study Activity 41.1 ——————

Find websites for ageing research institutions and identify commissioned work that relates to either promoting healthy ageing, centenarian studies, longevity or quality of life.

CONCERNS WITH AN AGEING SOCIETY

While an ageing society can be celebrated, there are concerns focused on the fact that advancing age is associated with diminishing decline of functional capacity and overall health, thus increasing the older person's dependency on society (Fries and Crapo, 1981; Guralnik and Schneider, 1987). Given this position it would seem right for governments, professional bodies and society to share their concerns about the effect an ageing society has on financial and human resources. In 1998/99 The National Health Service spent approximately 40% of its budget (£10 billion), and Social Service spent 50% (£5.2 billion), on older adults over the age of 65 years (Department of Health, 2001). In addition to the financial expenditure, 'two-thirds of general and acute hospital beds are used by people over 65', (Department of Health, 2001, p.1). Clearly, these percentages of total expenditure on health and social care illustrate the extent of the overall financial burden, suggesting an urgent need to review the nature of service provision and the ways in which professional agents provide care for older people.

In response to such illuminating information the UK government has seen fit to implement far-reaching reforms that will promote an integrated service model between health and social care. This is an attempt to provide a comprehensive service that increases access to services, encourages services that promote independent living in the communities in which older people live, promotes healthy living, improves older people's living conditions, improves the quality of care to older people and reduces duplicity of effort and ineffective use of resources (Department of Health, 2001).

On examination of these areas identified as part of the UK reform package for older people, the question arises as to why such initiatives are not already in place in affluent, caring societies. The answer lies in the evolution and disparate provision of health and social care for older people, society's views of older people, competing resources for other services, lack of understanding and empirically based evidence to underpin practice and a general lack of professional competence. The following will illustrate some of these issues to extend an understanding of the necessity for health and social care reforms.

Background

Up until recent times, providing care for the older person was not a fashionable option for health care professionals. It was viewed as a 'Cinderella' service, a low technological area, and one that was often a holding position until the person died. Within such a caring philosophy and environment it was customary to stereotype all older people in the same mould, reducing their individuality and respect for their personhood to a non-existent level. The predominant model of care was very regimented and passive, and did not encourage active participation, partnership approaches or indeed health promotion. Furthermore, the standard of care was often affected by negative staff attitudes and was deemed to be of poor quality. Within such frameworks of care discriminatory practices were the norm and often had the effect that the older person lost their sense of dignity, pride, respect and, as a consequence, their will to live.

Discrimination

Skeet (1985) found that in the western European countries older people who had served out their useful purpose were considered a burden on society and were uniformly given low status, an issue addressed in Chapter 22. While she found models of good practice towards the older person in some developing countries, such as Kenya and the Philippines, in the main she found evidence of discriminatory practice towards older people on a global scale. Skeet believed that the fundamental reason for such universal discrimination was centred on the fears of young members of society, who perceived that growing old inevitably meant reduced functional capacity with some degree of disability. Such perceptions portray a reminder of one's human frailty and that life from birth to death is a continuing process that is ultimately inevitable. Indeed, the media voice of modern societies places high value on youth and the maintenance of that youth, so it is easy to understand why ageing is something to be feared beyond all rational reasoning. Nonetheless, to deny or devalue the contribution to society that older people can bring is foolhardy, given their contribution to the development of societies in which they live. Many have a rich reservoir of intelligent wisdom, others are scientists, craftsmen or artists who have passed on their product or outcome for others to use and admire, and there are those who have dedicated their lives to caring for others.

Without recognising and respecting these valuable contributions of older people to society, it is questionable whether societies can be called civilised. Betrand Russell (cited in Wilson, 1973) suggests that, 'civilisation is concerned with values independent of utility'. This is a proposition contending that the older person should have equal status and respect in society, regardless of their present-day ability to contribute. Their societal position should be recognised and valued in the knowledge that they are heading towards the end of their journey in this life and their ability to contribute to society's needs should not be judged according to the degree of youthfulness and health they retain, but according to their overall contribution to society as a whole.

Discrimination in the NHS

Over the past few decades there has been much attention drawn to repeated service failures, discriminatory practice and poor quality of care given within the broad umbrella of health and social care services. Champions have persistently come forward to draw attention to governments, policy makers and professional bodies of the need to seek out ways of reforming and changing attitudes and disrespectful practices towards the older person.

In acknowledging the existence of discriminatory practice towards older people a 'flurry' of government recommendations and policy documents has emerged. In the main, the focus of these documents has been to eradicate discriminatory practice, change staff attitudes and provide a more comprehensive, cost-effective and integrated service for all older people. Added to this is a repeated request that health and social care

services for the older person should be removed from institutional settings and centre on the older person's own home environment, or at the very least within the community in which they live. It was conceived that such models of care would be more sensitive to the individual's needs, maintain the dignity and respect of the older person, improve standards of care and would be more efficient and cost-effective (DHSS, 1976, 1988). The Community Care Act (Department of Health, 1990) was instrumental in promoting major changes in health and social care services for older people, with the central theme of improving standards of care through the integration of services. Within the constructs of the Community Care Act, both the public and private sectors would be able to compete for service contracts, ensuring that services would be extended to give a wider range of community-based services supported by the private and public sectors. These would include private nursing homes, residential accommodation, sheltered accommodation and home care support services.

The policy documents identified above were indeed a beginning and some would argue a move in the right direction, but evidence has continued to identify repeated service failure and to reflect the position that the needs of older people have remained largely unserviced, unrecognised and disjointed. Legal investigations of service failure have identified quite convincingly that professionals giving care to older people fail to recognise their individualistic make-up, or to give appropriate respect for their personhood and have lacked the relevant knowledge and skill to assess older peoples' needs or give appropriate care. For example, acute medical and surgical services did not recognise the fact that the older person would take longer to recuperate after therapeutic or surgical interventions, or that they usually had a slower return to functional capacity than their younger counterparts. According to the Audit Commission (1992), these revelations have served to create tensions within a policy-driven service that called for a quick throughput of patients, based on increased economy and efficiency. In addition, evidence has continued to highlight that access and availability to health and social care services were unavailable in some authorities (Age Concern, 1999). Treatment was denied on age alone, and not on clinical reasons (Grant *et al.*, 2000), and cardio-pulmonary resuscitation services were also denied on this basis (Department of Health, 2000b).

Whichever way one looks at the evidence of discriminatory practice it is unethical and unreasonable and should no longer be tolerated in civilised societies, a view that has been embraced in the *National Service Framework (NSF) for Older People* (Department of Health, 2001), which states that discriminatory practice should be 'rooted out', and aims 'to ensure that older people are never unfairly discriminated against in accessing NHS or social care services as a result of their age' (p. 16). In supporting this aim, the NSF decrees that policy documents should not restrict care or access to provisions, as only clinical judgement is permissible.

THE NATIONAL SERVICE FRAMEWORK FOR OLDER PEOPLE (TEN-YEAR PLAN)

The National Service Framework for Older People (Department of Health, 2001) is part of the British Government's modernisation programme of health and social care services to ensure an efficient, effective and economic service that meets the demands of all its citizens in the twenty-first century. Currently, the government has provided a radical blueprint for change, which is incorporated in the *National Health Service Ten-Year Plan (NHSP)* (Department of Health, 2000a). Within this document there are major principles that refer to all age groups, genders and issues relating to peoples' cultures and diversity of needs. Chief among these principles are that the NHS will provide:

- A universal service based on clinical need, not ability to pay
- A comprehensive service to meet the complex needs of older people

- Individualised and culturally sensitive services for people and their carers
- Standards of service that will be audited and monitored
- A model for integrating health and social care services that will become 'seamless'
- Infrastructures that promote health and enhance the quality of life for older people.

The standards identified in the NHSP have recognised and reflected the changing nature and attitudes of society and the fact that the needs of older people are by no means uniform and require models of care to reflect their individualism.

It would be unfair to state that standards for older people do not already exist. During the 1990s there were some significant improvements. For instance, The Care Standards Act (2000) instigated an independent regulatory body that monitored care environments for older people outside the NHS local and national charters that are now available. Policy documents have highlighted adult abuse and steps have been taken to identify abusive behaviour towards old and vulnerable people. The NSF has acknowledged these developments and intends to advance further in some key areas of concern backed by evidence from research, clinical judgements and morbidity and mortality statistics for older people. In the first instance, the following areas have been identified as a priority:

- *Rooting out discrimination* – NHS services will be provided, regardless of age, based on clinical judgement, and social services will not use eligibility criteria to restrict access to services.
- *Person-centred care* – NHS and social services will respect older people's individualistic nature and allow them to make choices about their own care.
- *Intermediate care* – a new dimension of care service that will enable older people to have intermediate care within their own home environment or designated care setting, with the principal aim of promoting independent living.

779

- *General hospital care* – staff that have the relevant knowledge and skills to meet the needs of older people will provide specialist hospital care.
- *Stroke* – preventing strokes will be a priority for the NHS, but when stroke has occurred, specialist stroke services will be available.
- *Falls* – the NHS, working in partnership with councils, will seek to prevent falls and resultant fractures in the older population. When the older person has succumbed to a fall effective treatment will be given, followed by rehabilitation services if required.
- *Mental health in older people* – mental health services will be maximised to provide a comprehensive, integrated service for the older person suffering from mental ill health.
- *Promoting an active, healthy life* – promotion will be offered at all stages of the age span to encourage a healthy, active and independent life, thus reducing the need for support from families and health and social care services (Department of Health, 2000a, p. 14).

The scope of the NSF

There are many diseases and conditions that are more common in older people, such as cardiovascular conditions, stroke, respiratory disease, arthritis, diabetes, mental health problems and injuries and disabilities resulting from falls. In compiling the NSF standards for older people, these diseases and conditions have either been considered within the document at present, or will be considered at a later stage, with the exception of those disease entities such as cancer, coronary heart disease and diabetes that are within specific NSFs.

CHRONIC HEALTH CONDITIONS IN OLDER PEOPLE

Typically, older people face health issues that are chronic in nature, a fact that is claimed to have a significant correlation with increasing disability and premature death (Basford *et al.*, 2003). Hoffman *et al.* (1996) estimated that 88% of older people in the USA were affected by at least one chronic condition and 69% lived with more than one chronic condition. Currently, scientists are unable to find or offer cures for older people with chronic health conditions, but the effect of the diseases can be minimised through chronic disease management and health-promoting activities. This sometimes necessitates the older person altering their life style to manage or control symptoms and potentially life-threatening situations.

In addition to the loss of functional capacity, chronic conditions affect the individual's psychic and mental well-being, which can exacerbate the situation. It is therefore incumbent upon health and social care professionals to understand the prevalence and incidence of chronic disease and the nature of living with chronic health conditions so as to be able to implement the most effective intervention therapy for preventing health deterioration.

In a recent systematic review on older people living with multiple health conditions (Basford *et al.*, 2000), a list of 12 chronic health conditions was identified that predispose towards the following:

- A higher incidence of morbidity and mortality
- A higher burden of disease on the individual, caregiver and society
- Higher economic costs
- Reduction of the overall quality of life.

In addition, chronic health conditions were included that had an impact on the older person's ability to function independently or required profound changes in behaviour for them to effectively cope with the chronic condition. The list also gives indications as to whether the disease affected the cognitive, affective or physical systems and why the chronic disease was included, based on a coping rationale (*see* Table 41.1).

From the list in Table 41.1, it is clear that cardiovascular disease and stroke have a higher correlation with morbidity and mortality than any other chronic conditions. Cardiovascular disease is the leading cause of death in the USA (Monthly National Vital Statistics Report, 1999), and in 1997 accounted for the deaths of

Table 41.1 Prioritised list of chronic health conditions

Rank	Disease	Cognitive	Affective	Physical	Rationale for disease	Coping rationale
1	Cardio-vascular disease (CHD)	X	X	X	The estimated leading cause of mortality in the USA for 1998 The estimated leading cause of death in Europe for 1998 (WHO, 1999) The leading cause of work disability Eleven million Americans aged 65 years and older report disabilities caused by CHD (Centre for Disease Control, 1999)	Overwhelming evidence of mortality/morbidity indicates inclusion The nature of the disease (having to live with an imminent sudden attack) requires coping strategies
2	Stroke/ Hypertension	X	X	X	Ranked as the third most prevalent cause of death in people over 65 in the USA for 1994 with 134 340 deaths (Monthly Vital Statistics, **45**(3) (S), 1996) Accounts for 13.7% of predicted deaths in Europe for 1998 (WHO, 1999)	Affects an increasing aged population in greater numbers The coping strategies required are significant, even for a mild stroke A plethora of coping issues are raised in major stroke
3	Respiratory diseases	X (L)	X	X	Chronic obstructive pulmonary disease (COPD) and allied conditions are the fourth most common causes of death in the USA for those over 65, with 87 048 deaths (Monthly National Vital Statistics Report, 1999)	Requires coping strategies with progression of the disease process Affects cognition in later stages
4	Diabetes		X	X	Ranked as the sixth most prevalent cause of death in the USA in those over 65 (Monthly National Vital Statistics Report, 1999) An estimated 16 million Americans have diabetes (Centre for Disease Control, 1999)	If not managed, can lead to many comorbidities
5	Arthritis		X	X	Arthritis and related conditions affected nearly 43 million Americans in 1998 Nearly 50% of people over 65 have arthritis Second leading cause of work disability (Centre for Disease Control, 1999)	Large prevalence of disease Leads to loss of mobility/work/hobbies At advanced stage, results in comorbidity from development of other diseases

Continued

Table 41.1   Continued

Rank	Disease	Cognitive	Affective	Physical	Rationale for disease	Coping rationale
6	Lung cancer	X (L)	X	X	14 200 predicted deaths for the over-60s (Canadian Cancer Statistics, 1999) Lung cancer is the leading cause of cancer-related death among men in the USA (Centre for Disease Control, 1999)	Presented symptoms are the same as for respiratory diseases but treatment is different, therefore so are coping strategies (associated with chemo-radio-therapy) May affect cognition in tertiary stages of the disease and if secondary processes are involved (L)
7	Colorectal cancer		X	X	5300 predicted deaths for the over-60s (Canadian Cancer Statistics, 1999) Cancer of the colon or rectum is the second leading cause of cancer-related death in the USA	Incidence increases with advancing age Treatment of the disease requires traumatic surgery, which requires coping strategies
8	Prostate cancer		X	X	3990 predicted deaths for males over 60 years (Canadian Cancer Statistics, 1999) Prostate cancer is the second most commonly diagnosed form of cancer after skin cancer among men in the USA	About 80% of all men with clinically diagnosed prostate cancer fall into the age group of 65 and older Increases with age Surgical interventions require coping strategies Must cope with 'loss of manhood'
9	Breast cancer		X	X	3740 predicted deaths for women over 60 (Canadian Cancer Statistics, 1999) Breast cancer is the leading cancerous site in women	Incidence increases with age Surgical interventions/radio-therapy require coping strategies Radical mastectomy requires major adjustment in behaviour
10	Osteoporosis/ fractures		X	X	Osteoporosis is responsible for more than 1.5 million fractures annually, including 300 000 hip fractures, 700 000 vertebral fractures, 250 000 wrist fractures, 300 000 fractures at other sites White women 65 years or older have twice the incidence of fractures as African-American women (National Osteoporosis Foundation, 1999) Ten million individuals have the disease, while 18 million have low bone mass, placing them at increased risk for osteoporosis (National Osteoporosis Foundation, 1999)	Results in significant mobility loss and presents problems of mortality While we recognise that features are caused by multiple pathologies, fractures related to osteoporosis will be investigated based on statistics identified from the literature

Continued

Table 41.1 Continued

Rank	Disease	Cognitive	Affective	Physical	Rationale for disease	Coping rationale
11	Visual impairment		X	X	For individuals aged 65 or older, the rate of blindness is 135 per 1000 In the USA, an estimated 15 million people are blind or visually impaired 70% of severely visually impaired persons are aged 65 or over (Braille Institute, 1999)	More disabling with increasing age Significant behavioural adjustments are required to cope
12	Hearing impairment		X	X	An estimated 60% of people over 65 are affected Hearing loss is the third leading chronic disability in the USA (Hearing Alliance of America, 1997)	More disabling with increasing age Significant behavioural adjustments are required to cope

(From Basford et al., 2000)

726 974 older people (Monthly National Vital Statistics Reports, 1999). Correspondingly, in 1998 it was also the leading cause of death in Europe (World Health Organisation, 1999), while in Canada the incidence and prevalence of stroke was the leading cause of death, with almost two-thirds being over 65 years of age (Hodgson, 1998). The incidence of stroke is significant in most affluent societies, illustrated by the fact that the disease accounted for more that 13.7% of deaths in Europe in 1998 (World Health Organisation, 1999).

These two chronic conditions alone make alarming reading, but what is more disturbing is the increasing body of evidence that older people often suffer from more than one chronic health condition (DeMaria and Cohen, 1987; Verbrugge *et al.*, 1989). Guralnik and colleagues (1993) reported an increase in the reporting of two or more chronic health conditions from 50 to 70% among women of 60 years or older. Van den Akker *et al.* (1998) reported that there was a 78% prevalence of co-morbidity in a Dutch general practice population of older people over the age of 80.

The evidence suggests that as people age there is an increased correlation between multiple chronic health conditions and frailty. For example, with ageing there is an increasing loss of functional capacity due to loss of muscle mass and strength, decreased postural control, and a reduction in the capacity of the immune system to respond effectively. Internal organs lose their full functioning ability and energy levels decline. The accumulation of chronic health conditions affects the functional, physical and mental health of the older person (Angel and Angel 1995), often resulting in pain and suffering, which increases disability and difficulties with activities of daily living and results in loss of dependent living (Fried and Guralnik, 1997). The effect of all this is to reduce the quality of life. However, this situation can be alleviated through correct chronic disease management and the promotion of effective coping strategies that deal with chronic health conditions.

Coping with chronic health conditions

The ability to cope with chronic health conditions has a fundamental relationship with the older person's individuality and their perception of the illness. Scharloo *et al.* (1998) identified five dimensions within the literature on the structure of illness perceptions:

1 *Identity* refers to the label placed on the disease and its associated symptoms.
2 *Causes* refer to how the individual got the disease.
3 *Consequences* pertain to the expected outcome of the disease.
4 *Timescale* relates to expectations about the perseverance and characteristics of the illness.
5 *Controllability* refers to the beliefs the individual has about being able to control the disease.

Others have tried to identify coping strategies within a hierarchical framework. Four functions of coping have been described: prevention of stress from events or situations; alteration of the situation or problem; change in the meaning of the situation; and management of the symptoms or reactions to the stress. Nonetheless, Lazarus and Folkman's cognitive behavioural theory of stress describes coping as a process that involves two processes: appraisal and coping. Cognitive appraisal (also known as primary appraisal) involves the process by which an individual evaluates the degree of threat that is generated by the encounter with the environment. If the stressor is interpreted as positive (e.g. because the stressor is seen as a challenge), positive emotions result. Nonetheless, negative emotions result if the stressor threatens the physical and/or psychological self (a phenomenon that is commonly associated with chronic health conditions).

Following such negative developments, the cycle of negativity can be broken through secondary appraisal (assessment), which considers what might or can be done about the situation and whether a particular coping strategy will be effective. In this model, coping can be determined into two higher order constructs: problem-focused coping behavioural strategies, which aim at managing the external environmental aspects of the stressor; and emotion-focused coping or cognitive strategies, which regulate the individual's internal state or emotional reactions to the stressor.

A third coping dimension has been identified, which relates to avoidance (Viney and Westbrook, 1982; Mattlin *et al.*, 1990). Avoidance coping is demonstrated when an individual is confronted with a stressor but the confrontation is delayed through distracting mechanisms such as en-gaging in a substitute task, or through social diversion and behaviours such as denial and suppression.

Factors affecting coping with chronic health conditions

Experiences with illness throughout life will influence the older person's ability to effectively cope with chronic health conditions. Other factors relate to:

- *Gender differences* – which account for the ways in which men and women cope with the same situations. For example, women use more positive reappraisal than men (Brown *et al.*, 1989), while men use more self-control (keeping their feelings to themselves) (Folkman *et al.*, 1987).
- *The level of education* – the literature portrays the opinion that a poor level of education results in the use of ineffective coping strategies with chronic health conditions (Krough *et al.*, 1992; De Klerk *et al.*, 1997). Hubert identified that fewer years of education were reported to be associated with greater disability, a view supported by Verbrugge *et al.* (1991).
- *Cultural differences* – it has been reported that cultural differences and birth origins account for use of different coping strategies (Anderson *et al.*, 1995; Degazon, 1995).
- *Personality differences* – personality traits relate to coping choices, particularly so with chronic health conditions. For example, neuroticism is identified with coping behaviours that relate to wishful thinking, making events into catastrophes and emotional distress, while a hardy character relates to a set of attitudes towards challenge, commitment and control (Pollock, 1987).

Narsavage and Weaver (1994) reported that hardy people were more likely to use problem-solving coping strategies. Both types of strategies were considered to have a positive outcome.

- *Compliance with professional recommendations* – compliance describes the extent to which an individual follows a prescribed regimen of care in contrast to self-care, which can emphasise involvement in decision-making. It is estimated that non-compliance can range between 10 and 94% (Bradley, 1989; Taylor, 1990; Simons, 1992). Non-compliance is seen as a negative choice in maintaining health equilibrium throughout the life of the chronic disease condition. However, there are factors that assist a compliant behaviour, such as family support, the extent of the knowledge about the disease and mastery in self-management, as with diabetes mellitus and self-esteem (MacLean and Lo, 1998).
- *Age differences* – Aldwin *et al.* (1996) contend that 'with age', it is not coping strategies that change *per se*, but rather 'management strategies'. Older people can learn how to circumvent their problems through the use of effective management strategies. Aldwin continues to suggest that older people use less hostility and escapism, recognising the fact that these behaviours are ineffective.

Frequently occurring coping strategies used with chronic health conditions

The most frequently occurring coping strategies used with chronic health conditions can be classified under three umbrellas: cognitive; affective, and physical, or a combination of all three. Some of these strategies are deemed to have a positive effect and others negative within the overall management of chronic disease. Those of a more positive nature are centred upon:

- The patient having a high self-esteem and mastery of the situation (Penninx *et al.*, 1998)

- The ability to self-manage (Baker and Stern, 1993)
- Strong belief in cure and religiosity (Koeing *et al.*, 1992).

Conversely, negative coping strategies are focused on:

- Confrontational behaviour (Feifel, 1987)
- Defensiveness (Nyklicek *et al.*, 1998)
- Pessimism and certain types of social support (Powers and Jaloviec, 1987)
- Fatalism (Herbert and Gregor, 1997)
- Emotive behaviour (Downe Wambolt and Melanson, 1995)
- Taking abusive substances (Degazon, 1995)
- Self-blame (Revenson and Felton, 1989)
- Withdrawal
- Catastrophizing (Barkwell, 1991).

Study Activity 41.2

- In your reflective portfolio, write down positive and negative coping strategies used with chronic disease conditions.
- Consult your patients, identify ways in which they have coped over time and assess whether there are any similarities.
- If your patient is using negative health coping strategies, identify ways in which you could facilitate a change to positive ones.
- List the major incidence of chronic diseases in the Western communities. In your portfolio, reflect upon why these diseases should be preventable.
- What are the contributing factors leading to health failure in coronary heart disease and stroke?

THE ROLE OF THE NURSE

A review of the current job market for nursing positions indicates that there is a demand for specialist and consultant gerontological nurses working within primary care, acute hospitals, intermediate care, prison services and in the private sector, within areas such as residential and nursing homes. More specifically, gerontology is a broad umbrella, which can be broken down into further sub-sets of specialist nursing practice such as diabetes, respiratory care, palliative care, Alzheimer's disease and mental health, incontinence, rheumotology, cardiology, cancer, vision and hearing. Some of these services are increasingly nurse-led, working independently of medical practitioners but operating within defined medical protocols and with the availability of medical back-up should the need arise. While such services operated and delivered by nurses are in the minority, current changes in government legislation, such as extended nurse prescribing (Department of Health, 2001), offer much wider opportunities for nurses and eventually for other professional groups.

Inevitably, such changes reflect an increased accountability and responsibility for nurses, necessitating the need for further education and training to ensure that they are fit to practice in their new roles (Department of Health, 2001). Nurses who can prescribe treatment to older people need to be competent to assess, diagnose, manage and evaluate the care. The assessment will include diagnosing disease states not previously diagnosed by a medical practitioner (undifferentiated diagnosis). In gaining this competence nurses will have to learn 'physiology and altered physiology, health assessment and diagnostic skills, diagnostic reasoning, pharmacology and the effects of polypharmacy, ethical and legal issues and aspects of clinical governance' (Basford and Bowskill, 2001, p. 469).

It is assumed that nurse prescribing will effectively change the power relationships between doctors and nurses, at the same time developing a much stronger multi-professional team working to improve the overall quality of care to older people. In this sense, specialist and consultant gerontological nurses will be major players in ensuring that the needs of the older person are met. However, attention must be given to the education and training needs, clinical supervision and succession planning of nurses to secure the future workforce for working with older people in line with the increased responsibility and accountability bestowed upon them.

EDUCATION AND TRAINING

So often the nurse is taught to focus systematically on specific diagnosis; however, older people faced with managing chronic disease, disability and functional incapacity are not necessarily concerned with the disease itself. Often of more relevance to them is the range of symptoms that transcend any particular disability, chronic condition or a multiplicity of chronic conditions. These symptoms can include pain, depression, energy loss, sleep deprivation, altered nutrition, medication or attitudes, incontinence, memory loss, loss of independence and the ability to self-care. It is therefore the nurse's responsibility, through holistic assessment, to ascertain the actual and perceived priori of symptoms, or series of symptoms that greatly concern the older person, or their carers. For instance, incontinence can become a major problem for both the carer and patient. If badly managed, the burden can be exacerbated beyond what can be reasonably managed within the patient's own home environment. Promoting continence through health education can be effective in maintaining a degree of continence through correct pelvic floor exercises. Therefore the nurse should not just ascribe to a caring model that allows incontinence to be an accepted pattern of everyday life, but to one that can engage the patient and carer in a regime that promotes continence and will have the added bonus of preventing secondary urinary infections.

Other symptoms such as pain and depression also require a comprehensive understanding for the nurse to be able to assist the patient and their carers to cope more effectively and to improve the quality of life.

Pain

Pain is a common symptom associated with many diseases linked with old age; for example, both cancer and arthritis have a strong correlation with pain (Hampson *et al.*, 1994). Nevertheless, pain is often overlooked as being part of being old, although it significantly contributes to the person's distress and detracts from quality of life.

The difficulty with assessing pain intensity lies with the very nature of pain, which can incorporate sensory, emotional and cognitive components. For instance, there is a significant correlation between emotional distress and pain associated with rheumatoid arthritis (Brown *et al.*, 1989), while psychological distress such as anxiety, attention, and conditioning limit the effectiveness of pain treatment (Fry and Wong, 1991).

The ability of an older person with a chronic illness to withstand pain and reduce its impact on their quality of life depends upon their psychological coping mechanisms. Fry and Wong (1991) have identified that problem-focused interventions were of more benefit than emotion-focused interventions and had a sustained effect. By contrast, emotion-focused coping strategies encouraged dependency on others to control the pain and a predominance to engage in wishful thinking and catastrophizing that had a negative health outcome with regard to pain relief.

Other strategies for coping with and managing pain in a positive dimension are distraction activities, progressive muscular relaxation, compliance with medication, transcutaneous electrical nerve stimulation units or heat, acupuncture, acupressure, reflexology and aromatherapy.

Study Activity 41.3 _____

Jane, a 73-year-old woman, has suffered from rheumatoid arthritis for the past 15 years, but since her husband died she has not been able to control the intensity of her long-standing pain. She is often to be found in tears, and to date any change in pain medication has been to ill effect.

Consider the following:

- Did her pain symptoms increase at the time of her husband's death? What may be the reason for this? What psychological coping mechanisms do you think Jane uses?

- Now go to the journals and read around the management of pain with rheumatoid arthritis. What is the treatment regime prescribed? Is there any reference to identifying the patient's coping styles, or alternative pain relief methods other than medication?

- What is the nurse's role in alleviating Jane's pain?

Depression

Depression is a common co-morbid condition associated with the chronic ill health of older people. When present it has a serious effect on individual functional capacity (Lyness *et al.*, 1996) and increases dependency on others. In essence, the relationship of chronic illness and depression are cyclical in nature. For example, a chronic health condition that interferes with physical functioning causes difficulties in activities of daily living, making it difficult to maintain the social ties that protect individuals from depressive symptoms. Conversely, depressive symptoms reduce the ability of individuals to maintain functional capacity and assure their independence. In congruence with the interrelatedness of depression and chronic ill health, the following model has been devised:

- Physical disease increases the likelihood and subsequent onset of depression in the elderly only when it is associated with functional impairment.
- Functional impairment, whether associated with a particular chronic health condition or not, increases the probability of depression.
- The greater the degree of functional impairment, the greater is the risk of onset of depression.
- Depression can result in functional impairment at a greater level than is physically indicated by the severity of the disease, resulting in an excess disability.
- Depression can predispose an elderly individual to develop and/or exacerbate an illness.

While the evidence of depression and its relationship with chronic ill health in older people is overwhelming, there is a general lack of depression assessment by professionals. In consequence, there is very little evidence of preventative activity or suitable therapeutic interventions until the depressive symptom itself has proved to be a priority symptom.

Study Activity 41.4 _____

- Go back to your practice area and reassess your patient who has a chronic illness for any signs of depressive symptoms, mild or chronic. If depression is present, identify any intervention therapies already prescribed.
- Assess the patient's social networks and identify whether these have diminished over the period of deteriorating health.

SUMMARY

This chapter has defined the nature of the science of gerontology, focusing on the framework used in health care. Such a science is necessary if evidence of healthy living free from disability is to be identified. While scientific discovery is ongoing, there is also a need to find ways in which older people can live in relative comfort and health throughout long periods of chronic illness. Changing lifestyles to those deemed health-promoting lifestyles, and attention to living conditions and ways in which older people are coping effectively are important. In addition, organisations need to be more user-friendly, accessible, and patient-centred, features that are embraced within the *National Service Framework for Older People* (Department of Health, 2001), a template that will be used to make health and social care improvements over the next decade and beyond. Notwithstanding, the roles and responsibilities of nurses working in gerontological care environments are radically changing. This requires a focus on education and training to ensure that the nurse is fit and competent to practice.

Governments, professional bodies, scientists and communities have indeed cause to celebrate the arrival of an ageing society; however, the major point for celebration must be when all older people have medical and social care that is commensurate with their need, when discriminatory practice is totally abolished and when independent living with quality of life for all is an active aspiration.

REFERENCES

Age Concern (1999) *Turning Your Back on Us: Older people and the NHS*, Age Concern, London

Albert, M.S., Jones, K., Savage, C.R. *et al.* (1995) Predictors of cognitive changes in older persons: Mac Arthur studies of successful ageing. *Psychology and Ageing* 10, 578–89

Aldwin, C.M., Sutton, K.J., Chiara, G. *et al.* (1996). Age differences in stress, coping and appraisal: findings from the Normative Ageing study. *Journal of Gerontology: Series B: Psychological Sciences and Social Sciences* 51(4), 179–88

Alvarez, J.T. (1999) *Longevity, Longitude and Latitude: The Ambassador's statement*, The International Longevity Centre, Washington, DC *www.longevityworld.com/alvarez.html*.

Anderson, J.M., Wiggens, S., Rajwani, R. *et al.* (1995) Living with a chronic illness: Chinese-Canadian and Euro-Canadian women with diabetes – exploring factors that influence management. *Social and Scientific Medicine* 41, 181–95

Angel, R.J. and Angel, J.L. (1995) Mental and physical comorbidity among the elderly: the role of culture and social class. In: Padgett, D.K. (ed.) *Handbook on Ethnicity, Ageing and Mental Health*, Westport, CT, pp. 47–70.

Audit Commission (1992) *Homeward Bound: A new course to community health*, HMSO, London

Baker, C. and Stern, P.N. (1993) Finding meaning in chronic illness as the key to self-care. *Canadian Journal of Nursing Research* 25(2), 23–36

Barkwell, D.P. (1991) Ascribed meaning: a critical factor in coping and pain attenuation in patients with cancer-related pain. *Journal of Palliative Care* 7(3), 5–14

Basford, L. (2001) The future trends for nursing practice [Presidents' column, e-nursing]. *European Honours Society for Nursing and Midwifery* 1(1), 1–3

Basford, L. and Bowskill, D. (2001) Celebrating the present, challenging the future of nurse presenting. *British Journal of Community Nursing* 6(9), 467–71

Basford, L., Dowzer, C., Booth, A. *et al.* (2000) *Living with Multiple Health Conditions: A systematic search and literature review*, Scientific Report for the American Association of Retired Persons, Georgia

Basford, L., Poon, L., Dowzer, C. *et al.* (2003) The efficacy of health coping behaviours used by older adults for specific diseases. In: Poon, L., Hall Gueldner, S. and Sprouse, B. *Successful Aging and Adaptation with Chronic Diseases*, Springer, New York

Bradley, L. (1989) Adherence with treatment regimens among adult rheumatoid arthritis patients: current status and future directions. *Arthritis Care and Research* 2(3), 533–9

Braille Institute (1999) *General Statistics on Blindness*: www.Brailleinstitute.org/about/statistics.html

Brown, G.K., Nicassio, P.M., Wallston, K.A. *et al.* (1989) Pain coping strategies and depression in rheumatoid arthritis. *Journal of Consulting Clinical Psychology* 57, 652–7

Butler R.N. and Gleason, H.P. (eds) (1985) *Productive Ageing: Enhancing vitality in later life*, Springer, New York

Centre for Disease Control (1999) *Arthritis Online*: www.Edc.gov/nchs/fastats

Canadian Cancer Statistics (1999) *National Cancer Institute of Canada*: www.cancer.calstats

Darsavage, G.L. and Weaver, T.E. (1994) Physiologic statistics, coping and hardiness as predictors of outcomes in chronic obstructive pulmonary disease. *Nursing Research* 43(2), 90–4.

Degazon, C.E. (1995) Coping, diabetes and the older African American. *Nursing Outlook* 43(6), 254–9

DeMaria, L. and Cohen, H.J. (1987) Characteristics of lung cancer in elderly patients. *Journal of Gerontology* 42, 185–90

Department of Health (2000a) *The National Health Service Ten-Year Plan*, HMSO, London

Department of Health (2000b) *Resuscitation Policy*, HSC 028, HMSO, London

Department of Health (2001) *National Service Framework for Older People*, HMSO, London

DHSS (1976) *Priorities for Health and Personal Social Services: A consultative document*, HMSO, London

DHSS (1988) *Community Care: Agenda for Action*, HMSO, London

Downe Wambolt, B.L. and Mclanson, P.M. (1995) A casual model of coping and well-being in elderly spouse and empirical model. *Research of Ageing* 16, 167–90

Feifel, H., Strack, S. and Nafy, V.T. (1987) Coping strategies and associated features of medically ill patients. *Psychosomatic Medicine* 49, 616–25

Folkman, S., Lazerus, R.S., Pimley, S. *et al.* (1987) Age differences in stress and coping processes. *Psychological Ageing* 2(2), 171–84

Fried, L.P. and Guralnik, J.M. (1997) Disability in older adults: evidence regarding significance, etiology and risk. Journal of American Geriatric Society 45(1), 92–100

Fries, J.F. and Crapo, L.F. (1981) *Vitality and Ageing: Implications of the rectangular curve*, WH Freeman, San Francisco, CA

Fry, P.S. and Wong, T.P. (1991) Pain management training in the elderly: marking interventions with subjects coping styles. *Stress Medicine* 7, 93–8

Grant, P., Henry, J.M. and McNaughton, G.W. (2000) The management of elderly blunt trauma victims in Scotland: evidence against ageism. *Injury* 31, 519–29

Guralnik, J.M. and Schneider, E.L. (1987) The compression of morbidity: a dream, which may come true, someday. *Gerontological Perspective* 1, 8–14

Guralnik, J.M. Lacroix, A.L., Abbott, R.D. *et al.* (1993) Maintaining morbitity in later life: demographic characteristics and chronic conditions. *American Journal of Epidemology* 137, 845–57

Hampson, S.E., Glasgow, R.E. and Zeiss, A.M. (1994) Personal models of osteoarthritis and their relation to self-management abilities and quality of life. *Journal of Behavioural Medicine* 17(2), 312–16

Hearing Alliance of America (1997) *Statistics Online*: www.Hearingalliance.com

Herbert, R. and Gregor, F. (1997) Quality of life and coping strategies of clients with COPD. *Rehabilitation Nursing* 22(4), 182–7

Hodgson, C. (1998) Prevalence and disabilities of community living seniors who report the effects of stroke. *Canadian Medical Association Journal* 6 [supplement], Sp-514.

Hoffman, C., Rice, D. and Sung, H.Y. (1996) Persons with chronic conditions. Their prevalence and costs. JAMA 276(18), 1473–9

De Klerk, M.M., Huijsman, R. and Mcdonnell, J. (1997) The use of technical aids by elderly persons in The Netherlands: an application of Anderson and Newman model. *Gerontologist* 37(3), 365–73

Koeing, H.G., Cohen, H.J., Blazer, D.G. *et al.* (1992) Religious coping and depression among elderly, hospitalised medically ill men. *American Journal of Psychiatry* 149(12), 1693–1700

Krough, V., Trevisan, M., Jossa, F. *et al.* (1992) Coping and Blood pressure. *Journal of Human Hypertension* 6, 65–70

Lyness, J.M., Bruce, M.L., Koeing, H.G. *et al.* (1996) Depression and medical illness in late life: report of a symposium. *Journal of the American Geriatrics Society* 44(2), 198–203

MacLean, D. and Lo, R. (1998) The non-insulin pependent diabetic: success and failure compliance. *Australian Journal of Advanced Nursing* 14(4), 33–42

Maes, S., Leventhal, H. and De Ridder, D.T. (1996) Coping with chronic diseases. In: Zeidner, M. and Endler, N. (eds) *Handbook of Coping*, John Wiley, New York, pp. 221–51

Mattlin, J.A., Wetherington, E. and Kessler, R.C. (1990) Situational determinants of coping and coping effectiveness. *Journal of Health and Social Behaviour* 13(1), 103–22

Monthly National Vital Statistics Report (1999) *Centre for Disease Control Online*: www.Cdc.gov/nchs.html

National Osteoporosis Foundation (1999) *Osteoporosis Fast Facts Online*: www.nof.org/osteoporosis/stats/htm

Narsavage, G.L. and Weaver, T.E. (1994) Physiologic status, coping and hardiness as predictors of outcomes in chronic obstructive pulmonary disease. *Nursing Research* 43(2), 90–4

Nyklicek, I, Vingerhoets, A.J., Van Heck, G.L. *et al.* (1998). Defensive coping in relation to casual blood pressure and self-reported daily hassles and life events. *Journal of Behaviour Medicine* 21(2), 145–61

Penninx, B.W., Van Tilburg, T., Boeke, A.J. *et al.* (1998) Effects on social support and personal coping resources on depressive symptoms: different for various chronic health conditions. *Health Psychology* 17, 551–8

Pollock, S.E. (1987) Adaptation to chronic illness. *Nursing Clinics of North America*, 22(3), 631–44

Powers, M.J. and Jaloviec, A. (1987) Profile of the well controlled, well adjusted hypertensive patient. *Nursing Research* 36(2), 106–10

Revenson, T.A. and Felton, B.J. (1989) Disability and coping as predictors of psychological adjustments to rheumatoid arthritis. *Journal of Consulting and Clinical Psychology* 57(3), 344–8

Scharloo, M. Kaptein, A.A., Weinman, J. *et al.* (1998) Illness perceptions, coping and functioning in patients with rheumatoid arthritis, chronic obstructive pulmonary disease and psoriasis. *Journal of Psychosomatic Research* 44(5), 573–85

Seeman, T.E., Charpentier, P.A., Berkman, L.F. *et al.* (1995) Behavioural and psychosocial predictors of physical perfomance: MacArthur studies of successful ageing. *Journal of Gerontology* 50A, M177–83

Simons, M. (1992) Interventions related to compliance. *Nursing Clinics of North America* 27(2), 477–94

Taylor, S. (1990) Health psychology: the science and the field. *American Psychology* 45(1), 40–50

United States Bureau of the Census (1995) *Statistic Abstract of the United States: 1995* (115th edn), US Bureau of the Census, Washington DC

United States Bureau of the Census (1996) *Population Projections of the United States by Age, Sex, Race and Hispanic Origin: 1995 to 2050*, Current Population Reports, series P25–1130, US Bureau of the Census, Washington, DC

Van der Akker, M., Buntix, F, Metsemakers, J.F. *et al.* (1998) Multi-morbidity in general practice: prevalence, incidence and determinants of co-occuring chronic and recurrent disease. *Journal of Clinical Epidemiology* 51 (5), 367–75

Verbrugge, L.M., Lepkowski, J.M. and Imanaka, Y. (1989) Comorbidity and its impact on disability. *Milbank Quarterly* 67(3–4), 450–84

Verbrugge, L.M., Lepokowski, J.M. and Knoll, L.L. (1991) Levels of disability among US adults with arthritis. *Journal of Gerontology* 46(2), 571–83

Viney, L.L. and Westbrook, M.T. (1982) Coping with chronic illness: the mediating role of biographic and illness-related factors. *Journal of Death and Dying* 17(2), 169–81

Wilson, M. (1973) Caring for the aged population: the problem of society. *Nursing Times* 69(14), 486–91

World Health Organisation (1999) *The World Health Report 1999: Making a difference*, WHO, Geneva

MODULE 9: NURSING PERSPECTIVES

REFLECTIONS

Nursing has, over this last century, followed the paradigms of medicine, which has reduced health care into specialist areas of practice. In addition, it has been recognised that treating children and older adults with the same philosophies and models of care is unethical and does not serve the health needs of either group. Since 1989, educational preparation for nursing has been provided as four branches, which have been explored here. There remains much debate as to whether four branches is sufficient and it is speculated that six perspectives should now be considered, to include community care and gerontological care. Conversely, the debate challenges a specialised approach with proponents advocating a return to a generalist pre-registration programme in keeping with our European and North American colleagues. The debate is circular and therefore to date has no resolution. Nonetheless, exploring the perspectives on nursing in a discrete manner provides opportunities for you to gain a broad understanding of nursing.

By including gerontological nursing we have afforded you the opportunity to explore in-depth a grounding in the needs of older people and issues that are presented to nurses that require resolution and an increased knowledge base from which nursing should practice.

Unless you work with children only, you will come across older people in every care setting, be it acute care, intensive care, intermediate care, palliative care, secondary care, community care and tertiary care settings. Throughout the common foundation period you will have enjoyed the experience of nursing in all four branches, and across age ranges. You should, however, remember that health limitations do not follow a separate approach, and when someone has a physical dysfunction there is sometimes a mental impairment. Assessing patients' needs from a holistic perspective means that all human functioning is assessed regardless as to whether they are labelled mentally or physically ill.

MODULE 10:   INTO THE FUTURE

INTRODUCTION

This is the final module in this extensive textbook of nursing. Over 40 chapters have addressed important areas in the theory and practice of nursing. A significant theme that has frequently arisen is that of the constant change that confronts society as a whole and those involved in the delivery of health care in particular. Indeed, it is often stated that the only 'constant' left within our health services *is* change. In such circumstances it becomes difficult to consider with any degree of certainty how the future will unfold. By the same token, it is difficult to predict how our approaches to health care and nursing (as reflected in this book) will have validity in new and ever-changing worlds. This important consideration is the theme that runs through this final module.

The issues that are addressed in this module are problematic for nursing, but they reflect a level of uncertainty about the future that awaits society as a whole. Until the latter decades of the previous century, there was great faith in the advances of modernity, particularly in the scientific arena. Science and technology, it was hoped, would carry us forward to a new world wherein they would solve all the major problems that confronted humankind. As people in pre-modern times placed their hopes in religion, those in modernity gave their allegiance to the new religion of science, of which medicine was a major part. However, the new religion did not solve all our problems, and we now become aware of its shortcomings through a post-modern critique. In this new century we move forward into a new modernity or neo-modern era. While we continue to reap the benefits of science and technology, we are also now confronted by major risks emerging from the products of modernity that threaten us even at the global level. Thus, while we have radiotherapy and pharmaceutics, we also have the risks of nuclear armaments and germ and chemical warfare. And, while we have the benefits of modern technological health services, we also have the sense of depersonalisation and alienation that being treated within increasingly mechanistic and economics-driven services brings. To respond, in Chapter 43 Jean Watson suggests that we require ontological as well as technical competencies.

So how does nursing move forward in this changing world? This is the fundamental question addressed in this module. You must be careful not to interpret this simply as a rhetorical question of no practical value. If nursing is to make a difference in the future, we must address how our practice will best evolve to meet the demands of the future, and we must address where our profession will stand on the major issues that shape that future.

42 NURSING IN AN AGE OF CHANGE

Lynn Basford

LEARNING OUTCOMES

After studying this chapter, you will be able to:

- Discuss the influences of change
- Determine trends and key drivers that will influence change
- Understand why the nursing profession needs to be proactive and respond to change
- Critically review the impact of policy changes on the nursing profession
- Identify key components that should be within any 10-year strategic plans for the future of nursing
- Understand the influence of international trade markets
- Describe the moral and ethical issues in relation to the changing face of health care
- Discuss the need for working with others in the complex world of health care.

INTRODUCTION

The notion of a changed and constantly changing society with an array of health and social care needs is often spoken of by government ministers, professional bodies, the media and lay people alike. The impact of such changes for nurses and other health and social care workers are not always well articulated, or reflected in a coherent, logical, strategic plan that is owned by all.

Without any doubt, the twentieth century has seen a phenomenal amount of change within the context of the world order, societal expectations, norms and customs, communication systems, demography and epidemiology, and this has influenced the ways in which health and social care is organised and delivered. Change is in fact seen as a dynamic response to political directions, social trends, technological innovations, advancements in clinical practice (through new evidence), therapeutic modes and new professional roles and responsibilities. The need for constant change has become a normal state of living, which on one side of the coin can be viewed as a challenge, or, if ill managed, can have disastrous consequences on the individual, the profession and the organisation. It is therefore imperative that the nursing profession responds to the demands of change in a proactive and coherent manner, by recognising the major trends and key drivers for change, not only from a local position, but also nationally and globally. In doing so, nurses can assert a political voice influencing the direction of policy and cement the foundations for the future of nursing and health care.

In designing the future it is always wise to consider where nursing has been and the main influences for change along the way. In her editorial, Williams cited Isabel Hampton, who in 1893 wrote the following:

> *The social problems of human misery and suffering, and how best to relieve them, have wonderfully worked out since the days when Charles Dickens first began to exert the power of his genius upon the mind of the public in order to bring it into an active sense of its responsibility in such matters and perhaps in no branch, change be so marked as in the care of the sick, of all classes in all countries.*
>
> (Williams, 2001, p. 1)

It would somehow be a moment of true celebration if modern nurses could look back with a sense of collective pride in knowing that the profession had indeed responded and significantly changed all of human suffering and misery. Sadly, this is not the case, as much human suffering caused by disease, poverty, pestilence, war and economic deprivation still exists, even in those countries whose economic wealth has assured that comprehensive health and social care systems are available for all its citizens. Nonetheless, the profession of nursing can be proud of its individual and collective achievements around the globe in advancing the health and well-being of people and communities through responding to technological innovations, research findings and the increased understanding of the health paradigms and their relationships with nursing practice. Nursing should be applauded for its flexibility to change, to pioneer new ways of working, to respond to the changes needed in the educational curricula and government directions, to lead and direct others and, particularly importantly, to be the patient's advocate.

A quick review of the literature will clearly demonstrate that the art and science of nursing has evolved from the days when there were no antibiotic or antiviral agents, no immunisation programmes, no psychotropic medications, no media, no disposable equipment, no plastic, and no complex monitoring machines (Williams, 2001). In addition, there was no conscious awakening or empirical knowledge of the germ theory, with dire consequences to the health and well-being of patients

In the past, nursing, has often been labelled by feminist writers as an adjunct to the (male) medical profession, with nurses looked upon as 'hand maidens', with no rights to engage in clinical decision making, risk assessment, independent prescribing or ethical or moral debates about the patient's care. Furthermore, nurses did not have the rights to a political voice to direct health care and the future of the nursing profession. This picture portrays a clearly subservient role for nurses to the medical profession, one that has been difficult to change. Nonetheless, with the emancipation of women, which served to highlight the plight of women workers, and the increased professionalisation of nursing, nursing has been empowered to gain equal recognition for its contribution to the health and well-being of individuals and communities.

By contrast, the modern nurse is faced with making clinical decisions using evidence of practice and ethical and moral reasoning. Genome developments, in vitro fertilisation and abortion rights for women, risk assessment, transplantations, resource limitation and allocation of treatments and rights to life have brought about moral and ethical debates to which nurses are a party. In addition, the technological revolution in health care has called on the nursing profession to advance its knowledge and gain new skills with increasing sophistication and skill dexterity.

The increasing use of technology within everyday nursing practice has to some extent challenged paradigms of nursing that focused on caring as a central component of nursing within the healing context. It is therefore easy to see how the modern nurse fails to fully understand the fundamental value of caring as a healing commodity, but if nurses continue to disengage with this fundamental value it will be lost forever to others within the health care system. It remains necessary for all nurses, but especially nurse leaders and nurse theorists to re-examine nursing paradigms and seek new ways of explaining nursing within the new world order of care.

The future is intrinsically linked with the knowledge that health and social care is set to change within the context of major reforms. It is therefore difficult to predict with any accuracy what the future direction will hold. Nonetheless, there are some major trends and key driving forces that will at least inform the immediate future and from which hypotheses can be made.

NURSING PARADIGMS

In previous non-technological eras, the nurse was trained to use her hands, eyes, heart and intuition within the caring context (Williams,

2001). Skills that Benner (1984) has postulated are the attributes of being an expert and if we, as nurses, are not careful we can give away this inherent expertise as we increasingly engage with technological aspects of care. We should therefore not devalue these caring skills or overlook them as we cement plans for the future of nursing. Instead, we should revisit nursing paradigms, challenge their validity in the new world of nursing care and extend our understanding by seeking out new paradigms.

In her seminal work on nursing metaparadigms, Fawcett (1984) described four entities – person; environment; health; and nursing – which in her opinion constitute the areas that the discipline of nursing should be concerned about. Meleis (1991) has challenged this assumption, postulating the view that to include nursing in metaparadigms is a tautology since the metaparadigms are descriptors of nursing. Parse (1992) supports the view of Meleis by excluding nursing in her paradigm. Other nurse theorists have extolled different views, expressing the concepts of caring and the human health experience as part of their metaparadigm frameworks (Newman *et al.*, 1991). Caring values are seen as fundamental to the discipline of nursing and a body of knowledge that excludes the notion of caring within the human health experience is not deemed nursing knowledge. Kirby and Slevin (1992) expand on this theory by asserting that nursing involves the engagement of certain activities that are essentially metaparadigm elements, i.e. relationships, caring and health. Even from this small resumé of nursing theorist views on nursing paradigms we can see that there remains confusion and difference of opinion.

The caring component of nursing metaparadigms is an interesting one, given that care is not unique to the nursing profession. Nonetheless, if nurses can move their attention from the broad parameters of what caring is, or is not, within the healing context and start to explore what is actually happening within therapeutic relationships between the recipient and giver of care, then a greater appreciation and understanding can be gained. For example, we know that the human body transmits energy – energy that is both internal and external within the aura of the person. When there is blockage of this energy cycle the person is diseased, which can be transiently, as in an acute health situation, or as a chronic manifestation of ill health. The human body is capable of re-energising itself, but there may come a point when interventions are required to regain positive health equilibrium. Conversely, it can be argued that through the caring relationship healing energy is transmitted from the giver of care to the recipient through energy exchange, as in the quantum healing process (Chopra, 1990), which can be said to be part of the nursing relationship (Basford, 2001a).

THE IMPACT OF SCIENTIFIC DISCOVERIES AND RESEARCH FINDINGS

The global impact on research findings will inform nursing practice and nursing education and the interdependency of these three areas will form a pivotal pre-requisite for the future nurse. No longer will it be satisfactory for the nurse researcher to work in isolation from the world of practice, and neither will it be adequate for the nurse practitioner to ignore the evidence from research findings. Underpinning all of this is the continuous need for the nurse to advance her skills and knowledge base through the process of education and training. The constant flow between research, practice and education will be the norm for all nurses, not just for the elite within the profession.

Nurses must also recognise that evidence of practice will come from a much broader disciplinary base, which will drive new ways of evolving practice that may require totally different ways of viewing the world. For example, the Genome Projects will not only require new models of practice but have and will continue to advance debates within the psychological, sociological, spiritual, physical, ethical and moral arenas. It is therefore imperative that nurses engage with research and with these debates not only to direct clinical practice but also to influence policy.

POLITICS AND NURSING

Nothing in the world of health care is without political influence. Nurses are directed locally, nationally and globally to the politics of health. At the local level, the emergence of the newly formed primary care trusts will influence the direction of care, the commissioning of care and the manpower resources to undertake the caring activities. Implicit in this will be the assessment of education and training to meet the health care needs of the local people. Primary care trusts will endeavour to meet government targets and priorities, assessing and evaluating progress at each level of the operation. There will be a published list of health improvement programmes (HIMPs), which will be locally sensitive and will reflect the government's agendas through the published national service frameworks (NSFs) (Department of Health, 2001a) and the *NHS Ten-year Plan* (Department of Health, 2000).

From a global perspective, the changes occurring within demographics, epidemiology, the technological revolution, war, famine, poverty, and the speed of travel are all embraced within the political arena and are of concern to everyone (Oulton, 1999). The word 'globalisation' is a descriptive phrase suggesting that the boundaries that were once rigid are rapidly changing between individuals, societies and nations (International Federation of Trading and Development, 1998). This leads to the notion of a 'global village', where there are some commonalities between all societies; yet we must also recognise that there are some unique differences. It is essential that politicians and others clearly identify these commonalities and differences between countries and cultures so as to direct political frameworks that will address the health and social needs of all people. Nursing cannot be excused from entering these debates as countries and cultures become increasingly interdependent.

This increasing interdependence between all nations is influenced by the economic markets, natural resources, moral and political directives and exchange of human labour, all of which has an impact on the health and well-being of people within and between countries. For example, Clifford (2000) points out that the world markets have the capacity to increase trade, which includes both health care products and the trading of health care workers. What is of particular concern is the notion that human trade is more often from the developing countries with low economic national stability to those countries that are more affluent and have acute expert manpower shortages in health care. The moral dilemma here is the knowledge that these developing countries can ill afford to lose their trained expertise and that to poach such expertise is amoral (Salmon, 1999).

Clifford (2000) claims that in some countries the staffing crisis is so acute that up to 50% of the nursing unit will be from a different country. Abu-Zinahda (1999) points out that this diversity of the workforce may inadvertently reduce the political power of nurses. It is therefore important that his views are heard and the consequence of such actions fully appreciated. Meanwhile, it is important that the developed world seeks solutions to its own staffing crisis to keep pace with increasing demands on health care and diminish the need to disadvantage further those developing countries that have a great need for their own health care experts.

The increased mobility of health care workers is an acceptable position to take within the guise of reciprocity between nations, as within the European Union. Nevertheless, policy analysts and nurses must recognise that nursing is very diverse and it can be difficult to cross the international boundaries when the fiscal, management, political structures, language, education, training and environmental factors are very much different (Salmon, 1999). The nursing profession needs to recognise this while acknowledging that the movement of people from within and between countries creates multicultural societies whose health needs are diverse. Within the latter context nursing must move beyond insularity and the limitations of critical thought and in so doing widen the scope of its education and training.

Study Activity 42.1

Take a UK nurse and place her in the country of Kazakhstan, a former Russian state, where she is unaccustomed to the lack of running water, sewage disposal systems, no technological equipment to either give treatment or monitor conditions, no drugs, no disposable equipment and very little food. In addition, the nurse is required to care for people with infectious diseases such as bubonic plague, typhoid, diphtheria, polio myelitis, syphilis, tuberculosis and other sexually transmitted diseases.

- How do you think the nurse would cope? What skills could be transferred to these settings? What skills would be needed? What would be the health priorities in such countries? Are there any similarities with the nursing situation in the UK?
- Conversely, how would a nurse who was educated and trained in Kazakhstan perform if she were transported to a very busy high dependency ward in the UK? Would she be able to cope? What skills would she have that were transferable? What would be the skills deficit? What health priorities would she need to address in the UK?

You may think that the questions in Study Activity 1 are unrealistic because of the likelihood that diseases such as those identified in Kazakhstan will never be seen by the nurse in the UK. This is a false assumption, and a complacency nurses must not be allowed to adopt. If we are a global village by trade and transport then infectious diseases from other countries can and do very quickly transfer to people in the UK. A recent example of this occurred in 2001, where a school in Leicestershire had a spate of children infected with tuberculosis. It is evident from the reactions of such infectious disease outbreaks that people and nurses in the UK have forgotten the human distress such diseases cause. While this is understandable, what is of particular concern is the fact that in the UK there are several generations who do not have immunity from infectious diseases, either through natural exposure or through vaccination programmes, which makes each of us very vulnerable and exposed to epidemics. Today the nursing workforce in the UK is prepared to reduce the incidence of coronary heart disease, stroke and chronic illness, not the health issues associated with infectious diseases. The nursing profession must be mindful that yesterday's problems may be tomorrow's issues and the modern nurse needs to be prepared for such events (Basford, 2001b).

Study Activity 42.2

- Search the web to identify statistical information of the prevalence and incidence of the following diseases: tuberculosis; typhoid, paratyphoid; poliomyelitis; diphtheria, bubonic plague; syphilis; HIV and Aids; gonorrhoea; measles; chicken pox; mumps and rubella. (The World Health Data-base may be a good starting point.)
  - What is the effect on mortality and morbidity of the diseases?
  - What is the cause of the spread of these diseases?
  - What are the known treatments?
  - What can be done politically to reduce such incidence?
- Working in groups, discuss your findings and make recommendations.

Power and politics

The relationship between power and politics cannot be ignored, as health care teams across the globe are still dominated by the medical profession. Such models are even noted in the USA, which is surprising given that the Advanced Practitioner/Nurse Practitioner has roots in the USA (Whittle and Jester, 1998). The message resonates with the view that nursing is women's work and secondary to the work of men. In this sense, the politics of the women's movement and feminist emancipation cannot be divorced from the politics of nursing.

Drawing on Handy's (1993), work on the categorisations of power, we can see that power is identified as physical, resource, position, expert, personal and negative power. Nurses can draw on this model to usurp their own power in the new world orders of health care. For example, nurse leaders with personal power and expert power can clearly influence the political directives of an organisation. On the other hand, having negative power undermines their influential power. Robinson (1997) makes a plea for nurse leaders to use their power at national level debates so as to influence and change health policies. The first stage of political success is for nurses to be politically aware and to engage in politics locally prior to expanding their voice in the big political arenas of the world (Albarran, 1995).

DEMOGRAPHY

At the start of the twenty-first century, the demographic trend towards an ageing society has emerged, with a corresponding general lowering of birth rates. A glance at the gerontological literature and at government policy documents indicates a growing concern with the impact an ageing population will have on society as a whole. It is a double-edged sword in that health and social care systems encourage and support living a long, quality life that is sustained throughout the advancement of years. Nonetheless, there is no escaping the fact that an aged society is a growing drain on the economy by increasing demands on the health and social care systems (Basford, 2001a). In an attempt to change these trends recent health care policies have begun to address the phenomenon of an ageing society through the empowerment of older adults, preventative medicine, and careful management of chronic illness. Nurses are central in implementing these initiatives to ensure that a change in emphasis occurs from a dependent to an independent model, which supports older adults in their lifestyle and health choices (Department of Health, 2000). While such policy direction is admirable, nursing must be prepared to change antiquated practices that will enable and empower older adults to maintain their health status throughout every period of their life. The emergence of nurse-led services that support the management of chronic ill health are indeed a move in the right direction, but new services need to be developed. Such new initiatives require an educated and trained nursing workforce as the needs of the older adult are very much different to those of the young (Poon *et al.*, 2003).

In recognising the health and social needs of the older adult, there are also increasing needs associated with the young, who engage with 'risky behaviours' linked to drug and alcohol abuse. Such risky behaviours have serious consequences for their long-term health and safety. For example, the high levels of teenage pregnancies, sexually transmitted diseases and suicides have a direct correlation with 'risky' behaviours. In addition, funding these habits creates the need to engage with criminal behaviour that violates the values and norms of the society in which they live.

The reasons for 'risky behaviour' by the young are complex. Sociologists argue it is because of dysfunctional families and separated family life, while others contest that it is because of peer pressure and easier access to money. Whatever the reason, it is evident that 'risky' behaviours have a damaging effect on the health of the individual and on the wider community. In considering this nurses need to find solutions to support family life and family breakdowns, to consider the health and social needs of the young and to work proactively with community groups. It is important that the public health agendas meet the needs of both the young and old within a community.

AGEING WORKFORCE

Workforce planning has always used rather unsophisticated mechanisms to identify the workforce needs for the future. This has resulted in the formulation of a fragmented picture that has seemingly borne no resemblance to the realities of the national or global situation. The situation has improved at the regional level with the emergence of the Workforce Confederations, who have been charged with the responsibility to predict the workforce needs and match education contracts according to these findings.

It takes time to iron out the anomalies of years of miscalculation and it remains increasingly difficult to predict when an individual member of the workforce will take their retirement. This can occur anywhere between the ages 55 and 65 years. The statistical information received to date reflects a growing number of nurses who have reached or exceeded the age of 50, and in the next 15 years the NHS and the private sector are going to suffer acute shortages of skilled and experienced nurses working in all practice areas. This picture is not unique to the UK; indeed, a review of the situation in the USA reflects a similar picture, with 50% of the workforce over the age of 45 years (American Association of Registered Nurses, 1993). Williams (2001, p.2) has reported that 'nursing will suffer the most severe shortage in its history' at a time when there is a predicted growth for the Registered Nurse. On the one hand, we have an ageing workforce and on the other we have increasing demands for new nursing roles and new services such as Nurse Direct, walk-in centres, consultant nurses and triage nurses, who all come from the same pool of the established workforce. It is a situation that needs urgent attention if the future and direction of nursing is to be implemented by a sustained and skilled workforce.

TECHNOLOGY AND ITS IMPACT ON NURSING

The technological revolution has infiltrated every aspect of health care. Some of these changes have already called for radical shifts in practice, such as changes in surgical techniques to use both non-invasive and invasive imaging; pharmacological changes, which have stimulated target drug therapies; electronic data basing, which has driven the need for standards in universal language; the use of robotics, and hand-held biological instruments and smart materials; immunological advances; genetic and reproductive technologies, nanotechnology and e-learning for both staff and patient education (Flower, 1999).

Information technology and information management has become a core function of nurses and other health care workers, not only to access and store patient information but to ensure that practice is from an evidence base and that their own learning advances at the appropriate pace.

Indeed, the technological revolution has required new skills and competences along with a prevailing view that 'high tech, high trend' is central to nursing practice (Naisbitt, 1991). Of particular concern here is that nursing does not lose sight of the fact that technology and technological apparatus are tools through which the art of nursing is practiced, and the interface between the nurse and the patient is of paramount importance to the healing relationship. Furthermore, the power of the nurse–patient relationship should not be forgotten as technology continues to hurtle care within the paradigms of new thinking, which will require the nurse to be the moral and ethical agent of the patient in their pivotal role as the patient's advocate.

COLLABORATIVE HEALTH CARE

Collaborative practice and increased multi-disciplinary team working are buzzwords that have underpinned government policies over the past few decades. The reason for this is:

- The reporting of numerous service failures that have been the result of poor inter-professional communication within and between agents involved in the giving of health and social care
- Diversity, which has required continuity of care across care boundaries
- A policy drive to increase efficiency, effectiveness and economy of care provision
- Shared practice and shared clinical governance
- Reduction in expert human resources, such as GPs and junior doctors

● A review of occupational competence and the need to demonstrate transferability of skills (Basford *et al.*, 1998).

The notion of a seamless service demands interagency working and greater collaboration with others without attention to rigid demarcation of role boundaries (Department of Health, 1999a). Tribalistic professional behaviour has no role to play in the future of health care, where the patient journey and experience is central to all caring activity. Greater emphasis needs to be given to the design and competence of the teams, which focus specifically on the needs of the patient, and support workers may do health care tasks that were once the domain of specific professional groups. In addition, involvement of users and carers at all levels of the organisation's activities are now cemented in policy that cannot be ignored (Department of Health, 2000).

It is advocated that multi-professional teams need to understand each other's roles and speak a common language to enable effective communication and to have a single patient record spanning primary, secondary and social care boundaries. One way to expedite this thinking is the notion of shared learning in either the classroom or clinical setting. Models like this have been around for several decades but have been thwarted with barriers at the pre-qualifying level. New models of electronic learning or a greater emphasis on shared practice learning may resolve some of these early concerns.

Currently, there is a greater awareness by the professions that health and social care is a complex and sophisticated activity that cannot be undertaken by one discipline. The need to work together has never been so clear, particularly the understanding that there is shared clinical governance in all areas of the caring activity. Shared care must also mean shared responsibility with an ultimate aim to promote and advance the quality of care.

Study Activity 42.3 _____

● When out in practice examine how the members

of the multi-disciplinary team work together for the improvement of patient care.
● Identify similar skills and those that are very much different used by different health care professionals.
● Explore government policy documents and identify references to the notion of team working.

_____

New roles and new responsibilities

Within the context of social and health care reforms there is greater emphasis to change models of working. Nursing has already seen an influx of new roles and new responsibilities. For instance, take the role of the nurse consultant, the triage nurse, Nurse Direct, and walk-in centres, where the nurse is responsible for clinical decision-making, the assessment of need, prescribing treatment, evaluating the care and advice given, and managing others, including salaried doctors. The range of skills required may not be entirely new, but the accountability that goes with the new roles is so changed that there is a great need for nurses to be adequately prepared with the knowledge, skills, understanding and experience to fully engage with the new role. For example, the nurse will need to have a much more comprehensive knowledge of disease diagnosis, and diagnostic assessment, an advanced level of pathophysiology and altered physiology, pharmacology, the effects of polypharmacy, the ethical and legal issues that underpin clinical risk taking and clinical governance (Basford and Bowskill, 2001), and the management of budgets and people.

The influence of the changes in education and training relates to the level of expertise of nurses who already hold a degree of expertise after many years in the practical setting. Nonetheless, these new roles and responsibilities will be the tip of the iceberg when more and more nurses become extended Nurse Prescribers. To prepare the new work force, some of the knowledge and skill base will need to be undertaken at the pre-qualifying level, while at the other end of the spectrum advancements of this knowledge and skill will continue to keep pace with continued changes in the role of the modern nurse.

TRANSCULTURAL CARE

The UK is an ever-increasing multicultural society due to immigration and the migration of workers, predominantly from the commonwealth countries. While this is a known entity, very little has been done to address the spiritual, religious and cultural health needs, as opposed to those of the indigenous population. Of particular note is the general ignorance of health care workers, the lack of opportunities within the curriculum to gain insights and knowledge, and organisational policies that do not identify the health needs and differences of minority ethnic groups.

The emergence of the *Project 2000* curricula saw a slight change in educational patterns, which began to increase the awareness of student nurses in the knowledge that education is a powerful conduit to enable nursing to refocus itself and be more understanding of the multicultural and multi-religious needs of patients. What students saw in practice was a non-multicultural approach in the delivery of care, often excused by the 'business' of the care environment. In defence of this position it is sometimes very difficult to understand the needs of someone who comes from a very different culture and religious background and being busy can be a useful avoidance mechanism for nurses and others to employ.

Education is viewed as the key to the nurse's awakening towards providing multicultural health care and the process of awareness begins with spirituality. Narayanasamy (1999) suggests that spirituality is part of the essence of our humanity and provides a mechanism through which we manifest peace. This spiritual dimension of humans evokes feelings of love, joy, faith, hope, trust, awe and inspiration. When illness strikes people are keen to engage with their spiritual self, often asking the question 'What is the purpose of one's existence?' Many

use their religion for expressing their spirituality, but there are other ways. To deny individuals their right to express their spirituality in whichever mode is a denial of their basic health care needs. Nurses must therefore be sensitive to cultural and religious variations, particularly as society becomes more diverse. To do this Narayanasamy (1999) states that nursing requires:

- A database of information about culturally determined aspects of health and illness care
- Provision of culture-specific and sensitive nursing care
- Emphasis on caring acts as universal, but taking many forms and variations in many cultures
- An understanding that systems of treatment and care may already prevail in other cultures
- Attention to the significance of 'folk systems' and their need to be incorporated into professional approaches to care
- Self-awareness (subjecting self to challenges of assumptions)
- An understanding that one's own values, if imposed on others, can be offensive and unprofessional (and may lead to avoidance of carers) (Narayanasamy, 1999, pp. 274–85).

The future of nursing must incorporate a multicultural dimension if we are to provide quality health care for all and in moving in this direction nursing will contribute to the understanding of the differences and similarities between people and gain a broader understanding of health and illness (Leininger, 1978).

CHANGES IN THERAPEUTIC MODES

Health care in the UK has been modelled on a reductionistic medical model that viewed the patient as a disease entity rather than the sum of the whole. Nursing bought into this model, believing that the science of medicine was also the science and art of nursing until nurse theorists challenged this and offered models that were based around 'holism'. Holistic care is focused on the patient's physical, social, psychological and spiritual dimensions of health. Moving away from the medical model, nursing became linked to the philosophies akin to complementary and alternative therapies and began to embrace some of these therapies in everyday practice. Fifty years ago, the science and art of medicine was quite clearly opposite to the science and art of complementary and alternative therapies, creating a challenge for complementary therapists to provide evidence of their practice. While acknowledging that the empirical evidence of complementary therapy practice is weak, the growing body of evidence and the satisfaction and increased access made by the general public has seriously challenged traditional medicine, particularly with chronic and terminal health conditions. These factors have enabled a much more liberal approach towards therapeutic interventions used within the auspices of the NHS. Primary care trusts are increasingly expected to contract for complementary services along with traditional medical routes. These changes will impact greatly on the therapeutic modes patients will choose and the future of nursing depends on nurses either working with such practitioners or, as many do now, becoming complementary therapists themselves.

NURSING BUSINESS

For two decades the NHS, while remaining a recognised asset to the nation for the provision of health care, has increasingly been called to account for its human resource management, resource allocation and the total fiscal expenditure. More recently, policy direction has identified frameworks through which clinical governance will be monitored for its continual improvement and transparency throughout every level of the organisation's activities (Department of Health, 2001b). Quiet clearly this is a significant shift in the way in which a very large and complex organisation is managed. At face value this change can be viewed as a threat, creating feelings of anxiety within individuals and a sense of chaos for the organisation as a whole. On the

other hand, within this business ethos, nurses have risen to the challenge of a business culture, carving out their own niches or influencing change at all levels of the organisation. It is a particular opportunity for nurses, which will continue for a number of years. For example, nurses today employ salaried general practitioners, they lead on new services such as urology, rheumatology and chronic disease management services, they manage walk-in centres and Nurse Direct, they are members of the organisation's executive group and commissioning boards and the newly appointed consultant nurses are expected to make significant contributions to shaping local services (Department of Health, 1999b).

These new roles for nurses require the nurse to have expert clinical knowledge and a working knowledge of the business of health care. This includes activities such as budget management, resource management, strategic planning and clinical governance. It is no longer acceptable for the nurse practitioner, consultant nurse, health visitor, and district nurse or ward sister to be exempt from such involvement, as everything impinges on the quality of care. Quality of health care relies very heavily on the accurate prediction of skill mixing, sufficient availability of basic equipment, prescribing drugs, the provision of efficiently and economically run health care services, the predicted need of new services and the impact these will have on human and physical resources. We know that the world of health care business is diverse and nurses need to be able to respond to changes in the most efficient way. In the words of the Secretary of State (Department of Health, 1997) the NHS needs to continue to offer high-quality treatment and care when and where people need it in order to improve health and reduce inequalities.

The *NHS Ten-year Plan* (Department of Health, 2000) has endorsed these sentiments and we are set to see an active involvement of government to oversee health care reforms and give directions for change through government policy documents. In meeting government targets the business of health care requires a comprehensive and sophisticated mechanism for effective training and professional development. In addition, there is a need for information systems that are compatible with each other and a workforce who is able to feed data into the information systems and effectively interpret the outcome into effective clinical decision. There will also be a need to conduct estate management that is suitable for the delivery of modern treatments and caring activities. Underpinning all this is the notion that the business of the health care organisations must ensure financial viability and minimise risks to staff and the users of the health care service (Alderman, 2001).

Research indicates a sense of apathy and disillusionment within the health care workforce, which is associated with feelings of demotivation, being de-skilled and de-valued. Williams (1998) claims that such staff attitudes affect the quality of care and recommends that ways must be found in which staff (including nurses) have more control over their work and organisational and clinical decision-making.

In 1995, The National Health Service Executive formally recognised that nurses in clinical practice should be involved with the business of the health care organisation, particularly in helping to develop and review contracts. This is indeed a great opportunity for nurses, but the rejoicing must be tempered with a pragmatic realisation that not all nurses are ready and able to undertake these new roles and demands (Antrobus and Brown, 1997; Brocklehurst, 1999). Lacking in business skills and business acumen seriously disadvantages nurses to participate fully with their other medical colleagues. Antrobus and Brown (1997) clearly illustrated that doctors were more confident and assertive, with a longer history of being involved with management issues and making their demands for improved services known. In contrast, nurses were under-confident, hesitant and deferential, hiding behind hierarchy and lacking the ability to read and interpret data to best suit their own interest.

With such alarming evidence, great strides have been taken by government and regions to enable and empower nurses to gain the skills of leadership and management, which include strategic planning, clinical governance and fiscal management (Block, 1995; Greengard, 2000). Personal development plans are encouraged that address individual training needs, and each clinical speciality is encouraged to complete a business plan that links with the Departments of Health's key objectives and priorities for the future (Department of Health, 1999a).

Armed with this information, nurses must actively engage with the world of health care business, as indeed health care is the business of nursing. Having gained these skills, nurses will be juxtaposed to influence change at all levels of the organisation and effectively direct the future and the liberation of the nursing profession.

NURSE EDUCATION

The 1990s saw radical changes in the education and training of nurses, moving away dramatically from the apprenticeship model to a higher education that enables the student nurse to reflect in and on their practice. The result of such change was to ensure that the new practitioner would be knowledgeable and fit to practice.

The nurse's education does not finish upon registration. There is now a strong political directive for a nurse to continue to learn throughout the whole of her professional career, ensuring her continued competence to practice. This activity was cemented within the continuing professional development requirements for re-registration (United Kingdom Central Council, 1994), whereupon learning can be achieved through a variety of modes, which is evidenced through a professional portfolio. Flexible education has therefore become a buzzword not only with nursing, but within the broader framework of mainstream education. Models such as open and distance learning, e-learning, work-based learning and learning through teams are all modern approaches used to enhance the opportunities for everyone to learn on a continuous spiral throughout their professional life. The future of nursing education will change dramatically over the next decade and curriculum designers will be poised to reflect the new models of learning, which will be increasingly more flexible.

PUBLIC HEALTH

The notion of public health has been with nursing since the early years of Florence Nightingale, but only those nurses who had a distinct role in public health, such as health visitors and district nurses, were expected to fully embrace the philosophies underpinning the public health movement. Within the next decade this phenomenon is certainly going to change. Public health, as decreed by the Government's *NHS Ten-year Plan* (2000), is the business of everyone working in health care. Strategies and agendas are linked to this philosophy and the nursing profession will need to play a pivotal role, both at the strategic and clinical level of implementation.

SUMMARY

Nursing in an age of change is a phenomenon of evolving societies and should not be viewed as of major importance but as an accepted part of life. However, the pace and amount of change confronting the nursing profession as we move forward in the new millennium is so radical in nature that the nursing profession cannot either ignore or escape the influences of change. Indeed, the social, political and economic pressures in our world are placing great strains on health care systems, requiring radical changes that move away from traditional caring and organisational practices. Nurses are the largest group of health care workers and they are shaped by these reforms but they can also shape the reforms themselves by becoming political activists, or at least engaging in political debates.

To function in the new world of health care nurses must adapt to the demands of change, gaining new skills and knowledge along the way. They will lead others and in so doing will need to gain leadership skills and be clinical experts working from a strong evidence base. While many nurses' clinical competence will, of necessity, use technological therapies, there is a strong need to recognise and actively use the caring skills that are so intimate to the healing process as a central component of nursing care. In the words of the old adage, nurses should be constantly mindful not to 'throw the baby out with the bathwater'.

REFERENCES

American Association of Registered Nurses (1993) *Position Statement: Nursing education's agenda for the twenty-first century*, American Association of Registered Nurses, Washington DC

Abu-Zinahda, S. (1999) The relationship between staff and job characteristics to quality of work life, Paper presented at the ICN Centennial Celebration Conference, London

Albarran, J.W. (1995) Should nurses be politically aware? *British Journal of Nursing* 4(8), 461–5

Alderman, M.C. (2001) Nursing in the new millennium: challenges and opportunities. *Journal of Dermatology Nursing* 13(1), 44–5, 49–50

Antrobus, S. and Brown, S. (1997) The impact of commissioning agenda upon the nurse in practice: a proactive approach to influencing policy. *Journal of Advanced Nursing* 25, 309–15

Basford, L. (2001a) Quantum healing: nursing therapy [President's column, e-nursing]. *Journal of the European Honours Society for Nurses and Midwives* 2(2), 1–3

Basford, L. (2001b) Quantum healing: nursing therapy [President's column, e-nursing]. *Journal of the European Honours Society for Nurses and Midwives*, 1(1), 1–3

Basford, L. and Bowskill, D. (2001) Celebrating the present, challenging the future of nurse prescribing. *Journal of Community Nursing* 6(9), 467–71

Basford, L., Mathers, N. and Pirri, L. (1998) Lotus: a model for practice. *Multi-professional Learning* 15, 16–17

Benner, P. (1984) *From Novice to Expert: Excellence and power in clinical practice*, Addison-Wesley, Menlo Park, New York

Block, P. (1995) *Stewardship*, Berrett-Koehler, San Francisco, CA

Brocklehurst, J. (1999) Getting into business: how nurses can make a difference. *Nursing Standard* 14(2), 46–53

Chopra, D. (1990) *Quantum Healing: Exploring the frontiers of mind/body medicine*, Bantum Press, London

Clifford, C. (2000) International politics and nursing education: power and control. *Nurse Education Today* 20(1), 4–9

Department of Health (1997) *The New NHS: Modern, dependable*, The Stationery Office, London

Department of Health (1999a) *Saving Lives: Our healthier nation*, The Stationery Office, London

Department of Health (1999b) *Making a Difference: Strengthening the nursing, midwifery and health visiting contribution to health and health care*, The Stationery Office, London

Department of Health (2000) *The National Health Service Ten-year Plan*, DoH, London

Department of Health (2001a) *The National Service Framework for Older People*, HMSO, London

Department of Health (2001b) *The Commission for Health Improvement*, DoH, London

Fawcett, J. (1984) The metaparadigm of nursing: present status and future refinements. *IMAGE: Journal of Nursing Scholarship* 16, 84–7

Flower, J. (1999) Building the idea factory: a conversation with John Kao. *Health Forum Journal* 42, 12–15

Greengard, S. (2000) Business intelligence: creating strategic advantage. *Beyond Computing* 9, 18–23

Handy, C.(1993) *The Age of Unreason*, Harvard Business Review, Boston, MA

International Federation of Trading and Development (1998) The challenges of globalisation. *IFIDO News* 2, 2–4

Kirby, C. and Slevin, O. (1992) A new curriculum for care. In: Slevin, O. and Buckenham, M. (eds) *Project 2000: The teachers speak*, Campion Press, Edinburgh

Leininger, M. (1978) *Transcultural Nursing: Concepts, theories and practice*, John Wiley, New York

Meleis, A.I. (1991) *Theoretical Nursing: Development and progress* (2nd edition), J.B. Lippincott, New York

Naisbitt, J. (1991) *Megatrends: Ten new directions transforming our lives*, Warner Books, New York

Narayanasamy, A. (1999) ASSET: A model for actioning spirituality and spiritual care education and training. *Nurse Education Today* 19(4), 274–85

Newman, M.A., Sime, A.M. and Concoran-Perry, S.A. (1991) The focus of the discipline of nursing. *Advances In Nursing Science* 14(1), 1–6

Oulton J. (1999) Nursing's future. In: Maslin, A. (ed) *Nursing the World*, Nursing Times Books, London

Parse, R.R. (1992) Human becoming: Parse's theory of nursing. In: Riehl-Sisca, L. (ed.) *Conceptual Models for Nursing Practice* (3rd edition), Appleton and Lang, Norwalk, CN

Poon, L.W., Basford, L., Dowzer, C. *et al.* (2003) Living with multiple health problems: a coping perspective by older people. In: Poon, L.W., Hall Gueldner, S. and Spouse, B. (eds) *Successful Ageing and Adaptation with Chronic Diseases in Older People*, Springer, New York

Robinson, J. (1997) Power, politics and policy analysis in nursing. In: Perry, A. (ed.) *Nursing: A knowledge base for practice* (2nd edition), Arnold, London

Salmon, M. (1999) Nursing and midwifery at the crossroads: challenges and opportunities. In. Maslin, A. (ed.) *Nursing the World*, Nursing Times Books, London

United Kingdom Central Council (1994) *Professional Requirements for Educational Practice (PREP)*, UKCC, London

Williams, S. (1998) *Improving the Health of the NHS Workforce: Report of the partnership on the health of the NHS workforce*, The Nufield Trust, London

Williams, S. (2001) Nursing 2001: designing the future (presidential address). *Connecticut Nursing News* 7(4), 1, 3–4

Whittle, C. and Jester, R. (1998) *Health Assessment: A report on a visit to Denver, Colorado School of Health Sciences*, University of Birmingham, Birmingham

43

INTO THE FUTURE: POST-MODERN AND BEYOND*

Jean Watson

LEARNING OUTCOMES

After studying this chapter you will be able to:

- Appreciate the impact of modernity and post-modern influences upon nursing
- Recognise the value of looking to the past as a source of richness and depth for meeting the demands of the future
- Embrace human caring as a thread that extends from the past through the present to the future, as both the foundation upon which our practice rests and a beacon that lights pathways to our future
- Identify 'ontological competencies' that are equally important to technical competencies in our engagement in healing relations
- Reflect upon the post-modern condition as a space within which nursing can become a source of humanity and healing.

INTRODUCTION

Pre-modern, modern, post-modern: what are we to make of these changing worlds and times? As nursing and health care moves into another discourse in human history, related not only to its survival, but its integrity, how are we to consider our pre-modern roots, traditions, and rich history, in addressing the needs of humanity across worlds and time, while still being in the modern, post-modern world of complexity, techno-science, chaos, ambiguities and unknowns about the future? These are questions, issues and dilemmas that this chapter has sought to address.

LOOKING BACK TO PROJECT FORWARD

In more formally considering these futuristic concerns for a post-modern world of nursing, it seems that we have reached somewhat of a plateau, or an abyss, in trying to solve old problems through outmoded ways of thinking about what matters; about what nursing is all about; and about what and why we exist in the first place – now needing to 're-member' ourselves and our profession.

This chapter takes us back to the pre-modern values foundation, while projecting us forward into a renewed future that helps us survive with integrity and authenticity towards what truly matters. For it is only through such a journey towards personal–professional wholeness, which integrates past with the present – reconciles past and present with a new vision for the future – can we project any hope for healing: for self, for other, for the planet Earth, for human survival into this millennium.

What is this process of simultaneously propelling backwards and projecting forwards that we need at this moment in our present to make this journey into the future? First and foremost it begins with a centring and a 're-membering' why we are here; this 're-membering' returns us to our source, which is: *informed moral passion and basic values, knowledge and skills of human caring and healing*, but now we have to rediscover these, as if for the first time, for entirely new reasons: scientifically and spiritually (Watson, 1990).

The crisis in modern medicine, nursing and society itself, seems to lie in the lack of a mean-

---

*Parts of this chapter are adopted and adapted from Watson (2002a, b).

ingful philosophy about our own humanity, as well as the nature of our practices and the deeper dimensions of our work. It is as if our jobs have been too small for the nature of our work (Watson, 2002a). We have reached a point, a fault-line of sorts, whereby we now must treat ethical, philosophical, non-measurable aspects of our work, such as values, deep beliefs, intentions, consciousness, energy, spirit, and the artistry of our humanity, with the same attention we have given to physical disease, hospital–medical-orientated 'doing tasks', and institutional demands of the modern era (Watson, 2002b).

Nursing in the modern twentieth century world has been so confined and controlled by external, material physical realities, found within our institutions and Western medicine, that it and we have almost lost our way home to our heritage and *raison d'etre*. It seems at this crossroads we have reached a point where we have to return to our source for our survival. The source of humanity we seem to seek at this point is the core of human caring that comes from a deep dimension of our humanity, which in turn offers a spiritual basis for our practice and existence.

Study Activity 43.1 ⎯⎯⎯⎯⎯⎯

Reference is made in this chapter to the pre-modern, the modern, and the post-modern. It is suggested that in moving forward into a new, more complex world we need also to look to the past as a source that will enlighten the future.

● Carry out a library or Internet search using the three terms (pre-modern, modern and post-modern) as your search terms. The terms 'modernity' and 'modernisation' may also be helpful.
● Write brief explanations of the three terms and then relate these to the discussion in the first section of the chapter.

⎯⎯⎯⎯⎯⎯⎯⎯⎯⎯⎯⎯⎯⎯

SPIRIT AS SOURCE: TIMELESS, ENDURING, INFINITE

In considering pre-modern nursing perspectives, against the objectivist angst of the modern–post-modern crisis in science and society, nursing has always represented a rich spiritual tradition. Nursing leaders across time, as well as nurses in their intimate practices, have always refused to reduce the human to the moral status of object, and have rejected such practices that do so, in spite of being in systems where such practices are mainstream. Indeed, for Nightingale, nursing was considered a spiritual practice, a calling; spirituality was considered intrinsic to human nature and a potent source for healing. In this heritage, nursing and its caring-healing practices for humanity, in harmony with nature, form a values-based foundation that grounds nursing in creating and sustaining its post-modern future.

A tradition of human caring, of preserving human dignity, of preserving humanity itself, is a timeless, yet ironically futuristic, view of nursing, helping to re-establish old/new enduring relationships between such essentials in human nature as: caring, love, beauty, soul, related to inner healing, realigning us with the art and artistry of our being–becoming more human, more whole. This spirit-filled direction for nursing's future simultaneously intersects with the latest developments in mind–body medicine and new holistic medical practices and breakthroughs in so-called complementary-alternative medicine (Watson, 1999). Thus, there is a converging of paradigms and passions for new directions for science and self, of the practitioners and patients alike, as we make this collective turn towards a new future – a future we are co-creating in the present *now*.

It seems the convergence of consciousness which is emerging in health and healing practices is an awakened awareness that nursing's task in the world community coincides and intersects with the common tasks of humanity itself. These shared tasks are what I consider 'ontological competencies', in that they require developing our own humanity, and asking new questions about what it means to be fully human and humane.

These intersecting universal human pursuits include at least the following ontological dimensions and tasks related to living, being, and dying (Watson, 2002a, b):

- Healing our relationships with self and others and our place in the wider universe
- Understanding and transforming our own and other's suffering
- Deepening our understanding of death (the light–dark cycles of impermanence of all of life), including preparing for our own death
- Learning to open our hearts to infinite love, which allows us to find meaning in our own life, awakening to profound compassion, caring, and healing service in the world.

It is through entering into and engaging in these human tasks that we become healers; that we awaken to our own humanity and our shared humanity with all whom we touch in any given moment in time. It is here in these deeply intimate, timeless, transcendent human aspects of our work, and the personal–professional challenges they invoke, that we awaken to our source, our philosophical traditions and inspired/inspirited ideals. This connection with infinity of spirit returns us to our roots and our deepest ethical ideals for the future.

Nursing's tradition of caring and healing is, ironically, both historical and futuristic, in that it is guided by these timeless values. It is as if somewhere along the way in modern nursing's rise, we forgot that in taking care of people we are given the greatest honour one can have. It is here in this deeply subjective–intersubjective spirit-filled space of human caring relationships that nursing touches the sacred in the midst of the profane. To clarify and claim our deep human values and caring stance as the basis for nursing's future and past is a restoration of the heart and soul of nursing. For any profession that loses its values is soul-less; it becomes heartless and therefore becomes worthless. The worth of a profession is in clarifying, articulating, and manifesting its values through action. Our values renew our energy; they inspirit our commitment and purpose for compassionate service in the world. It is our values that unite us, rather than separate. When our values are congruent with our actions, we are in harmony. We may even say we are healthy; we are whole.

By cultivating mindfulness of values, such as loving, kindness, tenderness, caring, as our values become manifest in and through our actions, we recognise that we create the caring field in our life and world. Through our values we communicate an energy and consciousness that energetically begets these values back to our work and our world.

By not being mindful, intentional and conscious with respect to our values, we beget the opposite, which can be, and is, harmful to self, other, the system, and our world.

As our values become manifest in and through our actions, we recognise that we create the caring field in our life and world. In awakening to this new reality and newly acknowledged interrelationship between and among values, consciousness, intentionality, and actions, nursing is now invited, if not required, to re-pattern its energy field in the direction of an expanded caring–healing consciousness, moving towards deeper healing, and the spirit-filled aspects of our word (Quinn, 1992).

Nursing's values can now be named and claimed in this post-modern era as the very source for its survival in an age of despair and chaos. These timeless values offer nursing science and practice a meta-narrative that is human orientated, context sensitive, pattern focused, relational, participatory, and open to transformative possibilities for both self and other (Reed, 1995). Nursing, in this pre–post-modern sense can now be envisioned as the keeper of the common values that serve individuals, society, and civilisation, in that they help to sustain and preserve humanity.

Study Activity 43.2

The pre-modern or historical orientation that is also carried into our present and future includes at its heart a commitment to human caring.

- Review the statements about human caring by Kirby in Chapter 2. Identify the fundamental meaning of this term, including its characteristics in caring relations.

- In the current chapter, it is suggested that this is a timeless aspect of nursing, as important to our future as it was to our past. Reflect upon influences in modern health care systems that may make this human dimension of caring more difficult to sustain.
- In this chapter, a significant aspect of this dimension is described as infinite love, a spiritual source that enables us to find meaning and reach out to the other in compassionate, caring and healing ways. However, the use of the word 'love' is controversial within the caring professions. It seems to hold little value in modern, instrumental, high technological health care systems and, probably because of alternative erotic meanings of the term, is viewed with a high degree of discomfort and suspicion. Carry out a literature search of philosophical meanings of the term 'love', and its particular relevance in nursing and the wider therapeutic context. Search terms such as 'love', 'concern', 'compassion', 'passion', and 'agapé' may help. Write a brief account of your review that links to the discussion in the chapter.

SUMMARY

Finally, in this new post-modern time and space, we are called upon to create new space for nurses to enter into, yet become our own caring environment for self, other, and systems. Individually and collectively, nurses are being transformed, becoming the caring field, living the healing practices in their daily existence.

It is in this old/new space, grounded in our own philosophical and ethical heritage and extant theories, that nursing becomes what it ironically has been all along. It now embraces all aspects of its whole self – the deeply human dimensions of an energised, spirit-filled practice. By reconnecting with core values, knowledge, skills and traditions of caring and healing, nursing is charged with a call for a renewal of our professional ethic and ethos.

The future calls and waits for this old/new nursing. Where are we? Do we hear the call? Do we respond to the post-modern public cry for the sacred to manifest in the midst of science? Or will we go on acting as if nothing has happened?

Whichever road we choose, we now have new post-modern space to more fully embrace, articulate, and live out our holy, but firm, ground of being, with grace and dignity. Whether we choose to enter and dwell in this new territory remains a rhetorical and existential question. Each nurse is faced with this heart-felt challenge; if we choose wisely; the future opens to infinite possibilities for nursing's future.

Study Activity 43.3

On completion of this chapter, take some time for reflection in solitude. Do not look to other sources or literature, and do not indulge in analysis and note taking. Treat this reflection as a personal discourse between yourself and the chapter.

- Consider how what is said in the chapter fits with your own feelings about nursing.
- Identify any ways in which what is said in this chapter may influence your own approach to nursing in the future.

REFERENCES

Quinn, J. (1992) Holding sacred space: the nurse as healing environment. *Holistic Nursing Practice* 6(4), 26–36

Reed, P.G. (1995) A treatise on nursing knowledge development for the 21st century: beyond postmodernism. *Advances in Nursing Science* 17(3), 70–84

Watson, J. (1990) Caring knowledge and informed moral passion. *Advances in Nursing Science* 13(1), 15–24

Watson, J. (1999) *Postmodern Nursing and Beyond*, Churchill-Livingstone/Harcourt-Brace, Edinburgh

Watson, J. (2002a) Nursing: seeking its source and survival. *ICUs and Nursing Web Journal www.nursing.gr/J.W.editorial.pdf*

Watson, J. (2002b) Intentionality and caring-healing consciousness: a theory of transpersonal nursing. *Holistic Nursing Practice* 16(4), 12–19

44 GLOBAL DIMENSIONS: NURSING IN THE RISK SOCIETY

Oliver Slevin

> *The world is in agony. The agony is so pervasive and urgent that we are compelled to name its manifestations so that the depth of this pain may be made clear. Peace eludes us … the planet is being destroyed … neighbors live in fear … women and men are estranged from each other … children die! This is abhorrent!*
>
> (Parliament of the World's Religions, 1993)

LEARNING OUTCOMES

After studying this chapter you will be able to:

- Explain the process of globalisation as a social phenomenon *and* as a global consciousness
- Identify the new characteristics of globalisation in the modern era
- Describe the movement to a risk society and beyond this to a global risk society
- Discuss specific aspects of global risk, including disaster and terrorist attack
- Present a case for the emergence of a global ethic
- Discuss that particular aspect of globalisation that presents at local levels in the form of multicultural societies
- Present appropriate nursing responses and contributions in respect of the different aspects of globalisation discussed.

INTRODUCTION

In the earlier chapters of this final module we considered the impact of change upon nursing and considered how in a world of change we can look from the present both backwards and into the future. In one sense, this involved quite a dramatic change in perspective. From looking inwards to matters that concern us in the world of nursing, within health care systems, we turned to how the world as a whole impacts upon nursing. And not only this, but also how nursing can itself impact upon this world and upon these systems.

In the current chapter, we take this shift in perspective one step further. Here we consider issues on a *global* level that impact upon nursing. In doing so we address the positive impact upon humanity of globalisation, marked by international co-operation and sharing of wealth, technology and information in the service of humanity. But so too do we address the negative impact of a world gone wrong – war, famine, ecological disasters that are both natural and manmade. Importantly, we consider not only these 'impacts' but the part nursing can play in promoting the good and limiting the harm at a global level. As we consider key issues concerning global influences, in each instance we address in turn the implications of these issues for nursing.

GLOBALISATION IN THE MODERN ERA

Precedents

Globalisation is not a recent phenomenon. It commenced many centuries ago, well before Columbus and Brendan the Navigator sailed west in search of new worlds. Peoples move outwards and inwards, communicate, intermingle in the fields of international trade and politics. By such means, the web of social affiliations that we today term globalisation commenced at the level of nomadic groups and tribes, then nations and eventually continents. It is indeed part of humankind's nature that it will always look outwards to the world around it. But in doing so, a peculiar phenomenon occurs. Just as we reach out to the world, so too does it reach inwards, changing our way of thinking and feeling. There is thus in one sense a duality to globalisation: it is both an external coming together of people and environments and an internal change in how we think about the world that is in effect an altered state of consciousness.

Within the twentieth century and into this new millennium, globalisation has taken on a new meaning. Massive and rapid advances in technology have resulted in major developments, significant among which are the explosion of information, the significant advances in high technology communications, and the advances in rapid transit travel. Thus, it is now possible to communicate across the globe within seconds, to exchange large volumes of information by such channels, to travel to the extremes of the globe within a single day, and indeed to travel beyond Earth's bounds. The difference in the new globalisation phenomenon is essentially one of a transformation in consciousness. People now increasingly have an awareness of the totality of the Earth and its societies, and an increasing awareness of how circumstances at a global level impact on the local situation and vice versa. Such awareness emerged with the world wars of the previous century, including the pervasive impact of the Holocaust that spread across the civilised nations following the Second World War. This trend continued as, with mass communication advancements, awareness of major national and regional disasters became known as they were happening. Perhaps more significant in recent times, the 2001 attacks on the World Trade Center in New York, the 2003 Iraq war and the threat of global terrorism brought home to people how global influences reach not only into the nation-state but the very hearts and minds of individuals.

Benefits and challenges

The advantages of this new globalisation are numerous: the sharing of health technologies,

food, information, and expertise to name a few. However, part of the information exchange is an awareness of the plight of others, as referred to in the above opening quotation. The knowledge of war, famine, infringement of human rights, burgeon in upon us as never before. Significantly, we become aware that much of this human suffering is caused by that same globalisation that spreads good. Whatever the causes, the call from others in plight flash across the world on our television and computer screens, crash through national boundaries and stream in upon our consciousness. Governments respond, celebrities hold famine relief festivals, and some pack their bags and answer the call.

Just as there is a movement outwards, so too is there the movement inwards. What North America experienced in the previous centuries, other countries experienced in the twentieth century, as world-wide immigration led to increasingly multicultural societies. This trend brought with it not only the richness of cultural diversity, but also challenges in terms of such phenomena as integration and segregation, ethnicity and racialism, and changing demands upon health and social care services. These social migrations present challenges *for* nations and *between* nations.

Clearly, while global influences have the potential for great good, there are also major challenges involved. Indeed, as will be argued below, we are moving towards a situation wherein these challenges in some instances present major threats to the very existence of society, such that the phrase 'the risk society' (which we discuss below), has been coined. As indicated above, others grapple with the various challenges presented by globalisation – whether it be through government actions, the initiatives of voluntary agencies and transnational corporations, or the informal actions of groups and individuals. These global influences increasingly impact on every individual and no less on those who are nurses by profession. However, there is a need for a *nursing* response to global influences in the future, and this is the topic of the current chapter.

Study Activity 44.1

Carry out a library or Internet search for definitions of the term globalisation. Continue your search until you have four definitions or explanations that you understand. Make brief notes of these definitions/explanations and then re-read the previous section. Reflect upon how this activity has enhanced your capability to understand the points being made in the section.

Implications for nursing

A direct influence of this new globalisation phenomenon is the extent to which nursing itself attains a global dimension. That same feature of globalisation that relates to global communication networks encompasses within it a nursing global communication network. In its

inception, this has tended to be formal and as such perhaps of limited impact upon the general body of nurses world-wide. Significant in such formal developments has been the work of the World Health Organisation and specifically the World Health Assembly (established within the World Health Organisation framework). For example, the World Health Assembly Resolution WHA 49.1 made specific proposals for strengthening nursing and midwifery world-wide (World Health Assembly, 1996). These, as identified in Table 44.1, established aspirations for nursing developments at a global level. Significantly, the proposals identify a key role for a Global Advisory Group on Nursing and Midwifery (established by the Assembly in the early 1990s). The role of this group is clearly crucial to a global nursing impact, as indicated by its terms of reference:

Table 44.1   Strengthening nursing and midwifery 1996

The World Health Assembly

URGES Member States:

1   to involve nurses and midwives more closely in health care reform and in the development of national health policy;
2   to develop, where these do not exist, and carry out national action plans for health, including nursing/midwifery as an integral part of national health policy, outlining the steps necessary to bring about change in health care delivery, ensuring further development of policy, assessment of needs and utilisation of resources, legislation, management, working conditions, basic and continuing education, quality assurance and research;
3   to increase opportunities for nurses and midwives in the health teams when selecting candidates for fellowships in nursing and health-related fields;
4   to monitor and evaluate the progress towards attainment of national health and development targets and in particular the effective use of nurses and midwives in the priority areas of equitable access to health services, health protection and promotion, and prevention and control of specific health problems;
5   to strengthen nursing/midwifery education and practice in primary health care.

REQUESTS the Director-General:

1   to increase support to countries, where appropriate, in the development, implementation and evaluation of national plans for health development including nursing and midwifery;
2   to promote co-ordination between all agencies and collaborating centres and other organisations concerned in countries to support their health plan and make optimal use of available human and material resources;
3   to provide for the continued work of the Global Advisory Group on Nursing and Midwifery;
4   to promote and support the training of nursing/midwifery personnel in research methodology in order to facilitate their participation in health research programmes;
5   to keep the Health Assembly informed of progress made in the implementation of this resolution, and to report to the Fifty-fourth World Health Assembly in 2001.

(From: World Health Assembly, 1996)

- To advise the Director-General (of the World Health Assembly) on nursing and midwifery as an important resource for improving the health of all people, increasing equity of health outcomes and ensuring the right of all people to health.
- To guide the development of the Global Agenda for Nursing and Midwifery within the health agenda.
- To provide policy advice on how the responsiveness of health systems to people's health needs can be optimised through the effective use of nursing and midwifery services that are based on research as scientific evidence.
- To support the development and use of nursing and midwifery outcome indicators in relation to health gains and health status.
- To participate in resource mobilisation and efforts for the effective implementation of the Global Agenda for Nursing and Midwifery.
- To collaborate in establishing mechanisms for monitoring the progress of nursing and midwifery contributions to the health agenda and to the implementation of the Global Agenda for Nursing and Midwifery.

It will be clear from Table 44.1 that significant weight is given to the impact of nursing and midwifery in respect of health across a range of activities spanning health care policy, equitable access to services, public health, primary care, and research and development activities. It is important to note that this is in the context of a World Health Organisation, and that the push here is towards establishing standards at a *global* level. There is, of course, a question in respect of how such initiatives will make real world differences. The 'urges' and 'requests' contained in the resolution were to be revisited in 2001. The subsequent statement made in 2001 is informative in this respect (World Health Assembly, 2001). This is presented in Table 44.2.

While there is little evidence to indicate the progress over a 5 year period, it is at least possible to see a continuity of purpose here. Significantly, this continuity picks up on emerging problems that must be addressed at a

global level. As will be noted in Table 44.2 (overleaf), a significant trend emerging is the issue of human resources planning and the global shortage of nurses. Indeed, in a recent survey of Government Chief Nursing Officers, Salmon and Rambo (2002) found that the first ranked issue of concern was that of workforce difficulties and, in particular, the international shortage of nurses. This particular issue highlights one of the major difficulties within an increasingly global perspective, that of migration.

Where such global shortages occur there is a tendency for nurses to migrate from areas with fewer employment and career opportunities and lower pay to those areas where the employment and career opportunities and remuneration are significantly greater. Furthermore, as shortages become more critical in the more affluent Western countries, there are active recruitment drives to entice nurses away from areas where in fact the health needs are greater. Some years ago, Tudor Hart (1971) introduced the concept of the *inverse care law* that appeared to operate within the UK health care system. Essentially this states that those areas within that system where the health needs were greatest tended to receive lower quality of service, and that a significant factor in this was the tendency for doctors to choose to work in the more affluent areas. Thus, in Great Britain, health care was better in the south than in the north, and better in respectable suburbia than in inner city areas. Within the context of a global nursing shortage, a similar inverse care law would appear to be emerging, with richer countries with the lesser health care needs aggressively recruiting nurses from the poorer countries with greater health care needs.

While at first sight this would appear to advantage the more affluent Western societies, the situation is not without its problems. Kingmo (2001) has drawn attention to the vulnerability of migrant nurses, the potential for exploitation, and significant issues such as cultural and language barriers that may militate against such solutions being to the benefit of the recruiting state. It has been suggested that batch

Table 44.2   Strengthening nursing and midwifery 2001

The World Health Assembly

URGES Member States:

1   to further the development of their health systems and to pursue health sector reform by involving nurses and midwives in the framing, planning and implementation of health policy at all levels;
2   to review or develop and implement national action plans for health and models of education, legislation, regulation and practice for nurses and midwives, and to ensure that these adequately and appropriately reflect competencies and knowledge that enable nurses and midwives to meet the needs of the population they serve;
3   to establish comprehensive programmes for the development of human resources which support the training, recruitment and retention of a skilled and motivated nursing and midwifery workforce within health services;
4   to develop and implement policies and programmes which ensure healthy workplaces and quality of the work environment for nurses and midwives;
5   to underpin the above measures through continuing assessment of nursing and midwifery needs and by developing, reviewing regularly, and implementing national action plans for nursing and midwifery, as an integral part of national health policy;
6   to enhance the development of nursing and midwifery services that reduce risk factors and respond to health needs, on the basis of sound scientific and clinical evidence;
7   to prepare plans for evaluating nursing services.

REQUESTS the Director-General:

1   to provide support to Member States in setting up mechanisms for inquiry into the global shortage of nursing and midwifery personnel, including the impact of migration, and in developing human resources plans and programmes, including ethical international recruitment;
2   to provide support to Member States in their efforts to strengthen the contribution of nurses and midwives to the health of the populations and to take the necessary measures to increase the number of World Health Organisation collaborating centres for nursing and midwifery in developing countries;
3   to ensure the involvement of nursing and midwifery experts in the integrated planning of human resources for health, including support to Member States undertaking programmes of village skilled birth attendants, by developing guidelines and training modules, as an expanded role of nurses and in particular midwives;
4   to continue to co-operate with governments to promote effective co-ordination between all agencies and organisations concerned with the development of nursing and midwifery;
5   to provide continuing support for the work of the Global Advisory Group on Nursing and Midwifery, and to take account of the interest and contribution of nursing and midwifery in wider aspects of the development and implementation of the World Health Organisation's policy and programmes;
6   to develop and implement systems and uniform performance indicators at country, regional and global levels to monitor, measure, and report progress in achieving these goals;
7   to prepare rapidly a plan of action for the strengthening of nursing and midwifery and to provide for external evaluation at the conclusion thereof;
8   to keep the Health Assembly informed of progress made in the implementation of this resolution, and to report to the Fifty-sixth World Health Assembly in 2003.

(*From*: World Health Assembly, 2001)

recruitment of overseas recruits may produce short-term gains but possibly longer-term problems (Buchan and O'May, 1999). In addition, the International Council of Nurses (1999) cautions against such practices in countries where the reasons for poor recruitment or nurses leaving the profession have not been addressed in the first place.

It should be clear from the above comments that – at least in the context of more formal contexts such as the World Health Organisation – nursing has entered into and become influenced by the globalisation trend. While it may appear that there are some significant negative implications involved, it is at least important to note that the problems are being recognised on a global level and that global solutions are being considered.

A further positive aspect of the globalisation trend lies in the more informal developments. A cursory search of the Internet will display a large number of networks that are endeavouring to establish a global discourse between nurses across the globe. It is reasonable to assume that as such networking trends continue, the general body of nurses will establish a greater global consciousness, and that from this will emerge informal as well as formal collaboration. In essence, we can anticipate a global community of nurses with the potential for extending its influence on health across the full range of human endeavours, from the individual sick bed to the full expanses of the Earth.

Study Activity 44.2

Would you consider immigrating to another country to work as a nurse? Reflect upon such a move, and in doing so, list the possible advantages and disadvantages you might envisage. Consider what action you might take to overcome the disadvantages. If possible, discuss this issue with fellow students/peers.

THE NEW GLOBALISATION AS A SOURCE OF SOCIAL RISK

The economic drivers

A significant element of globalisation in the modern era is the extent to which the benefits of modernity have facilitated the process. A significant driver within this process, and one that some say is in fact the main driver, is that of economic globalisation. That is, the movement towards what is in fact an Earth-wide community within which the first citizens are multinational or transnational corporations. For centuries, globalisation has increasingly knitted together the world and created unity out of great diversity, but in the modern era we find the forces of modernity have finally facilitated an economic globalism. Products like Coca Cola, Hard Rock Cafe and McDonald's are the totems of the new globalisation, and corporations like Microsoft, Shell and IBM are its sources of power, often exceeding the power and wealth of whole nations. They are products known and consumed from Tasmania to Iceland, and also powerful companies that drive globalisation forward – establishing new markets for the 'wants' *they* have created; new ways to eat, drink and even live; and, new hopes and dreams.

It is important to recognise the importance of these economic drivers. The colonisation of poorer countries by the powerful in previous centuries was primarily in quest of profit. To this end, rich resources of poorer countries were plundered and human beings were sold into slavery. The Western powers who voiced protest and shock about the twentieth century Holocaust were the same nations that invented the concentration camp and the modern genocide of indigenous peoples in the colonial era.

Following the Second World War, colonisation was in decline and being replaced by a new globalism that still found its motive within economic drivers. However, now there was a recognition that a degree of co-operation rather than conflict was a more efficient way of amassing wealth. Immediately after the Second World War this was reflected in the famous international General Agreement on Tariffs and Trade (GATT), and in 1995 the GATT successor known as the World Trade Organisation (WTO) was established. Under GATT, and subsequently the WTO, agreements were reached on trade that would have the ultimate goal of improving the welfare of the peoples of the member nations. As this alliance grew and strengthened, it became increasingly clear that what affected one nation to a greater or lesser extent also affected all the others: globalisation had truly arrived. Significantly, a shift in emphasis occurred with the establishment of the WTO. What in GATT had originally been a 'marriage of convenience' now became one in which there was a consciousness of interconnectedness within which not only benefits but also risks were shared across nations.

Optimists look forward to a global village, linked by intercontinental communications, rapid transit travel and the Internet, and benefiting from ever-increasing material well-being through international co-operation and trade. At its extreme, this is the Utopian view. Pessimists see a frightful corporate tyranny destroying the environment, wasting rain forests and creating global warming, leaving behind a trail of toxic and nuclear waste, and sweeping away all that is healthy and meaningful to human existence. At its extreme, this is the Armageddon scenario. Between these two polarised positions lies the truth. For developments in insecticides and herbicides, we all pay the price of a toxic environment. For the benefits of nuclear energy, we suffer the risk of nuclear war. And with the benefits of international trade, we face the side-effects of industrialisation and technological advancement: carbon monoxide poisoning, pollution, deforestation and the longer-term consequences of these in the form of catastrophes such as flood and famine. Some of these side-effects could have been avoided, others can even yet be contained or reversed; but for others, it is too late.

The emergence of the risk society

The German social scientist Ulrich Beck (1992, 1997, 1999, 2000) and the British sociologist Anthony Giddens (1999, 2001; Giddens and Hutton, 2000) have been at the forefront of a critique of the extreme risks presented by the forces of late modernity – variously named neo-modernity or, the term coined by Beck, the risk society. For both Beck and Giddens, that reaction to modernity which is called post-modernism was a powerful critique of the ravages of late modernity. However, this move provided little in the way of proposals for a way forward. This is perhaps understandable, as the primary focus of post-modernism was a sceptical and critical questioning that not only cast doubt on modernity, but also on alternatives to it, even to the extent of turning in upon itself. Beck and Giddens do, conversely, present strong cases for confronting the problems. The premise under-lying this orientation is that while in the past our main concerns were advancement and its benefits to humankind, and with overcoming scarcity, the main concerns now are the risks created by this same advancement. Of this, Beck (1992) has said:

> *In advanced modernity the social production of wealth is systematically accompanied by the social production of risks ... How can the risks and hazards systematically produced as part of modernization be prevented, minimized, dramatized, or channelled? Where do they finally see the light of day in the shape of 'latent side effects', how can they be limited and distributed away so that they neither hamper the modernization process nor exceed the limits of that which is 'tolerable' – ecologically, medically, psychologically and socially? We are ... concerned no longer exclusively with making nature useful, or with releasing mankind from traditional constraints, but also and essentially with problems resulting from techno-economic development itself.*
>
> (Beck, 1992, p. 20)

A significant feature of this risk society lies in its essentially global dimensions that create an Earth-wide reflexivity in terms of the risks involved. Thus, we find that as tobacco manufacturers meet increasing attack in the West, they mount aggressive marketing strategies in developing countries. The fact that much of the health care in such countries depends on international aid, means that the health problems we currently endure and pay for in the West may also have to be paid for in such countries in the future, as we 'export' the risks of our affluence. This reflexivity extends even into apparent philanthropic strategies. As we export agricultural technology in the form of pesticides, herbicides and chemical fertilisers today, tomorrow we find DDT in the tea we drink. We are to a greater or lesser extent aware of many of the noxious substances that present risks and also the risks associated with such global influences as deforestation and global warming. However, there is a growing angst within societies about the hidden risks, such as the long-term use of nuclear power or the genetic modification of agricultural crops.

In a slightly different turn on the term reflexivity, Giddens (1999) refers to what he terms late modernity, where there is a sense that we are living in a 'runaway world'. Where the consequences of modernity intrude upon us, including risks that are known *and* risks that crash in upon us unexpectedly, the old modes of coping are no longer effective. We can no longer rely on traditional means of coping – the old tried and tested methods of religion, law and traditional science. These worked in a different time and in a more stable world. Now, we have to respond reflexively to new situations and new threats as they arise, by addressing them as emerging problems in a rational way when old solutions may no longer apply. In essence, modern society has moved towards a situation wherein we must respond to constant change; as Giddens terms it, we have entered an age of 'chronic revision'. What we find now is that this demand for reflexivity extends to a global plane, as increasingly events in one part of the globe affect peoples everywhere.

The globalisation of disaster

One particular example of such global impact is that of major disasters. We can think of these as phenomena with the following characteristics:

- They are events that usually emerge suddenly, as in earthquakes, but can emerge more gradually, as in drought and famine.
- They may be of natural origin (as in floods) or manmade (as in the Chernobyl atomic energy accident).
- Because of the global effects of some of the technological advances of modernity, some disasters classed as natural may be manmade in their origins (as when increases in world-wide flood disasters are argued to be linked to

global warming, which in turn is considered to be manmade).

- They are events that cause direct injury or death, and at the least affect the health and well-being of whole communities or populations.
- Populations that are more vulnerable (because of poverty, lack of civil defence infrastructures, or poorly developed health care systems) are more likely to be overwhelmed by such events, thus increasing the magnitude of the harm done.
- The extent of harm done is directly related to the degree of preparedness, and this is a significant factor where disasters are not anticipated as a possibility. (While in Russia there was little preparedness for the Chernobyl event, in San Francisco preparedness for earthquakes is a constant and conscious concern.)

The magnitude of such disasters can have transnational and even global impact. This is placed in perspective when it is noted that in the USA alone (which holds the economic balance of the world within its grasp), disasters cost in the region of $1 billion per day, and floods in China and Bangladesh alone have exceeded 700 000 recorded deaths. Disasters of such scale lead to a global response as well as global impact. The reasons for this can extend from a moral responsibility (which we discuss below) to the fact that, for global capitalism, disasters have profound economic effects: they drain development funding to such countries, and they impact directly on markets within them. In the past, such responses have tended to be in the nature of being almost reflex actions – airlifting in food, second-hand clothing, medical personnel and supplies, etc. However, more often than not, such aid was too late in arriving or was inappropriate in the context of local circumstances and cultural aspects of the disaster zone (as in the case of foodstuffs that were not palatable within the culture). In this respect, de Goyet (1999) has suggested that such well meaning but unhelpful interventions have contributed to what he described as 'disaster myths'. A more planned approach is needed, where attention is paid to the assessment of need extending across three main areas:

- the preparedness of vulnerable communities before disasters occur (Nyheim and Thielman, 1995)
- emergency intervention at the point of occurrence of the disaster
- programmes of recovery that assist communities in returning to their pre-disaster states.

The politics of risk

Another significant feature is the socio-political risk associated with the globalisation process. The seeds of discontent and resentment created by colonialism in the early stages of globalisation continue in the modern-day reactions to the foreign policies of superpowers and the sometimes unscrupulous behaviour of transnational corporations. As such influences continue to extend into global dimensions, so too does the resentment and opposition extend into becoming global risks. As a consequence, one of the newest risks emerging at the global level is that created by global terrorism. Whether these trends find their causes in the institutionalised terror of major powers and corporations, masquerading under the cover of humanitarian concerns and something that is called democratic principles, or the anarchic intentions of groupings that have evil intent, or some mixture of the two, is beyond the immediate concerns of this chapter. It is unlikely that such issues could be followed to their source in any case, such are the complexities of global currents and undercurrents. We find groups whose reactions against perceived injustices are in some circumstances twisted and prejudiced, but in other circumstances justified. We find the weapons of terror being brought into use to correct or revenge perceived injustices, and being properly condemned whatever the wrong that has been done. But we also find the voiced condemnations being made less valid when the government statesmen making them were even worse agents of terror in their time.

What is clear, and more so than ever before, is that since the tragic terrorist attacks on the World Trade Center in New York in September 2001, there is an unprecedented level of global anxiety in respect of the increase in such incidents. Contrary to the intentions of the perpetrators of such acts, this has resulted in alliances between nations that previously were entrenched in opposing viewpoints and even outright mistrust of one another. These nations are now becoming enjoined by necessity in a war against terrorism. The danger here is that such a war on terror may become a vehicle for other more covert political intentions as well as for its overt primary reasons. And in such situations, as is often the case, the innocent bystanders may be placed in the firing lines.

Such developments have resulted in unprecedented attention being paid to the capability to respond to such risk at both national and global levels. Within the UK, particular attention had been paid to this relatively new shift by the Government's influential Strategy Unit (2002). The Strategy Unit (2002) recognised that dealing with risk and uncertainty had become a central concern of Government and that there is a global dimension to this trend, stating:

> The second new factor is the greater connectedness of the world, through an integrated global economy and communication system and a shared environment. This has brought huge opportunities. But it also means that citizens in the UK are potentially more vulnerable to distant events – ranging from economic crises on the other side of the world, to attacks on IT networks, diseases carried by air travellers, or the indirect impact of civil wars and famines. Globally interconnected infrastructure brings with it increased exposure to catastrophic events elsewhere, as shown, for example, by the events of 11 September 2001. These systematic risks are now high on the policy agenda in many countries.
>
> (The Strategy Unit, 2002, p. 5)

Beck, whose earlier work was discussed above, had already anticipated this trend by extending his work on 'the risk society' into a consideration of 'the global risk society' (Beck, 1999). In this, he draws attention not only to the actual impact of such risk, but also to how it has affected the consciousness of such threat. More recently he stated:

> Terrorism operating on a global scale has opened a new chapter in world risk society. A clear distinction must be made between the attack itself and the terrorist threat which becomes universal as a result of it. What is politically crucial is not the risk itself but the perception of the risk. What men fear to be real is real in its consequences – fear creates its own reality. Capitalism requires optimism, which is destroyed by the collective belief in the terrorist threat, and that can plunge an already stumbling world economy into a state of crisis. Someone who sees the world as a terror risk, becomes incapable of action. That is the first trap the terrorists have set. The second trap: the perceived risk of terrorism, politically instrumentalised, unleashes security needs, which wipe out freedom and democracy, the very things which constitute the superiority of modernity. If we find ourselves faced with a choice between freedom or survival, then it is already too late, because most people will decide against freedom.
>
> (Beck, 2001)

By the later years of the twentieth century there was, as suggested earlier, an increasing consciousness of globalisation, as people everywhere moved towards an awareness of the global dimension and the interconnectedness of communities and nations. By the first years of this new millennium, this consciousness had extended into an awareness, and indeed increasingly universal anxiety, about the risks of modern global influences. Beck had, of course, been writing of such risks for more than a decade, and Greenpeace (the environmentalist organisation) had been highlighting the risks for much longer. But one was hidden within the academic undergrowth, and the other was contained by a constant labelling (sometimes by powerful nations, sometimes by powerful capitalist interests) as a fanatical fringe group. After the major terrorist incursions of the first years of the new millennium, and particularly the attack on the New York World Trade Center, all changed. This particular risk factor within the 'global risk society' could not be ignored and there was no way in which its presence could be questioned. Risk and its containment had, in the end, become a major feature of our existence.

Study Activity 44.3

In the previous section, we considered, among the various risks facing us at a global level, the risk of terrorist attack. In considering this, we addressed to some extent the traumatic effect that fear of terrorist attack imposes on people. There are also, of course, the after-effects of actual attacks, with injury, loss and post-traumatic stress syndrome. Using your library sources:

- Explore the possible impact of anticipating terrorist attacks on the health and well-being of individuals within a community.
- Explore the possible impact of actual terrorist attacks on the health and well-being of such individuals.
- Write brief accounts of the outcomes of your explorations. Reflect upon how such influences and the trauma they cause may be addressed at the political/government level. Note your main ideas for such political action.
- If fellow students have also completed this exercise, discuss these in seminar format.

Implications for nursing

It may seem that such matters are far removed from the day-to-day concerns of nurses. This is certainly the case in the context of the more insidious risks emerging from modernity. The fact that even in the far north, which might be reasonably assumed to be beyond the ravages of the harmful impact of modern technologies, over 75% of the plant life in Greenland is now endangered, may seem of little relevance to the nurse on a busy medical ward. However, it must be recognised that a significant aspect of globalisation is the way in which what happens across the world increasingly impacts upon all peoples in all places, at some stage. As nursing has at its core a concern for people and their health and well-being, we are unavoidably thrust into a need to respond to the risks emerging from global influences. Nursing must respond, in a genuine caring way, to the needs of the societies it serves. But to respond, there must be a recognition that while we live in an increasingly affluent and more comfortable world, this comfort has a cost in terms of risks that threaten not only the people but the entire planet.

If nurses cannot recognise these trends, cannot themselves experience the woundedness they incur, they will be ill placed to respond to a wounded and frightened people. It can be argued that there are a number of ways in which the nursing profession *can* make a difference in relation to the globalisation of risk. These may include:

- ensuring that, through our education and professional development processes, *all* nurses are aware of the influences of globalisation and, in particular, the risks it may present to health and well-being
- developing a greater sense of watchfulness in respect of potential or emerging risks and, in particular, the sudden threats of disaster or terrorist attacks
- establishing within nursing's repertoire of competencies the capacity to respond with skilled intervention where major disasters and catastrophes occur
- developing specialist preparation for *some* nurses, as advanced practitioners or nursing consultants who would take lead roles in responding to disasters in terms of prevention and preparedness, immediate emergency response, and recovery

- increasing political awareness and greater political influence at a global level through such agencies as the International Council of Nurses, government chief nurse networks, and emerging global nursing networks – this requires not only an awareness of the risks implicit in modernisation and globalisation, but also the courage to take stands where the health and well-being of people are threatened, and the capacity to act in a cohesive and politically effective way to further such interests
- including in public health and health promotion activities – the education of communities in actions that may be taken to avoid or contain such risks through community and political action; and, encouraging environment-friendly patterns of living
- recognising the risk of scapegoating ethnic groups in situations where such groups are associated with external threats, and treating such groups with compassion, sensitivity and understanding.

Study Activity 44.4

It may be expected that with the threat of major disaster having reached global dimensions, in our own society there is increasing attention to the need for preparedness. In this respect it can be expected that your own National Health Service or Health and Social Services Trust will have a disaster plan in place. Obtain or seek access to a copy of this plan (bearing in mind that some aspects of it may not be available for security reasons).

- Re-read the section on 'The new globalisation as a source of social risk'. Consider how the issues identified in this section have been covered in the disaster plan, and also any issues identified in the plan that are *not* included in the previous section. In particular, consider whether the plan includes the elements of: prevention and preparedness, emergency response, and recovery.
- Identify nursing involvement in the plan. Is there an indication that nurses participated in drawing up the

plan? Does the plan clearly identify the role of nurses in the disaster plan activities?

THE NEED FOR A GLOBAL ETHIC

Diversity

We opened this chapter with a quotation from the Parliament of the World's Religions that spoke of the world being in agony. In the final years of the previous century, this may have seemed to some an overreaction. However, the first years of the new millennium have emerged to present a world that is indeed in agony. What is perhaps particularly concerning is the fact that this is largely an agony visited on people by people, and the fact that this would appear to be of global dimensions. One reaction to this has been the call for what has become known as a global ethic.

We have already considered the issue of ethics in some detail in this book (in Chapter 13). In one sense, the call for a global ethic might be seen as a call for a global acceptance of the ethical precepts presented in that chapter. However, things are seldom so straightforward. It cannot be assumed that the ethical principles held to in one part of the globe will be readily accepted in another. Within our Western developed societies there are major differences across a wide range of issues, such as, for example, the sanctity of life. Even within our own society there are wide differences in respect of issues such as capital punishment, abortion and euthanasia. And barely 50 years after the fall of the Third Reich we have witnessed genocide, by its modern title of 'ethnic cleansing' in Europe and Africa, and chemical warfare in the Middle East.

The difficulty with establishing a global ethic is one of identifying moral values that can be globally accepted. Ethical positions are to a large extent contained within cultures, and develop through the articulation and acceptance into culture of ethical values. There are two important corollaries to this position:

- First, as Geertz (1973) has so effectively demonstrated, culture is a complex network of values and positions that extends throughout the culture to such an extent that each element becomes part of a cohesive whole: the world as a society knows it. In such circumstances, ethical values can be deeply embedded in a culture and as such are particularly difficult to shift. One example of this, pertinent to principles of health and well-being, is that of bodily mutilation. Within our Western culture, deliberate bodily mutilation is abhorrent. Yet, within some Middle Eastern cultures, bodily mutilation (such as severance of limbs as punishment for crime) is valued as a just action. Similarly, in some African and Asian countries, female circumcision is widely practised. This involves the surgical occlusion of the female genitalia of young girls, thus ensuring virginity until at marriage the occlusion is reversed through sexual intercourse. Within those cultures, such practices are deeply embedded in beliefs relating to guarantees of female purity. In our Western culture, such practices are adjudged mutilation and outlawed as extreme forms of child abuse. Horror is expressed at the ways in which this is achieved – often by unqualified women using no anaesthesia, and operating with the use of bush thorns and animal excreta pastes – and the pain and distress caused by brutal reversal through enforced and repeated sexual penetration at the point of marriage (*see*, for example, Dorkenoo, 1994).

- Second, while the *values and norms* associated with ethical standards within cultures are articulated, often to an elaborate degree, the *sources* of these are usually not so clearly articulated. Thus, we find that this or that course of action is defined as morally 'good', but the sources of this 'good' – its basis – are not clearly articulated. Charles Taylor (1989) speaks of this as the 'ethics of inarticulacy'. This phenomenon creates a paradox that makes it particularly difficult to argue for one ethical position or against another. While there may be a desire to argue against the ways in which ethical practices are articulated and enacted, this is difficult when the moral grounds upon which these are based remain unsaid, and sometimes even beyond words.

Towards a global consensus

Clearly, where circumstances such as those described above exist, the project of moving towards a global ethic is problematic. Yet it is also clear that as we move towards greater inter-connectedness, we must also establish the moral basis for how we will relate to one another at this global level. In a sense, the Parliament of the World's Religions (1993) attempted to arrive at what it felt could be accepted as a set of universal principles, enumerated as follows:

1 Commitment to a culture of non-violence and respect for life
2 Commitment to a culture of solidarity and a just economic order
3 Commitment to a culture of tolerance and a life of truthfulness
4 Commitment to a culture of equal rights and partnership between men and women.

It is of note that the statement of the Parliament was drafted by a distinguished theologian, Hans Küng. His parent university, Tübingen University in Germany, hosted a series of lectures on a global ethic, commencing in 2000. At the first of these, the British Prime Minister, Tony Blair (2000) proposed establishing a global ethic on the basis of the concept of community within which all are of equal worth as human beings. Explaining this position, he stated: 'Note: it is equal worth, not equality of income or outcome; or, simply, equality of opportunity. Rather, it affirms our equal right to dignity, liberty, freedom from discrimination as well as economic opportunity. The idea of community resolves the paradox of the modern world: it acknowledges our interdependence; it recognises our individual worth'. Some 2 years later, Mary Robinson (2002), the United Nations High Commissioner for Human Rights, delivered the

second lecture in this series. She similarly spoke of the possibility of a global ethic founded upon equal rights 'civil and political, social, economic and cultural, enjoyed without discrimination'. Whether this is viewed as a commitment to a common culture, or a sense of community, or a sense of human rights, all three of these assertions (by the Parliament, Blair and Robinson, respectively) rest upon a coming together of peoples and a dialogue within which at least a core of moral values may be accepted by all.

There is common ground between the above positions and the call by Etzioni (1997) for a New Golden Rule in ethics that does not oblige the individual to espouse the moral positions of the 'community', but does place upon the individual a responsibility to contribute, to attempt to convince the community of the right course. If all do this there is a genuine dialogue that seeks the right path. This has much in line with the communitarian or discourse ethics of Apel (1980) and Habermas (1990), discussed in Chapter 13. If such an orientation can be extended to the global community of nations, and if such moral discourse can be sustained as a valid concern *and* an ongoing commitment, then all will be aware of what has been achieved in terms of a global moral order, and what still has to be fought for. Indeed, it is not unreasonable to assume that, at least on the most important ethical issues, a consensus on global morals can be achieved. As suggested by Taylor (1989):

> We agree surprisingly well, across great differences of theological and metaphysical belief, about the demands of justice and benevolence, and their importance. There are differences, including the stridently debated one about abortion. But the very rarity of these cases, which contributes to their saliency, is eloquent testimony to the general agreement.
>
> (Taylor, 1989, p. 515)

Indeed, it may be that even attaining the agreement to which Taylor (1989) refers at a global level would be a significant step forward. That is, if all peoples subscribe to the position that they treat each other justly (with fairness, equity, and a respect for their autonomy) and with a concern for the well-being of their neighbours (not only by adopting a non-maleficent attitude, but also one of beneficence that reaches out in a helping and sustaining way), then we would have the foundations of a global ethic. Of course, in a rapidly changing world, constantly at risk and on the edge of chaos, new dilemmas will emerge to challenge global relationships. This is why, within a core set of universal morals, we also need the New Golden Rule that Etzioni (1997) has proposed. That is, a framework within which the global community becomes a space for dialogue in resolving global ethical problems.

Study Activity 44.5

'Charity begins at home'. We are all familiar with the old adage. In the context of the foregoing section, it may lead us to ask 'What moral obligation have we to other peoples?' Surely, such an argument runs, our first responsibility is to our immediate family and friends, then our local communities, and then our nation. We cannot be expected to right all the wrongs of the world.

- Consider the latter argument and then read through the main points of the above section. Reflect on these matters and then write two brief statements: an argument *for* a global ethic and an argument *against* a global ethic. Which argument holds sway for you?

Implications for nursing

Here, also, we find implications for nursing. In our profession we profess a caring for others. It is important to recall this fundamental meaning of the term profession, that at once places it upon the moral plane: we profess, make public the declaration, that we care for those we serve. In this new global era, nursing also moves towards a global community: a community of nurses that extends across and beyond nations. A question is raised, therefore, in respect of how nursing can acquit itself with ethical deportment on this global level.

In earlier chapters of this book we considered the problem confronting nursing in terms of arriving at an agreed body of knowledge, and indeed an agreed definition of nursing itself. These are issues that have grasped the imagination of nursing scholars, practitioners and managers alike. Thus, in the first four modules of the book we considered in some depth how knowledge and theory for nursing is constructed. In particular, we considered in great depth the evidence base for our practice. These emphases mirror the situation in the wider nursing literature. However, nursing also has a problem in arriving at an agreed position on what might constitute a nursing ethic. It is, of course, the case that in Chapter 13 we addressed the issue of ethics in some depth, and in so doing applied seminal thinking in the field of ethics and moral philosophy to the situation of health care and nursing. However, within our profession, and in a global context, there is much less space given to this matter than to the scientific basis of our practice.

It might be argued that on one level, the issue here is quite a straightforward one. That is, we might simply state that on a global, as well as a local, level nurses have a responsibility to ensure that their practice is founded on sound ethical principles. But this would be a simplification. A cursory review of Chapter 13, wherein we discussed ethics in general, will reveal that even an ethics based upon principles is open to question. There would be little advantage, and no space, for revisiting in this chapter the issues that are at stake in terms of the ethical foundations upon which a practice of nursing might be based. However, we can consider the extent to which nursing, in line with the wider global community, can move towards and contribute to the establishment and development of a global ethic. In doing so, we might address two broad areas: the values and principles we adopt and the global ethical discourse and how we might contribute to this.

Values and principles

In the earlier subsections, we considered factors or positions that might contribute to a global ethic. Drawing from the various positions reviewed, these can be summarised as:

- A commitment to a culture of non-violence and a respect for life; a just economic order; tolerance and a life of truthfulness; equal rights and partnership between men and women (Parliament of the World's Religions, 1993)
- A global ethic on the basis of the concept of community within which all are of equal worth as human beings (Blair, 2000)
- A global ethic founded upon equal rights 'civil and political, social, economic and cultural, enjoyed without discrimination' (Robinson, 2002)
- A responsibility to contribute, to attempt to convince the community of the right course as part of a framework, within which the global community becomes a space for dialogue in resolving global ethical problems (Etzioni, 1997).

The question we can beg here is: to what extent can nursing subscribe to, and contribute to the realisation of, such values and principles?

The nursing contribution to the global ethic discourse

We must recognise that the globalisation process encompasses a global consciousness, and that a part of this is an emerging sense of global responsibility. Such responsibility is by definition moral; it calls for a recognition of the ethical responsibility we carry beyond our immediate family and friends, local communities, and wider national societies, to a concern for peoples everywhere and indeed a concern for the global environment itself. In line with this, there is a concurrent global nursing consciousness, a recognition of a fellowship with nurses everywhere, that also encompasses this ethical responsibility. On a 'world stage', nursing is significant both numerically and in its capacity to influence.

It can make a valuable contribution by espousing global stands on ethical issues, and values and principles such as those listed above. And, nursing can participate actively in the discourses that might lead to a consensus on how we live together at the global level.

Beyond the above broad concerns with matters of value and principle, nursing can also bring a humane dimension to global ethics. Within individual modern health care structures, characterised by high technology interventions and economics-driven patterns of provision, it is often nursing that brings the human face of compassion to impersonal and dehumanising systems. As noted earlier, in Chapter 13, while not all nurses are committed to an ethic that is founded exclusively on compassionate care, this is at least an important dimension of nursing ethics (Noddings, 1984). It may be reasonable to regard a world dominated by economic and political concerns, being controlled primarily by men, as responding to ethical demands in a more problem-centred and rational way. Nurses (who are primarily women) can bring a feminist strength derived from compassion and caring into the arena of a global ethic.

Study Activity 44.6

As noted above, not everyone subscribes to the notion that an ethic can be wholly *based upon* care. Yet, it seems that caring is an essential aspect of all our moral choices: we might say, if we did not care, they would not even be moral choices as far as *we* were concerned. But how much can we care at a *global* level? Consider the following quotation:

> *Caring is an unquantifiable dimension to moral responsibility. But if we have a proper appreciation of the facts of world poverty, of our global moral identities, of the moral seriousness of responding to extreme suffering, of what quality of life really consists in, and of the duty of caring as much as we can consistent with our quality of life, then we will care as we ought.*
>
> (Dower, 1993, p. 282)

What is Dower getting at here? Is he saying that caring is a natural human condition, and that when we become aware of the plight of others, we will respond to the very limits that our circumstances allow? Or, is he saying that we are only required to care in so far as it does not require actions that would impinge in any way upon our own quality of life?

- Reflect upon the meaning Dower may be attempting to convey.
- Consider where you stand on this issue. Would *you* respond to the needs of others even if it had serious repercussions for your own quality of life, and if so under what circumstances would this occur?
- Do you see any difference between how you would respond in respect of your immediate family and friends, your patients, or on a wider global level? If so, what arguments would sustain the different positions? You might find it helpful to revisit Chapter 13 (Ethical knowing) when you are reflecting on these arguments.

THE MULTICULTURAL SOCIETY

Pushing down

One particularly important insight derived from the work of Giddens (1999), relates to how globalisation impacts upon the peoples of the Earth. He sees this as involving two processes: a 'pulling away from' and a 'pushing down' upon local communities *and* nation-states. In the previous sections of this chapter we have concentrated mainly on the former of these processes, the way in which we are all pulled out towards a global community that increasingly influences our lives. Indeed, in some instances this global pulling away even weakens the hold of the nation-state in some ways, as in the development of the European Union. However, it is important that in closing the chapter, we also recognise the 'pushing down' phenomenon and how it impacts upon our daily lives.

There are a number of senses in which this pushing down phenomenon impacts upon our lives:

1 The 'pulling away from' phenomenon creates in us a global consciousness, as referred to earlier. Therefore, as we live out our lives in our own communities, there is a reflexivity in the way we are constantly influenced by the wider world and events in it. The fisherman on the east coast of England may sit this evening with his wife, arranging for the payment of his gas and electricity services. His concerns this evening, as they were 50 years ago, centre upon his fishing and these domestic chores. But now, he is 'pulled away from' these to the knowledge that decisions at global levels may impose fishing sanctions; and 'pushing down' upon him is the knowledge that these may prevent him from fishing for cod next year. How he will pay these service bills next year depends on much more than his luck and skill as a fisherman. In this age, he may be destroyed by events outside of his control entirely. But on a grander scale, this 'pushing down' is perhaps most notable in our consciousness of major global risk, particularly in respect of terrorist attacks in recent times.

2 There is also a sense in which the wider world 'pushes down' upon us in actual or physical ways. This is particularly relevant in developing countries where even basic infrastructures such as health, energy, water and education are dependent on foreign aid. But it may also influence developed countries, as when, for example, diseases may be spread as a consequence of the vast increases in international travel. This is most recently witnessed in the severed Acute Respiratory Syndrome (SARS) that spread from China to other countries with dire consequences.

3 There is also a social impact occasioned by the increasing movement of peoples across national boundaries. One consequence of this is the way in which, particularly in developed countries, societies have become more multicultural. This may bring benefits in terms of cultural richness and diversity, including the possibility of strengthening knowledge bases and workforces. Of course, there are also

disadvantages. Issues of ethnic segregation and racism may arise, and for less developed countries there are the problems occasioned by the 'brain drain' of its most productive citizens to more affluent countries (the inverse care law referred to earlier).

It is this third pattern that we are specifically concerned with here. As globalisation has proceeded, there is a clear pattern whereby most developed countries have become increasingly multicultural. This is particularly witnessed as an outcome of the mass exoduses to North America in the past, and in those countries such as Great Britain, France, Holland and Portugal that were the great maritime trading nations. However, this trend has continued into the modern era. Most of the major cities of the developed world are now multicultural in the truest sense. Indeed, in the UK some towns and cities are characterised by the fact that the indigenous Anglo-Saxon population is in the minority.

We have noted above the ways in which such diversity can enrich a society. But we have noted also the difficulties that may arise. It is a part of this pattern that in times of growth and labour shortage, immigrants are welcomed, but in times of recession and unemployment resentment and racism can arise. It is also a part of this pattern that at times of increased concerns about global risk, anxiety and resentment can turn inwards to particular ethnic groups. There are, of course, historical examples of similar tendencies, as in the treatment of American citizens of Japanese descent during the Second World War (where whole families were incarcerated for most of the war years). However, there are modern-day equivalents. One such example is the fear, mistrust and sometimes overt resentment directed at Moslem communities following the attacks on New York's World Trade Center. In some instances this has attained the status of modern-day moral panics akin to the witch hunts of the Middle Ages and anti-Jewish pogroms.

The consequences of this situation are many, and certainly more than space in this chapter can

allow for. However, what is clear is that in the context of modern globalisation we must learn to live together, not only across nations and continents but also within our own communities. We are, of course, learning to live together on the global stage, to varying degrees of success. But we also must learn to live with the family next door, whose cultural spirit and way of life may originate many thousands of miles away.

Study Activity 44.7

People described as white, or Caucasian, or originating in the Occident (i.e. Europe or North America as opposed to the southern hemisphere or the Orient) sometimes discriminate against the other groups. In most parts of the world, being non-white can be problematic. We have already considered such matters in Module 5 of this book, but reflect now on why such racial disharmony is a *global* phenomenon, and the implications of this for the ongoing globalisation process.

Implications for nursing

These 'pushing down' trends have a number of implications for nursing. We have already considered issues such as global risk and major disaster, and nursing responses to these, earlier in this chapter. Such responses would have similar application in various settings. Clearly, in such circumstances the vulnerability of the affected population is a significant factor. Nurses who participate in disaster relief in developing countries must cope with the lack of preparedness caused by poverty and the lack of adequate infrastructures such as housing, water, sewage disposal, health services, etc. Within developed countries there is often the lack of preparedness caused by a failure to anticipate risk such as terrorist attack, and the immobilising shock caused when such instances occur. However, the response to such incidents would involve broadly similar principles based upon preparedness, emergency response, and recovery.

Similarly, we have also considered how the consciousness of risk can 'push down' on the communities we care for. There is, of course, the limited but nonetheless important risk occasioned by international travel, whereby diseases can be rapidly transmitted across borders. Of greater magnitude in recent times is the threat occasioned by attacks from international terrorist organisations. The fears and concern generated may sometimes lead to scapegoating of ethnic groups that are seen to be linked to the external threat. Here also, we noted that nursing has a role to play by treating people in such ethnic groupings equitably and with the same degree of compassion as for any other grouping. We have also noted the educative role of nurses, which may help to combat such ignorance and the persecution it may generate.

However, beyond such issues, there remain the demands placed upon nursing that are not necessarily associated with such 'pushing down' of perceived risk, but are essentially to do with the provision of care in a multiracial or multicultural society. For many nurses, working in major cities or densely populated conurbations, such circumstances are neither new nor unusual. Nurses working in London's East End, Leeds or Bradford, or New York's inner city boroughs, have been serving such diverse communities for decades. However, as globalisation proceeds, and as communities everywhere become more diverse, all nurses are increasingly called upon to care for persons from different cultural backgrounds. In addition, as noted above, with international travel, there are the demands of coping with tropical and other diseases that enter our health care systems through arriving travellers and returning international commuters.

The concern with culture as a phenomenon within nursing is not new. It finds its main exponent in American nurse Madeleine Leininger, who has been promoting her perspective of 'transcultural nursing' for several decades (Leininger, 1967, 1977, 1987, 2002). Fundamental to Leininger's views is the idea that if we are to care for people from diverse cultures, we need to understand those cultures. Care, Leininger claims, is embedded in culture and expressed in culturally defined ways. Thus, we need to be aware of these cultural patterns if we are to perceive the calls to care, and we need to be aware of the culturally defined ways in which a caring response must be framed. Leininger argues that while there are cultural differences, there are also universals, which include the essential compassionate call to care that is part of the human condition. In describing how her 'theory of culture care diversity and universality' emerged from her own practice extending back to the 1950s, Leininger (1996) reminisces:

> In a way, I experienced cultural shock and I felt helpless to assist children who so clearly expressed different cultural patterns and ways they wanted care ... The children were so expressive and persistent in what they wanted or needed, yet I was unable to respond appropriately to them (as) I did not understand their behavior. Later, I came to learn that their behavior (and care) were culturally constituted and influenced their mental health.
>
> (Leininger, 1996, p. 73)

From these early realisations, Leininger embarked upon a lengthy career of scholarly inquiry using social anthropological methods to explore cultural diversity using mainly ethnographic approaches. She in fact coined the term 'ethnonursing' to describe her research methods (Leininger, 1991). The purpose of her perspective is to ensure that there is cultural congruence between the nurse's understanding of and responses to patients or clients from different cultural backgrounds – what she terms 'culturally competent care'.

We have already considered this transcultural perspective in Module 5 of this book. But it is clear that these insights are now more important than they have been in the past. As we enter the new millennium, and what is in effect a new globalisation characterised by increasing awareness of risk from terrorism and other facets of this process, the issue of diversity within our own communities has the potential to erupt into hostility and defensiveness. There is a great need

829

for nurses to be capable of 'culturally *competent* care'. But, within this, there is in our present times a particularly vital need to be capable of 'culturally *sensitive* care'. Those who are in need of our care are always vulnerable. However, this vulnerability, and its negative impact on health, may be even greater where those we care for are from ethnic groups that feel devalued, mistrusted and alienated. In carrying this transcultural mission forward, it is important that:

- our nursing curricula and staff development programmes include transcultural nursing as an essential component
- where possible, nursing students gain supervised practice in different cultures
- as nurses, we share our knowledge and insights about culture care needs – at local levels, through our professional organisations, and via our global nursing networks
- within our increasingly diverse society, there are deliberate strategies to ensure that people from different ethnic groups are encouraged to enter nursing, so that our profession reflects the cultural diversity of our society and benefits from the richness of such diversity
- our care incorporates a dimension that includes attention to the cultural background of our patients, including the ethnic and culturally discrete groups within our own communities – the religious groupings and other indigenous people, such as those in traveller or Romany communities
- we are aware of the emergence of tropical and other diseases that enter our health care systems through international commuters and other international travellers, and develop the capability to respond to such unusual but periodically recurring instances.

Study Activity 44.8

Consider your recent practice experiences and identify a patient you were involved in caring for who came from an ethnic or religious grouping different to your own. Undertake a library and Internet search for information on the particular religion or ethnic group,

making notes of your findings. If possible, speak with someone from the particular group to try and obtain a more in-depth understanding of their culture, and the values and beliefs of the religion/ethnic group, and use this interview to extend your notes. Reflect upon the following questions:

- Was the information you collected new to you or were you already familiar with most of it?
- Do you think that the information you collected would have improved your care of the patient?
- If you feel it *would* have improved your care, list the main ways in which the care would have been improved.

SUMMARY

In this chapter we considered the emergence of globalisation in the modern era and its impact upon nursing. In so doing we reflected upon the benefits of modernity – of which globalisation is a part – but also upon the risks that emerge as a result of these developments. In following this path we drew particular attention to the emergence of a global consciousness that reflects not only an awareness of and concern for others across the Earth, but also an awareness of the risks that emerge. Significant among these are the modern manmade disasters and the deliberate threat to harm emerging from international terrorism. In addressing these developments and how they may be responded to, we considered the need for a global ethic that would assist us in ensuring that agreed moral standards are at the heart of our relations on a global plane. Finally, we recognised the ways in which globalisation not only 'pulls us away' from our local settings and the culture peculiar to them, but also 'pushes down' upon our local community life. One aspect of this that was given particular attention was the increasingly multicultural nature of our society, and in considering this we revisited the issues of race, ethnicity and transcultural understanding previously considered in Module 5.

In considering each of these important issues, we also attempted to address ways in which nursing can respond to the move towards globalisation. In each of the areas we addressed – modern-day new globalisation trends, risk, the need for a global ethic, and the cultural diversity within our own societies that emerges from global movements – we also considered the implications for nursing. It must be recognised in all of this that how globalisation extends into the future can only be predicted to a certain extent. While we know some of the emerging risks, others are predicted with varying degrees of uncertainty. But we must also acknowledge that there may be other risks of which we may not even yet be aware. If we are to survive on the planet, peoples everywhere must embrace a global commitment to living together in harmony, and working together to avoid, contain, or combat the risks that *will* emerge in the future. In nursing, we have a vital part to play in this. We are one of the groupings that are called upon when disasters occur or when needs of communities become critical. But we are also a global grouping, with an increasing global consciousness, and an already developed global professional network. In a world that may go wrong, or already emerging as a world *gone* wrong, nursing can be a powerful force for the good.

Of course, this may seem like some sort of empty mantra: statements such as 'a powerful force for the good' may seem to many to be not only meaningless, but also pompous and supercilious. Beck, whose work we have already referred to, presents an amusing anecdote that is of relevance here:

> *When I hear the word globalization, the following political caricature appears before my eyes: The Spanish conquerors. The Conquistadors appear in the New World in their shiny armor with horses and weapons. The thought bubble reads, "We have come to you to talk to you about God, civilization and the truth." And a group of bewildered native onlookers responds: "Of course, what would you like to know?"*
>
> (Beck, 2002)

Beck warns of the dangers of forcing *our* globalisation, with its standards, values and impositions on others who do not believe in them and do not want them. While we cannot condone violent responses, we should not be surprised by the terrorist consequences of such attitudes. Instead, there is a need to convince *each other* through dialogue that each of us is genuine in our respect for the other, and our commitment to working together to produce a safer and better world. There is much in this that requires a showing of compassion and care, a preparedness to listen, an acceptance of others and their values, a willingness to nurture relationships, and a capability to offer help as and when it is wanted with good will and without conditions that require the other to relinquish values and self-identity. These are the things that nurses do. These are the things that nurses may be able to encourage others to do, and this would indeed be a powerful force for the good.

REFERENCES

Apel, K.-O. (1980) The *a priori* of the communication community and the foundations of ethics: the problem of the rational foundation of ethics in the scientific age. In: Apel, K.-O. (ed.) *Towards a Transformation of Philosophy* (trans. G. Adey and D. Frisby), Routledge and Kegan Paul, London

Beck, U. (1992) *Risk Society: Towards a new modernity*, Sage, London

Beck, U. (1997) *The Reinvention of Politics: Rethinking modernity in the global social order*, Polity Press, Cambridge

Beck, U. (1999) *World Risk Society*, Polity Press, Malden, MA

Beck, U. (2000) *What is Globalization?* Polity Press, Malden, MA

Beck, U. (2001) The cosmopolitan state: towards a realistic utopia, *Eurozine* 2001-12-05

Beck, U. (2002) The silence of words and political dynamics in the World Risk Society. *Logos* 1, 4

Blair, A. (2000) *Values and the Power of Community*, University of Tübingen, Tübingen

Buchan, J. and O'May, F. (1999) Globalisation and healthcare labour markets: a case study from the United Kingdom. *Human Resources for Health Development Journal* 3(3), 100–209

De Goyet, C. de V. (1999) Stop propagating disaster myths. *DERA Newsletter* **October**, 1–3

Dorkenoo, E. (1994) *Cutting the Rose – Female genital mutilation: the practice and its prevention*, Minority Rights Publications, London

Dower, N. (1993) World poverty. In: Singer, P. (ed.) *A Companion to Ethics*, Blackwell, Oxford

Etzioni, A. (1997) *The New Golden Rule*, Profile Books, London

Geertz, C. (1973) *The Interpretation of Cultures*, Basic Books, New York

Giddens, A. (1999) *Runaway World: How globalisation is reshaping our lives*, Profile Books, London

Giddens, A. (2001) *The Global Third Way Debate*, Polity Press, Malden, MA

Giddens, A. and Hutton, W. (2000) *On the Edge: Living with global capitalism*, Jonathan Cape, London

Habermas, J. (1990) Discourse ethics. In: Habermas, J. (ed.), *Moral Consciousness and Communicative Action*, MIT Press, Boston, Mass

International Council of Nurses (1999) *Nurse Retention, Transfer, and Migration*, International Council of Nurses, Geneva

Kingmo, M. (2001) Nursing migration: global treasure hunt or disaster-in-the-making? *Nursing Inquiry* 8(4), 205–12

Leininger, M. (1967) The culture concept and its relevance to nursing. *Journal of Nursing Education* 6(2), 27–37

Leininger, M. (1977) Culture and transcultural nursing: meaning and significance for nurses, *NLN Publication,* (15-1662), 85–105

Leininger, M. (1987) A new generation of nurses discover transcultural nursing, *Nursing and Health Care* 8(5), 263

Leininger, M. (1991) Ethnonursing: a research method with enablers to study the theory of Culture Care *NLN Publication,* (15-2402), 73–117

Leininger, M. (1996) Culture care theory, research, and practice. *Nursing Science Quarterly* 9, 71–8

Leininger, M. (2002) Culture care theory: a major contribution to advance transcultural nursing knowledge and practices. *Journal of Transcultural Nursing* 13(3), 189–92; discussion 200–1

Noddings, N. (1984) *Caring: A feminine approach to ethics and moral education*, University of California Press, London

Nyheim, D. and Thielman, E. (1995) Disaster preparedness – European Union steps up its support. *D+C Development and Cooperation* 5, 16

Parliament of the World's Religions (1993) *Towards a Global Ethic*, Council of the Parliament of the World's Religions, Chicago, IL

Robinson, M. (2002) *Ethics, Human Rights and Globalization*, University of Tübingen, Tübingen

Salmon, M.E. and Rambo, K. (2002) Government Chief Nursing Officers: a study of key issues they face and the knowledge and skills required by their roles. *International Nursing Review* 49, 136–43

Strategy Unit (2002) *Risk: Improving Government's capability to handle risk and uncertainty*, Strategy Unit, Cabinet Office, London

Taylor, C. (1989) *Sources of the Self: The making of the modern identity*, Cambridge University Press, Cambridge

Tudor Hart, J. (1971) The inverse care law. *Lancet* **27 February**, 405–12

World Health Assembly (1996) *Strengthening Nursing and Midwifery. Forty-ninth World Health Assembly – Resolution WHA 49.1*, World Health Organisation, Geneva

World Health Assembly (2001) *Strengthening Nursing and Midwifery. Fifty-fourth World Health Assembly – Resolution WHA 54.12*, World Health Organisation, Geneva

Module 10: Into the future

Reflections

As you have progressed through the book, you will have noted that the earlier modules addressed the knowledge that might underpin practice, while later modules considered the practice circumstances within which such knowledge or theory is applied. At various points in the book it has been recognised that rapid change and burgeoning technological advancement is a constant in modern health care systems. However, these changes to a large extent mirror changes that are taking place in society as a whole. The arguments presented throughout this module share a common theme: the nature of change in our new century and how we in nursing may respond to an uncertain future.

In one sense, humankind has always been confronted with change as we have moved from pre-historic and primeval to modern times. However, the change phenomenon has taken on new dimensions in the short space of the last few decades. The progression through modern times has been characterised by a relinquishment of faith in old values and a new faith that science and technology would resolve our remaining problems. This did not happen, however, and has been highlighted, our now post-modern world is critically questioning that faith. As we move now through what is variously termed the new modernity or neo-modernity, we recognise that the benefits of modernity also bring with them extreme risks that are characterised by their global dimensions. Had there been any doubts about this line of argument, they have surely been dispelled by the terrorist bombings of the World Trade Center in New York in September 2001. As this book comes to publication we are into the third year since those events, and their impact on all facets of life, including health care systems, is still reverberating across our globe.

There are risks in attempting to see patterns in the present to form the future. Earlier we stated the oft-quoted mantra: The only thing that is constant in our modern world (and its health care systems) is change. That mantra could now be changed to: The only thing that is constant is uncertainty. The message emerging from this final module can be encapsulated in the following: We can no longer predict and *then* plan, beyond certain limits. We must instead plan for the unpredictable.

You may find it useful to reflect upon the above summary and how the points highlighted have been addressed in the chapters themselves. Having done this, reflect upon the possible implications for the future in the particular area of nursing or health care within which you work or train.

45 POSTSCRIPT

Lynn Basford and Oliver Slevin

The twenty-first century is an ideal time to celebrate nursing, given that the business of health care offers greater opportunities for the nursing profession than ever before imagined in modern history. The last century has seen nurses striving for professional recognition, for equality in the care/treatment setting and for educational opportunities that mirror our professional colleagues. To a large extent these aims have been achieved, or at the very least, frameworks have been put in place for the profession to capitalise on in the forthcoming years.

Today, the nurse is involved in every aspect of care delivery, managing care in all settings within multidisciplinary teams, commissioning and auditing multiprofessional care. To accommodate this, roles and responsibilities have changed, sometimes in radical ways that have allowed the nurse to take responsibility to diagnose, prescribe treatment, implement and evaluate care. Role changes have embraced consultant nurses, triage nurses, NHS Direct and nurses working in walk-in centres. In other instances, nurse-led clinics employ salaried doctors. Such reforms have required new knowledge and skills that enable the nurse to be fully competent and confident to practise within these new roles.

Of course, not all nurses work at such advanced levels at the beginning of their professional career, but the above illustrates a career trajectory that can be achieved. In the first instance the new nurse is required to consolidate her knowledge and skills within her chosen field of practice. Continuing professional education (a mandatory requirement) further facilitates the progression to expert nurse, highly competent and proficient in her domain. In achieving expertise, the nurse must work from an evidence-based position using skills of lifelong learning, information management, critical analysis and evaluation, and reflexivity. Fitness for practice and purpose embraces the notion that the nurse is able to demonstrate competence, which reflects the relevant knowledge, skill, understanding and experience.

While the need to work from the best possible source of evidence is of paramount importance, the reality of reading and synthesising the volume of information on a regular basis is a daunting task. This is especially so given that the business of health care is multifaceted and subject to change due to technological innovations, therapeutic and practice developments and scientific discoveries. Indeed, the nurse would need to read several articles per day just to keep abreast of her subject. Therefore, skills and techniques are required to assist this process, for example computerised literature searching skills, critical appraisal and evaluation techniques, examining systematic reviews or evidence-based journals, seeking information from other experts or pooling resources from peers and others, and discussing clinical events with a clinical supervisor.

Learning on the job is a necessary feature of modern-day practice, encouraged by the Government's political direction for lifelong learning which indicates that it should be centred on practice and near to the clinical setting. Lifelong learning and the notion of continuing professional development are synonymous with each other and are key factors in the Government's agenda for health and social care reform (Department of Health, 2001). The pivotal reason for this is to ensure that care is improved and enhanced so as to improve the quality of life (and life that is free from disabilities and chronic ill-health) for all people (Department of Health, 2000). From a lifelong learning perspective it is firmly believed that this will empower professionals to support changes in the clinical setting based on the best source of evidence, be able to transfer knowledge and skills to new fields of practice and develop personal and professional competence and confidence throughout their career. However, to meet the lifelong learning agenda, practitioners need skills to be able to reflect in and on practice in an attempt to eradicate uncertainty in the clinical setting using critical analysis of diagnostic interpretation and evaluation of the health outcome.

Given the enormity of change at every level of health and social care, it is tempting to think that much of what was known, or the skills that were used, are irrelevant to the nurse in the twenty-first century. This is clearly not the case, as our book has shown that concepts of care and caring are still a quintessential aspect of nursing today, as they have been throughout its past. Indeed, our first module is focused on care, from its historical roots, to the notion of self-care, informal care, and altruistic and organised care and finally, a modern phenomenon of empowered care. However, what nursing has failed to do is to find a universal explanation regarding the basic tenets of nursing care that is hopefully unique to the world of nursing and, if not, of such central importance that it formulates a basis for all nursing activity. This is not to say nurse theorists have not postulated their thoughts on nursing, but we argue that contemporary theorists need to re-examine these theories in the light of current practice and new knowledge.

Since 1995, nursing has entered the realms of higher education and this has been instrumental in providing sound education that is strongly linked to practice and is underpinned by a growing body of nursing research. The Quality Assurance Agency has been carrying out national assessments, an ongoing feature over these last few years, which have demonstrated that nursing, as a discipline, is highly committed to quality educational programmes, following a student-centred and student-sensitive philosophy. We have pioneered wider access and flexible opportunities within the curriculum for others to follow, having the knowledge that on the whole, many of our students are highly motivated and that they truly excel in their studies against all odds and previous educational exclusion. Many schools/departments of nursing scored maximum points from the Quality Assurance Agency, with nearly all achieving over 20 out of a possible 24. This was indeed a great achievement and something to be truly proud of. Of course, there are always lessons to be learned and nursing education has done just this.

Quality education provision has not been the only success story. From a very low research profile, the growth in research and scholarly activity since our move to higher education has been significant and needs to be commended, given the paucity of finances available for nursing research compared with medicine and other well-established disciplines. The dynamics of providing evidence of nursing practice through a rigorous scientific process are vital to secure nursing's future. This is not to say all nurses must be researchers, but all nurses must inform the research questions to be asked from practice and in addition implement sound research findings to their work. To this end, education is of central importance to enable practitioners to work in this manner. Thus, the triangulation between practice, research and education must be the way forward, formulating partnership working in all three domains to achieve this goal.

In the past, health and social care have organisationally been polar opposites to each other, evolving and developing on different trajectories that disable any opportunity for 'joined up' working between professional groups. After repeated service failures and the need to address duplication of effort, the Government has designed an action plan for major reforms. This plan will ensure that health and social care, and the professionals who work within these organisations, will work together to improve quality of care, and assure that the economics of caring are reduced. Therefore, working in multidisciplinary and multi-agency teams will be the norm. Working together–learning together is a Government slogan, but underpinning this is a directive for multiprofessional learning both in formal educational curricula and in the practice setting. The main emphasis is to make the learning meaningful for all professional groups with a focus on patient/client care. Thus, problem-solving ap-proaches to education are encouraged as a framework for future educational practice. This is not a new phenomenon as it has, in some guise or other, been around for four decades. Nonetheless, barriers previously given as legitimate excuses not to undertake such approaches have been surpassed by the arrival of new technology, e.g. E-learning, distance learning, practice-based learning and the arrival of virtual universities that will offer solutions to some of the old problems regarding a shared learning agenda.

A review of the press would have us believe that nursing is in crisis, as is the National Health Service, and, indeed, we cannot escape the fact that there is a real nursing shortage. However, look beyond the press headings and see each day how nursing finds its rewards, true job satisfaction and a deep sense of personal fulfilment. How often is another person privileged to enter people's lives, to share in their personal triumphs and tribulations, to share in birth and death, to be in the midst of all human suffering be it from famine, disease, pestilence, and war? Nursing can make this claim and in so doing we should not ignore our collective duty, which is not only to address individual, community and national health agendas, but also to look wider at the global health and welfare of all people, of all nations, races, religions and cultures.

Nursing in the twenty-first century is an exciting place to be and structures are in place for nurses to have a political voice that can really make a difference to the lives of many people. We offer you guidance in your career within this textbook and hope you find pride and fulfilment in your journey as a truly inspirational nurse.

REFERENCES

Department of Health (2000) *The National Health Service Ten-year Plan*, DoH, London

Department of Health (2001) *Working Together – Learning Together: A framework for lifelong learning for the NHS*, DoH, London

INDEX

Page references in italics indicate figures or tables.